Willard and Spackman's
Occupational Therapy

Willard and Spackman's Occupational Therapy

Seventh Edition

Edited by

Helen L. Hopkins, *Ed. D., O.T.R/L., F.A.O.T.A.*

Professor Emeritus of Occupational Therapy
College of Allied Health Professions
Temple University
Philadelphia, Pennsylvania

Helen D. Smith, *M.O.T., O.T.R/L., F.A.O.T.A.*

Associate Professor of Occupational Therapy
Tufts University — Boston School of Occupational Therapy
Medford, Massachusetts

36 Contributors

J. B. Lippincott Company
Philadelphia
London   Mexico City   New York
St. Louis   São Paulo   Sydney

Acquisition/Sponsoring Editor: Patricia Cleary
Developmental Editor: Eleanor Faven
Coordinating Editorial Assistant: Diana Merritt
Manuscript Editor: Brenda Lee Reed
Indexer: Catherine Battaglia
Design Coordinator: Paul Fry
Designer: William Boehm
Cover Designer: Donald Giordano
Production Manager: Kathleen P. Dunn
Production Coordinator: Ken Neimeister
Compositor: Progressive Typographers
Printer/Binder: The Murray Printing Company

7th Edition

3   5   6   4   2

Library of Congress Cataloging-in-Publication Data

Occupational therapy.
    Willard and Spackman's occupational therapy.

    Includes bibliographies and index.
    1. Occupational therapy.   I. Willard, Helen S.   II. Spackman,
Clare S.   III. Hopkins, Helen L.   IV. Smith, Helen D.   V. Title.
[DNLM: 1. Occupational Therapy. 2. Rehabilitation. WB 555
0141]
RM735.029   1988   615.8'5152   87-26258
ISBN 0-397-54679-3

Any procedure or practice described in this book should be applied by
the health-care practitioner under appropriate supervision in accordance with professional standards of care used with regard to the
unique circumstances that apply in each practice situation. Care has
been taken to confirm the accuracy of information presented and to
describe generally accepted practices. However, the authors, editors,
and publisher cannot accept any responsibility for errors or omissions
or for consequences from application of the information in this book
and make no warranty, express or implied, with respect to the contents
of the book.

    Every effort has been made to ensure drug selections and dosages
are in accordance with current recommendations and practice. Because of ongoing research, changes in government regulations, the
constant flow of information on drug therapy, and reactions and interactions, the reader is cautioned to check the package insert for each
drug for indications, dosages, warnings, and precautions, particularly
if the drug is new or infrequently used.

To Clare S. Spackman, M.S., O.T.R., F.A.O.T.A.
Occupational therapy clinician, educator, administrator,
leader, advocate—and our teacher, co-worker, and friend.

Give a man a fish, and you feed him for a day. Teach a man to fish, and you feed him for a lifetime. —Chinese proverb

CONTRIBUTORS

Abby Abildness, M.S., O.T.R.
Private practice
Hershey, Pennsylvania

Bonnie Sherry Almasy, B.S.
Rehabilitation Home Economist
Harmarville Rehabilitation Center
Pittsburgh, Pennsylvania

Carolyn M. Baum, M.A., O.T.R., F.A.O.T.A.
Clinical Director, OT Services
Washington University School Of Medicine
Irene Walter Johnson Institute of Rehabilitation
St. Louis, Missouri

Ellen S. Cohn, Ed. M., O.T.R.
Academic Fieldwork Coordinator
Tufts University — Boston School of Occupational
    Therapy
Medford, Massachusetts

Douglas M. Cole, B.S., O.T.R.
Director
Cole Center for Work Related Injuries
St. Louis, Missouri

Marianne Rozycka Dahl, M.B.A., O.T.R/L
Coordinator of Rehabilitation Services
Doylestown Hospital
Doylestown, Pennsylvania

Mary Margaret Daub, Ed. M., O.T.R/L
Associate Professor of Occupational Therapy
College of Allied Health Professions
Temple University
Philadelphia, Pennsylvania

Linda J. Davis, M.P.H., Ph. D., O.T.R.
Director, Pacific Geriatric Education Center
Health Sciences Campus
University of Southern California
Los Angeles, California

Elizabeth B. Devereaux, M.S.W., A.C.S.W., O.T.R/L,
    F.A.O.T.A.
Assistant Professor of Psychiatry
Department of Psychiatry
Marshall University, School of Medicine
Huntington, West Virginia

Judy Feinberg, M.S., O.T.R., F.A.O.T.A.
Assistant Director for Research and Administration
Occupational Therapy Department
Indiana University Hospitals;
Adjunct Assistant Professor
Occupational Therapy Program
Division of Allied Health Sciences
Indiana University
School of Medicine
Indianapolis, Indiana

Helen L. Hopkins, Ed. D., O.T.R/L, F.A.O.T.A.
Professor Emeritus
College of Allied Health Professions
Temple University
Philadelphia, Pennsylvania

Margaret Howison, B.S., O.T.R/L
Director of Occupational Therapy
The Pennsylvania State University
Elizabethtown Hospital and Rehabilitation Center;
Instructor of Occupational Therapy
Elizabethtown College
Elizabethtown, Pennsylvania

A. Joy Huss, M.S., O.T.R., R.P.T., F.A.O.T.A.
Associate Professor, Program in Occupational Therapy
University Hospitals
University of Minnesota
Minneapolis, Minnesota

Karen Jacobs, M.S., O.T.R/L
Instructor
Tufts University — Boston School of Occupational
    Therapy
Adjunct Clinical Instructor
Boston University;
Private practice
Boston, Massachusetts

Nancy Allen Kaufmann, Ed. M., O.T.R/L
Private practice
Newtown Square, Pennsylvania

Gary Kielhofner, D.P.H., O.T.R.
Assistant Professor and Chairman
Occupational Therapy Department
University of Illinois at Chicago
Chicago, Illinois

Ruth Ellen Levine, Ed. D., O.T.R/L, F.A.O.T.A.
Professor and Chairman
Department of Occupational Therapy
Thomas Jefferson University
Philadelphia, Pennsylvania

Linda L. Levy, M.A., O.T.R/L
Associate Professor
Department of Occupational Therapy
College of Allied Health Professions
Temple University
Philadelphia, Pennsylvania

Maude H. Malick, B.S., O.T.R/L
Assistant Administrator
Harmarville Rehabilitation Center
Pittsburgh, Pennsylvania

Sandra J. Malone, B.S., O.T.R/L, F.A.O.T.A.
Acting Special Assistant to the Assistant Secretary
    for Health
Maryland State Department of Health and Mental
    Hygiene
Baltimore, Maryland

Maureen Neistadt, M.S., O.T.R/L
Lecturer in Occupational Therapy
Tufts University — Boston School of Occupational
    Therapy
Medford, Massachusetts

Renee Okoye, M.S.H.S., O.T.R/L
Private practice
Massapequa, New York

Patricia Ostrow, M.A., O.T.R., F.A.O.T.A.
Director of Quality Review Division
American Occupational Therapy Association
Rockville, Maryland

Judith M. Perinchief, M.S., O.T.R/L
Assistant Professor of Occupational Therapy
College of Allied Health Professions
Temple University
Philadelphia, Pennsylvania

Patricia Ramm, M.A., O.T.R., F.A.O.T.A.
Private practice
Austin, Texas

Sharan L. Schwartzberg, Ed. D., O.T.R/L
Chairman
Department of Occupational Therapy
Tufts University — Boston School of Occupational
    Therapy
Medford, Massachusetts;
Associate Staff
Department of Psychiatry
Adjunct Staff
Occupational Therapy Department
Mount Auburn Hospital
Cambridge, Massachusetts

Reba M. Sebelist, M.A., O.T.R/L
Assistant Professor in Occupational Therapy — *Retired*
Elizabethtown College
Elizabethtown, Pennsylvania

Phillip Shannon, M.A., O.T.R.
Texas Operations Coordinator
Southwest Border Programs
Project Hope
Edinburg, Texas

Mary Silberzahn, M.A., O.T.R.
Sensory Integrative Specialist
Private practice;
Faculty Member, Center for the Study of Sensory
   Integrative Dysfunction
Los Angeles, California

Helen D. Smith, M.O.T., O.T.R/L, F.A.O.T.A.
Associate Professor of Occupational Therapy
Tufts University — Boston School of Occupational
   Therapy
Medford, Massachusetts

Elinor Anne Spencer, M.A., O.T.R., F.A.O.T.A.
Occupational Therapy Department
St. Joseph Hospital
Bangor, Maine

Maureen Moylan Syler, O.T.R.
Occupational Therapy Department
Austin Hand and Upper Extremity Rehabilitation
   Center
Austin, Texas

Sallie Elizabeth Taylor, M. Ed., O.T.R.
Clinical Specialist
Department of Preventive Medicine
Irene Walter Johnson Institute of Rehabilitation
Washington University School of Medicine
St. Louis, Missouri

Elizabeth Gordon Tiffany, M. Ed., O.T.R/L, F.A.O.T.A.
Chair and Associate Professor
College of Allied Health Professions
Temple University
Philadelphia, Pennsylvania

Ann Starnes Wade, M.A., O.T.R/L
Occupational Therapist
Colerain School
Columbus, Ohio

Elizabeth June Yerxa, Ed. D., O.T.R., F.A.O.T.A.
Chairperson, Department of Occupational Therapy
University of Southern California
Downey, California

PREFACE

Willard and Spackman's Occupational Therapy has, over the years, been a textbook written primarily for occupational therapy students. In preparation for this seventh edition, questionnaires were sent during the Fall of 1985 to all professional and technical occupational therapy educational programs in order to evaluate the textbook's usefulness for students. Detailed comments and constructive criticism were received from numerous programs and individual faculty members. As a result of the information received, changes and additions have been made in the *seventh edition.*

Existing chapters have been revised and updated and, when appropriate, information has been included about the role of the Certified Occupational Therapy Assistant.

Several new chapters have been added to address concerns identified through questionnaire responses. There is an introductory chapter that briefly addresses the occupational therapy definitions: the education, scope, and functions of occupational therapists and occupational therapy assistants; and accountability and the role of the professional organization and professional responsibility. A chapter has been added on the health-care delivery system and its influence on occupational therapy practice. The chapter on documentation has been enlarged. Additional new chapters cover the following topics: computers in occupational therapy, work hardening, and interpersonal relations and stress management. A chapter on acute care has replaced the chapter on general medicine and surgery.

The seventh edition is divided in six units. The first half of the book gives an overview of occupational therapy, while the second half concerns the implementation of occupational therapy in specific areas of practice.

There are five units in the overview. Unit I covers the history and philosophy of occupational therapy, and includes the introductory chapter; history of occupational therapy; the field's bases for practice in human development; occupation and activity; and frames of reference as organizing systems for practice. Unit II provides information on the health-care system. Unit III deals with research in occupational therapy. Unit IV presents the management aspect and includes information on documentation, uniform reporting, and quality assurance. Unit V covers the occupational therapy process, including the tools of practice: assessment and evaluation, activities of daily living, work assessment, leisure counseling, interpersonal relationships, orthotics, stress management, computers, biofeedback, and human sexuality.

Unit VI covers specific areas of practice: psychiatry and mental health; mental retardation; neurologic, arthritic, and orthopedic conditions; amputations; hand rehabilitation; blindness and deafness; specific pediatric conditions; cerebral palsy; the school system; gerontology, and home health care.

To provide background information, clarification of terminology, and assistance in the understanding of standards of practice, we have retained six appendices from the last edition, and have added three on documentation, delineation of the positions of OTR and COTA, and standardization of instruments and evaluation techniques. A directory of resources from various areas of practice rounds out the appendices. The directory has been compiled for the use of both students and practicing therapists. The glossary section has been updated to include new terminology.

We have worked to eliminate sexism in our terminology. In many cases we have used the phrases "he and she" or "his and her." In the cases where a female or male pronoun is used, it is because the sex of the client/patient has been mentioned, or for ease in reading the text.

Our attempt to provide comprehensive coverage of occupational therapy practice is evident in the choice of our thirty-six contributors. All are experts in their areas. Twelve are new to this edition. Thirty-five of the contributors are practicing occupational therapists and one is a rehabilitation home economist who works in an occupational therapy department. They represent nine universities and numerous clinics, community settings, and private practices in fourteen states. We thank them for their excellent contributions and for their assistance in providing a comprehensive overview of occupational therapy. Special thanks goes to Eleanor Faven of the J. B. Lippincott Company for her patience and assistance. Thanks is given also to our families and friends who provided moral support.

Helen L. Hopkins, Ed D., O.T.R/L, F.A.O.T.A.
Helen D. Smith, M.O.T., O.T.R/L, F.A.O.T.A.

CONTENTS

History and Philosophy

CHAPTER 1

An Introduction to Occupational Therapy

Scope of Occupational Therapy *Helen L. Hopkins*

Definition of Occupational Therapy

Over the course of the history of occupational therapy, the profession has been described and defined in many ways (see Chap. 2), but the earliest generally accepted definition was, "Occupational therapy is any activity, mental or physical, medically prescribed and professionally guided to aid a patient in recovery from disease or injury."[17]

As changes occurred in society and the demands for occupational therapy services grew, there were insufficient personnel to meet the needs. Thus other personnel assumed some of the aspects of treatment that once fell within the parameters of occupational therapy, including recreational therapy, art therapy, music therapy, and other therapies demanding specialized skills.

Attempts were made over the years to modify the definition of occupational therapy to reflect changes that had occurred both in our practice and in our relations with the medical profession. Today, occupational therapists generally receive referrals from physicians and have the prerogative of determining the course of treatment on the basis of their own assessments rather than having treatment prescribed and directed by the physician (as in our early definition). In 1972, a new definition of occupational therapy was accepted by the Delegate Assembly of the American Occupational Therapy Association (AOTA). The current official definition is:

> Occupational therapy is the art and science of directing man's participation in selected tasks to restore, reinforce and enhance performance, facilitate learning of those skills and functions essential for adaptation and productivity, diminish or correct pathology, and to promote and maintain health. Its fundamental concern is the capacity, throughout the life span, to perform with satisfaction to self and others those tasks and roles essential to productive living and to the mastery of self and the environment.[20]

The need for further clarification of the practice arose with the inception of licensure for occupational therapy in many states. Thus in 1981, a "Definition for the Purposes of Licensure"[19] was adopted by the Delegate Assembly (see Appendix A). As the field became better known and clarification of our practice was needed for the public, the following dictionary definition was adopted by the Representative Assembly in April 1986:

> Occupational Therapy: Therapeutic use of self-care, work and play activities to increase independent function, enhance development, and prevent disability. May include adaptation of task or environment to achieve maximum independence and to enhance quality of life.[13]

Location of Practice

Traditionally, most occupational therapists and occupational therapy assistants have practiced in institutional settings such as state hospitals, general hospitals, children's hospitals, rehabilitation centers, and schools for special children. With the passing of Public Law 94-142, which requires that all handicapped children receive free and "appropriate" education in the least restrictive setting and which includes occupational therapy as a "related service," many occupational therapists were hired to work in the public school system with children with developmental disabilities; learning disabilities; speech, language, and hearing impairment; and physical, emotional, and mental impairment. In addition, new positions have been created in neonatal units of hospitals where therapists work with "at-risk" infants. Thus the number of therapists working with children has increased, with the result that about one-third of all occupational therapists in the United States now work with children in public school systems, special schools, clinics, and hospitals.

As both mental hospitals and hospitals for the mentally retarded began to move patients out into community settings, many occupational therapists moved from hospitals to mental health–mental retardation centers in the community. Occupational therapy services were provided in free-standing community centers, in sheltered workshops, in store-front walk-in units, in shelters for the homeless, and in various community living arrangements.

With the inception of the Prospective Payment System and the introduction of diagnostic related groups (DRGs), which limit payment for a hospital stay according to a specified scale depending on the diagnosis, many patients were discharged to home sooner and "sicker," creating the need for more occupational therapy services in patients' homes or in long-term care facilities. Patients are admitted to rehabilitation centers before they are able to benefit from these services and are discharged to home before they are independent, thus requiring occupational therapy services in community agencies, outpatient work hardening units, or in patient's homes.

Currently, although occupational therapy services are available in more hospital settings than ever before, the greatest increase in services has been in the area of home care.[11] Many therapists work for corporations that provide occupational therapy services to hospitals, nursing homes, long-term care facilities, and home care. In addition, many therapists are working in private practice, not only in home care but also in physicians' offices and private practice agencies. There are also therapists working in industry, in correctional institutions, and in other nontraditional community settings.

Educational Requirements for Occupational Therapists and Occupational Therapy Assistants

Occupational Therapists

Over the years, the educational requirements for the registered occupational therapist (OTR) have expanded from a 6- to 12-week course in 1918 to the current requirement of at least a baccalaureate degree, including study of biological and behavioral sciences, pathological conditions, and specific occupational therapy techniques. The educational programs must comply with the 1983 "Essentials of an Academic Program for the Occupational Therapist"[3] in order to be accredited by the American Medical Association Committee on Allied Health Education and Accreditation (CAHEA) and the AOTA. After completing a minimum of 6 months of full-time fieldwork, graduates of accredited programs are eligible to take the AOTA Certification Examination to become registered occupational therapists (OTRs). All states that require licensure currently accept the AOTA's examination and educational requirements for state licensure. The required 6 months of full-time fieldwork is felt to provide the transition from the role of student to that of full-fledged professional practitioner. This will be discussed further in Section 2 of this chapter.

Occupational Therapy Assistants

The initial need for occupational therapy assistants grew out of a shortage of occupational therapy personnel in psychiatric facilities after World War II. At that time, assistants were trained on the job to compensate for the manpower shortage. In 1949, the Board of Management of the AOTA proposed the establishment of a 1-year educational program for occupational therapy assistants in psychiatric hospitals. This proposal was referred to the Committee on Psychiatry, Subcommittee on Research, for study.[8] In October 1956, the Board of Management approved a plan to recognize aide-level occupational therapy personnel, and a committee was appointed to develop a plan to recognize and train aides in occupational therapy.[7] In October 1957, the first set of standards for occupational therapy assistants, entitled "Requirements of an Acceptable Program and Curriculum Guide," was accepted. The plan was officially implemented 1 year later, and a grandfather clause was established to recognize previously trained assistants.[10,16] The training programs were established in those facilities requiring the services of an assistant such as state hospitals. The programs were 12 weeks in length and required 460 clock hours of training for working with psychiatric patients.[10,16] In 1960, similar programs were established for work in general practice. In 1963, the membership category of Certified Occupational Therapy Assistant (COTA) was established by the AOTA.[16] In 1964 and 1965, the first two associate degree programs for training COTAs were approved. At that time, educational programs trained students for practice in either psychiatry or general practice, but not in both. After a successful pilot program was conducted in 1966, which combined study in psychiatry and general practice, dual certification was established. By 1966, there were 12 programs for occupational therapy assistants, two of which granted associate degrees and ten of which granted certificates for work in both psychiatry and general practice.[1]

In 1971, it was proposed that occupational therapy assistants be required to take a national certification examination to be eligible to practice. This measure was adopted and the first occupational therapy assistants took new certification examination in 1977.[16] In the meantime, Resolution 311-71, passed by the Delegate Assembly in 1971, established criteria to enable the COTA to take the national certification examination to become an OTR. The first COTA took the examination in 1974 and became registered as an occupational therapist without meeting the regular educational requirements. Beginning in 1976, a COTA who wished to become an OTR had to meet the following criteria in addition to passing the OTR examination: current certification as a COTA, fieldwork experience comparable to that of the occupational therapy student, and 4 years of practice as a COTA.[6] This program was known as the *Career Mobility Program*. In 1984, it was determined by the policy-making body, now called the Representative Assembly, that COTAs could become OTRs through regular educational programs. The Career Mobility Program was no longer needed, so it was terminated. A motion passed by the Representative Assembly in April 1983 promoted the establishment of occupational therapy assistant programs at the associate degree level.[18] This motion became Association policy and discouraged the development of certificate programs for the occupational therapy assistant.

In 1983, the current "Essentials of an Approved Educational Program for the Occupational Therapy Assistant"[4] were adopted by the AOTA. Programs that meet these "Essentials" are approved by the Association. After completing the required 2 months of full-time fieldwork, graduates of these programs are eligible to take the AOTA Certification Examination to become COTAs. As with the OTR, the COTA certification examination and the educational and fieldwork requirements are acceptable for state licensure.

Roles and Functions of Registered Occupational Therapists and Certified Occupational Therapy Assistants

As the number of COTAs increased and the tasks delegated to them expanded, role and relationship problems and conflicts arose.[16] Thus, in 1963, it was determined that there was a need to clarify roles and functions of the occupational therapist and the occupational therapy assistant. In 1967, "A Guide for the Supervision of the COTA" was established which stated that the COTA was to be supervised by "an OTR, an experienced COTA or an OTR designate."[16] There was no further study until Ohio State University conducted a study on "Job Descriptions through Task Analysis" in 1972.[22] In 1973, the AOTA received a grant to "Delineate Roles and Functions of Occupational Therapy Personnel" to serve as a basis for proficiency examinations.[5] However, it was not until 1981 that the "Entry-Level Role Delineation for OTRs and COTAs" was approved by the Representative Assembly (see Appendix H). This Role Delineation was to be used to guide practice and as a basis for the scope of the "Essentials" for both levels of education and as a guide in the development of the certification examinations.

Because of major changes occurring in the health care delivery system, in 1985 the Commission on Education identified a need for revision of the 1981 Role Delineation. In addition, there was a need for the knowledge, skills, attitudes, and abilities to be specified for the functions identified within the role delineation. At the same time, the Certification Committee believed it was important to have an updated job analysis for entry-level practice to meet the requirement of the Equal Employment Opportunities Commission, which states that "professional associations offering examinations to state licensing agencies must use valid and job-related tests."[21]

The Role Delineation document was sent to the Intercommission Council, which was to develop a plan to address these concerns. The projected plan, which changed the name to the Professional and Technical Role Analysis (PATRA), will address the description of current roles and the knowledge, skills, attitudes, and abilities necessary to perform them. The PATRA committee is composed of both OTRs and COTAs representing both educators and practitioners. Once the PATRA task is completed, the results will be used for Essentials review and for development of a certification examination that evaluates the knowledge and skills needed for practice and delineates the roles of OTRs and COTAs.[21] This project is scheduled for completion and publication in 1988.

Accountability: Accreditation — Certification — Continuing Education

Because the demand for accountability is a driving force within the health care system today, the health care professions attempt to ensure the competence of practitioners in several ways. To ensure competence of entry-level practitioners, two processes are used to evaluate graduates of the educational programs: *accreditation* and *certification*. To maintain competence for practicing professionals, *continuing education programs* are perhaps the most widely used methods.

Accreditation

Accreditation is the process whereby educational programs are evaluated against a set of standards that represent the knowledge, skills, and attitudes needed for competent practice in a specified field. Every occupational therapy program and every occupational therapy assistant program must be accredited or approved every 5 to 7 years by demonstrating that its students are receiving an education that meets the standards specified in the "Essentials." Only those students who have graduated from an accredited occupational therapy program or an approved occupational therapy assistant program are permitted to take the certification examination that will allow them to practice in the field.

Certification

The certification process assures that each practitioner has the knowledge, skills, and attitudes required for competent practice in the field. It is assumed that passing a written comprehensive examination which covers all aspects of the education of the OTR or COTA will verify that the practitioner has the entry-level knowledge and thus is competent to practice. For this reason, certification examinations have been developed for both levels of practice. To assure that the practitioner

has the skills and attitudes as well as the knowledge, all students are also required to have practical experience (fieldwork) under the supervision of an experienced practitioner. Students from all schools are evaluated using the Fieldwork Evaluation Reports approved by the AOTA in 1983 and 1985.[14,15] Successful completion of the required fieldwork assignments, along with completion of the didactic and laboratory portions of the educational program, determine eligibility to take the certification examination. This examination is developed by a qualified testing agency, but questions are written and checked for accuracy by practicing occupational therapists and occupational therapy assistants. Recently, an independent Certification Board has been established by the Association to assure the public that the Association is not a "closed shop" and is, in fact, concerned for the welfare of the public. The Certification Board will be responsible for screening examination questions and assessing the breadth and depth of the test in order to evaluate the competence of applicants for practice in occupational therapy. When the PATRA task is completed, it will be used to analyze the quality and accuracy of the certification examinations and to provide guidance for updating the "Essentials." It is then hoped that through the accreditation and certification processes, the competence of entry-level practitioners can be ensured.

Continuing Education

Since accountability to the public is demanded not only of the entry-level practitioner but of all therapists and assistants in active practice, it is mandatory that practitioners keep pace with changes in society, in medicine, and in the practice of occupational therapy. It is, therefore, important that all occupational therapists acquire a commitment to life-long education.

The AOTA has recognized that opportunities for maintaining skills in traditional areas of practice as well as for gaining skills in new areas are often limited for practitioners because of the expense and availability of courses. For this reason, continuing education has been a high priority for the Association, and the Continuing Education Division was created in the national office to meet the needs of all practitioners. This division has provided resources for all members in many areas of practice through the development of "practice packets" which are updated constantly. In addition, the *Occupational Therapy News* publishes lists of continuing education programs being conducted throughout the country that are sponsored by the AOTA, state and regional occupational therapy associations, individuals, and private educational agencies.

In order to provide education for members in developing or expanding areas of practice, the Continuing Education Division of the AOTA has developed courses and training programs in several areas including: "Training: Occupational Therapy Educational Management in Schools" (TOTEMS); "Planning and Implementing Vocational Readiness in Occupational Therapy" (PIVOT); "Role of Occupational Therapy with the Elderly" (ROTE); and "Strategies, Concepts and Opportunities for Program Development and Evaluation in Mental Health" (SCOPE). These courses have been given at numerous locations throughout the country in an attempt to make this information available and affordable to all members. For each training course, manuals are available for purchase by members who are unable to attend the courses.

Educational opportunities also are available through many colleges and universities. Some of the programs are given as continuing education courses, whereas others are given as advanced degrees in special areas of practice or as advanced work in education, administration, or research.

Many books in specialty areas of occupational therapy practice are being published today. These, along with articles in journals such as the *American Journal of Occupational Therapy*, the *Occupational Therapy Journal of Research*, the special-interest newsletters, and the *Journal of Occupational Therapy in Health Care* make information available to all members and should help members keep cognizant of changes in occupational therapy and in society.

Licensure laws in many states require that each therapist acquire a specified number of continuing education units each year in order to retain a license. Some states have other requirements to assure that therapists retain competence. Whether because of state licensure requirements or because of feelings of professional obligation, it is vital that all practitioners maintain their competence using any or all of the resources available and develop an attitude favoring life-long learning.

Role of the Professional Organization

The AOTA is the official professional organization for occupational therapists and occupational therapy assistants. The Association was incorporated as the National Society for the Promotion of Occupational Therapy in March 1917. The present name was adopted in January 1923. The purposes of the Association, as indicated in the articles of incorporation as amended in 1976, are: "to advance the therapeutic value of occupation; to research the effects of occupation upon human beings and to disseminate that research; to promote the use of occupational therapy and to advance the standards of education and training in the field; to educate consumers about the effect of occupation upon their well-being; and to engage in such other activities as may be consid-

ered to be advantageous to the profession, its members and the consumer of occupational therapy services."[9]

The Association has its national headquarters in Rockville, Maryland, with a paid staff to conduct Association business. The volunteer sector of the Association is made up of all members, including the officers and representatives who are elected to develop policies and procedures. The Representative Assembly is the policy-making body and is composed of elected representatives from each state, the elected officers of the Assembly and the Association, the first alternate representative to the World Federation of Occupational Therapists, and the chair of the Student Committee. The Executive Board is the management body of the Association and directs its operations, with the national office staff conducting the day-to-day business.

There are three standing commissions of the Representative Assembly — Education, Practice, and Standards and Ethics — which recommend policies and procedures in their respective areas. The official bodies of the Association, composed of members from the volunteer sector, carry out business which enhances the education, research, and practice aspects of the profession. The standing committees of the Representative Assembly carry out the business of the Assembly. In addition, there now is an independent Certification Board which conducts affairs related to certification of occupational therapists and occupational therapy assistants. Figure 1-1 shows the organizational chart of the AOTA.

The national office is directed by an Executive Director, who has three Associate Directors to administer the operations of Professional Services, Membership Services, and Financial and Business Administration. The national office staff provides services for membership through the divisions of education, practice, continuing education, credentialling, government and legal affairs, publications, public information, conferences and meetings, membership, quality assurance, and finance and business.

Members of the Association receive numerous benefits. They receive a monthly journal and newspaper, a news weekly, a quarterly specialty section newspaper, continuing education information and opportunities, national conferences, support for education, practice and research, support for legislation at the national level, information on government and legal affairs, development and dissemination of information on standards of practice, position papers that define our areas of practice to the public, dissemination of public information to enhance our public image, and many others.

Professional Responsibility

As a member of a health care profession, each occupational therapist and occupational therapy assistant has

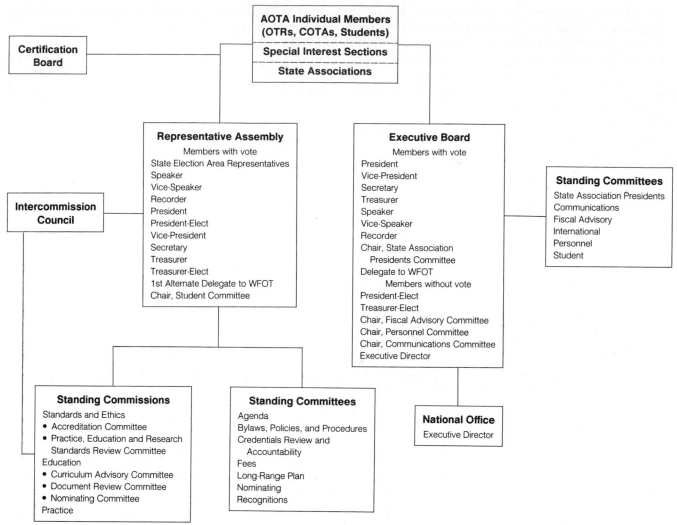

Figure 1-1. Organizational chart of The American Occupational Therapy Association, Inc.

professional responsibilities that must be met in order to enhance the public image of occupational therapy and to assure the viability of the profession. Each individual must take responsibility for his or her own competence as an occupational therapist or an occupational therapy assistant and must do whatever is needed to retain this competence. This can be done through reading of literature in the field; attendance at state, regional, and national meetings and conferences; and continuing or advanced education. Each occupational therapist, occupational therapy assistant, and occupational therapy student also has an obligation to be involved in district, state, and national association affairs to the highest extent possible in order to be informed of changes in the field and other health care concerns. It is also an obligation for the therapist, assistant, and student to maintain membership in the state and national association and to support their activities so that these associations can continue to provide services that will benefit members and the general public.

References

1. American Occupational Therapy Association Annual Business Meeting Minutes. Am J Occup Ther 21:95, 1967
2. American Occupational Therapy Association Annual Business Meeting Minutes. Am J Occup Ther 22:99, 1968
3. American Occupational Therapy Association: Essentials of an Accredited Educational Program for the Occupational Therapist. Am J Occup Ther 37:817, 1983
4. American Occupational Therapy Association: Essentials of an Approved Educational Program for the Occupational Therapy Assistant. Am J Occup Ther 37:824, 1983
5. American Occupational Therapy Association: Project to Delineate the Roles and Functions of Occupational Therapy Personnel in the Detail Needed to Serve as a Basis for the Construction of Proficiency Examinations. Department of Health, Education and Welfare, Public Health Services, National Institutes of Health, Bureau of Manpower Education, Division of Allied Health Manpower. Contract No. NO 1 AH 24172, Washington DC, 1973
6. American Occupational Therapy Association: Statement on Career Mobility. Am J Occup Ther 27:157, 1973

7. Board of Management Minutes, American Occupational Therapy Association. Am J Occup Ther 11:41, 1957

8. Committee Reports: Education Committee, American Occupational Therapy Association. Am J Occup Ther 4:221, 1949

9. Composite Articles of Incorporation of the American Occupational Therapy Association as Amended. In Reference Manual of the Official Documents of the American Occupational Therapy Association, Inc., p I-1. Rockville, MD, AOTA 1986

10. Crampton MW: The recognition of occupational therapy assistants. Am J Occup Ther 12:269, 1958

11. Dataline: Occupational therapy services increase in the nation's hospitals. Occup Ther News 40(4):6, 1986

12. Delegate Assembly Minutes, American Occupational Therapy Association. Am J Occup Ther 29:552, 1975

13. Dictionary Definition of Occupational Therapy, Representative Assembly Minutes. Am J Occup Ther 40:852, 1986

14. Fieldwork Evaluation Form for Occupational Therapy Students, Adopted 1983. In Reference Manual of the Official Documents of the American Occupational Ther-apy Association, Inc., p II-18-31. Rockville, MD, AOTA 1986

15. From FWPR to FWE. Occup Ther News 40(12):9, 1986

16. Hirama H: The COTA: A chronological review. In Ryan S: The Occupational Therapy Assistant: Roles and Responsibilities. pp 23–34. Thorofare, Slack, Inc., 1986

17. Mc Nary H: The scope of occupational therapy. In Willard HS, Spackman CS (eds): Occupational Therapy, p 10. Philadelphia, JB Lippincott, 1947

18. Minutes of the Representative Assembly, April 1983. Am J Occup Ther 37:834, 1983

19. Occupational Therapy Definition for Purposes of Licensure, Representative Assembly Minutes. Am J Occup Ther 35:798, 1981

20. Occupational Therapy: Its definition and functions. Am J Occup Ther 26:204, 1972

21. PATRA project: What it is and is not. Occup Ther News 40(12):9, 1986

22. Schoen KT: Development of Occupational Therapy Job Descriptions and Curricula Through Task Analysis. Department of Health Education and Welfare Grant #5 DO2 AH00964 01, 2, Columbus, Ohio State University, 1972

SECTION 2

Fieldwork Education: Applying Theory to Practice   *Ellen S. Cohn*

The consensus within the occupational therapy profession is that the fieldwork experience plays an integral role in an occupational therapist's professional development. In 1923, the first standards requiring fieldwork experiences were approved by the AOTA. Today, in addition to academic course work, 6 months of supervised fieldwork is a prerequisite for the national certification examination.[1] The process and content of fieldwork experiences have been debated over the years, yet the value of having an opportunity to apply theory to practice has never been denied. Christie, Joyce, and Moeller highlight that value by documenting the fieldwork experience as having the greatest impact on the development of a therapist's preference for a specific area of clinical practice. Of the 131 therapists surveyed, 55% indicated that clinical practice preferences were either formed or changed during the fieldwork experience, and another 24% noted that fieldwork experience expanded their interests to other areas of practice. Thus, the fieldwork experience can be rich and rewarding and will likely have a tremendous impact on students' career choices.[3]

While acknowledging that each student's fieldwork experience will be different, this chapter will provide an overview of the experience, including the roles and the responsibilities of the participants. The nature of the transition from the academic setting to the clinical world of practice, coupled with a description of the interview, supervisory, and evaluation processes, are intended to familiarze students with the expectations and procedures of fieldwork settings.

Purpose

The purpose of the fieldwork experience is to provide occupational therapy students with the opportunity to integrate academic knowledge with application skills at progressively higher levels of performance and responsibility. Students test firsthand the theories and facts learned in academic study and refine skills through interaction with patients under the supervision of qualified occupational therapists. Fieldwork provides students with situations in which to practice interpersonal skills with patients and staff and to develop characteristics essential to productive working relationships.[8] For students, the overall purpose of the fieldwork experience is to gain mastery of occupational therapy reasoning and techniques to develop entry-level competency. Upon completion of the fieldwork experience, students are expected to demonstrate competence in the areas of assessment, planning, treatment, problem-solving, administration, and professionalism.

Although the goals and objectives specific to each fieldwork setting will be initially delineated, students are expected to demonstrate competence in using the assessment tools and evaluative procedures routinely employed by occupational therapists. On the basis of the models and theories of occupational therapy practiced at the fieldwork centers, students should become proficient in implementing, justifying, and evaluating the effectiveness of treatment plans. Effective oral and written communication of ideas and objectives relevant to the roles and duties of an occupational therapist, including interaction with patients and staff in a professional manner, are also expected of occupational therapy students. Students are responsible for demonstrating a sensitivity to and respect for patient confidentiality. Finally, acquisition of professional characteristics that permit one to establish and sustain therapeutic relationships and to work collaboratively with others will be expected in all fieldwork centers.

The aforementioned competencies require specific skill development and the ability to interact with others. Another expectation, more internal to students' development of positive professional self-images, includes taking responsibility for maintaining, assessing, and improving self-competence. Students are responsible for articulating their understanding of theoretical information and identifying their abilities to implement assessment and treatment techniques. Moreover, the ability to benefit from supervision as a resource for self-directed learning is critical for professional development.[12]

Roles and Responsibilities

Upon completion of academic course work, occupational therapy students are eligible to begin their fieldwork experiences. Clearly defined objectives and guidelines provide students with the direction necessary for organizing their efforts toward achieving clinical competence. Considering the overall fieldwork objectives and the resources of the clinical facility, working toward mastery of the entry-level skills required for high-quality patient care is a mutual undertaking between the fieldwork educators and students. Both fieldwork educators and students are responsible for the process of evaluating student progress and modifying the learning experience within the environment. The roles and responsibilities of each of the participants in fieldwork education will be outlined.

Students

The responsibilities of the students are as follows:
1. Fulfilling all duties and responsibilities identified by the fieldwork educators and academic fieldwork coordinators within the designated times

2. Complying with the professional standards identified by the fieldwork facility, the university, and the Principles of Occupational Therapy Ethics as approved by the Representative Assembly of the American Occupational Therapy Association in 1979 (Appendix B)
3. Communicating with fieldwork educators to confirm the starting dates and other prerequisite information
4. Securing documentation of adequate medical and professional insurance for the duration of the fieldwork experience
5. Completing and presenting to the fieldwork educators one copy of the students' evaluation of the fieldwork experience[4]

Fieldwork Educators

The individuals responsible for the fieldwork education program in the clinic must be registered occupational therapists with a minimum of 1 year of experience in direct client services. As stated in the Essentials and Guidelines of an Accredited Education Program for the Occupational Therapist, these individuals are formally titled "fieldwork educators," although "clinical educators," "fieldwork supervisors," and "student supervisors" are interchangeable titles.[8]

Two areas of responsibility of fieldwork educators are administrative functions and direct day-to-day supervision. The administrative responsibilities of the fieldwork educator include, but are not limited to, the following:
1. Collaborating with the academic fieldwork coordinator in the development of a program that provides the best opportunity for the implementation of theoretical concepts offered as part of the academic educational program
2. Creating an environment that facilitates learning, clinical inquiry, and reflection on one's practice
3. Preparing, maintaining, and sending to the academic fieldwork coordinator current information about the fieldwork education center, including a statement of the conceptual models from which evaluation is derived and on which treatment is based
4. Scheduling students in collaboration with the academic fieldwork coordinator
5. Establishing objectives of the fieldwork experience and identifying the philosophy of the center
6. Contributing to the evaluation of each student at midpoint and termination. One copy of the terminal document must be signed by both the fieldwork educator and the student and sent to the fieldwork coordinator of the educational institution in which the student is enrolled
7. Being familiar with the policy regarding the withdrawal of students from fieldwork experience

of each educational institution from which students are accepted

8. Notifying the academic fieldwork coordinator of any student for whom the fieldwork center is requesting withdrawal or of other problems that may arise

9. Reviewing periodically the contractual agreement between the academic institution and the fieldwork center and ensuring that these agreements are signed

10. Providing regular and periodic supervision of students

The direct day-to-day supervisory responsibilities of the fieldwork educator include, but are not limited to:

1. Providing an adequate orientation to the fieldwork education center and to specific department policies and procedures

2. Assigning patients and clients to students and defining expectations clearly to students

3. Supervising the provision of occupational therapy services and the documentation and oral reporting of students

4. Assessing skills and knowledge of the students

5. Meeting with students regularly to review performance and to provide guidance using behavioral language and observable data. As a result of supervisor's feedback, goals for change are developed collaboratively by students and supervisors

6. Seeking out evaluation of own supervisory skills from appropriate people[8]

Academic Fieldwork Coordinator

Each academic program has an academic fieldwork coordinator who functions as a liaison between the academic setting, the fieldwork educators, and the students. The responsibilities of the academic fieldwork coordinator are:

1. Assigning eligible students to fieldwork experience and confirming the assignment in writing to each fieldwork educator

2. Assuring that all written contracts or letters of agreement between the educational institution and the fieldwork education center are signed and periodically reviewed

3. Making regular and periodic contacts with each fieldwork education center where students are placed

4. Maintaining a current information file on each fieldwork education center where students are placed

5. Identifying new sites for fieldwork education

6. Developing and implementing a policy for withdrawal of students from a fieldwork education center

7. Orienting students to the general purposes of fieldwork experience and providing them with necessary forms

8. Reassigning students who do not complete their original fieldwork assignments in accordance with the educational institution's policies

9. Developing fieldwork experience programs that provide the best opportunity for the implementation of theoretical concepts offered as part of the didactic curriculum

10. Maintaining a collaborative relationship with fieldwork education centers

11. Sending necessary information and forms for each student to the fieldwork educator[8]

Knowledge of the fieldwork education programs is an important aspect of the academic fieldwork coordinator's job. Periodic visits are made to the fieldwork centers, or when on-site visits are unrealistic, telephone communication is maintained. The academic fieldwork coordinator is available for consultation to both students and fieldwork educators.

Transition from Classroom to Clinic: Student to Professional

The shift from the academic setting to the clinical fieldwork setting is an obvious, yet potentially underestimated, life change. Occupational therapy students are making the environmental transition from the classroom to the clinic while simultaneously emerging from the role of students to the professional role of therapists. As with any transition, occupational therapy students leaving academia face a process of change from one structure, role, or sense of self to another. The struggle to assimilate into a new environment and to develop a new role may jolt students into disequilibrium, resulting in an inability to adjust. As is true of all life changes, the experience of disequilibrium can be an opportunity for growth, especially in the context of a supportive supervisory relationship. This time of transition results in changes in assumptions about oneself and the world and requires a corresponding change in one's behaviors and relationships. As students move into fieldwork settings, they develop new relationships, learning styles, behaviors, and self-perceptions. Students may begin to reassess their suppositions about occupational therapy, the theories learned in school, and their views of themselves as therapists, learners, and individuals. Since individuals differ in their ability to adapt to change, and because each student will be placed in a different fieldwork setting, the transition will have a different impact on each student.

The nature of the clinical fieldwork environment is fundamentally different from that of the academic environment. Knowing and acknowledging some of the distinctions between the two settings may ease the transition and provide students with support to accept the challenges of fieldwork experiences (Table 1-1). Within the fieldwork environment, the learning focus shifts to the application or implementation of mastered techniques in an applied interpersonal context. Techniques that were mastered in a simulated context now must be applied with attention to the patient's emotional needs. Abstract questions—appropriate in the academic environment—shift to pragmatic questions to reduce the possibility of error in one's thinking. Consequently, tolerance for ambiguity or uncertainty declines once students enter the fieldwork environment.

In the academic setting, students are accountable to themselves, and performance is evaluated on a summative basis through tests, assignments, and grades. Students choose whether to disclose grades to family or peers, and their performance does not affect others. In the fieldwork center, students' performance is evalu-

ated on a formative basis and may be observed by the entire health care term, especially at team meetings. Performance is no longer the private matter it was at school but is publicly observed, as it has a direct and critical impact on patients. Colleagues, patients, and their families then may offer meaningful feedback. Although all of these opportunities may create disequilibrium or tension, they likewise constitute new ways in which students learn about themselves and their profession. The broad and diverse experience within the fieldwork setting challenges students to redefine their sense of self.

From an educational perspective, fieldwork education likewise takes place in a situation in which fieldwork educators have little control. The organizational factors of the health care setting, coupled with patient care factors such as the nature and complexity of the patient's problem, the length of stay, and fluctuation in patient load make it difficult to make generalizations for planning. Conversely, in the academic setting, many of

Table 1-1. *Distinctions Between Academic and Clinical Settings*

	Academic Setting	*Clinical Setting*
Purpose	Facilitate dissemination of knowledge, development of creative thought and student growth, award degrees	Provide high-quality patient care
Faculty/supervisor accountability	1. To student 2. To university	1. To patient and family 2. To clinical center 3. To student
Student accountability	To self	To patients and families, supervisor, and clinical center
Pace	Adaptable to student and faculty needs	Dependent on patient needs; less adaptable
Student/educator ratio	Many students to one faculty member	One student to one supervisor
Source of feedback	Summative at midterm or at the end of term; provided by faculty	Provided by patients and families, supervisor, and other staff; formative
Degree of faculty/supervisor control of educational experience	Able to plan, controlled	Limited control; various diagnoses and lengths of patient stay
Primary learning tools	Books, lectures, audiovisual aids, case studies, simulation	Situation of practice; patients, families, and staff
Conceptual learning	Abstract, theoretical	Pragmatic, applied in interpersonal context
Learning process	Teacher-directed	Self-directed
Tolerance for ambiguity/uncertainty	High	Low
Life style	Flexible to plan time around class schedule	Structured; flexible time limited to evenings and weekends

the factors that operate as variables in the fieldwork setting are constant and inherently structured by faculty. The fieldwork eductors' primary responsibility is patient care, as they have an ethical imperative to ensure the welfare of patients. This appropriate professional ethic may constrain activities that may be desirable from the standpoint of education. One beneficial distinction between the academic environment and the clinic which allows fieldwork educators to adapt to the constraints of the clinic is the individualized supervisory relationship. This unique one-to-one relationship is a positive aspect of the fieldwork environment, as fieldwork educators have the luxury of adapting their styles to meet the needs of the learner.

Fieldwork Interviews

Most fieldwork educators require an interview to ensure that students understand the clinical expectations and the type of experience offered at their particular facility. The interview further serves to confirm the student's suitability for the particular fieldwork placement. Each academic program reserves fieldwork placements for a designated time, and students are then individually matched to the available placement. In most cases, only one student is scheduled to interview for a particular placement. Hence, the interview is usually noncompetitive and is designed for students and fieldwork educators to confirm assumptions. However, the fieldwork educators do have the right to decline acceptance of students based on the interview, just as students have the right to decline the particular fieldwork placement. The fieldwork educators notify either the students or the academic fieldwork coordinators of their intention to accept or deny the placement. In either case, the academic fieldwork coordinator serves as a liason and consultant.

As the interviews are designed to ensure a mutually agreeable match between students' career interests and fieldwork settings, a variety of professionally related questions may be generated by the fieldwork educators. For example, students may be asked to identify their clinical interests and long-term career goals, their expectations of the fieldwork experience, their frame of reference, or their experience in the academic setting. Additionally, some fieldwork educators will ask questions to ascertain why students chose occupational therapy as a profession or why students desire to train in the particular fieldwork setting. Therefore, it is useful for students to learn about the facility and to consider their professional goals before the interview. It is important to note that each interviewer will ask his or her own set of questions and probe different aspects of students' backgrounds.

The process of becoming an occupational therapist involves developing a sense of professional identity and utilizing the self as a therapeutic agent. Each student brings a unique composite of knowledge, skills, and personal style to the fieldwork experience. Therefore, depending on the type of facility, the role of occupational therapy, and the fieldwork educator's concept of supervision, the educator will ask different questions related to students' understanding of themselves. Students are commonly asked to identify experiences that may be relevant to fieldwork and to identify their strengths and weaknesses. Clarification of students' learning styles promotes an understanding of their preferred approach to learning and can assist both students and fieldwork educators in developing strategies to enhance the fieldwork experience. Since the fieldwork experience is a major life transition, the fieldwork educator may want to discuss a student's life style, social supports, and perceived ability to enter a new system, manage time, or handle stress. These questions are intended to appraise the potential influences on a student's performance, and students should be prepared to discuss these important issues. Students, in turn, may utilize their fieldwork interview to clarify their assumptions about the fieldwork requirements, the structure of supervision, the types of patients treated, the frame of reference of the occupational therapy department, and the philosophy of the entire facility.

Supervisory Relationship

In 1983, the AOTA defined supervision as a mutual understanding between supervisor and supervisee intended to promote growth and development while evaluating performance and maintaining standards.[2] Supervision is thus conceptualized as a dynamic teaching–learning relationship, an educational process that serves as a bridge between previously learned knowledge and clinical skill, and a mechanism that ensures an experiential learning environment. Since the goals and often the top priority in the clinical facility are directed toward providing high-quality care for patients, supervision will be structured to ensure such care for patients while simultaneously, but possibly secondarily, facilitating and managing the learning process for students. Within this framework, the fieldwork educator is a facilitator of learning who serves as a reflective model to be emulated as students progress toward greater responsibility in their role as occupational therapists.[6]

The importance of the relationship between fieldwork educators and students is inherent within the supervisory context. Christie, Joyce, and Moeller, in their study of 65 fieldwork centers, confirmed the longstanding belief that the relationship between students and fieldwork educators is the most significant aspect of the fieldwork experience. In the study, both students and educators perceived the supervisory process as the most critical element in distinguishing good from poor fieldwork experiences. Furthermore, communication and interpersonal skills were identified as distinguishing characteristics of effective supervision.[3]

Each member in the supervisory relationship enters with his or her own assumptions and expectations. These expectations are based on the student's past experiences with other supervisors, parents, or other authority figures. These experiences, coupled with student's emerging paradigms of occupational therapy and professional goals, provide the foundation for the supervisory relationship. Supervisors in turn have a notion of the behaviors, skills, and attitudes necessary for effective entry-level practice in their fieldwork settings. Initially, the delineation of expectations is a primary focus of supervision. Once the expectations of both supervisors and students are defined, the focus shifts to providing feedback related to the stated expectations.

The feedback provided by the fieldwork educators is critical to a student's development. Feedback, defined as "knowledge of the results of individual's performance to the extent that individual's behavior is changed in a desirable direction," refers to a particular aspect of behavior, to a total behavioral sequence or performance, or to the nature of the message itself; *e.g.*, the message may convey information about the student's attitudes toward patients. This definition connotes an expectation that "some change will occur in the student's understanding, attitude, or behavior in response to feedback."[11] In a direct manner, feedback can help to identify the next step in the change process, to clarify steps that have taken place, to evaluate whether a particular step meets performance criteria for a specific task and whether it relates to or achieves the overall goals, and to clarify or modify those goals or expectations as needed. One of the key sources for feedback during the fieldwork experience is the fieldwork educator. It is important for students to recognize that fieldwork educators are not judging the students' worth or goodness but rather assessing how well students are performing. Crist suggests that students "be willing to try new suggestions or ways, while evaluating their own biases and preferences."[10] Feedback, given honestly and sincerely, is often the most valuable change agent for students.

Fieldwork Evaluation

Frequently, students receive feedback informally during supervision meetings; however, formal mechanisms for providing feedback and evaluation of a student's performance, judgments, and attitudes are built into the fieldwork experience. There are two distinct purposes in fieldwork evaluation. One is the formative, ongoing process to direct student learning throughout the fieldwork experience and the other is summative to document the level of skills attained at the completion of the fieldwork experience. Although these two processes are different, they are not mutually exclusive. The formative process occurs throughout the fieldwork experience so students and fieldwork educators can compare perceptions, assess which student activities are important and which are less so, review objectives, plan new learning opportunities, and make necessary modifications in behaviors. As suggested by Yerxa, conseling students is an important component of evaluation: "Counseling means to give students an objective, specific view of performance in such a way that students can be assured of their strengths and strengthened to improve their weaknesses."[13] This is a continuing process throughout the fieldwork experience and is usually specific to the setting.

The second process, which is cumulative, requires documentation of students' performance upon completion of the fieldwork experience. The Fieldwork Evaluation (FWE) is the instrument adopted by the AOTA for evaluating performance of professional-level occupational therapy students in all fieldwork education centers.[9] The FWE is designed to assess students' performance of specific professional tasks. It is an evaluation tool and is not intended to serve as a tool for the counseling process described by Yerxa.

The FWE consists of two sections. The first section has 51 behavioral statements depicting competent performance in five areas: assessment, planning, treatment, problem solving, and administrative/professionalism. Each area is evaluated on the basis of performance, judgment, and attitude on a rating scale ranging from excellent to poor. The second section is a written summary of performance indicating particular strengths and weaknesses and any other information useful in documenting professional growth and learning. This form should serve as summary of what students already know of their performance. Completion, administration, and subsequent use of the FWE should be conducted with consideration of all legal and ethical implications regarding each student assessed. Such consideration includes the right to nonprejudicial evaluation, the right to privacy of information, and the right for students to appeal.[8]

The "Guidelines for an Occupational Therapy Fieldwork Experience — Level II" state that students should be evaluated at midterm and at completion of the fieldwork experience.[7] "When used at midterm, the recommended ratings for each of the 51-tasks are satisfactory plus (S+), satisfactory (S), and unsatisfactory (U)."[5] Numerical scores are avoided at midterm to separate evaluation from any association with grades and to help students view the feedback as an aid to the development of professionalism. Furthermore, the avoidance of scores at midterm prevents inflated terminal scores, as evaluators have a tendency to expect greater scores at the end of the fieldwork experience. As the AOTA suggests, "During the midterm review process, students and supervisors should collaboratively design a plan which would enable students to achieve entry level competence by the end of the fieldwork experience. This plan should include specific objectives and enabling activities to be used by students and supervisors in order to achieve the competence desired."[5]

Finally, the intent of the fieldwork evaluation is not to differentiate between students, but to measure their achievement of specific competencies. Future employers will want assurance that students satisfy the entry-level requirements. The FWE data may be synthesized to provide the foundation for employment references.

Summary

A profession usually defines its boundaries by setting up criteria for entry. In occupational therapy, the fieldwork experience is an essential component of the entry criteria. The purpose of fieldwork is to provide learning experiences that foster professional competence and personal growth. It is the beginning of a life-long process of connecting theory with practice. The depth of the experience will be highly dependent on the degree to which students and fieldwork educators share the responsibility for teaching and learning.

References

1. American Occupational Therapy Association: Essentials and guidelines of an accredited educational program for the occupational therapist. Am J Occup Ther 37:817, 1983
2. American Occupational Therapy Association: Reference Manual of the Official Documents of the American Occupational Therapy Association. Rockville, MD, American Occupational Therapy Association, 1983
3. Christie BA, Joyce PC, Moeller PL: Fieldwork experience I: Impact on practice preference. Am J Occup Ther 39:671, 1985
4. Cohn ES: Student Fieldwork Manual. Medford, MA, Tufts University–Boston School of Occupational Therapy, 1986
5. Commission on Education of the American Occupational Therapy Association: Fieldwork Evaluation for the Occupational Therapist. Rockville, MD, American Occupational Therapy Association, 1986
6. Commission on Education of the American Occupational Therapy Association: Fieldwork Experience Manual for Academic Fieldwork Coordinators, Fieldwork Supervisors and Students. Rockville, MD, American Occupational Therapy Association, 1977
7. Commission on Education of the American Occupational Therapy Association: Guidelines for an Occupational Therapy Fieldwork Experience — Level II. Rockville, MD, American Occupational Therapy Association, 1985
8. Commission on Education of the American Occupational Therapy Association: Guide to Fieldwork Education. Rockville, MD. American Occupational Therapy Association, 1985
9. Commission on Education of the American Occupational Therapy Association Resolution 584-82: Fieldwork Performance Report. Rockville, MD, American Occupational Therapy Association, 1986
10. Crist PAH: Contemporary Issues in Clinical Education. Thorofare, NJ, Slack, 1986
11. Freeman E: The importance of feedback in clinical supervision: Implications for direct practice. Clin Supervisor 3:5, 1985
12. Schwartz KB: Fieldwork Policies and Procedures. Medford, MA, Tufts University–Boston School of Occupational Therapy, 1980
13. Yerxa EJ: Problems of evaluating fieldwork students. Guide to Fieldwork Education, pp 178–183, Rockville, MD, American Occupational Therapy Association, 1985

CHAPTER 2

An Historical Perspective on Occupational Therapy *Helen L. Hopkins*

The term *occupation* has long been recognized as a requirement for survival and, to varying degrees, as a source of pleasure. The term *occupational therapy* may seem to indicate use of "work" as treatment, but those pioneers who fashioned the profession believed that the health of individuals was influenced by "the use of muscles and mind together in games, exercise and handicraft" as well as in work.[135] This, then, is the basis for the use of work, exercise, and play as modalities of treatment in occupational therapy.

In order to obtain a perspective on the profession of occupational therapy, it is necessary to trace the history of the use of "occupation" from its ancient origins until the present time. The origin and development of the profession will be traced through the description of the foci of those persons within the field upon whose efforts and ideas occupational therapy practice has been based.

Ancient Origins of Occupation for Treatment

Evidence can be found that the healing qualities of work, exercise, and play were recognized and utilized thousands of years ago. The interrelationships of these three aspects of occupational therapy were also recognized early in the history of civilization.

Exercise (Physical Training)

There is evidence that as early as 2600 BC the Chinese taught that disease was caused by organic inactivity and thus used physical training for the promotion of health. They came to utilize a series of medical gymnastics called *Cong Fu,* which they felt could not only prolong life but would ensure immortality of the soul.[54]

The ancient Persians also realized the beneficial effects of physical training and by about 1000 BC they began to use it to prepare their youth for military duty. They used a systematic course of physical training, which began at age 6 and continued through adult years. This resulted in the production of an army of physically fit, able-bodied fighters.

Among the ancient Greeks, physical training was developed to a high degree. Socrates (400 BC) and Plato (347 BC) understood the relation between physical status and mental health, and Aristotle (340 BC) felt that the "education of the body must precede that of the intellect."[54] The Athenians used physical training for its cultural and social aspects, whereas the Spartans used it to build military manpower.

Hippocrates, the father of medicine (359 BC), and Galen, his successor (200 AD), recommended that their patients exercise in the gymnasiums as a means of recovering from illness. The Roman Asclepiades (100 BC) advocated massage, therapeutic baths, and exercises for improving diseased conditions. Scientific medicine is indebted to the interest of the early Greeks and Romans in physical training.[55]

Recreation (Play)

Play, games, and pastimes were a part of the life of all primitive people, as evidenced by the toys, drawings, and sculptures found in excavations of ancient Egypt, Babylonia, and China as well as in the cultural remains of the Aztecs and Incas of the Western Hemisphere. The ancient Egyptians' inscriptions on stone depict the game of draughts, stately dances, the playing of the harp and lute, and children playing with balls, dolls, and jumping jacks.

The Egyptians in 2000 BC and the Greeks in 420 BC described diversion and recreation as a means of treating the sick.[40] One hundred years before Christ, Asclepiades, the Roman, recommended activity treatment for patients with mental diseases. This included diversions and entertainment, but only the diversional value was recognized.

In the 5th century AD, Caelius Aurelius of Sicca (Africa) recommended a careful regimen for convalescents that included walks, reading, theater performances, and throwing the discus. Traveling, especially sea voyages, was described as useful for treatment.

During the Dark Ages play was frowned upon by the Church and was regarded as evil, but its mental and physical influences were again recognized during the Renaissance.

Work

Records from 3400 BC indicate that in Egypt even men of leisure were involved in outdoor work and did not spend their days in idleness. The typical nobleman is pictured as being fond of nature and of working in his garden planting trees, "laying out arbors, excavating a pool, lining it with masonry, and filling it with fish."

The writings of the ancient Hebrews make reference to the beneficial effects of work on the body and mind. The ancient Greeks also recognized the value of work. Socrates said, "A man should inure himself to voluntary labor, and not give up to indulgence and pleasure, as they beget no good constitution of body nor knowledge of mind."

In 17 AD, Livy, the historian, wrote: "Toil and pleasure in their nature opposites are linked together in a kind of necessary connection." The value of alternating work and play was stressed by Phaedra, a writer of the

first century, who said "The mind ought sometimes to be diverted that it may return the better to thinking." Thus, the interrelatedness of work, exercise, and play was recognized 2,000 years ago.[54]

Therapy and Medicine in the 18th and 19th Centuries

Occupational therapy is intimately related to humane treatment. It was not until the last quarter of the 18th century, when people on both sides of the Atlantic began to regard others as equals and fought for this equality, that the practical application of occupational therapy was begun.[55] It was in the midst of the French Revolution (1786) that Philippe Pinel introduced work treatment in the Bicêtre Asylum for the Insane near Paris. In his book published in 1801, he describes his methods as "prescribed physical exercises and manual occupations." He said these should be employed in all mental hospitals because "rigorous executed manual labor is the best method of securing good morale and discipline. The return of convalescent patients to their previous interests, to the practice of their profession, to industriousness and perseverance have always been for me the best omen of final recovery."[71] This is the first reference in the literature to medically prescribed use of work for remediation.

On the other side of the Atlantic, where colonists were striving for equality and independence, the first hospital in the colonies, the Pennsylvania Hospital, was established in Philadelphia in 1752. Benjamin Franklin had been involved in drafting the petition for establishing this hospital, and it was probably at his suggestion that inmates who were able were provided with the light manual labor of spinning and carding wool and flax. In 1798 Benjamin Rush, M.D., one of the signers of the Declaration of Independence, advocated work as a remedial measure for patients in this hospital.[23] In an address to the Board of the Pennsylvania Hospital in 1810, Rush advised that "certain kinds of labor, exercise, and amusements be contrived for them, which should act at the same time, upon their bodies and minds. The advantages of labor have been evidenced in foreign hospitals as well as our own, in a greater number of recoveries taking place."[55]

In Germany, Johann Christian Reil recommended the use of work for treatment of the insane and also suggested the use of exercise and a special hospital gymnasium along with patient participation in dramatic productions and fine arts. Reil's writings give evidence of what was probably the first use of psychodrama in the treatment of the insane.[98]

In the early 1800s, Samuel Tuke, an English Quaker, established Retreat Asylum for the Insane at York, England. He used work or occupation therapy as Pinel did but placed special emphasis on humane treatment or treating patients as rational beings who have a capability of self-restraint. He called it *moral treatment.* Neither chains nor corporal punishment were used, and all patients wore clothes and were induced "to adopt orderly habits" and "participate in exercise and labour." [132]

In 1840, F. Leuret wrote a book entitled *On the Moral Treatment of Insanity.* He said all psychiatrists recommend diversions and work to prevent the effects of idleness and boredom. He stressed the improvement of habits and the development of a consciousness of society. He utilized exercise, drama, music, and reading along with manual labor. [53] Moral treatment was virtually synonymous with the principles and practice of occupational therapy; this was probably the first book entirely devoted to occupation therapy.

Many Americans visited Europe following the Revolutionary War and observed the treatment of the insane at European hospitals. Thomas Scattergood, a Quaker minister who visited Retreat, brought back to America the principles of "occupation and nonrestraint." These principles were used at Friends Asylum for the Insane in Philadelphia, a hospital that he had helped to estabish. The hospital was opened in May 1817 and continues to serve the mentally ill today. Thomas Eddy was another visitor to Retreat. A New York merchant and a member of the Society of Friends, he was so impressed with the improved care of the insane that he submitted suggestions for the "moral management" of the insane to the Governors of the Lunatic Asylum of the New York Hospital. As a result of his suggestions, the Bloomingdale Asylum was opened in 1821 in New York City and began moral management including occupation therapy. This hospital continues today as the Westchester Division of the New York Hospital. In 1818, McLean Asylum opened near Boston under the supervision of Rufus Wyman, M.D. He established, and was probably the first physician in this country to supervise, a program of occupation therapy. [53]

Around 1843, an innovation, regular classroom instruction, was introduced as a part of the care of the mentally ill in hospitals in both Europe and the United States. In 1844, Amariah Brigham, superintendent of the Utica State Hospital in New York, stated that "employment to be of benefit to the patient should not consider the question of gainful occupation, but should divert the patient from his morbid fancies, engage his attention, stimulate his interest, and lead him to resume natural and healthy methods of thought and occupation." [40] The idea that only the therapeutic value to the patient should be considered in selecting the activity was a new and important advance toward the more scientific use of occupation as therapy.

The period of maximum use of occupation therapy in the United States occurred during the lifetime of Thomas Story Kirkbride, M.D. He became superintendent of the Pennsylvania Hospital in 1840 and began a program of mental care that stressed occupation therapy. He said the value of occupation therapy cannot be measured in dollars and cents but must be judged in regard to the restoration of comfort to the inmates of the hospital. Crafts, amusements, and hospital occupations were used therapeutically. Kirkbride helped to organize the Association of Asylum Medical Superintendents, which later became the American Psychiatric Association. Through this association, Kirkbride influenced its members regarding the value of occupation therapy. [50]

During the 18th and 19th centuries, work or occupation therapy was utilized primarily in the care of mentally ill patients. The only mention in the literature of occupation therapy for the physically disabled was in a book published in 1780 in which a physician in the French cavalry, Clement-Joseph Tissot, gave detailed instructions for the use of crafts and recreational activities for disabilities of muscles and joints following disease or injury. [24]

The effective development of work or occupation therapy continued in the United States through 1860. Then it declined suddenly, and its emphasis on the therapeutic value of work was lost for more than a quarter of a century. There seem to be several causes for this period of disuse. Physicians became too busy with increasing responsibilities to take sufficient personal interest in work or occupation therapy. There was a lack of public interest and insight and an underestimation of the therapeutic value of occupation as well as "the real returns as compared to the incidental returns or possible economic proceeds from the treatment." [40] The economic pressures felt in all hospitals during and after the Civil War were also a cause for the decline of occupation therapy.

Genesis of the Occupational Therapy Profession in the United States

Forerunner of the Profession — Adolf Meyer's Philosophy

Toward the end of the 19th century, work as a therapeutic agent was again used in the treatment of the mentally ill in the United States. In a paper presented in December 1892, Adolf Meyer, a psychiatrist, reported that "the proper use of time in some helpful and gratifying activity appeared to be a fundamental issue in the treatment of the neuropsychiatric patient." [60] In 1895, Meyer's wife, Mary Potter Brooks Meyer, a social worker, introduced a systematic type of activity into the wards of a state institution in Worcester, Massachusetts. She was also the first social worker to provide a systematic program to help patients, their families, and the physician.

Meyer's philosophy of treatment and of occupational therapy had a marked impact on the philosophy and history of the profession. His philosophy, as stated in the first volume of the first official organ of the profession, published in 1922, was as follows:

> Our conception of man is that of an organism that maintains and balances itself in the world of reality and actuality by being in active life and active use, i.e. using and living and acting its time in harmony with its own nature and the nature about it. It is the use that we make of ourselves that gives the ultimate stamp to our every organ.[60]

Meyer described rhythms of life that must be kept in balance even under difficulty. These were work and play, rest and sleep. He said balance was attained by actual doing and practice, with a program of wholesome living as the basis for wholesome thinking, feeling, and interest. He felt that personality was fundamentally determined by performance.[40]

Meyer described mental illness as "a problem of living" and not merely as a disease of structure and function or of a toxic nature. He said because there was habit deterioration, systematic use of time and interest became both an obligation and a necessity. His statement from the yearbook of the Chicago School of Civics and Philanthropy (1908–1911) is the first reference in the literature that indicates that conflicts occur through poor adaptation and that occupation may influence and enhance human adaptiveness:

> During the last decade, we have come to realize more than ever that while some mental disorders are due to toxic conditions, others are rather due to conflicts in normal activities and a culturation of fruitful interests are the sanest and only efficient point of attack.[13]

Thus Meyer felt that the treatment of the mentally ill must be a blending of work and pleasure that included both recreation and productive activity. He said "the pleasure in achievement, a real pleasure in the use of one's hands and muscles and a happy appreciation of time" should be used as incentives in the management of patients and should replace the use of repressive rules. The goal for patients was to create an "orderly rhythm and sense of a day simply and naturally spent."[60]

Meyer said the philosophy of the occupational therapy worker should be "an awakening to the full meaning of time as the biggest wonder and asset of our lives and the valuation of opportunity and performance as the greatest measure of time."[60] Patients must have the realization of reality and a full sense of actuality. This was to be accomplished by providing opportunities rather than prescriptions, opportunities "to do, to plan and to create."[60]

Interpersonal relationships were also an important part of Meyer's philosophy of occupational therapy, for he felt that personal contact with instructors and helpers brought out an interchange of experiences and resources. Instructors had to be resourceful and respect the native capacities and interests of their patients.[60]

Adolf Meyer had thus provided the profession of occupational therapy with a philosophy upon which it could build.

Founders of the Profession

Susan E. Tracy

Susan E. Tracy probably can be called the first occupational therapist because, in 1905, during her training as a nurse, she noticed the benefits of occupation in relieving nervous tension and making bedrest more tolerable for patients. In working with orthopedic bedfast patients, she felt occupation was important because "happiness and contentment will certainly prove conducive to rest, and absolute rest is the foremost condition of recovery." She saw occupation as an important adjunct to drug treatment and also felt that instruction in self-help was important. Tracy believed that wholesome interests could be substituted for morbid ones and could carry over into the patient's life after discharge from the hospital. She also saw interpersonal relationships between the teacher or nurse and the patient as an important factor in the success of occupation treatment.[131]

Tracy began her work with the mentally ill when she became director of the Training School for Nurses at the Adams Nervine Asylum in Boston. It was here that in 1906 she developed the first systematic training course in occupation to prepare instructors for teaching patient activities. Up until this time, it was felt that craftsmen were probably the best teachers of patients in craft activities. However, since limitations were imposed on patients by illness or disease, it was determined that persons with medical training would be better qualified because they would recognize signs of fatigue or eyestrain and know the limitations caused by various diseases or injury. Thus the nurse seemed to be the most qualified person to teach occupation to patients. Tracy felt "Kindergarteners" (teachers of small children) could also qualify but would have to become nurses first. She also cautioned that the variety in activity choices must be great in order to meet individual patient requirements.

In 1910, the first book on occupations, *Studies in Invalid Occupations, A Manual for Nurses and Attendants,* was published.[131] This was a compilation of Tracy's lectures with an illustrated guide for the use of activities with patients. The book was primarily a craft book, giving methods of teaching and explaining the rationale for use of specific activities for many patient diagnoses in different types of settings (bed, ward, workshop, home). In this book, Tracy describes her concept of occupation by using a quote from John Dewey:

> By occupation is not meant any kind of "busy work" or exercise that may be given to a child to keep him out of mischief or idleness when seated at his desk. By occupation I mean a mode of activity on the part of the child which reproduces or runs parallel to some form of work carried on in the social life . . . The fundamental point of the psychology of an occupation is that it maintains a balance between the intellectual and the practical phases of experience.[19]

Tracy felt that occupations chosen can help retain connections with social life and provide tangible relations between the individual and other people and their needs, and thus "self-respect is preserved and ambition fostered."[131]

Tracy encouraged the use of occupation for treatment by conducting numerous training courses. In 1911, she conducted the first course in occupation at a general hospital, Massachusetts General Hospital Training School for Nurses. In 1914, as director of the Experiment Station for the Study of Invalid Occupations in Jamaica Plains, Massachusetts, she provided instruction for three classes of students: "(1) To invalids, whether inside or out of institutions, (2) To pupil nurses, in order to enlarge their practical equipment and (3) To Graduate Nurses who have felt the need of the work and may become teachers."[130] The description from a flier on the course is as follows:

> Each patient is considered in light of his threefold personality—body, mind and spirit.
>
> The Aim is likewise threefold:
> 1. The patient's physical improvement
> 2. His educational advancement
> 3. His financial betterment
>
> The Method is based upon a threefold principle:
> 1. The realization of resources
> 2. The ability to initiate activities
> 3. The participation in such activities of both sick and well subjects.[130]

Through her training courses, Tracy did much to disseminate knowledge of the use of occupation for treatment of both physically and mentally ill patients.

Herbert J. Hall

In 1904, Herbert J. Hall began to prescribe occupation for his patients as medicine to regulate life and direct interest. He called this the "work cure."[41]

In 1906, Harvard University became interested in work as a form of treatment and gave Hall a grant of $1000 "to assist in the study of the treatment of neurasthenia by progressive and graded manual occupation." Hall established a workshop in Marblehead, Massachu-

setts, where he used, as treatment, the crafts of hand-weaving, woodcarving, metalwork, and pottery "because of their universal appeal and the normalizing effect of suitable manual work." He said, "Suitable occupation of hand and mind is a very potent factor in the maintenance of the physical, mental and moral health in the individual and the community."[42]

Hall felt that nurses and social service workers should be trained in the use of work as treatment. Therefore, he began a training program for young women at Devereaux Mansion in Marblehead, Massachusetts, around 1908. In 1915, Hall and Buck published *The Work of Our Hands—A Study of Occupations for Invalids*.[43] They divided invalid occupation into "diversional" occupation for those patients in advanced stages of incurable diseases and "remedial" occupation for those patients for whom there was therapeutic and economic value in remedial work.

Eleanor Clarke Slagle

In 1908, a training course in occupations for hospital attendants was given at the Chicago School of Civics and Philanthropy, which was directed by Graham Taylor. Jane Addams, the director of Hull House, along with Julia Lanthrop and Taylor, influenced the development of a number of courses to meet the needs of the community. Lanthrop developed the course for hospital attendants with the purpose of substituting "the educational for the custodial idea in the daily care of the mentally unsound." "Attendants learned games, arts, crafts, and hobbies which they could use to reach their patients." The philosophy of the program was that the work of the attendant was educational and the "methods were those used by the best teachers of little children—teaching the use of muscles and mind together in games, exercises and handicraft."[58] These concepts were reinforced by Adolf Meyer who worked with Addams and Lanthrop and supported their work for the improvement of the care of the mentally ill in state hospitals in Illinois.

Up until this point in the development of occupational therapy, the persons most qualified to be occupation workers had fallen into the three categories of social workers, nurses, and kindergarten or crafts teachers. There were those who believed that nurses had the most desirable background because they had medical training and thus had higher qualifications for working with the sick and disabled. Lanthrop, however, believed that "occupational treatment was to have a large future in hospital treatment and that this service should be carried on by persons specifically educated for it."[116] This controversy continued for many years as courses designed for nurses or teachers were developed throughout the United States.

Eleanor Clarke Slagle, a social work student in the

Chicago School of Civics and Philanthropy, became concerned about the detrimental effects of idleness on the patients at Kankakee State Hospital. Consequently, she enrolled in Miss Lanthrop's first course in "curative occupations and recreations" for attendants and nurses in institutions for the insane given at the Chicago School of Civics and Philanthropy. Following her completion of the course in July 1911, she conducted a similar course at the State Hospital in Newberry, Michigan. She then went to Phipps Psychiatric Clinic in Johns Hopkins Hospital in Baltimore under Meyer, where she was the director of the Occupational Therapy Department for two years and conducted classes for nurses in "handiwork for dispensary patients."[31] In 1915, Slagle organized the first professional school for occupational therapists, the Henry B. Favill School of Occupations, in Chicago. She served as the director of this school from 1918 to 1922. At this school, Slagle used her background in social work. Special instruction was given in invalid occupations along with experience in working with mentally ill patients in order to develop the "habit training" method of treatment, based on the use of occupation. She based this method on the concept that "for the most part, our lives are made up of habit reactions" and "occupation usually remedially serves to overcome some habits, to modify others and to construct new ones to the end that habit reactions will be favorable to the restoration and maintenance of health."[117] Remedial occupation implied training in conduct, in habit training, and in the art of doing things in a socially acceptable manner. This method stressed the interdependence of mental and physical components; the need to build on the habit of attention; the need to analyze occupations; and the need to grade activity from simple to complex, to go from the known to the unknown, and to provide tasks that are of increasing interest and require increasing degrees of concentration. Included in the program were craft activities and preindustrial and vocational work as well as games, folk dancing, gymnastics, and playground activities. This type of rehabilitation program attempted to create a balanced program of work, rest, and play for mentally ill patients.

Slagle, in the development of her habit training program, built on the philosophy of Meyer and provided a model of treatment that was utilized in occupational therapy for mentally ill patients until the early 1950s.

William Rush Dunton, Jr — Father of the Profession

William Rush Dunton, Jr.'s endeavors on behalf of occupational therapy, as a practitioner, as a theoretician, as a philosopher, and as an officer of the national group, earned him the title of "father of occupational therapy." He was involved in the use of occupational therapy as treatment of mental patients as early as 1895. When he was staff psychiatrist at Sheppard and Enoch Pratt Asylum in Baltimore in 1895, a metalworking shop was fitted for treatment of patients. Later other crafts were added and, in 1908, a teacher in arts and crafts was engaged to instruct patients.[118] As Dunton observed his patients while they were engaged in occupations, he noted how important it was to have someone trained to direct their activities, and he became aware of the care required to place a patient in the right activity. Thus, in 1911, after studying Tracy's book on invalid occupations, he undertook the responsibility of conducting a series of classes on occupations and recreation for nurses at Sheppard and Enoch Pratt Asylum. In 1912, he was placed in charge of the occupations and recreation program at the hospital, and his classes for nurses became an ongoing program.[11]

In 1915, the first complete textbook on occupational therapy, *Occupational Therapy—A Manual for Nurses,*[22] written by Dunton, was published. This book outlined the basic tenets or cardinal rules in applying occupation therapy. He said occupation's primary purpose was "to divert the patient's attention from unpleasant subjects, to keep the patient's train of thought in more healthy channels, to control attention, to secure rest, to train in mental processes by educating hands, eyes, muscles, etc., to serve as a safety valve, to provide a new vocation."[22] The greatest part of this book dealt with simple activities that the nurse could use or adapt to treatment of patients.

George Edward Barton

Up until this time, the use of activity for therapy had been called by many titles such as moral treatment, work treatment, work therapy, occupation treatment, occupational reeducation, and ergotherapy. It was not until December 1914, at a meeting in Boston of hospital workers and the Massachusetts State Board of Insanity, that the term *occupational therapy* was introduced by a layman, George Edward Barton. Barton, an architect, became an advocate of this treatment after his own illness, during which he experienced the beneficial effects of directed occupation. He consequently organized an institution called Consolation House in Clifton Springs, New York, where, by means of occupations, people could be retrained or adjusted to gainful living. Barton described the purposes of occupational therapy as "to divert the patient's mind, to exercise some particular set of muscles or a limb, or perhaps merely to relieve the tedium of convalescence." He felt that "these activities may have little if any practical value beyond the immediate purpose they serve. . . . the idea is to give that sort [of activity] which will be preliminary to and dovetailed with the real vocational education which is to begin as soon as the patient is able to go farther along." He felt that the fundamental principle upon which occupational therapy rested was "not making of an object but the making of a man." He defined occupational therapy as the "science of instructing and encouraging the sick in such labors as will involve those energies and activities producing a beneficial therapeutic effect." [8]

Founding of the National Society for the Promotion of Occupational Therapy

Shortly before the United States entered World War I, a number of persons who were interested in providing occupation for patients decided that an association of workers to exchange views would be advantageous. Thus, in March 1917 at a meeting held at Consolation House, the National Society for the Promotion of Occupational Therapy was formed, incorporated, and chartered under the laws of the District of Columbia. The objectives of the association as noted in its constitution were "the advancement of occupation as a therapeutic measure, the study of the effects of occupation upon the human being, and the dissemination of scientific knowledge of this subject." [17] The title of the organization gives some indication of its character, for its membership included medical doctors, social workers, teachers, nurses, and artists whose main interests were in other areas. They did, however, recognize an inadequacy in the care of the sick and disabled that they felt might be filled by the technique called occupational therapy. The charter members of this society were George E. Barton, Eleanor Clarke Slagle, William Rush Dunton, Jr., Susan C. Johnson (occupational therapist at Montefiore Hospital in New York), Isabel G. Newton (Barton's secretary), and Thomas B. Kidner (vocational secretary of the Military Hospital Commission of Canada). Susan B. Tracy was unable to attend the meeting but was elected as an active member and incorporator of the society. A total of 14 active, 7 associate, and 26 sustaining members were elected to the society, and Barton became the first president.

The first annual meeting of the society was held in September 1917 in New York City.[46] The presentations at this conference centered on the theme "The Reconstruction of the Mentally and Physically Disabled." Dunton proposed a system of vocational education whereby the convalescent, while still in the hospital, could be evaluated and taught useful occupations that would be meaningful and useful on discharge.[95] His proposal included a plan for community action and canvassing of local businesses to determine if they would hire handicapped but trained persons.

Dunton was elected president of the society at this meeting, a post he held for two years. While he was president, it became apparent that there was a need for local organizations for exchange of ideas and concepts.

Dunton began organizing a cohesive group in the state of Maryland. Soon other states followed this lead, and a pattern of local organizations becoming affiliated with the national organization was established. This basic pattern remains today.[11]

This marked the beginning of the professional organization of occupational therapy in the United States. In 1923, the name was changed to its present title, the American Occupational Therapy Association.

In 1918, at the second annual meeting of the National Society for the Promotion of Occupational Therapy, Dunton delivered nine cardinal rules to guide practice. These were expanded to fifteen principles by a committee of therapists. Out of these fifteen principles came the first universal definition of occupational therapy: "A method of treatment by means of instruction and employment in productive occupation." The objectives were "To arouse interest, courage and confidence; to exercise the mind and body in healthy activities; to overcome functional disability; and to re-establish a capacity for industrial and social usefulness." [21]

In a second book, *Reconstruction Therapy*, published in 1919, Dunton further delineated the basic tenets upon which the profession of occupational therapy is based in the credo for occupational therapists:

> That occupation is as necessary to life as food and drink.
> That every human being should have both physical and mental occupation.
> That all should have occupations which they enjoy, or hobbies. These are the more necessary when the vocation is dull or distasteful. Every individual should have at least two hobbies, one outdoor and one indoor. A greater number will create wider interests, a broader intelligence.
> That sick minds, sick bodies, sick souls may be healed through occupation.[20]

The Maryland Psychiatric Quarterly, edited by Dunton, from its inception in 1911 published articles relating to occupations and amusement. This journal became the official organ of the National Society for the Promotion of Occupational Therapy when it was founded in 1917. In 1922, the *Archives of Occupational Therapy* was first published and became the official organ of the American Occupational Therapy Association. In 1925, the title of this journal was changed to *Occupational Therapy and Rehabilitation*. This was the official organ of the Association until 1947, when the American Occupational Therapy Association assumed the total responsibility for publication of its own organ and entitled it *American Journal of Occupational Therapy*.

Expansion During World War I

Shortly after the entrance of the United States into World War I, the nation was faced with wounded men in need of rehabilitation. Slagle approached the armed forces and pleaded the cause of therapy as a means of treating the wounded. After initial opposition, Surgeon General Gorgas of the Army authorized the appointment of Reconstruction Aides to serve in Army hospitals.[129] The National Committee for Mental Hygiene initially recruited four aides to serve in European-based hospitals of the American Expeditionary Forces. The success of this small group was such that in September 1917 General John J. Pershing cabled to Washington from Paris requesting 200 young women to serve in Army hospitals overseas.[47] Thus, directives from the Medical Department of the Army, dated January 1918 (Class 1) and March 1918 (Class 2), established training programs for two groups of reconstruction aides (Class 1, physiotherapy, and Class 2, occupational therapy). The physiotherapy aides were to be trained "to give massage and exercise and other remedial treatment to the returned soldiers," while the occupational therapy aides were to be trained "to furnish forms of occupation to convalescents in long illnesses and to give to patients the therapeutic benefit of activity." Rigid criteria were established for applicants including at least a high school education with experience in some profession such as social work or library science. Applicants had to be at least 25 years old, be citizens of the United States or one of its allies, and have theoretical knowledge and practical experience in various crafts. Initial intensive courses were given at the Henry B. Favill School in Chicago under Slagle and at the Teachers College of Columbia University in New York and the Boston School of Occupational Therapy (the Franklin Union) in Boston. The courses ranged from 6 to 12 weeks in length and included lectures on psychology of the handicapped, fatigue and the work cure, personal hygiene, anatomy, kinesiology, ethics, and hospital administration. Classes in the use and application of crafts included woodwork, weaving, cordwork, beadwork, basketry, and ceramics. Field work and practice in local hospitals were also a vital part of the training program.[14,127]

As requests for reconstruction aides increased, other emergency war courses were established throughout the country. Between April 1918 and July 1921, 25 schools had graduated 1685 reconstruction aides, of whom 460 served overseas.[46] Reconstruction aides were civilian employees who worked with patients in orthopedic and surgical wards as well as with those suffering from nervous or mental disorders.

Occupational therapy for the treatment of physical dysfunction gained impetus during this period, and the scientific approach to the treatment of physical disabilities was begun. In the *Army Manual on Occupational Therapy,* Bird T. Baldwin, a psychologist and director of Walter Reed General Hospital's Occupational Therapy Department, gives this explanation of occupational therapy:

Occupational therapy is based on the principle that the best type of remedial exercise is that which requires a series of specific voluntary movements involved in the ordinary trades and occupations, physical training, play or the daily routine activities of life. Our curative shops are now being organized and graduated on the principle which will enable us ultimately to isolate, classify, repeat and, to a limited degree, standardize and control the type of movements involved in the particular occupational and recreational operations. The patient's attention is repeatedly called to the particular remedial movements involved; at the same time the movements have the advantage of being initiated by the patient and of forming an integral and necessary part of the larger and more complex series of coordinated movements. The purposive nature of the movements and the end poduct of the work offer a direct incentive for sustained effort; the periodic measurement of the increase in range and strength of movement makes it possible for the patient to watch his recovery from day to day. . . . The records also enable the examiner to determine which mode of treatment leads to the greatest and most consistent gains in a particular case. . . .[7]

It was during this period that devices were developed to measure range of motion and strength; thus more scientific recording was made possible. The kinesiological analysis of activities begun during the war allowed activities to be chosen based on specific physical limitation. Adapted pieces of equipment were devised that provided specific motions for increasing range of motion and strength, and their use was then applied for the remediation of selected disabilities.

By the end of World War I, thousands of soldiers in the United States had received some form of occupational therapy, and the profession was beginning to gain public support.

Baldwin made a valuable contribution through the development of evaluation and treatment procedures for restoration of physical function and the dissemination of these methods through publication in the *Army Manual.*

Post-World War I to World War II

Many of the schools for training reconstruction aides closed permanently after World War I. The demand for trained occupational therapists in civilian hospitals caused the reopening of the Boston School of Occupational Therapy in the fall of 1919, followed shortly by the opening of the Philadelphia School of Occupational Therapy and the St. Louis School of Occupational Therapy. Two of these schools continue to function today: the Boston School is now located in Tufts University, and the St. Louis School is located in Washington University. The Philadelphia School (at the University of Pennsylvania) was phased out in 1981.

The American Occupational Therapy Association established "Minimum Standards for Courses of Training in Occupational Therapy" in 1923.[61] At this time, several war emergency schools were disbanded because of their inability to meet requirements. The minimum standards included a prerequisite of a high school education and a 12-month course of not less than 8 months of theoretical work and 3 months in practice. The establishment of standards did much to raise the status of the profession. However, the schools of occupational therapy trained therapists as teachers of crafts or occupations, which would help individuals move from acute illness to vocational training. Many therapists gained knowledge of anatomy, kinesiology, and medical conditions through postgraduate courses and developed principles of specific treatment to restore physical function on an empirical basis.[38]

The caliber of publications in the official journal of the Association, however, did not reflect a scientific basis for the profession. Articles generally were undocumented, unscientific, and inconclusive and fell into three categories: (1) description of occupational therapy as it was practiced at various hospitals, (2) helpful hints on crafts, and (3) the relationship of occupational therapy to other medical services.[38] Ethel Bowman, Associate Professor of Psychology at Goucher College, described the problem of the profession in 1922 as follows:

> Literally there is no psychology of occupational therapy today. Although there is abundant material for such, it is, at present, unorganized. In speaking of the psychology of a subject, we may mean that the known facts of scientific psychology have been given practical application, or that the peculiarly psychological aspects of the subject have been singled out and subjected to specific study by the methods which psychology has found applicable in its problems of pure science. In neither of these meanings have we a psychology of occupational therapy.[12]

In spite of the lack of scientific approach, occupational therapy was being utilized in both civilian and military hospitals throughout the United States. After their experiences during the war, physicians recognized the value of occupational therapy and established units in many general and children's hospitals. Treatment was based on the principles advocated by Dunton in 1915. These principles advocated that treatment should be prescribed and administered under constant medical supervision and correlated with other treatment of the patient; treatment should be directed to individual needs; treatment should arouse interest, courage, and confidence; treatment should exercise mind and body in healthy activity; treatment should overcome disability and reestablish capacity for industrial and social usefulness; occupation should be regulated and graded as a patient's strength and capabilities increased; employment in groups is advisable to provide opportunity for social adaptation; and the only reliable measure of the treatment is the effect on the patient.[93]

In 1923, the Federal Industrial Rehabilitation Act made it a requirement that every general hospital dealing with industrial accidents or illness provide occupational therapy as an integral part of its treatment. There was a demand for graduates of accredited schools in spite of budget cuts in hospitals during the Depression, demonstrating an increasing recognition of the necessity for constructive occupation in the maintenance of mental and physical health.[125] *

By 1928, there were six schools of occupational therapy. In addition to the Boston, Philadelphia, and St. Louis schools, Milwaukee Downer College, the University of Minnesota, and the University of Toronto in Canada had accredited programs. Each of these met the minimum standard of nine months' didactic and three months' clinical preparation. Each gave a diploma in occupational therapy, with the University of Minnesota giving a bachelor's degree as well. The Minnesota program was discontinued in 1931 because of low enrollment and the resignation of the director.[100]

In 1927, Everett Elwood recommended that the American Occupational Therapy Association safeguard the profession and maintain high standards by requiring all practitioners to be licensed and by utilizing a national examination to qualify graduates of the accredited schools.[26]

In 1931, a National Registry of all qualified occupational therapists was established "for the protection of hospitals and institutions from unqualified persons posing as occupational therapists." When the Association issued its first registry in 1932, 318 therapists were listed, all qualified by a rigid set of standards.[129] Registration required that therapists have one year of active practice under an experienced therapist and be recommended by that therapist.

In March 1931, the American Occupational Therapy Association requested that the American Medical Association undertake inspection and approval of the occupational therapy schools. Because the American Medical Association had experience in medical education and had investigated medical schools and teaching hospitals, the Council on Medical Education and Hospitals agreed to undertake the survey. The inspection began in November 1933. Following the inspection, meetings were held with representatives from the American Occupational Therapy Association, the Council on Physical Medicine, and the Council on Medical Education and Hospitals. The result of these meetings was the drafting of the "Essentials of an Acceptable School of Occupa-

---

* Personal discussion with Clare S. Spackman and Helen S. Willard.

tional Therapy." The "Essentials" were adopted by the Council on Medical Education and Hospitals in February 1935 and were ratified the following June by the House of Delegates of the American Medical Association at its Annual Meeting.[48]

The thirteen schools of occupational therapy in operation were evaluated in 1938, and only five schools met the essentials and were approved. They were the Boston, Philadelphia, and St. Louis Schools of Occupational Therapy and Milwaukee Downer College and the University of Toronto in Canada. Kalamazoo State Hospital School of Occupational Therapy received tentative approval. The "Essentials" increased the length of the program to 25 calendar months plus an additional 9 months of hospital practice training. The requirements expanded the theoretical basis of the profession by adding emphasis in biological and social sciences and clinical medicine. Clinical practice was expanded to include experience in mental, tuberculosis, children's, and orthopedic hospitals. Although degree courses were available at Milwaukee Downer and Kalamazoo, few students took advantage of this offering because a degree did not seem necessary. Therefore, most students received highly specialized training with no liberal arts input and received a diploma in occupational therapy in three years. Beginning in 1932, certificate programs for persons with bachelor's degrees were given at Boston, Philadelphia, and St. Louis. These courses required 1 year of didactic preparation plus 9 months of hospital practice. Graduates of the certificate program were permitted to become registered occupational therapists. There was no thought of graduate degrees in the field at this time, and there seemed to be no desire on the part of practitioners to write or publish literature for the field.[38] These schools graduated a total of 100 qualified therapists per year.

By 1938, 13% of the hospitals approved by the American Medical Association had qualified occupational therapists on their staffs. The majority of therapists were employed in mental hospitals.[125] The impetus given to the treatment of physical dysfunction through occupational therapy by World War I had diminished. The profession had been from its inception primarily one for women, and only one school, the St. Louis School of Occupational Therapy, accepted male students. Thus, only about 2½% of qualified therapists were men, and they were employed primarily in mental institutions, tuberculosis sanitoria, and penal institutions.[35,46] A few occupational therapists were in private practice in 1939, and five cities—Philadelphia, Hartford, Detroit, Milwaukee, and St. Louis—had visiting therapists, similar to visiting nurses, working with the homebound.[125]

In 1939, the first formal subjective registration examination developed by a committee of therapists was given. Those who failed were permitted to register on the basis of experience. About 1944, examinations were developed by each school and submitted for approval to the Registration Committee of the American Occupational Therapy Association.

During World War II and Immediately Following

World War I had given impetus to the new field of occupational therapy, but its development after the war was slow. After World War I, occupational therapy programs and personnel in all Army hospitals had been reduced to a minimum. There were five permanent Army general hospitals, only three of which had an occupational therapist employed.[49] At the beginning of World War II the total number of practicing occupational therapists in the United States was less than was needed by the military hospitals alone.[9]

Because of the need for therapists in both military and civilian hospitals, a number of new schools were organized. The number of approved schools increased from 5 in 1940 to 18 in 1945. At the request of the Surgeon General's Office, war emergency courses were started in a number of schools and prepared more than 500 qualified therapists for duty in the Army hospitals. These schools met American Medical Association minimum standards since they were intensive 1-year courses for college graduates who had basic psychology and at least 20 semester hours of fine, applied, or industrial arts or home economics. The course consisted of 4 months of theory in the civilian occupational therapy schools and 8 months of practical application and training under registered occupational therapists in Army hospitals.[10] Registration was acquired through passing of the Registration Examination approved by the American Occupational Therapy Association.

The critical personnel needs of the armed forces and war industries demanded maximum conservation of manpower. Thus a reconditioning program in the Armed Forces was established to

> accelerate the return to duty of convalescent patients in the highest state of physical and mental efficiency consistent with the capabilities and the type of duty to which they are being returned . . . or to provide for their return to civilian life in the highest possible degree of physical fitness, well oriented in the responsibilities of citizenship and prepared to adjust successfully to social and vocational pursuits.[67]

The reconditioning program included a coordinated program of educational reconditioning, physical reconditioning, and occupational therapy. Occupational therapists were civilians appointed to Army hospitals by the Surgeon General's Office. They supervised both the treatment programs and the volunteer Red Cross Arts and Skills, Recreational, and Diversional Programs.

By the end of World War II, more than 1000 occupational therapists were providing services in the military hospitals in the United States and abroad. Occupational therapists had to be prepared to work with persons having psychological and psychiatric problems as well as those having orthopedic and neurological problems. Techniques were developed for rapid total rehabilitation of patients in order to return them physically and mentally fit for service or work. The war had expanded the techniques and knowledge in occupational therapy, especially in the area of the treatment of the physically disabled.

In February 1947, the first National Objective Registration Examination was given. Very few men worked in the profession of occupational therapy, so it was looked upon as a woman's field. From 1941 to 1946 the number of registered occupational therapists almost doubled, from 1144 to 2265,[15] but the number of men in the profession remained at about 2½% of the total, or about 50.

Clare S. Spackman — Restoration of Physical Function

Because of increases in medical knowledge, discovery of new drugs, and improved medical care after World War II, the population of patients to be treated changed and increased. This placed new demands on therapists and required that new treatment procedures be developed. Other specialties were developed to satisfy unmet needs (*i.e.*, recreational therapy, educational therapy, and corrective therapy). Occupational therapists became specialized in the treatment of certain types of disabilities such as peripheral nerve injuries and amputations. This added to the base of knowledge and improved treatment techniques for these areas of practice.[119]

Occupational therapists had to be skilled in using constructive activities for treatment and also were required to utilize as treatment activities of daily living (ADL), work simplification, rehabilitation techniques for the handicapped homemaker, and training in the use of upper extremity prostheses. This expansion in techniques and knowledge in the area of physical dysfunction required extensive reorganization of the curricula of the accredited schools of occupational therapy. In order to assist schools in providing this new information to students, the first textbook in the United States on occupational therapy written primarily by occupational therapists, edited by Helen S. Willard and Clare S. Spackman, was published in 1947.[139] Spackman provided detailed information in this volume on the evaluation and treatment of patients with physical dysfunction.

Spackman believed that the exact function of occu-

pational therapy in the treatment of physical dysfunction should be specifically defined. In an article in which she traced the history of occupational therapy practice for restoration of physical function she says:

> Occupational therapy treats the patient by the use of constructive activity in a simulated, normal living and/or working situation. This is and always has been our function. Constructive activity is the Keynote of occupational therapy. . . . True occupational therapy cannot be used until the patient is capable not only of performing a given motion but of utilizing it to carry out a constructive activity. Occupational therapy's value lies in teaching the patient by use of constructive activities to transfer the motions and strength gained by corrective exercise in physical therapy into coordinated activity which will enable the patient to become personally independent and economically self-sufficient.[119]

Spackman made an impact on the treatment of patients physically disabled by disease or injury through publication of the book on occupational therapy and by the education of students utilizing the principles of evaluation and treatment.

Spackman represented the United States when the World Federation of Occupational Therapists was founded in 1954. She was elected to the position of Assistant Secretary-Treasurer at its first meeting, served as President of the organization from 1957 to 1962 and was Secretary-Treasurer from 1964 to 1972. Her interest and involvement with the World Federation did much to develop good relationships with member countries and encouraged expansion of the profession into many underdeveloped countries.

Formation of the World Federation of Occupational Therapists

The aftermath of World War II led to the rapid growth of allied medical services in many countries throughout the world. There was a need for exchange of information in regard to new methods of treatment, and many foreign therapists were seeking admission to take the registration examination of the American Occupational Therapy Association. The International Society for the Rehabilitation of the Disabled, concerned with the establishment of rehabilitation programs throughout the world, encouraged the formation of an International Association of Occupational Therapists, which would establish international standards for education and practice. In April 1952, representatives of six countries met in Liverpool, England, and drafted a constitution including qualifications of member associations and proposed "Minimum Educational Standards for Occupational Therapists" (revised in 1963). The American Occupational Therapy Association became one of the ten founding members of the World Federation of Occupational Therapists. The six countries represented at the founders' meeting were Canada, Denmark, Great Britain (England and Scotland), South Africa, Sweden, and the United States. Australia, New Zealand, Israel, and India were represented by written opinion and thus were included as founding members.

The first congress met in Edinburgh, Scotland, in 1954. Four hundred representatives from ten countries attended. The organization continued to grow, and by its second congress in 1958, there were 750 representatives from 38 countries.[120] In 1959, the World Federation of Occupational Therapists joined the World Health Organization and established a roster of expert advisors to work with countries trying to establish or develop their own occupational therapy programs. This roster has been maintained and continues to be used when therapists are needed to assist developing programs.

In 1960, the World Federation of Occupational Therapists formulated a code of "Ethics for Occupational Therapists" and "Functions of Occupational Therapy" (revised in 1962). The American Occupational Therapy Association also worked with the World Rehabilitation Fund, the Peace Corps, and the International Cooperation Administration. By the early 1960s, there was an active exchange of therapists among countries. Many American therapists worked abroad, and therapists from member countries worked in the United States. Members from countries meeting World Federation of Occupational Therapists standards were permitted to take the registration examination of the American Occupational Therapy Association.[120]

The World Federation of Occupational Therapists (WFOT) has continued to grow, and by 1986, there were 35 member countries. Delegates from these countries meet every two years as the "Council" and conduct business for the Federation. Every four years, there is a Congress which is sponsored by one of the member countries.

Committees of the Federation include: Education, Professional Practice, International Relations, Legislation, Congress, and Publications. Activities of note in 1986 were: the adoption of the 1984 "Minimum Standards for Education of Occupational Therapists"; development of contacts with countries who have occupational therapists but are not yet members of the Federation in an effort to share resources among members in each region; and representation at international meetings of the World Health Organization and the Nongovernmental Organizations Group on Aging. A pilot study on "Assessment of the Profession" has been started, which will examine the profession from the view of member countries as well as individual members. The *WFOT Bulletin*, published twice a year, is distributed to all Individual members of the Federation. Currently, there is a proposal for publication of an international journal of occupational therapy.[16]

Move Toward an "Exact" Science

The 1950s saw an increase in the development of rehabilitation techniques in physical dysfunction. The use of more exact methods of measuring physical function initiated a movement to make occupational therapy a more exact science. Advances were made in medical science for the control of diseases including poliomyelitis and tuberculosis. This caused a shift in emphasis in occupational therapy of physical dysfunction to the chronic conditions of arthritis, heart disease, stroke, traumatic injuries, and congenital defects. Federal legislation and the interest of insurance carriers and federal and state rehabilitation agencies gave added stimulus to the growth of occupational therapy in the treatment of physical dysfunction. New techniques were developed by therapists and biomedical engineers, and these new techniques influenced the procedures used in occupational therapy. The emphasis of treatment was to reduce defects related to the patient's pathological condition and to allow the individual to function at the highest level of which he or she was capable.[119] The occupational therapist functioned as a member of a team dedicated to the rehabilitation of the disabled.

During this period, the treatment of the psychiatric patient was also being examined by occupational therapists, with an increasing emphasis on the social adaptation of the patient or client and the individual's return to functioning in family and community. The concept of the "therapeutic use of self" became the primary focus of treatment and utilized psychotherapeutic techniques. This concept used social interactions as the tool for helping patients or clients deal with their emotional responses and with both the human and nonhuman environment.[115]

Gail S. Fidler—Psychiatric Occupational Therapy

The first comprehensive book on psychiatric occupational therapy was published in 1954. This book, *Introduction to Psychiatric Occupational Therapy*, by Gail S. Fidler and Jay W. Fidler, M.D., gave impetus to the psychodynamic approach to occupational therapy.[32] The Fidlers presented occupational therapy as a collaborative effort between the occupational therapist and the psychiatrist. Occupational therapy was the laboratory in which the patient or client could experiment in handling emotions and developing living skills through the use of productive activity. Guidelines for detailed activity analysis were developed. The book presented a process in which groups could be used to facilitate treatment; it also encouraged the study of projective techniques. In 1963, a second textbook on psychiatric occupational therapy was published by the Fidlers, *Occupational*

Therapy—A Communication Process in Psychiatry. This book presented occupational therapy as an important communication tool because activities could provide a means for understanding individuals through nonverbal communications during the activity process.[33]

From 1963 to 1964, Gail Fidler presented graduate courses in Occupational Therapy Supervision in Psychiatry at Columbia University. In 1967, she developed the master's program in Psychiatric Occupational Therapy at New York University, where she encouraged use of the scientific method in occupational therapy. Some of the leaders in the practice of psychiatric occupational therapy today are graduates of these programs.

Fidler has continued to be involved in clinical, academic, and administrative affairs of the profession because she sees importance in maintaining competence as an occupational therapist in all of these areas.

New Levels in Occupational Therapy Education

In spite of the fact that there was an increase in the number of occupational therapy schools, there continued to be a lack of qualified occupational therapists to fill the vacancies in both psychiatry and physical disability therapy. By 1960, there were 24 accredited schools of occupational therapy, all located in universities giving bachelor's degrees in conformance with the "Essentials" as revised in 1949.

With the dearth of qualified personnel, employers began to utilize persons trained in other fields to fill vacancies, thereby giving impetus to the expansion of related therapeutic groups such as recreational therapy, art therapy, music therapy, vocational rehabilitation counseling, manual arts therapy, and educational therapy. Development in these fields and the overlapping of roles caused some occupational therapists to question whether the profession was operating without a theoretical base.[36,136]

In 1947, the first program leading to a master's degree in occupational therapy was established at the University of Southern California. This course was for persons who were registered occupational therapists who had bachelor's degrees. Later in the same year, New York University began a similar graduate program. These programs were developed for therapists desiring advanced work in clinical specialty areas such as clinical psychopathology, physical disabilities, vocational rehabilitation, and special education.[38] It was hoped that graduate study on the part of occupational therapists would promote research, which was recognized as essential for increasing the knowledge and theoretical base of the profession.

At this same time, the profession began to examine the possibility of training a technical-level person to work as an assistant to the occupational therapist, thereby alleviating the lack of manpower in the field.[34] Criteria for the educational programs were determined, and standards for training assistants for general practice were implemented in October 1960.[18]

Changes in Focus— 1960s and 1970s

During the 1960s, psychiatric occupational therapists began to examine their role and function. Grant-funded consultants were hired by the American Occupational Therapy Association to help these therapists look at the impact of their treatment. Workshops were conducted throughout the country in group techniques and object relations. These workshops led psychiatric occupational therapists to examine neurobehavioral orientation to treatment, thus adding the dimension of perception to psychiatric treatment, which had previously had only a social and emotional base.[59]

During this same period, the basic master's program was introduced as a means of educating persons with bachelor's degrees in other fields in the basics of occupational therapy with advanced work in research methodology for the profession. The first program was a 2-year course conducted at the University of Southern California in 1964. Shortly thereafter, basic master's programs were begun at Boston University and Virginia Commonwealth University. These courses encouraged students to conduct research in the profession and to publish the results. This caused a gradual change in the articles published in the *American Journal of Occupational Therapy* and encouraged therapists to become involved in clinical research.

A. Jean Ayres—Neurobehavioral Orientation

A. Jean Ayres became interested in neurophysiological and developmental approaches to occupational therapy through her contacts with Margaret S. Rood, an occupational therapist and physical therapist who had investigated literature in these areas and developed the following basic principles:

1. Motor output is dependent upon sensory input. Thus sensory stimuli are utilized to activate and/or inhibit motor response.
2. Activation of motor response follows a normal developmental sequence. . . .
3. Since there is interaction within the nervous system between somatic, psychic and autonomic functions stimuli can be used to influence one or more directly or indirectly.[138]

In the early 1960s, Ayres began conducting research

that laid the foundation for a neurobehavioral orientation to occupational therapy. The basis of her work "is the recapitulation of the sequence of development."[6] This orientation was consequently termed "sensory integrative therapy" and accepted developmental stage concepts. Ayres proposed that the "principles that determined the direction of evolutionary development are manifested in the principles that govern the development of the capacity to perceive and learn by each child today." Therapy is based on the premise that the brain is a "self-organizing system" that integrates or coordinates "two or more functions or processes in a manner which enhances the adaptiveness of the brain's responses" and the fact that "one of the most powerful organizers of sensory input is movement which is adaptive to the organism." Treatment is based on purposeful movement that causes the individual to respond adaptively and requires a response that represents a "more mature or integrated action than previous performance."[5]

Mary Reilly — Occupational Behavior Orientation

In the 1960s, Mary Reilly suggested that the concern of occupational therapy should be patient achievement, since we are dealing with behavior that is subject to maturation and regression of illness. She suggests that we use the work–play continuum because "the play of childhood . . . contains a critical ability to transmit the adaptive skills necessary for complex work technology and urban living of today."[99] Thus, it would seem that Reilly is reemphasizing the need for habit training along with reduction of incapacity.

Reilly's orientation indicates recommitment to Meyer's and Slagle's philosophy of occupational therapy. Reilly stresses the importance of "examining the various life roles of the population relative to community adaptation, to identify the various skills that support these roles, and to create an environment where the relevant behavior could be evoked and practiced."[52] The occupational therapist's role is to facilitate achievement of competence. Emphasis is placed on the patient's or client's ability to cope with the community and with changes in life situations. Interpersonal relationships are essential factors in this process.

Wilma West — Prevention and Community Occupational Therapy

In 1966, Wilma West stated that the shift from medical to health concerns had implications for occupational therapy. She said that the profession must be involved in the new emphasis of "maintaining optimum health rather than an intermittent treatment of acute disease and disability" and that "health and medical care in the future . . . will emphasize human development by programs designed to promote better adaptation, rather than technologically oriented programs offering specific solutions to specific difficulties.[137] She described four emerging roles for the occupational therapist that would create new dimensions of function. These were evaluator, consultant, supervisor, and researcher. She suggested that the occupational therapist, to fulfill these roles in the prevention of disease, must move into and work in community settings.

Anne Cronin Mosey — Frames of Reference for Psychiatric Occupational Therapy

In 1970, Anne Mosey said that occupational therapy in psychiatry appeared to be functioning on the basis of intuition and without a theoretical base. She thought there should be a "conscious use of theoretical frames of reference as the basis for the treatment of psychosocial dysfunction." She categorized the three frames of reference available as analytical, acquisitional, and developmental. She said the *analytical* base "describes man as striving for need fulfillment, expression of primitive impulses or control of inherent drives." She described dysfunction as "symptom-producing unconscious content." Therapy attempts to bring the symptom-producing unconscious content to consciousness and integrate it with conscious content. The *acquisitional* base "focuses upon the various skills or abilities which the individual needs for adequate and satisfactory interaction in the environment." Human abilities are viewed as qualitative and nonstage specific. Dysfunction is described in terms of what behavior must be eliminated and what must be added in order for an individual to function in a normal environment. The *developmental* base is similar to the acquisitional in that it specifies the various skills and abilities which the individual needs for satisfactory interaction in the community. However, the abilities are considered to be interdependent, qualitative, and stage specific. The developmental base "assumes that the individual must go through incompleted stages in order to function in a mature manner." The individual's current adaptive skill, learning, and the expected environment must all be evaluated.[65] Mosey's developmental base is drawn from the theoretical formulations developed by Ayres.

In 1974, Mosey proposed an orientation to occupational therapy as an alternative to the medical and health model. She called it the "biopsychosocial model." She said this model "directs attention to the body, mind and environment of the client. It takes these facets into consideration without any sense of wellness or sickness on the part of the client." This model focuses on the individual as a "biological entity; a thinking and feeling person and a member of a community of others."[64] Although this model is described as an alternative, it seems to have been drawn from all previous orientations to occupational therapy.

Changes Within the Association — 1960s and 1970s

During the 1960s, the American Occupational Therapy Association was called on by its members to perform new functions such as providing administrative guidelines, suggesting treatment and consultative rates, and sponsoring a lobbyist for health legislation. These activities endangered the status of the professional organization as one of a "charitable, scientific, literary and educational nature." Therefore in 1965, the American Occupational Therapy Foundation was established under the laws of the state of Delaware as a philanthropic organization "to administer programs of a charitable, scientific, literary and educational nature." Its work aimed at "advancing the science of occupational therapy, supporting the education and research of its practitioners and increasing the public knowledge and understanding of the profession." This move allowed the American Occupational Therapy Association to serve as a "business league" and to perform the requested noneducational activities.[1]

The emphasis on accountability to consumers caused the Association to develop new standards for education and practice. In 1970, "Standards and Guidelines for an Occupational Therapy Affiliation Program" were drawn up.[121] In 1972, a new definition and statement of function was developed for the profession.[69] In 1973, "Standards for Occupational Therapists Providing Direct Service" were developed and published in the official journal of the Association.[122] That same year, the revised "Essentials of the Accredited Educational Programs for the Occupational Therapist" were adopted by the American Occupational Therapy Association and the House of Delegates of the American Medical Association.[28] These "Essentials" were approved by the Representative Assembly of the American Occupational Therapy Association in 1977. The "Essentials of an Approved Educational Program for the Occupational Therapy Assistant" were developed and adopted by the Council of Education of the American Occupational Therapy Association in 1975.[30] These were adopted by the Representative Assembly in 1977.

Since 1972, the Association has adopted numerous position papers, including ones on consumer involvement,[74] aging,[73] national system of certification for allied health personnel,[66] and national health issues.[72]

In October 1975, the Delegate Assembly adopted a resolution authorizing the development of a certification examination for occupational therapy assistants.[102] In April 1976, the Assembly passed a resolution authorizing the use of the certification examination as a partial fulfillment for certification of occupational therapy assistants.[103] The first certification examination was given in June 1977.

In September 1976, new bylaws were adopted by the Association; they became effective in November 1976.[2] These bylaws made many changes in the structure and organization of the Association. They identify the Representative Assembly as the policy-making body, which elects its own officers. Representatives from each state, the Association officers, the first alternate delegate of the World Federation of Occupational Therapists, and the president of the Student Association are voting members of the Assembly. The Executive Board became the management body, with Association officers, Representative Assembly officers, the World Federation delegate, and the president of the Association of Affiliate Presidents as members. The purpose of changes in the bylaws was to make the Association more responsive to the membership's needs and concerns.

In April 1977, the Representative Assembly adopted a "Definition of Occupational Therapy" for the purpose of licensure. The Assembly adopted a revised version of the definition in March 1981. This is to be used as a legal document and not as a philosophical definition for the profession (see Appendix A). At the same meeting, the Representative Assembly adopted the "Principles of Occupational Therapy Ethics." The Ethics Statements are to be used as guidelines for the profession and its practitioners but are not to be used as standards of expected care. Guidelines for Ethics Statements were developed and adopted by the Representative Assembly in April 1980[94] (see Appendix B).

Into the 1980s

With the adoption of the bylaws in 1976, the Association was committed to an advocacy position that included increased participation and involvement of members in Association activities. In order to obtain input from members, the *Occupational Therapy Newspaper* printed resolutions and other policy items along with a reply sheet for members to send opinions and comments to their representatives on the issues and resolutions that would establish policy for the Association. In 1978, Mae Hightower–Vandamm, president of the Association, introduced a plan whereby local task groups, chaired by members of the Executive Board, examined management issues and made recommendations for Executive Board decisions.[44] All meetings sponsored by the American Occupational Therapy Association were opened for membership audit except when material of confidential nature was under discussion.[62] The Association was thereby providing for as much membership participation and involvement as possible.

Because of changes occurring both within the Association and in society, the Representative Assembly, at their meeting in San Diego, California, in May 1978, authorized a Special Session of the Assembly to examine the status of the Association and the field as a whole. Concerns were identified relating to four areas within occupational therapy: *the philosophical base, practice, education,* and *credentialing.* Leaders from the field were invited to present papers and participate in this meeting.[68] This special session will probably "be recorded in the annals of the history of occupational therapy as one of the events that changed the future of our profession."[45] As a result of this meeting, the Association, for the first time, adopted a statement identifying the philosophical base of occupational therapy[107] and affirmed "occupation" as the common core of occupational therapy,[108] thereby providing the field with parameters within which to develop and grow.

Research

There was increased support of research by the membership because of the need to validate skills and substantiate the role of occupational therapy in health care. This support was evidenced by the establishment of a Committee on Research and a Research Advisory Council[114] within the Association, approval of a position of Research Coordinator in the National Office under the American Occupational Therapy Foundation (AOTF), and financial support for research activities within the field.[62] In April 1981, the AOTF published The *Occupational Therapy Journal of Research* for the first time.

Education

Because of changes occurring in the health care system and in the demands of the consumer of occupational therapy services, changes were required in the education of students and in the content of the educational programs. In 1983, new "Essentials of an Academic Program for the Occupational Therapist" were adopted by the Representative Assembly.[29] These "Essentials" increased the emphasis on professional competencies including research and problem-solving skills for entry-level practice. Since fieldwork is an integral part of the educational process, a new, validated "Fieldwork Evaluation" (FWE) was adopted in 1986.[113]

Programs for certified occupational therapy assistants (COTAs) had been developed as hospital-based certificate programs and two-year associate degree programs. Because of the need for more liberal arts in the education of occupational therapy assistants, a motion was passed by the Representative Assembly of the

AOTA in April 1983 which promoted the establishment of occupational therapy assistant programs at the associate degree level.[63] This motion became Association policy and resulted in discouragement of the development of certificate programs for the occupational therapy assistant. The number of programs for assistants has grown from 22 in 1970 to 58 in 1985, 49 of which grant associate degrees and five of which give certificates. Two schools have both types of programs. Enrollment in all programs tripled in this same 15-year period.[25]

During the same time, graduate education was thought to be necessary in order to advance the profession by developing a body of knowledge through research. A guide to graduate education in occupational therapy leading to a master's degree was endorsed,[39] and many post-baccalaureate programs were developed for registered occupational therapists to advance their knowledge. In addition, entry-level graduate programs were developed and were supported by the leadership of the profession as the entry level of professional education of the future. From 1970 to 1986, educational programs for the occupational therapist had grown from 37 to 64; five had only master's level programs and 59 had baccalaureate programs, with nine of these also having post-baccalaureate certificate programs, 15 also having professional (entry-level) master's degrees, and 20 also offering post-professional (advanced) master's degrees. Entry-level master's programs had increased from 10 in 1970 to 20 in 1986 with a fivefold increase in enrollment. In this same period, enrollment in baccalaureate programs increased by 56%.[25,57]

The need for scholarly activity in the profession was the impetus for the development of doctoral programs in occupational therapy. In 1974, New York University developed the first doctoral program in Occupational Therapy, with the first doctoral degree being awarded in the spring of 1984.[51]

A turning point in the profession's development occurred in June of 1986, when the Association supported a meeting of more than 300 educators from 111 schools to focus on the promotion of excellence in education (Target 2000). Topics discussed included: the role of education in the development of a profession; future trends and opportunities; purposes of academic and fieldwork education; linking theory, research and practice; and increasing research productivity.[128]

These trends in our educational patterns and the focus on excellence in education as demonstrated by Target 2000 have been in response to the proliferation of knowledge and technology in our society. It is only through education, research, and clinical competence that occupational therapy can be recognized as a viable health profession.

Support was given to students for development of a student organization in 1977.[104] Since that time, a student organization called the American Student Occupational Therapy Alliance has been founded.

Certification

Certification of occupational therapists and occupational therapy assistants has been considered a valid means of assuring the public that therapists and assistants are competent practitioners and that remaining certified assured this competence. Because continuing competence was of foremost concern to the profession, Resolution 540-79, adopted by the Representative Assembly in 1979, charged the AOTA to "design a recertification system that allows individual choice and alternative means to demonstrate continuing competence in the recertification process by offering a variety of options. . . ."[97, 101, 109] A task force developed several options which were, however, rejected by the Representative Assembly in 1982. As an alternative, specialty certification was proposed as a means of assuring competence. While the feasibility of this option continues to be studied, the issue of recertification is no longer being considered.

In April 1986, the Representative Assembly adopted Resolution 616-86, which is a policy for the development of an Autonomous Certification Board. This was done so that the Association could not be interpreted as a closed shop, in which the Association "controls entry into the profession to meet its own needs."[3] This policy separates membership and certification functions by "removing certification from direct control of the Association's policy formation, standard setting and the budget process."[3] Re-examination for expired certification was eliminated. It was determined that state licensure laws became the legal authority for assuring continuing competence requirements for practice. As of June 1986, 36 of the 50 states had licensure, registration, or trademark requirements for regulation and monitoring of practice in occupational therapy within their states.[124]

Practice

In the examination of practice, it was evident that there was much diversity within the field; the roles and functions of occupational therapists and occupational therapy assistants were unclear, and new areas of practice were being developed while some of our traditional areas of practice were being eroded. Because of the need for a unified identity and more uniform practice in the field, standards of practice were adopted by the Representative Assembly for Physical Disabilities, Mental Health, Developmental Disabilities and Home Health Care in 1978 and for practice in schools in 1980.[105,112] General "Standards of Practice for Occupational Therapy" were adopted by the Representative Assembly in 1983[123] (see Appendix C).

There was also a concern that not all practitioners were operating from the same baseline and that they were not using similar terminology and systems of evaluating and reporting progress. To assure more uniformity in communication, the document "Uniform Terminology System for Reporting OT Services" was developed and adopted by the Representative Assembly in 1979[134] (see Appendix D). This document identifies and describes the services that fall within the domain of occupational therapy, thereby placing some constraints on the field. There was also a need to place some type of value on our services in order to provide guidelines for determining fees for service; therefore, another document entitled "Occupational Therapy Product Output Reporting System" was developed and adopted by the Representative Assembly in 1980[70] (see Appendix E). This document provides guidelines for placing relative values on specific services provided by occupational therapists. In order to further clarify the role of occupational therapists in the health-care system, a generic guide for gathering baseline data was developed entitled "Uniform Occupational Therapy Evaluation Checklist,"[133] and this was adopted by the Representative Assembly in March 1981 (see Appendix F). This document was based on the Uniform Terminology document and indicates that all evaluation procedures used should reflect the philosophical base of occupational therapy. These three documents provide practicing therapists with guidance for their practice and give educational programs guidance for education of students.

The roles and functions of the occupational therapist and occupational therapy assistant had been examined for a number of years; however, there had been no consensus regarding differentiation in these roles and functions. An Entry Level/Role Delineation Committee was established by the Representative Assembly. The committee was charged with examining all previously developed documents concerned with roles and functions within occupational therapy and with developing a document that considered the concerns presented in all of the previous documents. A document entitled "Entry Level Role Delineation for OTRs and COTAs" was developed and adopted by the Representative Assembly in March 1981 (see Appendix H).[27] This was intended to assist members in their practice, to assist in the development of entry-level educational essentials and programs, and to assist in the development of certification criteria.

Occupational therapists seemed to be working in new areas of practice while abandoning some other areas where occupational therapy skills were traditionally used and valued. In order to verify our commitment to some of these areas of practice, position papers were adopted by the Representative Assembly which identified the various contributions of occupational therapy. Position papers were adopted on the role of occupational therapy in promotion of health and prevention of disability,[81] in the vocational rehabilitation process,[82] in independent living or alternate living situations,[80] as a related education service,[78] in home health care,[79] in sensory integrative dysfunction,[91] in long-term care occupational therapy and activity programs,[90] in services for the severely disabled,[89] in burn care delivery,[84] in hand rehabilitation,[86] in mental health,[87] in adult day care,[83] in services for Alzheimer's disease,[76] in rheumatoid disease,[88] in early childhood intervention,[85] in hospices,[75] in work hardening,[92] and in purposeful activity.[77] Additional areas of practice were being identified in such contexts as correctional institutions. In order to encourage and support the development of new areas of practice, the Commission on Practice was charged with identifying areas of occupational therapy practice that are in need of standards and guidelines, developing needed standards, and continuing to monitor ongoing and new parameters of practice.[111]

The concern for maintaining competency of practitioners was addressed by the Association in several ways. Support was given to continuing education institutes which were to be conducted throughout the country to meet the educational needs of practicing therapists.[110] Occupational therapists working in school systems were given the opportunity to develop their competence through a research and pilot training project called TOTEMS (Training: Occupational Therapy Educational Management in Schools).[37] Through this project, many therapists working in school systems throughout the country were given a special course for improving the quality of treatment in the school setting.

Due to the overwhelming success of the TOTEMS program, the AOTA decided to develop and conduct similar training programs in other areas of practice: PIVOT (Planning and Implementing Vocational Readiness in Occupational Therapy), ROTE (Role of Occupational Therapy with the Elderly), and SCOPE (Strategies, Concepts and Opportunities for Program Development and Evaluation in Mental Health). These training projects, along with institutes and workshops at the annual national, state, and regional conferences, have made continuing education opportunities available to meet the needs of practitioners for maintaining competence.

Accountability to health-care consumers has been of concern to all practitioners for many years. However, occupational therapists have not been involved in quality assurance projects until recently. The National Office Division of Quality Assurance has conducted pilot projects in this area that have demonstrated the need for and value of the involvement of occupational therapy departments in an ongoing quality-assurance process (see Chap. 14).

In addition to changes occurring within occupational therapy, changes taking place in society and in the government are affecting occupational therapy practice.

The Government and Legal Affairs Division (GLAD) of the National Office has been very active in keeping members informed and in soliciting help for passage of legislation through the publication of the *Federal Report* and the *GLAD Bulletin.* Through the efforts of this division and with membership support, the Medicare Bill was amended in October 1986. As a result of this amendment, occupational therapy will be reimbursed: (1) under Medicare Part B benefits to allow for uninterrupted service of patients in skilled nursing facilities; (2) for Medicare coverage in rehabilitation agencies such as Easter Seal Centers, public health departments, and physical therapy/speech therapy clinics, with service provided in an appropriate location such as a satellite center, skilled nursing facility, or a patient's home (occupational therapy can enter a case without the necessity of another skilled service); and (3) in private practice, where occupational therapy will become a new "provider" under Medicare, will be assigned a provider number and may bill Medicare directly for services in the office, skilled nursing facility, home, or any appropriate setting with a limit of $500 per beneficiary per year. Regulations and Guidelines issued by the Health Care Financing Administration were developed so that this amendment could be implemented. The amendment took effect as of July 1, 1987.[96]

Two other projects undertaken by the Association indicate we are coming of age. A Written History Committee was appointed in 1978 to produce a history for the Association. Help was solicited from the membership for this project. An Archives Committee was also established in 1978 to develop criteria and to process material for the archives and to find suitable storage for the historical documents of the Association.[106] The Archives of the Association are now located in the library of the University of Texas Medical Branch at Galveston.

In July 1980, the American Occupational Therapy Association moved into its first permanent home. Previously, the Association rented space for their national headquarters. In February 1980, an office building was purchased in Rockville, Maryland, as headquarters for the National Office. This was made possible through establishment of a Housing Reserve Account in 1974, which provided sufficient funds.

New bylaws were adopted by the membership of the Association in February 1981. These bylaws were written in outline format for easier use but did not change the overall organization of the Association. All policies of the Association were put into a standard format and collected into a policy manual. A committee has also developed a procedural guide for the Association.

Many of the issues and concerns discussed at the landmark meeting of the Representative Assembly in 1978 have been addressed. A philosophical base has been adopted; research is being conducted to verify practice; theoretical positions are being proposed; and practice is being conducted in new arenas. However, many issues and concerns remain to be addressed. In response to the many changes occurring in the health care arena, the Association developed a Strategic Integrated Management System (SIMS), which is used to forecast emerging issues, accommodate changes, integrate responses, and identify and analyze issues.[126] This system, along with the long-range plan of the Association, will be used as a tool for monitoring and working for achievement of the long-range goals of the Association.

Summary

In the first year of our Association's history, there were 40 members. By November 1985, this number had grown to 40,000.[4] Although our numbers have grown more than a thousand times and the focus within occupational therapy has changed, it is evident that there are at least four common propositions that have characterized the profession throughout its history:

1. The use of occupation or purposeful activity can influence the state of health of an individual.
2. Individuals and their adaptation and total functioning must be viewed with respect to their own environment, and remediation must take into consideration all the physical, psychological, and social factors.
3. Interpersonal relationships are an important factor in the occupational therapy process.
4. Occupational therapy is an adjunct to, and has its roots in medicine and must work in cooperation with medical professionals and other persons involved as health-care providers to ensure maximum benefits for clients.

Being founded on the principles and practices of moral treatment that value the quality of the daily life of disabled people, occupational therapy from its beginning has focused on health, adaptation, and function.

References

1. American Occupational Therapy Foundation—The First Decade 1965–1975. Am J Occup Ther 29:636, 1975
2. AOTA bylaws. Am J Occup Ther 31:111, 1977
3. AOTA certification structure changed. Occup Ther News 40(6): 1986
4. AOTA welcomes 40,000th member. Occup Ther News 39(11):1, 1985
5. Ayres AJ: Sensory Integration and Learning Disorders. p 8. Los Angeles, Western Psychological Services, 1972
6. Ayres AJ: The development of perceptual motor abilities: A theoretical basis for treatment of dysfunction. Eleanor Clarke Slagel Lecture. Presented at the AOTA Conference, October 1963, St. Louis. Am J Occup Ther 17:221, 1963
7. Baldwin BT: Occupational Therapy Applied to Restora-

tion of Function of Disabled Joints, pp 5–6. Washington DC, Walter Reed Monograph, April 1919
8. Barton GE: Teaching the Sick: A Manual of Occupational Therapy as Re-education, p 60. Philadelphia, WB Saunders, 1919
9. Barton WE: The challenge to occupational therapy. Occup Ther Rehabil 22:262, 1943
10. Barton WE: Training programs for occupational therapists in the US Army. Occup Ther Rehabil 23:282, 1944
11. Bing R: William Rush Dunton, Jr.—American Psychiatrist: A Study in Self. PhD dissertation, University of Maryland, 1961
12. Bowman E: Psychology of occupational therapy. Arch Occup Ther 1:172, 1922
13. Chicago School of Civics and Philanthropy Yearbook and Bulletin. p 98. August 1908–July 1911
14. Circulation of information concerning employment of reconstruction aides. Washington, Medical Department, US Army, January 22, 1918–March 27, 1918
15. Cobb MR: Report of the Executive Secretary to the Twenty-Sixth Annual Meeting of the American Occupational Therapy Association, August, 1946. Occup Ther Rehabil 25:259, 1946
16. Committee Reports. World Fed Occup Therap Bull 14:1, November 1986, and communication with Mae Hightower–VanDamm, WFOT delegate from the USA
17. Constitution of the National Society for the Promotion of Occupational Therapy, p 1. Baltimore, Sheppard Hospital Press, 1917
18. Crampton MW: Educational upheaval for occupational therapy assistants. Am J Occup Ther 21:317, 1967
19. Dewey J: The School and Society, pp 132–133. Chicago, University of Chicago Press, 1900. Paperback ed. 1956
20. Dunton WR, Jr: Credo. In Reconstruction Therapy, p 10. Philadelphia, WB Saunders, 1919
21. Dunton WR, Jr: Occupational therapy. In Barr, DP (ed): Barr's Modern Medical Therapy in General Practice, Vol 1, p 697. Baltimore, Williams & Wilkins, 1940
22. Dunton WR, Jr: Occupational Therapy—A Manual for Nurses. Philadelphia, WB Saunders, 1915
23. Dunton WR, Jr: Reconstruction Therapy, p 20. Philadelphia, WB Saunders, 1919
24. Dunton WR, Jr, Licht S: Occupational Therapy: Principles and Practice, 2nd ed, p 11. Springfield, IL, Charles C Thomas, 1957
25. 1986 Education Data Survey, pp 1, 6, 9, 12. Rockville, MD, American Occupational Therapy Association, 1986
26. Elwood ES: The National Board of Medical Examiners and medical education and the possible effect of the Board's program on the spread of occupational therapy. Occup Ther Rehabil 6:341, 1927
27. Entry level role delineation for OTR's and COTA's. Occup Ther News 35:8, 1981
28. Essentials of an accredited educational program for the occupational therapist. Am J Occup Ther 29:485, 1975
29. Essentials of an accredited program for the occupational therapist. Am J Occup Ther 37:817, 1983
30. Essentials of an approved educational program for the occupational therapy assistant. Am J Occup Ther 30:245, 1976
31. Experience of Eleanor Clark Slagle, 1910–1922. Docu-

ment from Archives, American Occupational Therapy Association, Bethesda, MD

32. Fidler GS, Fidler JW: Introduction to Psychiatric Occupational Therapy. New York, Macmillan, 1954
33. Fidler GS, Fidler JW: Occupational Therapy—A Communication Process in Psychiatry. New York; Macmillan, 1963
34. Final Report, Project Committee on Recognition of Occupational Therapy Assistants. Am J Occup Ther 13:269, 1958
35. Fish M: Occupational therapy in American colleges, pp 21–32. J Am Assoc Collegiate Registrars, October 1945
36. Gilette NR: Changing methods in the treatment of psychosocial dysfunction. Am J Occup Ther 21:230, 1967
37. Gilfoyle E: Training Occupational Therapy Educational Management in Schools. Rockville, MD, American Occupational Therapy Association, 1980
38. Greenman NB: The influence of the university setting on occupational therapy education. Master's thesis, Tufts College, Boston, 1953
39. Guide to graduate education leading to a master's degree. Adopted by Representative Assembly, May 1978. Am J Occup Ther 32:653, 1978
40. Haas LJ: Practical Occupational Therapy. pp 6, 11, 13. Milwaukee, Bruce Publishing Company, 1944
41. Hall HJ: Occupational Therapy, A New Profession. Concord: The Rumford Press, 1923
42. Hall HJ: Work cure, a report of five years' experience at an institution devoted to the therapeutic application of manual work. JAMA 54:12, 1910
43. Hall HJ, Buck Mertice MC: The Work of Our Hands—A Study of Occupations for Invalids. New York, Moffat, Yard and Co, 1915
44. Hightower–Vandamm M: Nationally speaking: Ah, faint glow of sunshine. Am J Occup Ther 33:219, 1979
45. Hightower–Vandamm M: Nationally speaking: Participation-treatment for survival. Am J Occup Ther 33:627, 1979
46. Historical Documents and Letters. Archives, American Occupational Therapy Association, Bethesda, MD
47. History. Occup Ther Rehabil 19:32, 1940
48. JAMA 104:1632, 1935; 105:690, 1935; 107:683, 1936
49. Kahmann WC, West W: Occupational therapy in the United States Army hospital, World War II. In Willard HS, Spackman CS (eds): Principles of Occupational Therapy, p 330. Philadelphia, JB Lippincott, 1947
50. Kirkbride TS: Report of the Pennsylvania Hospital for the Insane for the years 1841, 1842, and 1843, Philadelphia. Published by order of the Board of Managers, Pennsylvania Hospital, 1841, 1842, 1843
51. Labovitz D: First PhD in occupational therapy awarded. Occup Ther News 38(7):1, 1984
52. Laukaran VH: Toward a model of occupational therapy for community health. Am J Occup Ther 31:71, 1977
53. Leuret F: On the moral treatment of insanity, Paris, 1840. In Licht S: Occupational Therapy Source Book, pp 9, 63. Baltimore, Williams & Wilkins, 1948
54. Levin HL: Occupational and recreational therapy among the ancients. Occup Ther Rehabil 17:311, 1938
55. Licht S: Occupational Therapy Source Book, pp v, 1, 8. Baltimore, Williams & Wilkins, 1948

56. List of diagnostic related groups. Federal Register 49(171):34780, 1984
57. Listing Of Educational Programs in Occupational Therapy–November 1986. Am J Occup Ther 40:844, 1986
58. Loomis B, Wade BD: Chicago. Occupational Therapy Beginnings: Hull House, The Henry B. Favill School of Occupations and Eleanor Clark Slagle, p 2. Special Improvement Grant, US Public Health Services, Allied Health 50579-01, 1973
59. Mazer J: The occupational therapist as consultant. Am J Occup Ther 23:417, 1969
60. Meyer A: The philosophy of occupational therapy. Arch Occup Ther 1:1, 1922
61. Minimum standards for courses of training in occupational therapy. Arch Occup Ther 3:295, 1924
62. Minutes of representative assembly meeting, May 1978, San Diego, California. Am J Occup Ther 32:665, 1978; and Resolution 562-80: Minutes of representative assembly meeting, April 1980, Denver, Colorado. Am J Occup Ther 34: 859, 1980
63. Minutes of the representative assembly meeting, April 1983. Am J Occup Ther 37:834, 1983
64. Mosey AC: An alternative: the biopsychosocial model. Am J Occup Ther 23:140, 1974
65. Mosey AC: Three Frames of Reference for Mental Health, pp v, 15–17. Thorofare, NJ, Charles B. Slack, 1970
66. National system of certification of allied health personnel. Am J Occup Ther 30:50, 1976
67. Occupational Therapy. War Department Training Manual 8-291, p 1. Washington DC, US Government Printing Office, 1944
68. Occupational Therapy 2001. Rockville, MD, American Occupational Therapy Association, 1979
69. Occupational therapy: its definition and functions. Am J Occup Ther 26:204, 1972
70. Occupational therapy product output reporting system. Representative Assembly Minutes, April 1980, Denver, Colorado. Am J Occup Ther 34:865, 1980
71. Pinel P: Medical philosophical treatise on mental alienation, Paris, 1801. In Licht S: Occupational Therapy Source Book, p 19. Baltimore, Williams & Wilkins, 1948
72. Policy statement on national health issues. Delegate Assembly minutes. Am J Occup Ther 31:110, 1977
73. Position paper on aging. Am J Occup Ther 28: 564, 1974
74. Position paper on consumer involvement. Am J Occup Ther 27:48, 1972
75. Position paper on occupational therapy and hospice. Am J Occup Ther 40:839, 1986
76. Position paper on occupational therapy services for Alzheimer's disease and related disorders. Am J Occup Ther 40:822, 1986
77. Position paper on purposeful activities. Am J Occup Ther 37:805, 1983
78. Position paper on the role of occupational therapy as a related education service. Am J Occup Ther 35:811, 1981
79. Position paper on the role of occupational therapy in home health care. Am J Occup Ther 35:809, 1981
80. Position paper on the role of occupational therapy in

independent living or alternate living situations. Am J Occup Ther 35:812, 1981

81. Position paper on the role of occupational therapy in promotion of health and prevention of disabilities. Am J Occup Ther 33:50, 1979

82. Position paper on the role of occupational therapy in the vocational rehabilitation process. Am J Occup Ther 34:881, 1980

83. Position paper on the roles and functions of occupational therapy in adult day care. Am J Occup Ther 40:817, 1986

84. Position paper on the roles and functions of occupational therapy in burn care delivery. Am J Occup Ther 38:791, 1984

85. Position paper on the roles and functions of occupational therapy in early childhood intervention. Am J Occup Ther 40:835, 1986

86. Position paper on the roles and functions of occupational therapy in hand rehabilitation. Am J Occup Ther 38:795, 1984

87. Position paper on the roles and functions of occupational therapy in mental health. Am J Occup Ther 38:799, 1984

88. Position paper on the roles and functions of occupational therapy in the management of patients with rheumatic diseases. Am J Occup Ther 40:825, 1986

89. Position paper on the roles and functions of occupational therapy services for the severely disabled. Am J Occup Ther 37:811, 1983

90. Position paper on the roles and functions of the occupational therapist in long term care: Occupational therapy and activity programs. Am J Occup Ther 37:807, 1983

91. Position paper on the roles and functions of the occupational therapist in the treatment of sensory integrative dysfunction. Am J Occup Ther 35:831, 1982

92. Position paper on work hardening guidelines. Am J Occup Ther 40:841, 1986

93. Principles of Occupational Therapy. AOTA Bulletin No 4, 1923

94. Principles of occupational therapy ethics with guidelines. Am J Occup Ther 34:900, 1980

95. Proceedings of the National Society for the Promotion of Occupational Therapy: First Annual Meeting. Catonsville, MD, Spring Grove State Hospital, 1917

96. Provisions of Medicare amendment expand coverage for occupational therapy. Occup Ther News 40(12):4, 1986

97. Recertification: Your vote will count. Occup Ther News 35(5):1, 1981

98. Reil JC: Rhapsodies on the psychic treatment of the insane, Halle, 1803. In Licht S: Occupational Therapy Source Book, pp 25, 27. Baltimore, Williams & Wilkins, 1948

99. Reilly M: The educational process. Am J Occup Ther 23:303, 1969

100. Report of the Committee on Teaching Methods. Occup Ther Rehabil 7:287, 1928

101. Representative Assembly Minutes, April 1979, Detroit, Michigan. Am J Occup Ther 33:793, 1979

102. Resolution 465-75: Delegate Assembly minutes. Am J Occup Ther 30:177, 1976

103. Resolution 471-76: Delegate Assembly minutes. Am J Occup Ther 30:587, 1976

104. Resolution 516-77: Formation of a task force to establish guidelines for an occupational therapy student organization. Representative Assembly minutes, October 1977, Puerto Rico. Am J Occup Ther 32:251, 1978

105. Resolution 525-78: Standards of practice for mental health, developmental disabilities, physical disabilities and home health — Minutes of Representative Assembly, San Diego, California, May 1978. Am J Occup Ther 32:666, 1978

106. Resolution 526-78: Establishment of an archives task force of the AOTA. Representative Assembly Minutes, May 1978, San Diego, California. Am J Occup Ther 32:661, 1978

107. Resolution 531-79: Minutes of Representative Assembly, Detroit, Michigan, April 1979. Am J Occup Ther 33:785, 1979

108. Resolution 536-79: Minutes of Representative Assembly, Detroit, Michigan, April 1979. Am J Occup Ther 33:785, 1979

109. Resolution 540-79: Recertification as a means of assuring continuing competency for OTR's and COTA's. Am J Occup Ther 33: 793, 1979

110. Resolution 544-79: Delineation of the responsibilities of the AOTA continuing education program. Representative Assembly minutes, April 1979, Detroit, Michigan. Am J Occup Ther 33:796, 1979

111. Resolution 556-79: New areas of occupational therapy practice — identification and guidelines. Representative Assembly minutes, April 1979, Detroit, Michigan. Am J Occup Ther 33:806, 1979

112. Resolution 561-80: Standards of practice in schools. Am J Occup Ther 34:854, 1980

113. Resolution 584-82: Development of new validated fieldwork performance report. Am J Occup Ther 36:814, 1982

114. Resolution 587-82: Establishment of research advisery council. Am J Occup Ther 36:816, 1982

115. Semrad EV: The emotional needs of the disabled person. Proceedings of the Occupational Therapy Institute, New York, pp 28 – 38. American Occupational Therapy Association, 1956

116. Slagle EC: Occupational therapy. Trained Nurse Hosp Rev April 1938, p 380

117. Slagle EC: Training aides for mental patients. Papers on occupational therapy, p 40. Utica, NY, State Hospital Press, 1922

118. Slagle EC, Robeson HA: Syllabus for training of nurses in occupational therapy, p 10. Utica, NY, State Hospital Press, 1933

119. Spackman CS: A history of the practice of occupational therapy for restoration of physical function: 1917–1967. Am J Occup Ther 22:68, 1968

120. Spackman CS: The World Federation of Occupational Therapists 1952–1967. Am J Occup Ther 21:301, 1967

121. Standards and guidelines on occupational therapy affiliation program. AOTA Committee on Basic Professional Education. Am J Occup Ther 25:314, 1971

122. Standards for occupational therapists providing direct service. Am J Occup Ther 28:237, 1974

123. Standards of practice for occupational therapy. Am J Occup Ther 37:802, 1983

124. State regulation of occupational therapy personnel: Up-

date 1986. Occup Ther News 40(6):5, 1986

125. Stern EM: The work cure. Survey Graphic, April 1939, pp 1–4

126. Strategic Integrated Management System. Rockville, MD, American Occupational Therapy Association, 1983

127. Subjects and lectures for the first class (reconstruction aides) April 24, 1918, to July 13, 1918. Historical documents from Archives, Boston School of Occupational Therapy, Boston, 1918

128. Target 2000: A turning point in the profession's development. Occup Ther News 40(9):1, 1986, and Occupational Therapy Education: Target 2000 Proceedings, Rockville, MD, American Occupational Therapy Association, 1986

129. Then and Now, 1917–1967. Rockville, MD, American Occupational Therapy Association, 1967

130. Tracy SE: Flier on occupation course offered at Experiment Station for the Study of Invalid Occupations, Jamaica Plains, MA, 1914

131. Tracy SE: Studies in Invalid Occupations—A Manual for Nurses and Attendants. Boston, Whitcomb and Barrows, 1910

132. Tuke S: Description of the Retreat, an institution near York, for insane persons, York, 1816. In Licht S: Occupational Therapy Source Book, pp 41–56, Baltimore, Williams & Wilkins, 1948

133. Uniform occupational therapy evaluation checklist. Occup Ther News 35:11, 1981

134. Uniform terminology system for reporting occupational therapy services. Representative Assembly minutes, April 1979, Detroit, Michigan. Am J Occup Ther 33:805, 1979

135. Wade LC: Pioneer for Social Justice, 1851–1938: Graham Taylor, p 170. Chicago, University of Chicago Press, 1964

136. West W: Professional responsibility in times of change. Am J Occup Ther 22:9, 1968

137. West W: The occupational therapist's changing responsibility to the community. Am J Occup Ther 21:312, 1967

138. Willard HS, Spackman CS (eds): Occupational Therapy, 4th ed., p 380. Philadelphia, JB Lippincott, 1971

139. Willard HS, Spackman CS (eds): Principles of Occupational Therapy. Philadelphia, JB Lippincott, 1947

Current Basis for Theory and Philosophy of Occupational Therapy *Helen L. Hopkins*

Philosophical Base of Occupational Therapy

Philosophy is concerned "with the meaning of life and the significance of the world in which man finds himself."[3] Thus the philosophy of occupational therapy represents the profession's view of the nature of existence and gives meaning to and guides the actions of the profession. It also provides the fundamental set of values, beliefs, truths, and principles that guide the action of the profession's practitioners.[5]

The "Philosophical Base of Occupational Therapy," adoped in 1979, provides a foundation for the theory and practice of occupational therapy:

Man is an active being whose development is influenced by the use of purposeful activity. Using their capacity for intrinsic motivation, human beings are able to influence their physical and mental health and their social and physical environment through purposeful activity. Human life includes a process of continuous adaptation. Adaptation is a change in function that promotes survival and self-actualization. Biological, psychological, and enviromental factors may interrupt the adaptation process at any time throughout the life cycle. Dysfunction may occur when adaptation is impaired. Purposeful activity facilitates the adaptive process.

Occupational therapy is based on the belief that purposeful activity (occupation), including its interpersonal and environmental components, may be used to prevent and mediate dysfunction, and to elicit maximum adaptation. Activity as used by the occupational therapist includes both an intrinsic and a therapeutic purpose.*

As a further guide to education and practice, in April 1979, the Representative Assembly affirmed:

that there be a universal acceptance and implementation of the common core of occupational therapy as active participation of the patient/client in occupation for purposes of improving performance. The use of facilitating procedures is only acceptable as occupational therapy when used to prepare the patient/client for better performance and prevention of disability, through self-participation in occupation. . . . Increased emphasis should be placed "on more creative involvement of the patient/client in purposeful, motivating and constructive occupation based on individual behavioral evaluations and treatment."[4]

The definition of occupational therapy, the philosophical base statement, and the affirmation of occupation as the common core of occupational therapy place

_____

* Adopted by the Representative Assembly, April 1979, Detroit, Michigan.

parameters on the scope of occupational therapy. They provide guidance for education and practice and for the development and validation of theoretical propositions through research.

Theory Base

Throughout its history, the focus of the occupational therapy profession has been on the nature of the total individual in relation to society and the world in which the person lives. The body of knowledge in occupational therapy and its theoretical base are derived from several broad scientific areas, including biological and behavioral sciences, sociology, anthropology, and medicine. Knowledge in these areas is continually expanding and being modified, making it mandatory that occupational therapy change. Occupational therapy uses the broad knowledge areas as its theoretical underpinnings and can be effective only in proportion to the accuracy of these knowledge bases. Theoretical propositions are being built on these broad knowledge areas to form the beginning of occupational therapy's unique body of knowledge.

Theory and theoretical propositions are used to systematize known concepts and to describe, explain, and predict behavior. Using the concepts, assumptions, and principles from theories within our scientific base, theories must be reorganized in order to provide guidance for practice. The theories can then be used to describe, explain, and predict the behavior of our patients and can contribute to our understanding of function, dysfunction, evaluation, and treatment. In this way, theory can be linked to practice and a model for the profession can be developed.[1] According to Mosey, a model of a profession is broad in focus, gives unity and identity to the profession, and defines its relations to the society to which it is responsible. Thus, a model would include all of a profession's beliefs, philosophical assumptions, and knowledge.[2]

Frames of Reference

Frames of reference or approaches to treatment are derived from the model of the profession but are much narrower, using only those theoretical principles that are relevant to a specific area of human function. The frame of reference must, however, be consistent with the philosophical assumptions of the profession. The purpose of a frame of reference is to "formulate treatment strategies directed to specific areas of practice."[1] Frames of reference therefore include the particular theoretical formulations regarding the aspects of function/dysfunction that are specific to health problems encountered in practice. Each frame of reference will identify the theoretical propositions that are appropriate for dealing with a specific patient population; the nature

of the function/dysfunction of that population; and the behaviors that are indicative of function/dysfunction. These will then determine which evaluation procedures are appropriate, the long- and short-term goals, the sequencing of treatment, and the treatment modalities and techniques that are applicable. Figure 3-1 illustrates the relation of theory, philosophy, and frames of reference to practice.

Numerous theoretical vantage points are being used as frames of reference for practice. In this chapter, however, an overview of only nine major perspectives that have been published and are used by occupational therapy practitioners will be presented (Table 3-1). Each frame of reference presented has its merits and limitations, and it is vital that occupational therapists recognize these and choose the frame of reference that will best serve the particular patient population and setting. It is possible that in the course of treating a particular patient, more than one frame of reference could be used at different times. For example, in a patient with physical disabilities, the biomechanical frame of reference might be used in the acute stage of treatment, whereas after deficits have been reduced as much as possible, the rehabilitation or human occupation frame of reference might be more appropriate to the needs of the patient.

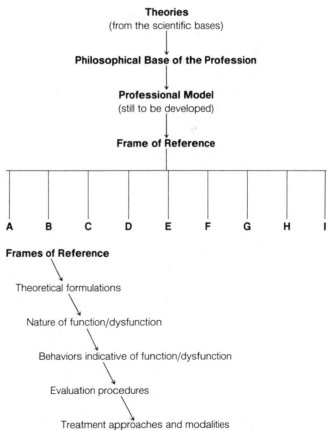

Figure 3-1. Relationship of theory, philosophy, and practice.

Table 3-1. Frames of Reference for Occupational Therapy Practice

Frame of Reference	Theoretical Base	Nature of Dysfunction	Evaluations	Treatment Modalities	Proponents
Behavioral	Psychology: learning occurs through interaction with a reinforcing environment	Lack of skills	Skills checklist, observation	Instruct in skills needed to promote learning; provided through reinforcement: shaping, chaining, task analysis, feedback	Watson, Skinner, Sullivan
Biomechanical	Physical sciences: kinetics, kinematics, medicine	Deficits in range of motion, strength, and endurance	Assessments of range of motion, manual muscle testing, endurance testing	Reduce deficits through direct cause-and-effect treatment process, exercise, and activity	Trombley
Cognitive	Biological psychiatry, neurosciences: behavior is self-regulated according to individual's purposes and cognitive abilities	Cognitive levels describe difference in task behavior, motor action, conscious awareness, purpose, process, and time	Task analysis: selection and modification in range of patient's ability	Provide tasks to match level of cognitive abilities—environmental compensations	Allen
Developmental	Psychology: human growth and maturation occur sequentially in a supporting environment	Developmental lag, stress-induced regression	Assess developmental levels, adaptive behaviors, and range of functions	Alter activity components of environment to achieve appropriate behavior. Create environment to promote development	Ayres, Llorens, Arieti, Piaget, Freud, Erickson
Neurodevelopmental	Psychology, neurosciences: normalization and integration of biological processes	Impairment of ability to process and act on information received from environment	Identify process deficits	Inhibit or excite neural mechanisms; special techniques and equipment to normalize biological processes	Ayres, Wilbarger, Bobath, Rood, King, Huss, Farber, Knickerbocker

Model	Theoretical base	Problem	Assessment	Intervention	Theorists
Sensorimotor	Development, neurosciences: relation between sensory input and neural integration	Perceptual motor deficits, inability to integrate sensory stimuli and produce motor response, abnormal motor and learning problems	Perceptual testing, observation	Body movement, gross motor and sensory integrative activities	Ayres, deQuiros
Human occupation — (Occupational behavior)	General systems theory, sociology: self-directed achievement of role requirements	Difficulties with roles, rules, habits, and skills needed to function in society, viewed in terms of volitional, habituation, and performance components	Interviews, time and activity inventory, observation in tasks, case analysis	Establish environment that allows exploration and development of competence and mastery; provide counseling and problem-solving to identify and alter maladaptive occupational lifestyle	Boulding, Bruner, von Bertolanffy, Reilly, Kielhofner, Shannon
Rehabilitation	Medicine, physical sciences: total capabilities of each individual based on examination of the parts	Deficits in physical, social, vocational, and economic aspects of life	Assess deficits and capabilities in activities of daily living, vocational and recreational activities, and access to the environment	Reduce effects of disability by learning to live with one's capabilities in all aspects of life. Adapt environment to obtain independence	Spackman, Trombly
Psychoanalytic	Psychiatry: striving for need fullfillment	Symptom-producing unconscious content	Identification of symptom-producing unconscious content	Bring symptom-producing content to consciousness and integrate with conscious content	Freud, Jung, Sullivan

It is important that practice in occupational therapy be based on theory, be rooted in the philosophical base of the profession, and be organized using a specified frame of reference to guide the choice of appropriate evaluation and treatment procedures so that our practice can be explained and refined.

The developmental, neurodevelopmental, sensorimotor, and human occupation (occupational behavior) frames of reference outlined in Table 3-1 are described more fully in Chapter 8.

Occupational Therapy Knowledge Base

The occupational therapy process requires that students have in-depth knowledge from the biological, behavioral, and medical sciences in order to identify theoretical formulations that will serve them in the development of frames of reference for practice. The nature of the individual and the function/dysfunction continuum, along with pathological processes that impinge on function, must be understood so that appropriate occupational therapy intervention procedures may be determined. Thus, one of the knowledge bases for occupational therapy must be identified as the basic sciences. Moreover, because occupational therapy is concerned both with human function throughout the life span and with the uniqueness of the individual, it is essential that practice be based on the normal development process. The impact of occupation or purposeful activity on the human organism also must be understood so that age-appropriate activities may be used. The next three chapters provide detailed explanations of the three major bases for the field of occupational therapy: human development, occupation, and activity.

References

1. Levy LL: Frames of reference for occupational therapy in mental health. In American Occupational Therapy Association: SCOPE. Rockville, MD, AOTA, 1986
2. Mosey AC: Occupational Therapy—Configuration of a Profession. New York, Raven Press, 1981
3. Randall TH, Buchler J: Philosophy: An Introduction, p 5. New York, Barnes & Noble, 1960
4. Resolution 532-79: Occupation as the common core of occupational therapy. Representative Assembly minutes, April 1979, Detroit, Michigan. Am J Occup Ther 33:785, 1979
5. Shannon PD: Philosophical considerations for the practice of occupational therapy. In Ryan SE (ed): The Occupational Therapy Assistant: Roles and Responsibilities, p 37. Thorofare, NJ, Slack, 1986

Bibliography

Ayres AJ: Sensory Integrative and Learning Disorders. Los Angeles, Western Psychological Services, 1972

Clark PN: Theoretical frameworks in contemporary occupational therapy practice 1. Am J Occup Ther 33:509, 1979

Clark PN: Human development through occupational therapy: A philosophy and conceptual model for practice 2. Am J Occup Ther 33:577, 1979

Fidler G, Fidler J: Doing and becoming: Purposeful action and self actualization. Am J Occup Ther 32:305, 1978

King LJ: A sensory-integrative approach to schizophrenia. Am J Occup Ther 28:529, 1974

Llorens LJ: Facilitating growth and development: The promise of occupational therapy. Am J Occup Ther 24:1, 1976

Moore JC: Behavior, bias and the limbic system. Am J Occup Ther 30:11, 1976

Mosey AC: Occupational Therapy: Theory and Practice. Medford, MA, Pothier Bros, 1968

Mosey AC: Recapitulation of ontogenesis: A theory for the practice of occupational therapy. Am J Occup Ther 22:426, 1968

Reed K, Sanderson SR: Concepts of Occupational Therapy. Baltimore, Williams & Wilkins, 1980

Reilly M: Occupational therapy can be one of the great ideas of 20th century medicine. Am J Occup Ther 16:1, 1962

CHAPTER 4

Occupational Therapy — Base in the Human Development Process

Introduction to Human Development *Mary Margaret Daub*

Human beings grow and mature, fulfilling their needs and striving to interact with their environment. They gain competence from this process of interaction and adaptation, gradually building a realistic sense of self-worth. Thus, each person becomes a unique individual with the potential of self-actualization.

Human development can be defined as changes in the structure, thought, or behavior of a person that occur as a function of both biological and environmental influences.[6] These changes may be quantitative or qualitative. Quantitative changes, such as height, physical skills, and vocabulary, are easily understood and measured. Qualitative changes are not so easily measured, because they include a subjective element: there is no scale on which to weigh the influence of social interactions, the significance of dreams, or the level of a child's self-awareness. These quantitative and qualitative, changes are part of a developmental continuum, an ongoing, orderly process that persists from conception to death.

Human Development

Biologists, psychologists, epistemologists, anthropologists, and others all investigate the principles and processes of human development, but from varied points of view and with different methods of study. Studies and experiments can be made through controlled situations, longitudinal study (observation of the same individual over time), cross-sectional study (observation of different individuals of different ages at one time), or cross-cultural patterns of behavior.

In this chapter, we view the following developmental aspects of a person that contribute and interrelate to make him or her a miraculous and complex entity: physical, sensory, perceptual, cognitive, emotional, social, and cultural. As the individual grows, these aspects mature and expand along a developmental continuum. Although the aspects differ from each other at one level, they are dynamically interrelated and interdependent.

Human Development and Occupational Therapy

Occupational therapists work with individuals who have had an interruption in one or more areas of development somewhere along the life continuum. In order to provide a meaningful service to these individuals, the therapist must understand the underlying principles of man's growth and function and the sequences of growth and behavior that are somewhat predictable for normal human development.

The occupational therapist is an agent of change. The client, often against severe odds, must change and adapt within his or her life situation. The therapist can directly influence the quality of that change. Therefore, the therapist must know the range and potential for change available and must have a working knowledge of those concepts of change and adaptation inherent in the study of human development.

The primary motivation is pragmatic: the normal must be learned in order to assist clients who have suffered a disruption in the normal pattern of development. But a second motivation inevitably lures us — the age-old curiosity about who we are, how we began, and how we can grow and change.

Factors that Influence Human Development

Biological and environmental influences act upon each individual making up that individual's unique gestalt. Biological influences include stages of growth, maturation, and aging. Growth is increase in size, function, or complexity up to some point of optimal maturity. Maturation is the emergence of an organism's genetic potential; it consists of a series of preprogrammed changes which comprise alterations not only in the organism's structure and form but also in its complexity, integration, organization, and function. Aging is biological evolution beyond the point of optimal maturity.[6]

General Principles of Human Development

There are some general principles and issues of human growth and development that must be understood before looking closer at specific areas of normal human growth.
1. *Development is orderly, predictable, sequential, and cumulative.*
2. *Each child develops at a different pace.* There is a wide range of individual differences along the normal continuum.
3. *The expectation of others affects a child's behavior.*

4. *At any one stage of development, a child might be placing particular emphasis on one aspect at the expense of another.*
5. *The behavior of a child does not consistently "improve"; it seems to alternate between periods of equilibrium (a good balance) and disequilibrium (less balance).*

Principles of Maturation

There are certain principles of maturation that tend to be relatively independent of environmental influences. They are:
1. *Cephalocaudal pattern of development.* Muscular development, control, and coordination progress from the head to the feet. That is, head control precedes that of the trunk and lower extremities.
2. *Proximal–distal and medial (rostral)–lateral patterns of development.* Parts of the body closest (proximal) to the spine tend to be controlled in a coordinated manner before the parts farthest away (distal) from it.
3. *Mass to specific pattern of development.* Initially, much of the motor activity of the infant consists of whole-body movement. With maturity, these undifferentiated and generalized mass responses become more specific.
4. *Gross motor to fine motor pattern of development.* Since control of proximal musculature precedes that of distal musculature, it follows that mastery of the larger muscles precedes mastery of the smaller muscles. This mastery must then become even more refined and definitive to permit acquisition of skills.

These four principles governing growth are not static but are continuously influencing motor development.

Theoretical Foundations

Theories of human development are important to the occupational therapist because:
1. Theories serve as an organizing mechanism: they attempt to sort out some of the complex factors in development.
2. Theories provide a basis for frames of reference from which one can develop therapeutic program objectives and treatment.
3. Theories are a basis for research that is needed in the field of occupational therapy.
4. Knowledge of different theories extends insight into human behavior, presenting alternative explanations of behavior on which to base treatment goals.
5. Theories provide the bases for justification and accountability. In essence, a theory becomes the rationale for our treatment process.

In adhering to a single theory to the exclusion of others, the therapist must keep the following in mind:

1. No one theory accounts for each and every aspect of the developmental process; therefore, the therapist must fully understand the parameters of any chosen theory.
2. The therapist must be able to translate the theory effectively into occupational therapy application.
3. Strict adherence to just one theory does not always allow for individual differences.
4. A single-theory approach may narrow a therapist's perspective and limit professional growth potential.

On the other hand, when a therapist chooses an eclectic approach; that is, bases a rationale on varied sources or theories, caution is advised because in order to be truly eclectic, the therapist must be thoroughly versed in each theory. The therapist must know the advantages and limitations of the theories so as to present a clearly defined rationale for client treatment.

No matter which approach is chosen, it is imperative that everyone involved in the treatment process: (1) know what rationale is being used, (2) understand how the rationale can be translated into occupational therapy practice, (3) be clear about how this treatment can be adapted to the individual client's needs, and (4) concur with the adoption of this rationale as a basis for treatment.

Learning Theory

Learning is the basic developmental process by which an individual's behavior is changed by the environment and is defined as a relatively permanent change in behavior or in the capacity for behavior resulting from either experience or practice.[6] This change occurs through experience and repetition. Psychologists have developed theories and paradigms to account for an individual's ability to adapt within his or her life space, and these theories serve as a framework for understanding varied aspects of human development.

Behavioral Theory

Some learning theorists view the individual as a purely responsive being, a mechanistic result of present and past environments. They observe the individual making responses to stimuli but give little regard to interpreting underlying reasons for those responses. Learning theorists view mankind within narrow parameters, assuming that behavior is a function of immediate stimuli. For them, learning takes place by means of respondent (classical) and/or operant conditioning.

In *classical* conditioning, two stimuli are presented *at the same time.* One is reinforcing (*e.g.,* food); the other is irrelevant (*e.g.,* sound of refrigerator door). This leads to the expectation of reinforcement and concomitant automatic response (*e.g.,* salivation) associated with the irrelevant stimulus (*i.e., learning has taken place*). Thus, even when the irrelevant stimulus is presented without the reinforcing stimulus, there is a response.

In *operant conditioning,* reinforcement (*e.g.,* praise or candy) is presented *following* behavior. Therefore, reinforcement is associated with the behavior (*i.e., learning has taken place*). Thus, behavior is repeated.

For the learning theorists, learning is a direct result of one or the other of these processes. In reality, even within the limitations of this theory, most learning would probably combine the two processes.

Social Learning Theory

The social learning theory is an outgrowth of learning theory. The proponents of social learning theory believe that most learning takes place through observing behavior and the effects of behavior. They attempt to explain why mankind uses models to learn social traits and how a socially acceptable repertoire of behaviors is developed.

Bandura's formulation of social learning theory adds an exciting extension to behavior theory. He maintains that:

1. Learning is acquired through observation and modeling.
2. There is a continuous reciprocal interaction between environmental, behavioral, and personal determinants of behavior.
3. The environment is not an autonomous force. It is regulated by its own contingencies, of which human behavior is only one.
4. Learning occurs by means of vicarious reinforcement (learning from observed positive and negative consequences of a model's behavior) and self-reinforcement.
5. Self-reinforcement yields self-efficacy or the ability of an individual to cope with stress.[2]
6. One's ability to judge how to deal with stress comes from:
   a. The performance mode—that is, how similar situations were handled in the past
   b. Vicarious information gained from observing the success or failure of others
   c. Social persuasion—that is, the undermining or reinforcement of one's sense of efficacy by others
   d. The person's perception of his or her physiology and its vulnerability in stressful situations[1,7]

Although the learning theorists have given developmentalists volumes of empirically based research explaining human behavior, the types of behavior that lend themselves to experimental methods are limited. These theorists cannot explain complex qualitative behaviors such as emotions or individual differences. Thus the social learning theory is best applied to specific behaviors rather than to the total area of development.

Psychoanalytic Theory

The theories of Sigmund Freud, Erik Erikson, and other neofreudians deal primarily with emotional and personality development. Their psychoanalytic approach to personality development stands in marked contrast to learning and biological theories. Like cognitive and developmental theories, psychoanalytic theory assumes that internal processes are as important as external experiences in shaping behavior.[3]

Sigmund Freud

Freud's theory sets forth basic assumptions about personality and psychosexual development:

1. All behavior is energized by fundamental instinctual drives: sexual drives or libido, life-preserving forces, and aggressive drives.
2. Throughout the lifespan, gratification and strategies to obtain gratification are the focal points of psychosexual development.
3. The type of gratification and the method of attaining it change with age, but the instinctual drive to obtain it remains constant.
4. Three basic structures of personality (id, ego, and superego) develop in childhood and function to assist in gratification of instincts.
5. If conflict arises between the different structures of personality, anxiety results. Defense mechanisms are automatic and unconscious strategies for dealing with anxiety.
6. A series of distinct psychosexual stages of personality development evolve during childhood. The first three, the *oral, anal,* and *phallic* stages, center on areas of the body that at each stage become a center for pleasure. These stages are followed by

the *latency* and *genital* stages, during which the personality is influenced by degrees of sexual interest, socialization, and an evolving focus on life goals. Freud sets the stage for the explanation of development of an individual's unconscious mind and its relationship to the ability to function.

Erik Erikson

A neofreudian, Erikson expanded Freud's theory to include the societal environment. His approach focuses on human psychosocial development. Erikson sees personality development as unfolding progressively throughout the life cycle. He does not place paramount importance on childhood experiences as Freud does. His eight stages of development are delineated by eight emotional crises or issues that must be resolved by the individual (Table 4-1). The resolution of these issues is the balance between the negative and positive poles of each stage. This resolution and its importance at any one point in life is a function of the individual's relationship to his place in his social and cultural environment. How a person resolves a crisis directly affects the quality of his or her ability to deal with a subsequent developmental issue. Further, Erikson believes that these crises may emerge throughout life.

The basic strength of theorists such as Freud and Erikson is their willingness to look at the whole person and at the conscious and unconscious factors of emotional development. They deal with interpersonal relationships, particularly as they relate to childhood experiences.

Other Psychoanalytical Theorists

Anna Freud

Freud's daughter's principal contribution was to extend the tenets of psychoanalysis to the study of children and education. She was concerned primarily with psycho-

Table 4-1. *Comparison of Erikson's and Freud's Stages of Psychosocial Development*

Erikson		Freud	
Stage	*Ages*	*Stage*	*Ages*
Trust–Mistrust	0–1	Oral	0–1
Autonomy–Shame	1–3	Anal	2–3
Initiative–Guilt	4–5	Phallic	4–5
Industry–Inferiority	6–11	Latency	6–12
Identity–Role diffusion	12–18	Genital	13–18 and adulthood
Intimacy–Isolation	Young adult		
Generativity–Stagnation	Middle adult		
Ego integrity–Despair	Later adult		

Table 4-2. *Sullivan's Stages of Personality Development*

Approximate Age	Stage	Child's Social Needs
Birth–2 years	Infancy	Security
2–6	Childhood	Adult attention and validation of experiences
6–10	Juvenile	Peer relationships
10–12	Pre-adolescent	Interpersonal intimacy in an isophilic relationship
12–16	Early adolescent	Intimacy; sexual gratification; personal security in heterophilic relationship
16–20	Late adolescent	"Special" heterophilic relationship and place in society

pathology rather than the normal sequences of personality development but focused much needed attention on the adolescent years.

Harry Stack Sullivan

Sullivan expanded the original psychoanalytic orientation to include an interpersonal theory of psychiatry, as he thought that it was through social interactions that the "self system" matures. This occurs through six stages of development (Table 4-2).

Peter Blos

Blos expanded psychoanalytic concepts, particularly in relation to adolescence. His theory centers on the process of individuation from parents and the development of significant relationships with others.

The weakness of psychoanalytical theory lies in the difficulty of defining parameters of development and of validating research. Most data are gleaned from adults whose subjective reconstruction of their childhood experiences may lead to invalid or vague conclusions.

Cognitive Theories

Jean Piaget

Piaget, a biologist–epistemologist, investigated the origin, nature, methods, and limits of human knowledge (Table 4-3). In contrast to the learning theorists, Piaget saw the human being as active, alert, and capable. That is, he believed that a person processes information rather than merely receiving it and does more than respond to stimuli; he gives structure and meaning to

stimuli. Piaget postulated that until a certain age, children form judgments through their perceptual world rather than by principles of logic: "What you see is what you get." If the child's perceptions and experiences fit a structure within his mind, they are assimilated or understood, whereas if the information received does not fit existing structure, the mind must change in order to accommodate the new experience. The schemata of a child—his or her methods of processing information—expand as the child grows. A person continuously adjusts his or her schemata in order to assimilate and accommodate new information. The human mind seeks equilibrium between assimilation and accommodation just as the human body seeks biological homeostasis.

As the child grows, his structural abilities to accommodate new information grow also. Piaget saw this as occurring in four major steps. The steps and mode of learning for each follow:

1. Sensorimotor period—body and movement
2. Preoperational period—imagery
3. Concrete operational period—concrete human/ nonhuman environment
4. Formal operational period—abstraction

Jerome Bruner

Bruner, also a cognitive theorist, investigates the individual as an artist (aesthetic being) and as a scientist (problem solver). Like Piaget, he sees the qualitative changes in the cognitive structures corresponding to biological growth. Both scientists also see the mind as developing in stages, but they differ on the role of language in development. Piaget views thought as preceding language skill, whereas Bruner sees language as a causative factor in acquiring problem-solving ability.

Unlike learning theorists, cognitive theorists attempt to show that the individual is motivated by his or her own basic competence and not merely by a stimulus–response reaction.[6] They also account for the role of such things as values, beliefs, and attitudes.

The major concern of cognitive theory is intellectual development; it does not explain all of human behavior (for example, social, emotional, and personality development). However, some of its proponents are now investigating these areas.

Humanistic Self-Theory of Self-Development

Humanistic psychologists react to the environmental determinism of learning and psychoanalytic theorists. Their primary focus is the individual's concept of *self*. They see man as self-determining and creative. Their aim is to maximize human potential. These theorists view each individual act optimistically as a function of the individual's self.

Table 4-3. *The Continuum of Cognitive Development*

Modality of Intelligence	Phase	Stage	Approximate Chronological Age
Sensorimotor	Sensorimotor	1. Use of reflexes	0–1 month
		2. First habits and primary circular reactions	1–4½ months
		3. Coordination of vision and prehension, secondary circular reactions	4½–9 months
		4. Coordination of secondary schemata and their application to new situations	9–12 months
		5. Differentiation of action schemata through tertiary circular reactions, discovery of new means	12–18 months
		6. First internalization of schemata and solution of some problems by deduction	18–24 months
Representative by means of concrete operations	Preconceptual	1. Appearance of symbolic function and the beginning of internalized actions accompanied by representation	2–4 years
	Intuitive thought	2. Representational organizations based on either static configurations or on assimilation to one's own action	4–5½ years
		3. Articulated representational regulations	5½–7 years
	Concrete operational	1. Simple operations (classifications, seriations, term-by-term correspondences, etc.)	7–9 years
		2. Whole systems (Euclidian coordinates, projective concepts, simultaneity)	9–11 years
Representative by means of formal operations	Formal operational	1. Hypothetico-deductive logic and combinatorial operations	11–14 years
		2. Structure of "lattice" and the group of 4 transformations	14 years+

From Maier HW (ed): *Three Theories of Child Development: The Contributions of Erik H. Erikson, Jean Piaget and Robert R. Sears,* rev ed, p 155. New York, Harper & Row, 1969. Reprinted with permission. The source was Piaget's paper: Les Stades du developpement intellectuel de l'enfant et de l'adolescent (1956). Adapted from Table 1, Intelligence is an ultimate goal, in Décarié TG: *Intelligence and Affectivity in Early Childhood,* p 15. New York, International Universities Press, 1965. Reprinted with permission.

Abraham Maslow

Maslow stresses that each person has an innate need for self-actualization. It is possible to attain this goal only when a well-integrated individual has satisfied "lower needs" such as safety, love, food, and shelter.

Carl Rogers

Rogers, another humanist, is concerned with helping each individual realize his or her potential by creating an interpersonal climate for growth with characteristics such as empathy, unconditional willingness to accept a person as he or she is, and a genuine involvement in the person's growth. The strength of this approach to human development is its concern with real-life situations. Humanistic theory is becoming an important consideration in educational programs for children, although its primary concern is adult adjustment. It does not, however, incorporate a method for achieving self-actualization.

Ethology

Ethologists study humans and animals in their natural environments and view them as having evolved similar behavior traits. They think it possible that humans, like other animals, have inherited behavior patterns. Ethologists do not ignore the history and the situation of behavior patterns, but essentially they look at behavior in terms of preserving the individual or the species within the evolution of civilization.

Ethology is an interesting and relatively new way of studying human behavior. It presupposes that animal behavior is a valid indicator of human behavior. A growing interest in its methods and principles indicates that ethology will play an increasing role in the study of human development.

Maturational Theory

Arnold Gesell

Gesell maintains that a baby's behavior is modified as a consequence of physiological maturation and feels that the child requires only general support and attention from the outside environment in order to develop normally. Gesell emphasizes the stability and conservatism of growth.

Gesell developed normative data about a child's gross motor, fine motor, adaptive skill, language, and social development as they relate to maturation of the central nervous system. He provides actual chronological scales for the parameters of normal development against which possible developmental delays can be detected. Such scales may serve the occupational therapist as a base line for setting occupational therapy goals and plans. Data collected from a large population of children evaluated by such scales may serve as a basis for research in child development.

Normative data are and must be updated continually. Scales must be used cautiously. A therapist has to know the type of population on which the scale was standardized and when it was developed. Many scales are not done cross-culturally and may be invalid for certain groups of children.

Ecological Theory

Urie Bronfenbrenner

Bronfenbrenner is credited with insisting that developmental psychology look beyond the dyad of mother and child into the cultural and personal relationships that form the ecological niche in which the child grows. He explored the ecology of development.

The totality of child development includes parental behaviors such as emotional tone, methods of discipline, patterns of communication, and type and extent of cognitive enrichment. Other major influences include the impact of other institutions on the child; the support systems available to the family; and the types of play activities, social interactions, and other forms of cognitive stimulation to which the child is exposed.[4,5]

References

1. Bandura A: Self-efficacy: Toward a unifying theory of behavioral change. Psychol Rev 84:191, 1977
2. Bandura A: Social Learning Theory. Englewood Cliffs, NJ, Prentice–Hall, 1977
3. Bee H: The Developing Child, 4th ed, p 29. New York, Harper & Row, 1985
4. Bronfenbrenner U: The Ecology of Human Development. Cambridge, MA: Harvard University Press, 1977
5. Bronfenbrenner U: Toward an experimental ecology of human development. Am Psychol 32:513, 1977
6. Craig GJ: Human Development, pp 11, 12, 32. Englewood Cliffs, NJ, Prentice–Hall, 1976
7. Davis I: Adolescents: Theoretical and Helping Perspectives, p 36. Boston, Kluwer–Hifhuff, 1985

Bibliography

Achenbach TM: Research in Developmental Psychology: Concepts, Strategies, Methods. New York, John Wiley & Sons, 1982

Brim OG Jr, Kagan J (eds): Constancy and Change in Human Development. Cambridge, MA, Harvard University Press, 1980

Craig G: Human Development, 4th ed. Englewood Cliffs, NJ, Prentice–Hall, 1985

Crain W: Theories of Development, 2nd ed. Englewood Cliffs, NJ, Prentice–Hall, 1985

Flavell JH: On cognitive development. Child Dev 53(a):1, 1982

Hergenhahn B: An Introduction to Theories of Personality, 2nd ed. Englewood Cliffs, NJ, Prentice–Hall, 1984

Kohlberg L: Essays on Moral Development, Vol 1, The Philosophy of Moral Development. New York, Harper & Row, 1981

Kuczaj SA II (ed): Language Development, Vol 2, Language, Thought, and Culture. Hillsdale, NJ, Erlbaum, 1982

Reese HW, Lipsitt LP (eds): Advances in Child Development and Behavior, Vol 16. New York, Academic Press, 1982

Prenatal Development Through Mid-Adulthood *Mary Margaret Daub*

Prenatal Development

Periods of Prenatal Development

Following fertilization of the ovum, there is a gestation period of 266 days (with a grace period of 11 days). The first phase (2 weeks) of prenatal growth is the *germinal period.* This is primarily a time of cell division and differentiation. Once the growing cell mass is fully implanted in the wall of the uterus, the *embryonic period* begins. During this period (8 weeks), structures and organs are formed and differentiated. Approximately 12 weeks following conception the *fetal period* begins: the first bone cells are developed, and growth continues until birth.

These first several weeks of development are marked by the emergence of physical characteristics. Approximately 26 days following conception, a body form is evolving, and there is the beginning of arm and leg buds. Two days later, the arms are developing at a greater rate than the legs. By the end of the first month, the details of the head — rudimentary eyes, ears, mouth, and brain — are seen faintly. The brain already shows primitive specialization. There is also a primitive heart and an umbilical cord as well as such organs as the liver, kidney, and stomach. The primitive embryo is now ¼ to ½ inch long, the size of half a pea. In one month's time the embryo is 10,000 times larger than the fertilized egg.

By the end of the second month, the embryo has familiar features: face, eyes, ears, nose, lips, tongue, muscles, and skin covering. The arms have discernible fingers and thumbs, and the legs have knees, ankles, and toes. All organs in the body are formed. The brain sends out impulses, the muscles and nerves are working together, and the heart is beating regularly and steadily. The endocrine system is functioning and so are the stomach, liver, and kidneys. Isolated reflexes can be elicited. In several months, these primitive systems will be truly functional.

The third month after conception traditionally marks the beginning of the fetal period. By the end of this month, the fetus has become active. In can kick, turn, close fingers, move its thumb into opposition, and open its mouth, although its eyelids are still closed. This period is marked by refinements of facial and extremity features. The palate and lips are formed and fused. Sexual differentiation is beginning.

The fourth month is a period in which the lower body parts develop more rapidly. The fetus weighs approximately 4 ounces and is 6 inches long. Its muscles and reflexive capabilities are maturing. The mother can now feel a "quickening" movement.

The fifth month is a stage of continued refinement. There is an increase in spontaneous activity. Fetal movements are markedly perceived by the mother. The fetus sleeps and wakes. However, its respiratory system is still too immature for life outside the uterus.

In the sixth month, the eyelids of the fetus open. Its eyes are formed and capable of movements (lateral and vertical). Taste buds have developed, as have eyelashes and brows. The fetus has a marked grasp reflex. It now weighs approximately 1½ pounds and is 12 to 14 inches long. But its breathing patterns are irregular; it can usually survive for only 24 hours outside the womb.

During the seventh month, the cerebral hemispheres cover almost all the brain, and the organism can make specialized responses. If born now, the child can survive in a sheltered environment.

The eighth and ninth months are periods of refinement of function. The immune system of the fetus begins to mature, enabling it to sustain independent life more safely when it is born.

Reflex development begins in the intrauterine environment. Reflexive behaviors are the building blocks of sensorimotor behaviors and the foundation of future sensorimotor patterns. As the central nervous system develops, reflexes/reflexive reactions are integrated and adapted in order for appropriate sensorimotor behaviors and skills to emerge. The absence or delay of reflex integration behaviors may indicate developmental delay or dysfunction. Reflexes are discussed further in Chapters 34 and 36.

Inherited and Environmental Influences

Genetic make-up delineates the parameters for development. Environmental factors influence the quality and extent to which heredity affects the potential for growth.

Although the uterus is a relatively safe and stable environment, it is not immune to environmental factors. The seriousness of the effect of these factors depends on the type of influence, the intensity of the influence, and the time the influence is introduced.

Since the germinal and embryonic stages are formation and differentiation periods, the first trimester of pregnancy (first 12 weeks) is critical in development. If normal growth is interrupted during this time, defects can arise.

Hereditary factors also contribute to the integrity of the growing organism. Therefore, it is imperative that the therapist understand the basis of genetic functioning, the implications of genetic malfunctioning for the developing organism, and those dysfunctions that are a direct result of genetic inheritance. Increased understanding of deoxyribonucleic acid (DNA) has shed light on those developmental traits that have specific hereditary components.

Childhood

The study of human development implies knowledge of the systems inherent in the developmental aspects (Fig. 4-1). It is essential that we as professionals have a view of the whole child as an evolving human being. The following sections will present an overview of the developmental systems and profiles of children at various stages of development.

Physical Development

In the first year, babies rapidly gain weight and length. The general rule being that the infant will triple his/her weight and add 10–12 inches in length within the first year. By age two, most toddlers are already half as tall as they will be as adults. After two, growth slows to a steady rate of 2–3 inches and 6 pounds a year until adolescence.

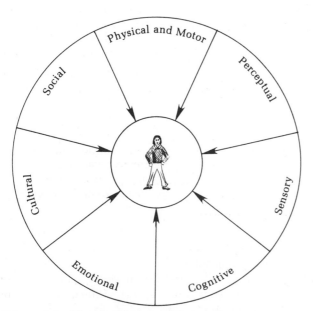

Figure 4-1. The developmental aspects.

Body shape and body parts do not grow at equal rates. Hands and feet mature earliest, followed by arms, legs and trunk. Bone growth follows a similar pattern, the most rapid development and ossification occurring within the first two years.

The development of the brain and central nervous system is incomplete at birth. The cortex is the least developed area: cortical development is about half complete at six months and 75% complete by age two.[4] Current thinking about hemispheric specialization is that the process is not complete until adolescence.[65] Likewise, although myelinization of the brain is thought to be almost complete by age two, the process probably continues into adolescence.

The endocrine system is functional from about the fourth month of gestation. Thyroxine and the pituitary growth hormone are most active in the early years, then level off until pubescence.[60]

Respiration and breathing follow a predictable and orderly progression. Breathing patterns affect not only the child's ability to survive outside the uterus but also his/her feeding and speech patterns.

Other physical attributes—facial features, teeth, hair, skin—develop and change at a slower and more steady pace. Changes are usually complete by the end of adolescence. It is important to note that some of these changes may affect sensory ability. For example, as the face broadens, auditory localization becomes more accurate.

Sensorimotor Development

At birth, the child demonstrates orderly and predictable movement patterns. The development of muscle tone, posture, and motor responses allows the child to survive and adapt within his/her environment. The child first gains control of the head, neck, and trunk. Gradually, he/she is able to roll, sit, crawl, creep, kneel, stand, and free himself/herself from the forces of gravity in locomotion. Fine-motor control begins with visual fixation, reaching, ulnar palmar, palmar, radial palmar, raking, radial grasp, release of objects and pincer grasp, followed by refinement of each skill (Table 4-4). The wonder of the developing child is that none of these developing patterns occurs in isolation; rather they are interactive and interdependent on all senses and developmental systems. The child learns and develops more motor patterns in the first year than he/she will develop over the rest of a lifetime.

Gross and fine motor development in early childhood involve the refinement of skills and equilibrium. Nearly all basic skills of motor behavior are complete by 6–7 years of age although refinement continues into adulthood.[41]

These changes occur at different rates with different children. But for every child, physical and sensorimotor

Table 4-4. *Fine Motor Development in the First Year*

Approximate Age (Months)	Vision	Hand Position	Grasp
1	Follows object to midline; regards object when brought to or just past midline when object is only 8–9 in from face	Hands fisted; forearm pronated; occasionally brings hand to mouth (primary circular reaction)	Grasp reflex; no release; object placed in hand drops immediately
2	Prolonged visual regard of objects; follows past midline; regards out-stretched arm (ATNR influence); follows object 180° in supine position	Brings hands to midline; hands may open at sight of object	Grasp reflex; no voluntary release
3	Glances at object in hand; shifts glance between two objects; regards object at midline	Holds hands loosely opened or closed; symmetrical arm/hand movement in supine position	Grasp reflex decreasing or absent; holds object briefly; attempts at swiping at object
4	Occular convergence; regards object held in hand; regards hand	Bilateral arm movement; waves arms and moves body at sight of object	Attempts to play with own fingers; palmar grasp emerges; temporary active grasp; attempts to reach object but misses target; object-to-mouth in supine position; lightly scratches or clutches at clothes
5	Looks momentarily after object dropped	Reaches for and grasps object with both hands; thumb to mouth	Holds block with one hand and regards second block; ulnar palmar grasp when given object
6	Eye-hand coordination emerges (arms used asymmetrically); prolonged regard of objects	Visually directed reaching; reaches for dropped object; supination of forearm in supine position	Radial palmar grasp with flexed wrist; rakes at pellet with fingers (no thumb); holds object in each hand; reaches for block beyond reach
7	Looks after object	Thumb opposition	Grasp in supine position with thumb adducted; poor active release; bangs, shakes, and pats objects; transfers one object hand to hand; retains one object when given another and regards both; radial palmar grasp with extended wrist; inferior scissors grasp with metacarpophalangeal joints flexed
8		Still rakes with entire arm	Inferior pincer (thumb, second and third fingers); continues to drop objects; scissor grasp with thumb (metacarpophalangeal joint joint extended)
9		Extended reach and grasp; forearm use between midposition and pronation	Pokes with extended index finger; neat pincer grasp between thumb and index finger emerging; voluntary release emerging

(continued)

Table 4-4. (continued)

Approximate Age (Months)	Vision	Hand Position	Grasp
10			Spontaneously notices pellet and pokes at it; voluntary release; good superior pincer; holds crayon with crude palmar grasp
12			Smooth grasp; precise release of object into cup of 2 inch diameter (concept of container and contained); pulls ¼ inch pegs from pegboard; removes and replaces pellet in bottle on command

Adapted from Gilfoyle EM, Grady AP: *Children Adapt,* Thorofare, NJ, Slack 1982; Clark PN, Allen AS: *Occupational Therapy for Children,* St. Louis, CV Mosby, 1985; The Mecklenburg Center of Human Development Motor Developmental Evaluation, Mecklenburg, NY, unpublished, 1970; Gesell A: *The First Five Years of Life,* New York, Harper and Row 1940.

development affects and is interrelated to all other aspects of development.

Sensory and Perceptual Development

The sensory system receives stimuli through the five senses. Perception is the mental process by which sensory, intellectual, and emotional data are organized meaningfully: it is the conscious recognition or interpretation of sensory stimuli. Perceptual awareness is the foundation of cognition.

Visual Development and Perception

Current research gives us some interesting information about visual attention and scanning. During the first two months of life, the infant focuses on *where* objects are in the world[51] and can even search for objects in the dark.[25] This process is termed the *secondary visual system.* When searching for objects, the baby generally demonstrates visual preference for their edges rather than their features. An exception to this rule is the human face: a child can and does attend to the features of the face. It also appears that the child can differentiate a photograph of a human face from the face itself.[24]

At approximately two months of age, the child shifts visual attention from where the object is to *what* it is. This is the foundation of object identity. At this stage, the child has evolved to use of the *primary visual system.* Fantz and Linn and their co-workers discovered that at this stage the infant prefers objects with large or multi-

ple pieces, with horizontal as opposed to vertical planes, and with curved as opposed to straight lines.[15,37]

Auditory Development

Auditory acuity develops and improves until adolescence. The infant's auditory acuity is better than his/her visual acuity. Current research suggests that within the general range of pitch and loudness of the human voice, infants hear as well as adults, although adults are more sensitive to quiet sounds.[54]

Development of the Other Senses

Gustatory and olfactory senses are less studied than are the others. These senses are interrelated and interdependent. Study of the development of the sense of taste (sweet, sour, bitter, and salt) indicates that infants react differently to at least three basic flavors and prefer sweet tastes to others. When given a variety of pleasant and noxious olfactory stimuli, the infant consistently responds more definitively to noxious smells.

Sensitivity to light touch is dramatically demonstrated by an infant's reflexive response. With maturation and experience, this sense of touch becomes more refined.

Cognitive Development
Major Views

There are three major views of cognitive development.

Intellectual Power Approach

This approach measures individual differences in intelligence by various tests. The intellectual quotient, originally a comparison of the child's chronological age with his/her mental age, is no longer used. Now, the child's performance is compared with the performance of a large group of children of the same age. The most commonly used tests are the Bayley Scales of Infants, the Stanford–Binet, and the Wechsler Intelligence Scales for Children. Both IQ tests and school achievement tests measure *performance*, not underlying intellectual ability or competence. These tests are discussed in Chapter 16.

Cognitive Developmental Approach

The focus here is on the development of cognitive structures rather than of intellectual power. Patterns of development that are common to all children rather than to individuals are studied.

Jean Piaget described four major stages of cognitive development (see the box "Summary of Piaget's Stages of Cognitive Development").

Current research concerning Piaget's stages indicates that imitation of behaviors may occur in substage I rather than substage II,[43] that deferred imitation may occur one year earlier than Piaget predicted,[33] and that infants remember what they see and organize their memory as early as age 8 to 10 months.[8]

Research on the preoperational period indicates that children from the age of 2 to 6 years are more skillful than Piaget originally thought. For example, a child as young as 2 or 3 years has at least some ability to understand that other people see or experience things differently.[17] The preoperational child may understand identities and do simple classification as early as three years.[4,42]

Summary of Piaget's Stages of Cognitive Development

The Sensorimotor Stage (Birth – 2 years)

The infant operates almost exclusively with overt schemes and actions. Learning occurs in six substages, as the child learns about the world in terms of what he/she can do with objects and with abundant new sensory information.

Substage 1 — Practice with reflexes. Reflex accommodation is a result of experience.

Substage 2 — Primary circular reactions. Chance movements lead to interesting results, which the child reproduces by trial and error. The infant does not distinguish between body and outside events.

Substage 3 — Secondary circular reactions. The child makes interesting things happen. He/she begins to coordinate two types of sensory information. The connections between actions and results are perceived and the actions are repeated.

Substage 4 — Coordination of secondary schemes. The infant combines actions to attain a goal. Familiar strategies are used in combination and in new situations.

Substage 5 — Experimentation. The infant tries new ways of playing, moving, and manipulating objects and begins to understand the concept of cause and effect.

Substage 6 — Beginning of thought. Objects now have permanence. The child uses images, words, or actions to represent objects.

The Preoperational Stage (2 – 6 Years)

The child uses symbols and internalized actions in everyday activity and thinks in images. The content of the thought is magical. In the beginning of the stage, the child is "centered": he/she can focus on only one aspect of a thought or situation at a time. Ginsburg and Opper summarized the preoperational child accurately:

> The [preoperational] child decenters his thought just as in the sensorimotor period the infant decentered his behavior. The newborn acts as if the world is centered about himself; and must learn to behave in more adaptive ways. Similarly, the young child thinks from a limited perspective and must widen it.[23]

Concrete Operational Stage (6 – 12 Years)

The child's logic is basic and inductive. He/she is still tied to specific experience but can do mental manipulations as well as physical ones.[4]

Formal Operations (12 Years)

Abstract and hypothetical deductive reasoning emerges. The child can manipulate images and objects in the mind and can think about things that have not been experienced or have not yet happened. The child can organize and systematize thought deductively.

The latest research on Piaget's concrete operational stage focuses on the sequence of the development of concrete operations and on whether the child's skills are consistent across tasks. Carol Tomlinson–Keasey and others found that there are definitive sequences in operational thought and that a child in the concrete operational stage performs at or about the same level consistently on a wide series of tasks.[63]

Information Processing Approach

In the last few years, a third approach, known as information processing, has emerged.[56,57] This approach searches for the fundamental processes or strategies that constitute cognition. Once these processes are known, one can investigate whether they change with age and whether children differ in their speed of acquiring cognitive skills. This approach seems to skillfully combine concepts of cognitive power with structural approaches to cognitive development.

Language Development

An overview of cognition would be incomplete without a discussion of the acquisition of language skills. Language is the expression of the child's thoughts and the understanding of the world. Children's language is complex, productive, creative, and governed by rules. It is an arbitrary system of symbols that allows one to understand myriad messages. During the first year of the child's life, he/she goes through several prelinguistic phases: crying, cooing, babbling (see the box "Sequences of Language Development").

At approximately 1 year of age the first words emerge. After the first word is spoken, it takes 3 to 4 months to add the next ten words.[44] Vocabulary increases rapidly thereafter, and by 2 years of age, the child typically has a 300-word vocabulary. Language becomes more complex with the addition of plurals, past tense, auxiliary verbs, and prepositions. There appears to be a language sequencing in a predictable order, as the child progressively adds questions, negatives, superlatives, and so forth. Semantic development follows a predictable course. A child seems to have concepts or categories before he/she has words for them. By the time a child is 5 or 6 years old, his/her language is much like an adult's, but the child does not develop language skill fully until 8 or 9 years of age. The meaning of words for children seems to center on the function and the perceptual properties of objects and people.

There are individual differences in rate of language and grammar development, as well as in language style, that are influenced by both heredity and environment. Current theory focuses on the child's general cognitive development and the impact of the language heard by the child.[4]

Emotional Development and Theories of Personality

The emotional responses of children are related to the development of personality; that is, the person's unique, individual, relatively enduring pattern of relating to others and responding to the world.[4] Several theories have been used to describe the development of personality.

Temperament Theory

Temperament theory is predominantly, but not exclusively, a biological theory of personality development. Some basic concepts of this theory are:
1. Each individual is born with characteristic patterns of responding to the environment.
2. These temperamental characteristics affect the way the child responds to people and things around him/her.
3. The child's temperament also affects the way others respond to him/her.

Social Learning Theory

This theory says that the patterns of social behavior (what we normally call personality) are learned through modeling and can be specific to particular situations. If these patterns of personality are situation-specific, then personality patterns may not be consistent across situations or over time. The child's cognitive capacity may affect his/her ability to understand or attend to a model's behavior.

Psychoanalytic Theory

Psychoanalytic theory takes account both of inborn qualities and of particular environmental needs. The best known of the psychoanalytic theorists, Freud and Erikson, dealt with the developmental aspects of the origins of personality in childhood.

The concepts of Freud's theory were outlined earlier in this chapter. Freud identified three basic structures of personality in childhood: the id, ego, and superego. The *id* is the storehouse of basic energy, continually pushing for immediate gratification. The *ego* organizes, plans, and reality-tests the personality. Thought and language are ego functions. The *superego* is the conscience portion of personality; it contains parental and societal values

Sequences of Language Development*

Prelinguistic Speech

Before a child says his first real word, he goes through the following six, and perhaps seven, stages of speech:

1. *Undifferentiated crying.* With "no language but a cry," babies come into this world. Early crying is a reflexive reaction to the environment produced by the expiration of breath.
2. *Differentiated crying.* After the first month of life (and of crying), the close listener can often discriminate differences in a baby's cries and can identify their causes.
3. *Cooing.* At about six weeks, chance movements of the child's mechanisms produce a variety of simple sounds called cooing. These squeals, gurgles, and bleats are usually emitted when he is happy and contented. The first sounds are vowels, and the first consonant is h.
4. *Babbling.* These vocal gymnastics begin at about three or four months, as a child playfully repeats a variety of sounds. Again, he is most likely to babble when he is contented and when he is alone. As he lies in his crib or sits in his infant seat, he loquaciously, and often loudly, spouts forth a variety of simple consonant and vowel sounds: "ma-ma-ma-ma-ma," "da-da-da-da-da," "bi-bi-bi-bi-bi-bi," and so forth. While most children babble, a few seem to skip this stage. Deaf children babble normally for the first few months of life, but then appear to lose interest when they cannot hear themselves.
5. *Lallation or imperfect imitation.* Some time during the second half of the first year, a child seems to become more aware of the sounds around him. He will become quiet as he listens to some sound. When it stops, he babbles in excitement, accidentally repeating the sounds and syllables he has heard. Then he imitates his own sounds.
6. *Echolalia or imitation of the sounds of others.* At about the age of nine or ten months, a child seems to consciously imitate the sounds made by others, even though he still does not understand them.
7. *Expressive jargon.* During the second year, many children use *expressive jargon.* This term, coined by Gesell, refers to a string of utterances that *sound* like sentences, with pauses, inflections, and rhythms. However, speech is not yet communicated verbally on a consistent basis.

Linguistic Speech

1. *One-word sentence (holophrase).* At about a year, a child points to a cracker, a toy, a pacifier, and says "da." His parents correctly interpret the command as "Give me that" or "I want that." He points to the door and says, "out." His single word thus expresses a complete thought, even though his listeners may not always be able to divine what that complete thought may be.
2. *Multiword sentence.* Some time about the age of two, a child strings together two or more words to make a sentence. When he wants to feed himself with no interference, he says imperiously, "Mommy 'way."

The child may develop a combination of sounds that mean something to him but may not necessarily be understood by the listener. Usually this communication style occurs at the time the child is learning nouns. The sounds or syllables are attached to the newly learned nouns.

The earliest multiword sentences are combinations of nouns and verbs. Other parts of speech, such as articles, prepositions, and adjectives, are lacking. Although these sentences are far from grammatical, they do communicate. This is *telegraphic speech;* it contains only words that carry meaning.

3. *Grammatically correct verbal utterances.* At about the age of three, the child has an impressive command of the language. He now has a vocabulary of some 900 words; he speaks in longer sentences that include all the parts of speech; and he has a good grasp of grammatical principles. His grammar is not the same one used by adults because he makes little allowance for exceptions to the linguistic rules he has assimilated. So, he says, "We goed to the store."

* Adapted from Eisenson J et al: The Psychology of Communication. New York, Appleton-Century-Crofts, 1963; Lenneberg EH: Biological Function of Language. New York, John Wiley & Sons, 1967; Clifton C: Language acquisition. In Spencer TD, Kass N (eds): Perspectives in Child Psychology: Research & Review. New York, McGraw-Hill, 1970

and is developed by means of the identification process. When conflict arises between the id, ego, and superego, anxiety results. The child develops defense mechanisms (normal automatic and unconscious strategies) for reducing stress when faced with intense anxiety. He/she also goes through distinct psychosexual stages, each of which focuses on sexual gratification in a specific erogenous zone.

Erik Erikson, also a psychoanalytic theorist, concentrated on ego development throughout the life span. He was concerned with societal and social demands on the child and refered to "psychosocial" stages of development. The four stages in childhood are summarized below.

Basic Trust versus Mistrust

The first ego challenge occurs during the first year of life within the context of the relationship with the primary caregiver (usually the mother). The challenge is to establish a sense of *basic trust* in the world and in oneself. This sense develops when the caregiver accommodates herself to the needs of the infant. The infant then learns that the caregiver is separate from the self but can be counted on to reappear even if she leaves temporarily. To the extent that the caregiver is unreliable and mutual regulation does not occur, a sense of *basic mistrust* may develop. In the adult, residues of basic mistrust may show up as extreme denial of needing anyone else or an inability to tolerate separation from those one depends on. The favorable outcome of this challenge to trust is the development of drive and hope.[29]

Autonomy versus Doubt and Shame

The second challenge emerges from the increasing capacities for cognitive discrimination and self-control and is confronted during the second and third years of life. The young child relates importantly with both parents and can differentiate them from each other and from himself. The ego challenge is to establish a firm sense of *autonomy*, and of self as a distinct person capable of internal self-regulation and not ruled only by external forces. The risk at this stage is that the child will be incapable of self-regulation or will be given too little opportunity for self-regulation; in this case, a sense of *doubt* about the self and *shame* in one's impulses may overwhelm one's sense of autonomy. Adult manifestations of the sense of doubt and shame include an excessive preoccupation with issues of control — either keeping too much control over oneself or yielding too much control and direction to others. Establishing the right balance between autonomy and doubt results in the development of self-control and willpower.[26]

Initiative versus Guilt

The third challenge is to establish a sense of *initiative* and overcome excessive *guilt*. These issues are most crucial between the ages of 3 and 6 years, and they link the child in mutual regulation to the wider family unit. A special challenge involves the competition between the child and the same-sex parent for the attention and affection of the opposite-sex parent; this is traditionally referred to as the *Oedipal situation,* or the *family romance.* The favorable outcome of this period is to become capable of direction and purpose.

Industry versus Inferiority

The fourth ego challenge links the child to the wider world of peers and adults outside the family. This phase usually begins with entrance into formal education at the age of 6 or 7 years and ends with puberty. The challenge is to establish a sense of *industry* — the sense that one is a worker who can develop whatever skills and competencies are needed to be productive and admired in that particular culture. The risk is that the child will not acquire the necessary skills to relate effectively outside the family and will develop a sense of *inferiority.* Some adults have a lingering sense of incompetence; they fear they cannot achieve anything well enough to be evaluated by an impartial judge. They may have great difficulties in work settings that are not "familial."

The emotional world of the child is a complex interaction of personality development, self-concept, bonding, attachment, family interactions, and personal relationships. Childhood is the testing ground for emotions and behaviors that will be the cornerstones of adaptive behaviors.

Social Development

The Concept of Self

Any discussion of children's social relationships must proceed from an understanding of the concept of self and how it develops. The emerging concept of self has several elements, including:

1. The *I* or *existential self:* awareness of self as separate. This sense of self occurs with self-recognition at approximately 15 to 18 months of age.
2. The *me* or *categorical self,* arrived at by comparing the self to others in one or more categories.
3. *Self-esteem:* the dimension of self-concept that includes a negative and/or positive sense of self. Studies have demonstrated that the child with high self-esteem does somewhat better on school achievement tests; sees himself/herself as respon-

sible for success or failure; has more friends; and has a positive view of parental relationships.[12]

Sex-Role Development

By the age of 2 or 3 years, the child generally identifies himself/herself as a boy or girl (gender identity). By age 4, he/she understands that gender is stable throughout life; and by age 5 or 6, the child has the concept of gender constancy (gender does not change by appearance change). Sex-role concepts and stereotyping appear to be strongest at 6 to 7 years of age.

There are many theories of sex-role development. Mischel, a social learning theorist, emphasizes the role of reinforcement and modeling as the basis of sex-role acquisition. Freud's explanation rests on the concept of identification, by which the child imitates the same-sex parent. Kohlberg proposed a cognitive-developmental model: the child imitates the same-sex model only after gender constancy is confirmed. Current research proposes that the child begins to develop rules about what a boy or girl does after he/she understands gender differences.[4]

Social Relationships

As the child develops a sense of self, he/she interacts with others to form social relationships. Bowlby and Ainsworth describe the basic sense of attachment in infancy. They describe attachment as an invisible, internal affectional bond demonstrated by attachment behaviors that allow the child to retain closeness to a significant person. Attachment begins with initial bonding and continues with mutual attachment behaviors. Although research by Klaus and Kennel suggested that initial bonding (12 – 24 hours after birth) and early contact were vital for the development of parent–child relationships, more current research indicates that early contact may be only partially potent or cirtical for long-term parent–child relationships.[35]

The meshing of attachment behaviors is much more critical for parent attachment. The child develops attachment to both the mother and father. The child sends out signals and the parent responds. By 4 to 5 months of age, most infants have formed strong attachment to a primary caretaker (usually the mother). A father who was present at the birth of his baby indicates stronger bonding to the child than a father who was not present.

The attachment process occurs in several phases, according to Ainsworth:

Phase 1—Initial Attachment. During the first four months, the infant displays proximity-promoting behaviors (behaviors that bring people closer). There is no consistent attachment to one parent or the other.

Phase 2—Attachment-in-the-making. At about 3 months of age, the infant can distinguish between familiar and unfamiliar faces and dispenses attachment behaviors more discriminatingly. There is no complete attachment to a single person.

Phase 3—Clear-cut attachment. By about 6 to 7 months, attachment is directed toward one person. The mode of attachment changes—it becomes proximity-seeking. The child literally moves toward the caretaker.

Phase 4—Multiple attachments. Single attachment occurs between 6 and 12 months. After that time, attachments spread to others.[2]

Patterns of Attachment

In general, from 7 to 8 months of age, the child shows strong attachment to either the father or the mother in preference to a stranger. He/she typically turns to the mother rather than the father when under stress. The older child seems to form a stronger attachment and identification with the same-sex parent. The securely attached child uses the adult as a safe base for exploration. Secure attachment is fostered by attentive and loving interaction between child and parent.

Relationships with Other Children

Relationships with other children become more central from the age of 1 to 2 years. By 4 to 5 years, children have formed individual relationships. Friendships become stable in elementary school. Peer interaction becomes increasingly important, reaching a climax during adolescence.

Development of Social Cognition

The child's thinking has an impact on his/her relationships with people and objects. In particular, the child's perspective-taking ability is central to his/her emerging understanding of other people and relationships. Selman's theory of social understanding indicates the relation of social perspective thinking to the development of social relationships. The level of social understanding can be seen in the child's understanding of friendships, groups, and parent–child relationships. The two key levels in early childhood are the reciprocal level (7 to 12 years) and the mutual level (10 to 15 years). In the reciprocal level, the child understands that others either feel and see things differently than he/she does or that others feel and see things in the same way. Relationships are seen as two-way interactions. In the mutual level, the youngster understands that relationships require constant mutual adjustment.[4]

Moral Development

Social understanding also requires the child to think about and explain other people's actions. The child must develop a sense of morality. Kohlberg has delineated six stages of moral reasoning (see the box "Summary of Kohlberg's Six Stages of Moral Reasoning.").

Summary of Kohlberg's Six Stages of Moral Reasoning*

Level I

Pre-Moral (4–10 years). Primary emphasis is on external control and ideas of others. These standards are followed either to avoid punishment or to gain reward.

Type I—Punishment and obedience. The child obeys to avoid punishment.

Type II—Naive instrumental hedonism. Conformity to rules is out of self-interest.

Level II

Morality of Conventional Role Conformity (10–13 years). The child wishes to please others and internalizes some of the standards of those persons deemed important to him or her. The child now decides if some action is good by his or her standards.

Type III—Maintaining approval of others. The child judges the intentions of others and yields an opinion.

Type IV—Authority maintaining morality. The child shows respect for authority and maintenance of social order.

Level III

Morality of Self-Accepted Moral Principles (13 years to adulthood). True morality: the individual recognizes the possible conflict between standards and realizes that conduct and reasoning about right and wrong are a result of internal control.

Type V—Morality of contract, of individual rights, and of accepted democratic law. People think in logical terms, valuing the will of society as a whole. These values are for the most part substantiated by obeying the law.

Type VI—Morality of individual principles of conscience. The individual does what he/she thinks is right as a result of his/her internalized values.

* Adapted from Kohlberg L: The child as a moral philosopher. Psychol Today 2:25, 1968

The development of the social world of the child is a complex process. Self-concept, bonding, attachment, social relationships with others, the understanding of social interactions—as well as the broader world of judgment and morality—all interact in order for the child to become socially competent.

Cultural Development

It is impossible to include all aspects and nuances of cultural influences in this overview of development. Instead, we will look beyond the primary attachments of mother and child to the family and the intricate network of relationships that form the child's ecological system or niche.

1. The family, with parental behavior, control, and emotional tone, has a most significant effect on the child's adaptive response. It appears that parents who are warm and affectionate foster in the child more secure attachments and peer relationships.[4]

2. Parents who are autocratic instead of authoritarian or permissive in expressing parental control tend to influence positive self-esteem and competence. This positive sense of self extends to school and to a variety of social situations.[3,46]

3. Parents who provide a rich nonhuman environment, enriched language, and developmentally appropriate play activities seem to have a closer relationship with their child. The child also tends to show more rapid growth in cognitive ability.[64]

There are myriad institutional and societal influences on a child's development. For example, the socioeconomic level influences family interaction, degree of stress tolerance, health, and availability of support systems to the family. Parents living in poverty tend to talk less frequently to children; they provide a less stimulating or age-appropriate learning environment. Poverty often causes the parent to be less available to the child. The parenting style appears to be more authoritarian and more physical in the approach to discipline.[3] A child from this lower economic situation also tends to do less well in school and to have lower IQ scores. Fewer students from poor families participate in higher education.

Research also points to the importance of a secure support system for parents. For example, Hetherington found that children of divorced parents tend to have closer and more secure relationships with the parent who had continued support from friends and family.[27] A social network takes time to cultivate, but the outcome for both child and parents seems positive.

Beyond family and social networks, the type and method of education have a major impact on the developing child. Attending school fosters information processing, but it is the qualities of the school and the teacher that affect the child's attitude toward school, academic achievement, and future educational pursuits. Effective schools and teachers are authoritative and they demonstrate excellent communication skills, shared goals, and high levels of control without strong punitive responses. They also emphasize academic importance and achievement.[50]

The play environment, television, and the types of aggressive activities engaged in also influence the effectiveness of the child's adaptation.

Throughout all the transitions of childhood, the child who experiences excitement, joy, pleasure, and mastery of developmental tasks shows positive adaptive behaviors. Parents also experience a feeling of self-satisfaction and delight in watching their children's development. The result can only be positive personal growth for child and parent.

Play in Child Development

As a child progresses from infant to adult, his/her major focus of activity evolves along a play-work continuum. At each developmental period, the balance between play and work shifts. For the preschool child, play is the central activity. The structure of the early school years teaches the child to balance work and play activities. As a child approaches adolescence, he/she becomes increasingly involved in structured and work-oriented activity. This work focus increases through the teen years. For adults, work and career development are balanced with either active or passive leisure time activities.

Over the years, educators and developmentalists have developed many definitions for the word *play*, but inherent in all of these definitions is the concept that play is an activity voluntarily engaged in for pleasure. This activity is significant because it assists the child to adapt within his/her environment or culture. A child's play develops through several stages from passive observation to cooperative, purposeful activity (see the box "Play Behavior").

Play Behavior*

Unoccupied Play Behavior. The child seems not to be playing but momentarily watches activity in the environment. When not attending, the child plays with his/her body, engages in gross motor behavior (*e.g.,* climbing up or down from chairs, following people around) or just sits looking around the room.

Onlooker Play. The child watches others play and engages in conversation with those playing. He/she definitely is observing the children rather than events, although he/she does not engage in actual play.

Solitary Independent Play. The child pursues play activities alone and independently from the other children playing. Although the child often positions himself close to others, he/she makes no reference to what they are doing.

Parallel Play. The child plays with toys similar to those used by other children near him/her but plays beside rather than with the children.

Associative Play. The child plays with others. There is no organization of play activities in his/her peer group, no division of labor, and no product. Each child acts individually; his/her interest focusing on the association rather than the play activity.

Cooperative or Organized Supplementary Play. The child plays with other children in an organized manner for a purpose (*e.g.,* making something, formal games). There is a marked sense of belonging to the group, which is now directed by one or two leaders. Each child finds some role in the new organization, his efforts augmented by the other members of the group.

* Adapted from Parten MB: Social play among preschool children. J Abnorm Soc Pyschol 27:243, 1932.

Functions of Play

Through play, the child learns to explore, develop, and master physical and social skills.

Social

During play, the young child tests family, adult, and gender roles at his/her own pace, free from the limits of the adult world. Play teaches a child to relate to others, first as an observer and later as a participant in cooperative and/or competitive and group endeavors. Play provides a means by which the child gains an insight into the mores of his/her culture. As the child comes to an understanding of what is "acceptable" and what is "not acceptable," the child begins to develop a sense of social morality.

Physical/Sensory/Perceptual

Children love to repeat activity. They will engage in seemingly endless repetition of both gross and fine motor skills for the pure joy of mastery. As his/her skills proliferate, a child can integrate more complex and coordinated activities. Sensory and motor activity teach the child the physical realities of the world as well as the capabilities and limitations of his/her own body. Play also provides a release for excess energy which restores body equilibrium, freeing the child for new endeavors. It heightens a child's perceptual ability: events or objects in the play environment allow the child to perceive forms and spatial and temporal relationships. He/she begins to classify objects and relate them to other objects, forming the basis for logical thought.

Emotional

Play allows the child to discover a sense of self, an internal stability. The child begins to trust the constancy and consistency of the environment. This trust forms the basis for ego identity. Play lets a child test the reality of inner and outer worlds. It enables him to express feelings without fear of punishment and, conversely, helps him learn to control his frustrations and impulses. This control provides the basis for ego strength, self-confidence, and potential adaptation to future needs. Play is fun—it opens to the child a world of joy, humor, and creativity.

Cognitive

Play activities are closely related to the child's level of cognitive development. Through play, the child learns to manipulate events and objects in the internal and external environment. This manipulation and combination of novel events lay the foundation for problem solving. Representational thought emerges as the child engages in symbolic and dramatic play; abstract thought has its basis in activities that allow for classification and problem-solving ability. The concrete experiences of play allow the child to make a more accurate assessment of the environment and his/her role in it.

Content and Structure of Play

To gain a real insight into a child's world, we must look intently at his/her play. The classifications that follow are descriptive rather than theoretical.

Elizabeth Hurlock delineates four general stages of play:

1. *The exploratory stage* (infant). Once control of the upper extremities is attained, the infant can more determinedly explore his body and the objects within his environment.
2. *The toy stage* (1 to 7–8 years). Constructive play begins at 3 years and culminates in the development of hobbies. During the school years, hobbies and collections serve as social and status agents.
3. *The play stage* (school years). In this period, which overlaps with Stages 2 and 4, the development of productive construction, games, and sports occurs.
4. *Adolescent play/work stage.* Preadolescent play and work activities become more complex. The young person begins to project future goals and activity plans into his/her creative endeavors. The elements of introspection and daydreaming reach a peak.[52]

Sara Smilansky[55] focuses only on dramatic play, defining four specific types:

1. *Functional play.* This includes all simple verbal and behavioral play and allows the child to explore the immediate environment.
2. *Constructive play.* At about 2 years of age, a child begins to demonstrate dramatic skill. "Making believe" in reality-oriented play helps the child make the link between his/her world and the adult world.
3. *Dramatic play.* The two main elements of dramatic play are imitation of an adult (the real world) and a "pretend" situation (the unreal world). The highest level of dramatic play is sociodramatic play, in which at least two children engage in play-acting activity, imitating the real speech and gestures of others in an imaginery situation.
4. *Games with rules.* This stage begins during the school years and culminates in adulthood.

Piaget identified the structure of play according to the cognitive complexity of activities[48] as follows (refer to the box "Summary of Piaget's Stages of Cognitive Development, p. 54 for listing of Sensorimotor substages):

Practice Games

Practice games include any activity that the child repeats for pure pleasure, such as pure sensorimotor practice and mental exercise.

These practice games appear in Piaget's Substage 2 of the sensorimotor period.

Symbolic Games

Symbolic games appear in Substage 6 of the sensorimotor period. Symbolic games are difficult to differentiate from practice games; the main difference is the introduction of make-believe.

Games With Rules

As the child grows and interacts with peers, sensorimotor and symbolic games become "games with rules." These games require mental organization and operations.

Constructional Games

This fourth category is identified by Piaget, although he specifies that it does not occupy its own space. Constructional games are found in all three structural types, but they occupy space "half-way between play and intelligent work, or between play and imitation."[48]

Theories of Play

Erikson

I Med D

Erikson discusses play as a sequential unfolding of psychosocial relationships.[52]

Stage 1 — the Auto-Cosmic Stage. From birth to 15 months, the child focuses on his own body. During the first phase of this stage, the self is the center of exploration. Kinesthetic sensations and sensual perceptions are repeated. In the second phase, the child starts to explore other people or objects. Although the focus of his/her actions is still sensual pleasure, the actions may now be directed to cause and effect (for example, crying for attention).

Stage 2 — the Microcosmic Stage. From 15 months to 3 years, the child uses small toys and objects to play out themes, and he begins to master the environment.

Stage 3 — the Macrosphere Stage. From nursery school to 7 years, the child's play revolves around other children. This interaction begins with minimal communication. Initially, a child may view other children as objects, but as his experiences increase, the child learns to participate in cooperative role taking.

Stage 4 — Industry versus Inferiority. From 7 years to preadolescence, the school-age child learns the skills and tools of his/her culture. Mastery of tasks and the development of competency are intrinsic rewards.

Stage 5 — Identity versus Role Confusion. During the adolescent years, the focus of play and activities is role identification. Work-oriented tasks play a major role in the child's life situation.[52]

Anna Freud

To Anna Freud, the ability to work is related to the pleasure of achievement, which has a basis in early play activity. A person's ability to work is related to his/her ego development and ability to (1) control and modify impulses, (2) delay gratification, (3) carry out preconceived plans even when frustration intervenes, (4) neutralize energies of instinctual drives through sublimated pleasures, and (5) be governed by a reality principle rather than a pleasure principle.[21]

Jean Piaget

Piaget believed that activity or play may be an end product for a child. What is play at one stage may be work at another. Once the child learns an activity, it is repeated for the sheer joy of mastery. Piaget defined play as pure assimilation — the repetition of a behavior or a scheme solely for the pleasure of conquering a skill.[49] He believed that the types and evolution of play activities a child chooses reflect the child's level of cognitive development. To Piaget, play and cognitive development are parallel and interdependent. Play fosters the child's ability to master and to become competent within his/her world.

Reilly

Reilly believes that in play, children require rules that give meaning to the environment.[9] The three phases of play behavior that follow facilitate imagination, curiosity, and need fulfillment:

1. Exploratory behavior: The child's attempt to test reality; satisfy his/her basic needs; and search for the meaning of movements, objects, and people within his/her environment.
2. Competency behavior: Environmental feedback and developmental sequences that facilitate acquisition of competence. The child learns to adapt behavior in order to develop a sense of mastery and self-confidence.
3. Achievement behavior: Guided by societal standards, this behavior facilitates risk-taking ability and the development of a sense of competition.

Reilly believes that through play, the child acquires a variety of role behaviors and masters many skills. The play behavior of the child is an antecedent of adult competence.

Role of Play in the Occupational Therapy Process

Play is the "occupational" performance of childhood and thus is the medium of intervention in the pediatric occupational therapy process. The occupational therapist must understand the developmental sequences of play in order to facilitate appropriate play behavior. Observational skills, a play history, knowledge of developmental sequences, and activity analysis provide a baseline for pediatric assessment. Play serves as the main modality to facilitate change in the developmental level(s) of children. Roles and adaptive behaviors can be learned through the play process. The total life experiences of self care, family, school performance, and social interaction can be enhanced by use of play in the treatment process. The occupational therapist adapts play activities to facilitate appropriate developmental sequences.

Takata[59] and Florey[18] provided a taxonomy and classification of play which forms a basis for establishing play history and developmental sequences of play behaviors. These schema provide a basis for organizing and assessing play behavior.

Adolescence

Adolescence is derived from a Latin word meaning *to come to maturity*. It begins at pubescence, a period of about 2 years prior to the onset of puberty. Pubescence is a time of physiological changes: a growth spurt, a synchronous growth of body systems, and increased hormonal activity which triggers the emergence of primary and secondary sex characteristics. Pubescence culminates at puberty, when sexual maturity and reproductive capacity are complete.

It is not as easy to determine when adolescence ends and adulthood begins. This depends on a combination of physical, emotional, social, legal, and cultural determinants.

Theories of Adolescent Behavior

At present, there is no single unified or comprehensive theory of adolescent behavior. Many theorists view adolescence from a specific aspect(s) of the developmental continuum. Table 4-5 summarizes the theoretical orientations.

Developmental Stages

Physical Development

Bodily growth and sexual maturation are gradual processes brought about by androgens, estrogens, and other hormones. The first sign of puberty in girls is the appearance of "breast buds" (age 8–13 years). Puberty is completed within 3 years. Menarche (10–16½ years) occurs at the end of this time after the peak of height spurt. Puberty in boys starts approximately two years later than girls. Pubic hair appears between 10 and 15 years; penis growth starts between 11 and 14½, with ejaculation taking place a year after accelerated penis growth.

In addition to primary and secondary sex characteristics, other changes include:
1. Lungs and heart increase in size. The heart rate drops. This change is more pronounced in boys than in girls.

2. Boys experience greater growth in muscle and muscle mass in relation to body weight; girls have an increased ratio of fat tissue to body weight.
3. Facial structures begin to take on adult features.
4. Sex differences in the shape and proportions of the trunk become obvious.
5. Sex differences in strength (boys greater than girls) appear that seem to be related to the increase in muscle size, skeletal growth, body weight and neural organization.[38,61,62]
6. Motor coordination shows little sex difference until approximately age 14. Boys continue to develop coordination after 14 years, whereas girls do not demonstrate marked changes after this age.[40]
7. Some body organs and structures do not change appreciably during adolescence. For example, the brain reaches 95% of adult size and weight by age 10.[61]

There is evidence that puberty is beginning earlier. This change is thought to be a result of better nutrition and a decrease in diseases. Another interesting hypothesis is the stimulation and stress factor theory which states that such factors as stimulation, noise, crowding, and artificial light may effect these changes.[1]

Sensory and Perceptual Development

The sensory and perceptual capabilities of the adolescent are negligible in contrast to his/her physical and cognitive changes. The perceptual world of the adolescent is enhanced by its interrelationship with expanding cognitive skill.

I read

Cognitive Development

Adolescence ushers in changes in cognitive processes. Piaget's period of formal operations emerges. Inhelder and Piaget characterize the adolescent's formal operational thought process as follows:
1. The capability of dealing logically with many factors at once.
2. The ability to utilize a secondary system, for example, trigonometry. This ability to manipulate symbols makes the adolescent's thought processes more flexible. He/she is now able to introspect and reflect on his/her own mental capacities.
3. The ability to construct ideal or contrary-to-fact situations.
4. The ability to deal with the possible as well as the real.[30]

One of the significant outcomes of formal operational thought is that the adolescent is freed from the

Table 4-5. Theories of Adolescence

Theorist	Theory and Hypothesis	Assumption(s)	View of Adolescence
C. Darwin	Evolutionary–Laws of nature uniform throughout time	Natural selection, species variability adaptation	Maturation is result of adaptation; sexual behavior is influenced by learning
S. Hall	Evolutionary–Theory of recapitulation of development	Simultaneous evolution of developmental aspects of adolescence with particular emphasis on biological factor	Two distinct periods of adolescence (early, late) usually characterized by storm/stress. Adolescence is period of potential personal and societal changes
A. Gesell	Maturational–Development is natural biological unfolding	Predictable sequences and cycles of development (ages and stages)	Adolescence is transition toward maturity. There are specific descriptions of aspects of development during years 10–16
R. Havighurst	Normative–Human behavior is learning	Each stage of development has specific learned tasks and there are teachable moments or sensitive periods for learning these tasks	The adolescent years (12–18) focus on eight developmental tasks: 1. Achieving new and mature relations with agemates of both sexes 2. Achieving appropriate sex-role development 3. Accepting one's physical development and using the body effectively 4. Emotional independence from primary caretakers 5. Preparing for marriage and family life 6. Career development 7. Value acquisition and development of personal ideology 8. Developing and achieving socially responsible behavior
S. Freud	Psychoanalytic–Fundamental biological instincts; focus is on gratification of basic instincts in psychosexual stages of development	The unconscious; shifting sexual energy from the mouth to the anus to the genital area; id, ego, and superego as the three basic mental functions. Defense mechanisms, which protect ego from unacceptable wishes	Final stage of personality development in pre-adolescence; puberty results in reemergence of infantile themes, especially Oedipal or Electra conflicts; patterns of impulse expression, defensive style, and sublimation crystallize into a life orientation; the genital stage
A. Freud	Same as S. Freud	Same as S. Freud	Time of increased libidinal energy associated with biological maturation; ego is in danger of being overwhelmed by instinct; emphasizes asceticism and intellectuality as two powerful adolescent defenses

(continued)

Table 4-5.   *(continued)*

Theorist	*Theory and Hypothesis*	*Assumption(s)*	*View of Adolescence*
P. Blos	Same as Freud	Adolescence is psychological adaptation to biological maturation; the coping system	Three phases of adolescence: (1) early—the onset of puberty; (2) adolescence proper—autonomy from earlier objects of cathexis; (3) late—development of judgment, interests, and intellect; sexual identity established; consolidation of personal identity
E. Erikson	Neofreudian—Focus on conscious self (ego development); psychosocial stages; social and cultural influences affect behavior	Eight stages of psychosocial development from infancy throughout adult life, with a psychosocial crisis or bipolar situation to be resolved during each stage. Developmental periods are defined partly by maturation	Identity *versus* role diffusion or confusion; adolescent reexamines identity and roles (sexual and occupational identities); resolution of crisis or task results ideally in reintegrated sense of self
H.S. Sullivan	Psychoanalytic/Social Psychology—All people exist in an interpersonal field with specific determinants of its own	Three kinds of experience: (1) sensations, perceptions, and emotions experienced before language; (2) private symbols, including fantasies and daydreams; (3) shared symbols. Dymanisms—patterns of interaction	Three phases of adolescence: (1) preadolescence—need for a close relationship with another person of the same sex; (2) early—interest in heterosexual relationships, conflict between needs for intimacy and needs for sexual gratification; (3) late—establishment of mature repertoire of interpersonal relationships, emergence of self-respect (Also see Table 4-2)
J. Piaget	Cognitive/developmental—Knowledge is based on action; structural properties of human brain, sense receptors, and nervous system provide universal bases for human cognition	Scheme: adaptation, which consists of assimilation and accommodation; stages of development: sensorimotor, preoperational, concrete operations, formal operations	Adult reasoning achieved during adolescence; thought governed by principles of logic; hypothesis raising and testing; simultaneous manipulation of more than two variables; consequences of actions anticipated; logical inconsistencies recognized; future computeralized
L. Kohlberg	Cognitive/developmental—Moral reasoning is reflection of level of cognitive development	Levels of moral reasoning: preconventional (ages 4–10); conventional (ages 10–16); postconventional (ages 16 on)	Period during which personal morality emerges; transition between conventional and postconventional levels may bring doubt, personal reflection, and confusion; period when new moral code or moral philosophy can emerge
K. Lewin	Social psychology—All behavior must be understood in context of field in which it occurs; every psychological concept can be expressed by a mathematical formula	Behavior is function of life space, which includes person and all facts or events in environment of which person is aware; person has a perceptual–motor region and an interpersonal	Adolescent as "marginal man" straddling of boundary between childhood and adulthood unstable; Greater uncertainty about regions of environment and about

(continued)

Table 4-5. (continued)

Theorist	Theory and Hypothesis	Assumption(s)	View of Adolescence
		region; environment is divided into regions that represent settings, relationships, and barriers to access	interpersonal and perceptual–motor regions
D. Ausubel	Integrated psychology of adolescence – Adolescence is distinct developmental phase with changes that are biological and social in origin	Adolescence is period of reorganization; biosocial changes are evident and discontinuous; changes are cross-cultural	Uniform elements of common psychological reactions, sexual maturation, sex roles combined with personality traits, changed states, and emerging adult roles
M. Mead and R. Benedict	Cultural anthropology	Degree of continuity between child and adult roles is central focus in cultural impact on personality development (Benedict). Relation between biological and cultural determinants studied by Mead; was known as cultural determinants, which implied that culture was dominant factor in personality development	Gave cross-cultural perspective on adolescent behavior. Delineated operations of biology and culture in adolescent development and gave increased insight into our own and other cultures.
U. Brofenbrenner	Ecological theory – Child develops within context of ecological systems	There is hierarchy of ecological microsystems mesosystems, and exosystems overarched by macrosystem; these systems affect child's development and manner in which child perceives and deals with his/her environment; basis units of analysis are dyad, triad, etc.	Adolescent is seen individually in context of systems in which he/she is involved

Adapted from Bee H: *The Developing Child,* pp 330–339. New York, Harper & Row, 1985; Bronfenbrenner U, Crouter AC: The evolution of environmental models in developmental research. In Mussen P (ed): *Handbook of Child Psychology,* 4th ed, Vol 1, *History, Theory and Methods.* New York, John Wiley & Sons, 1983; Davis I: *Adolescence: Theoretical and Helping Perspectives,* pp 25–40. Boston, Kluwer & Nijhoff, 1985; Lloyd M: *Adolescence,* pp 9–26. New York, Harper & Row, 1985.

cognitive limitations of the present. He/she now has a view of what is possible, of the future. This mode of thought is linked to the idealism of youth.

Social Cognition

Social cognition is the development of observations, information, and conceptualizations about our own and others' social roles and about relationships, thoughts, feelings, intentions, and moral or religious judgments. The adolescent's ability to make moral judgments seems to be related to his/her ability to see another's point of view and to relate it to him/herself. Flavell and Ailman's view of social cognition parallels the adolescent's ability to reach formal operational thought.[16]

Adolescent Egocentricism

The concept of egocentricism is of special interest because it seems to be an important link between personality dynamics and cognitive processes. The freedom and flexibility of thought that come with formal operations can also cause the adolescent to be overly conscious of his/her thoughts, appearance, and feelings. He/she realizes that other people have their own thoughts and perceptions, but the adolescents' self-preoccupation persuades him/her that their thoughts are focused on him/her. Elkind[14] describes manifestations of this egocentrism as follows:

1. *Imaginary audience.* The adolescent is constructing or reacting to an imagined audience. For example, when the student catches the eye of the teacher he

wonders what the teacher is thinking about him at that moment.

2. *Personal fable.* The adolescent imagines that because so many people are interested in him/her, then he/she must be very special. For example, the adolescent knows that "no one ever has felt the way I do."

3. *Pseudostupidity.* The adolescent tends to interpret situations at a more complex level than is warranted. The obvious tends to elude him. For example, he may look for a lost sock, shoe, or book in the places he is least likely to find it.

Emotional Development

Emotional responses are particularly significant in adolescence. Childhood feelings, coupled with new life experiences, affect personality and emotional development. Hormonal changes that accompany physical maturation cause frequent emotional lability. Cognitive changes allow for personal introspection and enable the young person to think about himself/herself in a more abstract manner. The focus of thought shifts inward. The adolescent is concerned with his/her own feelings as he/she responds to others and to his/her expanding world. This emotional awakening affects the evolving self-image and esteem of the adolescent. The teen must also adapt to new role behaviors and expectations within his/her environment. These changes often evoke strong emotional responses.

Concept of Self

Changes in self-concept are a reflection not only of physical and cognitive maturation but also of the search for a new understanding of self. Self-esteem (or how one perceives how others see him/her) is rooted in early family interactions. Self-esteem tends to increase from youth through late adolescence.

Sex Roles

Sex-role concepts are formed in early childhood. The adolescent's view of sexual identity depends a great deal on the kinds of models encountered. During adolescence, the young person's self concept becomes more abstract and less dependent on external physical qualities. By late adolescence, the self concept undergoes a kind of reorganization. The result is a new and future-oriented personal and ideological identity.

Social Development

Peer relationships in adolescence are an essential part of the transition from dependent child to independent adult. Interaction with equals allows the teen to practice aspects of relationships that are critical to later role development. The influence of the group seems to peak in the early adolescent years (12–14) and declines in later adolescence.[6]

The structure of groups changes in adolescence. Early cliques or small cohesive groups evolve into larger crowds made up of several cliques. At 13 to 15 years, the young person begins to try out new heterosexual skills in the protected environment of the crowd. Once feelings of self confidence develop, heterosexual pair relationships begin. Individual friendships take on importance in the adolescent years. With his/her increased cognitive skill, the teen is able to understand more fully the viewpoints and feelings of others. This ability fosters more intimate sharing of feelings between friends. The development of close friendships evolves through adolescence, and, as Erikson suggests, peaks in the early adult years.

Family relationships in early adolescence are more complex than friendships. The teen now understands and desires the concept of a more intimate relationship based on mutual tolerance.[53] However, he/she is also keenly aware of the fact that adults possess more power. Conflict is a natural consequence of these polarized concepts. This cycle of intimacy, interdependence, and autonomy causes fluctuations and continued struggle between the family and child throughout the life cycle.[53]

Cultural Development

Developmental psychologists have been struggling with the question: "Is adolescence a culture unto itself or just a subculture within society?" The evidence suggests that it is a subculture. There seems to be only a broad transmission of values and traditions from one generation of teens to another; for instance, dress customs, behaviors, and mutual leisure activities provide a superficial "shared culture." But the behavior of teens does not consistently influence their adult life. The peer subculture appears, instead, to be a vehicle for transition into the adult world.

Issues in Adolescence

Need for and Development of Independence

The adolescent's need for and development of independence is often manifested in parent–child conflict. Elkind interprets this conflict as a function of the age of the adolescent and the maturity of the parent.[14] He states that conflicts arise as a result of three kinds of arrangements: bargains, agreements, and contracts.

For Elkind, the parent-adolescent conflict is a stage

in the process of self-differentiation. He hypothesizes that each arrangement has three complementary "invariant clauses" whose content varies with age level:

Responsibility–freedom. The parent demands that the adolescent fulfill certain social responsibilities in return for complementary freedoms. The content of this clause changes with age.

Achievement–support. This clause functions in the development of a sense of competence: in the adolescent's ability to meet social and academic standards and in the parent's ability to instruct, supervise, and reinforce his/her accomplishments.

Loyalty–commitment. This clause is closely related to the development of a value system. The parent expects the adolescent to give primary allegiance to the family, and the young person expects the parent to support him/her and make a commitment to his/her values and beliefs.

Group interactions and peer relationships provide the transient feedback necessary for the adolescent's development of social independence and self-worth. Peer interaction teaches the adolescent the norms of society, as well as how to contribute to and establish group goals. In peer relationships he/she tests and begins to understand various social roles while reinforcing his/her own identity.

Awakening of Sexuality— Need for and Development of Intimacy

Physical changes in the young adolescent force him/her to face or identify his concept of sexuality and body image. Sexuality is the totality of the individual's attitudes, values, goals, and behaviors (both internal and external) based on, or determined by, his/her perception of his/her gender.

Sexual awareness begins in and develops from early childhood. But adolescence brings a heightened, often acute, awareness of gender difference, erotic sensations, sexual relationships, potential adult roles, and the need for intimacy.

Though there is no significant intellectual difference between a male and female adolescent, there are cultural and social pressures which may influence his/her self-concept.[52]

Emotionally, adolescents must attempt to come to terms with both their ideal and their real selves. They are forced to evaluate their masculine/feminine roles, reviewing their gender identity, orientation, and gender preference.

As the young person resolves the issues of the adolescent period, a feeling of well-being and self-identity emerges. This process of identity formation does not evolve smoothly for all adolescents. If the crisis is not resolved, role diffusion results. The young person is unable to respond to the demands of various role expectations. The youth beset by role diffusion wanders from one goal to another. Instead of constructive experimentation with options, this adolescent makes aimless and vague attempts at problem solving.

In a predominantly peer environment, charged with sexual curiosity, adolescents confront two major types of relationships: homosexual and heterosexual. Evidence suggests that a homosexual relationship is not uncommon in adolescence. Possibly this stems from the adolescent's sexual insecurity—the need to compare himself/herself with someone nonthreatening and sexually similar. The encounter, conducted in a "safe" and comfortable environment, may be his/her first extrafamilial attachment. The development of a meaningful heterosexual relationship is based on both physical and psychosocial intimacy. In order to develop true intimacy, the adolescent must be aware of his/her abilities and be able to share himself/herself with others. It is critical that his/her internal identity be secure in order to prevent identity diffusion and stress on his/her sexuality.

Development of a Philosophy of Life, a Value System, and a Humanistic Attitude

According to Piaget, the adolescent (12+ years) develops a "morality of reciprocity." When a child reaches formal operational thought, he/she is able to engage in the abstract thinking and introspection which help him/her to develop an internally monitored value system. The adolescent's ability to interpret and internalize rules enables him/her to "discover the boundaries that separate his self from the other person, but (he) will learn to understand the other person and be understood by him."[47] Through this process the adolescent begins to develop an empathetic attitude toward others.

Many factors influence the development of an ideology—parents, peers, significant others, religious training, and cultural and social background. Some theorists speculate that from the time of adolescence the person is dealing with the "child of the past"; that each early experience in the child's social life and culture directly and indirectly affect his/her development of a philosophy of life. This philosophy comes about, finally, as a result of the interaction between the individual's society and culture and his/her internal learned responses.

Consistency of attitude is the most valuable commodity a parent can transmit to a child in order to help him/her form an intact value system. High self-esteem, internalization of expectations, and self-discipline are linked with parental style and are crucial for the formation of adult moral standards.[5,10]

Peers and significant others (family members, teachers, friends) provide an avenue by which the adolescent can identify and test his/her capabilities and ideas. Through testing, he/she will eventually crystallize his/her self-image and value system. Religious training and experience add another dimension to the young person's ability to internalize and reinforce value systems. Religious exposure seems to be most effective when both parents follow similar standards and reinforce their value system.

Different cultures produce different value orientations. There are differences in values both within a culture and between cultures. The expectations of the individual are determined by the way people in a given culture view life roles. Some of the issues around which individual roles are determined include:

1. Responsibility *versus* nonresponsibility
2. Authority figures *versus* nonauthority figures
3. Dominance *versus* submission

Development of a Career Choice

From approximately 15 through 65 years of age, work occupies a large part of a person's life. The vocational decisions an adolescent makes affect his/her future social relationships, leisure-time activities, material gains, and marital and child-rearing attitudes.

Major influences on career choice include ability, gender, community (rural vs. urban), parental occupation, expectations, and occupational attractiveness.

Planning for work is difficult for a young person, whose aspirations tend to be more idealistic than realistic. With increased maturity, the adolescent gains a more realistic view of career choice and his/her abilities and needs.

One might surmise that minority students, who sometimes encounter stiff barriers and resistance as they move toward status roles, would tend to lower their career expectations. However, studies have proven that the opposite is true.[11,34] This increase in vocational aspiration may reflect three attitudes: (1) their efforts to conform to the American cultural emphasis on occupational success and status; (2) their substitution of future projections for their inability to move ahead in a success-oriented society; or (3) their exaggerated perception of the new horizons open to minority groups.

Gender also plays an important role in career decisions. In the last few years, the feminist movement has had a strong impact on society's view of women's career options. Introduced early in the socialization process, these new attitudes toward female career possibilities can extend a girl's job scope. Even a girl with traditional expectations should take the time to explore her real career potential.

Brief summaries of three theories concerning career choice and development are discussed below.

Self-Concept Theory (Super)

Super states that as a person grows, he/she must integrate self-images into a self-concept that prevails in all daily activities, including his/her job. Occupational experiences culminate in work roles and career patterns that are consistent with the maturation of self-concept. Super identifies five vocational developmental tasks:

1. *Crystallization of vocational preference (14–18 years).* As their self-concept matures, adolescents develop ideas about work, and they begin to make educational decisions based on these ideas.
2. *Specification of vocational program (18–21 years).* Detailed vocational plans are set forth.
3. *Implementation of vocational preferences (21–24 years).* The young adult has completed his/her initial training phase and has secured a job.
4. *Stabilization of career (25–35 years).* The individual enhances his/her talents, narrows his/her field of interest, and finds personal satisfaction in work.
5. *Consolidation of career role (35 upward).* The person develops expertise, strengthens his/her skills, and acquires status.[58]

This developmental theory is valid only in that there is a progression of vocational tasks. The age range varies with socioeconomic conditions.

Cognitive Social Theory (Ginsberg)

Ginsberg believes that vocational choice is related to a developmental process of decision making. A person makes continuous choices "between career preparation and goals and the reality of the world of work."[22] This process is open-ended and is continuous throughout life; it is not confined to the adolescent and young adult.

Life-Style Orientation (Holland)

Holland focuses on the relationship between personality characteristics and vocational choice (a trait-factor theory). He believes that job choice is a reflection of personality—that a person chooses work environments that foster his/her personal orientation.

Adulthood

Developmental progression reaches its height in adulthood. As the individual grows beyond childhood, he/she refines his/her self-image, develops sexual and psychosocial intimacy, becomes productive and effective in the world of work and family, and finally reaches an integrity and a sense of fulfillment which affirms life as a meaningful adventure.

The complexity of the modern world, society, and culture inhibit the smooth resolution of many issues of adulthood.

Issues in Young Adulthood

Psychological Issues

Our society designates young adulthood (the ages between 20 and 40) as prime time—when life is most satisfying and rewarding. Those persons considered "happiest" by others are the middle-aged! Cameron concludes that happiness is not determined by, or closely related to, age as such; it is relatively constant across the life span. In another study, Lowenthal also concludes that neither age nor life stage is relevant in measuring life satisfaction, although the sense of well-being is different for men than for women. Women tend to express more complex stages of feelings. The "happiest" women in the study are those who have both positive and negative experiences, especially in the recent past; the "happiest" men relate only positive experiences in the recent past.[39]

Erikson believed that young adults are involved in working toward the development of intimacy with others as opposed to isolation from them. This intimacy includes a sense of commitment to concrete affiliations and partnerships, the ability to abide by such commitments, and the experience of cooperating and sharing with others even when this necessitates sacrifice and compromise.[32] A person who is unable to develop a sense of intimacy lives in a world apart, absorbed by himself/herself.

Stress is one factor that does seem relative to age and stage in adult life. Young newlyweds, for example, reported 2½ times the number of stressful situations than did middle-aged and older adults, though the type of stress encountered varies with sex. For men, stress is usually related to occupation; for women, it stems more often from health issues (their own and others) and interpersonal conflicts. Middle-aged and older adults seem to experience less stress than the young.

Physical Issues

In early adulthood most of the growth processes have run their course. But the body never remains static: the bright-eyed and sharp-eared young adult is already undergoing decremental changes in vision and hearing. The earliest change is in visual accommodation ability, which peaks in grade school and begins to decline even before a person's "prime." Other aspects of vision tend to remain unchanged.

The ability to hear high-frequency sounds begins to diminish in adolescence, whereas pitch discrimination (high tones) begins to decline in the midtwenties. These slight negative changes in early adulthood usually have little or no effect on the daily functioning of the young adult.

Cognitive Issues

Intellectual development peaks in the early adult years. Catell proposes two levels of mental ability: fluid and crystallized intelligence. *Fluid intelligence* refers to capabilities such as associative memory, inductive reasoning, and figural relationships. *Crystallized intelligence* refers to skills such as verbal comprehension and the handling of word relationships. The former skills are closely aligned to innate intellect; the latter are more dependent on learning and experience. Horn presented evidence that suggests that fluid intelligence may diminish slightly following adolescence, whereas crystallized intelligence increases with age.[28]

Creativity seems to peak in the early thirties. In a historical study of thousands of creative men and women, Lehman found that the peak years of most people's creative ventures have been in their thirties. For example, the mean years for symphony writing were 30–34 years of age. Dennis found that creative persons usually continue to produce creative endeavors throughout their lives.[13]

In Piaget's description of cognitive development, formal operational thought is acquired unevenly during adolescence and early adulthood. The ability to use interpropositional thought, combinational analysis, and hypothetical deductive reasoning are a result of innate intelligence, education, and life experiences. Some adults never attain formal operational thought. When this level of cognitive development is reached in early adulthood, the young adult relies heavily on it in all areas of life.[48]

Vocational and Life Goal Issues

Career choice remains a paramount issue in the twenties. A high school graduate usually experiments with several jobs before settling into stable employment. Those young persons who choose careers that require further education tend to remain on the job longer and feel more secure in their commitment.

Most employment in our culture involves some level of on-the-job training. The process of establishing a career involves the development of job skills and interpersonal working relationships between employer and other employees. Job changes are most frequent during the early adult years, the average duration of employment for the young adult is two years.

Life-Style Issues

As the young person enters adulthood, he/she usually leaves his/her family of origin and establishes a new nuclear family.

Blood suggests five prerequisites for a successful marriage: compatibility, skill, effort, commitment, and support.[7] Folkman and Clatworthy add two more characteristics: flexibility and love.[19] Americans tend to choose mates with similar backgrounds. Studies indicate that race is the most critical factor in this choice, followed by social class, educational group, religious affiliation, and ethnic origin.[52]

Alternatives to marriage began to emerge in the 1960s and 1970s. More permissive sexual attitudes and greater social acceptance together with the advent of the feminist movement brought about an increase in the practice of cohabitation. In many ways, "live-in" relationships appear to be similar to marriage. However, the marriage license seems to have a subtle psychological effect on such a commitment.

Many individuals are choosing single life as an alternative to marriage. A primary reason is career development. Single persons have the advantage of freedom in decision making, though they often spend a large amount of time seeking companions and nurturing relationships.[52]

Other types of relationships, including homosexual bonding, communal living, and being a "swinging single," exist as alternatives to traditional life styles. Choosing the direction of one's personal life pattern is a major decision of early adulthood.

Another major issue in the young adult's life is parenthood. Both cultural and personal influences affect this decision. The reasons for choosing parenthood are as varied as the couples involved in the choice. Children may be viewed as another outlet for one's creativity, as an opportunity to fulfill a life goal, or as another opportunity to share oneself with others. A growing number of young couples are opting not to become parents. Some reasons cited include complete fulfillment with a mate, career development, and socioeconomic factors. Maternal instinct is a myth: not all women experience loving and protective feelings toward children. Yarrow *et al* found that women who have good self-concepts and who enjoy their roles in life are more likely to be good mothers than are those who are dissatisfied with what they are doing.[20] Children can be enriching and exciting additions to the young adult's life when he/she is ready for the responsibility of rearing them.

Social Issues

During adolescence, a person uses the peer group as a sounding board for developing a self-concept. Once this concept becomes stable, the young adult usually develops a few meaningful relationships—friends who usually have parallel interests and who compliment his/her uniqueness and need system.

When the young adult leaves home, the relationship with his/her family of origin may either weaken or grow stronger. The direction this relationship takes strongly depends on his/her ability to understand and react to other value systems and life styles.

Many young adults today have a variety of options available that were not available to their parents and grandparents—more vocational opportunities, more leisure time, and many more life choice possibilities.

Today's young adults are conscious of the need for a balance in the work–play continuum, and they establish meaningful life goals that balance their physical and psychosocial needs.

Issues in Mid Adulthood

Physical Issues

There are vast differences among people in mid-adulthood (the ages between 40 and 60) in terms of physical changes. After a person is 40 years of age, physiological changes occur in all body systems, but the extent of their manifestation depends a great deal on individual genetic and environmental influences.

Menopause refers to all the physiological changes that occur when a woman's monthly menstrual function ceases. The female reproductive system changes with advancing age, and childbearing usually ceases during the late thirties or forties. American women reach menopause at approximately 40 to 54 years of age.[20] As the levels of estrogen decrease, some women experience vasomotor and other physical changes. The psychological changes associated with menopause are often exaggerated.

There is a great deal of debate about whether men undergo a parallel experience (the male climateric). Most social scientists believe that men do experience a transition. The time of onset is variable, and the period may be accompanied by both physical and psychological changes.

Cognitive Issues

As mentioned previously, fluid intelligence may diminish gradually from middle to later years, whereas crystallized intelligence may increase. Cross-sectional studies comparing people of different ages show generational differences in intelligence. Recent generations tend to be taller, heavier, stronger, and more intelligent.[52] This generational shift is known as the secular trend. Other studies indicate that intellectual ability peaks during the middle years and then remains stable throughout this period and into the beginning of old age.[52]

Psychological Issues

Erikson sees midlife as a crisis of *generativity versus stagnation.* Unless a person continues to grow and change, he/she stagnates and regresses emotionally. This growth is evidenced in his/her creativity, interest in others, and concern with the next generation. Generativity is fostered through positive reciprocal contacts with the younger generation.

Social Issues

Certain social issues are paramount during middle age. Havighurst identifies seven developmental tasks with this period:
1. Achieving adult civic and social responsibility
2. Establishing and maintaining an economic standard of living
3. Assisting young people to become responsible adults
4. Developing leisure time activities
5. Relating to one's spouse as a person
6. Accepting the physiological changes of middle age
7. Adjusting to aging parents[26]

Levinson and Gould find significant differences between the developmental adjustments of the forties and the fifties: whereas the forties are often years of unrest, toward 50, adults settle down again.[36]

During his/her forties, a person may experience many transitions. Parents who are undergoing physiological and psychological changes themselves may be confronted by children in the throes of adolescent conflict. Reaching a psychological half-way point sets off reflection on past achievements and concern for future goals. The stress of this midlife transition can be an impetus for developmental growth and change, or it can cause a crisis of discontent.

Midlife is often a time when people redefine relationships with parents. Researchers indicate that the middle-aged adult seems to become more empathetic and sympathetic toward his aging parents. He/she begins to feel that he/she understands his/her parents' life situation. But when aging parents become physically or economically dependent on their children, problems may arise.

For women, midlife may be the beginning of a second career, an exciting renewal. For men, midlife is often the time of highest financial security. Their career power and prestige is usually at a peak. Men seldom make radical shifts or impulsive moves at this stage. Generally, they remain in the same job until retirement. Usually, the years between 50 and 65 are the most satisfying of a man's career.

Leisure activities expand during midlife. It is common for adults to pursue activities that they had established early in their adult lives. Neugarten notes an interesting change in the concept of leisure in America. A hundred years ago, the higher one's education and income, the more leisure one had. Now, the best educated and most skilled professionals put in 60- to 80-hour work weeks, and it is the blue collar workers who have the most leisure time.[45]

The postparental period for some couples is a time to enjoy the fruits of the hard work of earlier years. These couples find a new pleasure in marriage and a new intensity in their relationship.[31] But while marital happiness increases for some, it evaporates for others. Some couples seek divorce soon after their children leave home, though they have long since lost contact with each other.

When children leave home, one or both parents may experience the empty-nest phenomenon—a feeling of loss. This syndrome usually coincides with the marriage (or a comparable declaration of independence) of the last child at home. The crisis is usually resolved through expanding nurturing experiences (parents, pets, etc.). But the "empty nest" can lead, eventually, to sexual problems or divorce.

As their children establish new nuclear families, parents take on new roles as grandparents and in-laws. These new roles bring to midlife another potential for satisfaction and happiness or for frustration and despair.

The middle years do more than reflect the accomplishments of earlier years. They are characterized by development and change. The physical and psychological crises which occur hold out tremendous potential for growth. Middle age rings with productivity, generativity, and a high satisfaction with life.

References

1. Adams JF: Earlier menarche, greater height and weight: A stimulation stress factor hypothesis. Genet Psychol Monogr 104:3, 1981
2. Ainsworth M: Attachment: Retrospect and prospect. In Parkes CM, Stevenson–Hind M (eds): The Place of Attachment in Human Behavior. New York, Basic Books, 1982
3. Baumrind D: The development of instrumental competence through socialization. In Pick AD (ed): Minnesota Symposium on Child Psychology, Vol 7. Minneapolis, University of Minnesota Press, 1973

4. Bee H: The Developing Child, 4th ed, pp 119, 124, 228, 240, 320, 340, 372, 446, 465–470. New York, Harper & Row, 1985

5. Berkowitz L: The Development of Motives and Values in the Child. New York, Basic Books, 1964

6. Berndt T: Developmental changes in conformity to peers and family. Dev Psychol 15:658, 1979

7. Blood RO: Marriage, 3rd ed, p 40. New York, Free Press, 1978

8. Caron AJ, Caron RF: Cognitive development in early infancy. In Field TM, (ed): Review of Human Development. New York, John Wiley & Sons, 1982

9. Clark P, Allen A: Occupational Therapy for Children, p 38. St Louis, CV Mosby, 1985

10. Coppersmith S: The Antecedents of Self Esteem. San Francisco, Freeman, 1967

11. Cosby A: Occupational expectations and the hypothesis of increasing realism of choice. J Voc Behav 5:53, 1974

12. Damon W, Hart D: The development of self understanding from infancy through adolescence. Child Dev 53:841, 1982

13. Dennis W: Creative productivity between the ages of twenty and eighty years. J Gerontol 21:1, 1966

14. Elkind D: Egocentrism in adolescence. Child Dev 38:1025, 1967

15. Fantz RI, Fagan JF III: Visual attention to size and number of pattern details by term and preterm infants during the first six months. Child Dev 46:3, 1975

16. Flavell JH: Cognitive Development. Englewood Cliffs, NJ, Prentice–Hall, 1977

17. Flavell JH: Structures, stages and sequences in cognitive development. In Collins WA (ed): The Concept of Development. Minnesota Symposium in Child Psychology, Vol 15. Hillsdale, NJ, Erlbaum, 1982

18. Florey L: An approach to play and play development. Am J Occup Ther 25:275, 1971

19. Folkman JD, Clatworthy NM: Marriage Has Many Faces, p 80. Columbus, Merrill, 1970

20. Freiberg K: Human Development: A Life Span Approach, pp 359–361. Belmont, Calfornia, Wadsworth, 1979

21. Freud A: The concept of developmental lines. In Normality and Pathology in Childhood: Assessment of Development. New York, International Universities Press, 1965

22. Ginsberg E: Toward a theory of occupational choice as a restatement. Voc Guidance Quart 20:169, 1972

23. Ginsberg H, Opper S: Piaget's Theory of Intellectual Development, p 111. Englewood Cliffs, NJ, Prentice–Hall, 1969

24. Goren CC, Sart M, Wu PK: Visual following and pattern discrimination of face-like stimuli by newborn infants. Pediatrics 56:544, 1975

25. Haith MM: Rules that Babies Look By, pp 65, 84. Hillsdale, NJ, Erlbaum, 1980

26. Havighurst R: Developmental Tasks and Education, 3rd ed. New York, McKay Publishers, 1972

27. Hetherington EM: Divorce: A child's perspective. Am Psychol 34:851, 1979

28. Horn J: Organization of data on life span development of human abilities. In Goulet L, Baltes P (eds): Life Span Developmental Psychology. New York, Academic Press, 1970

29. Huyok MH, Hoyer WJ: Adulthood and Aging, pp 207–211. Belmont, CA: Wadsworth, 1982

30. Inhelder B, Piaget J: The Growth of Logical Thinking from Childhood to Adolescence. New York, Basic Books, 1958

31. Isaacson L: Career Information in Counseling and Teaching, pp 36–38. Boston, Allyn & Bacon, 1968

32. Kastenbaum R: Humans Developing: A Life Span Perspective, pp 518–522. Boston, Allyn & Bacon, 1972

33. Kaye K, Marcus J: Infant imitations: The sensorimotor agenda. Dev Psychol 17:258, 1981

34. Kuvlesky W, Wright D, Juarez R: Status projections and ethnicity: A comparison of Mexican American, Negro, and Anglo youths. J Voc Behav 1:137, 1971

35. Lamb ME (ed): The Development of Attachment and Affiliative Systems. New York, Plenum Press, 1982

36. Levinson D: The psychological development of man in early adulthood and midlife transition. In Ricks D, Thomas A, Roff M (eds): Life History Research in Psychopathology III, p 254. Minneapolis, University of Minnesota Press, 1974

37. Linn S, Reznick JS, Kagan J, Hans S: Salience of visual patterns in the human infant. Dev Psychol 18:651, 1982

38. Lloyd M: Adolescence, pp 4–42. New York, Harper & Row, 1985

39. Lowenthal MT: Four Stages of Life, p 100. San Francisco, Jassey and Bass, 1975

40. Malina RM: Adolescent changes in size, build, composition and performance. In Human Biology, pp 46, 117–131. Washington, DC, National Center of Health Statistics, 1975

41. Malina RM: Motor development in the early years. In Moore SG, Cooper CR (eds): The Young Child: Review of Research, Vol 3. Washington, DC, National Association for the Education of Young Children, 1982

42. Markham EM, Cox B, Machida S: The standard object sorting task as a measure of conceptual organization. Dev Psychol 17:115, 1981

43. Meltzoff AN, Moore MH: Newborn infants imitate adult facial gestures. Child Dev 54:702, 1983

44. Nelson K: Structure and Strategy in Learning to Talk. Monogr Soc Res Child Dev 38(149), 1973

45. Neugarten B: The roles we play. In Quality of Life: The Middle Years. Acton, MA, Publishing Sciences Group, 1974

46. Patterson GR: Families: Applications of Social Learning to Family Life. Champaign, IL, Research Press, 1975

47. Piaget J: The Moral Judgement of the Child. Gaban M (trans). Glencoe, IL, Free Press, 1948

48. Piaget J: The Origins of Intelligence, pp 68, 150. Cook M (trans). New York, International Universities Press, 1953

49. Piaget J: Play, Dreams, and Imitation in Childhood, p 6. Gatteango C, Hudson FM (trans). New York: WW Norton Press, 1965

50. Rutter M: School effects on pupil progress: Research findings and policy implications. Child Dev 54:1, 1983

51. Salapatek P: Pattern perception in early infancy. In Cohen LB, Salapatek P (eds): Infant Perception: From Sensation to Cognition, Vol 1. New York, Academic Press, 1975

52. Schuster C, Ashburn S: The Process of Human Development: A Holistic Approach, pp 291, 299, 309, 623–624, 772–773. Boston, Little, Brown & Co., 1980

53. Selman RL: The Growth of Interpersonal Understanding. New York, Academic Press, 1980

54. Sinnott JM, Pisoni DB, Aslin RN: Comparison of pure auditory behavior in human infants and adults. Infant Behav Dev 6:3, 1983

55. Smilansky G: The Effect of Sociodramatic Play on Disadvantaged Youth, Chaps 1–3. New York, John Wiley & Sons, 1968

56. Sternberg RJ: The evolution of theories of intelligence. Intelligence 5:149, 1981

57. Sternberg RJ (ed): Handbook of Human Intelligence. Cambridge, Cambridge University Press, 1982

58. Super D: Vocational development in adolescence and early childhood: Tasks and behaviors. In Super D, Starishevsky R, Matlin J (eds): Career Development: Self Concept Theory. New York, College Examination Board, 1963

59. Takata N: Introduction to a series: Occupational behavior research for pediatric process. Am J Occup Ther 34:11, 1980

60. Tanner JM: Fetus into Man: Physical Growth from Conception to Maturity, p 108. Cambridge, MA, Harvard University Press, 1978

61. Tanner JM: Physical growth. In Mussen PH (ed): Carmichael's Manual of Child Psychology, 3rd ed, Vol 2, pp 95–96. New York, John Wiley & Sons, 1970

62. Tanner JM: Sequence, tempo and individual variation in growth and development of boys and girls aged 12–16. In Harrison SJ, McDermott JF Jr (eds): New Directions in Childhood Psychopathology, Vol 1. Developmental Considerations, pp 182–202. New York, International University Press, 1980

63. Tomlinson–Keasey C, Eisert DC, Kahle LR, Hardy–Brown K, Keasey B: The structure of concrete operational thought. Child Dev 50:1153, 1978

64. Wachs TD, Gruen GE: Early Experience and Human Development. New York, Plenum Press, 1982

65. Wolff PH: Normal variation in human maturation. In Connelly KJ, Prechtl HRF (eds): Maturation and Development: Biological and Psychological Perspectives. Clin Dev Med 77/78. London, Heinemann, 1981

Bibliography

Infancy and Childhood

Berndt TJ: Effects of friendship on prosocial intentions and behavior. Child Dev 52:636, 1981

Capute AJ: Early neuromotor reflexes in infancy. Pediatr Ann 15:217, 1986

Clark PN, Allen AS: Occupational Therapy for Children. St Louis, CV Mosby, 1985

Cullen R, Harrison RF: Behavioral assessment of the neonate. Irish J Med Sci 155:6, 1986

Flower MJ: Neuromaturation of the human fetus. J Med Philos 10:237, 1985

Frankenburg WK, Emde RN, Sullivan JW (eds): Early Identification of Children at Risk. New York, Plenum, 1985

Harris J, Liebert R: Child: The Development from Birth Through Adolescence. Englewood Cliffs, NJ, Prentice–Hall, 1984

Jacklin CN, Dipietro JA, Maccoby EE: Sex-typing behavior and sex-typing pressure in child/parent interaction. Arch Sex Behav 13:413, 1984

Kline RB, Lachar D, Sprague DJ: The Personality Inventory for Children (PIC): An unbiased predictor of cognition and academic status. J Pediatr Psychol 10:461, 1985

Lamke LK: Adjustment and sex-role orientation. J Youth Adolescence 11:247, 1982

Sharp JT: Development of gross motor skills in the normal child. Clin Podiatr 1:447, 1984

Skinner L: Motor Development in the Preschool Years. Springfield, IL: Charles C Thomas, 1979

Play

Cotton NS: Childhood play as an analog to adult capacity to work. Child Psychiatr Human Dev 14:135, 1984

Field TM, DeStefano L, Koewler JH III: Fantasy play of toddlers and preschoolers. Dev Psychol 18:503, 1982

Florey L: Studies of play: Implications for growth development and for clinical practice. Am J Occup Ther 35:519, 1981

Ungerer JA, Sigman M: The relation of play and sensorimotor behavior to language in the second year. Child Dev 55:1448, 1984

Watson MW: Agents and recipient objects in the development of early symbolic play. Child Dev 55:1091, 1984

Adolescence

Conger J: Adolescence: Generation under Pressure. New York, Harper & Row, 1980

Conger J, Peterson AC: Adolescence & Youth: Psychological Development in a Changing World, 3rd ed. New York, Harper & Row, 1983

Davis IP: Adolescents: Theoretical and Helping Perspectives. Boston: Kluwer Academic Publications, 1985

Ford ME: Social cognition and social competence in adolescence. Dev Psychol 18:323, 1982

Kimmel DC, Weiner IB: Adolescence: A Developmental Transition. New York, Erlbaum, 1985

Massad CM: Sex role identity and adjustment during adolescence. Child Dev 52:1290, 1981

McKinney JP: Developmental Psychology: The Adolescent and Young Adult. New York, Dorsey, 1982

Muuss RE: Theories of Adolescence, 4th ed. New York, Random House, 1982

Rice FP: The Adolescent: Development, Relationships, and Culture, 4th ed. New York, Allyn & Bacon, 1984

Rowe I, Marcia JE: Ego identity status, formal operations, and moral development. J Youth Adolescence 9:87, 1980

Adulthood

Baruch G, Brooks–Gunn J: Women in Midlife. New York, Plenum Press, 1984

Blank TO: A Social Psychology of Developing Adults. New York, John Wiley & Sons, 1982

Bourne B: Effects of aging on work satisfaction, performance and motivation. Aging Work 5:37, 1982

Bumagin VE, Hirn KF: Observations on changing relationships for older women. Am J Psychoanal 42:133, 1982

Chinin AB: Modal logic: A new paradigm of development and late-life potential. Human Dev 27:42, 1984

Donohugh D: The Middle Years. Philadelphia, WB Saunders, 1981

Eichorn DH, Clausen JA, Haan N, Honzik MP, Mussen PH (eds): Present and Past in Middle Life. New York, Academic Press, 1981

Farrell MP, Rosenberg S: Men at Midlife. Boston, Auburn House, 1981

Gowdy WJ, Gaudeau JF: Social ties and life satisfaction of older persons: Another evaluation. J Gerontol Social Work 4:35, 1981

Gross H, Sussman MB (eds): Alternatives to Traditional Family Living. New York, Haworth Press, 1982

Kaufert PA: Women and their health in middle years: A Manitoba project. Social Sci Med 18:279, 1984

Madonia J: The trauma of unemployment and its consequences. J Appl Psychol 52:884, 1984

McPherson B: Aging as a Social Process. Toronto: Butterworth & Co., 1983

Moss MS, Moss S: The impact of parental death on middle aged children. Omega J Death Dying 14:65, 1983–84

Rogers D: Adult Years: An Introduction to Aging, 3rd ed. Englewood Cliffs, NJ, Prentice–Hall, 1986

Sanstock JW: Life Span Development. Iowa City, WC Brown, 1983

SECTION 3
Late Adulthood *Linda L. Levy*

The aging process is difficult to define because it connotes three distinct phenomena: the biological capacity for survival, the psychological capacity for adaptation, and the sociological capacity for the fulfillment of social roles.[4] Within these three spheres, developmental challenges are presented to older adults which rarely occur simultaneously but rather at different times and different rates. For example, a 60-year-old who is unable to establish intimate relationships would be considered "young" psychologically, whereas a 70-year-old who is still employed would be considered "young"—and a 40-year-old grandmother "older"—in terms of social age. As a result, there are vast variations in biological, psychological, and social aging, which are only roughly related to one's chronological age. One's "age," then, is best conceptualized in terms of one's health and diverse psychological and sociological challenges rather than by one's chronological age. This perspective is aptly expressed by the adage, "You are only as old as you feel."

At the same time, it cannot be overemphasized that any of the challenges of aging are approached by individuals whose life experiences in confronting developmental crises have provided them with a rich and complex variety of coping mechanisms. Hence, it would be inaccurate to characterize any but a broad and heterogeneous view of "normal" aging. In fact, older adults vary more in patterns of normal functioning than do individuals at any other stage in the life span, and one of the few generalizations that researchers are willing to make

about older adults is that they tend to become less like each other and more like themselves—that is, they become increasingly individualistic as they age. It is only with this appreciation of the tremendous variability that exists among older people that we can begin to explore the developmental challenges that are presented by the aging process.

Biological Aging

Biological aging refers to the condition of the biological organism with respect to his potential life span[4] and is closely connected to physical health. The physical changes that occur with aging are a continuation of the decline that, most researchers agree, begins as soon as physical maturity is reached at approximately age 18 to 22. It is not yet possible to distinguish which changes are truly a result of aging (those that are determined by heredity) and which are a result of disease or a variety of environmental and physical factors. However, one of the most consistently documented changes is a diminished capacity to maintain or regain homeostasis, an internal steady state that normally is maintained in the face of changing environmental circumstances. Although there is little change in homeostatic mechanisms under resting conditions, the rate of readjustment to normal equilibrium *after stress* is slower in older individuals than in young. For example, the capacity of the kidneys for removing waste, the ability to maintain body temperature during exposure to heat or cold, and the efficiency of blood-sugar regulation decrease with age. Similarly, when an older person develops an infection, the body temperature does not rise as rapidly or as markedly as in younger people, and, having risen, takes longer to return to normal. The stressors that disrupt these processes can be either physical (*e.g.,* a virus or exercise) or psychosocial (*e.g.,* loss of spouse or relocation). In either case, with advancing age, the capacity for homeostasis gradually declines, and the range of adjustment and adaptation becomes smaller and narrower. Accordingly, biological aging results in increased vulnerability. For reasons that are not yet fully understood, it also results in decreases in the efficiency and function of a number of organs.

Before we address these diverse changes, there are a number of issues to be kept in mind. First, it should be emphasized that within individuals, biological changes occur at different times and rates in different organs, tissues, and cells; and within different individuals, these changes occur at vastly different times and rates. For example, visible signs of aging such as graying or baldness can occur at age 30 in one individual and at age 70 in another. Second, whereas some biological aging occurs naturally in body organs, biochemical pathways, musculoskeletal systems, and the central nervous system, what is largely unappreciated is the fact that the health and physical ability of most older persons do not decline precipitously, nor are the changes quickly disabling. Limitations in the activities of daily living are reported by only 13% of those aged 65 and 74, 25% of those between 75 and 84, and 46% of those 85 years and older.[27] Hence, most who live into their 80s do so without experiencing difficulties in carrying out major tasks and without changes in their normal functioning due to biological aging. However, 85% of the population over 65 years of age experience at least one chronic condition, with multiple chronic conditions such as arthritis, hypertension, and impaired hearing commonplace.[27] A key implication here is that despite the prevalence of chronic impairments, most older individuals have developed coping mechanisms that enable them to lead well-functioning lives.[15] At the same time, it becomes apparent that criteria such as "absence of disease" are not useful when addressing the question of what it means for the aged to be healthy. Finally, it should be acknowledged that there is not necessarily a direct cause and effect relationship between the degree of structural impairment within an organ and the presence of impaired function or disease. For example, it is not unusual at autopsy to discover extensive changes in the blood vessels in the brain even in elderly persons who had little clinical evidence of mental impairment.[26]

Having considered these issues, we can begin to summarize some of the major biological changes associated with aging.

Age-related changes in the **sensory systems** include:

Vision. Decreased pupil size and loss of transparency, and increased thickness of the lens allow less light to reach the retina; hence, older people need twice as much illumination as younger people. Decreased elasticity of the lens results in presbyopia (farsightedness). Visual acuity and the ability to discriminate colors also decrease progressively with age.
Hearing. Decreased auditory acuity at high frequencies impairs the ability to discriminate words and to understand normal conversation.
Taste and smell. Decreased sensitivity in discriminating salty, sweet, and sour tastes as well as in the ability to discriminate food odors is typical.

For a comprehensive discussion of these sensory changes and their critical implications for the practice of occupational therapy, see Levy.[13]

Age-related changes in the **organ systems** include:
Muscular structure. Muscle weight and strength decrease, the number and diameter of muscle fibers decrease, and hypertrophy occurs. The valves of the heart become thicker and less flexible. Atrophy increases.
Skeletal system. Skeletal mass decreases, bones become more porous and brittle as demineralization occurs, and the synovium in joints degenerates, resulting in decreased flexibility.
Cardiovascular system. The heart and blood vessels become more rigid due to collagen changes, and blood vessels narrow due to arteriosclerotic changes. A decline is evident in the maximal heart rate, exercise stroke volume, cardiac output, maximal oxygen consumption, and capacity for responding to extra work. Peripheral vascular resistance increases.
Respiratory system. Expiration and inspiration decrease as a result of atrophy of the intercostal muscles and diaphragm and decreased expandability of intercostal bone, muscle, and pulmonary tissue. There is thickening of pulmonary arterial walls and thinning of the alveolar walls. Consequently, there is a 10% to 15% decrease in the oxygen content of the blood, and emphysema becomes common in very old age.
Excretory systems. In the urinary system, there is a decrease in kidney weight and ability to eliminate waste products. Urinary frequency increases. In the digestive system, ability to secrete adequate digestive juices is reduced and there is atrophy of gastrointestinal mucosa, decreased absorption from the gastrointestinal tract, and decreased muscle tone and peristalsis, resulting in indigestion and constipation.
Gallbladder/liver. There is an increased prevalence of gallstones and decreased size and efficiency of the liver.

Psychological Aging

Psychological aging refers to a person's ability to adapt to changing environments and is primarily reflected in an individual's intellectual skills and emotional well-being. As we have seen, some degree of biological decline is virtually inevitable as we age. However, this is not the case with psychological aging: there is great potential for continuing growth and development, and most older people get "better" as they get older.

In regard to intellectual skills, the relationship between age and intelligence is insignificant. Any relationship that does occur involves memory, speed of response, and perceptual–integrative functions (reflecting, perhaps, decreased efficiency of the central nervous system) rather than overall intelligence.[5] In crystallized aspects of intellectual functioning, older people continue to improve until at least age 55 or 60, with little apparent decline until their mid-70s or beyond.[22] On the Wechsler Adult Intelligence Scale (WAIS), this would be reflected on the information, vocabulary, and comprehension subtests—those which involve verbal abilities and are influenced by both experience and education. Palmore provides data from seven long-term investigations that older people with advanced education who are working without time pressure show little or no cognitive deterioration with age.[20] Memory, in particular, short-term and recent memory, shows some decline with age, but people who exercise their memories are able to maintain both remote and recent memory well into old age.[2] And, although older people often require somewhat longer to learn material, when given extra time, they learn as well as younger people.[6]

In addition, many older people continue to be creative in later life.[7] Dennis found that creativity remained high in many older people who were creative in their earlier years[11]: literary scholars, historians, and philosophers were as productive in their 70s as they were in their 40s. The productivity of most scientists in their 70s declined from 25% to 50% from its peak, but inventors were most productive from ages 60 to 80. There are numerous examples of creative contributions that were made in old age. For example, Tolstoy wrote *Resurrection* when he was in his 70s, Ben Franklin invented bifocals when he was 78, and both Georgia O'Keeffe and Pablo Picasso were creating important works of art at 90. Michelangelo completed the dome of St. Peter's in Rome when he was 70, Goethe was 82 when he finished *Faust,* and Verdi produced *Otello* at 74 and *Falstaff* at 80. A number of reviewers note that works of late life typically have a maturity, a complexity, and an insight into the interrelationships of things that the works of younger people lack.[23]

At the same time, late adulthood provides a number of opportunities for psychological growth and expansion. Older people may come to accept and understand both themselves and others better as they age. This insight is key to the development of a number of the intervention strategies used with dysfunctional older individuals.

A brief review of Erikson's epigenetic principle[12] may begin to shed light on this issue. This principle states that human growth and development progresses through a number of stages which are invariant, each stage being a necessary precursor to its succeeding stage. Within any stage, age-specific psychological conflicts emerge and assume priority in accordance with normal physiological maturity and psychological awareness. This is not to say that the conflict is ever fully resolved within the stage where it assumes priority; rather, resolution becomes a continuing process which proceeds at different paces within each individual in response to changing environmental circumstances. And so, as an individual's relation to his environment changes, so does his experience of each of the conflicts. Notwithstanding, conflicts within each stage of development must be dealt with to a certain degree for further psychological development to occur. Simply stated, the issue becomes one of the ratio between the favorable and unfavorable qualities of any given conflict that become integrated within the personality structure at any given stage. If the preponderance of integration is directed toward the favorable components of the conflict, then a firm basis is laid for the development of succeeding components of the personality. Conversely, if the preponderance of integration is directed toward the unfavorable components of the conflict, a weak and vulnerable base is laid for further psychological development. To reiterate, however, these conflicts are never resolved once and for all. Remnants of both components of each conflict (**trust** and **mistrust**, for example) remain as important personality determinants within each of us.

The epigenetic principle is of particular importance for understanding psychological aging because it underscores the unceasing potential for personality growth and development throughout the lifespan. It proposes that the individual continues to work through each of these conflicts to a greater or lesser degree throughout the life cycle, as his or her environmental context changes; and it conceptualizes the healthy personality as continually in the process of growth, expansion, and development even until death. This principle also maintains that an individual's psychological resources are intimately connected to the levels of integration he has attained thus far within stage-specific conflicts. An important corollary here is that there are more chances to integrate the favorable qualities of a given conflict inadequately as time goes on, which inevitably impairs development in each succeeding stage. As a result, the pleasures inherent in the last phase of life—**Integrity**

Erickson's Analysis of Life Stages

1. In the first stage of development, the individual faces the conflict between **trust** and **mistrust.** The task is to learn that the world is a good place and that others are trustworthy and to acquire a sense of trustworthiness as far as the self is concerned. Out of trust develops *hope*, the ego strength of infancy. In the older adult, this is reflected as *faith* in personal religious beliefs or in ethical and moral systems. A successful resolution of this conflict becomes manifest as a sense of peace within the context of dying. A well-loved child will retain that sense of infantile omnipotence which trusts that the world ultimately has satisfying things to offer, even those that are unknown.

The impairment of basic trust is expressed in a basic mistrust: a tendency toward withdrawal, alienation, fear of strangers, and lack of affiliation, as well as a belief in being controlled by fate or chance. This is a conflict that is often revived in the face of chronic illness when the individual places his life in the care of others. The struggle of helpless dependency and allowing oneself to be cared for is recreated and must be worked through.

2. In the second stage, the individual first experiences the impact of socialization and begins to adapt his or her wishes and needs to those of society. The developmental crisis is the struggle of **autonomy** (or self-control) against **doubt** and **shame,** and the critical learning tasks become those of "holding on" *versus* "letting go." From a sense of self-control not associated with loss of self-esteem comes a lasting sense of dignity and pride. If autonomy predominates over shame, the basic strength of early childhood, a rudimentary *will* develops. Failure to reach such autonomy results in a sense of doubt and shame, a loss of face and dignity, and a tenuous capacity for self-control. The individual compensates by becoming "overcontrolled;" *i.e.,* compulsive, in matters of time, money, and affection.

This struggle is highlighted by the process of leaving a legacy (letting go) when one's physical or mental capacities require it. Letting go without loss of dignity involves the critical element of *free will* —of *choosing* to let go—as well as **trust** that others will carry on with what one has created. Difficulties in letting go of money or possessions is especially reflective of difficulties derived from this stage.

3. In the third developmental stage, the individual builds on his/her sense of autonomy and is ready to develop **initiative,** a sense of direction or *purpose* derived from his experiences of venturing out, exploring, and discovering what potential the world has to offer. Feelings of **guilt** (versus shame) are now possible because of the maturation of the child's conscience. (Shame is externally induced, whereas guilt is internal.) Hence, failure in this developmental stage leads to an undue sense of doing wrong and guilt. The adult overburdened with guilt—essentially for "having dared to dream"—may become excessively inhibited, vindictive, or self-righteous. Rather than seeing possibilities in life, he/she becomes concerned with what cannot or should not be done.

In the older adult, failure within this stage will undermine the individual's ability to conceptualize and create new alternatives. This skill is critical to successful adjustment to changing environmental circumstances or increasing disability.

4. In the fourth developmental stage, the individual learns to gain recognition by learning specific skills and acquiring knowledge and is ready to develop a sense of **industry.** If industry predominates, the individual will derive a basic sense that he/she can master the environment—*competence.* If he/she feels that his/her skills are not up to the requirements of the physical and social world, a sense of **inferiority** develops.

In the older adult, a sense of competence is likewise required in the face of disability. Healthy adjustment is derived from the ability to compensate for disabilities by creatively manipulating the environment to permit maximum levels of functioning.

5. Adolescence, the fifth stage, is particularly critical because it is during this period that a sense of **identity** develops. The task of this difficult period is to discover "who one is": what kind of man or woman to be, what career and roles to pursue, and what one's individual outlook on society and the world is. Once a basic sense of identity is established, *fidelity* can emerge. The individual is able to commit himself/herself to some desired goal or cause. Failure in this stage leads to **identity diffusion**: the individual does not attain a feeling of security about who he/she is or would like to be, his/her gender identity, ability to master drives, attractiveness to others, and his/her ability to make the right decisions.

The search for identity continues throughout life. As Butler phrases it, "When identity is established or maintained, I find it an ominous sign rather than a favorable one. A continuing life-long identity crisis seems to be a sign of good health." [1] An individual's new identity in old age comes from finding new uses for what has been learned during previous years and from developing new ways of coming to terms with reality. That reality consists of personal strengths and weaknesses as well as a changing world that is not always to one's liking.[1]

6. In young adulthood, the task is to develop **intimacy,** a development that necessarily requires the prior establishment of some sense of identity or self. In intimacy, the individual is able to fuse his identity with another and commit himself to relationships that demand sacrifice and compromise. Successful resolution of this stage results in *love,* where the individual comes to see himself as worthy of love as well as capable of loving. When the stage is not resolved successfully, a sense of **isolation** and self-absorption predominates. The individual's relationships lack warmth, spontaneity, and deep emotional commitment. There may also be fear that fusion with another will weaken one's own sense of identity.

For the older adult, research has amply demonstrated that the maintenance of a stable intimate relationship serves a critical function in protecting the individual's morale and mental stability against the various social losses (*e.g.,* widowhood, retirement) that are associated with aging.[16]

7. In middle adulthood, the struggle is between **generativity** and the forces of **self-absorption** and **stagnation.** Generativity relates primarily to establishing and guiding the next generation and can be expressed in the bearing and rearing of children, in contributing to the well-being of others, and in creating products and ideas of value to society. Giving must assume priority over getting. In addition, this stage requires a reappraisal of work and relationship goals in order to focus one's efforts in directions consistent with one's inner values. It also requires an elemental *faith* that the species should be preserved and that one's contributions are valuable and can ultimately make a difference. When generativity fails to predominate, a sense of stagnation pervades the individual's life: the individual has failed to come to terms with his values and priorities, and his efforts lose their meaning.

Generative acts are characterized by *care,* and for care to develop, an individual must have attained strengths from all the previous stages: *hope, will, purpose, competence, fidelity,* and *love.* Erikson sees generativity as the driving power of human organization. Perhaps if more individuals were able to attain it, then world peace might become a political reality.

8. The final stage of the life cycle is later adulthood, when the task is to develop **integrity,** a sense of the coherence and wholeness of one's life. A person accepts that life, sees meaning in it, believes that he or she did the best that could be done under the circumstances, and feels satisfied with the wisdom attained thus far. When integrity predominates, *wisdom,* the virtue of old age, can emerge. Again, this presupposes the more or less successful resolution of the previous stages and builds on all the previously developed strengths of *hope, will, purpose, competence, fidelity, love,* and *care.* With wisdom comes a shift in identity: out of the sense of identity developed in adolescence emerges an existential identity, which comes from facing the border of one's life, realizing the relativity of one's own identity, and coming to terms with the world outside the self and with one's connection to the universe. It also enables a reconciliation with, and acceptance of, death. Stern offers the thesis that "adaptation to death is necessary for full personality maturation, and deficiency in this adaptation is an integral factor in neurosis."[24] It is a key developmental task—then, to come to view one's own death as the appropriate outcome of one's life. At age 80, Bertrand Russell beautifully characterized the successful negotiation of this stage when he wrote:

> Psychologically, there are two dangers to be guarded against in old age. One of these is undue absorption with the past. . . . The other . . . is clinging to youth in the hope of sucking vigor from vitality. . . . The best way to overcome it—so it seems to me—is to make your interests gradually wider and more impersonal, until bit by bit the walls of the ego recede and your life becomes increasingly merged with the universal life. An individual human existence should be like a river—small at first, narrowly contained within its banks, and rushing passionately . . . Gradually, the river grows wider, the banks recede, the waters flow more quietly, and in the end, without any visible break, they become merged in the sea.[10]

When integrity fails to predominate, a sense of **despair** pervades. A person fears death and wishes desperately for another chance, or he may withdraw from all involvement with others in a gesture of defeat.

It should be emphasized that the development of integrity is very much undermined by stresses inherent to the aging process. The multiple physical and social losses which occur must be worked through in relation to their relevant developmental conflicts, so there is much psychologically to be learned. Otherwise, the losses of aging can indeed become overwhelming contributors to despair.

—are necessarily the most difficult ones to attain. The displayed material, an adaptation of Erikson's Analysis of Life Stages, presents the implications of his analysis for the older adult.

In summary, Erikson's developmental tasks, if successfully negotiated, result in emotional maturity, integrity, and profound life satisfaction. Mature psychological development is reflected in an autonomous individual who is able to value himself/herself while achieving closeness and relatedness to others, who is able to look realistically at successes and failures and feel that life has been worthwhile, and who has come to a sense of peace with the prospect of death. This state is attained by a continuing process of progressive synthesis and integration of a number of personality components. However, conflicts are never resolved once and for all; rather, they are continually in the *process* of resolution. The aging individual, then, is ever-learning, ever-adjusting, and ever-developing. Indeed, he or she can be working through conflicts derived from deficient learning early in life even up to death.

Sociological Aging

A dynamic interaction between individuals and society is also inherent to the aging process. Social aging occurs as the roles and functions of an individual change within society. It refers to the age-specific roles an individual assumes within the context of the society in which he lives and is reflected largely in how the individual behaves in light of the expectations of his social group. As will be seen, some of the most significant challenges of aging are presented by the social aging process.

Before we proceed, an overview of some basic sociological concepts is in order. *Roles* are the social structures through which individuals are given opportunities to make contributions to society. Role opportunities are provided in the institutional spheres of the society: the economic, religious, educational, and family systems. Roles also prescribe specific *norms* and *standards* for appropriate and expected behaviors. In addition, all societies use *age-grading systems* to define and classify who is young, middle-aged, and old. *Age-specific roles* and expectations for behavior are ascribed in terms of these classifications.[9] Hence, "young," "middle-aged," and "old" people are expected to behave and to be treated differently from people in other age classes within a society. This serves to create predictable age-related patterns of behavior and social interaction. The oft-heard exhortation to "act one's age" means precisely to conform to these age-specific role expectations.

Age roles and the associated expectations for appropriate behavior differ from culture to culture and from era to era. However, all individuals are effectively so-cialized to the particular role prescribed for their age group in their society. Therefore, when they reach later adulthood, their attitudes and behavior reflect their earlier expectations regarding appropriate behavior for older people. An individual who lives in a society that considers the elderly useless and expendable is likely to have a negative view of his/her own aging and would be given limited role opportunities to make meaningful contributions; conversely, an individual who lives in a society that considers the elderly valuable and useful citizens is likely to have positive feelings about his/her own aging and would be given ample role opportunities to make meaningful contributions. In similar fashion, a person may be made to feel old because society expects him/her to be or may act older than he/she feels to avoid violating social norms and expectation. Hence, the subjective experience of social aging is to a large extent determined by the expectations of society.

As indicated earlier, age-specific roles are largely determined by the age-grading system which all societies use to classify their members into various categories. The criteria that societies use for age grading vary widely and often relate to a specific organization or activity. For example, in some societies, one becomes old when one becomes the oldest member of a family or when one is no longer able to hunt. However, in industrial societies, there appear to be no specific criteria such as social categories or ability to function.[3] Instead, people are arbitrarily assigned to an age category. In the United States, this is usually done by chronological age; *i.e.*, when one reaches 65, the age of retirement that was arbitrarily selected in 1935 under the Social Security Act.

A significant problem with this arbitrary designation is that when most Americans think of old age, they think of stereotypical (and, as we shall see, "ageist") characteristics, such as declining health, energy, or mental capacities. They also are led to believe that older people are a homogeneous group, yet, as was discussed earlier, the reality is that chronological age is an especially poor indicator of the characteristics of aging for individuals. The older a group of individuals gets, the more *dissimilar* they become in terms of abilities. In recognition of this misperception, a number of sociologists maintain that many of the problems that older people experience in American society can be attributed to the injustices of an arbitrary system that implies that everyone over 65 is physically and mentally old.[3] Rosow states the problem another way: that older people have two kinds of problems—the kind they really have, and the kind that other people think they have.[21]

Both of these perspectives underscore the unfortunate reality that societies ascribe to their aged those roles and privileges commensurate with its underlying philosophy irrespective of the facts. In particular, our society promotes significant stereotypes and negative attitudes that serve to age individuals prematurely and unfairly. This is tantamount to discrimination against older people on the basis of age, a phenomenon that Butler has aptly describd as "ageism." [8] Butler conceptualizes ageism as the protective mechanism that society uses to avoid confronting the difficult issues of aging, illness, and death. It is, then, merely a poorly masked innate fear of our own aging and death. Although largely unconscious, ageism results in a perception of aging as a period of powerlessness, uselessness, disability, and disease.[8] This problem is accentuated by the fact that older people have already been socialized into accepting these negative stereotypes at the same time that others are perceiving them negatively. As a result, these stereotypes and attitudes cannot help but undermine the self-concepts and sense of self-worth of older people.

A closely related effect of ageist attitudes is the role restrictions that our society imposes on older people. Our society devalues older people and assumes them to be nonproductive and noncontributing. Consequently, older people are provided with few role opportunities and are not given the prerogative of selecting new roles even if they are physically and mentally able to fill them. In our society, the age role of older people has oftentimes been characterized as a "roleless role," meaning that there are few if any roles expected of or provided for older people that would enable them to make meaningful contributions. Instead, older people are expected to defer their acquired positions of power and leadership within the community to the young. Perhaps one of the most blatant examples of these restrictions is mandatory retirement. Conceptually, mandatory retirement is a form of age discrimination, because it imposes retirement purely on the basis of age.[3] The law prohibits age discrimination in employment for people between the ages of 40 and 64, but older people are denied such protection.

The problem of restrictions in role opportunities for older people is compounded by the fact that it occurs at a time they are already experiencing a diminished opportunity to engage in many of their most meaningful roles owing to, for example, reduction in income because of loss of job, the death of family and friends, and mobility of children. The grandparent role is one of the few new roles that becomes open to them, and it takes on special significance because so many other areas of role performance have become closed. It also is a role that has many positive connotations, in contrast to the few other new roles that are available, such as "widow," "new resident" (special living conditions often become necessary, requiring relocation to unfamiliar environments), "volunteer," and "retiree."

A word on retirement: most older adults are pleased to discover that, despite the social obstacles discussed above, the role of retiree can have pleasant connota-

tions.[25] This outcome depends on factors such as the work *versus* leisure orientation of the individual, as well as whether they have health and money and are able to find meaningful ways to occupy their time, again, in spite of the restrictions imposed by our social system.

The tragedy is that when such restricted role opportunities are provided to older people, both society and older people lose. Society loses the talents of older people, and older people are excluded from significant social participation and deprived of their social identity. The responses of older people to these injustices range from complete resignation to militant resistance. Yet to intervene effectively in the process by which older people find themselves less useful to society will require a reorganization of the social system and its underlying values. Only then will older individuals be provided with opportunities to make meaningful contributions.

As is apparent, the social aging process is fraught with undue hardships and significant challenges. This is not to say that older people have not been able to find ways to cope with the difficulties. It is indeed testimony to the adaptability of older people that so many of them continue to report high life satisfaction and high morale despite the despiriting social restrictions that they encounter in their day-to-day lives. In fact, successful adaptation in old age is the rule rather than the exception.[14] Research in this area reveals that there are essentially two key variables in retaining high morale and a feeling of life satisfaction: health and meaningful activity.[19] It also suggests that successful adaptation to social aging is to a large extent determined by the ability to compensate; *e.g.*, by finding ways to increase activity in other areas, when roles are taken away; *e.g.*, through retirement or loss of a spouse. Obviously, people can and do survive in our restricted social environment: the larger question to be addressed is whether they *must*.

Nonetheless, there is room for optimism. There is evidence that the age-grading system, which has led to the restrictions in the social-role allocation experienced by older people, may be breaking down. Neugarten proposes that the United States is becoming an "age-irrelevant" society, in which chronological age is losing much of the meaning it once had.[18] Middle-aged and older adults are returning to school; middle-aged adults may divorce, remarry, and start new families; and both men and women are starting new careers during middle and retirement age. It is unclear how the age-grading system will adjust to these changes, but one would hope that society might begin to recognize that there are many different but equally acceptable ways for people to behave at all ages. Neugarten and Hagestad also caution, however, that our age-grading system appears to be going in contradictory directions. On the one hand, chronological age is being used increasingly as an index for benefits such as medicare and social security. On the other hand, this trend is counterbalanced by efforts to do away with the notion that age itself should be the determining factor in how roles and privileges are allocated in adulthood.[19]

Not incidentally, this rethinking of age roles is occurring at a time when American society is seriously questioning its ability to financially support a growing population of nonworking individuals over the age of 65. The age at which individuals can be required to retire has already been raised to 70 years, and it is likely that further efforts will be made to maintain older people in the economic sector. This economic imperative may well be the impetus required to force society's recognition that older people are able to make contributions that were previously thought inappropriate or even impossible. Now that their productivity is needed, older people may finally be provided with role opportunities to make meaningful contributions that they were always entitled to by virtue of their many capabilities. Consequently, the status, self-identity, and life satisfaction of all older people may be enhanced, and the stresses inherent in social aging might be significantly eased for future generations.

Conclusion

Aging is a dynamic process, which cannot be understood without an appreciation of the ways in which biological, psychological, and social aspects interact over the course of the life cycle. The changes that older people experience are mediated by their health, their own psychology, and their interactions with society. Biological decline is inevitable, but it may not affect the functioning of older people to a great extent until some threshold has passed, usually in late old age. By contrast, psychological growth is not restricted: there is no point where the psychological growth of older people ceases. There may also be considerable social growth in old age. Despite stereotypic beliefs about older people which may restrict new learning opportunities and obstruct participation, a significant number of older people succeed in leading productive and worthwhile lives.

Aging, then, is not without its difficulties, but there are also a number of redeeming features. This perspective has been validated by a number of researchers who, like Maas and Kuypers, find that:

> Old age merely continues what earlier years have launched. Finally, even when young adulthood is too narrowly lived or painfully overburdened, the later years may offer new opportunities. Different ways of living may be developed as our social environments change with time — and as we change them. In our study, we have found that *old age can provide a second and better chance at life* [17] (author's italics).

Nor can we forget that truly, it is only if we're lucky, that we, too, will be old someday. After all, as George Bernard Shaw adeptly reminds us, there is only one alternative!

References

1. Aiken L: Later Life. Philadelphia, WB Saunders, 1976
2. Atchley R: The Social Forces in Later Life, 2nd ed. Belmont, CA, Wadsworth Publishing, 1977
3. Atchley R: Aging as a social problem: An overview. In Seltzer M, Corbett S, Atchley R (eds): Social Problems of the Aging. Belmont, CA, Wadsworth Publishing, 1978
4. Birren J, Renner V: Research on the psychology of aging: Principles and experimentation. In Birren J, Schaie K (eds): Handbook of the Psychology of Aging. New York, Von Nostrand Reinhold, 1977
5. Botwinick J: Intellectual Abilities. In Birren J, Schaie K (eds): Handbook of the Psychology of Aging. New York, Von Nostrand Reinhold, 1977
6. Botwinick J, Thompson L: Components of reaction time in relation to age and sex. J Gen Psychol 108:175, 1966
7. Butler R: The destiny of creativity in later life. In Levin B, Kahana R (eds): Psychodynamic Studies on Aging. New York, International Universities Press, 1967
8. Butler R: Why Survive? Being Old in America. New York, Harper & Row, 1975
9. Cowgill D, Holmes L: Aging and Modernization. New York, Appleton–Century–Crofts, 1972
10. Dangott L, Kalish R: A Time to Enjoy: The Pleasures of Aging. Englewood Cliffs, NJ, Prentice–Hall, 1979
11. Dennis W: Creative productivity between 20 and 80 years. J Gerontol 21:1, 1966
12. Erikson E: Identity and the life cycle. In Klein G (ed): Psychological Issues, Vol 1, No 1. New York, International Universities Press, 1959
13. Levy L: Sensory change and compensation. In Davis L, Kirkland M (eds): Role of Occupational Therapy With the Elderly. Rockville, MD, American Occupational Therapy Association, 1986
14. Lieberman M: Social and psychological determinants of adaptation. Int J Aging Human Dev 9:115, 1978
15. Lowenthal MF, Chiriboga D: Social stress and adaptation: Toward a life course perspective. In Eisdorfer C, Lawton M (eds): The Psychology of Adult Development and Aging. Washington, DC, American Psychological Association, 1973
16. Lowenthal M, Haven C: Interaction and adaptation: Intimacy as a critical variable. Am Sociol Rev 33:20, 1968
17. Maas H, Kuypers J: From Thirty to Seventy. San Francisco, Jossey–Bass, 1974
18. Neugarten B: The future and the young–old. Gerontologist 15:4, 1975
19. Neugarten B, Hagestad G: Age and the life course. In Binstock R, Shanas E (eds): Handbook of Aging and the Social Sciences. New York, Von Nostrand Reinhold, 1976
20. Palmore E: Normal Aging II. Durham, NC, Duke University Press, 1974
21. Rosow I: Social Integration of the Aged. New York, Free Press, 1967

22. Schaie K: The Seattle longitudinal study: A twenty-one year exploration of psychometric intelligence in adulthood. In Schaie K (ed): Longitudinal Studies of Adult Psychological Development. New York, Guilford Press, 1982

23. Schaie K, Geiwitz J: Late life. In Adult Development and Aging. Boston, Little, Brown & Co, 1982

24. Stern M: Fear of death and neuroses. J Am Psychoanal Assoc 16:3, 1968

25. Streib G, Schneider C: Retirement in American Society: Impact and Process. Ithaca, NY, Cornell University Press, 1971

26. Tomlinson B, Blessed G, Roth M: Observations of the brain of demented old people. J Neurological Sci 11:205, 1970

27. US Senate Special Committee on Aging: Aging America: Trends and Projections, 1985–1986. Washington, DC, US Government Printing Office, 1986

CHAPTER 5

Occupational Therapy— Base in Occupation   *Gary Kielhofner*

In 1910, occupational therapy was defined as the "science of healing by occupation."[32] Though many other definitions have since been proposed to elaborate this simple theme and to reflect growing knowledge in occupational therapy, it still stands as the best reminder of what the occupational therapist is—an expert in the influence of occupation on health.

Although early occupational therapy leaders saw the necessity of understanding occupation,[15,19] it is only more recently that occupational therapists have begun to recognize the necessity of having a clearer and deeper conceptualization of occupation and its influence on health.[10,26,38] Reilly and many of her students began developing the thesis that successful application of occupation as a therapeutic medium required a thorough understanding of the nature of occupation.[11,20,23,25,26,36,39] Yerxa placed this relationship in perspective when she identified the study of occupation as the basic science of the field and the study of occupational therapy as the field's applied science.[40]

Responding to the need for a science of occupation, this chapter draws together relevant information to conceptualize the nature of occupation in human life. It takes an interdisciplinary view of occupation; knowledge that has been accumulated in various fields to explain occupation is organized around the following proposed definition:

> Occupation is the dominant activity of human beings that includes serious, productive pursuits and playful, creative, and festive behaviors. It is the result of evolutionary processes culminating in a biological, psychological, and social need for both playful and productive activity.

This definition points out some characteristics of occupation and opens possibilities for further elaboration. As knowledge accumulates, the definition should expand and become more comprehensive and integrated.

Occupation as the Major Activity of Human Beings

Occupation refers to human activity; however, not all activity is occupation: Humans engage in survival, sexual, spiritual, and social activities in addition to those acivities that are specifically occupational in nature. Survival and sexual activities are rooted in the biological requirements of the individual and the species. Survival functions are those that preserve the basic integrity of the organism; they include such activities as eating and avoiding pain and danger. Sexual activities bond relationships and serve the perpetuation of the species. Social activities refer to the forms of interaction and relations between individuals and their patterned order. The social characteristic of human beings involves the affiliative or affective bond between members of the species, their ability to share meanings, and their capacity for integration of action. Social activities have their genesis in the requirement of a group for coordinated activities between members. Language is probably the most important dimension of social activity, as it is the medium for most human interaction. Spiritual activities are also a fundamental part of human existence. Every civilization has some expression of human belief in an incomprehensible and ultimate dimension and related ethical codes.

It would be incorrect to suggest that one could clearly categorize all human activities. Social relations and sexuality overlap, spiritual activities involve coordinated human interaction, and social processes are often deeply infused with the spirituality of the cultural group. However, just as one can observe human activities that fulfill certain needs and that are primarily or uniquely spiritual, social, or sexual, there are those that are primarily occupational. Occupation can be seen to fulfill the basic need of human beings, individually and collectively, to explore and master their world.[20]

In everyday life, occupation is often interrelated with sexual, survival, social, and spiritual activities. On the other hand, many work, play, and self-care activities, although they may indirectly serve survival or other needs, are primarily occupational in nature. Further, human beings clearly work and play far beyond the immediate demands for survival. Such activities, done for their own sake, serve a basic urge for exploration and mastery. Thus, some activities have an occupational dimension whereas other activities are solely or primarily occupational in nature.

To say that occupation is a major human activity does not mean it is more important than other areas of human behavior but rather denotes that occupation ordinarily entails the majority of human time. Most waking hours are spent in play, self-care, and work. For all their other characteristics, human beings are most definitely occupational creatures.

Forms of Occupation

The study of occupation begins with identification and classification of different forms of occupation. Further, to guide treatment, occupational therapy needs to develop its own system of classifying occupational dysfunctions.[28] Such a classification of dysfunction must be built on a previous taxonomy of healthy occupation. For example, the concept of a patient having a work or play

dysfunction implies that "work" and "play" are defined behaviors for which there are criteria of adaptive and maladaptive functioning.

In occupational therapy, three areas of occupation are generally recognized: work, play, and self-care.[24] These categories appear to have inherent validity and will serve as a starting place for defining different forms of occupational behavior. These occupational behaviors form an interrelated gestalt. For example, work and play exist in an important dynamic balance throughout life, self-care is a necessary part of having a work role, and adult leisure is earned through work. These examples demonstrate the interdependence of these activities, which supports the argument that they form a common domain of behavior.

Work

Work may be conceptualized to include all forms of productive activities, whether or not they are reimbursed. Productive activities are those that provide a service or commodity needed by another or that add new abilities, ideas, knowledge, objects, or performances to the cultural tradition. The productive activity of work thus maintains and advances society. An activity considered to be one's work is generally organized into a major life role. Life roles are positions in life recognized by the social environment and by the role incumbant. Roles are not merely a means of organizing one's activity into a position within society; they also are an important source of identity. Thus, activities engaged in to fulfill one's duties as a student, housewife, or volunteer are properly considered work. According to this definition, work is not limited to adults; it extends to school-age children and the elderly. Such a broad definition of work is relevant to occupational therapy, since many of the field's clients and patients do not have access to roles in marketplace labor.

Daily Living Tasks

The concept of self-care is expanded here to encompass a larger collection of daily living tasks. They include self-care, chores, maintenance of one's living space, and those behaviors required for access to resources (traveling, shopping, and so forth). Daily living tasks are expected of all capable members of the social group; however, they seldom form a significant part of one's identity. Unlike work, daily living tasks do not contribute directly to the services or commodities of the social group, and they are not publicly valued like work. However, when an individual cannot perform them, the productivity of another social member such as a family member or a caretaker is required. Thus, daily living tasks are indirectly productive for the social group.

Play

The whole range of behaviors from childhood to old age constitute play. In youth, play predominates in daily life and involves exploratory, creative, and game behaviors. In adolescence and adulthood, it decreases in amount and transforms into hobbies, social recreation, sports, cultural celebration, and ritual. In old age, play once again becomes a predominant occupational behavior; it is generally referred to as leisure—a way of life earned through the labor of adulthood.

Continua of Occupational Behaviors

Occupational behaviors can be conceptualized as existing along continua. For instance, they range from serious to frivolous, from overtly productive to apparently useless, from private to public, and from formal to informal. On the one end of the continua, we find playful behaviors that are typically perceived as frivolous, private, and apparently not productive, though it will be shown later that they serve a very important utility for individuals and social groups. On the other end of the continua, we find the more serious, overtly useful, and public behaviors of work. Daily living tasks fall somewhere in between (Fig. 5-1). Although this schema reveals something about the differences in these occupations, it also demonstrates that their characteristics may overlap. This points out the difficulty in establishing clear criteria to differentiate occupational behaviors. Additionally, some occupational behaviors such as hobbies or amateur pursuits appear to exist on the border between work and play. Thus, it is helpful not only to recognize the continua of characteristics but also to note that the concepts of work, play, and daily living tasks are not always discrete and mutually exclusive.

The range of serious and frivolous activities and the formal and informal aspects of occupation can be a useful indication of someone's occupational adaptation. For instance, a person whose work is formal, serious, and highly productive may require play of the opposite character to counterbalance it.

Understanding more about the forms that occupations take would enhance the ability of therapists to deal with the occupational problems of clients and patients as well as their ability to use occupation therapeutically.

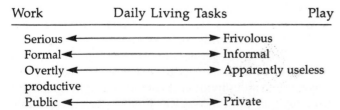

Figure 5-1. Continua of occupational behaviors.

Further theory and research are needed to augment the field's understanding of occupation through the life span, its various forms in culture, and the overall dynamics of occupation in an individual's life.

Occupation as an Evolutionary Trait

Human behavior is a product of a long period of biological and social–technical evolution. From the beginning of evolution, action was basic to survival; even the simplest organism is fundamentally spontaneous and active. The process of evolution, reflected in the phylogenetic scale, demonstrates a progressive increase in organisms' requirements and capacities for more and more complex actions.[34] With advanced nervous systems came an increase in the amount and diversity of action needed. This need first appears in the young, where spontaneous playful action is a means of learning basic skills that are biologically transmitted to members of lower, simpler species.[33] As the nervous system of a species advances to a more complex and adaptable form, the rigidity of biologically encoded ability is progressively left behind. Thus, behavior that is innate in simpler species' members must be learned by the individuals of higher species. That is, animals that have very specialized behavior acquire much of it through genetic inheritance, whereas more complex animals that adapt through their behavioral variability are less endowed with inherent programming but rather have brains with a greater capacity to organize the information from experience. Many theorists agree that play is the prerequisite for learning this flexible behavior. The play of the young of these more adaptable species is characterized by a greater urge to use capacity and by an exploratory urge that arises from the nervous system's requirement for experience as a learning process. Most mammals, in their immature period, romp, jump, run, engage in rough and tumble play, and explore objects and places, all with no apparent motive except the playing itself. Studies have supported the hypothesis that these animals must learn to use their bodies and to deal with their environment through this early form of play.[5]

In primate species and in humans, play is more elaborate and includes social acts, fine motor manipulation, tool use, and imitation.[2] In these play forms, the individual learns complex behaviors that are part of the retinue of skills making up its species' typical approach to adaptation. Play enables this learning because it is a nonserious practice in which the organism can make mistakes, engage in trial and error, and try out new behaviors without serious consequences.[2]

Human beings are at the apex of the evolutionary trend toward adaptation through flexible rather than specialized behaviors. The evolution of flexibility in human activity requires a highly plastic nervous system in the young, a behavioral mechanism to provide experience, a social system that supports and protects the young, and a process for storing the collective experience of members to provide a pool of information for the young to acquire.

The route to generalization (that is, adaptation through flexibility rather than specialization) that human beings followed in evolution is also reflected in the highly adaptive human hand and its intimate relationship with the brain. Together with the visual sense, they form a complex that greatly enhances the ability of the organism to explore and master its environment. The human hand is morphologically suited for extensive manipulation and exploration of objects in the environment. Consequently, there is a greatly enhanced capacity for gaining technological control over the environment by using and elaborating this eye–hand–brain complex. This is first represented in the emergence of tool use and later in tool making. Tools are primarily entensions of the hand,[35] and they represent elaboration of the urge to explore and to have effects on the world. While many species exhibit some primitive kinds of tool use, human beings alone are spontaneous and extensive tool makers and inventors. The invention of tools, which is a central component of the tremendous growth of technology characterizing human work throughout history, is, almost paradoxically, an outgrowth or product of play.[3] Behavioral flexibility that is gained in play[33] includes the production of extensions of biological equipment; that is, tool production.

Observations on semidomesticated monkeys provide a model for how play was responsible for the evolution of tool making in human life.[17] In free-ranging monkey troups that have a sufficient food supply provided by caretakers (hence the term semidomesticated), play becomes more prevalent in the young. From this play emerges a plethora of new behavior forms. Most are idiosyncratic and eventually die out, but some of these behaviors, which include forms of tool use, prove adaptive. Older monkeys learn the new behavior by imitating it, and eventually the behavior is spread through the troup and is learned by successive generations in their play as they imitate older monkeys. This is a primitive version of the evolutionary complex of humans (including a plastic nervous system, a behavioral mechanism for learning, a pressure-free social group, and imitation as a means of spreading and preserving individual experience in the group). In addition to these primate studies, investigations of children have found evidence that play with objects is an important precursor to the inventive use of objects as tools.[7,31] Thus, play is centrally important for the technological abilities of both individual members and the entire social group.

Play, tool use, the human hand, and the brain are all important and interrelated factors in human evolution where both behavior and physical morphology are changed in concert. Each interrelates with and influences the selective advantage of the other. Bruner[2] and Washburn[35] propose the following explanation for how human evolution took place. As prehominids left the jungle for the savannas, they gained adaptive advantage by standing upright on the tall grassy plains. Eventually, they relinquished brachiation for ambulation as a mode of locomotion. Simultaneously, the pressures of hunting and of surviving predators on the savanna required coordinated group efforts and individuals with more complex brains to initiate and interpret the communications. These had adaptive advantage.

This evolving animal with a larger brain had to be born through the smaller birth canal of the ambulator's stockier pelvis. Thus, the progeny of the changing prehominid were born more immature, with brains that would grow and mature substantially after birth. This more immature brain was, consequently, more plastic and suited to learning. Concurrently, the growing complexity of the social group included a division of labor, with some individuals serving as caretakers of helpless infants. This created an ideal environment for the emergence of more and more elaborate play forms. Young prehominids, protected by their mothers and having survival needs met by the work of the troup, were freed to engage in whatever nonserious pursuits they wished. Unlike the young of other species, who had to learn locomotion and other adult skills soon after birth or in a very short period of development, these individuals remained immature for years, during which they played and acquired more and more behavioral flexibility. In time, this youthful play produced a more creative and inventive adult likely to contribute technical or social advancement to the group. Since group members could readily communicate, they could also acquire and impart advances.

The end results of this evolutionary trend are the creative, aesthetic, and playful characteristics of the human being and the flexible behavior that characterizes the species. Human beings play more than any other animal. In addition, human beings have the unusual characteristic of elaborating their behavior far beyond that required by survival. For instance, hunting and gathering societies that require only about 18 hours of weekly labor for food gathering and other survival needs manage a long week spent in ritual and festive behaviors that require substantial energy and investment. By evolving a more complex culture, and thereby requiring members to acquire it, human societies are constantly advancing the demands on individuals for adaptation. This is poignantly demonstrataed when persons who manage to fulfill their basic survival needs, but violate social norms of conduct, are judged to be maladaptive.

Not only has the human brain evolved to be able to learn these cultural behaviors, but its very structure and processes are intimately interrelated with these varied behavior forms. The human being must acquire the complex behavior of culture to function at all.[17] In the course of evolution, the brain was programmed for exploration and mastery; consequently, individuals must engage in a wide range of occupational activities, especially early play, to use their biological inheritance properly.

As human culture becomes more elaborate, its demands for all forms of occupation increase. Accumulated technology and knowledge make the requirement for learning to work ever more demanding. In human history, simple imitation was replaced by apprenticeship. More recently, the explosion of human knowledge and technique expanded apprenticeship to a long period of public tutelage beginning with common knowledge and culminating (sometimes 20 or more years later) in specialized training. This process continues; just as mathematics and reading have become, in a few generations, almost essential for self-care and work, computer fluency will likely emerge as the new requirement for coming generations.

Thus, it can be seen that the process of human evolution has intimately involved occupation. Through evolution, the demands for both play and work have increased. Changes in the organism thrust the human species more and more toward both the capacity and the need for occupation. The human trait of occupation emerged in this evolutionary concatenation of a nervous system of growing complexity, increased playfulness, tool use, an increasing urge for action, and technical–social change and growth. The occupational nature of human beings is reflected throughout the modern human situation. Humans life begin as players, go through a long period of preparation for productivity, enter worker roles, and eventually return to a play-dominated phase in retirement. This schema of daily human life has its origins in a complex interrelated set of factors that have unfolded over eons. It is not by chance that human beings work, play, and care for themselves; it is biologically and socially encoded in the species.

Because occupation has been a central feature of human evolution, it fills an important place in the adaptive capacity of the species and its individual members. Without occupational activities, individuals would regress and be disorganized, if they survived at all. Without the playful and productive contributions of members, social and cultural life would cease. Occupation is so central to adaptation that when it is absent or distorted in the individual or culture, there is great cause for alarm. Importantly, the role of the occupational ther-apist centers on situations where individuals or groups have lost their occupational capabilities.

Occupation and the Biological Dimension

The complex nervous system of human beings requires rich and varied stimuli achievable only through active engagement of the world.[25] Occupation is centrally important in the development of biological features in childhood and their maintenance in adulthood. The nervous and musculoskeletal system of the child receives constant use through the childhood occupation of play. Play is an important arena for the neurological "programming" that the child's developing nervous system requires. Development is not just a predetermined change in the structures of the body but includes the effects of experiences that become imprinted into those biological structures.[3,34] All those neurological and musculoskeletal features that make possible such functions as coordinated movement and perception have much of their genesis in play.

In adulthood and in old age, occupation is important for maintaining biological functions. For instance, a severe restriction of occupational activities is associated with the impairment of strength, endurance, mobility, cardiovascular function, metabolism and nervous system function. Stress has long been recognized to be a major etiological factor in many biological problems. It has also been recognized that boredom or a lack of satisfying and meaningful occupations produces stress and thus ranks as a physiological threat. Along these same lines, longevity and health in old age are related to maintaining meaningful work and leisure throughout adulthood and old age.[6]

The mechanism by which occupation maintains healthy biological functioning is complex; only a little is understood about it. New relationships between occupation and biological well-being are constantly being discovered. For example, it was noted that running seemed to have a positive effect on depressed persons. Later it was discovered that such physical exertion is a catalyst for the release of catacholamines in the brain, which are the organism's natural antidepressants.[22]

It is theorized that the conscious functions of human beings engaged in the purposeful activity of occupation have direct controlling effects on the brain's physiology.[13,30] Such proposals, which attempt to bridge the mind–body dichotomy, are paving the way to a deeper understanding of how a human being's goal-directed use of time and energy reverberates throughout the organism, affecting basic biological processes. In sum, it may be argued that when a human being engages in meaningful occupation, mind and body function in an integrated and resonating manner. Thus, occupation plays a role in maintaining the biological organization of the organism.

The Psychological Dimension of Occupation

There is an intimate relationship between occupation and the psychological aspect of human beings. For the present discussion, the latter is defined as the symbolic (*i.e.,* temporal, meaningful, and purposive) and affective experience of the self and the world.

Childhood is an important determinant of children's growing sense of control over their world and their destiny; it is a source of their feeling of well-being. Children become aware of the effects they can have on the world, and they begin to develop a sense of personal causation —the belief that they have skills, can control events, and will succeed.[22] Without positive play experiences, this image of personal competence will not develop.

Play is also central to children's symbolic development.[3] Their growing awareness of time and its role in structuring activities and their growing sense of meaning or purpose, which can define positive existence, all accrue from play experience.[27]

In play, children learn the basic symbolic skills that enable them to deal with motion, objects, people, and events. These have been referred to as the rules that children internalize about their actions and their environment.[27] These rules form an internal map of external reality and its potentials for action. Children deprived of play experiences are poorer practical problem solvers, are less creative, have less information about their environment, and exhibit less flexible and adaptive approaches to their environment.[7,32] In play, children learn a growing sense of time as they sequence events, take turns, and compartmentalize activities into meaningful episodes. Eventually, as the child's sense of time grows, there is an increasing future orientation. Children, in their fantasy, begin to bridge the transition to the future and, in so doing, create purposes and meanings for themselves about their own existence. The simple dramatic play of a child serves a deep purpose of allowing the child to experience some of the meaning of being a parent, firefighter, nurse, or other adult figure. Paradoxically, the fantasy of childhood is an important process for developing a healthy sense of reality and of how one can competently face and master the requirements of life.

As the child develops, the growing necessity of being productive slowly emerges. The child first learns tasks of self-care, advances to chores, and by adolescence begins entry into work situations. The less serious productive roles that children and adolescents perform in the home are important precursers of competence in adult life.[18] In the transition from childhood to adulthood, the individual also undergoes the important process of occupational choice.[37] The combined experiences of dramatic play, childhood activities yielding interests, a growing sense of meaning and value, and realistic experiences of older childhood and adolescence culminate in the consequential choice to enter or begin preparation for a kind of work. As might be expected, children with poor play experiences and little opportunity for chores and recognition by adults may fail in this occupational choice process, and they may enter into a vicious cycle of dissatisfaction and failure in their adult work careers.[8]

Daily living tasks and work are critical adult activities. For most individuals, they are a means of earning a living and contributing to the maintenance of a household. The work role is valued by society, so that working is often the primary source of self-esteem and feelings of control and competence. Work is a means of pursuing personal interests and of developing personal abilities. Many persons who find they cannot meet these needs in work will seek to do so in their recreation or in a more serious amateur pursuit. This reflects the fact that human beings have a need for occupation far beyond that dictated by sheer survival.

Work is a major factor in the structuring of time throughout adult life. Daily and weekly routines are often dictated by the work schedule. The work career may imply a structured sequence of years of advancement through steps or positions in a given line of work. Individuals measure their own growth, and they progress by their advancement in time through a series of jobs, positions, or work titles. Failure to meet socially normative patterns of advancement can result in a loss of self-esteem and a sense of being out of control.

Satisfaction in work ordinarily requires that the person be able to exercise and develop skills he or she values, to find work interesting, and to see tangible results of his or her efforts. The satisfaction and sense of personal mastery that comes from work of whatever type is an important source of mental health in the adult. When persons begin to fail in their work roles, or when they cannot meet their needs for satisfaction in work, they can become candidates for mental illness.[29] The stress of not being able to find meaning in one's existence is being recognized increasingly as a significant etiological factor in mental illness.[12] The growing trend in modern industrial societies toward impersonal, mechanized, and noncreative work has already initiated an epidemic of persons who exhibit maladaptive lifestyles. As people become disengaged from the meaning of work and its potential for self-satisfaction, they become alienated from society, demonstrate deviant behaviors, and lead unhappy and often disorganized lives.

As this trend continues, occupational therapy will have to address a whole new area of health problems that come directly from the disintegration of normal occupation. Such a demand will require occupational therapists to compel and encourage institutions and workplaces to make changes that would restore the health of individuals.[16]

Although adult life is still largely dominated by work, there has been a growing trend toward more leisure in modern society. Today, the leisure or recreational period of an adult's life is likely to be substantial and to have a large impact on life-satisfaction. Vacations, weekends, and retirement are life spaces that the individual literally earns through work. Adult life involves a dynamic balance of work, play, and sleep patterns. If balance is not preserved, the individual may have a dysfunction of his or her occupational life with other consequences, such as a loss of life satisfaction and erosion of competence.[29]

Old age in modern society is marked by a major transition from working to enjoying leisure. This is often a period of adjustment; persons who have a well-developed leisure role before retirement (those who have hobbies, or other avocational interests) generally have less difficulty adjusting to retirement. However, for many elderly persons, physical problems, lack of resources, and environmental constraints limit opportunities for engaging in sufficient occupational activities; when this is true, life satisfaction is less.[14]

The Social Dimension of Occupation

The role of occupation in social life can be described in terms of the contributions of both work and play. As already noted, play was a central mechanism in the evolution of the human species, having been responsible for the elaboration and creation of new behaviors that eventually entered the cultural repertoire of the social group. It also served to initiate the immature into the demands of the physical and social environment. In modern society, play still prepares the young for adult life in a particular social group. The special beliefs, values, ways of interacting, and technology of the social group are reflected in the play of the young who are thereby inducted into a way of living. For instance, social groups that stress competition in adult interaction have young who play competitive games, whereas social groups that stress cooperation in social interaction have a remarkable absence of competitive games in childhood[4]; instead, children play to maximize everyone's status. In primitive tribes, children play with bows and arrows and the artifacts of that group; children in modern societies play with toy trucks, stoves, and other implements of modern culture. Play also keeps pace with the changes in the culture's technology. For instance, the appearance of electronic games in the play of today's young is an important precurser of a new generation for whom computer fluency will be highly desirable in adult adaptation. The games of each culture thus reflect its requirements so that the young learn how to participate in the culture through their play. The simple and seemingly unimportant play activities of children serve a vital function of maintaining the continuity of social knowledge and of bringing to the young the technology of the social system.

In human social life, play serves a vital role well beyond the childhood years. Adult play is important for reaffirming the culture's values,[9] a way of stepping back and of affirming the fundamental tenets of a culture. For instance, the football game has been analyzed as a metaphor for the competition, teamwork, and technical precision that characterize American work.[1] Adult players and spectators become intensely involved in the emotion and meaning of the game at a symbolic level; this serves in subtle ways to cement their commitment to the way of life of their social group. The celebrative or festive and ritual forms of adult play are critical for the maintenance of social life. Graduation ceremonies, the Fourth of July, religious rituals, Thanksgiving dinner, and other forms of celebration allow the individual to take account of accomplishments, worthwhile things in life, and central values. These forms of play are critical to the spirit of the culture.

When adult play forms begin to change, it may signal that cultural change is on the way.[21] When such play becomes disrupted or when members of a group lose their affinity to such play forms, a culture may be in deep trouble. It is notable that individuals who find themselves alienated from social life (for example, the mentally ill) often find holidays intolerable and have difficulty celebrating. Despite its often frivolous and unproductive facade, the play of adult life is an important process in social life. It is a dynamic that maintains the morale, commitment, and value structure of the social group. Although its contributions to the social group are less apparent than those of work, it should never be construed as less important.

Work is a basic fact of all social groups. Human societies are characterized by a division in labor in which individuals take on specialized functions. Rarely do individual human beings perform the whole range of labor necessary for self-preservation. Rather, tasks are traditionally divided according to age, sex, social position, and aptitude. Each worker depends in some important way on the contributions of others. In modern society, there is greater specialization of work than at any other time. The network of productive contributions in American society is almost unfathomable. From the perspective of social life, important contributions extend beyond paid labor. In fact, marketplace waged productivity is only a small portion of the actual work that keeps a society functioning. Everything from the household chores done by the young through volunteer work, homemaking, and mutual assistance in families and neighborhoods to the leadership jobs in government are necessary for the maintenance of social life. It is for this reason that societies value the productive contributions of their members. The young are inducted into an ethic that defines social expectations for their work. In response, adults feel a sense of self-worth and affiliation with the social group by virtue of making productive contributions.

Some trends in modern life raise questions about the future of work in society. The substitution of mechanical and electronic processes for human labor and thinking, as well as economic processes that do not demand everyone's contribution, may have ill effects for both the group and the individual. The social group not only needs the work of its members, but it owes them the opportunity to work. The reciprocity of the individual and the social group in productive exchange is a central feature of human life. Without work, neither the social group nor the individual is adaptive.

One possibility for modern society is the emergence of new valued and valuable work forms. Volunteerism is an important factor in social life today, and it serves both individual and group needs. Hobbies have often been turned into productive pursuits that benefit others. In a society with increasing numbers of disabled, elderly, and unemployed individuals, such emerging nontraditional work forms may well be a useful answer. However, to function, they must become part of the cultural fabric; thus, social change is required. For occupational therapists, the implication is involvement in social action as well as individual assistance. Functions such as organizing volunteer groups of disabled persons or running hobby shops for the elderly could be important types of socially based occupational therapy in the future.

Occupation and Therapy

The previous sections examine several facets of the proposed definition of occupation. This final part will discuss the consequences of these characteristics of occupation for therapy. Basically, there are two implications: (1) since occupation is so central to human adaptation, its absence or disruption (irrespective of any other medical or social problem) is a threat to health, and (2) when illness, trauma, or social conditions have affected the biological or psychological health of an individual, occupation is an effective means for reorganizing behavior.

Although these two statements separate disruption of occupation from medical illness for conceptual clarity, it should be realized that many clients seen by occupational therapists show a complex of interrelated problems involving both a medical problem and a loss or disruption of occupation. Often the picture is compli-

cated when the disorder is a developmental or long-standing one. For instance, children with minimal brain dysfunction may be poor players because of the damaged equipment they have for play. The paucity of play, in turn, slows the developmental process, exacerbating the original problem. Another example is the elderly person whose waning physical abilities force confinement to an institution where there are no opportunities to pursue some lifelong occupation; this may cause depression and lead to physical deterioration.

Sometimes a medical problem is not involved initially, as when a person loses an occupation by virtue of social circumstances; for instance, loss of a job or rearing in an environment that failed to nurture play. However, such disruption of occupation can lead to psychological and biological dysfunctions. Depression, physiological correlates of the stress of boredom, and manifold other medical problems may have their etiology in the lack of normal occupation.

Occupational therapists intervene with carefully guided and organized activities. These occupational activities often influence both the occupational dysfunction and any extant medical problem. Since the two are likely to be intermingled to begin with, the use of occupation as therapy is often an especially efficacious approach. To use the previous examples, engagement of children in more rich and varied play will not only allow them to acquire normal play behaviors but will have an organizing and maturing effect on their nervous systems. Providing opportunities for elderly persons to pursue valued occupations will not only restore morale but will provide exercise of their physical capacities.

As the organizing influence of occupation is more fully understood, occupational therapists will become increasingly able to expand its therapeutic use. This will require careful study and the development of theories that explain the dynamics and characteristic of occupation. One must have a thorough understanding of any tool to use it effectively. Since an occupational therapist's unique and powerful tool is occupation, it behooves the field and the individual therapist to achieve a deep understanding of it.

References

1. Arens W: Playing with aggression. In Cherfas J, Lewin R: Not Work Alone: A Cross-Cultural View of Activities Superfluous to Survival. Beverly Hills, Sage Publications. 1980
2. Bruner J: Nature and uses of immaturity. Am Psychol 27:687, 1972
3. Bruner J: The organization of early skilled action. Child Dev 44:1, 1973
4. Cherfas J: It's only a game. In Cherfas J, Lewin R: Not Work Alone: A Cross-Cultural View of Activities Superfluous to Survival. Beverly Hills: Sage Publications, 1980
5. Cherfas J, Lewin R: Not Work Alone: A Cross-Cultural

View of Activities Superfluous to Survival. Beverly Hills, Sage Publications, 1980

6. Cousins N: Anatomy of an Illness. New York, Bantam, 1981
7. Dansky J, Silverman I: Effects of play on associate fluency in preschool children. In Bruner J, Jolly A, Sylva K (eds): Play—Its Role in Development and Evolution. New York, Basic Books, 1976
8. de Renne–Stephen C: Imitation: A mechanism of play behavior. Am J Occup Ther 34:95, 1980
9. Duthie J: The ritual of a technological society? In Schwartzman HB (ed): Play and Culture. West Point, NY Leisure Press, 1980
10. Finn G: The occupational therapist in prevention programs. Am J Occup Ther 31:658, 1977
11. Florey L: Intrinsic motivation: The dynamics of occupational therapy theory. Am J Occup Ther 23:319, 1969
12. Frankl V: Man's Search for Meaning: An Introduction to Logotherapy. New York, Washington Square Press, 1982
13. Furst C: Origins of the Mind: Mind–Brain Connections. Englewood Cliffs, NJ, Prentice–Hall, 1979
14. Gregory M: Occupation behavior and life satisfaction among retirees, Master's thesis, Virginia Commonwealth University, 1981
15. Johnson J: Old values—new directions: Competence, adaptation, integration. Am J Occup Ther 35:589, 1981
16. Johnson J, Kielhofner G: The role of occupational therapy in the health care system of the future. In Kielhofner G (ed): Health Through Occupation: Theory and Practice in Occupational Therapy. Philadelphia, FA Davis, 1983
17. Kawai M: Newly acquired pre-cultural behavior of the natural troop of Japanese monkeys on the Koshima Islet. Primates 6:1, 1956
18. Kielhofner G: A model of human occupation 2: Ontogenesis from the perspective of temporal adaptation. Am J Occup Ther 34:657, 1980
19. Kielhofner G, Burke J: Occupational therapy after 60 years: An account of changing identity and knowledge. Am J Occup Ther 31:675, 1977
20. Kielhofner G, Burke J: A model of human occupation 1: Framework and content. Am J Occup Ther 34:572, 1980
21. Lavenda R: From festival of progress to masque of degradation: Carnival in Carcas as a changing metaphor for social reality. In Schwartzman HB (ed): Play and Culture. West Point, NY, Leisure Press, 1980
22. Leer F: Running as an adjunct to psychotherapy. Social Work, January 1980, pp 20–25
23. Matsutsuyu J: Occupational behavior—a perspective on work and play. Am J Occup Ther 25:291, 1971
24. Meyer A: The philosophy of occupational therapy. Am J Occup Ther 31:639, 1977
25. Reilly M: Occupational therapy can be one of the great ideas of 20th century medicine. Am J Occup Ther 16:1, 1962
26. Reilly M: Occupational therapy—a historical perspective: The modernization of occupational therapy. Am J Occup Ther 25:243, 1971
27. Robinson A: Play: The arena for the acquisition of rules of competent behavior. Am J Occup Ther 31:248, 1977
28. Rogers J: Order and disorder in occupational therapy and in medicine. Am J Occup Ther 36:29, 1982
29. Shannon P: The work–play model: A basis for occupational therapy programming. Am J Occup Ther 24:215, 1970
30. Sperry R: An objective approach to subjective experience: Further evaluation of a hypothesis. Psychol Rev 77:585, 1970
31. Sylva K, Bruner J, Genova P: The role of play in the problem-solving of children 3–5 years old. In Bruner J, Jolly A, Sylva K (eds): Play—Its Role in Development and Evolution. New York, Basic Books, 1976
32. Training Teachers for Occupational Therapy for the Rehabilitation of Disabled Soldiers and Sailors. Federal Board for Vocations Education Bulletin No. 6, p 13. Washington DC, US Government Printing Office, 1918
33. Vandenberg B, Kielhofner G: Play in evolution, culture, and individual adaptation: Implications for therapy. Am J Occup Ther 36:20, 1982
34. von Bertalanffy L: General systems theory and psychiatry. In Arieti S (ed): American Handbook of Psychiatry, Vol 3, New York, Basic Books, 1969
35. Washburn S: Tools and evolution. Sci Am 203(2):63, 1960
36. Watanabe S: Four concepts basic to the occupational therapy process. Am J Occup Ther 22:339, 1968
37. Webster PS: Occupational role development in the young adult with mild mental retardation. Am J Occup Ther 34:13, 1980
38. Weimer R: Traditional and Nontraditional Practice Arenas in Occupational Therapy: 2001 AD, pp 42–53. Rockville, MD, American Occupational Therapy Association, 1979
39. Woodside H: Dimensions of the occupational behavior model. Can J Occup Ther 43:11, 1976
40. Yerxa E: Oversimplification: The hobgoblin of occupational therapy. Presented at the American Occupational Therapy Association Conference, Portland, OR, 1983

CHAPTER 6

Occupational Therapy – Base in Activity

Helen L. Hopkins
and
Elizabeth G. Tiffany

The things human beings do and the objects they make provide a bridge between their inner reality and their external world. In their activities they show their concern with how to survive, be comfortable, have pleasure, solve problems, express themselves, and be related with others and the wider world of society. They experience themselves and come to know their strengths and weaknesses or limits through the things they do. The roles they assume have inherent functions, skills, and behaviors that are necessary to support them. There are, for example, characteristic activities that are necessary for the student, parent, store manager, beach bum, and so forth. It is probably for these reasons, more than for any others, that occupational therapy, with its emphasis on the use of activity to promote function, came into being.

Characteristics of Occupational Therapy Activity

In occupational therapy, the term *occupation* is used "in the context of man's goal-directed use of time, energy, interest and attention."[6] Thus occupation consists of being occupied productively in activities that "are primary agents for learning and development and an es-

sential source of satisfaction"[3] (see Chap. 5). Activities as used in occupational therapy should have at least eight characteristics:

1. *Be goal directed.* Activities should have some purpose or reason for their use to be considered occupational therapy activity. "Busy work," or just keeping the hands occupied, may be of some value to the client, but generally it is not chosen with a specific goal in mind.

2. *Have significance at some level to the client.* Activities should have value and usefulness to the client, even though the value may be realized only at some future date. That is, the activity may seem to have no immediate value in reaching a specified goal but will make it possible to reach that goal in a week, a month, or some time later. The activity should have some relationship to the roles the individual plays in society.

3. *Require client involvement at some level* (either mental or physical). Activities require "doing" or participation on the part of the client. The individual engaged in the activity should be involved in selecting the activity as well as in the performance of it and thus receives self-gratification from the results. He or she is not a recipient but rather a participant. Participation may be active or passive.

4. *Be geared to prevention of malfunction and/or maintenance or improvement of function and quality of life.* The choice and type of activity is dependent on the client's level of function and ability to participate; however, the goal is clear.

5. *Reflect client involvement in life task situations* (ADL, play, work). Activities are used to acquire or redevelop those skills essential for fulfillment of life roles. Activities develop competence in the performance of those tasks essential to the life roles of each individual.

6. *Relate to the interests of the client.* Involvement in the choice of activity is vital. Commitment to the tasks will be attained only if client goals and interests are considered and met.

7. *Be adaptable and gradable.* Activity must be age appropriate, be able to be increased or decreased in complexity, and be graded in time and strength required.

8. *Be determined through the occupational therapist's professional judgment based on knowledge.* Knowledge of human development, medical pathology, interpersonal relationships, and value of activity to the person are required to make the match between client problems and the activities that will be most meaningful and serviceable in reaching the therapeutic goals of occupational therapy.

These eight characteristics are among the fundamental precepts that define occupational therapy. It is in the *application* of the activity that the effectiveness of occupational therapy as a mode of treatment for dysfunction or as a promoter of well-being is experienced.

Some element of volition is involved in mental, physical, and social activities. It is the volitional aspect of activities that is important in the occupational therapy process. The use of carefully planned activity to facilitate change is a unique characteristic of occupational therapy. Activities to be used are influenced, of course, by the total treatment context but may also be significant in determining the nature of that context. Limitations on the kinds of activities to be used are often imposed by the environment, materials, or resources available as well as by the therapist's knowledge, skill, interests, and creativity.

In 1981, Fidler referred to the concept of purposefulness in activities as fundamental to the occupational therapy process.[2] She suggested that two assumptions are made about the meaning and use of activities:

One assumption fundamental to the use of purposeful activity may be expressed as: A society's values and norms *weight* certain tasks and activities. Mastery and competence in those activities and tasks that are valued and given priority by one's society or social group have greater meaning in *describing* and *defining* one's social efficacy than mastery and competence in activities carrying less

social significance. This assumption speaks to the social relevance of an activity.

A second assumption may be framed as: An individual's unique neurobiology and psychology *weight* certain tasks and activities so that mastery and competence in these are more readily achieved and have greater meaning to that individual in terms of intrinsic gratification, personal pleasure, and satisfaction. This assumption relates to matching an activity to the person.

She went on to refer to the idea that every activity has social, cultural, and personal meanings that are both real and symbolic.

With these ideas in mind, occupational therapists have used activities in a number of ways. General categories into which occupational therapy activities may fall include body movement, individual and team sports, games, crafts, personal hygiene and grooming, activities of daily living or life skills, prevocational practice, horticulture, work, and creative activity. Activities may be used as part of the initial assessment and have, inherently, a function in the ongoing evaluation process. Observation or measurement of the client's performance, behavior, and end product in the execution of an activity can yield much information valuable in determining the directions of treatment. The relatively objective nature of data obtained in the activity process is valuable to the therapist and to other members of the treatment team. Most importantly, it is valuable to the client.

A difficult problem sometimes encountered with clients is their inability to understand their personal assets and limitations. Often, activities that involve manipulating objects, tools, and materials and producing something finished at the end provide concrete evidence that can be used to help the client test reality about himself or herself.

Activities used within a group context may provide opportunities to explore and practice dimensions of interpersonal relationships, to give and receive support, and to experience cooperative working on an individual or a collective task. Freely creative activities can provide communication links between the therapist and the client on deeper levels than may be experienced in structured tasks.

Activities can provide the basis for *exploration* and *learning, practicing,* and *achieving mastery.* They permit participation from the simplest, developmentally earliest, and nonverbal levels. It is the task of the occupational therapist to understand the meaning of activity and to know how to determine the potential of each given activity for promoting performance.

Activity Analysis

The first consideration in the use of activity therapeutically is understanding the activity and its *explicit* components; that is, the aspects of the activity which are evident and will be present regardless of the context, the therapeutic goals, or the frame of reference within which the activity is to be used. The dimensions of any activity include: the *analysis* of the adaptive skills required; the *skill level* needed to accomplish the activity at a minimal level; the *gradability* of the activity in terms of skill levels, time to accomplish, and repetition; its *flexibility* in terms of space, equipment, and supplies; its *cultural implications; age-appropriateness; safety considerations;* and *cost.*

The accompanying sample form focuses on general activity analysis based on explicit data. It is presented here primarily as an indicator of the range of considerations that might be attended to in planning the use of a specific activity.

The application of an activity, or the making of the *match* between the activity and the client, is critical to the process. Mosey defines the process as *activity synthesis,* "combining component parts of the human and nonhuman environment so as to design an activity suitable for evaluation or intervention."[5] It is at this point that the data collected regarding the activity and the client must be seen within the perspective of a *frame of reference.* The frame of reference defines the choice of activity and the aspects of that activity that will promote the goals of the intervention. The frame of reference will determine which dimensions of the activity are to be emphasized and the depth to which some of the dimensions are to be explored and exploited. For example, a biomechanical frame of reference will be most concerned with the motor aspects of the activity, where as a psychoanalytic frame of reference will be concerned with its symbolic potential. Activity analysis based on a behavioral frame of reference will be concerned especially with the specification and seriation of the component parts of the activity, their potential as, or the need for, reinforcement contingencies, and the measurability of the data. A sensory-integrative frame of reference will focus on the sensory, perceptual, and physical aspects of the activity. A developmental perspective will be concerned with the parallels between the levels of functioning required or expected and developmental levels. Within an occupational behavior perspective, the concern will be for the potential of the activity to promote competence and balance within the individual's life roles in society.

The Therapeutic Application of Activity

Keeping in mind the importance of the frame of reference in determining the specific ways in which activity synthesis is to take place, there are general considerations which may be applied to most situations.

Therapeutic application of activity to meet the specific needs of each client requires that the choice of activity be made on the basis of those activity properties that seem to have an impact on the previously identified problems. Consideration must be given to all factors that may have an impact on the individual's ability to function, including physical, psychosocial, cultural, and economic factors. The activity may need to be adapted to provide the desired amount of complexity, the correct exercise, or the desired amount of social interaction. Successful completion of the activity promotes development of competence. Clients' interest and involvement may be enhanced by providing feedback on their progress. Some activities utilized in the treatment of physical dysfunction allow the use of biofeedback to indicate correct use of muscles and adequate performance. Interaction between the therapist and the client, which provides reassurance and encouragement as well as accurate perception of function, is vital to the therapeutic process.

In conditions involving physical dysfunction, the activities are selected for their physical restorative powers as well as for their psychological and psychosocial properties. They must be constructive and provide the desired exercise. This enables the client to translate the motion, strength, and coordination gained to normal activity, thus providing the additional psychological value of success in achievement. Activities used for treatment of physical disabilities must be adaptable so they can provide specific exercise for affected joints or muscles. Activities should be in accord with the following criteria to meet physical restoration requirements[8]:

1. *Provide action rather than position.* Activity should provide for alternate contraction and relaxation of muscles. Activities should be analyzed from a kinesiological point of view to determine their components, the motions required, the muscle power required, and the range of motion and strengthening the activity can provide.

2. *Require repetition of the motion.* Activity should permit repetition of the desired motion for an indefinite but controllable number of times.

3. *Permit gradation in the range of motion, resistance, and coordination.* Activity should allow a greater range of motion than is permitted by the limitation in the joint so the activity can allow for increase in *joint range. Resistance* is required in order to strengthen a muscle. Thus the activity should be gradable in the amount of resistance it provides so that resistance can be increased as power returns. When *coordination* is affected, the activity should be graded so that it provides exercise requiring gross coordination and working toward fine coordination. The activity may also be varied or adapted through positioning or by changing the way the task is performed.

(Text continues on page 98)

ACTIVITY ANALYSIS FORM

Activity analyzed:
Average time required for completion:
Average number of sessions required to complete:
Brief description: (include criteria for determining success)

Activity Characteristics   *Explanations*

	Skill required ✓	Degree Low Medium High	Is activity gradable? How?
A. MOTOR			
1. Position:			
a. activity			
b. patient/client			
2. Motion(s) components			
a. joints involved			
b. motion(s) involved			
3. Muscles utilized			
4. Direction of resistance			
5. Action rather than position			
6. Repetition of motion(s)			
7. Rhythm developed			
8. Maintained contraction (static)			
9. Manual dexterity			
10. Gross motor			
11. Fine motor			
12. Bilateral			
13. Unilateral			
14. Endurance			
15. Rate of performance			
16. Grading adaptability			
a. R.O.M.			
b. resistance			
c. coordination			
d. substitution			
B. SENSORY			
1. Visual			
2. Auditory (impact on)			
3. Gustatory			
4. Olfactory			
5. Tactile			
a. temperature of material			
b. texture of material			
c. heavy to light touch			
C. COGNITIVE			
1. Organizational ability			
2. Problem solving ability			
a. planning			
b. trial and error			
3. Logical thinking			
4. Concentration			
5. Attention span			
6. Written/oral/demonstration directions			
a. complex			
b. simple			
7. Reading			
8. Seriation			
9. Interpret signs & symbols			
10. Multiple processing/steps involved			
11. Creativity			
12. Use of imagination			
13. Establish goal & carry out means to attain it			
14. Causal relationships involved (perceive cause & effect)			
15. Centering			

Activity Characteristics	Skill required ✓	Degree Low Medium High	Is activity gradable? How?
16. Perceive viewpoint of others			
17. Test reality			
D. PERCEPTUAL			
1. Sensory integration required			
2. Differentiation			
a. Figure-ground			
b. Space relationships			
c. Object constancy			
d. Kinesthesia			
e. Proprioception			
f. Stereognosis			
g. Form constancy			
h. Color perception			
i. Auditory perception			
3. Tactile integration			
4. Motor planning			
5. Bilateral integration			
6. Body scheme			
7. Vestibular			
E. EMOTIONAL			
1. Passive or aggressive motion			
2. Destructive			
3. Gratification			
a. immediate			
b. delayed			
4. Structured			
5. Unstructured			
6. Allows control			
7. Success/failure possibility			
8. Independence			
9. Dependence			
10. Symbolism involved			
11. Reality testing			
12. Handle feelings			
13. Impulse control			
F. SOCIAL			
1. Interaction required			
2. Isolating activity			
3. Group activity			
4. Competition			
5. Responsibility involved			
6. Communication necessary			
7. Work in small groups			
8. Work in large groups			
9. Work with one other person			
10. Test reality			
11. Control—lead			
12. Follow—cooperate			
G. CULTURAL			
1. Relevancy to personal			
a. Value system			
b. Life situations			
H. COMMON TO ALL			
1. Age appropriateness			
2. Safety precautions & hazards			
3. Sexual identification			
4. Space required			
5. Equipment needed			
6. Vocational application			
7. Cost			
8. Adaptability			

The psychosocial aspects of activities need to be considered in the treatment of clients with all kinds of disabilities, but certain psychodynamic properties are of primary consideration in psychiatric occupational therapy. These include[1]:

1. Property of materials—resistive, pliable, controlled, or messy, as well as the sensory input they provide (tactile, auditory, olfactory, visual, proprioceptive)
2. Complexity of the activity—number of steps in the activity and the repetition required
3. Preparation required—arrangement of supplies, adaptation of environment
4. Amount and type of directions—oral or written directions, diagrams, demonstration
5. Inherent structure and controls (rules)
6. Predictability of results
7. Type of learning required—old learning, adapted old learning, or new learning
8. Decision making required on part of patient
9. Attention span—minutes or hours
10. Interaction—solitary; parallel; with peers, small group, large group; cooperation
11. Communication—nonverbal, little, oral directions, reading, writing
12. Motivation—creative, gratifying, intellectually challenging, effect on others, relevance to life space and roles
13. Time—completion of activity in one session or sessions, quick success, delayed gratification

In working with children, a combination of psychosocial, psychodynamic, physical, and developmental factors must be considered. The activities may be required to provide specific aspects relating to normal growth and development and must be age-appropriate in complexity and the dexterity required, yet may need to provide some aspects that promote physical function and that promote psychological well-being.

Prevocational activities are selected on the basis of their ability to contribute to work-related skills. They must be selected for their relationship to the components of the actual work requirements such as physical performance, coordination, concentration, speed and accuracy, endurance, routinization and boredom factors, initiative, and decision making.

For individuals with sensory-integration problems (cognitive-perceptual-motor dysfunction), the sensory stimuli presented by the activity must be analyzed along with the "intersensory-integrative mechanisms involved and the motor response required."[4] Thus tactile, kinesthetic, visual, auditory, and olfactory sensations must be analyzed for each activity along with the type of response required (motor, visual, and verbal). Activity analysis in this area requires analysis of the neurological integration of the input from the senses and the muscu-

lar response to this stimulation and integration, and it is therefore called the neurobehavioral approach to activity analysis. Activities must be analyzed with all the components in mind in order to choose the one most appropriate to meet all therapeutic requirements.[4]

In selecting an activity to be used in the therapeutic process, the therapist must answer five basic questions:

1. *How* do you do the activity? The therapist must know the components of the activity, the process involved, and the tools, equipment, and supplies needed, and he/she must know how to do it well enough to be able to teach it.
2. *What* activity is most appropriate for the requirements of the situation? The therapist must assess the problems involved; the needs, interests, and preferences of the patient/client; and, with the individual, determine the activity that best meets the requirements for therapeutic intervention.
3. *Why* was a specific activity chosen? The therapist must be able to determine the reason for the choice of activity on the basis of a frame of reference that is consistent with the overall treatment rationale.
4. *Where* will the activity be performed? The therapist may be constrained in the choice of an activity by the location or situation within which the activity will be carried out. For example, if the activity is to be done by an individual in bed, it cannot be too messy or require large tools or equipment.
5. *When* will the activity be carried out? The time of day or season of the year may influence the type of activity that is relevant. For example, self-care activities are most logically carried out at the time of day when they are usually done; for example, bathing and dressing before breakfast. Relevance may be dictated by the time of year; for example, making decorations or presents at Christmas.

The Nonhuman Environment

Any discussion of the use of activities in occupational therapy is a discussion designed to raise one's consciousness of the value of the nonhuman environment in providing tools for therapeutic intervention. The importance of the nonhuman world has been eloquently addressed by Searles,[7] who describes the impact of human–nonhuman relationships in normal development and in the treatment of individuals whose lives were disordered.

The term "nonhuman environment" refers to objects, such as tools, furniture, toys, pets, plants, cars, art, dishes, wood, yarn, and clay and to places, such as a room, a stairwell, a swimming pool, a beach, a crowded street, or a forest. In essence, the nonhuman environment includes all those things that are part of the human experience but are not men, women, or children. The nonhuman environment is characterized by such features as colors, temperature, smells, textures, movement, stillness, physical dimensions, and degrees of predictability.

Occupational therapists have long been aware of Searles' discussions of the nonhuman environment. Much of the treatment planning in occupational therapy has either deliberately or intuitively relied on the use of tools, supplies, equipment, and space to further the goals of treatment. The use of a hammock, a big beach ball, bright toys, bells, music, and scents, for instance, relates to the earliest and most enduring human experience of the nonhuman world as *stimulation*. Early in life, the nonhuman world allows the individual to experience the *difference between self and not-self*. By getting to know that the teddy bear is separate from himself, the child begins to be aware of his own separate entity. Throughout life, the nonhuman world clearly has the potential of providing a sense of *security* and *predictability*. Security, experienced physically through warm clothing, food, a piece of furniture, or a favorite spot in the woods, gets translated into symbolic terms identified with caring and being nurtured. The sense of "all rightness" is fostered by the experience of textures, pressure, and the unchanging nature of an object. The nonhuman world allows human beings to *express feelings* in ways and with objects that may seem safer than would other human beings. For example, the teddy bear can be spanked or cuddled; the golf ball can be driven across the green; the clay can be wedged. The nonhuman world thus can provide a *practice ground* for human-to-human interactions. It also provides a challenge for the *development of skills* and *experiences of competence and mastery*. Learning to ride a bike, to drive a car, to read a book, to knit a scarf, to bake a cake, or to work a computer are examples of the infinite number of experiences that are part of the process of living.

Consideration of the nonhuman environment is of paramount importance because of the richness of its potential for influencing change and promoting growth. Awareness of less-than-positive experiences with the nonhuman environment that may be described in a client's history may give clues to deficit areas for which remediation can be planned. Examples of this might be lack of play objects or of predictable living space or presentation of the nonhuman world in a place where war is a fact of life. The occupational therapy repertoire of possibilities is big. In using supplies, equipment, space, and tangible objects as tools, occupational therapy has a wide range of nonhuman possibilities to incorporate into the treatment process.

The Teaching–Learning Process

In order to use activity therapeutically, each occupational therapist must become adept in giving individuals or groups instructions in the processes involved. Therapists must also learn to make astute observations regarding how the activity is approached, the way it is carried out, and the work habits exhibited in the performance of the activity. These nonverbal cues can assist the therapist in determining the functional level of the individual.

Occupational therapists must know how to teach the processes involved in an activity so that the client understands clearly what is to be done, yet requires a minimum amount of correction and supervision. The better the instruction, the greater the chance of success, and the more successful the experiences, the greater the competency gained. It is therefore vital that the therapist determine the complexity of the activity to be certain it is within the ability of the individual.

Preparation for Instruction

Successful instruction requires preparation by the therapist. The therapist should analyze the processes and the steps along with the key points involved in the performance of the activity. This is called the *breakdown of the activity*. The *important steps* are the component parts of the total activity, while the *key points* are the specific steps involved in performance of the activity (Table 6-1).

The therapist should have the proper tools, necessary materials, and equipment ready for use before beginning instruction. The work area should be arranged

Table 6-1. *Example of Breakdown of an Activity (Typing on Standard Typewriter)*

Important Steps	*Key Points*
1. Insert paper in typewriter	1. Pick up paper
	2. Insert paper at back of platen
	3. Pull paper release lever forward
	4. Slide paper to typing level and adjust
	5. Snap paper release into place
2. Type	1. Place fingers on "home" keys
	2. Type to end of line
	3. Push carriage return lever to return carriage and move paper to next line
3. Take paper out of typewriter	1. Pull paper release forward
	2. Remove paper
	3. Snap paper release into place

properly with a minimum of clutter so that work can be conducted safely and without strain. Before beginning, consideration must be given to how much of the activity may be accomplished in one session. A simple activity with few steps may be taught in a half-hour session, whereas a more complex activity with many steps may require several sessions to accomplish. The activity of typing, for example, with three steps, may be accomplished in one session with many individuals and might be considered to be one unit of learning. However, becoming adept in typing is not possible in one session. Activities such as dressing may have several units of learning such as (1) put on shirt and button it, (2) put on slacks and fasten, (3) put on socks, and (4) put on shoes and tie them. Each unit may need to be taught in one or more sessions with repetition required for competence.

Steps in Instruction[8]

After the therapist has made all preparations, instruction may begin using a combination of verbal directions and demonstration. There are four basic steps in instruction: (1) preparation of the patient/client, (2) presentation of the activity, (3) try out performance, and (4) follow-up.

Step 1. Preparation of the Patient/Client

1. Establish rapport with the individual to be instructed in order to allay fear and encourage participation.
2. Find out how much the individual knows about the activity so that instruction may be geared accordingly.
3. Involve the individual in the activity in order to assure interest in it. Be sure the individual understands the purpose and value of performance of the activity.
4. Place the individual in a comfortable and correct position for performance of the activity. When demonstrating, work at the side of the individual so that the process may easily be seen. In most cases, do *not* work opposite, as this may create a reverse mental image. However, when teaching an individual with hand dominance opposite that of the therapist, it may be appropriate to instruct while sitting opposite the individual.

Step 2. Presentation of the Activity

1. Give oral directions and demonstrate the process. Written directions and diagrams may be helpful, depending on the complexity of the activity and the learning ability and preferences of the patient/client.
2. Present the instruction slowly and patiently.
3. Teach the process step by step, stressing key points.
4. Teach no more than can be mastered at one time.

Step 3. Try Out Performance

1. The individual should perform the activity either step by step with the therapist or immediately after being shown.
2. Correct errors as they occur. If possible, they should be anticipated so they can be avoided.
3. Have the individual explain the process.
4. Have the individual repeat the activity several times to be sure he or she can perform it correctly.

Step 4. Follow-Up

1. Put the individual on his or her own to work independently.
2. Designate a person who can help if difficulties arise.
3. Check progress frequently to correct errors and to assure success in performance. Less frequent checks are sufficient as competence increases.

Adaptation of Instruction

Adaptation of the method of instruction and preparation for it may be required for persons having special problems. The visually handicapped, for example, must have the work area precisely and consistently arranged, with every tool or piece of equipment in the same place for each session. Since use of sensation is vital to learning by the visually handicapped, opportunity must be provided and emphasized for tactile input in every step of the process. Oral instructions must be more specific and very clearly stated.

Individuals with cognitive problems, or those who have difficulty following directions, require modification in the instructions. The activity must be simplified as much as possible so that only one- or two-step operations are required. Directions must be given one step at a time and must be clear, concise, consistent, and concrete.

Special adaptations also must be made for those individuals having any physical dysfunction. For example, an individual who can use only one hand should be instructed by the therapist who demonstrates using only one hand. This requires that the therapist learn to do the activity with one hand.

Summary

Activity, as a base for occupational therapy, has been described in regard to its value to human functioning and the occupational therapy process. Eight characteristics of activities provide fundamental precepts that define occupational therapy, and the ability to analyze an activity in regard to all these aspects is an essential skill for an occupational therapist and is vital to the effective application of activity as a means of evaluation and treatment. It is critical, however, that the activity be utilized within the perspective of the frame of reference chosen to guide treatment. Having analyzed the activity and chosen the frame of reference, the therapist must match the activity and provide those dimensions that are most appropriate to meet each client's specific needs. In addition to being able to analyze an activity and utilize it for evaluation and treatment, the occupational therapist must be skilled in giving instructions in the processes involved and be able to adapt the activity and the instruction to suit the circumstances. The use of activity, activity analysis, activity synthesis, and adaptation are vital in the occupational therapy process.

References

1. Activity analysis. Occupational Therapy Dept., Norristown State Hospital, Norristown PA, 1977
2. Fidler GS: From crafts to competence. Am J Occup Ther 35:568, 1981
3. Kielhofner G: Occupation. In Hopkins HL, Smith HD (eds): Willard and Spackman's Occupational Therapy, 6th ed. Philadelphia, JB Lippincott, 1983
4. Llorens L: Activity analysis for cognitive-perceptual-motor dysfunction. Am J Occup Ther 27:453, 1973
5. Mosey AC: Psychosocial Components of Occupational Therapy. New York, Raven Press, 1985
6. Occupational therapy—its definition and functions. Am J Occup Ther 20:204, 1976
7. Searles H: The Nonhuman Environment. New York, International Universities Press, 1960
8. Willard HS, Spackman CS (eds): Occupational Therapy, 4th ed, pp 171–182. Philadelphia, JB Lippincott, 1971

CHAPTER 7

Occupational Therapy — A Problem-Solving Process

Helen L. Hopkins
and
Elizabeth G. Tiffany

The occupational therapy process seeks to help individuals who are ill or disabled and to provide conditions that will promote their optimal health and functioning. Occupational therapists work within a number of structures to achieve those purposes. In addition to providing treatment, therapists must be prepared to deal with issues such as scheduling, budget, staff supervision, and interdisciplinary relationships. At each level of functioning, the therapist needs to be prepared to carry out measures to effect change, to nurture growth, and to establish systems that will promote and support health. Skill in problem-solving is basic to success.

Generic Approach to Problem-Solving

A generic approach to problem-solving may prove useful to the therapist at all levels: administrative, supervisory, and clinical. This approach consists of five critical steps: problem identification, solution development, development of a plan of action, implementation of the plan, and assessment of the results.[11] In the initial step, *problem identification,* an effort is made to identify, spec-ify, and clarify the nature of the problem and to analyze its elements and components. *Solution development* involves scrutiny of the information collected in the first step. On the basis of this scrutiny, alternatives are explored, and broad goals and objectives are set. From among the possible alternatives and goals, one choice is made at a time. The problem-solver next undertakes the *development of a plan of action,* a realistic and sometimes detailed description of the activities that will be used to accomplish the goal selected. In the *implementation of the plan,* those activities are carried out. The final step listed, *assessment of results,* is in fact undertaken during, as well as at the end of, implementation. Often, a fine-tuning of the plan or a second exploration of alternatives or choice of a different goal may be indicated.

Examples of administrative, supervisory, or interdisciplinary team problems for which the problem-solving steps would prove useful are providing wheelchair accessibility in an old building, enabling a reticent student to overcome difficulty in giving oral reports in staff meetings, and communicatin˜ the importance of proper positioning to a teacher of a cerebral palsied child. Many such problems are solved intuitively and smoothly, but occasionally, if one of the five steps is omitted, problems are magnified rather than diminished.

Adapting Problem-Solving to Clinical Treatment

In the clinical treatment situation, the problem-solving steps become translated into the whole process of intervention. To provide valid and effective treatment for the disabled client, the occupational therapist must address a number of questions: On what basis do I understand this person? How do I conceptualize human personality, human behavior, physical function, and the ways in which human beings learn, grow, and change? How do I understand pathology or the disease process? What about its etiologic factors and its prognosis? What do I know about the external factors which now impinge on this person? What about the social and work worlds in which he/she must function now and in the future? What do I know about the methods of treatment or frames of reference for treatment currently being used with this person? How can I best communicate with this person so that we build a mutual understanding of reality that is as clear as possible?

In addressing these questions, the therapist is laying the groundwork for the problem-solving process to follow, a process that can be organized as a series of logical steps which parallel the steps of the generic approach to problem-solving: initial assessment, setting treatment objectives, development of a treatment plan, implementation of the plan, and periodic or continual evaluation. A sixth step is added to the treatment process: treatment termination.

The *initial assessment* step requires collection of data which describe the client objectively. These data should include information about the existing pathology or disability and its effects on the person's life. They should also include information about the client's existing skills and strengths and educational and vocational background. They may include information about the client's personal history, developmental level, social and cultural world, and value systems.

Setting *treatment objectives* is the step in which reasonable predicted outcomes of the occupational therapy process are explored and named and in which realistic and objectively identifiable long- and short-term goals are stated. When the initial evaluation has been concluded, the therapist should have a clear picture of the client, of his/her assets and limitations, and of realistic expectations for future performance. In the evaluation, certain basic ingredients should have been contributing to setting both long-term and short-term goals for treatment:

1. *The client's needs and goals.* However obliquely they may be communicated, the wishes and needs of the client are there. Unless the goals of treatment are mutually understood by therapist and client on some level, they probably cannot be achieved.

2. *The treatment goals, the treatment approach, and the frame of reference for treatment used by the total team.* Again, coherence between the client's own goals and those of the team is important. The goals of occupational therapy must fit with both.

3. *Knowledge of the individual's disease process and the possible residual physical or psychological limitations.*

4. *Knowledge of the treatment methods and approaches being used.* What medications is the client receiving?

5. *Knowledge about the world in which the client is expected to live.* What skills are needed to cope with the demands of life at home, in the community, at work, at play, or in the institution?

6. *Knowledge about the client's value system and what is important to him/her.*

The therapist analyzes the evaluation data in the light of the potential situation for occupational therapy. What does the therapist know about the prognosis for recovery or maintenance of function for people having a specific disease? Who are the other members of the treatment team and what is the potential for collaborative efforts among them? Can the therapist expect professional and community support for efforts made in occupational therapy? What are the realistic limits of the occupational therapy setting? To what extent will it be possible to manipulate objects and the environment to provide the best opportunities for the patient to grow and function to maximum capabilities? In what ways can we measure the success of the plan? These are hard but vital questions that must be faced in setting objectives and planning treatment.

Long-term objectives in occupational therapy usually represent a part of the long-term treatment objectives of the team. A long-term objective may be stated, "the patient will be able to function well enough to go back to his job." A long-term objective related to this in occupational therapy might be stated, "the patient will be able to organize his thoughts and actions to carry out a task from beginning to end." Short-term objectives contribute to the achievement of long-term objectives. A short-term objective related to the above might be stated, "the patient will be able to maintain attention to a given task for 15 minutes." Short-term objectives, then, represent the steps of achievement which will facilitate the attainment of the long-term objective.

Depending on the treatment situation and the pathology of the client, there may be either multiple or single sets of objectives. The results of the evaluation may also indicate that occupational therapy is not needed or relevant for a client at a given time. If attainable treatment objectives for occupational therapy cannot be determined, it is probably not appropriate for the client to be referred to occupational therapy.

It is on the basis of selected objectives that a *treat-*

ment plan is developed. A description of the methods to be used to meet the treatment objectives constitutes the treatment plan. Just as the objectives represent an action-oriented summary of the client's evaluation, the plan represents a synthesis of the therapist's knowledge of the potential of activites and relationships as facilitators of growth and performance. It is a nuts and bolts statement of such things as the tools, materials, and equipment; the kinds of direction or guidance; the structure of the activity; the times and places in which the activity will take place; whether treatment will be accomplished individually or in a group; and the extent to which the family or the community is to be involved. A treatment plan is first stated in reference to each short-term objective, and it needs to be flexible enough to permit changes if re-evaluation suggests that the plan is not working.

It is probably in the development of a treatment plan that the therapist is most often faced with the responsibility for sound professional judgment. The plan needs to be reasonable and possible and to show a clear relationship to the objectives of treatment.

The *implementation* of the treatment plan connects action and the performance of activities with the goals of treatment and acts on the implicit contract which has been developed between the therapist and the client. Implementation consists of three distinct phases: (1) the orientation phase, when the therapist and client define the parameters and expectations of the activities that will be used and the therapist may describe or demonstrate the procedures that are involved; (2) the development phase, during which the therapist guides the client through exploration or practice in doing the activities; and (3) the termination phase, when the client has completed the plan, re-evaluation takes place, and the need for the setting of further objectives is considered.

During the development phase, there should be continual evaluation to check the effectiveness of the plan and the relevance of the objectives. During this time, it is likely that new objectives and new treatment plans will evolve. Indeed, periodic or continual *evaluation* is essential in all three phases of treatment in order to assess the validity of the objectives and the efficacy of the treatment plan and process, to identify the need for changes in aproach, and to determine when treatment can be terminated.

It is most satisfying when *treatment termination* takes place with a final assessment and clear indications for the future performance of the client. Termination can be an affirmation of the success of the plan and the process. For this reason, termination is a critical step in the occupational therapy process and deserves thoughtful planning. In reality, the termination phase is not always achieved. Clients may be discharged before objectives are met. In some situations, particularly with chronically ill patients, the treatment goal is maintenance of func-

tion, and therefore short-term objectives are so numerous that the occupational therapy process may continue for a long time.

The use of the problem-solving process in occupational therapy requires creativity and imagination on the part of the therapist. The therapist must use knowledge, skills, and good professional judgment to find the best possible solution for each client.[10,14]

It is important for the patient or client to be involved in the process of problem identification so that the assets as well as liabilities of the situation may be determined. The goals that are established, the alternative chosen, and the plan of action must reflect what is desired by and acceptable to the patient or client. In order to be successful, moreover, the plan of action and the approach must be compatible with those of other professionals working with the individual. The values and lifestyle of the client's family should also be taken into consideration.

Each plan of action must be examined for its probable value and the potential outcomes of treatment or intervention. If the plan appears feasible, and if it offers a promising solution, it can be implemented. Short-term goals with manageable elements contribute to the achievement of long-term goals. The therapist needs to be clear about the relationship between the long-term and short-term goals and their sequencing. There must be periodic reevaluation to determine progress, the goals reached and the problems solved. It may be necessary to make modifications or to adapt goals and plans as changes occur. There are occasions when abandonment of an unsuccessful plan is necessary, requiring a determination of another course of action. As new knowledge develops and as new viewpoints evolve, new alternatives arise that provide different approaches for intervention in occupational therapy.

Approaches to Intervention

The selection of the issues and data that will be given attention in the problem-solving process and the choices among treatment plan alternatives are determined by the frame of reference within which the therapist is working. In occupational therapy today there are several alternative approaches to intervention that may be chosen, depending on the therapist's orientation and rationale for treatment. Each approach has a specific knowledge base, each is built on stated concepts, and each utilizes a rationale that constrains the occupational therapy program by specifying the type of appropriate activities. Among the currently identified approaches to treatment are rehabilitation/habilitation[7]; acquisitional or behavioral; developmental (including a variety of special foci, such as neurodevelopmental, adaptive skills, and sensory-integration); psychoanalytic; and occupational behavior.[8,9,13,17] These approaches overlap in some areas. Their importance lies in the fact that they provide the therapist with specific guidelines within which to apply knowledge and skills. The experience, values, sociocultural assumptions, points of view, and concept of reality inherent in an agency's philosophy promote the choice of a specific frame of reference.[2] For example, within the developmental approach, one occupational therapist, a group of therapists, or agency may favor a neurodevelopmental perspective for treatment of children with cerebral palsy and may utilize the Bobath frame of reference, whereas others may favor a neurophysiological perspective and may use a Rood frame of reference. Some agencies use more than one approach to intervention, depending on the type of clients as well as on the preferences, biases, and expertise of the therapists. This increases the number and variety of frames of reference that may be used. The rationale and basis for choosing an approach and frame of reference, as well as the knowledge base and concepts inherent in that approach, must be understood by the therapist.

The occupational therapy intervention process will differ according to the approach and frame of reference chosen, but the overall goals of the process can be described as *prevention* of conditions causing or resulting in loss of function; *remediation, treatment,* or *rehabilitation* for restoration of function and performance; and *promotion and maintenance* of health and optimal functioning.

Basis for Treatment Approaches: The Four Elements

In the application of the problem-solving process to occupational therapy intervention, regardless of the frame of reference chosen, four elements are considered, and it is in the use and dynamic interplay of these elements that occupational therapy can claim its uniqueness. The four elements are the *patient or client,* the *therapist and the therapeutic relationship,* the *activity,* and the *context for treatment.* A brief discussion of each of the four elements is presented here; the reader is encouraged to "flesh out" the many important pieces that are part of clinical problem-solving.

The Patient or Client

Problems in a client's ability to adapt and function are multifaceted, and it is critical that the therapist understand as much as possible about the specific motor, cognitive, emotional, or social difficulties the individual may be experiencing. Clinical diagnoses or clinical impressions are only a starting point in this understanding; it must be couched in a broader sense of the human and nonhuman factors involved. There are a great many

ways in which human personality and behavior may be conceptualized. For the purpose of establishing a baseline, we will consider here a few factors which are especially important in the occupational therapy process. These are in no way exclusive, and the reader is referred to the bibliography and is encouraged to search the literatures of the social and biological sciences for other perspectives.

Stress

Any consideration of disability or dysfunction must include attention to the role that stress plays in the development and exacerbation of problems. In 1956, Hans Selye wrote *The Stress of Life,*[21] in which he described the interrelations of the body systems and the extensive effects of stress on the whole organism. In the years which have followed the publication of Selye's work, interest in the nature of stress has spurred a great deal of research as well as much public speculation. During the 1960s and 1970s, we saw a proliferation of popular movements and literature dealing with methods of coping with stress and tension. Stress is often viewed in the context of technological advances and ideational changes, such as those described by Toffler in *Future Shock.*[22]

Coleman broadly defines stress as the "adjustive demands made upon the individual." He points out that stress may occur on physiological or psychological levels.[1] On the physiological level, examples of stressors are a broken limb, invasion by a virus, ingestion of poison, blood sugar imbalance, or an arthritic condition. On the psychological level, stressors may be the loss of a loved one, failure in an important test, the necessity of choosing between two highly desirable (or undesirable) alternatives, or bombardment with too many things to do. The effects of stress, regardless of the original stressful event, are felt in various degrees throughout the body. Data on autonomic system responses, cortical changes, muscle tension, and subjective experience indicate clearly that mind, emotions, and body are inseparably involved in reactions to stress.

Coleman further points out that the severity of stress depends on three factors: (1) the characteristics of the demand; (2) the characteristics of the individual; and (3) the external resources and supports available to the individual. Demands may be brief or long-lasting. The threat to the individual's actual survival may in reality be great or small. The stressful event may occur alone or in combination with other stressful factors. Stressful reactions may predispose an individual to further negative stress reactions.

According to Coleman, the longer stress continues, the more severe it becomes. Many small stresses occurring simultaneously may create a stress overload, and the gradual building up of insignificant events over a long period of time may add up to greater stress than a single severe incident.

On the other hand, stress, as "the adjustive demands made upon the individual," may be viewed as having the potential for positive effects. It is in the last two factors mentioned by Coleman — the characteristics of the individual and the external resources and supports available — that there exist possibilities for change, growth, and strengthening of coping mechanisms to deal with inevitable future stresses. A crisis may combine danger with opportunity, and recognition of these possibilities is important in occupational therapy.

Characteristics of the individual include genetic predispositions; intelligence; temperament; body type; structural strengths and weaknesses of the body systems; basic environmental influences such as nutrition, clothing, and housing; parental nurturance; discipline; the cumulative effects of interactions with significant people in school, church, and the neighborhood; and the mores and cultural factors that impinge on the development of personalilty. The individual is a total being, a composite of physical, sensory, perceptual, emotional, cognitive, social, and cultural behaviors and skills. The extent to which this composite is elastic (able to rebound), flexible (able to bend, compromise, and change), and strong (able to stand firm) is significant in determining the extent to which individuals can meet the demands made on them. The characteristics of the individual, although basically established by adulthood, may be considered dynamic and alterable in some measure throughout life. If this were not so, there would be no reason for therapy.

External resources for coping with stress are multidimensional. They include family, neighborhood, religious group, friends, money, educational opportunities, the possibility of a vacation, and even the climate.

The therapeutic process is inherently one of change. It is hoped that occupational therapy intervention will lead the client to new and more effective ways of functioning. Sometimes, change can be frightening, and the therapist must be conscious of this as an additional element or stressor in the problem-solving process. For example, independence and a sense of autonomy are not cheaply gained. Often, though highly desired, they pose a sense of risk for individuals whose physical or emotional difficulties have rendered them dependent for a time. Within the problem-solving process, the therapist must address the question of risk *versus* gain. Clients sometimes need reassurance with regard to the efforts they are investing in the therapeutic process. Sometimes they may *feel they are losing more than they are gaining by giving up dysfunction,* and this can become a significant consideration, if not a determinant, in the therapeutic outcome. One problem for the therapist is the fact that change as a stressor is frequently not recognized, even by the client.

For the health professional whose commitment is to facilitate competence on the part of the dysfunctional, the careful consideration of Coleman's three aspects is essential. It is important to be sensitive to the possibility that stress, regardless of its nature, may be responsible for regression and a lessened ability to perceive realistically or to behave adaptively. This in itself contributes to further stress and further regression, and a vicious downward spiral has been started. On the other hand, true coping behavior in which an individual is able to feel competent and to experience success or mastery seems to lead to further strengths, more adaptive skills, and additional successes.

Motivation

The key to success in a program of occupational therapy often lies in the extent to which the patient or client may be motivated to participate in it. Human motivation has been much studied and seems to be one of the most important areas to which the occupational therapist should give attention. Motivation may be defined as an arousal to action, initiating, molding, and sustaining specific action patterns.[3] The task of the occupational therapist requires that the client be motivated, first to participate in treatment and second to sustain the healthy patterns one hopes to establish in the process.

One may consider that behavior is motivated by principles of drive reduction, need satisfaction, and the pleasure principle. The role of reinforcement as a basic motivator has been much studied, and one needs to look carefully at the many aspects of reinforcement and aversive conditioning approaches to achieving motivation. Other theories suggest that behavior, beyond those aspects related to survival, is motivated by innate curiosity and in a need to interact with the environment.

The examination of the range of "normal" behavior reveals that people are motivated by many factors; for example, novelty, complexity, surprise, competition, and cooperation. Personality types have been characterized in terms of dominant social motivational patterns: (1) *affiliation* — liking people; (2) *aggression* — moving against people; (3) *dominance* — trying to dominate people; and (4) *cognizance* — exploring and asking questions.

McClelland has studied factors related to "need for achievement," defined as the extent to which a person enjoys competition against a standard of excellence. Individuals may be characterized as falling somewhere along a continuum: at the low end, the individual tends to prefer no-risk situations where competition is minimal. This personality variable appears to be dynamic and powerful and seems to be set at a very early age.[12]

Related to achievement motivation as a personality factor is the issue of field dependence. Some people demonstrate unique, integrated, individual, internal schemes; those who do tend to be less conforming to social pressure and more in conformity to standards that are internalized and personal. Such individuals are characterized as *field-independent.* Those individuals who seem to be highly motivated to conform to standards or pressures that are external are characterized as *field-dependent.*[19]

Another related and powerful factor is *locus of control*—the extent to which individuals perceive that the events and situations of their lives are controlled by themselves *versus* chance or luck. This variable is, again, measured on a continuum that goes from an extreme internal locus of control to an extreme external locus of control. Those who perceive control as being internal feel that they are responsible and are able to direct and control their life situations; whereas those who perceive control as being external see themselves as the recipients or victims of fate. Extremes in either direction, obviously, are unrealistic.[4,19,24]

Two factors may be critical in determining the nature of an individual's orientation with regard to achievement motivation, field dependence, and locus of control. First, there are the quality and quantity of experiences that the individual had as a child and the extent to which they were pleasurable, reinforcing, or satisfying. Second, and perhaps more basic, is the consideration of the individual's ability to process the information received from the external world. Both of these considerations appear to be of great importance. There is a need for continuing research into their complex relations with human motivation and basic self-concept.

Piaget[15] and White[23] have spoken eloquently of the importance of the experience of success in promoting feelings of efficacy and motivating further performance. What seems to be of great importance is that the individual clearly understands, experiences, and owns the behaviors and their effects. Those situational variables that are not, in fact, related to an individual's behavior or control need to be understood as such.

Another factor very powerful in determining motivation is anxiety. Anxiety may be a strong motivator for performance up to a point but this varies with individuals and with specific situations. Beyond that point, anxiety inhibits motivation, tends to render the individual rigid and unable to adapt to new situations, and reduces integrative mechanisms.

All of these considerations are of great importance to the occupational therapist because of the need to elicit the cooperation and participation of the patient or client. The results of illness and disability may be perceived differently by different individuals with regard to their sense of responsibility and efficacy. The extent to which standards of achievement must be internalized to be motivating to an individual varies. Clarity of feedback, awareness of anxiety levels, and the ability to identify what may be uniquely reinforcing to an individual may be critical to the success or failure of a treatment program.

The Nonhuman World

From the moment of birth, human beings become part of a world of things to be experienced—to be seen, felt, heard, smelled, tasted, feared, and enjoyed.

For infants and growing children, the human and nonhuman objects of their worlds are crucial in determining the kinds of people they will become. For the occupational therapist, understanding the ways in which a person interacts with the nonhuman world is important. Harold Searles, in his book *The Nonhuman Environment,*[20] explores in depth the kinds and qualities of meanings that human beings invest in their worlds of things, places, and spaces. He refers to kinds of relationships that characterize human interactions with their nonhuman worlds as they grow up. People are able to use the nonhuman world to gain a sense of stability and continuity, to practice skills in relating, to assuage strong feelings, to foster self-realization, to deepen the awareness of reality, and to foster appreciation and acceptance of fellow human beings.

The healthy adult has learned to live in some degree of adaptation with the things and places of his or her world. What is the range of feelings inherent in the experiences of the nonhuman world? There are experiences of pleasure in fixing the engine of a car, pride in baking a cake, excitement in riding a roller coaster, frustration in coping with a machine that will not work, discomfort in being wet and cold in a storm, power in moving a heavy object, helplessness in not being able to move a heavy object, catharsis in housecleaning, wholeness in being beside the ocean, or comfort in being in a warm bed on a cold night.

The things and places of the world offer sources of pleasure and pain, opportunities to practice skills and to express ourselves, challenges to survive, and chances to live well. There is a continual and intimate relatedness with the nonhuman world.

The arts and artifacts that human beings come to treasure become symbolically invested with the values of the people who produce and use them. This goes far beyond things like dishes, vases, furniture, books, toys, and paintings. It goes into the uses of space and the kinds of personal privacy that may be fostered and the extent to which the world of nature is regarded and incorporated into an individual's living space.

What does all this mean to the occupational therapist? It has everything to do with attention to the potential meanings of the tools and materials of the activities used in treatment and the kinds of environments in which the therapist practices. It means the therapist can help the patient or client develop ways of trusting and *using* the nonhuman world; that this may have primary importance all by itself. The use of the nonhuman world is significant in providing a bridge for human relationships. It means the articles used and treasured by a person give clues not only to that person's private gestalt but also to the culture of the society in which he/she lives. It means that when a patient or client has permitted himself to invest in creating or producing something tangible or ideational in occupational therapy, the therapist needs to respect the person's ownership of that product.

Cultural Implications

Much is said about the need to understand the family and community to which each patient or client belongs. The rich literatures of sociology and anthropology on the subject of cultural influences are worth studying. There is little doubt that social systems are a powerful, although often subtle, influence on basic ways of perceiving, thinking, feeling, and behaving. Learning begins at conception and continues through interactions with both human and nonhuman environments; therefore, cultural values, biases, and customs are powerful in the formation of personalities. The kinds of toys, games, foods, and other objects that are presented; the kinds of music and stories; the humor; the behavior that is encouraged and the behavior that is discouraged; the quality and quantity of parenting experienced; and the amount of touching and closeness between people are just some of the ways in which children are influenced by the culture of their families. Cultural influences are deep. As Edward Hall says:

> Most of culture lies hidden and is outside voluntary control, making up the warp and weft of human existence. Even when small fragments of culture are elevated to awareness, they are difficult to change, not only because they are so personally experienced but because people cannot act or interact at all in any meaningful way except through the medium of culture.[6]

Both the therapist's perceptions and behavior and the client's perceptions and behavior are filtered through the screen of culture.

The occupational therapist must be concerned about values. Values determine how individuals feel about people, ideas, and things and how they act toward them. Value conflicts, both within the self and between individuals and groups, are responsible for many of the difficulties which are part of everyone's living experience. In today's society, with rapid mass communication and mobility, the potential for value conflicts seems to be increasing.

Among the daily behaviors to be considered are the ways in which a client views and manages time, space (personal distance and territory), objects, dress, daily self-care activities, money, work, play, and study. How does the client respond to pain, loss, illness, and death? What is considered rude? How important is the family? What constitutes friendship? What about religious beliefs, rituals, and observances? Is anxiety handled by laughing and talking or by withdrawing? What is the significance of food and mealtimes? How is anger dealt with? What are the characteristic support systems of the group? Certain Asian groups laugh when they are confronted with danger. Some groups consider manual occupations degrading. The average American is more scheduled and time-bound than individuals from most cultural groups. In a culturally heterogeneous population, there will be a wide range of behaviors and lifestyles which may be considered normal. To help the client function within his/her own world, the therapist needs to understand that world.

The Therapist

The therapist in a treatment setting is, by definition, a helper. The roles a therapist assumes may vary. The therapist may legitimately be a teacher or a facilitator who brings knowledge and skills to the client's unique situation. The most important prerequisite to being an effective helper is self-knowledge: the helper needs to be aware of his/her own needs, perceptual biases, and capabilities.

The relationship that is established between the therapist and the client may well determine the success or failure of the treatment plan. The establishment of effective and clear communication both ways is the first essential part of the relationship. Sensitivity to the level and mode of communication that will work with a given client and skill in using this knowledge may be the critical factor. For example, if a patient is functioning on a preverbal level of understanding, one must think of nonverbal ways of communicating meaning. If a patient thinks in concrete terms and understands only tangible things, one must think of concrete and tangible ways to explain feelings, meanings, and actions. With a patient who is severely regressed, it may be important to use the process of *naming* and showing as the purposes and processes of the activities are explained.

Frank has pointed out that one must be aware, also, that in any encounter between two people, there may be at least six selves communicating; each party possesses an idealized self, a self perceived by the other person, and the actual self.[5] The transactional analysis model describes the parent self, child self, and adult self. Discrepancies between the individuals' perceptions of one another lead to complex distortions. Transference and countertransference phenomena may also be encountered. When one is working within the psychoanalytic frame of reference, these phenomena are used as part of the therapeutic process, but most other frames of reference used in the occupational therapy process tend to deemphasize transference when it occurs and instead work toward the conscious perception of the therapist as a new person, different from past significant persons. The therapist can accomplish this by acting as a "total, reacting, feeling person."[13]

Without the establishment of trust between the client and therapist, it is unlikely that a truly collaborative effort will be possible. For some people, the trust issue may be powerful, and the establishment of trust may take a long time. The therapist's own self confidence and ability to be honest and open in the relationship and the extent to which he/she is able to communicate "unconditional positive regard" and empathy for the client will affect the client's ability to invest trust in the relationship.[18] Purtilo[16] has identified some of the issues and factors which are vital in the therapeutic relationship (see the box below, "The Personal–Professional Self").

The Personal–Professional Self

He decides whether to use the first or last name of each new patient; he is cautious, knowing the casual use of the first name may be harmful; he is relaxed in using the last names of patients.

He incorporates actions that communicate caring into the patient–health professional interaction; he recognizes efficiency as a trait which can express caring when it does not impose rigid limits on the interaction.

He recognizes that wearing a uniform does not necessarily make a patient feel *less* cared for nor does the more casual appearance of street clothes make a patient feel *more* cared for.

He combines a pleasant approach with professional competence.

He is interested in the patient as a person with values, needs, and beliefs, but does not encourage a relationship that will lead to over-dependence (detrimental dependence).

He is respected by the patient who recognizes his integrity. He acknowledges that complete, open, mutual sharing with each other is not conducive to the functioning of a public-sector relationship.

He maintains a balance between sound health care and effective patient–health professional interaction.

He does not need to overprotect himself or to take unnecessary risks; he knows his limits.

From Purtilo R: *The Allied Health Professional and the Patient* © 1973 by WB Saunders, Philadelphia. Reprinted with permission.

Interpersonal issues such as dependency, aggressiveness or passivity, and personal need gratification or control are often challenges to the therapeutic relationship. They need to be identified for what they are and resolved as realistically and honestly as possible. When these behaviors emerge, they are often manifestations of the maladaptive modes of thinking, feeling, and acting that have interfered with the person's ability to function. If efforts between the therapist and client to identify and change what may be occurring are unsuccessful, the therapist may wish to find another professional with whom to discuss and objectify the situation.

One of the ways of conceptualizing the progress of a therapeutic relationship is to think of phases. The first phase is an affective one in which the therapist elicits the trust of the client by demonstrating empathy or understanding for his/her feelings and plight. This, depending on the client's need state or pathology, may be accomplished in a few words, a nod, or touch of the hand. It may, however, take a long time. The second phase is one of gathering facts and information, identifying the problems to be solved, and sorting out the realistic levels of solution that may be worked toward. In the third phase, the period of developing an action plan to work on resolving the problems, some form of contract or agreement is made with the patient or client. This is implicit in what has been, on some level at least, a cooperative effort. The contract is an understanding on the part of both the therapist and the client of what the process will be and of what expectations each person may have of the other. In the fourth phase, the period of implementation of the plan, the conditions of the contract are tested. The issues of trust may emerge again, and it is important for the therapist to meet his/her responsibilities as planned and to communicate clearly the expectation that the client will follow through in meeting responsibilities also.

In the final phase, the termination period, when separation becomes imminent, new issues may arise. If the therapeutic relationship has been important and helpful, the termination of the relationship may feel difficult to both the therapist and the client. On the other hand, all of the focus of treatment in occupational therapy has been directed toward increasingly independent functioning and, thus, the termination of treatment may evoke celebrative feelings.

The Activity

Purpose

Activities are used as facilitators for transactions between people. The focus on doing, not merely talking, is useful in both one-to-one and group interactions. It allows for nonverbal communication, confrontations around interpersonal issues, and safe withdrawal when needed.

The activities with which occupational therapy is primarily concerned are those that help to promote competence and achievement in the client's ability to function in his/her own world. The three categories of self-care, work, and play, and the maintenance of a healthy balance in the individual's activity life, provide important foci for occupational therapy. This emphasis requires consideration of the client's developmental levels of functioning and of demands placed on the client by daily activities. Activities used as treatment are limited only by the constraints of the treatment context, which includes time, space, cost, the support of other team members, and the preferences and skills of the therapist.

Achieving a scientific understanding of the nature of activities and of their ability to promote performance is a monumental task and continues to be a significant challenge to occupational therapy. We have intuitive notions about activities and have experienced some degree of empirical success in their use through the years. However, scientific research data still are lacking. The importance of understanding the elements of activity cannot be overemphasized.

Choice

The art of occupational therapy is in finding and using activities that are relevant to meeting the treatment objectives and that have meaning to the patient or client. It seems a simple, almost glib, statement to say that one matches the activity (which has been carefully analyzed) with the needs of the client (who has been carefully evaluated). This process is far from simple. The choice of activity, within the scope and limitations of a program, remains crucial to the success of the treatment. Decisions need to be made: Should the activity be done on a one-to-one basis or in a group? How important is the process and how important is an end product? How much of the activity should rely on verbal communication? How much physical or sensory involvement should be planned? What is the range within which time requirements may be graded? In what ways will the patient experience exploration, mastery, and achievement?

To use crafts or not to use crafts? The early occupational therapists used a wide range of activities of which crafts were an important part. In recent times, except in some segments of the population, crafts became less well respected and less frequently used. The basketweaver image of the occupational therapist is a ludicrous one that ignores the possibilities for learning and growth which are inherent in crafts. It ignores basic anthropological and physiological data relating hand use with cognitive functioning. From the perspective of modern mechanistic achievement and production-oriented society, simple handcrafts are viewed as quaint, childish, or primitive. This attitude is a pervasive one and affects how both the therapist and the client may feel about a given craft activity. Crafts, however, offer a highly flexible, easily controlled modality through which an individual may explore, practice, and develop a wide range of basic physical, perceptual, and cognitive skills. One experiences the tools and materials through the senses. One also experiences the effects of one's actions on something that is visible and tangible. For the patient or client who is unable to cope with many social variables or verbal interactions, the craft still may be the modality of choice.

The Context

When we speak of the context for treatment, we mean much more than the setting in which treatment is to take place. Context here has a dimension of time: today with an awareness of yesterday and a deliberate plan for tomorrow. In terms of place, it designates all those areas a treatment plan utilizes; for example, a shop, a ward, a home, a work setting, Main Street, and the baseball diamond. It also includes some sense of the treatment objectives and plan and the efforts and thinking of all of the people engaged in the helping process. The context for treatment has parts that are controllable and parts that are not controllable. In proceeding with treatment, we may wish to move from a highly controlled context; *e.g.*, the hospital, with a professional team, planned treatment procedures, set schedules, to a gradually less controlled and more realistic context; *e.g.*, the community where the client experiences semiautonomy or the home where the client is autonomous. In modern occupational therapy, contexts for treatment have become highly varied and far more complex than they were when occupational therapy began.

Factors that are considered in identifying contexts for treatment include:
1. The characteristics, issues, needs, and objectives of the client population
2. The kind of setting and its means of support
3. Frames of reference for treatment and the nature of the treatment team
4. Kinds of evaluative procedures that are used
5. Kinds of treatment objectives that are set
6. Kinds of treatment plans that are developed
7. Kinds of records and reports that are made—to whom the treatment team is accountable and how this is accomplished

Summary

The clinical problem-solver, in making plans and carrying out a therapeutic or preventive program, will wish to consider the many aspects of the four elements. Only some aspects have been suggested in this chapter. The choice of information and the issues to which attention will be drawn as well as the emphasis placed on each item will be influenced by the frame of reference used. It is important, in the problem-solving process, that a clear focus be maintained, and the frame of reference helps to make that possible. This is true whether the issues are clinical or administrative ones. The four elements addressed in this chapter are translatable into administrative and supervisory terms, and the need for a frame of reference is important in administrative and supervisory areas, too. The problem-solving process, with its five steps of problem identification, solution development, development of a plan of action, implementation of the plan, and assessment of results is applicable to the many arenas in which occupational therapists work. The development of the problem-solving approach and skill in its use can be the key to success as a clinical therapist, a supervisor, or an administrator or in any of the other roles which occupational therapists may take.

References

1. Coleman JC: Life stress and maladaptive behavior. Am J Occup Ther 27:169, 1973
2. Conte JR, Conte WR: The use of conceptual models in occupational therapy. Am J Occup Ther 31:262, 1977
3. Cratty BJ: Movement Behavior and Motor Learning. Philadelphia, Lea & Febiger, 1967
4. Ducette J, Wolk S: Cognitive and motivational correlates of generalized expectancies for control. J Pers Soc Psychol 26:420, 1973
5. Frank J: The therapeutic use of self. Am J Occup Ther 12:215, 1958
6. Hall ET: The Hidden Dimension. p 188. Garden City, NY, Doubleday & Co, 1966
7. Hopkins HL, Smith H (eds): Willard and Spackman's Occupational Therapy, 5th ed, p 110. Philadelphia, JB Lippincott, 1978
8. Huss AJ: Sensorimotor approaches. In Hopkins HL, Smith H (eds): Willard and Spackman's Occupational Therapy, 5th ed, pp 125–134. Philadelphia, JB Lippincott, 1978
9. King LJ: A sensori-integrative approach to schizophrenia. Am J Occup Ther 28:529, 1974
10. Marshall E: A problem solving method of learning, measured against a rote memory method. Am J Occup Ther 19:60, 1965
11. May BJ, Newman J: Developing competence in problem-solving: A behavioral model. Phys Ther 60:1140, 1980
12. McClelland D: The Achieving Society. New York, Free Press, 1967
13. Mosey A: Three Frames of Reference for Mental Health. Thorofare, NJ, Charles B Slack, 1971
14. Parnes SJ: Creative Behavior Guidebook. New York, Charles Scribner's Sons, 1967
15. Piaget J: The Origins of Intelligence in Children. New York, International Universities Press, 1966
16. Purtilo R: The Allied Health Professional and the Patient. Philadelphia, WB Saunders, 1973
17. Reilly M: Occupational therapy can be one of the greatest ideas of twentieth century medicine. Am J Occup Ther 16:1, 1962
18. Rogers C: Client Centered Therapy. Boston, Houghton Mifflin, 1951
19. Rotter JB: Clinical Psychology. Englewood Cliffs, NJ, Prentice–Hall, 1971
20. Searles H: The Nonhuman Environment, pp 78–120. New York, International Universities Press, 1960
21. Selye H: The Stress of Life. New York, McGraw–Hill, 1956
22. Toffler A: Future Shock. New York, Random House, 1970
23. White RW: The urge towards competence. Am J Occup Ther 25:271, 1971
24. Wolk S, Ducette J: The motivating effect of locus of control on achievement motivation. J Pers 41:59, 1973

CHAPTER 8

Frames of Reference— Organizing Systems for Occupational Therapy Practice

Developmental Frame of Reference *Elizabeth G. Tiffany*

Change is continuous in the human condition. To examine the ways in which people change in their lives is to look at four processes: (1) genetically programmed *maturation*; (2) *development* based on the interaction between the individual's maturation level and factors in the external environment; (3) *conscious choice* based on the individual's abilities (maturationally and developmentally) to assess the risks and the gains involved in making a choice and (4) *chance* based on external factors over which the individual may have little or no control but which may effect profound changes in the individual's life. The four processes are obviously interrelated and mutually dependent.

A developmental approach to treatment in occupational therapy attends to all four processes: to maturation as a given which must be understood and carefully assessed in the provision of treatment, in the planning for prevention, and in the promotion of wellness; to development as the primary area within which the manipulation of conditions external to the patient can be

made to facilitate positive adaptation and functioning; to conscious choice, or degrees of autonomy, as a goal to be achieved; and to chance as a given which must be understood in terms of the adjustive demands which may be placed on the individual.

Translating this further into occupational therapy terms, the therapist needs to consider developmental aspects from at least three vantage points: (1) the client's unique levels of functioning and adaptation; (2) the level of function that can be reasonably expected at the client's level of development; and (3) the age-specific crises and vulnerabilities the client might be subject to.

Theorists and spokespeople for the significance of human development include Piaget,[10] Maslow,[8] Erikson,[5] Freud,[3] Arieti,[1] and Searles.[11] Their contribution has included the definition of stages and structures that relate to the unfolding of the human personality. Although each of these theorists has chosen to view development from a unique perspective, there is fundamental agreement on certain points regarding the directions and growth of human capacities for functioning. Human feelings and behavior are the products of exceedingly complex interactions between internal and external factors. Internal factors include physiological, anatomical, sensory, and perceptual structures and functions; biochemistry, metabolism, response to pain; and the experiences of joy, balance, and remembering, as well as associating and integrating those experiences. External factors include the people, places, and things of life; the kinds of stimuli that impinge upon the senses; the nuances of interpersonal experiences; and the subtle, intangible, but pervasive ambience of the nonhuman environment. Growth and development occur within the limits and horizons effected in the dynamic interplay between an individual's basic equipment and the external world. Human potential is profoundly influenced and shaped by this interplay. It is from this perspective that a developmental approach to occupational therapy has evolved.

Many occupational therapists have chosen to focus primarily on the developmental process as a base upon which to build treatment. Some, like Llorens,[7] have studied and written extensively, describing a comprehensive approach to occupational therapy as a process through which positive human growth can be fostered. King,[6] building on the works of Ayres,[2] recognized sensory integration as one of the fundamental adaptive skills, underlying the quality and direction of cognitive and social adaptive skills.

Mosey,[9] in 1968, also acknowledged the importance of recognizing the individual's levels of adaptation and functioning in the performance of life tasks and in human relationships. At that time, Mosey proposed that a useful organization on which occupational therapy intervention could be based would consider seven adaptive skills: *perceptual–motor; cognitive; drive-object; dyadic interaction; group interaction; self-identity;* and *sexual identity.* The sequential mastery of these skills within this scheme is seen as prerequisite to the achievement of optimal adaptation.

In 1979, Clark published *Analysis of Four Theoretical Frameworks for Occupational Therapy* in which she compared four prevalent approaches to occupational therapy in terms of their significance to a developmental approach.[4] She identified the four frameworks as *adaptive performance, biodevelopmental, facilitating growth and development,* and *occupational behavior.* Each of these frameworks has a unique emphasis, and each has emerged as significant and important in occupational therapy practice. They share a basic concern for identifying clearly the individual's levels of functioning and for providing opportunities for overcoming dysfunction through attention to developmentally appropriate activities.

Briefly described, the developmental approach is based on the following premises:

1. Human beings normally develop in a sequential way.
2. Each new gain in structure (physical or mental) enables the individual to gain in function.
3. Each new gain in functional ability makes further development and adaptation possible.
4. Physical, sensory, perceptual, cognitive, social, and emotional aspects of the individual are intimately connected and affect the developmental state of the *whole* individual.
5. Conditions of stress cause the individual to regress to earlier levels of adaptation.
6. Successful experiences foster a sense of wholeness and competence.

Human beings tend to be facilitated toward positive development or reintegration of their adaptive abilities when their experiences are successful ones.

The developmental approach to treatment requires that the therapist assess and understand the levels of adaptation on which the client is functioning, and, as much as possible, the conditions which tend to make the client function at the highest and at the lowest levels. The therapist then needs to think in terms of providing opportunities for the client to have experiences that (1) provide success experiences by meeting his/her levels of adaptation; (2) encourage "safe" exploration and practice as the client is enabled to move to more mature levels of adaptation; and (3) provide opportunities for challenge, surprise, and novelty when the client is ready.

This approach may be applied in a number of therapeutic situations: with infants and children where there is evidence of delay or interruption in the normal process of development; with psychiatrically ill clients whose behaviors show regression to earlier stages of adaptation; with the mentally retarded; and with any clients who, because of the stress of physical pain, illness, loss of function, or some disabling condition, may be unable to think, feel, or act at a normal level.

The reader is referred to Chapter 4 for important background information and further resources on human development.

References

1. Arieti S: The Intrapsychic Self. New York, Basic Books, 1967
2. Ayres AJ: The development of perceptual motor abilities: A theoretical basis for treatment of dysfunction. Am J Occup Ther 17:221, 1963
3. Brill AA (ed): Basic Writings of Sigmund Freud. New York, Modern Library, 1958
4. Clark PN: Human development through occupational therapy: Theoretical Frameworks in occupational therapy practice 1. Am J Occup Ther 33:8, 1979

5. Erikson E: Identity and Psychosocial Development of the Child. In Discussions on Child Development, Vol 30. New York, International Universities Press, 1958

6. King LJ: Toward a science of adaptive responses. Am J Occup Ther 32:429, 1979

7. Llorens L: Facilitating growth and development. Am J Occup Ther 24:93, 1970

8. Maslow A: Toward a Psychology of Being. Princeton, NJ, Van Nostrand, 1962

9. Mosey AC: Three Frames of Reference for Mental Health. Thorofare, NJ, Charles B. Slack, 1970

10. Piaget J: Origins of Intelligence in Children. New York, International Universities Press, 1952

11. Searles H: The Nonhuman Environment. New York, International Universities Press, 1960

SECTION 2
Sensorimotor and Neurodevelopmental Frames of Reference   *A. Joy Huss*

Neuroanatomy and Neurophysiology — Bases for Sensorimotor Approaches*

In order to understand human behavior and function, it is necessary to have a basic knowledge of the structure and function of the nervous system. This system is responsible for control not only of the skeletal and smooth muscles but also of the emotions, memory, and intellect. Thus it becomes important for the occupational therapist, regardless of specialty area, to have a basic understanding of the nervous system. Since knowledge of the nervous system is not yet complete, it is the professional's responsibility to stay abreast of current information.

The Nervous System

The nervous system is divided arbitrarily into three divisions: central (CNS); peripheral (PNS); and autonomic (ANS). The ANS has two subdivisions, the sympathetic (SNS) and parasympathetic (PSNS).

The CNS consists of those structures located inside the skull and vertebral column: the brain and spinal cord. The PNS structures are located outside of the bony cavities and carry sensory and motor information from and to the peripheral structures and sensory information from smooth and cardiac muscles and glands to the CNS.

The ANS is an efferent (motor) system supplying information to the smooth muscles, cardiac muscle, and glands. The SNS (thoracolumbar system) is located at spinal cord levels T_1 to L_2. The PSNS anatomically surrounds the SNS, being found in cranial nerves 3, 7, 9, and 10 and in sacral levels 2, 3, and 4 (craniosacral system). The SNS supplies both axial and appendicular structures, while the PSNS supplies only axial structures. Thus, axially the two systems work synergistically. The SNS provides an adrenalin response which is a generalized, fast-acting, excitatory reaction. The PSNS is a specific, slower-acting system which tends to conserve energy. In the appendicular areas, the SNS provides its own synergistic action. For example, it can either increase or decrease the blood flow to the extremities, depending on the needs of the organism.

Functionally, all three divisions (CNS, PNS, ANS), are interrelated and cannot be isolated. What occurs in one division will have an effect on the other divisions. Even though a given treatment may be said to affect a certain part of the system, it will ultimately have an effect, either positive or negative, on the entire system and thus on the individual's behavior, because the nervous system functions holistically.

The CNS contains more than 50 billion neurons of various sizes, cell body sizes and shapes, and degrees of axonal myelination. Generally, the larger the axon diameter, the more heavily myelinated it becomes with nervous system maturation and the faster it will conduct an impulse. Conversely, the smaller the axonal diameter, the less myelin and the slower the conduction rate will be. Neurons can thus be classified according to axon diameter and myelin covering (Table 8-1). Although the smallest fibers are classified as nonmyelinated, a single Schwann cell may envelop several of these fibers with a single layer of myelin. The heavier the myelin sheath, the longer it takes to develop. Therefore, it may be years

* Appreciation is extended to Josephine C. Moore, Ph.D., O.T.R., for her continuing efforts to assist all of us in the understanding of the neuroanatomical and neurophysiological aspects of human function.

Table 8-1. *Nerve Fiber Classification in Descending Order of Myelin Thickness and Conduction Velocity*

General Classification	Dorsal Root Classification	Ventral Root Classification	
A. Large axonal diameter with heaviest myelin wrap	I. 70–120 m/sec Ia—primary sensory ending from neuromuscular spindle Ib—from Golgi tendon organ	Alpha (α)	Motoneurons to extrafusal somatic muscles; 15–120 m/sec
	II. 30–70 m/sec Encapsulated receptors: secondary sensory ending from neuromuscular spindle; cutaneous touch pressure; joint receptors; dermal receptors	Beta (β) Gamma (γ)	Few; innervate both extrafusal and intrafusal fibers Motoneurons to intrafusal fibers of neuromuscular spindles; 10–45 m/sec
	III. Delta (δ)—12–30 m/sec Nonencapsulated nerve endings: mechanoreceptors; cold-sensitive thermoreceptors; some nociceptors		
B. Intermediate axonal diameter and myelin wrap	Visceral afferents—3–15 m/sec		Preganglionic autonomic fibers; 3–15 m/sec
C. Small axonal diameter and essentially unmyelinated	IV. Free nerve endings. Probably serve all sensory modalities; 0.6–2 m/sec. Sometimes referred to as dorsal root C (drC) fibers		Postganglionic sympathetic axons of ANS; 0.7–2.3 m/sec. Sometimes referred to as sympathetic C (sC) fibers

Adapted from Barr ML: The Human Nervous System: An Anatomic Viewpoint, 3rd ed, pp 25–36. Hagerstown, Harper & Row, 1979; Noback CR, Demarest RJ: The Human Nervous System: Basic Principles of Neurobiology, 3rd ed, pp 165–169. New York, McGraw–Hill, 1981.

before full functional capacity is reached. Generally, the larger fibers process the more discriminative, exploratory, or epicritic functions, while the intermediate-size fibers process the protective or protopathic functions, and the smaller fibers process the more primitive functions of the ANS and reticular formation.

In the spinal cord, the A fibers (largest) are found predominately in the dorsolateral portion and will cross over in the medulla. They serve such functions as conscious proprioception, discriminatory tactile, two-point discrimination, vibratory sense, and voluntary motor activity. The B fibers (intermediate) are found predominately in the ventro lateral portion of the spinal cord, and they cross at spinal levels. Functions served include pain, temperature, light touch, vibratory sense, and nonvoluntary motor activity. The C fibers (smallest) are generally found in the area surrounding the gray matter of the cord, and they have a bilateral effect.

Phylogenetically, the nervous system has developed from the most primitive, bilateral functions such as ANS and reticular, referred to as *archi*, to intermediate protective functions known as *paleo*, to the discriminative functions called *neo*. The neo functions, because they involve larger cell bodies and nerve fibers that require more oxygen, are more vulnerable to trauma, whereas

the archi systems are the least vulnerable. Although it depends to some degree on the location and nature of the trauma, the nervous system tends to protect the archi systems the longest. This, then, has implications for rehabilitation. If the system has been damaged, one should first integrate the archi systems, progress through the paleo functions, and finally attempt to rehabilitate the neo functions such as speech and fine manipulation. It is extremely difficult, for example, to use the hands for fine control if the background base of postural stability is deficient.

Excitation and Inhibition

At birth, the individual operates on an excitatory basis: the slightest stimulus sets off a mass reaction. At this time the nervous system is essentially immature. With maturity of the system a base of inhibition is laid down because of the myelination of higher centers that tend to be inhibitory. Normal functioning is dependent on a balance of excitatory and inhibitory influences on the lower motoneurons of the spinal cord and cranial nerves. In order for excitation and inhibition to be mediated by the CNS, there are two basic types of neurons: excitatory and inhibitory. Histologically, the two are similar. The difference is the chemical secreted at the synapse and the effect of that chemical on the postsynaptic neuron. Since a given neuron can have synaptic input from 1000 to 100,000 other neurons, whether or not the firing threshold is reached for propagation of an impulse depends on the total balance between excitatory and inhibitory synapses. For example, if the ratio is 2 : 1 inhibitory/facilitory, then the excitatory impulse will be blocked. If the total system balance is more toward excitation, then the clinical picture may be one of hyperactivity or hypertonicity. If the balance is more toward inhibition, then the clinical picture will be hypotonicity. Depending on the area of trauma and the moment-to-moment state of the individual, which is based in part on the amount and type of sensory input being received and processed, the tonal picture may fluctuate. One can see such fluctuations even in the normal individual.

Excitation and inhibition within the CNS is a complex interaction of presynaptic and postsynaptic inhibition via interneurons and inhibitory centers. For a more thorough understanding of this process, two of the better references are Noback and Williams and Warwick.[16,18]

The balance of excitation and inhibition ultimately affects the threshold levels of postsynaptic neurons within the CNS and the lower motoneurons. Generally speaking, the normal resting threshold is −70 mV and the firing potential is −50 mV. With repeated excitation the resting potential may shift toward −60 mV, which means that a lesser amount of additional excitation is needed to reach firing potential. On the other hand, if the system is receiving more inhibitory overlay, the resting potential may be close to −80 mV so that additional excitation is needed to reach the firing potential. The hypertonic or hyperactive individual may have an overall balance of too much excitation, so that resting potentials are very close to firing potentials, while conversely the hypotonic individual may have a greater discrepancy between resting and firing potentials. The aim of treatment thus becomes an *appropriate* use of sensory input to change the overall balance of the system toward a more normal range of −70 mV resting potential.

Sensory Receptors

One way this can be accomplished is through the use of the sensory receptors. *Exteroceptors* are located in the skin, eyes, and ears. They respond to changes in the external environment such as the general senses of pain, temperature, light touch or light pressure, tactile or touch pressure, and the special senses of vision and hearing. *Proprioceptors* are concerned with vibration, deep pressure, and the position and movements of the body. These receptors are located in the muscles (neuromuscular spindles), tendons (Golgi tendon organs), fas-

cia, joint capsules, ligaments, and the vestibular or equilibrium mechanisms of the inner ear. *Interoceptors*, also called visceroceptors, mediate sensations from the viscera. They play a role in digestion, control of blood pressure, cardiac function, respiration, and so forth. The sensations of fullness of the stomach and bladder or pain from excessive distention are the result of stimulation of these receptors. Visceral sensations are diffuse and poorly localized. The sensations of olfaction and taste have been variously classified as exteroceptors or interoceptors.

Since the nervous system acts as a sensorimotor–sensory feedback system with integration provided by the CNS, various treatment approaches, discussed later in this book, have been developed to excite or dampen these sensory receptors which in turn will have an effect on motor control. If the system is deprived of appropriate sensory input and its integration, disorganized behaviors will result. Sensory deprivation affects synaptic growth and development as well as delaying myelination. An enriched environment will have the opposite effect. Appropriate input includes not only stimulation of the suitable receptors (exteroceptors, proprioceptors, interoceptors) but must also be meaningful to the individual's system, be of the correct intensity and duration, and be applied with tender loving care (TLC) for concurrent emotional integration.

Each of us is bombarded constantly with a multiplicity of sensory inputs, most of which do not evoke a response at a conscious level but are filtered by the reticular system and integrated subcortically. The reticular system extends throughout the spinal cord, brainstem, and diencephalic nuclei of the thalamus and hypothalamus with indirect connections with the cerebral cortex and limbic system.[18] The entire system is polysynaptic.

Reticular Activating System

The reticular activating system (RAS), or ascending portion, provides a generalized bombardment of the cerebral cortex for the purposes of providing the level of consciousness or "awakeness" and the level of alertness to what is most important in the environment. Olfactory and cutaneous stimuli have a profound effect on the level of consciousness. Psychic, auditory, and visual stimuli affect the level of alertness and attention. Damage to this system may result in prolonged coma.[3]

The descending fibers of the reticular system, having received information from the motor centers of the cortex, basal ganglia, and cerebellum, significantly influence the threshold levels of both alpha and gamma motoneurons of the spinal cord and cranial nerves. Since the nuclear centers of this system in the brainstem consist of both excitatory and inhibitory centers, the effect on the motoneurons can be either facilitory or inhibitory. Control centers of the ANS of the brainstem are also affected by this system with effects on respiration, circulation, and heart rate.[3,16,18]

Thus, this entire reticular system has implications for treatment not only of the individual with CNS dysfunction, but also for those with other types of problems, as well as for dealings with students, peers, and others. The type and amount of stimuli being received in relation to the individual's present state will have an effect on his/her responses to the environment and his/her ability to learn.

Limbic System

The limbic system consists of structures found deep within the cerebral hemispheres such as the cingulate, hippocampal, and parahippocampal gyri; the mammillary bodies of the hypothalamus; the fornix, uncus, amygdala, and the medial aspect of the thalamus. According to Moore, the limbic system, because of its location and the structures involved integrates the older sensorimotor, visceral, and reticular systems with the newer, higher-level cognitive functions.[13] In lower animals, these structures serve the olfactory functions and are called the rhinencephalon.

Moore indicates that in human beings, the limbic system is that which drives us to act for survival as individuals and as a species. She uses the mnemonic *MOVE* to outline the functions:

M—memory. Although memory is probably stored in many areas of the CNS, certain parts of the limbic system such as the hippocampus and mammillary bodies appear to be a necessary part of the circuitry for both long-term and short-term memory.
O—olfaction. Although human beings no longer depend on the sense of smell for survival, it still has an influence on the sense of taste, recall of past experiences, emotional responses, and visceral functions.
V—visceral functions related to behavior in conjunction with sensorimotor, cognitive, and emotional responses. The system helps maintain the homeostatic balance. Excessive emotional or physical stress may disturb this balance, with resultant alerting of the SNS for "fight or flight" responses. If continued for too long, the response to distress may disturb the entire balance of the nervous system, leading to disintegration of the individual's behavior.
E—emotional tone or drive. These have been referred to as the "3 Fs": feeding, fighting, and reproduction.[11] The feeding drive involves not only the food, water, and air needed for physical survival, but also, and probably even more important, of the need for love or TLC or, as Broadbent has called it, the "belonging instinct."[7] This drive must be met in order to assure the survival of the individual and the species.[7,9,13]

Since the limbic system is so complex, made up of

fiber connections not only within the system but also with adjacent areas including the reticular system, any stimulation causes long-lasting afterdischarges. Many of its pathways are circular as well as reciprocal in nature. Thus stimulation of one area has an effect on all other areas, which then give feedback both directly and indirectly to the site of original stimulation. Emotional learning thus has strong reinforcement. We are all familiar with an event or song that continually replays itself within our own mind, and with the patient with a cerebrovascular accident who still retains emotional language such as swearing, singing, laughter, and crying although the higher cortical functions of language are lost.[13] Therefore, as therapists we cannot ignore the effects of what we do on the limbic system and the implications for affecting the entire balance of the client.

Corticobulbar System

The corticobulbar system, which innervates the motor nuclei of the cranial nerves, and the corticospinal system, both of which are commonly referred to as the pyramidal system, originate in several areas of the cortex. The figures vary from author to author, but, contrary to popular belief, this system does not originate only in Brodmann's area 4 or the motor strip of the frontal lobe.[3,8,16] Noback indicates that approximately 60% of the fibers originate in areas 4 and 6 of the frontal lobe, whereas the remaining 40% come from areas 3, 1, 2, and 5 of the parietal lobe. Barr indicates that 40% are from area 4; 20% from 3, 1, and 2; and the remainder are predominantly from 6 and 8 of the frontal lobe with the rest being from areas 5 and 7 of the parietal lobe. Approximately 90% of the fibers in this system are small fibers with 2% to 3% being the large fibers from the Betz cells of area 4. Of the more than one million fibers making up the corticospinal system, 85% to 90% cross over in the medullary pyramidal decussation to form the lateral corticospinal tract. Most of the remaining fibers, which do not cross over, make up the anterior corticospinal tract, while a few enter the ipsilateral lateral corticospinal tract. Most of these uncrossed fibers, however, do cross in the spinal cord at their level of function. The lateral corticospinal tracts extend throughout the spinal cord. Approximately 50% of the fibers terminate in the cervical region, 20% in the thoracic area, with the remaining 30% extending to the lumbosacral segments.[16] Barr's figures are 55%, 20%, and 25% respectively.[3] The anterior corticospinal tracts terminate primarily in the cervical area.

Both the corticobulbar and corticospinal fibers traverse the posterior portion of the internal capsule that is supplied primarily by branches of the middle cerebral artery. This is probably the most common area of occlusion in a cerebral vascular accident. Also traversing this area of the internal capsule are sensory projection fibers from the thalamus to the parietal lobe and fibers from the optic and auditory radiations.

At spinal cord levels, it is estimated that at least 90% of the corticospinal fibers synapse with interneurons before exerting their influence on both alpha gamma motoneurons. Some fibers may synapse directly on alpha motoneurons, especially for fine control of the digits. The remainder of the fibers synapse via interneurons in the sensory relay nuclei of the posterior horn of the spinal cord and the brainstem nuclei for the pathways of conscious proprioception.[3,16]

Pyramidal System

Thus the pyramidal system, which was once thought to be *the* direct, monosynaptic pathway for voluntary control of all musculature, is now thought by some observers to be a system for control of speed and agility of voluntary movement and especially significant in the ability to use the digits independently for fine skill.[17]

Extrapyramidal System

The extrapyramidal system includes all of the motor systems other than the corticobulbar and corticospinal (pyramidal) system. The extrapyramidal systems originates from the same cortical areas as the pyramidal, the basal ganglia of the telencephalon, red nucleus, reticular system, substantia nigra of the brainstem, and certain thalamic nuclei of the diencephalon. There is considerable interaction between the pyramidal and extrapyramidal systems via collaterals and feedback circuits. Thus the extrapyramidal system also plays a role in voluntary movement and may provide the background base necessary for postural control.[3,16] With a pure lesion of the pyramidal system, which is relatively rare, there will be flaccidity. However, if any extrapyramidal areas are also involved, there will be hypertonicity. The automatic components of movement and posture are controlled subcortically, whereas the volitional component is controlled primarily at the cortical level. It is difficult, if not impossible, to control more than one act at a time on a cortical level. Therefore, it is necessary for these two systems to act together in order that one may perform a skilled activity on a solid postural base. For example, one can consciously direct the necessary finger movements to perform a Beethoven sonata, but the necessary wrist, forearm, arm, shoulder, trunk, and lower extremity movements are directed simultaneously by subcortical extrapyramidal centers. It is probable that more than 90% of the activities that one performs daily are subcortically controlled.

The circuitry is extremely complex, and a breakdown in one area will affect the functioning of other areas. Thus, the clinical picture will vary considerably from one individual to another. This also makes it extremely difficult to localize the exact area of trauma on the basis of the clinical picture.

Vestibulocochlear System

The connections and pathways of the vestibulocochlear system are many and very intricate. Any of the newer neuroanatomy texts reviews this information. At one time, the vestibular or equilibrium mechanisms were considered separate from the cochlear or auditory processes, but the newer evidence from both the clinical and laboratory research areas now indicates that there are many interactions between these two senses. Enhancement of one will affect the other. Input to this total system assists in the integration of brainstem functions, which then releases the higher centers to perform their functions better.[1] Vestibular therapy is now an accepted method of treatment. However, its various methods and effects, both positive and negative, should be understood by the clinician before being used with any client. Ayres is an excellent reference for this understanding. Basically, any movement that is done slowly and repetitively will dampen the system, whereas movement that is rapid will enhance the system. Many techniques based on this premise are discussed elsewhere in this volume.

Conclusion

As research continues into the structure and function of the neuromuscular spindle and the neurotendinous organ (Golgi tendon organ, GTO), these sensory receptors become more complex and thus more difficult to understand. Moore provided an update on this complexity.[14,15] At present, it appears that the primary sensory ending of the neuromuscular spindle is highly sensitive to vibration, which is why vibrators are being used in treatment. Bishop has written three articles on this subject.[4-6] Noback, Nolte, and Barr[3,16,17] provide an understanding of the structure and possible functions of both of these sensory receptors.

It is important to remember that stimulation of these sensory organs is only *one* way to provide input to the CNS and *may* be an appropriate treatment technique if used in conjunction with other types of input. Used in isolation, it may not be appropriate.

Basic information at this time seems to indicate that the neuromuscular spindle provides autogenic excitation, whereas the neurotendinous organ provides autogenic inhibition. These two structures work closely together and are influenced by higher CNS structures as well as by the present state of the individual.

Overview of Sensorimotor Approaches

Fay–Doman–Delacato: Neuromuscular Reflex Therapy

Temple Fay, neurosurgeon, was the forerunner of the sensorimotor approaches, beginning in the early 1940s. For nearly two decades, he observed , discussed, demonstrated, and wrote about neuromuscular reflex therapy, which he defined as the "utilization of reflex levels of response to the highest level possible."[1] Much of his work was done without present knowledge and understanding of the central nervous system, and it was based on the work of Sherrington. His basic premise was that ontogeny recapitulates phylogeny. Therefore, an individual's neurological development parallels the evolution from fish to amphibian to reptile to anthropoid. Since human movement is based on patterns of muscle activity, not on individual muscle response, Fay believed that if reflex patterns were elicited and utilized properly, functional movement could be established. As a result, his treatment program involved the following six concepts:

1. After careful observation of the patient's level of functioning, including existing reflexes and automatic responses, treatment began with simple patterns of movement utilizing these reflexes.
2. Because in normal development each stage lays the foundation for the next stage, so in treatment it is essential that lower levels of mobility be developed before expecting higher levels.
3. Reflexes in and of themselves are not abnormal but may indicate pathology if they interfere with refined coordinated movement. Therefore, reflexes can be utilized to develop muscle tone, inhibit antagonists, and lead to higher levels of coordinated movement.
4. Passive exercise patterns which involve the total extremity, not isolated joints, can enhance the sensory feedback mechanisms important for movement.
5. Active or passive patterns done repeatedly will in time lead to the spontaneous development of higher-level patterns.
6. The patterns utilized are prone patterns of forward propulsion that can be observed in normal human infants as well as in amphibian and reptilitan life forms.

The three basic patterns used are homologous (bunny hop), homolateral (camel walk), and crossed-diagonal (reciprocal).

Homologous is a bilateral symmetrical pattern. With the head in midline with extension of the neck, the upper extremities are flexed at the shoulder while the lower extremities are extended at the hip. The extremities are then reversed rhythmically with neck flexion. In prone, this is not too effective for propulsion, but in the all-fours position, it is commonly called the bunny hop.

Homolateral is an ipsilateral pattern with the head, thorax, and pelvis turned toward the flexing upper and lower extremities with extension of the contralateral extremities. The pattern is then reversed, leading with the head. In the all-fours position, this provides a gait similar to that of a camel.

Crossed-diagonal is a more highly integrated pattern with flexion of the upper extremity and extension of the lower extremity on the face side and extension of the upper limb with flexion of the lower limb on the opposite side. In the all-fours position, this provides the typical reciprocal gait pattern seen in higher mammals and human infants.

Following the prone position are the all-fours (hands and knees), plantigrade (hands and feet), and erect postures. All three patterns are utilized in the first three positions. Homolateral and crossed-diagonal are utilized in the erect position. Depending on the level of development, patterns are done passively, active-assistively, or actively. The key elements in planning the program for a patient are intellectual and functional motor development levels. Chronological age is less important.

Fay's work has provided the foundation for the approach now advocated by Carl Delacato, Ed.D., Robert Doman, M.D., and Glenn Doman, physical therapist. The same patterns of movement are utilized. In addition, the program includes selective use of sensory stimulation procedures such as heat, cold, brushing, and pinching to establish hand dominance and a breathing exercise routine to increase the vital capacity.

The program for any given patient is administered at least four times per day for 5 minutes, 7 days a week. Each treatment requires at least three adults, because each extremity must be manipulated smoothly and rhythmically in the proper pattern.

Bobath: Neurodevelopmental Treatment

The neurodevelopmental treatment approach has been developed in England by Berta Bobath, physical therapist, and Karel Bobath, neuropsychiatrist. Their work was begun in the 1940s as they observed and worked with patients with cerebral palsy or adult-acquired hemiplegia. However, the treatment is appropriate to a wide variety of other dysfunctions of the central nervous system. Treatment foundations are based on the experimental works of Magnus, Sherrington, deKleijn, Rademaker, Schaltenbrand, Walshe, and Weisz.

The concept of neurodevelopment treatment is based on two fundamental principles about the nature of the central nervous system dysfunction: (1) the arrest or retardation of normal movement is caused by the interference with normal brain maturation resulting from brain lesion, and (2) the resultant release of abnormal or immature postural reflex activity causes the observed abnormal patterns of posture and movement. On the basis of these concepts, treatment techniques have been developed by the Bobaths and others and are continually being added to and refined. Kong, Quilan, Finnie, Mueller, Reye, Mohr, and Morris are names often associated with neurodevelopmental treatment.

The primary aim of treatment handling is the inhibition of abnormal movement patterns with the simultaneous facilitation of normal righting and equilibrium reactions and other appropriate normal movement patterns. The patient is so handled that the abnormal patterns are blocked and higher-level reactions are elicited to give the patient more normal sensory experience. The therapist takes the patient through a series of graded sensory and motor experiences which set the stage for learning new, less stereotyped movement patterns. Through preparation activities, the therapist normalizes the muscle tone (increasing it in the individuals or body parts where tone is too low and decreasing it in the individuals or body parts where it is too high), moves the patient passively to provide sensory experience of unfamiliar movement patterns, encourages active movement from the patient while still providing guidance control and, eventually, encourages the patient to move actively without control. This sequence may take place in one treatment session or may involve weeks or months of therapy.

Movement is a physiological necessity. It allows us to maintain normal muscle tone and yet to be prepared to change that tone instantaneously in response to environmental demand. Movement is the primary modality in neurodevelopmental treatment. Normal movement inhibits abnormal movement; thus normal movement becomes both the process and the goal of therapy. Key points of control are used to influence the movement and balance of tone in the rest of the body. Key points of control are body parts, usually proximal; for example, the trunk and shoulders may be used to prepare the arms for weight bearing and the rest of the body for sidesitting. In addition to facilitation of movement, techniques of tapping, placing and holding, and compression may be used to change the muscle tone when appropriate.[12]

The primary success of neurodevelopmental treatment is contingent on the therapist's ability to make changes in the muscle tone. Prolonged bracing, extensive surgery, and static positioning are usually incompatible with this treatment, becuause they do not allow for changes in muscle tone.

As in all systems of therapy, a thorough initial assessment and frequent reassessment are necessary. The evaluation includes the following: type, strength, and distribution of muscle tone in all positions; abnormal patterns of posture and movement; basic automatic (normal) reactions; general stage of development with awareness of important gaps; contractures and deformities; and other associated handicaps. Readers not familiar with the basic reflex and developmental information are referred to Bobath, Fiorentino, Gesell, and Peiper. On the basis of the initial assessment, a plan of therapy is individualized appropriate to the present level of development and needs of the patient.

Teamwork among occupational therapist, physical therapist, speech therapist, physicians, classroom teacher, and parents is considered an essential aspect of treatment. Therapy is a 24-hour-a-day process when the whole patient and his/her perceptual systems, learning capabilities, personality, and motor system are influenced by the damage to the central nervous system. Close communication and cooperation in the whole treatment plan are essential to prevent disagreement in approach and confusion for the patient and his/her family.

Rood: Neurophysiological Approach

Margaret S. Rood, occupational therapist and physical therapist, frustrated by the slow improvement of patients with cerebral palsy, began to study the neurophysiological and developmental literature in the late 1930s. Based on the works of Sherrington, Gesell, Denny-Brown, Eldred, Hooker, Magoun, Cooper, Boyd, and others, a method of treatment has evolved since the 1940s. The basic principles utilized are as follows[1]:

1. Motor output is dependent on sensory input. Thus sensory stimuli are used to activate and/or inhibit motor responses.
2. Activation of motor responses follows a normal developmental sequence. All muscles progress through the following stages of development:
   a. Full range of shortening and lengthening with the antagonist. Phasic movement — reciprocal innervation
   b. A pattern of cocontraction in which antagonistic muscles of one or more joints work together for a holding action. Stability — tonic postural set
   c. A pattern of heavy work movement superimposed on the cocontraction. Movement in weight-bearing position
   d. Skill or coordinate movement. Movement in non–weight-bearing position with stabilization at the proximal joints

Table 8-2. *Developmental Sequence Neurophysiological Approach (based on Work of Margaret Rood)*

Reciprocal Motion	*Co-Contraction* *(Stability)*	*Heavy Work** *(Movement on Stability)*	*Light Work†* *(Skill)*
1. Inspiration			
2. Expiration			
3. Withdrawal pattern— flexion toward T_{10}			
4. Rolling			
5. Pivot: prone extension except for elbows, which are flexed with arms externally rotated and adducted	6. Neck co-contraction		
	7. Prone on elbows	8. Weight shift: forward; backward; turn (side/side)	9. Belly crawl
	10. All fours	11. Weight shift (rocking): forward/backward; side/side; diagonal	12. Creeping: homologous (bunny hop); homolateral (camel walk); reciprocal
	13. Sitting	14. Weight shift	15. Sit without hand support
	16. Kneeling	17. Weight shift	18. Kneel walk
	19. Half kneel	20. Weight shift	
		21. Assuming standing from half kneel	
	22. Standing	23. Weight shift	24. Walking
			25. Hand skills perfected

* Movement occurs proximally while the distal part of the segment is fixed to the surface (being used for support).

† The distal part of the extremity is free and moving in space while stability is occurring proximally.

3. Since there is interaction within the nervous system between somatic, psychic, and autonomic functions, stimuli can be used to influence one or more directly or indirectly.

This treatment approach can thus be defined as "the activation, facilitation, and inhibition of muscle action, voluntary and involuntary, through the reflex arc" *

This treatment approach assumes that an exercise per se is not treatment unless the pattern of response is correct and results in feedback which enhances learning of that response. Treatment or therapy is not in the form of a motor act alone, but rather is the application of stimuli to activate a response, followed by sensory input from a correct response with additional stimuli given to facilitate or inhibit elements in the pattern. The use of stimuli is an integral part of treatment, since sensory factors are essential for the achievement and maintenance of normal motor functions.[1]

Developmental sequences are outlined in Tables 8-2 and 8-3. These patterns are used to evaluate the patient's level of development which in turn determines the level of treatment.

Sensory stimulation is provided first for the proprioceptors, utilizing vibration, rubbing pressure into the muscle bellies, joint compression, quick stretch of the muscle to be facilitated, and appropriate vestivular input. If necessary, this is followed by exteroceptive input of light touch and/or rapid brushing. Ice, if used at all, is applied with great caution and only to the extremities. If exteroceptive input is used, there should be a careful follow-up of the patient by the therapist for several hours. Since cutaneous stimuli have a profound effect on the reticular system, there may be adverse rebound effects if exteroceptive stimulation is not used appropriately.

Inhibitory procedures used by Rood include slow stroking, neutral warmth, and slow rolling for overall relaxation and pressure to the muscle insertion for specific relaxation. Slow stroking is an alternate stroking of the posterior primary rami with a firm but light pressure.

---

* Rood MS: Personal communication, 1975

Table 8-3.   *Vital Function Developmental Sequences*

Reciprocal Innervation	Stability or Co-innervation	Movement Superimposed on Stability	Skill
1. Inspiration			
2. Expiration	3. Sucking	4. Swallowing fluids	5. Phonation
		6. Chewing	
		7. Swallowing solids	8. Speech

One hand starts at the cervical area and progresses to the lower lumbar region. As the first hand finishes, the second hand starts. Thus, there is always contact with the patient. This is done for no more than 3 minutes. If the hair growth pattern is irregular, this may be irritating to the patient. Neutral warmth is the wrapping of part or all of the patient in a cotton towel or blanket until the appropriate amount of relaxation is observed. Slow rolling from supine to side and return is also generally inhibitory. The rolling continues until relaxation is seen.

Depending on the type of muscle tone and developmental level of the patient, a treatment program may be all-inhibitory, inhibitory and facilitory, or all-facilitory.

Cortical demand for voluntary effort on the part of the patient is directed through activities that utilize the patterns that have been stimulated. The patient's attention is thus directed to the activity and not to specific movement or stabilizing patterns.

Kabat–Knott–Voss: Proprioceptive Neuromuscular Facilitation

Around 1946, Herman Kabat, physiatrist and neurophysiologist, began the development of a therapy system based on neurophysiological principles outlined by Sherrington, Coghill, McGraw, Gesell, Hellebrandt, and Pavlov. The major emphasis is stimulation of the proprioceptors with active participation by the patient. These principles were expanded and utilized in treatment by Margaret Knott and Dorothy Voss, both physical therapists. "Proprioceptive neuromuscular facilitation enlists the less involved parts, to promote a balanced antagonism of reflex activity, of muscle groups and of components of motion." [10]

As stated by Knott and Voss in the second edition of *Proprioceptive Neuromuscular Facilitation,* the philosophy of treatment is:

> . . . based upon the ideas that all human beings respond in accordance with demand; that existing potentials may be developed more fully; that movements must be specific and directed toward a goal; that activity is necessary to the best development of coordination, strength, and endurance; and that the stronger body parts strengthening

weaker parts through cooperaction lead toward a goal of optimum function.[2]

The technique is therefore defined as "methods of promoting or hastening the response of the neuromuscular mechanism through stimulation of the proprioceptors." [10]

There has been a gradual evolution of the technique since the 1940s. Initially, greatest emphasis was placed on the use of maximal resistance throughout the range of motion. Patterns of movement were utilized that allowed action at two or more joints and that required two component actions of a given muscle. Other factors considered important were stretch for proprioceptive stimulation, positioning to enhance contraction, motion beginning in the strongest part of the range progressing to the weaker part, incorporation of reflexes, and reinforcement through resistance.

In 1949, based on Sherrington's law of successive induction, rhythmic stabilization and slow reversal procedures were added to enhance facilitation of the weaker muscles. In 1951, the patterns of movement were analyzed more thoroughly. In order to apply stretch to maximally elongated muscles, it was found that patterns that were spiral and diagonal were most effective and that they also corresponded more nearly to normal functional patterns of movement.

Since that time, the above principles have been incorporated into mat, gait, and self-care activities to assist in motor learning and the development of strength and balance.

Current techniques being used are maximal, but not overpowering resistance; quick stretch; postural and righting reflexes; mass movement patterns with spiral and diagonal components; reversal of antagonists (rhythmic stabilization and slow reversal); and ice (generally used for inhibition and occasionally for facilitation).

The patient is evaluated developmentally, and treatment begun appropriately. In all cases, beginning treatment utilizes the strongest groups of muscles and the most coordinated movements the patient has for reciprocal innervation, irradiation, and summation. Movement patterns are reinforced through simple verbal commands which utilize the patient's voluntary control.

Brunnstrom's Approach

Around 1951, Signe Brunnstrom, physical therapist, became concerned with the lack of rehabilitation of the upper extremity in acquired hemiplegia. She studied the research on reflex responses in decerebrate cats and hemiplegia in man. From the research efforts of Riddoch and Buzzard, Magnus and deKleijn, and Simons, Brunnstrom selected the effects of associated reactions initiated either by voluntary effort on the noninvolved side or by reflex stimulation, postural reactions resulting from tonic neck, and tonic labyrinthine reflexes, and the flexion and extension synergies. After careful observation of more than 100 hemiplegic patients, she delineated the stages of recovery and techniques to facilitate the patient's progression from one stage to the next. Thus, treatment consists of developing the potential for "coordinate movement with reflexlike mechanisms, sensory cues, volitional effort and gradation of demand through the stages of recovery."[1]

The stages of recovery follow a definite sequence, and the patient never skips a stage. However, he or she may plateau at any one of the following six stages:

1. Immediately after the vascular insult there appears to be flaccidity with no voluntary movement in the affected extremities.
2. Spasticity begins to develop. The flexion and extension synergies can be stimulated reflexively. They first appear with cocontraction but gradually become more distinct with the flexion synergy dominating the upper extremity and the extension synergy dominating the lower extremity.
3. Spasticity becomes quite severe. However, the synergies can now be voluntarily initiated with some range of motion. Any attempt to use the extremity voluntarily results in a synergy pattern.
4. Spasticity begins to decrease. Simple uncoordinated movements that differ from the basic synergies can be performed slowly and deliberately. Also, reciprocal movements within the synergies are beginning to develop.
5. Spasticity continues to decrease until the patient can perform some functional activities although still slowly and deliberately without eliciting synergies. Some independence of the synergy patterns is achieved, and isolated individual joint movement is possible.
6. Spasticity has almost disappeared. Individual joint motion is freer and has controlled speed and direction. With rapid, reciprocal movement, some incoordination may still be present.

Because of the degree of cortical control necessary for hand control, recovery of function in the hand is more difficult and less predictable. Mass grasp does precede mass extension, and thumb motion precedes finger motion.

After evaluation of the patient's stage of recovery and sensory status, treatment aimed at reflex training follows. The steps of treatment are:

1. Motion synergies are elicited on a reflex level. Reflexes used include:
   a. Tonic neck reflex
   b. Tonic labyrinthine reflex
   c. Tonic lumbar reflex
   d. Resistance to voluntary contraction of noninvolved limb. (It is important to note that in the upper extremities, resistance to flexion of the noninvolved extremity facilitates flexion in the involved extremity and vice versa. In the lower extremities, resistance to flexion in the noninvolved extremity facilitates extension of the involved extremity and vice versa.)
   e. Sensory stimulation, which includes quick stretch, passive movement, tapping over a muscle belly, surface stroking, positioning, and pressure on the muscle belly or tendon.
2. Motion synergies are captured, that is, an effort is made to establish voluntary control of the synergies. This is accomplished by utilization of the following stages:
   a. Repetition using facilitation
   b. Repetition without facilitation
   c. Working from proximal to distal, concentrating on various components of the synergy with and without the use of facilitation. Reciprocal motion between the two synergies is started with a goal of diminishing the time lag between contraction and relaxation of antagonistic muscles.
3. Motion synergies are conditioned by combining elements of antagonistic synergies starting with the stronger components. At this point, time is also spent on muscles that do not participate in the synergies, such as the serratus anterior and the peroneal muscles. As progress occurs, more complex motions with rapid reciprocation are initiated.
4. The most difficult step is the elicitation of voluntary hand and finger function. Maneuvers such as Souque's phenomenon and imitation synkinesis are helpful.[1]

Postures and positions used during treatment include supine, sitting, and standing. Visual and verbal cues are used throughout. Volitional effort and functional activities are initiated early, and they are considered necessary if there is to be carry-over by the patient.

Ayres: Sensory Integration Approach to Learning Disorders

A. Jean Ayres, Ph.D., O.T.R., began her studies of children with learning disabilities in the 1950s. She and others observed that the cognitive approach to treatment of such children had led to dissatisfaction with skill training as an end in and of itself, because too many children were still unable to generalize and respond adaptively to their environment. Study of the approaches of Knott, Bobath, Fay, and especially Rood for the physically handicapped, which emphasized integration of the nervous system at subcortical levels, seemed to have some application to those with learning problems.

Ayres' intensive and extensive research studies of these latter problems, along with intense study of the integrative functions of the nervous system, led to her present and still evolving theoretical framework from which treatment procedures are devised. This is discussed further in the next section.

Fuchs: Orthokinetics

Julius Fuchs, orthopedic surgeon, dissatisfied with the static approach of braces, casts, and splints, created devices that provided immediate mobilization as well as support. His work was done in the 1920s and published in German in 1927; however, a description in English was not published until 1955. The principles originally were applied to fractures, scoliosis, and other orthopedic problems. The application to neurological and arthritic dyskinesias was made in the 1950s by Manfred Blashy, physiatrist, and Elsbeth Harrison and Ernest Fuchs, both occupational therapists.

The basic idea in orthokinetics is the use of a segment or cuff composed of elastic and inelastic parts. Several of these put together form the orthokinetic tube. The inelastic or inactive fields cover those parts where support and muscle inactivity are desired. The elastic or active fields cover those parts where muscle activity is desired. The inactive field thus becomes the inhibitory field and the active field the facilitory field.

Originally, these cuffs were made of leather and molded directly to the patient. Currently, they are made of Ace bandages or sewing elastic 1 to 6 inches wide, depending on the size of the area of application. The device is usually two or three layers thick for the active field and three to four layers thick in the inactive field. The layers are stitched firmly together to provide the inactive field and left free for the active field. The cuff can be fastened with Velcro.

Among the results claimed by Fuchs and others are (1) rapid relief of pain, (2) increase of muscle strength, (3) increased range of motion, (4) muscle re-education,

and (5) improvement of coordination. I have also noted an increase in girth as muscle bulk fills in.

The cuffs are worn repeatedly to increase the effects. They can be worn all day while the individual is active. This provides continuous sensory input. The greater the imbalance initially between agonist and antagonist muscle groups, the quicker the effects will be noticed.

This is an effective, inexpensive procedure that supplies continuous input when the patient is not "in therapy." It should be further investigated by occupational and physical therapists for its value as an adjunct to treatment.

Summary

In looking at the various sensorimotor treatment approaches, it is helpful to place them in a continuum of control needed by the patient.

The Fay–Doman–Delacato approach is initially one of passive movements superimposed on the patient; only later does this call for active participation on the part of the patient.

Rood uses a strong mixture of exteroceptive and proprioceptive input in developmental patterns followed by activity utilizing the stability and mobility components of the patterns. The individual's attention is directed to the activity and not to the patterns per se.

Orthokinetics provides a continuous exteroceptive input followed by proprioceptive feedback as muscles are facilitated and inhibited. The individual is able to use the resultant muscle function in activities of daily living.

Bobath inhibits primitive patterns and then facilitates righting and equilibrium reactions, controlling at key points, so that the nervous system receives feedback only from more normal movement. Whenever possible, cortical control of movement is demanded.

Brunnstrom uses the initial synergy patterns seen in recovery from cerebral vascular insult on both a reflexive level and with conscious control by the patient. Using exteroceptive and proprioceptive input as well as cortical control, these patterns are then broken up and lead to functional movement.

Kabot, Knott, and Voss place primary emphasis on proprioceptive input reinforced by visual and verbal cues that demand cortical control by the client. Exteroceptive stimulation is considered primarily in the placement of the therapist's hands.

Thus, when the client is at a level in which cortical control hinders movement, approaches such as the Rood, Fuchs, Bobath, and Fay can be utilized. Once cortical control begins to develop and strengthening is needed, the Brunnstrom and Kabat-Knott-Voss approaches become appropriate.

Many of the techniques of the various approaches are quite similar. Often, it is feasible to employ techniques from various approaches at any given time with any individual. The therapist must know and understand normal human development, neurophysiology, and techniques of evaluation in order to use these treatment approaches effectively.

At present, there is controversy whether these approaches to the treatment of CNS dysfunction should be used by occupational therapists or whether they are strictly a physical therapy approach. Being certified in both professions, I firmly believe that occupational therapists should know and utilize the underlying principles and techniques of the sensorimotor approaches. It takes appropriate input to organize the CNS for output, and the motor output must be purposeful, goal-directed activity in order for it to be retained and built upon by the CNS. Occupational therapists are in a unique position to utilize purposeful, goal-directed activity on a subcortical level. These approaches will not be effective unless the client is allowed to actively respond to the input in a meaningful way.

References

1. Am J Phys Med: NUSTEP, 46:1, 1967
2. Ayres AJ: Sensory Integration and Learning Disorders. Los Angeles, Western Psychological Services, 1972
3. Barr ML: The Human Nervous System: An Anatomic Viewpoint, 3rd ed. Hagerstown, Harper & Row, 1979
4. Bishop B: Vibratory stimulation I: Neurophysiology of motor responses. Phys Ther 54:1273, 1974
5. Bishop B: Vibratory stimulation II: Vibratory stimulation as an evaluation tool. Phys Ther 55:28, 1975
6. Bishop B: Vibratory stimulation III: Possible applications of vibration in treatment of motor dysfunction. Phys Ther 55:139, 1975
7. Broadbent WW: How To Be Loved. Englewood Cliffs, Prentice–Hall, 1976
8. Gilman S, Newman SW: Manter and Gatz's Essentials of Clinical Neuroanatomy & Neurophysiology, 7th ed. Philadelphia, FA Davis, 1987
9. Huss AJ: Touch with care or a caring touch? Am J Occup Ther 31:11, 1977
10. Knott M, Voss DE: Proprioceptive Neuromuscular Facilitation: Patterns and Techniques, 2nd ed. New York, Harper & Row, 1968
11. MacLean PD: The limbic system with respect to self-preservation and the preservation of the species. J Nerv Ment Dis 127:1, 1958
12. Manning J: Facilitation of movement—the Bobath approach. Physiotherapy (Eng) 58:403, 1972
13. Moore JC: Behavior, bias, and the limbic system. Am J Occup Ther 30:11, 1976
14. Moore JC: The Golgi tendon organ: A review and update. Am J Occup Ther 38:227, 1984
15. Moore JC: The Golgi tendon organ and the muscle spindle. Am J Occup Ther 28:415, 1974
16. Noback CR, Demarest RJ: The Human Nervous System: Basic Principles of Neurobiology, 3rd ed. New York, McGraw–Hill, 1981
17. Nolte J: The Human Brain: An Introduction to Its Functional Anatomy. St Louis, CV Mosby, 1981
18. Williams PL, Warwick R: Functional Neuroanatomy of Man. Philadelphia, WB Saunders, 1975

Bibliography

Bailey DM: The effects of vestibular stimulation on verbalization in chronic schizophrenics. Am J Occup Ther 32:445, 1978

Blashy M: Manipulation of the neuromuscular unit in the periphery of the central nervous system. J South Med Assoc 54:873, 1961

Blashy M, Fuchs R: Orthokinetics: A new receptor facilitation method. Am J Occup Ther 13:226, 1959

Blashy M, Harrison HE, Fuchs EM: Orthokinetics—a preliminary report on recent experiences with a little known rehabilitation therapy. VA Bull, 1955

Bobath B: Abnormal Postural Reflex Activity Caused by Brain Lesions, 2nd ed. London, Wm Hemann, 1971

Bobath B: Motor development, its effect on general development and application to the treatment of cerebral palsy. Physiotherapy (Eng) 57:526, 1971

Bobath B: Adult Hemiplegia: Evaluation and Treatment, 2nd ed. London, Wm Heinemann, 197: A Neurophysiological Basis for the Treatment of Cerebral Palsy. Philadelphia, JB Lippincott, 1980

Bobath K, Bobath B: The facilitation of normal postural reactions and movements in the treatment of cerebral palsy. Physiotherapy (Eng) 50:246, 1964

Bobath K, Bobath B: The importance of memory traces of motor efferent discharges for learning skilled movements. Dev Med Child Neurol 16:837, 1974

Brunnstrom S: Movement Therapy in Hemiplegia: A Neurophysiological Approach. New York, Harper & Row, 1970

Carlson SJ: A neurophysiological analysis of inhibitive casting. Phys Occup Ther Pediatr 4:31, 1984

Carpenter MB: Core Text of Neuroanatomy, 3rd ed. Baltimore, Williams & Wilkins, 1985

Curry EL, Clelland JA: Effects of the asymmetric tonic neck reflex and high-frequency muscle vibration on isometric wrist extension strength in normal adults. Phys Ther 61:487, 1981

Dayhoff N: Rethinking stroke: Soft or hard devices to position hands. Am J Nurs 7:1142, 1975

Desmedt JE: Motor Unit Types, Recruitment and Plasticity in Health and Disease. Progress in Clinical Neurophysiology series, Vol 9. New York, S Karger, 1981

Doman G, Delacato C: Children with severe brain injuries. JAMA 174:257, 1960

Farber SD: Olfaction in health and disease. Am J Occup Ther 32:155, 1978

Farber SD: Neurorehabilitation: A Multi-Sensory Approach. Philadelphia, WB Saunders, 1982

Fay T: Basic considerations regarding neuromuscular and reflex therapy. Spastics Quart 3, 1954

Fay T: Neuromuscular reflex therapy for spastic disorders. J Florida Med Assoc 44, 1958

Fiorentino M: Reflex Testing Methods for Evaluating CNS

Development, 2nd ed. Springfield, Charles C Thomas, 1976

Fiorentino M: A Basis for Sensorimotor Development— Normal and Abnormal: The Influence of Primitive, Postural Reflexes on the Development and Distribution of Tone. Springfield, Charles C Thomas, 1981

Fox JVD: The olfactory system: Implications for the occupational therapist. Am J Occup Ther 20:173, 1966

Gellhorn E: Principles of Autonomic-Somatic Integrations. Minneapolis, University of Minnesota Press, 1967

Gilfoyle EM, Grady AP, Moore JC: Children Adapt, 2nd ed. Thorofare, NJ, Charles B Slack, 1986

Goff B: The application of recent advances in neurophysiology to Miss M. Rood's concept of neuromuscular facilitation. Physiotherapy (Eng) 58:409, 1972

Granit R: The functional role of the muscle spindles—facts and hypotheses. Brain 98:531, 1975

Hagbarth KE: Effects of the Jendrassik manoeuvre on muscle spindle activity in man. J Neurol Neurosurg Psych 38:1143, 1975

Harlowe D, VanDuesen J: Brief: Evaluating cutaneous sensation following CVA: Relationships among touch, pain, temperature tests. Occup Ther J Res 5:70, 1985

Haron M, Henderson A: Active and passive touch in developmentally dyspraxic and normal boys. Occup Ther J Res 5:101, 1985

Harris FA: Multiple-loop modulation of motor outflow: A physiological basis for facilitation techniques. Phys Ther 51:391, 1971

Harris FA: Facilitation techniques in therapeutic exercise. In Basmajian JW (ed): Therapeutic Exercise, Student Ed. Baltimore, Williams & Wilkins, 1980

Heiniger MC, Randolph SL: Neurophysiological Concepts in Human Behavior: The Tree of Learning. St Louis, CV Mosby, 1981

Huss AJ: Application of Rood technique to treatment of the physically handicapped child. In West W (ed): Occupational Therapy for the Multiply Handicapped Child. Chicago, University of Chicago Press, 1965

Huss AJ: Clinical application of sensorimotor treatment techniques in physical dysfunction, and controversy and confusion in physical dysfunction treatment techniques— clinical aspects. In Zamir L (ed): Expanding Dimensions in Rehabilitation. Springfield, Charles C Thomas, 1969

Kabot H: Central facilitation: The basis of treatment for paralysis. Permanente Fnd Med Bull 10, 1962

Keshner EA: Reevaluating the theoretical model underlying the neurodevelopmental theroy: A literature review. Phys Ther 61:1035, 1981

King LJ: Toward a science of adaptive responses. Am J Occup Ther 32:429, 1978

Knott M: Bulbar involvement with good recovery. JAPTA 46:721, 1966

Knott M: Neuromuscular facilitation in the treatment of rheumatoid arthritis. JAPTA 44:737, 1964

Koczwara H: Use of a vibrator to facilitate motor and kinesthetic behavior in children. Phys Ther 55:510, 1975

Kukulka CG, Beckman SM, Holte JB et al: Effects of intermittent tendon pressure on alpha motoneuron excitability. Phys Ther 66:1091, 1986

Leiper CI, Miller A, Lang J et al: Sensory feedback for head control in cerebral palsy. Phys Ther 61:512, 1981

Loomis J: Facilitation techniques in hemiplegia—treatment of the arm. J Can Physiother Assoc 25:283, 1973

Magoun HW: The Waking Brain, 2nd ed. Springfield, Charles C Thomas, 1963

Mason CR: One melthod for assessing the effectiveness of fast brushing. Phys Ther 65:1197, 1985

McClannahan C: Feeding & Caring for Infants and Children with Special Needs, 2nd ed. Rockville, MD. AOTA Products, 1987

McPherson JJ: Objective evaluation of a splint designed to reduce hypertonicity. Am J Occup Ther 35:189, 1981

Montgomery P, Richter E: Sensorimotor Integration for Developmentally Disabled Children: A Handbook. Los Angeles, Western Psychological Services, 1977

Moore JC: Concepts from the Neurobehavioral Sciences. Dubuque, Kendall–Hunt, 1973

Moore JC: Recovery potentials following CNS lesions: A brief historical perspective in relation to modern research data on neuroplasticity. Am J Occup Ther 40:459, 1986

Neeman R: Techniques of preparing effective orthokinetic cuffs. AOTA Bull 6:1, 1971

Neuhaus BE, Ascher ER, Coullon BA et al: A survey of rationales for and against hand splinting in hemiplegia. Am J Occup Ther 35:83, 1981

Noback CR, Demerest RJ: The Nervous System: Introduction and Review, 3rd ed. New York, McGraw–Hill, 1986

Ottenbacher KJ, Biocca Z, DeCremer G, et al: Quantitative analysis of the effectiveness of pediatric therapy: Emphasis on the neurodevelopmental treatment approach. Phys Ther 66:1095, 1986

Payton OD, Hirt S, Newton RA: Scientific Bases for Neurophysiologic Approaches to Therapeutic Exercise. Philadelphia, FA Davis, 1977

Pink M: Contralateral effects of upper extremity proprioceptive neuromuscular facilitation patterns. Phys Ther 61:1158, 1981

Ray SA, Bundy AC, Nelson DL: Decreasing drooling through techniques to facilitate mouth closure. Am J Occup Ther 37:749, 1983

Resman MKH: Effect of sensory stimulation on eye contact in a profoundly retarded adult. Am J Occup Ther 35:31, 1981

Rheault W, Derleth M, Casey M et al: Effects of an inverted position on blood pressure, pulse rate, and deep tendon reflexes of healthy young adults. Phys Ther 65:1358, 1985

Romero-Sierra C: Neuroanatomy: A Conceptual Approach. New York, Churchill Livingstone, 1986

Rood MS: Proprioceptive neuromuscular facilitation and demonstration physiotherapy and occupational therapy. S Afr Cerebral Palsy J 13:3, 1969

Rood MS: The use of sensory receptors to activate, facilitate, and inhibit motor response, autonomic and somatic, in developmental sequence. In Sattely C, Kandel D: Approaches to the Treatment of Patients with Neuromuscular Dysfunction. Study Course VI. Dubuque, Wm C Brown, 1962

Rood MS: Use of Reflexes as an Aid in Occupational Therapy. Speech delivered at World Federation of Occupational Therapy Meeting, Copenhagen, 1958

Scratton D: Management of the Motor Disorders of Children with Cerebral Palsy. Clin Dev Med Monogr Ser 90. Philadelphia, JB Lippincott, 1984

Sherrington C: The Integrative Action of the Nervous System. New Haven, Yale University Press, 1961

Springer SP, Deutsch G: Left Brain, Right Brain, rev ed. New York, WH Freeman, 1985

Tokizane T: Electromyographic studies on tonic neck, lumbar and labyrinthine reflexes in normal persons. Jap J Physiol 2:130, 1951

Trombly CA: Occupational Therapy for Physical Dysfunction, 2nd ed. Baltimore, Williams & Wilkins, 1983

Umphred DA: Neurological Rehabilitation. St Louis, CV Mosby, 1985

Voss DE: Proprioceptive neuromuscular facilitation: Application of patterns and technics in occupational therapy. Am J Occup Ther 13:191, 1959

Voss DE, Ionta MK, Myers BJ: Proprioceptive Neuromuscular Facilitation: Patterns and Techniques, 3rd ed. Philadelphia, Harper & Row, 1985

Weeks ZR: Effects of the vestibular system on human development I: Overview of functions and effects of stimulation. Am J Occup Ther 33:376, 1979

Whelan JK: Effects of orthokinetics on upper extremity function adult hemiplegic patient. Am J Occup Ther 18:141, 1964

Zelle RS, Coyner AB: Developmentally Disabled Infants and Toddlers: Assessment and Intervention. Philadelphia, FA Davis, 1983

SECTION 3

Integration in Sensorimotor Therapy   *Mary Silberzahn*

The continuing development of sensorimotor theory and practice in occupational therapy is closely associated with current research and advancements in the neurosciences. Neurology began as a science which dealt with abnormalities and disease related to central nervous system (CNS) damage or lesions. Sensorimotor therapies were developed beginning in the 1940s to alleviate impaired motor function resulting from CNS abnormalities and can be viewed as a compatible, even complementary, continuum of neuromuscular, neurodevelopmental, and neurophysiological approaches. Rood, followed by Ayres, introduced the concept of integration based on the recognition that the CNS not only directs motor action but also uses sensory feedback from motor activity for coordinating motor function. In 1963, Ayres suggested that it is more useful to think of the primary task of the CNS as one of integration: "Thoughts, previous experience, sensory input and motor output are all integrated continuously."[1] A therapeutic approach that utilizes concepts of integration promotes generalized motor ability as opposed to skill in a single task.

During the second half of this century, the idea that discrete parts of matter could be studied meaningfully in isolation from the whole began to be seriously challenged by some researchers. Findings of modern physics led to the recognition that the universe is a dynamic system whose natural forces and physical laws influence all substance including human life, and these findings led the way to the change which is evolving in scientific thinking. Capra has described the need to study matter in terms of interaction and interrelationships:

The properties of a particle can be understood only in terms of its activity—of its interaction with the surrounding environment . . . the particle, therefore, cannot be seen as an isolated entity, but has to be understood as an integrated part of the whole.[7]

The new direction investigators in the neurosciences must adopt is clearly stated by Walsh:

. . . to understand neural structures and function fully we need to examine the brain when it is engaged in meaningful activity, function and behavior, and in terms of its relationship to the environment.[32]

There are indications of change. Neuroscience has expanded to include neurobehavior and the study of nondiscrete lesions observable only when the individual interacts with the environment. The focus of sensorimotor therapy has shifted from a model of neuropathology to a model of functional relationships both within the brain and between the individual and the environment. New models designed to study the relationship of parts to the whole can be found in general systems theory and in Luria's neurobehavioral approach to the study of higher cortical functions. Specific to occupational therapy is the theoretical model of sensory integration and learning disabilities constructed by Ayres in the late 1960s. This theory has influenced the occupational therapist's role in evaluation and treatment of children and adults, many of whose problems in behavior and learning cannot be related directly to discrete pathology within the nervous system.

A. Jean Ayres and Julio B. de Quiros were among the first researchers to recognize human learning as a meaningful activity dependent on a system of dynamic interaction between the brain and the environment. Both of these investigators, working independently, studied learning disabilities as systemic dysfunctions. They reasoned that dysfunction in neural integration (*i.e.,* in the way in which the brain combines and interprets sensations from different sensory modalities for coordinated, intentional motor acts) may explain some idiopathic childhood learning disorders. Although the work of each investigator reflects their professional orientation — Ayres as an occupational therapist with a doctorate in educational psychology and de Quiros, a doctor of medicine with additional doctorates in communication disorders — their published works are complementary. Ayres stresses the importance of the integration of sensations for learning: "It is the nature and sequence of sensory integration that is the *sine qua non* to understanding perception and the requirements of early academic learning."[4] De Quiros emphasizes the motor activity basis of knowledge: "Postural systems permit the development of motor activity," then "intentional and coordinated motor activity allows the presence of learning processes."[9]

The primary purpose of this discussion is to present an overview of current theoretical concepts of integration which support the role of occupational therapy in treating persons with learning disorders related to sensorimotor dysfunction. Although the subject is approached from a developmental point of view, the underlying idea — that the brain is a dynamic and complex system whose functions depend on the influence of the environment — has significance for all areas of occupational therapy practice in which impaired function is evidenced by inability to adapt and learn in the environment. According to the concept of a functional system, a problem in any area of the brain will lead to disintegration of the entire system. As Luria has pointed out, "a lesion of a particular part of the brain in early childhood had a systemic effect on the *higher* cortical areas superposed above it, whereas a lesion of the same region in adult life affects *lower* zones of the cortex, which now begin to depend on them."[20]

Integration and Learning

Development, a process of continuous change throughout the life cycle, is the result of the interaction of evolution, maturation, and learning.[9] It is the interaction of these processes and of the environmental influences on which they depend that is of major concern to the occupational therapist.

Evolution is defined as the "biological development of inherited behaviors"[9] and includes all predetermined changes which occur within the organism during the life span. Studies in brain evolution include the sequence and rate of myelination; the interconnections of neural pathways, structures, and functions; and the potential interrelations with human behavior and learning. Inherent within the brain are genetically programmed behaviors such as species-specific positions and patterns of movement which, according to ideas of species evolution, are "behavioral reflections of genetic memories about the experiences of earlier brains."[6]

Maturation is the outward manifestation of biological and environmental changes.[9] Species-specific patterns such as sitting, crawling, standing, and walking which depend on central programs of the nervous system become evident.

Evolution and maturation make *learning* possible but cannot be equated with it. The biological child will grow; pass through the cycles of infancy, childhood, puberty, and adulthood; and experience the effects of aging yet may remain limited in the acquisition of human learning. Learning unique to humankind is established on symbolic abilities. These abilities demand sufficient bioneurological development, adequate environmental influences, and noninterference by the body itself with higher cortical levels.[9]

Species evolutionary theory proposes that the changes in brain structure and function are directly related to environmental change. The innate drive for homeostasis and survival requires that the organism adapt to the demands of the environment. Adaptation requires changes in the nervous system which permit more complex sensory reception and interpretation of sensory data for information about the self in space and the environment. The ability to use the negative feedback from sensorimotor activity for functional reorganization within the nervous system, and thus permit adaptation at a higher level, appears to be critical to the idea that only the most adaptable survive. When the necessary sensory and motor units were functionally organized according to survival needs, the species was established. Species-specific programs for behavior are genetically transmitted to each member of the species. However, each member must undergo, to a lesser or greater degree, a period of biological learning which involves sensory and motor activity organized for adaptive behavior in order to actualize the genetic potential for species learning.

A continual dynamic balance between evolution and maturation supports the inner drive toward goal-directed sensory and motor activity and facilitates the neural integration of these experiences. The normal child will immediately begin to use what is available for learning to control the body in space and for exploration or manipulation of the physical/object world.

Human learning is a function that becomes evident only through the help of the human environment, whereas biological learning emerges from the bioneural capacities of the child for purposeful action and progressive integration. De Quiros and Schrager[9] have distinguished four developmentally acquired learning processes. The first two depend mainly on the biological child interacting with the natural environment and can be acquired by both children and animals with the guidance of caretakers. The last two processes depend on higher cortical functions and represent human acquisitions which must have the help of human tutors and appropriate tools. In *primary learning processes,* the child learns adaptation and survival in the natural environment. As postures and equilibrium are acquired, the child learns to use species-specific behaviors to act in space and to learn the position and location of the body in space and in relation to environmental forces and objects. The child learns to use motion for body competency. In *secondary learning processes,* the child learns from his own sensory and motor experiences and from the experiences of others. Through the use of his physical abilities and body knowledge, he learns behaviors appropriate to the human environment, such as self-dressing and self-feeding and learns to recognize environmental dangers and to take precautionary measures; *i.e.,* the stove is hot, how to cross the street, what to do in case of fire. He also begins to learn emotional–social behaviors. In *tertiary learning processes,* action gives way to perception, the acquisition and use of concrete knowledge about location and position and properties of the spatial/object world. The child develops lingua, the use of words to express his concrete perceptual knowledge and to direct motor ability. Lingua is a learned ability and is the basis for language as symbolic communication. In *quaternary learning processes,* the child learns to mentally manipulate percepts formed earlier. Symbols are used to transmit and receive information. The ability to think abstractly and creatively, to formulate plans to direct actions, and to use language as an expression of ideas and concepts becomes evident.

Learning Disabilities

Learning disabilities are disturbances in the acquisition of specific human skills: a dysfunction of cortical processes.[9] The presenting problems are in reading, writing, mathematics, or language. De Quiros maintains that learning disabilities are systemic dysfunctions: "that which generates a learning disability is not an assumed central nervous system dysfunction but the interaction between neurological disturbances and environmental influences."[9] If early systemic integration fails, higher, more complex systems cannot be formed adequately. Learning disabilities can begin between ages three and five years when the cerebellum should become active in postural integration and the child begins to learn through adaptive involvement with the environment.[9]

Learning disabilities are not a diagnostic category, because the etiologies of various disabilities differ. De Quiros has categorized learning problems as a primary disability when the etiology is unknown and as a sec-

ondary disability when related to other abnormalities such as brain damage, hearing or visual impairment, or psychic or environmental problems. Primary learning disabilities are further divided into those resulting from compensated brain damage or dysfunction manifested by developmental dysphasia, dyslexia, or apractognosia; from perceptual handicaps, especially auditory and visual discrimination deficits; and from faulty postural afferences, mainly vestibular and proprioceptive.

Those children whose learning problems can be related to inadequate integration of vestibular and proprioceptive inputs are of special concern to the occupational therapist because their problems stem from lower levels of the brain and involve the integration of sensory and motor functions. Reading disabilities may result from vestibular–oculomotor dysfunction when visual fixation and sequencing are inadequate. Lack of postural control and the failure to acquire skilled movement may generate disturbances in attention span and in writing when vestibular–spinal pathways are not functioning adequately.[9] De Quiros proposes the use of past pathology to clarify the confusion surrounding the term "minimal brain dysfunction." Past pathology is associated with developmental lags and can explain many symptoms that commonly result from brain damage in the learning-disabled child such as hypertonia or hypotonia, poor attention span, disinhibition, and perseveration. According to the concept of past pathology, brain damage occurred early in life and was "successfully" treated medically so that asymmetries disappear during dynamic situations. However, earlier damage can be detected through the observation of static responses such as an asymmetrical tonic neck reflex and asymmetries observed in the maintained prone extension or supine flexion position and in the one-foot-stand position.

Systemic Integration

The human nervous system, comprising the brain structures and pathways, is a system of nature and, as such, has wholeness that cannot be reduced to parts, self-maintenance in a changing environment, self-creation in response to environmental challenges, and participation in the hierarchical order of nature.[32] The nervous system is also a system for information processing and has the characteristics of cybernetics, "the science of control mechanisms and their associated information systems."[9] In this sense, a system has a source of input of energy or information, a means for internally organizing or integrating this input into units of energy or information, and a means of releasing the energy or information as output. The output is returned to the input through feedback mechanisms, and the system is modified to incorporate change and to maintain balance. If one part of the system is in dysfunction, the whole system will be disrupted.

Russian psychologists, beginning in the 1920s, proposed that higher mental abilities depend on a "functional system" that includes not only the function of a particular neural structure but also a dynamic interaction between parts within the nervous system and between the organism and the environment.[20] They believed that a function expressed as behavior depends on neural subsystems functionally organized according to the task demand. Although the function (*e.g.,* movement) remains the same, the neural combinations will vary according to the sensorimotor feedback for monitoring performance. Thus, the task and the feedback both influence the neural combinations or subsystems serving the function.

The idea of integrative functions of the nervous system was first introduced to the neurosciences in 1870 by Hughlings Jackson. As a result of Jackson's work, it is now recognized that the nervous system is organized in vertical hierarchical levels of function: the low (spinal) level; the intermediate (brain stem–cerebellar) level; and the higher (cortical) levels. Neural integrative levels are most helpful in studying the progressive functional organization of sensory and motor activity below the level of the cortex. When integrated into the whole of neural activity for behavior and learning, efferent and afferent impulses at lower levels act as an integrated whole to subserve cerebral cortex functions.

During the child's development, both the structure and the "interfunctional organization" of higher mental processes change.[20] Sensory input from the external environment and feedback from purposeful motor activity are progressively integrated, and functional systems are reorganized within the developing brain. As existing subsystems are integrated into a higher functional whole, entirely new systemic properties are originated. This idea is expressed in gestalt theory as "the whole is greater than the sum of the parts."

Schematically, in every motor function a low intermediate, and higher level of activity can be recognized beginning with the regulation of posture and tone and permitting environmental exploration and, later, participation in higher cortical learning. When lower-level functions such as posture maintenance are not established and integrated so that they contribute to, but do not interfere with, higher cortical functions, learning possibilities are decreased. According to de Quiros and Schrager, progressive integration permits the exclusion of body efferent and afferent impulses from consciousness through the transfer of some brain functions to automatic levels.[9]

Schrager, on the basis of his work with de Quiros, has delineated a hierarchy of systemic integration for human learning: tonic–postural–antigravitational integration, sensory integration, motor integration, corporal integration, spatial integration, symbolic integration, volitional integration, and psychosocio-cultural integration.[25] As the need for integration becomes less demanding in one area through the establishment of new neural subsystems, the brain is gradually freed to integrate sensorimotor activity at progressively higher levels and, finally, to exclude afferent and efferent impulses from consciousness. Not only is this process efficient in preventing fragmentation of brain function, but it also permits the specialized functions of the cerebral hemispheres to emerge.

Ayres focuses on the events between the sensation and the response, which she has identified as sensory integration, in relation to the acquisition of human learning.[4] She emphasizes the need for sensations to be processed and integrated as information from the enviroment and from the body and interpreted for the planning and execution of motor acts. Purposeful, goal-directed motor acts, important to learning, arise from meaningful sensory stimuli, that is, an accurate interpretation of environmental demands. The neural integration of sensory stimuli depends on the convergence of efferent impulses at common integration structures for intermodality association and thus for coordinating several types of information. Other neurophysiological regulators of sensory integration are the central control of centrifugal flow, interrelations between depressing and facilitating impulses, sensorimotor feedback, and inhibitory processes. The tracing of sensory systems and their possible sites of integration and the functional significance of the integrative action are essential to understanding the relation between sensory integration and learning. The sensorimotor approach to the treatment of learning disabilities requires that the therapist have a working knowledge of the interaction between neurological functions and environmental influences.

Tonic–Postural–Antigravitational Integration

The drive to obtain and maintain the upright position is innate in the human species. Control of the body in space is essential to survival and, even in adulthood, supersedes other cortical functions when threatened. The control and integration of the postural system is also basic to human learning. "To achieve postural control is to develop attention span, to open exteroceptors (particularly eyes and ears), and to allow more skilled movements."[9] According to evolution theory, human learning began when a species obtained an upright, antigravity position and the upper extremeties were freed for tool use.

Tone refers to the tension state or activity level of the nervous system which provides the background energy for action. Posture is the "reflex activity of the body in relation to space"[9] based on muscle tone for the flexed or extended tonic posture. Equilibrium is the "interplay between various forces, particularly gravity, and the motor power of the skeletal muscles."[9] Equilibrium is the interrelation of the body to the environment and is based on the interaction of vestibular, somatosensory, and visual functions coordinated by the cerebellum. Posture and equilibrium comprise the postural system, which maintains relationships within the body itself and within space so that body positions appropriate to goal-directed activity can be obtained and maintained. The brain is continuously receiving information about the body through sensory input to higher centers. These higher cortical levels can be used to control the postural system but, in order for human learning to occur at higher levels, sensorimotor activity from the body must be inhibited (*i.e.*, excluded from consciousness). De Quiros uses the term "corporal potentiality" to express the possibility of excluding body information from conscious awareness in order to obtain human learning.[9]

Primary postural integration at the brainstem–cerebellar level, which should be achieved during the first three or four years of life, coordinates species-specific positions and patterns of movement at levels below consciousness. The child has automatic control of sitting, standing, walking in space; balance is perfectly controlled. However, in order to engage in goal-directed activities, the child needs "purposeful equilibrium," the postural background for purposeful action in the space/object world. Purposeful equilibrium is both dependent on and contributes to body laterality, according to de Quiros.

Dysfunction in primary postural integration is manifested by low muscle tone, poor extraocular responses, and poor equilibrium reactions. A similar dysfunction has been identified and described by Ayres as the syndrome of "postural and bilateral integration,"[4] and more recently referred to as "vestibular–bilateral integration."[5] The clinical parameters are poorly integrated primitive postural reflexes, immature equilibrium reactions, poor ocular control, and a variety of observable deficits in bilateral and symmetrical functions. The distinguishing feature of Ayres' syndrome is the emphasis she places on integration of the function of the two sides of the body as related to interhemispheric communication.

Sensory Integration

Sensory integration is defined by Ayres as:

> the organization of sensory input for use. The "use" may be a perception of the body or the world, or an adaptive response or a learning process, or the development of some neural function. Through sensory integration, the many parts of the nervous system work together so that a person can interact with the environment effectively and experience appropriate satisfaction.[5]

Progressive postural control permits increasing freedom for the child to be actively and purposefully involved in motor interactions with the environment. During the establishment of purposeful equilibrium, the child is continuously changing the intensity and frequency of sensory input from vestibular, somatosensory, and visual as well as auditory and tactile channels. Through adaptation to change in sensory input, various new combinations are established by the nervous system as information about constancy and change of position and location of the self and objects in the spatial world. All discriminative senses require normal movements for function, and the processing of information takes place within the general mechanisms of perceptual adaptation to the environment.[9] An example of auditory–visual–kinesthetic behavior cited by de Quiros and Schrager is: a baby turns its head toward a sound source, looks for an object (auditory–visual association), and then attempts to grasp it (visual–kinesthetic association). Sherrington recognized the importance of movement to perception as he described tactile and visual perception as the relation between the tactile–muscular labyrinth and the visuo–muscular labyrinth.[9]

Memory of movement from these adaptive behaviors is available to guide similar or more complex movements. Meaningful motor experiences give rise to body laterality, developing with purposeful equilibrium, motor skills, and body scheme connected with cortical representation, registration, and formation of engrams at higher cortical levels.[9]

De Quiros and Schrager clearly stated the significance of sensory integration: "There is no doubt that the knowledge we have from ourselves and from our environment, as well as the recognition of what we could do—with all that information—depends mainly on sensory integration."[9] They also point out that: "If sensory integration fails, all sequences (maturation, functional, experimental) will be disrupted according to the degree of the handicap, thus determining an unusual developmental pattern."[9]

Ayres has divided sensory integration into levels which must be sequentially attained for body–brain specialization, abstract thinking, concentration, academic learning, and self-organization, self-esteem, self-control, and self-confidence.[5] The primary level consists of organization from vestibular and proprioceptive sensory input for postural and ocular control and gravitational security and from tactile input for maternal bonding, comforting, and feeding. The secondary level permits body percept, coordinated use of the two sides of the body, and motor planning. Activity level, attention span, and emotional stability are organized at this level. The third integrative level establishes relationships for eye–hand coordination, visual perception, and purposeful activity.

Motor Integration

All new voluntary motor acts involve intention and thus cortical participation, sensory integration, and postural control. Afferent synthesis of information-producing sensations at the cortical level allows adequate motor responses. Thus, as Ayres points out, skilled motor action is an integrator of cortically received sensory flow, including visual input.[4] Motor skills acquired through synthesis of afferent impulses can be excluded from consciousness but remain as automatic habitual behaviors.

Continual sensory feedback and adequate integration and interpretation of these sensations are necessary for a response to be adaptive. Learning from body movement depends on sensory feedback from purposeful motor action and the integration of this feedback. In his discussion of feedback as a cybernetic principle, de Quiros notes that Wiener, a mathematician, described feedback as, "the perceptual reactions of a person to his own responses; as a process by which goal directed responses are checked and corrected." De Quiros then defines feedback as "the arrival at the central nervous system of the information from any action performed by the individual or produced within the individual."[9] Feedback, then, provides information about goal achievement. But goal achievement cannot always be equated with sensory integration and learning: the manner in which the goal is achieved must be examined.

Feedback of a general nature is supplied by all receptors which participate in the action. During early learning, the very young child must depend on external feedback from vision, tactile, and auditory input in coordination with internal feedback from body movement. When the specific feedback as kinesthetic information from the proprioceptors is continuously monitored and checked by higher centers to assure the kinetic order of the movement, motor activities can be performed without the input from vision, touch, and hearing.

The importance of kinesthesia in the performance of goal-directed motor acts re-emphasizes the role of the vestibular–proprioceptive system. Proprioceptive information from muscles, joints, and tendons is related more to body position, whereas kinesthesia, the sensitivity produced by proprioceptors, is related more to body movements. Kinesthesia is important to dynamic equilibrium in association with vestibular and visual inputs and in intentional movements as movement perception for feedback information.[9]

Praxis is "a learned ability to plan and direct a temporal series of coordinated movements toward achieving a result–usually a skilled and non-habitual act."[4] The major neural substrate for praxis is diencephalic and cortical. Postural, sensory, and motor integration contribute to the ability to formulate a plan for use of the body as a motor tool. Body scheme, when defined as a postural model (as by Schilder[24]), arises from an integration of optic, kinesthetic, and tactile sensations producing a flexible model of the body that is a major factor in promoting praxis.

Apraxia in children, according to Ayres, is a "disorder of sensory integration interfering with ability to plan and execute skilled or non-habitual motor tasks."[4] Problems in motor sequencing are frequently included in this disorder. The dysfunction lies in the processing of sensory integration, planning, and motion rather than in sensory input or motor output. Developmental apraxia apparently "arises from a neurodevelopmental deviation that prevents the maturation of the inhibitory mechanisms and the development of the integrative mechanisms."[4] Ayres also suggests another possibility: the reduction of the brain's receptivity to the inhibiting stimuli.

The tactile system particularly concerned with the ability to "progam" a skilled motor act is considered by Ayres and others to be the critical system for the development of praxis. A disorder in integration of somatosensory stimuli, especially as identified by low scores on most, but usually not all, Southern California Sensory Integration Tactile Tests, has led Ayres to hypothesize a relationship between dysfunction in the tactile system and apraxia. Apraxia is currently being studied more extensively by Ayres, and identification of more specific parameters of this disorder should be forthcoming.

Corporal Integration

The way body parts work together influences the way the developing brain receives, codes, and integrates sensory input for purposeful motor activity. The quality and quantity of motor activity is an external manifestation of neural integration which subserves hemispheric specialization.

During the development of primary postural control, both sides of the body need to be involved in maintaining posture and equilibrium. Ayres proposes that brainstem postural mechanisms are important for interhemispheric integration. She emphasizes the relationship between observations of the coordinated use of two sides of the body and neural bilateral integration at lower levels.[4]

Lateralization of body motor functions depends on primary postural integration. After three years of age, when myelination of pontocerebellar pathways is completed, the body begins to "divide" vertically so that each side can assume independent functions. Lateral integration of sensory input from peripheral receptors and feedback mechanisms occurs at several neural levels. This functional reorganization at lower brain levels is important to exclude some parts of the body which intervened during the period of primary postural integration in order to permit planning of a series of motor activities. Body lateralization cannot be equated with cerebral specialization but serves as a step in the exclusion of sensorimotor functions. As speech begins to control motor functions, the left cerebral hemisphere begins to exclude postural activity in order to develop symbolic functions. The right cerebral hemisphere retains postural control.[9]

Cortical Integration

Progressive integration of space, symbolism, volition, and psychosocio-cultural experiences at the cortical level depends on integration at lower brain levels. What is integrated is influenced by variables within each member of the human species and within the environment to a much greater degree than at subcortical levels.

Luria described three basic functional units of the human brain, each making a specific contribution, working together for complex forms of mental activity.[20] Each unit is arranged in a vertical hierarchy of brainstem and subcortical structures and, within the cortex, primary projection area, projection–association area, and zones of overlapping. These units are functionally organized to regulate tone and the waking state; to obtain, process, and store information; and to program, regulate, and verify mental activity.

The first unit, which regulates tone, waking, and mental states, is a function of the reticular formation, the ascending and descending system, located in the medial region of the cortex. Its principal function is to regulate and modify the general activity state of the whole nervous system, cortical tone, muscle tone, and emotional tone, through gradual changes in the level of excitation according to functional needs. As such, it provides a background for stimuli, a stable base for organization of the brain's various processes such as arousal, orienting, vital functions, and emotions and for strengthening motor reactions to stimuli. The reticular formation receives nonspecific input from all sensory receptors at the brainstem level and transmits excitatory impulses to the cortex which, in turn, modulates and regulates the neural activity of the reticular formation.

The second unit, located in the posterior zones of the cortex, receives specific sensory input according to the "all or nothing" law from visual, auditory, vestibular, and somatosensory receptors. Input is combined in a hierarchical manner in the three zones of the cortex for specific modality analysis and integrated for perception and for symbolic processes.

All behavior becomes subordinated to the third unit, located in the prefrontal regions of the brain. This area is functionally organized for creating intentions, forming plans, programming actions, regulating behavior for goal attainment, verifying conscious activity, and correcting errors. The role in regulating the activity states that are the background for behavior and changing the states according to conscious intent and plans is important to the organization of human behavior. This region has rich two-way connections with all lower brain levels and virtually all parts of the cortex. It receives energy from the first unit and exerts inhibitory, activating, and modulating influences on the reticular formation.

Spatial Integration

Continuous motion in space is broken up by objects, words, and body movement in space. The integration of space begins with sensorimotor feedback from intentional motor activities. The body moves in space and thus breaks up the continuous motion of internal space. The vestibular, proprioceptive, and cutaneous sensory input from purposeful self-motion is important for body awareness (body concept, scheme, and image) and establishes the basis for concepts of motion such as direction, distance, pressure, and weight.

The organization of space, according to Luria, is a function of the second brain unit.[20] The primary zone, identical in each hemisphere, processes modality-specific stimuli. The secondary zone is a transition area in which sensory-specific input is functionally organized as information. Hemispheric specialization begins in this zone and depends on both body lateralization and the emergence of speech. The tertiary zone is the multisensory integrative zone for spatial organization of movement as well as mathematical operations and understanding of complex language structure.

The structural organization of the human nervous system strongly implies that nature intended body information to precede space information. The structures and pathways most directly related to body tone and movement are more medial and less specific and develop earliest. Lateral structures and pathways for discrimination and skilled motor functions develop later. It has also been established that insults to the nervous system during development are most likely to negatively affect the older structures.[23]

Deficits in these older, more primitive areas may go undetected, perhaps because of the social emphasis on technology and the object world and because early neurological dysfunction is more difficult to identify and the findings do not easily lend themselves to behavioral measurements. The child will use that which is available to maintain posture and equilibrium, to act motorically, to know the object world, and to communicate. Vision and audition and tactile functions specialized for information about object space can be used to monitor body position in relation to space as well as to gather information about object space and therefore attempt to compensate for vestibular–proprioceptive dysfunction. This neural organization problem may be masked until school age, when the child is expected to use perception and symbolism for academic learning. The probability of a learning disability is high. Remediation limited to eliciting behavior which must be organized at higher cortical levels, when the dysfunctioning part of the system can be identified at lower brain levels, may not be sufficient to facilitate the child's attainment of optimal potential.

Motion is used to act in space and to learn about the object physical world. The relationship of postural development to the acquisition of spacial/object knowledge has been described by de Quiros and Schrager.[9] During the first quarter year of life, the vestibular–proprioceptive system determines asymmetrical positions; head control is achieved. During the second quarter year, visual perception and coordinated movements are available, and sitting balance is achieved. With head control and sitting balance, the child is able to "face space" in the third quarter year of life and begin knowing the object world through auditory, visual, and kinesthetic modalities. During the fourth quarter year, the child begins to walk and to explore "surrounding space." "Limiting space" begins in the second year as the child begins to interact with the environment through purposeful equilibrium and adaptive motor behavior and speech. Integration of the postural system between the third and fourth years and functional reorganization for body lateralization permits knowing "environmental space," as evidenced by the use of lingua or concrete speech. Reading and writing are possible during the fifth and sixth years as the child achieves "corporal potentiality" or the ability to exclude from consciousness the sensorimotor activity of the body. The ability to use language as symbolic expression and to use skilled voluntary coordinated movements to control the physical world begins to be possible in the sixth and seventh years.

Symbolic Integration

As the cerebral hemispheres continue to differentiate in secondary and tertiary zones, sensory integration, spatial organization, and postural control develop as functions of the right hemisphere. The left hemisphere becomes specialized for cognitive activity connected with speech, perceptions organized into logical schemas as symbols, active verbal memory, and logical thought. According to de Quiros' schema, the exclusion of body afferent and efferent impulses through the attainment of purposeful equilibrium, the establishment of body laterality, and right cerebral hemispheric control of posture frees the left hemisphere for symbolic activity and language.

Volitive Integration

Between the ages of four and seven years, the frontal lobes become prepared for action, and it becomes possi-

ble for the child to have increasing control over his/her behavior. Language begins to control motor activity. Symbols are used as tools for communication and thinking: for internalizing one's world, controlling and assessing one's behavior, planning, and benefiting from the transmission of accumulated generations of learning. Symbols allow abstract thinking and mental manipulation of ideas, creativity, and complex thoughts. The child is considered ready for formal academic education at seven years of age. Human tutors and sociocultural tools must be available to provide information which the child uses for symbolic organization and for all higher cortical functions. The prefrontal lobes are functionally organized by ten years of age.[20] The achievement of Piagetian operational thought coincides with the establishment of symbolism in the left cerebral hemisphere and the completion of prefrontal lobe maturation.

Psychosocio-Cultural Integration

The use of symbolism for abstract thinking and inner language permits continual development of the psychic life. Through expressive language, relations are established with the sociocultural world. Play and work experiences and the impact of the vast variety and quality of human connections during the life cycle are important factors in the system of each life.

Sensorimotor Evaluation

Up to this time, empirical evidence of direct relationships between sensory input, neural integration at lower brain levels, and human learning have been difficult to establish. At least some of the problems may arise from the use of procedures designed to identify and measure functions as static conditions isolated from the system rather than behavior as dynamic interrelationships between the body/brain and the environment. More investigators are realizing that a dynamic system such as the brain transcends direct relationships between cause and effect.[32] New methods of investigation must be devised which evaluate the individual's ability to adapt and function within a changing environment.[9,32] Evaluation of sensorimotor levels of function contributes to differential diagnosis when human behavior and learning are viewed as a functional system, a complex interaction between the body/brain and the environment depending on progressive systemic integration.

Clinical assessment continues to be a principal method of identifying sensory and motor symptoms that interfere with the acquisition of learning. The challenge lies in the need to observe signs and interpret test results for information about the nature of the interaction between bioneural factors and the environment and the impact of this relationship on behavior and the learning process. Tests and clinical observations traditionally used by occupational therapists in pediatric assessments can contribute important data for early detection of factors that can disrupt the process of human learning. "It is undeniable that all postural or motor delay disturbs the acquisition of adequate connections with the environment and hence, with the acquisition of lingua and language."[9] Developmental screening and developmental tests measure a variety of parameters which are not necessarily additive but rather may be interactive so that the final outcome cannot be predicted in simple additive fashion.[32] Discrepancies between parameter evolution and maturation evidenced by sensorimotor function in the infant and young child deserve further investigation.

Test procedures are described by Ayres and by de Quiros in the context of their theoretical models and cannot be presented in isolation nor be used properly without an understanding of the theories which support their use. The sequence of systemic integration proposed by Schrager can be a useful guide in the organization of data for interpretation.

Symptoms of poor tonic–postural–antigravitational integration include low muscle tone, evidence of inadequate inhibition of primitive postural reflexes, poor ocular control, and inadequate equilibrium reactions including postural background control, as well as deficits in bilateral coordination. Dysfunction in these areas can be associated with the vestibular system, but in young children, vestibular inputs act together with proprioception and the cerebellum and influence ocular movements, so all these factors must be examined.[9] De Quiros points out the need to assess the postural system under both static and dynamic conditions to differentiate between existing pathology, past pathology, and abnormal postural afferents. He recommends evaluation procedures which use hard *versus* soft surfaces and vision *versus* occluded vision. Tests in the static situation provide data on organic or "structural" conditions, whereas those in the dynamic situation provide information on functional compensations.[9]

A number of traditional tests are clinically useful for obtaining data but the ability to observe signs and interpret test results pertinent to understanding the nature of the problem depends on the orientation of the evaluator. For example, the ability to stand on one foot and hop in place on one foot is a frequently used observation which becomes a test when time is measured. De Quiros gives this procedure new value in that through observations of the quality of the response he has interpreted the data to differentiate vestibular, proprioceptive, and ocular dysfunction. An inference from this example is that the value of a technique lies in the knowledge of the user.

The goal in assessing sensory integration is to determine if sensations have been organized for information about the body, perception of the object world, and, later, for symbolic communication. Irregularities in the postural systems can be important indicators of sensory-integrative dysfunction, as they interfere with the ability to act in space. In addition, the vestibular influence on the extraocular muscles is important to the gathering and organizing of information about the position and location of the body in space, in relation to objects in space, and in object–space relations. A sensory history can provide useful data about arousal reactions to vestibular and somatosensory stimuli. Lack of response, hypersensitive or defensive responses, or sensory avoiding or sensory seeking behaviors suggest that sensations are not available for use as information.

The Southern California Sensory Integration Tests[2] and the Southern California Postrotary Nystagmus Test,[3] a standardized battery of 18 tests, were constructed by Ayres in the 1970s to detect and to determine the nature of sensory-integrative dysfunction. Interpretation of test data by comparing one area of performance that comprises a meaningful cluster (*e.g.,* visual) with other areas of performance (*e.g.,* tactile) yields information about the child's sensory functions and functional relationships. This battery of tests is being revised as the Southern California Sensory Integration and Praxis Tests.

Deficits in motor integration may be observed as clumsiness, awkwardness, poor coordination, and a limited repertoire of available motor combinations for flexibility and skill. Traditional tests can be useful in identifying deficits at this level, but when deficits in motor skills are associated with a learning disability, the evaluator will need to interpret the test data in relation to observations and to data obtained from assessment of postural mechanisms and sensory integrative functions.

Although the apraxic child may have symptoms of inadequate motor functions, the syndrome of developmental apraxia can be differentiated by observations of trouble with constructive, manipulative play; difficulty in learning skills such as self-dressing, drawing, cutting, pasting, and assembling objects; and problems in learning to write and to use tools. The child will have difficulty initiating nonhabitual motor acts but may be able to learn a skill and perform in a coordinated manner.[7] Standardized evaluation procedures for developmental apraxia are a part of the Southern California Sensory Integration Tests. The assessment of this area of dysfunction will be expanded in the Southern California Sensory Integration and Praxis Tests.

Observations of corporal integration are based on how body parts work together in both the static and the dynamic situation. Many pertinent observations can be made in conjunction with evaluation of the postural system and during administration of the Southern California Sensory Integration Tests. Ayres has stressed the need to observe and to evaluate through standardized procedures the coordinated use of the two sides of the body.[4] Evidence of dysfunction may include a tendency to ipsilateral hand usage and avoidance of midline crossing, difficulty in using the two hands or two eyes in a coordinated manner and, frequently, in poorly established hand dominance. The ability of a child of four years to use one side of the body independently of the other (*i.e.*, to stand and hop in place on one foot or to develop a dominant hand for skill) are indicators of body lateralization.[9]

Three behavioral symptoms that commonly appear in learning disabilities—hyperactivity, hypoactivity, and restlessness—can be related to different types of neural dysfunction, according to de Quiros.[9] Hyperactivity is a lack of central inhibition of external stimuli, mainly associated with minimal brain dysfunction. Hypoactivity may be related to too much cortical inhibition. Restlessness is a failure to inhibit the postural system and is related to vestibular—proprioceptive dissociation.

Therapeutic Considerations

When learning disabilities are viewed as systemic dysfunctions, the goal of sensorimotor therapy must be, as Ayres states, "to improve the way the brain processes and organizes sensations."[5] Therapeutic procedures must be devised on the basis of the therapist's understanding of the nature of the disorder which has interfered with the learning system of the child. Treatment techniques can become therapeutic tools when used by a qualified therapist.

Sensory-integrative therapy for the child emphasizes somatosensory and vestibular input, usually through whole-body movements in space which facilitate sensory stimulation and adaptive responses. Ayres describes the central idea of sensory-integrative therapy as: "to provide and control sensory input, especially the input from the vestibular system, muscles and joints, and skin in such a way that the child spontaneously forms the adaptive responses that integrate those sensations."[5] Integration, according to Ayres, "most often occurs when the child wants the stimulus and initiates an activity to get those sensations."[5] In sensory-integrative therapy, then, the therapist manipulates the environment to activate the child. The innate drive of the child, the natural environment of motion supplemented with equipment that invites self-direction and organization of internal motion, should promote the adaptive responses necessary for sensory integration.

Sensory integration depends on postural control; that is, the control of body reflexes and of the body in space. Therapeutic procedures to enhance postural development and the motor functions which contribute to it have been established in occupational therapy and are discussed elsewhere in this book. Underlying de Quiros' notion of purposeful equilibrium is the association of

vestibular–proprioceptive inputs elicited by experiences on unstable surfaces such as a rocking board and changing-consistency surfaces such as hard to soft surfaces. De Quiros' idea of purposeful equilibrium may be the link between traditional sensorimotor therapy to enhance neuromuscular functions for postural control and Ayres' notion of an adaptive response to facilitate integration of sensory input for use.

Ayres includes in her therapeutic considerations the need to prepare the child's nervous system to make an adaptive response through the use of sensory facilitation and inhibition procedures. The importance of the need to modulate or balance the activity level within the nervous system will be discussed in the following section.

Motion in Sensorimotor Therapy

The focus of this section so far has been on the child's use of space, that is, on the ability to relate the self to the surrounding physical/object and to acquire information from this interaction. During early development, the child must establish a place in space and learn about the spatial coordinates of the self and of objects and about the physical properties of the body and the objects around him/her in order to function in the world. Less attention has been given to the use of motion (*i.e.*, the child's ability to establish a relationship between the motion within and that around him). All of these factors contribute to human behavior and the process of learning. The child must be able to use motion to act in space and to learn from purposeful action.

Theorists from diverse areas are now beginning to recognize that the system of life is part of the universal system of motion and space.[15,19,22,26,32] The human connection with the physical/object world depends on human connection with the universe and the natural environment. Motion as a phenomenon of the universe is a force in time which penetrates, unifies, and energizes all that exists. Life is embodied motion, a dynamic process of change subject to physical laws as determined by the nature of the universe. The design of the living organism enables each life to use motion and the laws of motion for its own survival and advancement. Each human life, through the nervous system, self-regulates and self-organizes the forces and flow of motion to maintain harmony and unity between the self and the universal whole; to adapt to and to know, and sometimes to control, the physical world; and to transform percepts into symbols for mental activity. The relationship between motion and human thinking became evident to Schwenk while scientifically observing movement of flowing elements and the forms which arise through these movements. He concludes:

> The activity of thinking is essentially an expression of flowing movement . . . Every idea—like every organic

form—arises in a process of flow, until the movement congeals into a form.[26]

The implications of this recently recognized relationship between human life and the universe are yet to be clearly defined in the psychological and neurosciences. However, it is becoming apparent to some investigators that the foundations of human behavior and learning must lie in the inseparable relationship between life and the universe. This relationship, as Walsh states, is established by the nervous system:

It is now apparent that the brain, the organ clearly designed to know the universe (and hence itself), cannot be fully described independently of the universe it is designed to know . . . The history of their interaction is engraved in neural pathways, neural structures, chemical reactions, and molecular configurations.[32]

The implications for occupational therapy perhaps may be more easily recognized because as a profession, we have resisted the separation of body from mind; feelings from action and skill; and adaptation to the environment from academic learning. The relationship of gravity, coordinated movement, self-regulation and organization, balance, and harmony to human function is basic to the development of occupational therapy goals and therapeutic modalities. The recent focus on human life as part of the universal whole with the potential for differentiation of function into increasingly complex forms while maintaining balance and unity within can add depth and breadth to existing theory and practice.

In the remainder of this section sensorimotor functions will be shown to be important to the relationship between universe and life forces as a means of integrating the self according to the plan of the universal system. Rhythm, gravity, and other universal energies influence the state of the organism. The organism organizes this motion to act in space, which is known because of the objects positioned and located in it. Arousal to change in the external environment is a change in state and is one of the factors which makes learning about the object world possible. The vestibular system is now recognized as critical to the establishment of the self–universe relationship as well as to the self–self and self–object relationships as the foundation for all aspects of human behavior.

The literature which supports such a relationship is just beginning to be developed but may lead the way to an interdisciplinary approach to the study of human behavior and to methods of intervention when behavior is disrupted. As scientists continue to probe the secrets of the universe, the rationale for therapeutic intervention using principles of motion may become more clearly stated. This overview is presented as an introduction and is by no means inclusive of the issues related to each area.

Dysfunction in Use of Motion

Since the introduction of Ayres' theory of sensory integration, occupational therapy practice has expanded to include children who appear to be unable to regulate the flow and organize the energies of motion—to use motion to act in space. The ability of these children to reach out to the external world and to benefit from experiences available in that world is dramatically impaired. The autistic are most representative of this group, but symptoms also can be seen in many children with sensorimotor dysfunction. The problem may be viewed as a motion dysfunction as opposed to an object/space dysfunction—impairment in the use of nonspecific sensations of motion which must precede the use of specific sensations for information.

Although these problems frequently interfere with learning, their impact is even greater and more debilitating to development of the sense of self and to emotional life. Clinical manifestations include, but are not limited to, inability to acquire and maintain a steady state, lack of response or abnormal response to specific sensory stimuli and to gravity and movement experiences, and lack of locomotion fluency and flexibility in changing activity levels or tension states and body positions. Some of these problems have been discussed by Ayres as tactile defensiveness, gravitational insecurity, and intolerance for rapid or spinning movement, which she relates to inadequate neural inhibition.[5]

Gravity

Gravity is one of the energies of the universe; it is the force and the "glue of the universe." It pulls everything toward the center and holds things in place. It forces the body parts and organs toward a center for the sense of self and from which all body motion takes place. The use of gravity is important in maintaining a steady state. According to the laws of physics, the object is in a steady state when on the ground. Thus, the upright position defies the steady state and threatens survival. However, within each brain is the primal drive and mechanisms to use the internal force of motion to counter the external forces and thus re-establish balance in space. The postural system reacts to the downward pull of gravity to establish antigravity positions, to move in space, and, later, to act purposefully in space. As the child begins to move against gravity, the pressure solidifies muscles and other tissues and organs.

Deficits in this interaction between the self and the universe disrupt the process of life. Insecurity and fear of motion in space counter the natural drive to use motion to act in space. Postural integration as well as emotional stability and flexibility will be negatively influenced. Ayres has described children who are reluctant to move because they feel the pull of gravity so intensely that they fear falling.[5] She has termed this hypersensitivity to gravitational pressure "gravitational insecurity." The problem, according to Ayres, is "an abnormal anxiety and distress caused by inadequate modulation of inhibition of sensations that arise when the gravity receptors of the vestibular system are stimulated by head position or movement."[5]

Weisberg, working from Ayres' theory, designed a pilot study to examine the emotional response in gravitational insecurity by measuring galvanic skin response and skin temperature.[33] On the basis of her findings, she posits a basic difference between the autonomic nervous system functioning of developmentally delayed children and that of normal children.

Rhythm

Rhythm began to be recognized more clearly in the 1950s as a phenomenon of motion important to the life process. Writing at that time, Gooddy pointed out that principles of clinical neurology, neuroanatomy, and neurophysiology were limited to the spatial aspects of human function.[14] The temporal aspects, he believed, were equally important and could be explored as the time sense. He proposed that the nervous system be viewed as a complex clock-system which transmits and regulates time information. A clock allows one to see intervals of space equivalent to intervals of time, and thus one can conceptualize the continuous motion of the universe and of the self as broken up into equal intervals in time. Gooddy quoted Einstein and Infield on the clock as a means of ordering motion: "The primitive subjective feeling of time flow enables us to order our impressions, to judge that one event takes place earlier, another later."[14] The serial ordering of motion flow is a factor in visual, auditory, and tactile perception. For instance, one feels nothing, one feels a pin prick, one feels nothing. Perception, then, is an event in time as well as in space. Gooddy also referred to the perceptual ability to judge motion as the "motion sense."[13] Timed motion is a factor in writing, in phrases for speech and reading, and in the symbols of mathematics. In his later writings, Gooddy discussed the time sense in relation to a variety of physiological and pathological disorders.[12]

The qualities of rhythm have been recognized as inherent in motor functions. Automatic motor functions such as sucking, chewing, swallowing, and patterns of locomotion are regulated by central oscillators in rhythmic patterns of fluency, coordination, and sequencing. Thelan suggests that a fundamental characteristic of all levels of gross and fine motor control and postural maintenance may be the intrinsic rhythmic patterning of motion.[31] Wolff noted that spontaneous motor discharges of infants occur during sleep in rhythmic sequence and that each type of discharge has its specific rhythm.[34] He concluded that rhythm must be involved in the serial ordering of gait, speech, and other complex functions as

well as in the anticipatory functions in early development such as flapping of the extremities to be picked up or to express joy.

More recently, E. Roy John's studies led him to state that the brain's rhythms count for as much as or more than the connections between its parts.[17] According to John, during learning many parts of the brain acquire a new rhythm of firing which corresponds to the learning. That is, it is the unique cell-firing rhythm which is important to learning and memory; small groups of cells do not form new connections, but rather new firing patterns. From studying electrical rhythms from many parts of the brain, John found that the more a brain region senses an event, the more it remembers. The implications of John's work for sensorimotor therapy deserve further investigation but do seem to support use of rhythmic repetition as a therapeutic modality under appropriate conditions.

Rhythm or time, according to Condon, "must be seen as a fundamental aspect of the organization of behavior and not as something added to it."[8] He suggests that the function of a part, such as eye movements, may more profitably be studied as part of the total rhythmic activity of the body. Through the use of microfilm of body movements, Condon discovered a precise pattern of order sustained between simultaneously moving parts which gives rise to a "process unit . . . a distinguishable, recurring form of order within the organized process of behavior."[8] Condon postulated that multiple integrated levels of organization comprise behavior and that within each individual behavior, there appears to be a "rhythmic hierarchy . . . where suborganizations are unified aspects of wider and wider circumscribing organization."[8]

Condon has demonstrated that linguistic–kinetic behavior is inseparable, that body motion is internally organized with speech.[8] Among his findings are precise synchronization of the micromovements of the speaker's body with the microunits of his speech (self-synchrony); entrainment of movement between speaker and listener (interactional synchrony); and lack of this synchrony in children with learning problems. Some children, especially the autistic, not only respond to the original sound but seem to have a delayed response also, as though they hear the sound again.

Condon's work has made motion visible and gives validity to the frequently used term of "orchestrated movements." Music makes rhythm audible and demonstrates the emotional influence of motion as rhythmic vibrations of the universe.[35]

When space is conceived of as emptiness filled with the motion of the universe, of vibrations, music can be considered as universal vibrations brought to conscious awareness through sound. The influence of continuous motion can be analyzed and studied through music. As Leonard points out: "The way that music works . . . is also the way the world of objects and events works, for it is all vibration."[19] Music is a rhythmic force, a power, which affects heart beat, blood pressure, digestion, respiration, and emotions. In brief, music acts on the cells and organs and through the emotions and influences bodily processes, including muscle activity. Both language and music affect awareness and perception of time. Music creates order out of chaos. The rhythms create unity; the melody, continuity; and the harmony, compatibility and balance.[30] When music is equated with vibration and with the motion of universal forces which penetrate the body, the importance of continuous rhythmic experiences through total body movement and rhythmic motor activities becomes evident.

The effects of continuous rhythmic experiences on neural maturation in the premature infant have been well documented and include cessation of crying, significant weight gains, more and longer periods of quiet sleep, calming and alerting, a decrease in heart rate and irregular breathing, and greater visual and auditory and motor maturity.[10] The therapeutic benefits of horseback riding, walking and jogging, music, and controlled alternating linear motion have recently been recognized.[28]

Studies suggest that the rhythmic ordering of sensations of motion at the sensorimotor level is important to neural organization and thus to behavior and learning. However, the full potential of the therapeutic use of rhythmic experiences is yet to be explored. The analysis of the child's rhythmic patterning, both in static and dynamic situations, as well as analysis of activities and experiences which facilitate rhythmic responses are worthy of further consideration.

Steady State and Arousal

The organism strives to maintain a state of rhythmic stability and energy constancy according to the universal plan yet has an inner drive and need to use energy for its own survival, goal-directed behavior, and learning in the physical world. It is now recognized that the steady state in a complex organism is a dynamic state in which the organism is continuously adapting to change.[15,32] The concept of balance, then, may not be limited to postural balance but may include balance of the life system within the universe and with the physical/object world.

Children with sensorimotor dysfunction demonstrate a variety of balance problems. The hyperactive, hypoactive, or restless child has difficulty acquiring a calm and alert state for attending to learning experiences. Inappropriate or abnormal use of motion as energy is manifested by low muscle tone, low or labile emotional activity, and a generalized low activity level. Some children tend to fatigue easily—to run out of energy—whereas others are "too tired" to participate actively in a therapy program. These problems

are related to neural inhibition and vestibular–proprioceptive association, as discussed by Ayres and de Quiros.

The nervous system is designed for balance: to acquire and to maintain a dynamic steady state. Of particular importance to this discussion is the continuous background discharge used to maintain a baseline for change, arousal for conscious awareness of external events, and feedback within the nervous system to use sensations as energy and information for the organism's own advancement.

Autonomic Nervous System

The autonomic nervous system, according to Gooddy, is the "nervous system of rhythmicity," the regulator of rhythms essential to volitional activity.[14] Furthermore, "only when the *rates* of functioning of these metabolic systems which maintain life and health are normal does living matter (human being or plant or single cell) prosper."[14] The autonomic nervous system maintains an internal steady rhythm, a resting state, which can be accelerated, decelerated, or altered according to emotional change, body movement, or external influences as well as to physiological factors. The concept of homeostasis refers to physiological stability—the tendency of the body to maintain a steady state despite external changes.[27]

A continuous rhythmic background discharge from afferent fibers even in the absence of obvious stimulation of the receptor organs is associated with certain slowly adapting receptors such as those which respond continuously for as long as several minutes to pressure on the skin; with thermoreceptors; and with pain, vestibular, and retinal receptors. The physiological importance of background discharge is that the excitability of various pathways remains high and thus contributes to maintaining the waking state. This provides a background for change; in the presence of an ongoing background discharge, a decrease as well as an increase in stimuli can be signaled. In contrast, there are fast-adapting (phasic) receptors which respond immediately with a burst of energy to a change in the intensity of stimuli. These receptors are found in touch endings, joint receptors, and endings around hair follicles. They provide information about change in the environment.[21] Occupational therapists influence these receptors to change the arousal level. For example, touch pressure will lower the level of excitation, whereas light touch will increase the excitatory state.

Arousal

Reafferent stimuli, novel stimuli, and stimuli that are of special significance to the organism elicit an arousal reaction which breaks up existing rhythmic patterns. The organism strives to maintain or re-establish a steady state either through behavior which seeks or avoids stimuli, through neurological processes such as habituation and integration, or through the endocrine system, especially the adrenal hormones.[32] Sokolov suggests that stimulus matching may be important in adaptation and learning.[29] According to this model, each stimulus which is attended to is registered as a neural model; restimulation activates a matching of the new stimuli with a previous model. If matching does not occur, orienting and searching processes are needed before a steady state can be re-established.

Stimulus deprivation has been shown to be related to hyperarousal when the organism does not have the opportunity to form a variety of models and thus does not have a store of neuronal models available for matching.[32] The frequently observed hyperarousal state of the autistic person may be related to an inability to register stimuli so that the orienting and searching process must continue.[5] Therapeutic intervention would depend on the nature of the problem such as a need for sensory stimulation, for activities which facilitate negative feedback, or for establishment of a steady state from which change could occur.

Neural Feedback

To adapt to change requires energy. To avoid energy loss, the nervous system has automatic control systems —servomechanisms. The nervous system is arranged in open loops for exchange of energy within the environment and in closed loops for functional organization to maintain or restore internal balance. The closed loops feed energy back into the system which can be utilized to maintain the system; output can control input. Positive feedback adds to the input and thus to the energy of the system. But the energy can become explosive if not needed or regulated. The therapeutic use of direct sensory stimulation to increase the general activity level is an example of the use of positive feedback, but the possibilities for overstimulation cannot be overlooked. Negative feedback occurs during adaptive motor activity and permits self-correcting adjustments by giving immediate information about the prior performance so that a predetermined goal can be met. Integrative centers are crucial control centers of the negative feedback systems, as energy must be continuously processed as information.[21] Negative feedback is essential to the process of learning, as discussed in the first part of this section.

The control systems concept is used by therapists to facilitate modulation of the child's nervous system and to promote sensory processing as information. Although the therapist may use direct sensory stimuli to raise the activity level (positive feedback), these proce-dures should be followed by activities that require an adaptive response (negative feedback) at the appropriate level to regulate energy and to organize it more efficiently within the brain. Direct sensory input and adaptive responses can be used to lower the activity level, but the modalities will be used differently.

Vestibular System

The most primal relations to be established are those that connect the self in motion with the world of motion and facilitate the organization of the motion within the self to act in the spatial environment. The vestibular organ and its extensive system of influence throughout the brain is now recognized as the essential influence in fetal and early development.

The vestibular system is unique in that its receptors respond to the continuous motion of the universe and to the change in head position and motion (gravity and movement) rather than to the tangible, physical/object world. It is a major connection between the self and the universal system of motion, harmony and unity, and order. It is concerned with orientation of the self in space: obtaining and maintaining the self in universal space using the laws of motion to maintain posture and equilibrium. The peripheral receptors receive the constant force of gravity and maintain a vestibular tone in the absence of stimuli. They detect change in this force as a result of changes in the relation of the head to space and of acceleration or deceleration of movement of the head in space such as occurs in turning the head to one side.[16,21]

The vestibular system is involved in many functions of the human nervous system, including ocular, cerebellar, spinal, reticular, and cortical functions as well as some autonomic functions. It is related to behavior both as a gravity receptor and as part of the cerebellar influence on the limbic system.[11] It contributes to the general activity level of the brain and to nonspecific sensory information through the reticular system. The vestibular system has a primary influence on the extraocular muscles and the proprioceptors for early postural control, for locomotion, and for orientation in space.[4,9]

The importance of the vestibular system can be traced to early species evolution when an organ for sensing motion and space orientation permitted organisms to move freely in the environment.[23] Vestibular receptors develop early in intrauterine life and send impulses to oculomotor nerves, spinal cord motor cells, and the cerebellum and other brain centers, facilitating fetal movements and position changes. Toxins and other factors that cause anomalies of nervous system development often selectively affect those structures developing earliest.[18] A disturbance of vestibular functions by any factor will be reflected in the formation and function of the entire nervous system. Thus, the vestibular system is a primary target for evaluation and therapeutic intervention during early development.

Summary

The change in sensorimotor theory and practice since they were introduced into occupational therapy in the 1940s reflects increased understanding of human nature in all scientific areas. The concept of systems of function and the recognition of the universe as a system from which all other systems are developed have led to a more holistic interpretation of human behavior.

The concept of "functional systems", that is, that a function of any organ, body part, or brain structure can be realized only in an environment that permits, supports, and promotes function, has influenced the shift of focus in sensorimotor therapy from brain pathology to dysfunction in the individual's ability to use available function to interact optimally with the environment. The system is open to environmental exchanges through its sensory and motor mechanisms; it regulates input through feedback mechanisms for energy and information (integration of sensations) and releases this energy as appropriate motor behaviors. Human behavior and learning as end products of a complex functional system of neural mechanisms and environmental influences will be interfered with if any part of this functioning unit is unable to contribute to the whole. Sensorimotor therapy is concerned with systems that organize and reorganize during early development and do not depend on human learning and abstract thinking but rather subserve the development of these human processes.

A more recent "discovery"—that the universe is a dynamic system and that all life is part of this system—has expanded the environment's availability for use in sensorimotor therapy to include the universal forces, energies, and rhythm as well as the natural environment subject to physical laws of the universe and the object/human environment that influences the process of human learning.

The philosophy underlying this section is that human development depends on relationships established with motion and with object space and that the ways in which these relationships are formed differ but can be viewed as a developmental continuum. Motion is the penetrating environmental influence for the system of life, whereas the space/object world supports the system of learning. The system of life uses the energies and rhythms of universal motion to develop and maintain the life force, the tone, and the activity level in harmony and unity according to the universal plan. All living organisms use motion to overcome the forces of motion and to move in the physical world. As the postural system develops, the child begins to control motion to adapt to the physical and object world and to integrate the sensations from these experiences as information. This period of sensorimotor development permits perception of the object world and facilitates the transformation of this concrete knowledge into symbolic activity for language and abstract thinking.

Sensorimotor functions are inherent in the process of human learning and the development of occupational behaviors of play and work. Occupational therapy practice depends on theory and validation of theoretical constructs. The possibilities for expansion in this area are increasing as science, as a study of parts, becomes the study of dynamic systems of function.

References

1. Ayres AJ: Occupational therapy directed toward neuromuscular integration. In Willard HS, Spackman CS (eds): Occupational Therapy, 3rd ed, p 360. Philadelphia: JB Lippincott, 1963
2. Ayres AJ: Southern California Sensory Integrative Tests Manual. Los Angeles, Western Psychological Services, 1972
3. Ayres AJ: Southern California Sensory Integration Interpretation Manual. Los Angeles, Western Psychological Services, 1977
4. Ayres AJ: Sensory Integration and Learning Disorders, pp 150, 165, 176. Los Angeles, Western Psychological Services, 1979
5. Ayres AJ: Sensory Integration and the Child, pp 140, 182, 184. Los Angeles, Western Psychological Services, 1979
6. Blakemore C: Mechanics of the Mind, p 112. Cambridge, Cambridge University Press, 1977
7. Capra F: The Tao of Physics, p 63. Berkeley, Shambhala, 1975
8. Condon WS: Multiple response to sound in dysfunctional children. J Autism Childh Schizophrenia 5:37, 1975
9. De Quiros JB,* Schrager OL: Neuropsychological Fundamentals in Learning Disabilities, pp 30, 32, 35, 55, 74, 82, 147, 206, 245, 247, 252. San Rafael, Academic Therapy Publications, 1978
10. Field T: Supplemental stimulation of preterm neonates. Early Human Dev 4:301, 1980
11. Frick RB: The ego and the vestibulocerebellar system. Psychoanal Quart 11:93, 1982
12. Gooddy W: Disorders of the time sense. In Vinken PJ, Bruyn GW (eds): Handbook of Clinical Neurology, vol 3, pp 229–250. Amsterdam: North-Holland Publishing, 1969
13. Gooddy W: Some aspects of human orientation in space. Brain 76:3, September 1953
14. Gooddy W: Time and the nervous system. Lancet 1:1139, 1958

---

* Literature in english by this author will be found under "De Quiros"; his book in english is referenced, "Quiros JB de"; his works in spanish can be found under the entry, "Quiros."

15. Hanna T: The Body of Life. New York, Alfred A Knopf, 1983
16. Hunt CC (ed): Neurophysiology. MTP Int Rev Sci. Baltimore, University Park Press, 1975
17. John ER: How the brain works—A new theory. Psychol Today 9(12):48, 1976
18. Klosovski BN: The Development of the Brain and Its Disturbance by Harmful Factors. London, Pergamon Press, 1963
19. Leonard G: The Silent Pulse. New York, Bantam, 1981
20. Luria AR: The Working Brain, p 33, Haigh B (trans): New York, Basic Books, 1973
21. Noback CR: The Human Nervous System. New York, McGraw–Hill, 1967
22. Pearce JD: Magical Child. New York, Bantam, 1980
23. Sarnat HB, Netsky MG: Evolution of the Nervous System. New York, Oxford University Press, 1974
24. Schilder P: The Image and Appearance of the Human Body. New York, John Wiley & Sons, 1964
25. Schrager OL: Systemic integration processes: Basis for human learning. Buenos Aires, unpublished, 1979
26. Schwenk T: Sensitive Chaos. New York, Schocken, 1978
27. Selye H: The Stress of LifNew York, McGraw–Hill, 1956
28. Silberzahn M: CALM: A therapeutic device. AOTA Sensory Integrative Specialty Sec Newslett 3:1, 1980
29. Sokolov EN: Neuronal models and the orienting reflex. In Brazier MA (ed): The Central Nervous System and Behavio, G Macey, 1960
30. Tame D: The Secret Power of Music. New York, Destiny Books, 1984
31. Thelan E: Rhythmical behavior in infancy. Dev Psychol 17:237, 1981
32. Walsh R: Toward an Ecology of Brain, pp 2, 139. New York, Spectrum Publications, 1981
33. Weisberg A: The role of psychophysiology in defining gravitational insecurity: A pilot study. AOTA Sensory Integration Specialty Sec Newslett 7:4, 1984
34. Wolff PH: The role of biological rhythms in early psychological development. Bull Menninger Clin 31(4):197, 1967
35. Zuckerkandl V: Sound and Symbol. Princeton, Princeton University Press, 1956

SECTION 4

Occupational Behavior Frame of Reference *Phillip D. Shannon*

Occupational behavior represents, in part, a recommitment to the philosophy of Adolph Meyer. From this recommitment, time, and how one occupies time, emerged as one of the major themes of occupational behavior.

Meyer's philosophical teachings about time and what one does with one's time were based on a common-sense logic derived from his observations of everyday living. Time, he said, is the "biggest wonder and asset of our lives."[14] What one does with one's time is called occupation, or work, and any form of pleasureable or enjoyable activity.[14] It is the quality of one's occupation that determines one's adaptiveness in the general sense; what determines one's adaptiveness in the temporal sense is the capacity to manage time effectively with regard to the nature of one's occupation.

How one organizes one's time to facilitate one's adaptiveness in the temporal sense is directed by the requirements of role. It is within the context of role, a second major theme of occupational behavior, that one organizes time for work, play, rest, and sleep—occupation, what one does with one's time.

Reilly maintains that organizing one's time and one's behavior to meet the demands of daily living is a complex process that evolves hierarchically from rules to skills to roles.[15] For example, to become socially competent, one must first learn the rules for social interaction. These rules, when combined and sequenced properly, are transformed into skills.[18] Skills, or the tools one uses to interact with the environment, are incorporated into roles. Without skills, competency, in the service of role performance, will not emerge.

Competency, a third major theme of occupational behavior, is the key to successful living. The specific competency behaviors that emerge in the evolution of one's occupational behavior are guided by the requirements of role. In acquiring these competency behaviors, one is able to have an impact on the environment.

These three major themes of occupational behavior—temporal adaptation, role, and competency—will be presented in greater detail in this section. First, however, logic dictates a discussion of occupational behavior from the perspective of paradigm so that its complexity and scope can be appreciated.

Paradigm

Paradigm "is a global construct that is not easily defined."[10] Basically, however, a paradigm represents the values and beliefs that are shared by the members of a professional community.[10] These values and beliefs provide philosophical direction for a profession, and they are primary in distinguishing one paradigm from another.

A paradigm offers more than philosophical direction, however, it delineates the nature and scope of the services that will be provided by a profession; it determines what will be included and what excluded in the educational preparation of the professional; and will also guide a profession's research interests.[22] (See Shannon for a description of the process by which paradigms evolve).

Not all of the members of a professional community necessarily share the same values and beliefs, which is why none of the health care professions can lay claim to a paradigm in the true meaning of the construct. At most, all that can be claimed by a profession is a set of emergent paradigms competing for acceptance.

To swear allegiance to a paradigm is to swear allegiance also to a particular set of philosophical values and beliefs. It is in taking this oath of loyalty to a paradigm that various subgroups within a profession are distinguished from one another in terms of what they believe and what they do. In occupational therapy, for example, those individuals who subscribe to a psychoanalytic paradigm *versus* a sensory-integration paradigm *versus* an occupational behavior paradigm differ in their beliefs and actions.

The emergent paradigms in occupational therapy, which are not limited to those just mentioned, represent two categorical types of paradigms that are descriptive of the practice of occupational therapy, past and present. Each has its own set of characteristics, and each exemplifies a type of thought and action that limit or expand practice. The first of these categorical types of paradigms is biomedical; the second is biosocial.

Biomedical Paradigms

Biomedical paradigms are distinguished by the following:

1. The human organism is perceived in isolation from the environment, and interest is demonstrated only in the internal system of the body and mind.
2. Intervention occurs in the presence of internal systems dysfunctions caused by disease or disability.
3. The purpose of intervention is to minimize or eliminate internal systems dysfunctions through the process of symptom reduction.

The operative principle in a biomedical approach to the practice of occupational therapy is simply this: if the pathology is corrected, the individual will be able to function. The question raised by the application of this principle is this: what constitutes function? Essentially, function is perceived as the ability to care for one's self,

typically described in terms that refer to one's physical independence and psychological stability.

Biosocial Paradigms

In contrast to biomedical paradigms, biosocial paradigms are characterized by the following:

1. The human organism is perceived as a complex system interacting with another complex system, the environment.
2. Intervention occurs in the presence of disease or disability and also in the presence of deprivation.
3. The purpose of intervention is to expand the individual's capacities for interacting with the environment, subsequent to biomedical intervention, through the process of skill development.

The guiding principle in a biosocial approach to the practice of occupational therapy is this: biomedical intervention is a necessary, but not necessarily sufficient, condition for producing competent behavior. Biomedical intervention increases one's functional capacities for becoming competent. Biosocial intervention, the necessarily sufficient condition for producing competent behavior, builds on these functional capacities by developing or redeveloping the skills that one needs for environmental mastery and achievement.

What constitutes function with regard to a biosocial approach to practice? The ability to care for one's self and the capacity to interact with the environment in such a way that one can experience productivity and satisfaction in life and therefore achieve a sense of quality to one's life.

Occupational Behavior: A Biosocial Paradigm

Occupational behavior is a biosocial approach to the practice of occupational therapy that recognizes and addresses the complex interaction of two complex systems, organism and environment. Indeed, organism and environment are perceived as inseparable. As a biosocial approach to the practice of occupational therapy, occupational behavior incorporates all that is characteristic of a biomedical approach. However, it transcends biomedical concerns to address the larger concerns related to the performance of roles. Responding to the biomedical needs of the patient is viewed as the first step, not the last, in the intervention process.

In the process of intervening, attention is directed toward the disorganized behaviors produced by disease, disability, or deprivation. The primary goal of intervention is to transform disorganized behavior into organized behavior for meeting the demands of daily living. It is in this transformation process that the development of competence is emphasized in the service of role performance and temporal adaptation.

It was mentioned previously that occupational behavior represents, in part, a recommitment to the philosophy of Adolph Meyer. However, this is not all that occupational behavior represents. In practice, occupational behavior is occupational therapy applied in its most comprehensive form. As education, it is the study of occupational therapy at higher levels of complexity.

For example, when attending to the leisure needs of a patient, a typical approach is to expose the patient to a variety of activities hoping that his or her interest in an activity will be sufficiently aroused to continue the activity when treatment is terminated. This approach, if at all successful, is successful by chance and not by design.

An approach that is designed to improve one's leisure life will consider one's values, interests, goals, attitudes, motivations, and roles—a whole set of factors that are ignored in the simplistic approach described above. Intervention directed toward improving one's leisure life is a complex process that cannot be undertaken without first understanding the complexities of leisure itself. Occupational behavior addresses these complexities and the complexity of human behavior in general.

Certainly, the three major themes of occupational behavior that were introduced earlier are part of this complexity, as are such subthemes as motivation, occupational choice, work, and play.[12] Unfortunately, these subthemes are too extensive to be discussed in the space of a single chapter. Instead, emphasis is placed on the major themes of temporal adaptation, role, and competency, with the intent of providing a perspective on the relationship among these three themes.

Temporal Adaptation

It was not very long ago, historically speaking, that the mentally ill were housed in large asylums, "insane asylums," where they were locked away, sometimes locked up (shackled), and most certainly locked out as members of the human species. They were treated as they were perceived, as subhuman creatures fit only for confinement to a cage. They were stripped of their human dignity and denied any hope of a future beyond the walls of the asylum.

It was not until the 1800s that a change in attitude toward the mentally ill occurred, prompted by the moral conviction that all people, regardless of circumstance, should be treated with respect and that their human dignity should be preserved. This change in attitude ushered in the era of moral treatment, when caring replaced controlling and when the random activity of the mentally ill was replaced by guided activity in the form of occupation.[1,5]

The notion of providing "occupations" for the men-
tally ill was slow to gain momentum; after all, this was a novel, if not revolutionary, idea, and those who worked in the insane asylums were not at all convinced that the mentally ill could be trusted to engage in occupations without harming themselves, or more importantly, someone else.

Adolph Meyer was instrumental in convincing his colleagues and others that mental illness was not incurable in the sense of a terminal cancer, and that the disorganized behaviors of the mentally ill could be transformed into organized behaviors. The mechanism for this transformation process was the proper use of time —occupation.[5,14]

Although Meyer's work was concentrated in the area of psychiatry, the application of his ideas extends far beyond psychiatry. Indeed, his ideas are as applicable to persons with developmental and physical disabilities as they are to the mentally ill. Certainly the proper use of time has an organizing effect on the disorganized behaviors of those with learning deficits and those faced with the residual effects of a disabling condition.

It is this issue that Kielhofner addresses in an article where he introduces seven propositions concerning temporal function and dysfunction.[8] The first five of these propositions will be reviewed collectively; the remaining two propositions are discussed individually and expanded on as a matter of emphasis.

According to Kielhofner, how one perceives and uses time is determined by one's culture, which is transmitted to new generations through the socialization process. One is, therefore, predisposed to organize one's time according to cultural norms. Among these norms is the rule for organizing one's daily living activities in such a way that there is a temporal order to one's occupation. The form that one's occupation takes, and the ensuing arrangements that one makes to establish and maintain this temporal order, is guided by the requirements of role and by one's values, interests, and goals.[8]

These five propositions suggest some obvious clinical concerns. First, the practitioner must be sensitive to cultural differences, and particularly subcultural differences, regarding one's perceptions and use of time. There are, for example, subcultural differences in peoples' perceptions and use of time among ethnic groups, age groups, work groups, and so forth. If these differences did not exist among these subcultures, neither would nondiscriminatory laws exist to protect these differences.

Second, the practitioner must identify the extent to which these cultural or subcultural norms regarding one's perceptions and use of time influence, or fail to influence, one's behavior with regard to the degree of order or disorder in one's temporal function. Third, the practitioner must recognize also that institutions, such as hospitals, are subcultures that prescribe a set of norms regarding the patient's use of time.[17] These norms may act as a deterrent to one's efforts to establish or re-establish a temporal order in one's life.

In another publication by Kielhofner, two concepts are presented with regard to the mentally retarded and their perceptions of time, concepts that can be generalized to other institutionalized populations as well. The first concept, that of "time tracks," suggests that people perceive themselves as being on a continuum of time that extends from the present into the future, with major milestones to be achieved as one progresses along this continuum. What Kielhofner emphasizes in terms of the mentally retarded is that they are on a different time track than mainstream America. Consequently, they see themselves as "frozen in time," which is the second concept, with little or no control over their temporal function.[9]

These two concepts are descriptive also of other institutionalized populations. In terms of their temporal function, they also are off-track, so to speak; they, too, are frozen in time, unable to progress along a well-defined path into the future. How are these frozen images in time unfrozen, and how is the individual redirected toward his or her path into the future?

Answers to these questions are provided by Reilly. First, the institution must be flexible enough to allow for individual differences regarding one's normal use of time. Second, opportunities must be provided for choice in organizing one's daily routine.[17] Lacking these specifications, one's path into the future is blocked, and dependency on others for organizing one's daily routine may become a way of life.[9]

A fourth clinical concern suggested by Kielhofner's first five propositions is that organizing one's time around the requirements of role is complicated by the fact that roles are dynamic, not static.[4] As roles change, how one organizes time in support of role must also change. This is particularly important when a role change is forced; for example, in the presence of a disabling condition, unemployment, mandatory retirement, and so forth. The individual's temporal behaviors must be reorganized to meet the requirements of role.

Finally, in organizing one's time for occupation, consideration must be given to a balanced life in the quantitative sense (*i.e.*, time for work, play, rest, and sleep) and in the qualitative sense (*i.e.*, opportunities to pursue one's interests and goals in the service of need satisfaction).[20] The extent to which the environment limits or expands these opportunities will determine the degree to which a balanced life is possible and therefore the quality of one's temporal adaptation.

The influence of one's values, interests, and goals in determining the nature of one's occupation cannot be underestimated. From one's value system, interests emerge which are transformed into goals. Without goals, one cannot organize one's daily life. When an individual's goals are not apparent, or when the person has difficulty establishing goals, clarifying one's values and interests is a necessary first step.

The sixth proposition that Kielhofner presents regarding one's temporal function or dysfunction is that "habits are the basic structures by which daily behavior is ordered in time."[8] Surely, without habits, one's life cannot be organized to meet the demands of daily living. However, habits are comprised of skills that with practice become automatic routines. Consequently, skills are the point of intervention in transforming disorganized behavior into organized behavior. More is said about this later in the section on competency.

The seventh proposition developed by Kielhofner is that "temporal dysfunction may occur as an integral part of some mental illness, or as a consequence of imposed physical disability."[8] The validity of this statement, which should include also "as a consequence of mental illness," is clearly evident in the case histories of individuals with physical and mental disorders. Also, common sense suggests that one's inability to manage time effectively might, given a different set of conditions, progress into a mental illness.

On the other hand, the inability to manage time effectively might not evolve into a mental illness, nor evolve from an associated mental or physical disorder. It may, however, stand in the way of achieving one's goals in life. Perhaps an example is needed to clarify this point: Work and play are mutually influential in that a negative work life can have a negative impact on play and *vice versa*.[20,21] An individual with whom I was associated was faced with the problem of not knowing how to use his free time. This inability to use free time in ways that were satisfying was having a negative impact on his work life and his relationships with other people; in short, he was miserable. In exploring his past and present interests, and in developing and implementing some strategies for reactivating and activating some of these interests, the change in behavior was remarkable. The goal was to enrich this individual's play life and thereby to improve the quality of his work life. This indeed occurred when he was able to involve himself in free-time activities offering him a degree of enjoyment and satisfaction.

It is these marginal people, those on the fringe, the ones whose temporal adaptation is at risk but whose problems in managing their time effectively may never grow into a mental illness, who are often overlooked in terms of professional intervention. Examples of these people are those who are late for appointments; those who cannot get to work on time; those who cannot seem to organize their time to "earn a day's pay for a day's work"; those who sit in boredom in the evening and on weekends because there is nothing to do, nowhere to go. If the term "prevention" is to have meaning, it must be defined in new ways so that the underserved in society, those whose temporal adaptation is at risk, receive the attention needed to improve their daily lives regardless of whether the threat of mental illness lurks on the horizon.

In summary, temporal adaptation refers to how one occupies time, not only within the context of a day, a week, or a month, but across the life span. Time is spent or used in work, play, rest, and sleep; and the capacity to use time effectively, proportional to each individual's needs, is a measure of one's adaptiveness.

The illustration provided above with regard to Kielhofner's seventh proposition is an example of temporal function and dysfunction within the context of a day, a week, a month. Temporal adaptation, as it applies to time used across the life span, is translated into the concept of role, a second major theme of occupational behavior.

Role

It should be obvious that people occupy their time performing roles that provide the context within which one organizes time for work, play, rest, and sleep — occupation. Briefly defined, role refers to the expected behaviors associated with a particular status or position that one occupies in a social system.[4] These expected behaviors are both externally and internally determined.

It was mentioned previously that roles are dynamic, not static. What this means is that role is the behavioral aspect of status. Status, by itself, is a static concept that takes on meaning only when accompanied by a set of behaviors. These are the everyday behaviors that one demonstrates as a spouse, a worker, or a friend, the specific role behaviors associated with each of these statuses.

That roles are dynamic, not static, has another meaning, however. Roles are dynamic in the sense that within time and across time, meaning the transition from one role to another, the requirements of role change. Therefore, the expected behaviors associated with these roles also change. This dynamic aspect of role is exemplified by two parallel developmental continuums.

First, there is a developmental continuum that is maturational in nature: That focuses on age-appropriate behaviors; that corresponds to the developmental stages of childhood, adolescence, adulthood, and aging. Second, there is a developmental continuum that is occupational in nature: that focuses on role-appropriate behaviors; that corresponds to the occupational roles of preschooler, student, worker and/or homemaker, and retiree. These two developmental continuums are illustrated in Figure 8-1 as they correspond to each other.

Inherent in these two developmental continuums are three categories of roles: (1) familial roles, which are roles of relationships such as mother–son; (2) sexual

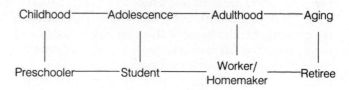

Maturational Continuum

Occupational Role Continuum

Figure 8-1. Correspondence of maturational continuum and occupational role continuum.

roles, which are roles of identity such as boy, girl; and (3) occupational roles, which are roles of performance such as student, retiree.[4,13] Familial and sexual roles evolve along the first continuum; occupational roles evolve along the second continuum.

The concept of occupational role accounts for those major life roles that extend across the life span, life roles that provide the direction for organizing one's time. From an occupational behavior perspective, occupational roles, in contrast to familial and sexual roles, are seen as the most amenable to occupational therapy intervention, considering that occupational roles are performance-oriented. Familial and sexual roles are not ignored, and intervention is considered to the extent that problems with the performance of familial or sexual roles interfere with the performance of occupational roles.

The enactment of role is an ongoing complex process as described by Katz and Kahn in their system model of the role episode (Fig. 8-2), which also provides an explanation for the statement made earlier — that role behaviors are externally and internally determined.[7] What the model illustrates is the following:

Considering the relationship between an employer and an employee, Box I represents the employer's expectations of the employee (focal person) in terms of role performance. Box II represents what the employer communicates, or fails to communicate, to the employee in the attempt to bring the employee's performance into compliance with the employer's expectations. These verbal and nonverbal messages are communicated to the employee as indicated by arrow 1.

These messages are received by the employee, as represented by Box III. The employee interprets the employer's communications, taking into consideration also his or her own internal perceptions of the job relative to role performance. This blend of external and internal expectations culminates in role behavior, as indicated by Box IV, with its quantitative and qualitative aspects. This role behavior, as demonstrated by the employee's job performance, is evaluated by the employer, indicated by the feedback loop (number 2). The cycle begins again to either sustain or modify the performance of the employee.

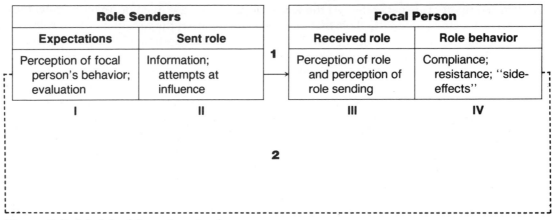

Figure 8-2. Model of the role episode.

As oversimplified as this illustration might appear, what complicates the role episode is that the focal person rarely receives messages from a single role sender. Rather, messages are received from multiple role senders at the same time. In other words, the role episode is an ongoing process of sending, receiving, interpreting, and responding to role expectations communicated by all of the people in a particular setting—home, workplace, school, hospital—with whom the focal person is associated.

What this suggests with regard to role function and dysfunction is that the assessment of role must be performed within an environmental context. Consideration must be given to the multiple environments that influence a person's role behavior to identify the external expectancies of role and not just the internal expectations of the individual. This is particularly important when there are problems resulting in or leading to role dysfunction.

Problems in role, as described primarily in the management literature, include (1) role overload (excessive demands); (2) role ambiguity (unclear or confusing expectations); and (3) role conflict (conflict between internal and external role expectations).[6,7] Role conflict refers not only to conflict situations involving the performance of a single role but also to conflict among roles, such as the conflict that might occur from the combined occupational roles of student–worker or homemaker–worker where one set of role expectations is in conflict with another. Also, there may be conflict between role types; for example, between an occupational role and a familial role. The occupational role of worker might conflict with the familial role of father, for example, in terms of the time and effort devoted to each of these roles.

What the management literature does not discuss is a fourth type of role dysfunction, given the label here of role interference. Role interference refers to those situations where a person lacks the abilities or skills (*i.e.*, the person never acquired them) for role performance or to

the inability to perform roles due to some trauma or to the residual effects of disease or disability.

In any of these instances, as well as in their absence, the problems in role described in the management literature may exist simultaneously. Intervention in situations of role dysfunction is, consequently, complicated by the possibility of problems in role being multiple and simultaneous.

From the perspective of occupational behavior, patients are viewed not in the limited context of disease or disability, but as occupying roles.[21] This perspective does not ignore disease or disability; on the contrary, disease and disability, as they affect role performance, are high priorities for occupational therapy intervention. However, occupational behavior transcends the perspective of the medical model to include a concern also for the requirements or expectations of role.

Prerequisite to performing roles effectively are two sets of competency behaviors that will be discussed. First, however, it is necessary to understand what competency means.

Competency

Competency, as defined by Robert White, is the "capacity to interact effectively with the environment."[23] In more practical terms, "to be competent means to be sufficient or adequate to meet the demands of a situation or task."[24]

From his studies of animals and small children, White offers evidence for a type of motivation to explain the force behind competence, which he calls the "effectance motive." What evolves when the effectance motive is operating, in contrast to when innate drives are operating to satisfy tissue needs, is effectance. Effectance, or having an impact on the environment, produces a sense of efficacy or "joy in being a cause."[23,24]

There are two sets of competency behaviors, or two levels of competence. At the first level, the capacities for becoming competent are generated. At the second level, attention is directed toward the skills that one needs for environmental mastery and achievement. The first level addresses biomedical concerns, the preconditions for competency; the second level addresses biosocial concerns, the conditions for competency.

Intervention at the biomedical level is concerned with the internal systems of the body and mind where (1) the physical, psychological, and social capacities of the individual must be nurtured and protected in the interest of promoting and maintaining competence, or (2) where, in the case of the emotionally or physically disabled, dysfunctional internal systems must be restored to their maximum limits of function.

Restoring function at the biomedical level, however, does not guarantee competency. Indeed, reducing the symptoms of an emotional or physical disorder does not ensure that the person will be able to work, to play, or to interact effectively with the environment. What is needed, in addition to biomedical intervention, is intervention at the biosocial level. Intervention at this level concentrates on the development of skills in preparation for the resumption of role or the transition from one role to another.

Earlier, when discussing Kielhofner's sixth proposition that "habits are the basic structures by which behavior is ordered in time," the point was made that skills, not habits, are the focus of intervention for transforming disorganized behavior into organized behavior.[8] Habits are indeed the basic structures by which behavior is ordered in time, but what supports these structures are skills. One cannot approach habits directly in terms of correcting faulty or bad habits but only indirectly through skills.

What is important clinically when developing or redeveloping one's skills for daily living is suggested by Burke. When teaching skills to an individual, Burke maintains that what is taught must be valued by the individual. In other words, what is taught must be seen as having some utility in terms of one's ability to interact with the environment. Otherwise, the person will see himself or herself as ill-equipped to meet the demands of daily living.[3]

Commenting on this same issue, but addressing his comments to education in general, Bruner suggests the consideration of two principles when teaching skills. First, the principle of social relevance states that what is taught must have some social value. Second, the principle of personal relevance states that what is taught should have some benefit to the individual in terms of his or her personal values and needs.[2]

Translated to the practice of occupational therapy, these ideas mean that skills that are taught should have social relevance, that is, they should involve the ability to perform roles and therefore to participate as a productive member of society. In other words, skills that are

taught must be linked to role; they must not be isolated from the requirements of role, or their social value will be questionable. Also, skills that are taught should have personal relevance in terms of increasing the person's capacity to have an impact on the environment. Skills are the means by which one achieves effectance, the means by which one becomes competent. As skills are acquired and applied, a sense of control is generated, a sense of efficacy develops to serve as an intrinsic motivator for one's present and continued strivings toward competence.[3]

Postscript

As a postscript to this discussion of three of the major themes of occupational behavior, an example illustrating the clinical value of occupational behavior seems appropriate.

A couple of years ago, a workshop was organized by a group of people with multiple sclerosis, not by professionals, for themselves and for their families. Approximately 130 people attended the workshop, and one could quickly sense the disappointment, anger, and frustration that these people were experiencing in their lives. The major problem that they were experiencing, which obviously created problems for their families as well, was that they were having difficulty organizing their time to meet the demands of daily living. The biomedical needs of these individuals had been addressed by professionals, but their biosocial needs were being ignored. As a consequence of their disabling condition, time had to be restructured: it took them longer to dress themselves, to perform their chores, to prepare a meal. Since they tended to fatigue easily, the old routines that had served them prior to the onset of multiple sclerosis no longer worked. However, they had difficulty abandoning these routines, as inefficient as they had become, because they were not aware of any alternatives. Also, because so much time was spent maintaining themselves and their homes, opportunities to be productive in work or leisure were almost nonexistent. They desperately wanted these oportunities to be productive, but they did not know how to go about providing them.

The appropriateness and value of occupational behavior was clearly evident when these people shared their problems. Had the professionals who responded to their biomedical needs also addressed their biosocial needs, these people might not have been in the predicament in which they found themselves. They could not organize their time; no new skills were provided to replace those that had eroded, except for those associated with mobility and self-care; they had accepted the role of patient in the absence of a viable alternative; they were hungry for leisure activities, but they did not know where to start. Some could no longer work or felt that they could no longer work, and unfortunately, they did not know that leisure could be an alternative to work in terms of a productive, satisfying life. In fact, one gentleman, whose satisfactions in life were derived primarily from work, made the following comment in response to the frustration that he felt from not being able to work: "If leisure could do for me what work did for me, I would be a happy man."

What is sad about this man's situation and the situation in which all of these individuals found themselves is that much of their disappointment, anger, and frustration could have been avoided had the professionals who attended to their biomedical needs approached treatment from a broader perspective. Instead, these patients had to organize themselves to receive a level of care that should have been provided when under the care of professionals.

Summary

In the Report on the American Occupational Therapy Association Project To Identify the Philosophical Base of Occupational Therapy, occupation is defined as "goal-directed behavior aimed at the development of play, work, and life skills for optimal time management." [19] Included in this report also are three explanations of why man engages in occupation: (1) to acquire the skills and behaviors necessary for ensuring one's survival; (2) to achieve a sense of quality in one's life; and (3) to contribute to the progress and well-being of society by being a productive member of that society.[19]

It was the issue of man's need for occupation that Reilly addressed in her Eleanor Clarke Slagle Lecture when she challenged the profession to identify the vital need of man that it would serve, if not man's vital need for occupation.[16] Convinced that man's need for occupation was indeed the vital need that should be served by occupational therapy, and committed as she was to her profession, her studies, her writings, and her lectures concentrated on addressing this issue. What evolved from her work and from the work of her associates, was an emergent paradigm for the profession: the paradigm of occupational behavior.

References

1. Bockoven JS: Legacy of moral treatment — 1800's to 1910. Am J Occup Ther 25:223, 1971
2. Bruner J: The skill of relevance or the relevance of skills. Saturday Review April:66, 1970
3. Burke JP: A clinical perspective on motivation: Pawn versus origin. Am J Occup Ther 31:254, 1977
4. Heard C: Occupational role acquisition: A perspective on the chronically disabled. Am J Occup Ther 31:243, 1977
5. Hopkins HL: An historical perspective on occupational therapy. In Hopkins HL, Smith HD (eds): Willard and Spackman's Occupational Therapy, 6th ed. Philadelphia, JB Lippincott, 1983
6. Kahn RL: Conflict, ambiguity, and overload: Three elements in job stress. Occup Ment Health 3:2, 1973
7. Katz D, Kahn RL: The Social Psychology Of Organizations. New York, John Wiley & Sons, 1966
8. Kielhofner G: Temporal adaptation: A conceptual framework for occupational therapy. Am J Occup Ther 31:235, 1977
9. Kielhofner G: The temporal dimension in the lives of retarded adults: A problem of interaction and intervention. Am J Occup Ther 33:161, 1979
10. Kuhn TS: The Structure Of Scientific Revolutions, 2nd ed. Chicago, University of Chicago Press, 1970
11. Kuhn TS: The Essential Tension. Chicago, University of Chicago Press, 1977
12. Matsutsuyu J: Occupational behavior approach. In Hopkins HL, Smith HD (eds): Willard and Spackman's Occupational Therapy, 6th ed. Philadelphia, JB Lippincott, 1983
13. Matsutsuyu J: Occupational behavior: A perspective on work And play. Am J Occup Ther 25:291, 1971
14. Meyer A: The philosophy of occupation therapy. Arch Occup Ther 1:1, 1922. Reprinted in Am J Occup Ther 31:639, 1977
15. Reilly M: Defining a cobweb, and an explanation of play. In Reilly M (ed): Play As Exploratory Learning. Beverly Hills, Sage Publications, 1974
16. Reilly M: Occupational therapy can be one of the great ideas of 20th century medicine. Am J Occup Ther 16:1, 1962
17. Reilly M: A psychiatric occupational therapy program as a teaching model. Am J Occup Ther 20:61, 1966
18. Robinson AL: Play: The arena for acquisition of rules for competent behavior. Am J Occup Ther 31:248, 1977
19. Shannon PD: Report On The AOTA Project To Identify The Philisophical Base Of Occupational Therapy, January 1983. Condensed under the title: Toward A Philosophy Of Occupational Therapy, August 1983. Bethesda, American Occupational Therapy Association (in press)
20. Shannon PD: The work–play model: A basis for occupational therapy programming in psychiatry. Am J Occup Ther 24:215, 1970
21. Shannon PD: Work–Play theory and the occupational therapy process. Am J Occup Ther 26:169, 1972
22. Shannon PD: The derailment of occupational therapy. Am J Occup Ther 31:229, 1977
23. White RW: Motivation reconsidered: The concept of competence. Psychol Rev 66:297, 1959
24. White RW: The urge towards competence. Am J Occup Ther 25:271, 1971

The Health Care System

CHAPTER 9

Occupational Therapy's Place in the Health Care System

SECTION **1**

The Health Care Delivery System Today   *Linda L. Levy*

A revolution is occurring in our health care delivery system. Within the past two decades, social, economic, and political pressures have been added to those of science and technology, producing a demand for a new concept of health care, a new ethic of responsibility for both consumers and providers, and a new structuring of health care institutions to deliver broader, better, and more cost-effective care. As a result, the health care delivery system has become not a changed system, but rather a perpetually changing one. In light of the rapid changes that are occurring, the practice of occupational therapy a few years hence will likely be significantly different from what it is today.

In order to understand some of these changes, it is necessary to have a basic understanding of the system's function and structure. At the outset, it should be acknowledged that the term "system" is a misnomer. In reality, the United States does not have a single comprehensible system for delivering health care. Instead, the system is a conglomeration of many often-independent components which overlap and interact in a variety of ways.

Function of the Health Care Delivery System

The function of the health care delivery system is to deliver equitable, efficient, and effective services to the population. The services are derived from the veritable explosion in medical research and technology in the last decade, which has produced profound effects on the state of medicine and what it is capable of doing. And yet, paradoxically perhaps, there are serious concerns about health care and its delivery in the United States. The system by which these magnificent medical advances are made available to the public has been described as a "no-system system," or "push-cart vending in the age of supermarkets." That is, for all its technological sophistication, it does not provide the health care the population needs, and the health care it does deliver it delivers inefficiently.

These views are gaining credibility. Our research and technology are unequalled by any other nation, and yet the United States is hardly a leader in the delivery of health care. Indicators of health status, such as infant mortality, maternal mortality, life expectancy, and death rates for middle-aged citizens, reveal that the United States lags far behind almost every nation in Western Europe. To make matters worse, few countries in the world spend as much as the United States does on health care either in absolute terms or as a percentage of the gross national product. And, as is reflected in indicators of health status, the benefits do not appear to be justifying the costs. Furthermore, health costs are rising faster than practically any other segment of the nation's economy, which is draining resources from equally essential sectors, such as housing, education, and national defense and contributing significantly to the national deficit.

There are also mounting concerns about the availability, accessibility, and quality of health care services. It has become apparent that good health care is simply not available to many Americans. People seeking health care face many geographic and economic barriers. Wide geographic variations exist in the distribution of physicians and other health care workers. As a result, in many rural areas and in the poor parts of large cities, it is difficult, if not impossible, for many people to obtain proper health care. Americans are also denied access to health care because they cannot afford insurance or have health problems that make them uninsurable. In fact, very few are covered against the costs of catastrophic illness. To complicate the issue further, the quality of care varies greatly, particularly when one's eligibility for care is determined by one's insurance coverage rather than by one's need. Moreover, even when citizens have adequate insurance coverage, there are still vast differences in the quality of care available in different geographic regions and even in different sections of the same city.

Increasingly, critics contend that we have all but ignored the delivery of health care in our preoccupation with developing technology to treat diseases. They further question how such inequities can be tolerated in a society with so much know-how. One conclusion is little disputed, however: in the United States, there is a crisis in health care.

Origins of the Problem

The health care crisis in America affects all people financially and in terms of the availability and quality of care they receive. Simply stated, the crisis is due to the fact that our knowledge of health care (*i.e.,* our technology) has evolved at a much greater rate than our ability to

deliver that care. This has created a large discrepancy between the demand for health care and the supply of services, which—true to market principles—results in sharply increasing costs. To understand how this situation came about, some historical background is necessary.

At the turn of the present century, all health care was provided by general fee-for-service family physicians engaged in solo practice. It was a time when medicine had few effective remedies, and, as historians note, patients who went to physicians had only a fifty–fifty chance of benefitting from the encounter.[15] However, in 1910, as a result of the Flexner report, medical education became a university undertaking, and health care began to be firmly rooted in medical science. Thereafter, knowledge about the workings of the human body and the causes of disease developed rapidly, which led to a need for highly trained specialists who were better equipped to handle the new technologies. General family physicians were gradually replaced on medical school faculties with full-time specialist physicians, so, medical students had little contact with those who were practicing general medicine, and specialists became their only role models. This trend away from the general physician toward the more narrowly oriented specialist was further reinforced in World War II, when specialists were rewarded with higher rank and pay in the armed forces than general physicians.

Thus, by the late 1940s, general physicians began to disappear, replaced by an ever-increasing variety of specialists with more prestige and higher incomes. The problem for the health care delivery system was that no resources were developed to take the place of the family doctor who heretofore had been central to health care delivery, providing the general medical care needed by most of the population. Furthermore, family doctors could coordinate the diverse services of the emerging specialities and were willing to provide continuing care. Now, the more expensive specialists dominated the health care system. At times, internists, pediatricians, and obstetrician–gynecologists would assume responsibility for the general medical care that was most needed by the population. More often, however, Americans had to forego general medical care or had to depend on hospital emergency rooms and clinics for diagnostic assistance and care. In either case, general medical care became increasingly unavailable (*i.e.,* the supply decreased). Concurrently, the costs began to rise.

The now-predominant specialists adopted the same solo practice model for the delivery of health care used by the general physician at a time when illness could be managed by a single family doctor. They continued to operate relatively independently, notwithstanding consultation agreements with other physicians, laboratories, and hospitals. This was another unfortunate development for the health care system, because no mechanisms were designed to coordinate their specialized services. The linkages among specialists were informal and difficult to maintain and became inefficient and inconvenient to consumers. It was not unusual for patients to go to a number of different specialists and hospitals for one disease episode, and there were few general physicians available to provide the requisite continuing care. To this day, most patients receive fragmented specialized care without a general family physician to provide continuity of care. This situation has become especially problematic given the changing nature of the diseases that the health system currently confronts—diseases that are more chronic, complicated, and difficult to defeat (an issue to be discussed in more detail later). Thus, with the rise in specialist technology, health care became fragmented as well as more costly.

The specialization of physicians was accompanied by an increasing variety and number of allied health practitioners. In addition, an increasing complexity developed in the services provided by hospitals, the essential "workshops" of many of the new specialists.[12] A technological gap developed between the care that could be provided in physicians' offices and the care provided in hospitals by highly specialized medical personnel using complex equipment. Consequently, hospitals were elevated to the central position in health care delivery. Note that prior to this century, hospitals were places to avoid, because they were notorious for filth and overcrowding as well as for high rates of mortality. The postoperative infection rate, for instance, was 100% and the postoperative mortality rate, 80%.[9] Wealthier patients were treated at home by their family physician. Now, the role and function of the hospital in health care delivery was completely reversed.

The central position of hospitals in the health care delivery system became reinforced and solidified in the Depression era by the development of health insurance. The providers of care, first hospitals and then physicians, were concerned about the increasing inability of many consumers to pay their rising health care bills. Health insurance (*e.g.*, Blue Cross and Blue Shield) was created to spread the risk of health costs among consumers and to assure that the hospitals themselves would be paid. It became an enormously popular benefit for American employees after World War II because the premiums were tax deductible for the employer and not taxable to the employee. As unions found it increasingly difficult to obtain wage increases, health insurance became a desirable benefit to bargain for during negotiations. Today, health insurance has become one of the benefits employers are expected to offer employees.

Although health insurance did help provide for the consumer's need for protection, at the same time it produced untoward effects on the delivery of health services. The plan that the hospitals and physicians created largely served their interests and was inevitably inflationary. It clearly favored inpatient acute hospital care and specifically excluded equally important and less expensive non–hospital-based services. There were no cost-control measures built into the plan that would restrain the use of high-cost facilities and procedures. In fact, the plan was based on a cost plus fee-for-service system which rewarded hospitals and physicians for providing more services rather than fewer. In addition, it became economically favorable for both patients and physicians to use hospitals, since hospital services were covered whereas less-expensive alternatives were not. We know that increased demand results in increased costs. In this case, it is important to recognize that health insurance increased the demand for the most expensive of medical services (*i.e.*, hospital services) rather than for the less expensive alternatives. As a result, insurance served to increase overall health care costs rather than to offset them.

To complicate matters further, the federal government adopted this hospital-based fee-for-service model of health insurance with the introduction of Medicare and Medicaid in 1965. These entitlement programs were enacted in the era of the "Great Society" to address the problems of lack of health care for the elderly and the poor. Subsequently, the demands on the health care system increased dramatically. Billions of federal dollars were spent—virtually without control—on hospital services. Hospitals flourished and became the heart of the health care system. As a result, high-cost hospital-based services became the primary focus of the health care delivery system. As we shall see, this occurred to the unfortunate neglect of the general medical, long-term care, rehabilitation, and preventive services that are needed to serve the dominant health problems of our population today.

Some final points about health insurance are important. Not only did it promote the rapid growth of hospitals, its taken-for-granted nature led to the development of a political philosophy which considered health care an entitlement in this country; that is, a right rather than a privilege. This philosophical change produced even more powerful demands on the health care delivery system. Insurance provided unlimited access to health care, and the costs of that care were no longer checked by one's ability to pay; nor was anyone really concerned about excessive use of services or rising costs when everyone knew the bill would be paid. Costs and demand, then, rose sharply. Moreover, with the increase in utilization of health services, the system has become crowded. As a result, health care has become not only more costly but harder to get (*i.e.*, the demand has far surpassed the supply.)

We are only beginning to realize the unfortunate effects of both this shift in political philosophy and our inflationary model of health insurance. The costs of health insurance have risen dramatically, which has made it inaccessible to the near poor (those ineligible for Medicaid) and to a growing number of middle-income families. Also, unions and industry are beginning to recognize that making private health insurance coverage universal and passing health insurance costs on to consumers has made it difficult for the United States to compete with other countries. For example, General Motors Corporation spends more for health insurance benefits for its employees and their families than it pays for steel to manufacture its automobiles; and in 1983, health insurance premiums added an estimated $600 to the price of every new American car.[7] This cost clearly has a serious impact on the nation's economy.

There was another consequence of specialist technology that for all practical purposes, decreased the supply of health services: the geographic maldistribution of physicians. The distribution of physicians in this country is weighted heavily toward metropolitan areas, yet, poverty-stricken areas of the cities are unable to attract the services of private physicians. Specialists, in particular, tend to cluster around hospitals in big cities, partly to keep up with their specialties, partly to have the sophisticated equipment and hospital support services they need, and partly to have access to a population large enough to provide sufficient incidence of the diseases for which their services are needed. They also tend to practice in those communities that can best afford their services. The geographic maldistribution has become worse, not better, in the last decade, and it contributes to the lack of availability of health care in many sections of the country (*i.e.*, the supply) and, consequently, to the increased costs of health care.

The costs of health care as well as its quality are also affected by the distinctive nature of the medical market place. It should be recognized that with the purchase of health care services, a great deal of information is hidden from the consumer. Most consumers are not knowledgeable about what services are available, what costs are involved, and what alternatives are available. They are not in a position to evaluate the quality of care they receive, nor are they able— especially in times of emergency—to shop around for the best service at the best price. This, too, translates into large variations in quality and into higher and higher costs.

There is a final factor that contributes substantially to the crisis in health care. We have witnessed medical miracles such as organ transplants and open heart surgery and expect that these sophisticated methods will be available for all diseases. Ironically, these increased expectations about what medicine ought to be able to accomplish are contributing to the health care crisis, because people have come to expect more from the health care system than it can provide. As was mentioned earlier, there is profound national concern that despite massive health expenditures, the nation's health has improved less than expected. There is a critical assumption underlying this expectation; that is, that "health care makes people healthy." The problem for the health care system is that, contrary to this popular belief, health care will *not* make people healthy. A brief overview of the leading causes of death and disability in this country may shed light on this issue.

Prior to this century, the major causes of illness and death were infectious diseases, such as pneumonia, influenza, tuberculosis, diptheria, cholera, and smallpox. Cures such as antibiotics and immunizations were not available, and unsophisticated public health standards, such as the lack of safe water and milk and inadequate sewage disposal, contributed to widespread infection of the population. Today, improvements in sanitation, breakthroughs in antibiotic therapy, and immunization have greatly reduced the role of infectious diseases as causes of deaths, and other disease categories are taking their place. Specifically, diseases of the heart and circulation now account for more than half of all deaths and disability. Cancers account for about half of the remainder, with the other primary causes of death being cirrhosis of the liver, diabetes, and accidents. These diseases plus arthritis and musculoskeletal impairments, are also the primary causes of disability.

Ironically, the prevalence of these more chronic diseases is testimony to our success in eliminating infectious diseases. (Accidents, the one nondisease cited, have become a major cause of death in this century because of the use of the automobile). Survival from the diseases that used to kill early in life dramatically increased life expectancy and thereby allowed the illnesses that occur later in life to increase in frequency. Consequently, the present-day health care system is faced with an older, more illness-prone population, whose disabilities are much more difficult and costly to treat. Concomitantly, this age shift in the population has dramatically increased the demand for health services. The key questions to be asked are:

For how many of today's diseases do we now have an effective technology for cure or prevention, comparable to antibiotics for the treatment of pneumonia?
Are we failing to treat these diseases effectively because of deficiencies in the health care delivery system?
Or do present mortality and disability rates from these diseases merely reflect the absence of any known technology that works?

The unfortunate reality is that with the present state of our knowledge, there is no medical treatment that will prevent heart disease, stroke, diabetes, cirrhosis, arthritis, or injuries, nor do we possess any effective technology for cure of these diseases. The medical treatment that we do possess will relieve pain, stabilize the patient's condition, arrest deterioration, provide support, and reduce disability to some degree, yet there is little evidence that our technology has contributed substantially to improved health or longevity. In other words, even if we had the best health care delivery system in the world, there are very real limits to the impact it could have on the major health problems that Americans face today.

This is not to say that nothing can be done to increase the health of the American people. There may well be little hope for prevention or cure of these diseases through medical intervention, yet there is much to suggest that these diseases occur prematurely, that many have significantly more damaging effects than are necessary, and, in some cases, that they are avoidable through control of unhealthy life styles and behaviors. In fact, the whole "Health Promotion and Disease Prevention" movement is based on the recognition that the most useful solutions to the most prominent health problems of our time are prevention and control of the progress of these diseases. To illustrate:

Heart disease is the most common cause of disability of Americans over the age of 40, yet it has been estimated that 80% of all deaths from heart disease occur prematurely and are facilitated by unhealthy habits, primarily cigarette smoking, overweight, and sedentary lifestyle.

Lung cancer is our most common lethal malignancy, yet it is estimated that 80% of all lung cancer deaths are directly caused by cigarette smoking. Other types of cancer are also related to, and worsened by, smoking (oral and bladder cancer), the ingestion of food additives and certain drugs, and the inhaling of a wide variety of noxious agents.

Cirrhosis is directly related to, and worsened by, excessive ingestion of alcohol together with poor nutrition.

Accident fatalities are directly related to alcohol ingestion, excessive speed, and refusal to use seat belts.[19]

Anywhere from 4% to 100% of patients with diabetes, hypertension, ulcers, rheumatic fever, or tuberculosis fail to comply with medical/rehabilitative recommendations designed to lessen the effects of their diseases.[20]

A recurring theme in these examples is that the diseases that most threaten the health of the American public have a number of well-established risk factors. By removing the risk factors associated with the progress of these diseases, one can postpone their occurrence, lessen their debilitating effects, and, in some cases, even prevent them from occurring at all. To a large extent, control of present major health problems entails modification of individual behaviors and life styles.

In light of these observations, convincing arguments have been made that the next major advances in the health of the American people will be made not by what the health care system is able to provide, but rather by what individuals are willing to do for themselves. More attention is being paid to studies that reveal that good health and longevity are as much related to a self-enforced regimen of sufficient sleep, regular well-balanced meals, moderate exercise and weight, no smoking, and little or no drinking as they are to professionally delivered services.[6] If individuals were willing to do these things, the impact on the nation's health would be enormous, and billions of health care dollars would be saved. If they are not willing, we probably should stop complaining about the steadily rising costs of health care and the lack of expected results.[19] We must realize that more medical care will not, in itself, result in better health.

The tragedy is, however, that this insight is little promoted by the health care system. In addition, it requires a rejection of an assumption that is widely accepted (*i.e.*, that "health care makes people healthy"), as well as modifications of behaviors that are notoriously difficult to change. Although reorganization of our health care system is undoubtedly needed to improve accessibility and quality and to contain costs, the fact is that improving the health care system is not necessarily the most effective way of improving health. This is not to say that the health care system is good for nothing; rather, it is not good for everything.

In summary, we have inherited our present health care delivery system from nearly a century of haphazard growth. It was derived from a family doctor–centered health care system that worked reasonably well at a time when medical science and education were less sophisticated, health problems were more straightforward, delivery of health care was simpler, and society, correctly doubting the benefits anyway, was less demanding. The system is now proving inadequate in the face of new demographic, epidemiologic, and social problems that are largely the result of medicine's technological success.[12]

The most striking characteristic of the health care system, as Freymann[12] notes, is perhaps *imbalance*. We have gone from no science to little but science, from no specialists to practically all specialists, from widespread fear of hospitals to widespread idolization of them, from insufficient funding to financing that overloaded the system, from life familiar with death to a long lifespan that is almost guaranteed, from lavish support of one fragment of the system (acute care) to neglect of the others (chronic, psychiatric, and preventive services), from an abundance of inadequate doctors to a maldistribution of good ones, from no faith in medicine to unrealistic faith in it.[12] Yet, it is the imbalance that has developed between the *supply* of health services and the *demand* for health services that has created the most devastating impact on the delivery of health services today. There are a number of forces that have contributed to this imbalance. These include changes in:

Research and technology which fostered specialization
The status of hospitals
The methods of financing care
The role played by government
Public values and expectations
The nature of disease
The age composition of the population

All of these forces have caused demand to increase faster than supply can increase. The result has been continuing rapid rises in health care costs.

Reform of the Health Care System: Past, Present, and Future

The frequent frustration of unmet demands as well as concern about costs have created increasing political pressure for major changes in the health care delivery system. Notable examples of efforts at reform include the following:

National health insurance proposals, which attempt to ensure that all Americans are covered by a more comprehensive (less "hospital-based") model of health insurance and which would also protect them in the event of catastrophic illness
Social Security Amendments of 1972 (P.L. 92-603), which provided for the establishment of Professional Standard Review Organizations to ensure that federally funded programs, such as Medicare and Medicaid, were used in an efficient and effective manner
Health Maintenance Organization Act of 1973 (P.L. 93-222), which provided for the planning and development of HMOs to encourage less costly ambulatory care outside the hospital, including preventive, diagnostic, therapeutic, and rehabilitative services
National Health Planning and Resources Development Act of 1974 (P.L. 93-641), which established regional health systems agencies to assume responsibility for health care planning for community needs and for cost containment. It required hospitals that wished to engage in major construction or to change service programs to be reviewed
The National Consumer Health Information and Health Promotion Act of 1976, which attempted to set rational goals for health information and education
Health Professions Educational Assistance Act (P.L. 94-484), which provided incentives for medical schools to increase the number of family practice physicians to 50% of their graduates and also attempts to attract physicians to underserved areas by subsidizing their medical education
Title VII of the Medicare Prospective Payment Legislation (P.L. 98-21), which provided incentives for cost containment and better management of resources by a reimbursement structure based on a patient's diagnosis rather than the direct costs of care

Any proposals for reform of the health care system — in the past, present, or the future — bring with them hopes to contain costs, to provide accessibility of services for all, and to improve the quality and continuity of health care. They also hope to encourage a more effective and rational utilization of services by both provider and consumers; that is, by modifying the demand for the most expensive of health services, as well as by structural reform of the delivery system, to make our hospital-dominated system more comprehensive. It is, however, fair to suggest that in the present environment of sluggish economic growth, low productivity growth, and inflation, it is the cost of health care that is moving politicians to basic reform of the health care delivery system, rather than any concerns they have about the performance, structure, and efficiency of that system. As we have seen, basic market principles dictate that any proposal aimed at containing costs will have to increase supply more than demand.

The Structure of the Health Care System

The structure of the health care system is based on the historic precedents and economic incentives discussed above. It is comprised of many independent components affiliated in a variety of ways and of many smaller systems serving specific groups of people. We will begin to explore its structural components by looking at its two major divisions.

There are two basic divisions for delivering health care in the United States: a *public system* and a *private system.* The *public* system is operated by federal, state, and local governments and has two major concerns. The first is primary prevention services provided at the public health level to prevent disease. Examples include sanitation systems, water purification and fluoridation, and immunization programs for children of low-income families. The second major concern of the public system is the operation of a series of smaller subsystems to provide health care to specific groups of entitled individuals. For example, the military operates its own health care system for people in the armed services, the Veterans Administration takes care of many of the nation's veterans, and the Indian Health Service is responsible for caring for persons on reservations. In addition, there has been a long tradition that care of the developmentally disabled child and the severely or chronically mentally ill adult is provided by a public system developed at the state level.

The *private* health system consists of a loose association of independent health professionals who provide personal health care services on a fee-for-service basis. Most health care expenditures—more than 90%—occur within the private system.[15] Because of its predominance, the rest of this discussion will focus on the private health system.

The major components of the private health care system include:

1. Financing
2. Payment mechanism
3. Health care personnel
4. Institutions for delivering care
5. System regulation

A brief description of each component follows.

Financing

The health care system accounts for more than $350 billion in national expenditures, an average of $1500 per person per year.[14] (By contrast, *per capita* expenditures per year for health care in Third World countries are $1.50.) Of these funds, approximately 42% is spent on hospital care, 19% on physician services, 6% on dentist services, 7% on drugs, 8% on nursing home care, and the remainder on a wide variety of other activities, including research and prevention.[14] Health care costs are increasing faster than practically any other aspect of the nation's economy. The percentage of the gross national product (all economic activity) spent on health care in the United States has increased from about 5% in the 1960s to 11% now.[14]

This doubling of the resources devoted to health care is of great concern to those who finance it from two perspectives. The first is reflected in questions about whether the economy can afford such large expenditures for health care when there are so many other needs to be met from the same funds. As we spend more for medicine, there is necessarily less available for other critical sectors of the economy, including education, housing, nutrition, transportation, income supplementation, and defense. The second perspective is reflected in questions about what we are getting for our health care dollar. Critics note that for all our increased expenditures, there has been no statistically significant change in the health of the American population.[11] Thus, valid arguments are being raised that we would be healthier if we spent the money on education, better public housing, or better highways.

Another important trend in financing health care is the increasing share of the health care bill that is paid by federal or state governments (*i.e.*, the taxpayer). In the early 1960s, governments paid for 25% of all health care; now, governments pay more than 40% of the nation's health care bill.[14] The two publicly financed national entitlement programs, Medicaid and Medicare, account for most of these funds. The costs of these programs have increased so dramatically that taxpayers and governments are beginning to reassess their abilities to pay for services for the poor and the elderly.

Ultimately, the people pay all health care costs. However, there are two sources of income for the health care system. The first is individuals and families. They pay directly for services and also pay indirectly through their own health insurance premiums; through federal, state and local taxes; and through the purchase of goods and services (a portion of domestic consumer prices reflects the costs of the workers' health insurance premiums). The other income source is the employer. Employers pay an equal share of Social Security taxes as well as health insurance premiums and corporate income taxes. Funds from these two sources, individuals and employers, are transferred to private insurers and governments who purchase health services. Private and public insurance have become the major form of financing medical care, accounting for 75% of expenditures for all personal health care and 90% of all hospital care expenditures.[13]

Payment Mechanisms

As noted above, both public funds (approximately 40%) and private funds pay for the health care received in the United States. Within each sector, there are a variety of spending sources. Public funds, for example, come through such diverse programs as temporary disability insurance, workmens' compensation, public assistance, Veteran's Administration, Office of Economic Opportunity, Defense Department, public health services, maternal and child health services, school health, and vocational rehabilitation. However, as indicated earlier, the major sources of public funding of health care are Medicare and Medicaid. Private health expenditures consist of direct payments by consumers for health care and, more commonly, insurance payments made on their behalf. Private insurance is sold largely through employers. There are three major types: Blue Cross, commercial insurance, and health maintenance organizations (HMO's).

Before proceeding, it should be recognized that in the United States, access to health care is dependent on the availability of insurance, and 85% of the population has some form of health insurance protection, either public or private.[22] This means that 15% of all Americans have no insurance protection, a problem which has become worse in the last decade.

The principal insurance plans are presented below.

Medicare

Medicare consists of a basic program of hospitalization insurance under which most persons aged 65 and over are protected against the major costs of hospital and related care (Part A); and a supplementary insurance program through which persons aged 65 and over are aided in paying physician, home health, and other health care bills. Coverage under the basic (Part A) program of hospital insurance is automatically available to all aged individuals covered by the Social Security system. Part B requires a premium payment from the beneficiary to cover part of the costs. Medicare is a single federal program administered by the Social Security Administration.

Medicaid

Medicaid provides federal assistance to states to cover certain medical expenses of specified groups of low-income people (the needy aged, the blind, the disabled) and welfare recipients. The size and the scope of the program is determined by the individual states, but participating states are required to cover the following basic services for the welfare population: inpatient hospital services, outpatient hospital services, skilled nursing home services, physician services, and limited home health services. In addition, a number of services can be supplied at state option, including, for example, clinic services, dental care, occupational therapy and physical therapy services, drugs, vision care, prosthetic devices, and skilled nursing home services. As a result, Medicaid provides widely varying coverages and might best be conceptualized as a series of 50 separate programs, each administered by individual state welfare departments.

As indicated earlier, health care costs under Medicaid and Medicare have increased rapidly, which has led to cutbacks in both eligibility and benefits, as well as in payments to providers. In some states, Medicaid now pays as little as 40% of physician charges. Consequently, providers are becoming more reluctant to treat Medicaid patients. Accessibility to health care for the poor and the elderly may then decline as the government finds it increasingly difficult to pay the bills.

Blue Cross

Blue Cross is the largest private financier of hospital care in the United States. Even though there are actually 75 independent Blue Cross plans, these plans are linked by the National Blue Cross Association, which represents them in national affairs and provides services in marketing, education, research, and public relations. Blue Cross plans are primarily nonprofit voluntary organizations which operate under enabling legislation specifi-

cally enacted to cover nonprofit prepayment plans. Therefore, they are often subject to state regulation of their rates and benefits, usually by the insurance department of the state in which the plan operates.

In general, Blue Cross coverage is designed to provide reasonably full payment of the total bill for most hospitalizations. Other than that, there is no standard plan. Employers can buy any package of benefits and other plan characteristics that they want, and the insurer "costs out" the benefit package that is selected to determine the premiums. Individual policies may also cover, for example, outpatient physician services, prescription drugs, or services provided by psychologists, chiropractors, podiatrists, and nurse practitioners.

It is important to recognize that the predominance of Blue Cross plans for private insurance coverage was reinforced by the federal government with the passage of Medicare and Medicaid legislation, because Blue Cross was designated as the fiscal intermediary between hospitals and Medicare.

Commercial Insurance

From the consumer's point of view, commercial insurance is not noticeably different from Blue Cross. However, insurance contracts in this area are indemnity contracts, offered by for-profit insurance companies through employers. Under indemnity insurance, when the enrollee uses health care services that are covered by the benefits of his specific plan, the insurance company pays the individual a certain amount of money, and he is responsible for paying the provider. Hence, this method of insurance involves more administrative paper work than Blue Cross, because the enrollee must file claims for benefits. In contrast to Blue Cross, commercial insurance companies are profit-making businesses which can provide similar benefits to individuals in different states. This is advantageous for large employers, who are able to obtain uniform benefits for employees in different states by access to only one company.

Health Maintenance Organizations (HMOs)

In the early 1970s, the federal government promoted prepaid group practice through HMO's. A prepaid group practice is an organization that agrees to provide most or all the care that enrollees need in return for an established monthly fee. The organization, in turn, hires or contracts with physicians and hospitals for enrollees' care. The HMO thus has an incentive to contain health care costs, since its income is fixed regardless of how much care is provided. HMOs often provide a wider range of services at less cost than traditional insurance programs. They also provide more preventive care, since it is in their interests for enrollees to stay healthy.

Indeed, HMOs achieve their savings through lower rates of hospitalization despite higher rates of ambulatory care. There is considerable national interest in HMOs because they are 10% to 40% less expensive than the conventional system for delivering health care.[4]

Who Is Excluded?

Although insurance coverage provided by both the private and the public sectors for health care is extensive, there are still many Americans who have no coverage. These include the unemployed, the independently employed (health insurance is very costly for individuals who cannot obtain group coverage), those employed in transient jobs, those who change jobs frequently or changed jobs recently, those with "bad" diagnoses, and the chronically sick. In addition, there are employers of low-income workers who offer either no insurance plans or plans that cover workers but not their dependents. It is also expected that the Reagan administration health care cutbacks will worsen access for large parts of the population.[18]

One final note. Health policy is very much determined by the manner in which health care is purchased. As a result, the power to change the system rests in large part with those who control Medicare, Medicaid, Blue Cross, and other insurance monies. When the government entered the financing health care with Medicare and Medicaid, the central debate in Congress became, not whether the federal government would intervene in the system, but the nature and extent of the direction it would impose in return for its massive investment. In relationship to the determination of health care policy, private insurers are following the lead of the federal government.

Health Care Personnel

At present, almost eight million people are employed directly or indirectly in the health care delivery system,[25] making health care the second largest employer in the United States, exceeded only by the construction industry. Health care is also one of the fastest growing industries: between 1970 and 1980, the number of persons employed increased 70%.[25] This rapid growth of manpower is mainly the result of the rapid advances in technology and the need for more specialized personnel. It should be recognized that health care personnel were rarely scrutinized in the past for the efficiency, efficacy, or cost effectiveness of their services because of the open-ended flow (until recently) of third-party payments for many services.[17] However, times are changing rapidly, and health care rationing has become a major concern. This will undoubtedly affect the health care work force.

The number of physicians has also increased dramatically. In 1970, approximately 11,000 students entered medical schools in the United States; by 1984, this number had doubled.[2] Although in the 1960s there was fear about a doctor shortage, there now are questions about a doctor surplus. While debate continues about how many physicians and what types are actually needed, we know that an increase in the supply of doctors means more medical care and, ultimately, higher costs, because physicians create their own demand for services by ordering tests, hospitalizations, and referrals. This is also the case with other types of health professionals. An increase in the supply of health providers will increase the supply and ofttimes the demand for their services. That is, more occupational therapists means more services, which tends to increase the demand for their services. Again, this translates into higher costs.

In terms of practice type, approximately 85% of physicians in the United States are specialists,[25] and the need for more general practitioners is well recognized. As indicated earlier, one of the key provisions of the Health Professions Educational Assistance Act of 1976 was to require medical schools with teaching hospitals to provide a greater proportion of their medical residencies in family practice medicine. Another major problem with our supply of physicians has also been mentioned; that is, most physicians want to practice in metropolitan areas where the potential for peer interaction, for working in the best hospitals, and for higher incomes has been the greatest. As a result, many inner-city and rural areas have shortages of physicians, while other parts of the country have surpluses. Federal programs have attempted to attract physicians to shortage areas, such as through the National Health Corps (P.L. 94-484), which subsidized medical education in return for a commitment to practice in medically underserved areas. However, just as we cannot force physicians to choose family practice instead of a specialty, there is no way to force physicians to practice where they are most needed. Similar maldistribution occurs for all other health professionals, including occupational therapists.

Physicians exert the most powerful influence over the health care industry because they control hospital utilization, drug prescriptions, and referral for services reimbursed by Medicare, Medicaid, and other insurance plans. In fact, this dominance is guaranteed by law. Hence, the ability of other health care professionals to influence the health care system is limited. And yet, physicians represent only a minority (9%) of professionals involved in the delivery of health care. Nurses represent the majority of health care professionals (nearly 55%).[23] With 40,000 practitioners, occupational therapists represent approximately 0.5% of the persons employed in health-related activities.

Health Institutions

Hospitals

The hospital is the center of our health care delivery system, accounting for the highest percentage of health care expenditures. Of the approximately 7,000 hospitals in the country, nearly 6,000 are community hospitals,[1] most of which focus on the provision of short-term acute care. However, this total includes hospitals with specialized missions, such as children's rehabilitation, as well as hospitals owned and operated by the federal government (*e.g.*, Veterans Administration or military hospitals). Most private hospitals in this country are owned by nonprofit corporations, such as religious groups and city/county corporations, although increasingly private hospitals are being bought by chains, most of which are for-profit companies.

There are large geographical disparities in hospital distribution. The number of hospital beds per 1,000 population is on the average 60% greater in the industrial New England and Mid-Atlantic states than in the Rocky Mountain states.[25] This reflects too many beds in metropolitan areas as well as too few in rural areas.

The most significant trends in the hospital industry over the past decade have been the development of multihospital systems and the proliferation of for-profit hospitals. Multihospital systems are being organized largely by for-profit corporations, although nonprofit hospitals are beginning to affiliate with each other as well. Hospitals are attempting to coordinate and consolidate services to allow them to compete more aggressively, increase efficiency, and remain financially viable. As a result, it is likely that independent nonprofit community hospitals will be forced out in the near future.

In addition to the growth of multihospital systems, there has been rapid growth in the number of for-profit (proprietary) hospitals. Today, proprietary hospitals are owned and operated by large national or international corporations that can buy supplies and equipment in bulk and who employ a wide range of experts in financing, marketing, and planning to manage the hospital.

There are trends that bear watching. In 1983, Medicare Prospective Payment legislation was enacted which changed the way hospitals are reimbursed for Medicare bills. Under the new system, diagnoses are divided into diagnostic-related groups (DRGs), and the government has set a fixed price for treatment of each diagnosis, regardless of what services are provided. If hospitals spend less, they make money; if they spend more, they lose money. Clearly, this offers a financial incentive to limit treatment and discharge patients as early as possible. And, as one might predict, the average length of hospital stay has declined continuously since 1983. The DRG reimbursement policy also encourages hospitals to change the mix of services they provide in favor of those that are most profitable. Consequently, there is concern that low-profit but essential services — such as head trauma and burn care — may be eliminated by hospitals seeking to maximize their overal reimbursement.

Nursing Homes

The fastest growing category of health care spending in the United States is nursing home care. There are about 18,000 nursing homes in the United States,[24] a total which by all estimates falls far short of the national need. Moreover, it is estimated that an additional 1.2 million nursing home beds will be needed by the year 2000 just to maintain present levels of service.[24] Nursing homes provide both inpatient care which is less intense than that provided in hospitals and care for the permanently dependent, such as the severely affected Alzheimer's disease victim. The vast majority of nursing homes are small proprietary institutions with fewer than 100 beds. Less than 20% are nonprofit or owned by government.[24] Increasingly, however, nursing homes are being bought or built by large health care corporations.

It is important to recognize that nursing home care is subject to severe financial restrictions that affect the availability of nursing homes as well as the quality and scope of services they can provide. Medicare provides minimal assistance in paying for nursing home care. Reimbursement is available under Medicaid, but individuals must exhaust both Medicare benefits and their personal financial resources to become eligible for Medicaid reimbursement. Even then, as mentioned earlier, levels of reimbursement under Medicaid are typically low. If sufficient political pressure were exerted to increase funding for nursing home care, the quantity, quality, and range of services offered would undoubtedly improve. As of this writing, a Medicare amendment has been proposed by the Reagan administration that would provide coverage for extended nursing home care.

Home Health Care and Hospice Care

There are two additional institutions for the delivery of health care to be mentioned which have grown rapidly within the last decade: home health care and hospice care.

Home care has been called the sleeping giant of the health care industry.[5] Although it is still in its infancy compared to hospitals and nursing homes, it is rapidly expanding as a result of pressure from an aging population, skyrocketing Medicare and Medicaid expenditures, a hospital and provider industry experiencing financial stress, and a business community searching for more cost-effective health care benefits for its employees.[3] Home care services have also become a preferred method of providing health care to a large segment of our population. Bringing services to people in their own homes is seen as a realistic and more humane approach for all but the most complex of health care services. The major goals of home care have been to prevent hospitalization and to delay or avoid residential health care placement. However, home care, a less costly method of service delivery, has become especially attractive to institutions attempting to make the DRG system profitable by sending patients home quicker and sicker.[8]

Home health care is generally considered to include the provision of skilled nursing services; occupational, physical, and speech therapy; medical social services; dietary services; homemaker services; home health aide services; respiratory therapy; and medical supplies, drugs and appliances. They are provided through public agencies; nonprofit agencies such as visiting nurses associations (VNAs); agencies operated by hospitals, skilled nursing facilities, or rehabilitation facilities; and proprietary organizations. Many hospitals are responding to the advent of DRGs by establishing their own agencies to replenish revenues lost under prospective payment. Reimbursements for services vary but are derived most commonly from Medicare and Medicaid, as well as from the Veterans Administration; the Civilian Health and Medical Program of the Uniformed Services (CHAMPUS); Title III of the Older Americans Act; Social Services Block Grants to states (formerly Title XX); private health insurance; and private payment by patients.

Hospice is both a philosophy and an organized program of care designed for terminally ill patients and their families. It has only recently become a significant component of the health care delivery system. The overall goal is to minimize suffering and heroic intervention while offering palliative care to the patient and support to the patient and family during the process of dying. As such, it is viewed as an organized reaction to a significant social problem: the depersonalization of care for the terminally ill and the failure of the existing medical care system to meet the needs of the dying.[21] It is also being seen as a cost-saving alternative in health care delivery.

A variety of organizational structures deliver hospice care, including free-standing or independent programs, hospital-based programs, home health agency-based programs, and community-based (or "volunteer") programs. Hospices provide or arrange for the following services: nursing, physician services, social work, pastoral care, bereavement counseling, nutrition, physical and occupational therapy, psychological services, pharmacy services, medical supplies, laboratory services, home health aide services, personal care, housekeeping and homemaker services, and short-term inpatient services.[21]

Reimbursement for hospice care has increased dramatically in the past few years. In 1981, Blue Cross initiated coverage for hospice care. Shortly thereafter, a number of commercial insurers followed their lead. Medicare reimbursement was established in 1983 within the Tax Equity and Fiscal Responsibility Act (TEFRA), and in 1986, the Omnibus Budget Reconciliation Act sanctioned the addition of a hospice benefit to the list of services which states may choose to add to their Medicaid plans. With these reimbursement mechanisms, hospice care has been placed in the mainstream of the health care delivery system.

System Regulation

The private health care system functions under a complex set of rules and regulations. The law has assumed a steadily increasing role in health care, given its interests in protecting the public health, safety, and welfare and in protecting the rights of providers and patients in the health care process.

Traditionally, the primary responsibility for formulating health care policy has rested within individual states. For example, licensure of health personnel; accreditation of hospitals, nursing homes, and other health facilities; the protection of patients' rights; statutes which define criteria for pronouncing death; and the negligence, liability, and malpractice system are operated primarily by the states. However, the federal government is assuming more of a role over health care issues in order to protect its increased stake in the system, primarily through regulations that are attached to the use of Medicare and Medicaid funds. Further, the federal courts have become significantly involved in bioethical questions, especially those bearing on abortion, the definition of death, and human subject research.

In addition, the private health care system functions under a set of professional regulations. The involvement of individual professions in the regulatory process acknowledges that specific professional competence is needed to evaluate the quality of care given by health providers. Consequently, accreditation of medical, dental, and allied health professional schools; requirements for certification examinations; certification of the qualifications of health providers; and malpractice criteria have become the responsibility of professional associations.

Health Promotion and Disease Prevention

Within the last decade, there has been a growing trend toward wellness-oriented health care, disease prevention, and health promotion. A number of the social and demographic factors discussed previously have sparked this interest, including the change in focus from acute infectious diseases to chronic degenerative diseases, the recognition of lifestyle and individual behaviors as significant factors in the disease process, the increasing shortcomings of traditional medicine, the age shifts in our population, and the unbearable economic prospect of maintaining an ailing elder population.[10] In 1974, the government cited "the promotion of activities for the prevention of disease" as one of the ten national health priorities (P.L. 93-641, Section 1502). This law acknowledged the importance of taking action either to avoid illness or to reduce the premature occurrence of disabilities attending the chronic diseases that medicine today is unable to cure as a way of reducing the cost of treatment. Beyond this acknowledgment, however, lie more important issues, chief among them being the actual resources we are willing to commit to this effort. Of the $355 billion spent annually on health care in the United States, only about 3% ($11 billion) is spent on prevention services.[14]

However, a number of hospitals are beginning to establish their own health promotion/disease prevention (HP/DP) programs, in large part to make money and also to improve their images in the community. The American Hospital Association's Center for Health Promotion has been a major stimulus and guide for hospitals in developing these programs.[16] The HD/DP programs include one or more elements of primary prevention (the prevention of disease before any symptoms are present), secondary prevention (screening, early detection, and early treatment of clinically inapparent disease in a person who has been defined as at risk), and tertiary prevention (the treatment of acquired disease in a manner designed to minimize the development of complications). The recommended core HP/DP programs[16] include:

1. In primary prevention, the "basic seven" personal preventive interventions:
   Exercise promotion
   Smoking cessation
   Weight loss
   Stress management
   Nutrition counseling
   Substance abuse control
   Personal accident prevention
2. In secondary prevention, screening and early detection of:
   Cancer
   Hypertension
   Diabetes
   Heart Disease
   Glaucoma
3. In tertiary prevention:
   Cardiac rehabilitation
   Pulmonary rehabilitation
   Musculoskeletal rehabilitation

References

1. American Hospital Association: Hospital Statistics, 1984, Appendix I, A 10, City, American Hospital Association, 1984
2. American Medical Association: 84th Annual report on medical education in the United States, 1983–84. JAMA 252:1505, 1984
3. Arbeiter J: The big shift to home health nursing. RN 147(11):38, 1984
4. Arnould R: Do HMOs produce services more efficiently? Inquiry 21:3, 1984
5. Balinksky W: Home care: Current trends and future prospects, New York Bus Group Health Newslett 5, 1985
6. Breslow L: Research in a strategy for health improvement. Int J Health Serv 3:7, 1973
7. Califano JA: America's Health Care Revolution. New York, Random House, 1986
8. Coleman J, Smith D: DRGs and the growth of home health care. Nursing Econ 2:391, 1984
9. Crichton M: Five Patients: The Hospital Explained. New York, Alfred E. Knopf, 1970
10. Dychtwald K: Wellness and Health Promotion for the Elderly. Rockville, MD, Aspen Publications, 1986
11. Eisenberg L: The Search for Care. Daedalus Winter: 235, 1977
12. Freymann JG: The American Health Care System: Its Genesis and Trajectory, pp 96–97. Huntington, NY: Robert Krieger Publishing, 1977
13. Gibson RM, Fisher CR: National Health Expenditures, Fiscal Year 1977. Social Security Bull 41:3, 1978
14. Gibson RM, Levi HK, Lazenby H, et al: National Health Care Expenditures, 1983. Health Care Financing Rev 6 (Winter): Tables 1 and 2, 1984
15. Henderson LJ: The Study of Man. Philadelphia, University of Pennsylvania Press, 1941
16. Jonas S: Health manpower. In Jonas S (ed): Health Care Delivery in the United States. New York, Springer, 1986
17. Jonas S, Rosenberg S: Health Manpower and Ambulatory care. In Jonas S (ed): Health Care Delivery in the United States, p 53. New York, Springer, 1986
18. Kinzer D: Care of the poor revisited. Inquiry 21:5, 1984
19. Knowles JH: The responsibility of the individual. Daedalus Winter: 57, 1977
20. Marston MV: Compliance with medical regimens: A review of the literature. Nursing Res 19:312, 1970
21. Paradis LF: Hospice Handbook, Germantown, MD, Aspen Publications, 1985
22. Swartz K: Testimony before the Subcommittee on Health of the Committee on Finance, US Senate, April 27, 1984. Washington, DC, US Government Printing Office, 1984
23. US Bureau of the Census: Statistical Abstract of the United States: 1985, Table 156. Washington, DC, US Government Printing Office, 1986
24. US Bureau of Census: 1976 Survey of Institutionalized Persons: A Study of Persons Receiving Long Term Care. Current Population Reports, Series P-23, No. 69. Washington, DC, US Government Printing Office, 1978
25. US Department of Health and Human Services: Health United States, 1984, Tables 59, 61, and 66. US Dept. of Health and Human Services Pub. No. PHS 85-1232. Washington, DC, US Government Printing Office, 1984

SECTION 2

Influences of the Health Care System on Occupational Therapy Practice *Judith M. Perinchief*

The intent of health care in the United States is to provide equitable, efficient, and effective care to the population. This care should be available and accessible to all and of assured quality. As a provider within the health care system, the occupational therapist is confronted with numerous issues and dilemmas.

Issues

Environment and Society

Traditionally, the occupational therapist practiced in institutionally based service areas, and coverage for service was of little concern. The cost of service was frequently incorporated in the *per diem* charge for hospitalization and occasionally covered by selling projects made by patients. Philanthropic gifts and funds from volunteer organizations were often used to augment the budget.

In the 1960s, with the expansion of national health insurance programs on a private and federal government basis, financial support from the above sources greatly diminished, and occupational therapy managers were suddenly involved in extensive budgeting for their departments. Previously, providers had been shielded from price competition. Now, all allied health practitioners were competing for a controlled if not shrinking health care dollar. The practitioner was confronted with situations that limited occupational therapy services or made them inaccessible under a given insurance program. In the past, occupational therapists had not had to consider the importance of their services in relation to others; suddenly, reimbursement sources were determining the provision of care, and occupational therapy was not necessarily among the services recognized for coverage. For the most part, occupational therapy had not been represented in the political arena when the determination regarding coverage was made on a national level. The practitioner now had to justify service and validate practice previously taken for granted by the system at large. The consumer, who had acquired power in demanding care, had little knowledge or understanding of the services of the occupational therapist, as previously, the consumer had relied on the physician to determine which services were required. The physicians had become occupied with protecting their own practice and had little concern for the plight of other health care professionals. In sum, the power began to shift from the provider to the consumer.

Profession

In order for the occupational therapist to provide service, methods had to be instituted to educate consumers, legislators, reimbursement agencies, and other practitioners. The occupational therapy profession was confronted with significant public relations issues and was placed in the position of having to explain, defend, and validate services. The American Occupational Therapy Association (AOTA) began to take steps in the national office at the direction of the Representative Assembly. Public relations efforts increased, position papers were drafted and published, and the Government and Legal Affairs Division was instituted. To facilitate occupational therapists' negotiations with commercial insurance companies for coverage of service, a handbook on third-party reimbursement was prepared in 1976 by the Government and Legal Affairs Division.

Twenty years ago, public discussion of the quality of occupational therapy services barely existed, but within a decade, quality assurance became a major issue for the profession. The AOTA Division of Practice launched workshops and initiated publications to disperse information and knowledge to the practitioner within hospital-based programs requiring quality assurance and peer review. Increasingly, materials became available on utilization review, quality assurance, program evaluation, and performance appraisal of employees. By 1982, the government had instituted a massive effort to develop a nationwide quality assurance system. In the future, it is expected that the quality assurance system will encompass nonhospital institutional care, ambulatory care, and care reimbursed by private health insurers.

Education

Educational programs in occupational therapy have continued to prepare generalists for practice while the health care system shifted emphasis to the specialist in practice. The occupational therapist became a specialist through experience in practice, and this is still the method open to most practicing therapists. Contrary to former employment habits, the occupational therapist today does not move from one area of practice to another but rather refines skills and knowledge in a specific area of practice; for example, hand therapy, drug and alcohol programs, head injury, burn treatment, and early intervention programs. These choices, unintentional though they may be, tend to favor programs recognized as necessary and reimbursable by funding sources. The profession had made a commitment to high-quality educational programs at the entry level, but the needs of practitioners to be prepared for the marketplace were largely ignored.

In answer to this problem, continuing education training programs were developed by the Association to provide competence in special areas of practice such as TOTEMS, PIVOT, ROTE, and SCOPE (see Chapter 2). In addition, position papers describing the role and function of occupational therapy in specialty areas of practice were developed, and free packets of literature in specialty areas were made available to the members of AOTA.

Personnel

Occupational therapy has been identified by the Bureau of Health Professions as having significant manpower shortages.[3] This statistic is noted in spite of a 230% growth in occupational therapy between 1966 and 1978.[2] The growth of the profession can be traced to the overall expansion of the health care system and to an increased awareness of the value of rehabilitation services. A manpower study by the profession in 1985 also indicated a geographic maldistribution of occupational therapists which was related to location of other health care providers, of delivery systems, and of educational programs.[1]

In 1984, 18% of surveyed hospitals indicated that they would be adding or expanding occupational therapy departments over the next 2 years.[4] This is an interesting fact in light of the institution of the medicare prospective payment system that was then facing the health care industry. With the development of new and alternative health care programs, the demand for occupational therapy services should increase proportionally. Although there have been efforts to encourage migration of occupational therapists to less professionally populated areas, there is no way to force occupational therapists to choose a specific practice area or geographic location.

Practice

With the onset of the medicare prospective payment system and diagnostic-related groups, the decreased length of stay and limitations on treatment for cost/profit purposes, occupational therapists began to look for alternative ways to provide service. Occupational therapy service was limited when lengths of stay were shortened, and therapists were heard to comment that patients were "discharged too soon" or "sicker" at the next level of care under the new system. This was particularly evident in moves from acute care to rehabilitation or home care settings. Therapists practicing in nursing homes talked about an increase in the number of patients referred who required intensive intervention within that setting. The economics of the system rather than the need or condition of the patient dictated the amount and level of occupational therapy service. Now, the therapist must examine alternatives for the well-being of the patient. Occupational therapy was frequently not covered at the next level of care to which the patient would be transferred or the coverage was time limited for a patient who actually needed a greater length of service as a result of shortened service at the previous level of care.

As a result, occupational therapy services provided within the hospital have been streamlined to maintain quality yet provide vital services in a shorter time. The evaluation process has become more efficient to allow more time for intervention. The occupational therapist prioritizes goals and treatment in accordance with the estimated length of stay and anticipated intervention at succeeding levels of care. This increases the demand for effective communication between the occupational therapists practicing at various levels within the health care system, not only to avoid duplication of effort but also to allow for cost-effective service to meet the needs of the patient.

The occupational therapist today must be acutely aware of and extremely knowledgeable about health care reimbursement as the therapist plans and implements treatment programs for the individual patient. It is not sufficient to know that a given patient has private insurance coverage; the therapist must be aware of the limitations of that coverage and of the alternatives for coverage should the need arise. This frequently becomes part of patient education during the treatment process.

Over the last 10 years, occupational therapists have witnessed an increase in independent practice opportunities. There has been a redistribution of jobs toward outpatient facilities, home health agencies, and nontraditional settings. The allied health personnel as a group have been striving for professional status and thus have become very competitive in the health care marketplace. The occupational therapist as a member of this group has sought recognition as an independent practitioner. Home care has become a major area of practice for increasing numbers of occupational therapists. Despite the fact that reimbursement has been difficult until the passage of recent legislation (Reconciliation Act of 1986), the profession recognized the need for and potential growth of service in home care. This is also true of the therapist who practiced in a nursing home. Maintenance of health, prevention of further disabling conditions, and promotion of independence within the community are major issues for the population receiving service through home health agencies. In providing service at this level, the occupational therapist helps the patient avoid a more costly level of care; that is, the hospital or the skilled nursing facility.

Implications for the Future

The profession must change with changing times. Target components of the health care system include multihospital systems, health maintenance organizations (HMOs), home health providers, proprietary sections, and integrated health service systems. Clinical areas to be considered should include health promotion, wellness and disease prevention, hospice care, gerontology, drug abuse and addiction programs, terminal disease, stress management, and vocational issues. The occupational therapist possesses the tools of health promotion and disease prevention in the teaching as well as the treatment of the patient. This will require an expansion of traditional patient education roles.

In shifting from institutional care to other settings, occupational therapists must examine their traditional roles and methods in the context of the changes within the overall system. For example, the therapist interested in employment in an HMO-type setting must market occupational therapy services. This will require written proposals describing the service to be provided and how these services would benefit the health plan by decreasing institutional care and overall costs. This is knowledge that the individual might not have acquired through previous educational experience or on-the-job experience.

Occupational therapists have demonstrated strengths in home care, designing living space and adapting environments, adapting toys, working in prisons, designing programs for the homeless, and teaching life skills to young unwed mothers.[5] These represent some of the emerging nontraditional settings for practice. It is important that the profession be prepared to change rapidly, to adapt or modify delivery of service in accord with the health care system demands, and to educate personnel to practice in these emerging settings.

The total impact of the prospective payment system (P.L. 98-21, 1983) is still emerging. However, there is strong evidence of increased demands for productivity, cost effectiveness, and new sites of delivery of service. Current trends can be interpreted for future areas of programming based on societal emphasis on health promotion; survival of individuals with previously life-threatening disabilities or disease processes as the result of improved technology; increases in health maintenance programs in the workplace and among the older population; and the mainstreaming of mental health patients into the community. The occupational therapists has the expertise to offer programs for each of these areas; the profession must be prepared to meet the need, or others will fill the positions.

The profession has identified several goals as the result of the manpower study. These include the promotion of new educational programs in underserved states; development of nontraditional educational and recruitment programs to meet the demand for qualified professionals; expansion of continuing education programs to increase the skills of the practicing therapist; examination of the opportunities available in occupational therapy educational programs to expand exposure to nontraditional practice settings; ensuring that future therapists are equipped with knowledge and skill in management, systems behavior, health economics, and marketing; development of promotional materials for use in marketing services; and increasing research and promotional activities to meet the needs of persons unserved or underserved. As a result of the changes in the health care delivery system over the last few years, the profession has adopted a strategic intergrated management system (SIMS) approach in order to identify changes that will impact on the profession and to enable the profession to adapt to these changes.

As individuals within the profession, each occupational therapist must become self confident, assertive, and risk taking and a critical thinker[5] because he/she is a participant in the provision of health care in a time of increased competition for status, recognition, and reimbursement. Occupational therapy service must be developed as a scientific discipline to gain a stronger position with a strong professional identity. There must be increased dialogue between educators and clinicians toward common goals. An expansion of the acute-care model of practice to include ambulatory and prevention aspects of treatment will provide greater service to the population. Finally, the occupational therapist must assist individuals to gain control over their health through new programming, technological advances, and expanded education programs.

References

1. Ad Hoc Commission on Occupational Therapy Manpower: Occupational Therapy Manpower: A Plan for Progress. Rockville, MD, American Occupational Therapy Association, 1985
2. Bezold C: Health care in the US: Four alternative futures. The Futurist 16(4):14, 1982
3. Bureau of Health Manpower, Health Resources Administration: A Report on Allied Health Personnel. Dept. of Health, Education and Welfare Pub. No. HRA 80-28. Washington, DC, US Government Printing Office, 1979
4. Freeland MS, Schendler CE: Health spending in the 1980's: Integration of clinical practice patterns of management. Health Care Financing Rev 5(3):1, 1984
5. Labovitz D: Meeting the challenge: Occupational therapy survival, 2000 and beyond. Keynote address, New York State Occupational Therapy Association, October 1986

UNIT III

Research

CHAPTER 10

Research in Occupational Therapy *Elizabeth J. Yerxa*

A significant characteristic of professional persons is that they are able to work with a considerable degree of autonomy.[11] An example of such professional autonomy is the characteristic of being able to conceptualize, implement, evaluate, and report the results of a research study. Occupational therapy researchers possess a high degree of autonomy. Being a researcher is an exciting new role for occupational therapists because it affords opportunities to make creative and self-directed contributions to the quality of life for persons served by the profession through the generation of new knowledge.

In its quality of autonomy, the researcher role both represents and enhances occupational therapy's progress toward a more fully developed profession. In exploring the researcher role in occupational therapy, this chapter discusses the nature of research, the relationship of research to occupational therapy theory and practice, the importance of theory, the status of occupational therapy research, the characteristics of researchers who have published their work, the content of research, current and past research efforts, research needs and how they might be met, a model of an occupational therapy researcher—A. Jean Ayres, and ethical considerations in conducting research.

The Nature of Research

Alfred North Whitehead called research a "welcoming attitude toward change." Kerlinger has a much more formal definition: "Systematic, controlled, empirical and critical investigation of hypothetical propositions about the presumed relationships among natural phenomena."[5] "To see what everyone else has seen and to think what no one else has thought" is the research process according to Wandelt, a nursing researcher.[15] Whatever definition might be proposed, research is the process by which knowledge is developed, tested, and made public.

Relationship of Research to Theory and Practice

Occupational therapy is concerned with helping people. Its practitioners make decisions which result in a goal being attained for another person, a goal which is perceived as "good" by that person and the therapist together. The profession exists for clinical practice, and all occupational therapy knowledge flows from practice, generated from what each occupational therapist sees, hears, and feels while working with patients.

As occupational therapists observe, they begin to develop hypotheses which when validated become theories. Theories are statements that suggest relationships between the things seen so that they can be controlled, understood, or explained.[12] Making the right things happen in predictable ways is the gift received from theory. When theoretical statements have been formulated, they are tested to see if, in fact, they enable occupational therapists to predict and control phenomena. That phase of the process is *research,* and the goal is to determine to what degree data from the senses confirm or fail to confirm the theoretical statements. Knowledge is developed in this way—knowledge that flows back into practice so that a better job can be done. Practice to theory to research and back to practice is the unending cycle that generates knowledge.

The Importance of Theory

The abstract statements that constitute theories are the source of life for practice and research, for they enable generalizations to be made from direct experience in order to control future events. Imagine a world without theory. Practice would have to be based on trial and error or on tradition or intuition. Since there would be no abstract conceptualization, there would be no knowledge. If there were no knowledge, universities could be closed and persons taught all they need to know by apprenticeship. However, there would be no way to store knowledge or test it or improve upon it. There would be no sense of understanding as to how and why things happen, because such a sense can be conveyed only by theory.[12] If there were no sense of understanding, then there would be no way of expanding or improving practice, nor any way to assure occupational therapists that what they did for their patients was truly "good."

Theories consist of statements that relate concepts. A concept is a way of classifying the world according to some criterion: small, medium, and large are concepts, as are play, work, and rest or apraxia, tactile defensiveness, and form perception. Concepts are the bricks from which theory is constructed. Occupational therapy concepts are often either unclearly defined or not defined at all. Thus, it is extremely difficult to agree on their meanings. Occupational therapy knowledge has very few concepts that have operational definitions; that is, definitions that will allow the concept to be applied or tested in the real world. As one scientist put it, the clearest ideas are the ones that are the easiest to falsify.[12] Occupational therapy needs clear definitions with agreed upon meanings that can be tested in the real world in order to determine not only what is true but also what is false.

Typologies are classification systems based on sets of concepts. Ayres' sensory–integrative syndromes constitute a sensory–integrative dysfunction typology. The few other typologies that have been published are not generally useful for the purposes of science, because the concepts are often vague and unclear. Typologies allow theoretical statements that relate concepts to be generated. For example, "if a patient has apraxia, then he will have difficulty imitating postures" is a theoretical statement relating the concept of apraxia to the concept of imitating postures, a theoretical statement using the sensory–integration typology. A collection of such statements constitutes a theory.

In occupational therapy today, few theories exist that allow knowledge to be developed and tested. Thus, little basis is available for scientifically predicting, controlling, or even explaining what occurs in practice. Moreover, little confidence can be held in the theories that do exist, since few data support the statements constituting the theory. Occupational therapy practice, for the most part, is based on tradition and untested hypotheses.

It is proposed that occupational therapy's lack of research activity is directly related to its lack of theory and, paradoxically, that its lack of theory is directly related to the profession's lack of research. What does exist is clinical practice, standing alone, teeming with opportunities to observe, to theorize, and to conduct research in concrete settings.

Status of Research in Occupational Therapy

Research in occupational therapy is in its infancy. Many leaders in the profession emphasize that research should have the highest priority in order to develop the knowledge base of the profession,[16] but what, in fact, is being done?

In 1974, a paper presented at the World Federation of Occupational Therapy Conference in Vancouver was titled "Occupational Therapy Research in 1974: Models of Enlightenment." [16] In it, all papers published in the *American Journal of Occupational Therapy* for the year 1973 were surveyed, with the following findings: of a total of 57 articles, 25 (44%) were concerned with research. Of these 25, 17 involved descriptive research; that is, they were concerned with describing selected characteristics of a sample with no attempt to manipulate variables; one was philosophical, that is, it discussed the *need* for research; and the remaining seven were experimental, that is, they involved the systematic and controlled manipulation of variables in order to test hypotheses. Three of these experimental studies concerned the outcomes or results of occupational therapy, and only two (or 3% of the total papers) employed statistical tools. The author concluded, "Since the editorial board of the *Journal* is eager to publish research reports which will help substantiate the validity of the profession, we can only conclude that scientific research is rare in occupational therapy at present."[16]

In preparation for writing this chapter, a similar survey was conducted, this time assessing the research content of the *American Journal of Occupational Therapy* for the full calendar year of 1979. In 1979, the *Journal* was published monthly, so this sample was based on a review of 12 issues, whereas the 1973 survey covered only eight issues. Seventy-one papers were published in 1979 (excluding regular feature articles such as "Nationally Speaking"). Of these, 31 (44%) concerned research. Twenty-six, or 37%, of all the papers reported descriptive research, none was philosophical, one provided education about the research process, and four (6%) were experimental, with two of these, or 3% of all the papers, assessing the effects or outcomes of occupational therapy.

Comparing the quantity and categories of research papers between 1973 and 1979, one is struck by the fact that the percentages of research papers published and the percentages within each category, although 6 years apart, were almost identical. This finding becomes even more striking when one remembers that only eight issues were published in 1973. If a projection of 3.1 research papers per journal (based on the average number published per issue in 1973) is extended to a twelve-issue year, 1973 would have produced 37.5 research articles compared to only 31 for 1979. In interpreting this result, it is important to realize that six of the 1973 articles were part of the special series on research in sensory–integrative development, which might have inflated the research productivity for 1973. However, taking all of these factors into account, the comparison of these two periods makes it appear that the quantity and type of research reported in the *Journal* has remained approximately the same, with 44% of the papers being research papers and the majority of these reporting descriptive surveys.

Ottenbacher and Short also studied the types of research published in the *American Journal of Occupational Therapy*, but their data base included articles published from January 1970 through May 1980.[9] They concluded that a significant increase in "quasi-experimental" studies occurred after 1978, with a corresponding decrease in descriptive research ($p < 0.001$). Correlational, case, and field studies remained approximately the same in number. These authors also noted that since so few studies could be classified as true experiments, no such category could be formed. This finding was explained on the basis of the practical and ethical constraints on research performed with human subjects.

Another comparison, by Ottenbacher and Petersen, focused on quantitative analyses in research articles published in the *American Journal of Occupational Therapy* during the entire year of 1973 (Volume 27) *versus* 1983 (Volume 37).[8] A 21% increase in the use of advanced statistical tools was observed along with a 25% decrease in articles employing no statistical analysis ($p < 0.008$).

Researcher Characteristics

Author characteristics were assessed in order to determine the source of research productivity. In 1979, 77% of the papers were authored by persons with a Master's degree or above, whereas in 1973, only 52% of the authors held postgraduate degrees. Ottenbacher and Petersen's comparison of 1973 and 1983 revealed that 85% of the senior authors in 1983 held postgraduate degrees.[8] The professional roles of authors also demonstrated a dramatic shift. In 1973, only 35% of the authors of research papers were academic faculty members, whereas in 1979, 58% of the authors came from academia. Thus, a trend toward increasing research productivity among those with postgraduate degrees and faculty appointments might be occurring, perhaps in recognition of the "publish or perish" admonition in academia along with increasing awareness of the vital role of occupational therapy university faculty in generating knowledge.

Research Content

The content of the research papers reported in 1979 will now be looked at more closely. The largest number of papers dealt with characteristics of the disabled, followed by studies concerning occupational therapy education and those focusing on the characteristics of occupational therapy practice. The 12 remaining papers defied categorization, except that two concerned sensory–integrative theory. It appears that a majority of research in 1979 was concerned with describing and operationalizing concepts that characterized those aspects of disabled persons considered particularly significant to occupational therapy.

The instrumentation, or the measuring tools, employed will now be analyzed. How many 1979 papers employed new instruments designed to operationalize occupational therapy concepts? Seventeen, or 24%, of the papers reported developing a new instrument in order to gather data. Of these 17, only three, or 18% of the total using new instruments, mentioned procedures designed to estimate their reliability. No papers reported the development of an instrument for use primarily as a research tool, and only one reported the formulation of a new clinical instrument.

Thus, if 1979 is a valid example, it appears that the quantity and type of occupational therapy research have not changed much since 1973. However, more persons with postgraduate degrees and academic appointments are producing the research. A paucity of papers concerned with the development of research instruments exists, and most papers that discussed new instruments for data gathering failed to establish the reliability of those instruments.

My conclusion about research in occupational therapy is different now from what it was in 1973. Occupational therapy research today is highly varied in content, represents myriad fragmented theoretical perspectives, is primarily descriptive, and has an urgent need for valid and reliable instruments that operationalize theoretical concepts.

Research Needed

Much of the research done in occupational therapy thus far is descriptive of patient or occupational therapist characteristics or is concerned with the outcomes of occupational therapy education. Many political and economic pressures are being exerted from both within and outside the profession for occupational therapy to prove its efficacy. Occupational therapy is not alone in experiencing these pressures, since all of the health professions are expected to be accountable in delivering the service they say they are delivering.[13] The current state of research in occupational therapy represents a stage in the normal evolution of professional knowledge, which proceeds from the intuitive practice of an untested art to the logically rigorous practice of a science. As will be seen below, *descriptive* rather than experimental research appears to be appropriate for the development of occupational therapy knowledge at its current state. Where should the occupational therapy researcher begin?

Occupational therapists should take a good, hard look at what they are doing. Clinical observation is the beginning of all research. Some scientists suggest that all theory begins with *criticism* that goes on to identify the components of the criticized situation and to suggest solutions or better ways of doing things.[15] Occupational therapy research needs more published in-depth case studies that are carefully described. An individual patient, looked at precisely, can suggest significant variables to be isolated and generate innumerable questions to be tested in later studies involving groups. The careful observation of individuals can lead researchers to classify important characteristics, to give those characteristics names, and to define, in words and in operations, what those concepts mean. Later, the characteristics can be used in typologies to generate questions about whole groups of persons and can then be tested by gathering and analyzing data. *All research begins with giving things names.*

Description is the mother of theory. Unfortunately, occupational therapists sometimes are given the impression that only experimental research is true and valuable research (as was my belief in 1974). By experi-

mental is meant research that manipulates variables (causes) to produce a predetermined outcome (effect). Such research tests the effects of occupational therapy; for instance, study of the effects of a play intervention program on the developmental skills of children with mental retardation is experimental research.

In my opinion, occupational therapy concepts generally are so nonspecific that the profession needs to give far greater emphasis to descriptive research than to experimental research at this stage. Descriptive research sets forth what is in the here and now. It enables researchers to catalogue the important characteristics of reality as seen from the unique perspective of a therapist. Researchers cannot begin to manipulate variables until the important variables have been clearly defined and described. Some examples of descriptive research possibilities that could contribute knowledge development are the following:

> Who are occupational therapy's patients? What characteristics do these patients have that are particularly pertinent to occupational therapy's perspective of human beings as self-directed, active organisms seeking meaning through activity? What is the nature of occupational therapy practice? What sort of intervention is used, with what kinds of patients, under what conditions? For example, Bissell and Mailloux published the results of a study describing the frequency and extent of the use of crafts by occupational therapists working with patients who have physical disabilities.[2]
>
> How do patients respond to the occupational therapy process and setting? What do they perceive as their need for occupational therapy services? Under what conditions do occupational therapists provide service; that is, one-to-one, in groups, daily, monthly? Who provides it: OTRs, COTAs? When is it provided in relation to the onset of pathology? Where is it provided? What evaluation methods are used and what do they show about specific groups of patients? To what extent are patients satisfied with the occupational therapy service they receive? Over time, to what extent do patients maintain the status they had achieved when occupational therapy services were terminated?
>
> What can be learned about "normal" persons? How do happy, productive persons use their time in everyday activity? How much time do "normal" persons spend on self-maintenance, leisure, work? What about retired persons? What is a "balanced" life, and how is it related to other measures of health or healthfulness?

These descriptions would contribute knowledge, not only to occupational therapy, but also to a science of *occupation* and how it relates to health. Both are needed.

Descriptive research enables investigators to isolate variables of interest as abstract concepts such as community adjustment, independence in self-maintenance activities, and solitary play. Once these concepts have been identified, they need to be operationalized; that is, defined in measurable terms. When that has been done, instruments can be constructed to measure characteristics of groups of people so that researchers can begin to make comparisons.

There is a pressing need to develop reliable and valid occupational therapy instruments, for the majority of instruments that the profession has are designed for clinical use, not for research. It is not known whether they test what they say they test, nor is it known whether they measure phenomena consistently. Thus, they are of little use for knowledge development. Clinical instruments may be refined into research instruments, but instruments that operationalize the concepts constituting occupational therapy theories are also needed. As happened with sensory–integrative theory, when standardized tests become available, torrents of research will burst forth utilizing them to evaluate a theory.

Test development and standardization are complex and sophisticated processes, and it is my belief that the profession will not have the instruments it desperately needs until students in occupational therapy doctoral programs produce them. At any rate, until researchers define and measure concepts, the profession will not be able to develop and test occupational therapy knowledge or to make it public. Instruments are needed that will accurately measure work behavior, play, leisure pursuits, habits, skills, body scheme, attitudes, precision of motor control, social role behaviors, responses to crafts, goal setting, and successful community adjustment, to name a few.

Once concepts have been defined, conceptually and operationally, on the basis of observation and description, relationships between concepts can be explored. These relationships reflect associations rather than causation and are often expressed as correlations. Some examples of association are such relationships as self-care independence to self-esteem and employment, developmental delays to environmental bleakness, and play behavior to social skill development.

Only after occupational therapy concepts have been defined, operationalized, and related will researchers be prepared to conduct studies which manipulate variables to produce both a predictable and a "good" result; that is, experiments which assess the effects of occupational therapy. Until researchers define treatment as it is generated from a theory and develop valid and reliable ways of measuring outcomes with groups of people, the profession will not be ready to conduct the experimental or quasi-experimental research it needs.

Meeting Research Needs

How can individual therapists contribute to knowledge development for the practice of occupational therapy? First, remember that all theory and research are generated from practice and begin with *observation*. Look at your patients and environments, yes, even yourselves, with fresh and careful eyes, clearly describing and recording what you see.

Criticize what you see, but do not let yourself stop with criticism. Research and theory are generated when you are dissatisfied with what you are doing and care enough to think of ways to make things better. Theory is generated from events that frustrate people.

Explore the variety of research approaches that lend themselves to the kinds of complexity encountered in the theory and practice of occupational therapy. Single-system research,[7] employing repeated measures of treatment effects on a single patient, institution, or system, may provide a new research approach that is practical for use in clinical settings and which lends itself particularly to exploring single-treatment outcomes. In contrast, other research approaches, such as participant observation,[14] qualitative evaluation methods,[10] and the life-history method,[6] may have a goodness of fit with the complexity of the problems occupational therapists encounter and the richness of the patient/environmental interaction involved in occupation. There is no research approach or method that has been stamped "approved" by the scientific community in occupational therapy. Cox and West explicated some of the advantages and disadvantages of a variety of research methods but emphasized the importance of selecting an area of study which is of great interest to the researcher.[3] Often such burning interest is related to criticism of the status quo.

Occupational therapy needs to treasure its young people and those who are new to the profession by helping them saturate themselves with its current knowledge, incomplete though it is, and by welcoming their criticism. Considerable evidence exists that the people who invent the truly new ideas or create new theories are usually new to a field and deeply immersed in it without preconceptions or vested interest in what is the "true" or "right" theory. Having nothing to give up or lose, they invent new theories to explain the old reality that the rest of the profession has lived with for decades. It is comforting to know that these persons are usually bright, but not necessarily geniuses!

If occupational therapy is to develop and test a unique configuration of knowledge, much hard work needs to be done by dedicated and well-trained people. Think of the road, from observation in practice, to concepts, to definitions, to relational statements, to instruments, to experiments. Who is going to do all these things? Such an effort can best be accomplished by graduate students who work with knowledgeable faculty and clinicians. For this reason, the potential for knowledge development will be attained only when this profession makes the conscious decision to focus its graduate programs on the development of research competence by students and faculty. A consensus is needed for knowledge generation as is a willingness to focus all of occupational therapy's graduate educational resources along with the rich intellectual resources of its young people on one goal, *knowledge* that enables occupational therapists to do the best for patients, be they persons with chronic schizophrenia, spinal cord injury, or mental retardation.

Occupational therapy researchers need to work closely with the clinicians who have the criticisms and frustrations and who also have access to patients. This can be accomplished by developing consortia or by formalized relationships between academic and clinical programs. Such relationships can provide strong bonds between practice and theory, generating knowledge and improving the quality of practice simultaneously.

Model of an Occupational Therapy Researcher

Ayres provides a current model of an occupational therapy clinical researcher. In 1963, she published her first papers describing the discovery of a previously unidentified group of perceptual motor syndromes.[1] These syndromes had been identified through a period of painstaking clinical observation followed by conceptualization, descriptions, hypothesis formation, controlled testing of the hypothetical observations, careful analysis of the data gathered, and, finally, the drawing of tentative conclusions about the hypotheses. One occupational therapist plans a treatment program for an individual patient; Ayres extended the thought process to apply to whole groups of individuals in a scientifically rigorous way. She presented her data for the scrutiny of the disinterested scientific community so that her observations could be tested by others. Occupational therapy theory is developed and tested through this process. Isolated and meaningless facts must be interrelated and rendered meaningful in the fabric of a theory, just as isolated threads must be woven into the fabric of a garment to create a design. Each new experiment tests a theory and either supports its validity or fails to support it. Ayres developed and validated a battery of objective tests in order to evaluate her theory. At present, occupational therapy possesses few such standardized tests for theory testing. This lack of objective instrumentation for the measurement of change constitutes a significant barrier to research productivity.

Ayres serves as an example of an occupational therapist and researcher who was motivated by a desire to improve the lives of children handicapped by the inability to process and use sensorimotor information. Her long and sometimes arduous path toward developing theory began with simple clinical observation. Her interest in determining relationships between the clinical facts she discovered, so they could be organized into a coherent whole, was based on wanting to do a better job as an occupational therapist. The clinical researcher in occupational therapy obtains the reward of serving patients or clients in numbers far beyond those reached in a one-to-one clinical therapy program. The researcher also enjoys the excitement that comes from the discovery of new knowledge and the pride that emanates from contributing to the future development of the profession.

Ethical Considerations

The clinical researcher must maintain a high level of consciousness of the ethics involved in protecting the rights of human subjects. All human beings who take part in occupational therapy research have the right to give or withhold their informed consent for participation in the project. Subjects need to know what, if any, risks could accrue to them, as well as any benefits to be obtained for themselves or humanity from participating in the research. They must be informed that they can withdraw from a project at any time without fear of reprisal. They need to be assured that privacy and anonymity will be preserved by the researcher.[4] Signed instruments of informed consent must be retained by the researcher as evidence of the subject's willingness to participate in the research project.

Conclusion

For those who seek a career that requires a deep personal commitment and provides substantial rewards from the excitement of discovery and the generation of new knowledge, the role of occupational therapy researcher is offered as a road to unlimited growth with the opportunity to become a self-directed pioneer and a leader in determining the future direction of the profession.

References

1. Ayres AJ: The development of perceptual–motor abilities: A theoretical basis for treatment of dysfunction. The Eleanor Clark Slagle Lectures. Rockville, MD, American Occupational Therapy Association, 1973
2. Bissell J, Mailloux Z: The use of crafts in occupational therapy for the physically disabled. Am J Occup Ther 35:369, 1981
3. Cox R, West W: Fundamentals of Research for Health Professionals, pp 25–45. Rockville, MD, Ramsco, 1982
4. Fox D: The Research Process in Education. New York, Holt, Rinehart and Winston, 1969
5. Kerlinger F: Foundations of Behavioral Research. New York, Holt, Rinehart and Winston, 1967
6. Langness L, Frank G: Lives: An Anthropological Approach to Biography, pp 31–61. Novato, CA, Chandler and Sharp, 1981

7. Ottenbacher K: Evaluating Clinical Change: Strategies for Occupational and Physical Therapists, pp 44–45. Baltimore, Williams & Wilkins, 1986

8. Ottenbacher K, Petersen P: Quantitative trends in occupational therapy research: Implications for practice and education. Am J Occup Ther 39:240, 1985

9. Ottenbacher K, Short P: Publication trends in occupational therapy. Occup Ther J Res 2:80, 1982

10. Patton M: Qualitative Evaluation Methods, pp 21–38. Beverly Hills, Sage, 1980

11. Pavalko R: Sociology of Occupations and Professions, pp 33–36. Itasca, IL, FT Peacock Publications, 1971

12. Reynolds PD: A Primer in Theory Construction, pp 3–11, 116. Indianapolis, Bobbs–Merrill, 1971

13. Somers A: Health Care in Transition. Chicago, Hospital Research and Education Trust, 1971

14. Spradley J: Participant Observation, pp 13–25. New York, Holt, Rinehart and Winston, 1980

15. Wandelt M: Guide for the Beginning Researcher. pp 8–9. New York, Appleton–Century–Crofts, 1970

16. Yerxa E: Occupational therapy research in 1974: Models of enlightenment. Proc World Fed Occup Therap, pp 674–680, 1974

17. Yerxa E, Gilfoyle E: AOTF research seminar. Am J Occup Ther 30:509, 1976

Management

CHAPTER 11

General Perspectives on Management and Planning

Carolyn M. Baum and Elizabeth Devereaux

The last decade brought many challenges to the health professional. Several years ago, it was not necessary to introduce the entry-level professional, or for that matter, the practicing clinician, to finance and marketing concepts and practices. Now, basic management is critical to occupational therapy practice.

The complexity of the environments in which occupational therapists work mandates that every therapist possess management skills and, more importantly, view themselves as managers. The tasks may be managing a patient's program, managing a class of students, managing a research protocol, or managing a program, a department, or even a facility or an educational program. Although the tasks differ, the functions all require that management concepts and principles be employed.

Systems Approach to Management

In order to be effective in implementing services in today's health care environment, the occupational therapist must be acquainted with systems theory. This section is intended to provide a clinically oriented introduction to systems theory. It is hoped that this general introduction will encourage further study of the subject.

The main objective of a general systems approach is to develop a framework for communications. Communication is the process which allows a system to function in an organized fashion to meet its objective.

"General systems theory" is the name that has come into use to describe a level of theoretical model building that falls somewhere between the highly generalized construction of pure mathematics and the specific theories of the specialized discipline. "Each discipline corresponds to a certain section of the empirical world and each develops theories which have particular application to its own empirical segment." [3] "Since the early 1950s, it is felt that there needs to be a process to discuss the general relationship of empirical models; this process is general systems theory." [6] General systems theory has no specific methodology. Rather, it outlines a way of thinking about relationships of parts and wholes. [7]

There are two ways of dealing with complex problems. One is to introduce arbitrary techniques to analyze the system: the mathematical approach. The other is to accept the complexities of the system and to search for the structural patterns that will enable one to examine the problem as a whole: a systems approach. A systems approach allows integration of diverse programs and values into a unity of action. Each of the components of the system must work in its own way, within its own logic, and according to its own theories in order to be effective, yet all components must work together toward a common goal. Each must accept, understand, and carry out its own function as a part of a whole.

The problem in a systems approach is that it lacks clarity. Communication is a continuing problem, and a lack of communication causes breakdowns. There is constant need for arbitration of conflicts between members of the organization. A successful systems approach demands the following:

1. Absolute clarity of objectives
2. Objectives for each program derived from the objectives as a whole
3. Each person in the system fully understanding the missions, objectives, and strategies of the organization
4. Each person in the system making an effort to know what goes on throughout the entire system
5. A strong manager taking responsibility for relationships and communication
6. A manager functioning to integrate the activities and tasks of the personnel to accomplish the goals of the organization.[1]

Systems Theory Terminology

Some key terms in the vocabulary of general systems theory include[1]:

System: an organized whole consisting of interrelated, interdependent parts
Open system: the individual and the environment mutually influence one another, and there is an exchange of information, matter, and energy[2]
Closed system: a system isolated from its environment, in that information, matter, and energy are not exchanged.[2]

The open system develops relationships between programs or departments and is directed to a common goal. A closed system emphasizes on its own objectives, not the objectives of the organization. In today's environment of external competition, it is critically important for organizational units within a facility to employ an open systems approach for the benefit of patients. A closed systems approach that isolates one component of the organization from another often creates gaps between services, and makes it impossible for a patient to feel that the program or the facility is organized to serve his or her needs. As we note the importance of consumer satisfaction in a changing health care environment, it is obvious that an open systems approach is needed to satisfy the consumer and keep the consumer at the center of the activities.

Other important terms are[1]:

Input: information taken into a system through transformation or recognition of energy, matter, or information (*e.g.,* admission to a facility or referral for rehabilitation services)
Output: information flowing from the system (*e.g.,* a patient trained and educated to accomplish activities to support independence or a family member educated to act as a caregiver for an individual)
Feedback loop: the output returned to the input to modify the system. This process can be positive or negative (*e.g.,* the quality assurance activities of a department or the results of an audit after a patient has been discharged)
Equifinality: a state of stability in spite of a continuous flow and exchange of information (Equifinality is something we all strive for as we operate in complex systems, continuing to move toward objectives and goals despite changes that could distract us from those activities.)

General System Principles

Principle: The entire system is changed when any part of the system or any related system is changed. This basic systems principle is often discussed in the context of a void being created in a system and something moving in to fill that void. It is particularly important for the occupational therapist to understand this principle, because we can see in our history some very important changes in the way health care has been managed when there has been a shortage of occupational therapy manpower. For example, following World War II, when there were not enough occupational therapists to provide services to a growing population of disabled, other disciplines evolved to manage the activity-based programs (*i.e.,* recreational therapy, music therapy, art therapy). Additionally, we saw major changes in vocational programming at this time, because occupational therapists did not have the manpower to cover the entire aspect of programming to serve the disabled population.

Principle: By looking at one part of the system in isolation, one gets a distorted view of the system and of any related system. It is critical that the system be viewed as a whole and that the relationship of the parts be viewed as a process. One must not look specifically at one segment and profess to understand the whole. "General systems theory . . . enables the therapist to identify the possibilities among a vast number of variables."[7]

Systems Skills

A general systems approach is valuable to the occupational therapist in viewing patients, programs, and organizations. It gives a framework for understanding the following:

1. Where occupational therapy fits into more complex structures

2. That change is an element of the whole and that it has a ripple effect
3. The complexity of interactions
4. The values inherent in the system
5. The formal and informal structures of the system
6. The culture of the system
7. The behaviors that create an imbalance in the system.

It is impossible to list all the skills and knowledge needed to cope with complex systems. However, some of the most important will be identified. The following list has been adapted from Hall.[9]

1. *Recognize the values of the institution in which one works and the values of the other departments that are contributing to the management of one's patients.*

All institutions have values, and those values usually encompass patient service, patient education, community development, and research. It important for the occupational therapist to know the priorities an institution places on these values. It also is important that the personal values of the occupational therapist match the values of the organization to support the growth of both the institution and the individual.

2. *Know the plans of the organization.*

Each organization, in order to survive in a changing marketplace, must plan for at least 10 years and have a strategic management plan directed toward the next 3-year period. It is critical that the occupational therapist manager communicate those plans to the staff so they will know how occupational therapy activities can contribute to the growth of the organization. Additionally, it is important for the manager to direct the department activities to enhance the overall activities of the institution.

3. *Define a personal role for oneself that will contribute to that organization.*

Occupational therapists who contribute to the overall activities of an organization will define a personal role for themselves in the system and thus be recognized as a valuable member of the organization.

4. *Contribute to the development of goals for the institution as well as motivate other staff members to establish and achieve goals for the organization.*

The occupational therapist who makes a contribution to the development of the organization has made a contribution that will be noticed and therefore will achieve influence and power.

5. *Analyze those tasks needed to achieve the objectives of the organization.*

The occupational therapist who has a background in task analysis can responsibly identify directions for departments and programs, identifying the specific activities that must be accomplished and proceeding with the accomplishment of those tasks to achieve organization objectives.

6. *Distinguish between the myths and the reality of the system and the behaviors represented in it.*

Often, organizations take on a certain communication system. Some communication is positive, and some has a more negative effect. It is important to avoid unquestioning acceptance of the perceptions of others, as they may be different from yours. Many problems exist in a system because people's actions are based on another person's interpretation of problems or situations rather than on the individual's own determination.

7. *Understand the structure of the institution and recognize who has authority and power.*

It is very important for occupational therapists to understand the structure of the institution in which they are working and to position themselves within the system to be known by the people within it.

8. *Understand what knowledge is necessary to implement a comprehensive occupational therapy program for the system.*

The health care system is changing rapidly, and the body of knowledge that occupational therapists must utilize to influence performance is changing just as quickly. Within the last 5 years, the basic science information relating to human capacity to attain performance and to overcome disability has changed greatly. Additionally, technology had a major impact on how an individual can function. It is the occupational therapist's responsibility to maintain current knowledge of occupational therapy practice and to further develop occupational therapy programs to meet the needs of the consumer and the full needs for services in the institution.

By developing behaviors that ensure that you are using system skills in your approach in your professional situation, it is possible to exert control over your environment and to make changes that are beneficial to patients, to your program and to your organization.

Establishing Power and Influence in a System

The system skills defined in this chapter assist the occupational therapy manager and the individual clinician in gaining power. Sometimes, the person with authority is not the one with power. It is important to realize that both formal and informal power structures exist. According to Kantor, "power issues occupy center stage, not because individuals are greedy for more power, but because some people are incapacitated without it."[11] Whenever an individual is to be held accountable, he or she must have the authority, power, influence, and control to enable the desired event to happen. Generally, the total amount of those elements needed to get the job done is not ascribed to the responsible individual or position but rather is a combination of elements ascribed to the position and those assumed by the individual.

Authority is defined as the right to give commands or to take action, whereas *power* is influence built through carefully planned means.[13] In order to accomplish objectives, it must be determined who has the authority to make the necessary decisions and who has the power to influence those decisions. Most people work in a hierarchical organization, where the power flows from the top down and each person except the highest and the lowest in a superior position is also in a subordinate position.[10] "The hallmark of power is the ability to get things done and to influence the internal and external environments."[8] Power is often as much a function of individual personalities as it is of titles, and people seldom share it willingly.[5]

Power groups may shift, depending on who has the skills to meet the current demands of the system. For example, the group with marketing skills may acquire greater power as hospitals search for expanded markets to fill empty beds. Occupational therapy has the potential to be viewed as a power group as the health care field places more emphasis on the functional capabilities of individuals and expects them to be more responsible for their own status.

In today's health care systems, the influence an occupational therapist has is enhanced by the relationships he or she has developed. There appears to be a fascination with the person who symbolizes or exercises power, an overestimation of the powerful person's qualities, that carries immense influence with those around; Freud called this phenomenon "transference."[2] The identification with a manager with power makes co-workers feel that they share that power, as opposed to the feeling of powerlessness and helplessness that can accompany feeling alone.[4] This interdependence of relationships can enhance the power of the manager while sustaining the feeling of community with co-workers.

It is important for the occupational therapist to have both authority and power. Authority normally is delegated to the position, whereas power is developed through the ways the individual uses that authority. In her article "The Extra Edge," Cherie Burns describes personal power skills that high achievers have used to increase their influence beyond the clout that came with the job: likeability, connections, reciprocity, expert power, and rewards combined with excellent job performance.[4] Through developing collaborative relationships both internal and external to the system, a wide area of influence and, therefore, power is created. If occupational therapists are to accomplish their objectives, they need to gain influence with those persons who control services. Examples of those in controlling positions are insurance companies and other third-party payers, regulatory agencies, referral services, and the administration of the facility. The occupational therapist with power has more opportunity to be creative and to explore, while the therapist without power really has no choice but to maintain control over activities within his or her jurisdiction.

"[We] must learn to deal with the subtleties of life and organizations—it comes from practice, learning what your resources are, how you can win support for an issue by changing labels under which you bring it up, or calling in favors that are owed to you—these are skills. How you develop your backing is critical. It is not through independent goal development and education, but through focusing on the organization and sharing with others . . . successes and failures."[12]

Management Skills Needed by the Entry-Level Clinician

Occupational therapists entering practice today must have basic knowledge and skills to function responsibly within their job situation and to contribute to the development of the profession of occupational therapy. Some specific knowledge and skills must be developed to ensure successful performance, not only as a member of a profession that is undergoing great change, but also as a professional working in a health care system that is undergoing the most dramatic change in its history. To help the clinician recognize the importance of this knowledge and these skills, an inventory was developed with the hope that the educator or the clinician who recognizes a void in any of these skills will look to other resources for knowledge in these areas to lay the groundwork for further professional development and growth (see box).

Resources for Managers

The American Occupational Therapy Association can provide the clinician with copies of current standards, model job descriptions, example of procedures, current laws that affect the manager–clinician's performance, and potential contacts to assist in problem solving. The clinician can contact the federal government either through regional offices or through the Association member hotline 1-800-THE-AOTA for help in obtaining resources to solve problems.

The clinician's greatest ally is the administrator, who can provide assistance and support for developing effective management skills. The manager of occupational therapy is an important link in the administrative management system, because it is through the managers of an organization that the objectives of the facility are accomplished.

Resources that can be very helpful in meeting the challenge of the changing health care system are listed in the Bibliography, and in Appendix J.

Behaviors and Management Skills Needed by the Entry-Level Clinician

This is designed as a self-assessment tool. Use the following as a guide to determine if further study would be helpful.

Code:

1—I have a working knowledge and have kept current on changes.

2—I need assistance in accessing resources and information.

3—I have no need for knowledge of these issues and I do not need assistance.

1	2	3	
___	___	___	Responsibly function within the standards and ethics of the profession
___	___	___	Understand and use established models of OT service to meet the expectations of the facility and program and the needs of the patients
___	___	___	Implement programs using current knowledge and modify programs to remain current and within the defined market of the facility or institution
___	___	___	Am aware of the official positions of the profession on disability and health-related issues
___	___	___	Access the resources of the American Occupational Therapy Association and the local and state association
___	___	___	Understand the environmental forces affecting health care
___	___	___	Recognize general health issues and their impact on current and future occupational therapy programming, as well as on the patients or students served by the program
___	___	___	Understand the implications of regulations and major legislation on occupational therapy services

1	2	3	
___	___	___	Inform legislators of issues that require legislative action to promote health and protect consumers, as well as the public in general
___	___	___	Establish relationships with referral sources, colleagues, and management
___	___	___	Build confidence and skill to ensure a growing role for myself in the system and prepare for new responsibilities
___	___	___	Understand the reimbursement mechanisms and procedures that support payment for services
___	___	___	Know how to record clinical data to meet standards of the program or institution
___	___	___	Follow procedures for documentation, and contribute to quality assurance activities
___	___	___	Provide direction for specific tasks to volunteers and aides and provide supervision and program planning assistance to certified occupational therapy assistant
___	___	___	Use technology to achieve productivity in reports and communication
___	___	___	Contribute to goal setting and program planning
___	___	___	Follow institutional budget plans and procedures
___	___	___	Know how costs for services are determined
___	___	___	Negotiate with peers and colleagues to achieve the goals of the occupational therapy program and the patient
___	___	___	Market occupational therapy services within the institution or system

References

1. Baker F: Symposium on Systems and Medicare Care, pp 10, 14, 22. Boston, Harvard University Press, 1968
2. Becker E: The Denial of Death, pp 127–129, 133. New York, Free Press, 1973
3. Boulding KE: General systems theory: The skeleton of science. Management Sci 2(3):197, 1956
4. Burns C: The extra edge. Savvy 3(12):38, 1982
5. Doudna C, Rupp C: Up the masthead: The push for power in the press. Savvy 1(9):25, 1980
6. Gaudinski MA: Intangibles facilitating or inhibiting

health care delivery systems. Aviat Space Environ Med 49:1111, 1978

7. Grinker RR Sr: In memory of Ludwig von Bertalanffy's contribution to psychiatry. Behav Sci 21:211, 1976

8. Haiman S: Directing. In: Bair J, Gray M (eds): The Occupational Therapy Manager, p 187. Rockville, MD, American Occupational Association, 1985

9. Hall BP: The Development of Consciousness: A Confluent Theory of Values, p 145. New York, Paulist Press, 1976

10. Harragan BL: Games Mother Never Taught You: Corporate Gamesmanship for Women, pp 47–48. New York, Warner Books, 1977

11. Kantor RM: Men and Women of the Corporation, p 205. New York, Basic Books, 1977

12. Kantor RM: You don't have to play by their rules. Ms. Magazine p 63 October 1979

13. Thompson AM, Wood MD: Management Strategies for Women, or Now That I'm Boss How Do I Run This Place? pp 44–45. New York, Simon and Schuster, 1980

Bibliography

Articles and Books

Baum CM, Luebben AJ: Prospective Payment Systems: A Handbook for Health Care Clinicians. Thorafare, NJ, Charles B Slack, 1986

Cassak D: Restructuring the health care system: A report on the Robert S. First Conference on Home Health Care and Alternate Site Delivery Systems. Health Industry Today pp 24–37, March 1984

Coddington DC, Palmquist LE, Trollinger WV: Strategies for survival in the hospital industry. Harvard Bus Rev 63:129, 1985

Coile RC Jr: Strategies for Survival in the Hospital Industry. Rockville, MD, Aspen Publishers, 1986

Drucker PF: Managing in Turbulent Times. New York, Harper and Row, 1982

Environmental Assessment (annual). Chicago, Hospital Research and Educational Trust

Environmental Impact Statement (annual). Rockville, MD, American Occupational Therapy Association

Evashwick CJ, Read WA: Hospitals and LTC: Options, alternatives, implications. Health Care Finan Manage pp 60–70, June 1984

Greenberg W, Southby RMF: Health Care Institutes in Flux. Arlington, Information Resources Press, 1984

Johnson EA, Johnson RL: Hospitals Under Fire. Rockville, MD, Aspen Publishers, 1986

Lesko M: Information U.S.A. Crawfordsville, IN, RR Donnelley and Sons, 1983

Mackey FG: Comprehensive rehabilitation care will take prominent place in delivery system. Hospitals pp 59–75, October 1981

Somers AR: Long-term care for the elderly and disabled. N Engl J Med 307:221, 1982

The Occupational Therapy Manager. Rockville, MD, American Occupational Therapy Association, 1985

Uniform Terminology for Reporting Occupational Therapy Services. The Representative Assembly, American Occupational Therapy Association, March 1979

Winston S: The Organized Executive. New York, WW Norton, 1983

Winston S: Getting Organized. New York, Warner Books, 1978

Periodicals

Government and Legal Affairs Division: Federal Report. Rockville, MD, American Occupational Therapy Association

Harvard Business Review, Boston, Massachusetts 20850

Business and Health, Washington, DC 20003

CHAPTER 12

Documentation *Douglas M. Cole*

One of the most important functions performed by occupational therapists is to describe clearly, concisely, and accurately, the data and rationale that support their specific treatment methods in the clinic. Therapy by itself does not describe its frame of reference, theory base, purpose, or benefit to the patient. These things must be explained.

Through various structured note-writing techniques, therapists can provide effective documentation of treatment methods and of the patient's response in a clear, logical format. Note writing allows the therapist to convey information about occupational therapy to other professionals, to report its effect on the patient's status, and to project information regarding the patient's rehabilitation prognosis and future functional role in the community. It is senseless to provide effective, functionally oriented, successful, and cost-effective treatment only to document the results in nebulous, uninformative, and rote fashion. Documentation, therefore, is the key to effectively describing occupational therapy services to the medical and rehabilitation communities.

Rationale

Next to treatment itself, documentation of treatment accounts for a major percentage of time in an occupa-

tional therapist's daily activities. Although the purpose of note writing is inherently clear, such writing is often looked upon as a chore or a burden and in some cases is neglected. The purpose of this chapter is to convey the importance of note writing as a sophisticated tool for establishing clear communication, providing effective case management, implementing research, and even marketing. With recent cutbacks and regulation changes in the health care system, it becomes more and more evident that occupational therapy services must show that they are effective and necessary. Good note writing can prove that occupational therapy services promote a more functional return of the patient to independent daily living, community involvement, and work. Documentation cannot be looked upon as a chore and must be undertaken with a fresh outlook and diligence.

Documentation for Communication

The basic purposes of note writing are to record patient status, to implement a plan for treatment, to provide patient goals, and to record progress in therapy. The therapy note stands as documentation of occupational therapy services rendered to the patient and communicates directly with the various health care professionals and third-party payers involved. The therapist's note may be the only means by which a physician, nurse, insurance carrier, or social worker can evaluate the therapy provided, since in most cases, these professionals are not present during the occupational therapy sessions. Poorly organized notes, long narrative sections, or even poor handwriting can interfere with understanding of the services provided. The note must be organized, concise, and legible. In other words, the note must be readable.

Readability also requires that the therapist take care in the use of abbreviations and jargon familiar to occupational therapists but possibly not clear to other professionals. For example, ROM is an abbreviation not only for "range of motion," but also for "rupture of membrane." Of course, the context in which the abbreviation is used is extremely important. However, therapists need to remember that abbreviations that may save time for the note writer may not communicate treatment strategies or other information effectively.

The first rule in developing effective team relationships with other medical professionals is to open clean lines of communication. An easy-to-read note is an effective beginning. This is true with both inpatient populations, where several physicians and nurses may read therapy notes daily to obtain information about the patient, and with outpatient populations, where the referring physician, rehabilitation nurse, and insurance carrier communicate solely through the mail with the occupational therapist. In both situations, the note stands alone, to be evaluated by other professionals in the absence of the occupational therapist.

Documentation for Case Management

When team approaches to patient treatment are used within a facility, it is necessary and beneficial that the team members effectively communicate their respective treatments and case plans. This decreases overlap or duplication of services, ensures that all aspects of the patient's condition are considered, improves the efficiency of the services provided, and educates the various team members about each service. Often, case management occurs in team meetings or patient rounds, in which individual services report their treatment plans and the patient's progress. Presentation of information in a clear and logical way facilitates communication at these meetings. It is most helpful if the therapist can refer to an updated, concise, and organized note during this presentation. In the absence of team meetings, each team member should be able to read the progress notes of the other services and obtain the information necessary to coordinate rehabilitation plans.

Lastly, some facilities use a case management coordinator or senior therapist who reviews multidisciplinary cases and must then prepare an individualized reha-

bilitation plan (IRP). This coordinator must read and synthesize various notes into an overall case plan. In this situation, structured note writing can improve the efficiency of the coordinator, especially in facilities where several team members (*e.g.*, occupational therapist, physical therapist, speech therapist) write notes using the same basic format. Consistency between services in documentation styles adds to the readability of notes and to the organization of the IRP.

Documentation for Research

A further argument for consistency of note writing within a particular service or between services in a facility is the potential for collecting and analyzing research data from patient files. For example, an audit of all the total-hip-replacement patients seen in the past year within a facility could be helpful to the occupational therapy director for analyzing such things as average length of hospital stay, similarity of problem lists, type and cost of equipment provided, follow-up services, and discharge status. This audit would be exceedingly difficult if the various therapists documented their discharge status in different styles, time frames, and terminology. Furthermore, the data would not be meaningful if each therapist happened to omit or neglect to consider various findings in a note. For example, the researcher would not be able to assume that because "shoe and sock donning" was not reported in the note that the patient could dress himself independently; "shoe and sock donning" may not have been evaluated at all. On the other hand, if the treating therapists had followed a consistent format for their documentation, the researcher could refer to similar sections of each note and collect information in consistent terminology from each therapist. Research protocols can be established which require identical documentation of patient's functional status in a given diagnostic group using specific terminology or functional measurement scales. An example would be the consistent reporting of dressing status using only the terms "unable," "poor," "fair," and "good." Each term would have an established operational definition related to dressing skills, and different treatment techniques could then be compared for their effectiveness in improving dressing.

The key point here is that a consistent documentation format can easily lend itself to meaningful and practical clinical research if therapists are informed about and comply with a given note-writing style.

Documentation for Marketing

Generally, in both outpatient and inpatient treatment settings, the need for communicating with third-party payers, physicians, and rehabilitation agencies allows a therapist to educate these professionals about occupational therapy services. This education can easily be considered a form of marketing. As medical professionals and third-party payers become better informed about effective occupational therapy services, the likelihood that they will continue to refer patients to those programs increases. Note-writing formats, therefore, should be developed with consideration for the information requirements and documentation needs of the various professionals receiving the notes. This is especially true for outpatient vendors or purchasers of occupational therapy services such as workman's compensation carriers, vocational rehabilitation counselors, private insurance carriers, rehabilitation nurses (case managers), and community physicians. These purchasers are keenly interested in the presence, timeliness, and content of the notes provided to them. Notes which are not received or are received late or which provide little information are meaningless. Ultimately, the occupational therapy service itself can be judged or perceived to be noneffective when in fact effective treatment is provided. Poor documentation affects the vendor's view of the occupational therapy service provided and possibly of the entire facility.

Phone communication with these referring agencies is equally important. The time spent on the phone establishing contact and rapport with individual medical and rehabilitation professionals can be a beneficial investment, especially when the occupational therapist can obtain constructive criticism about notes he or she sends into the community. The result of this communication should enhance the therapist's reporting style and the effectiveness of documentation.

Legal Aspects of Note Writing

Occupational therapy documentation and the medical record often play an important role in patients' litigation, Social Security appeals, disability ratings, or malpractice suits. Therefore, it is extremely important that each record contain information that accurately and completely describes the therapy intervention, treatment techniques, and patient responses. The medical record, and often the individual treatment notes, can be subpoenaed or submitted during depositions. There, the note must stand alone as evidence of events and patient outcomes during treatment. Obviously, effective documentation is important, especially when court decisions can significantly affect people's lives. Sometimes, such decisions are made on the basis of what is present or absent or even misunderstood due to incomplete writing in a note.

Another point that underscores the importance of clear note writing is that often a therapist will be called on to present, clarify, or defend a note written several years earlier. The therapist may be asked to recall information about the patient relying solely on the treatment note.

It is crucial that therapists review and understand the rationale and rules of their facility pertaining to note writing. Each facility is required to address the documentation guidelines provided by agencies which accredit them and to comply with legal requirements from the risk management or business office of their administration. Very often, facilities adopt specific criteria for monitoring note writing and establish standards for their therapists to follow.

Examples of how individual accrediting agencies can provide guidelines are the Joint Commission on Accreditation of Hospitals (JCAH)[3] and Commission on the Accreditation of Rehabilitation Facilities (CARF)[1] guidelines requiring a statement in the initial note about the patient's understanding or acceptance of the treatment plan. CARF guidelines require a statement about the patient's medical history in the initial note and a statement of whether each goal was achieved in the discharge note. Also required are the plans to be utilized for continued treatment or follow-up after discharge in the discharge note. Another accrediting agency, the Comprehensive Outpatient Rehabilitation Facility (CORF),[2] provides Medicare guidelines for the information necessary in the initial note. In addition to specifying standard note-writing policies, CORF requires that the patient's referring physician, the diagnosis, the treatment requested by the physician, the date of onset of the disease or injury, and date of referral by the physician be included in each initial note. CORF guidelines also require that short-term and long-term goals be stated in behavioral terminology, that a specific treatment plan be included in the note, and that a patient's rehabilitation potential or prognosis be included in the assessment. Failure to include this information could result in denial of payment for therapy services and possibly reconsideration of CORF accreditation for the facility. Also, on the basis of CORF audits of a facility's medical records that show consistently poor documentation, money can be *reclaimed* from previous payments. In these cases, proper documentation on the part of the therapist can affect financial reimbursement or the status of the facility within the community.

These guidelines should not be looked on as a burden but as a mechanism to ensure effective documentation and protect the rights of the patient, the therapist, and the facility. Almost always, these guidelines can be addressed with simple structured or "canned" statements. For example,

In the "Objective" section of the note, include: "Patient with (diagnosis) since (date of onset) was referred on (date) by (physician) for (specific treatment)." (*Example:* "Patient with right carpal tunnel syndrome since 5/2/86 was referred on 5/31/86 by Dr. Black for splinting and daily living skills assessment.")
In the "Plan" section of the note, include: "Patient (family) was informed of above plan and concurred." *or* "Patient was unable to concur with the plan due to

senile dementia. Patient's family was informed of and concurred with the plan.''

Each of these statements addresses guidelines intended to facilitate communication with and to convey appropriate information to professionals working with the patient. The guidelines also ensure that the therapist has adequate information regarding the case prior to treatment, conveys his or her treatment plan to the patient or family, and documents the course of therapy.

Various requirements also exist for the frequency with which notes must be written to ensure effective updating of the patient's progress. Again, therapists should refer to the guidelines established by each facility and its accrediting agencies. However, one rule-of-thumb for writing progress notes is once a week and any time significant increases or decreases in a patient's status are identified. A week is usually sufficient time to provide treatment and to document progress on every problem being addressed in the therapy plan. Of course, if a client were to show significant gains in range of motion or daily living skills, or suddenly became listless and less responsive, immediate documentation should be placed in the medical record.

The required frequency of note writing can vary among accrediting agencies and third-party payers. Various Medicare guidelines require a daily record of attendance and response to treatment to be included in the medical record. Likewise, many workman's compensation guidelines require daily documentation and may deny payment in the absence of specific progress notes or poor documentation.

Lastly, the style and frequency of documentation which addresses the legal requirements of a facility must be taken in the context of the environment in which treatment is provided. For example, treatment rendered to patients seen as outpatients once every 2 weeks in hospital clinics will differ significantly from that given acute care patients receiving treatment two or three times a day, and requirements in such settings will differ significantly from those in psychiatric or long-term care facilities. Each facility, and possibly even individual occupational therapy services within a facility, must design its documentation style and frequency of reporting to provide the most accurate medical record possible.

The Problem-Oriented Medical Record

The problem-oriented medical record (POMR),[4] developed by Lawrence Weed, M.D., provides an excellent basic structure for note writing. Better known as the SOAP system, the POMR format structures the note into four sections.

The first section is *subjective,* where the therapist records the patient's and family's report of limitations, concerns, and problems. Subjective information is data that are reported and cannot be verified or measured during the evaluation.

The second section is *objective,* where the therapist records all measurable, quantifiable, and observable data obtained during the evaluation. This section also can contain reports of medical history from other medical professionals. The therapist must be sure not to confuse subjective and objective information or to omit either. Together, the subjective and objective portions of the note make up the data base from which treatment plans are derived.

The third section of the note is the *assessment,* where the therapist reports his or her professional opinions and judgments as to the patient's functional limitations and expected benefit from rehabilitation and the problem list. The problem list is the key to the POMR system. Problems are numbered and referred to by number later in the progress notes. (*e.g.,* Problem 1 — Decreased orientation; Problem 2 — Decreased upper extremity range of motion.) Reporting these problems by number in the progress note indexes the entire medical record from the initial note to the discharge note. This enhances readability, as a medical professional can then track the course of a particular problem by referring to the specific problem number in each note.

The last section of the POMR format is the *Plan,* where the therapist sets forth the specific treatment plan, the short- and long-term goals, and the frequency and duration of treatment. This section of the note will be critically evaluated by rehabilitation professionals and third-party payers in regard to the pertinence and necessity of the stated treatment.

The POMR system can provide the foundation for developing a structured documentation format in any facility. Further guidelines and terminology can then be used to enhance, individualize, and address the specific needs of the programs within a facility.

How to Establish an Individualized Note-Writing Format

A note-writing format for a given facility is simply an outline provided to structure the information obtained by each therapist into a consistent document. The POMR system can be used as a start. Individual note formats or outlines can then be created that are specific for an individual patient population or are more generic to address a patient population that is more diverse or variable. The individualized format should be established after considering the facility's services, its goals within the hospital and community, its patient populations, and the requirements of the agencies which accredit it. Reviewing the policy manuals referenced at the end of this chapter will provide some guidance in preparing most documentation formats.

Another consideration in the development of a note format is the frame of reference or specific protocols for therapy used in a given facility. Again, the format can be specific, requiring detailed and standardized documentation of various tests and measures, or it can be generic. A generic format requires that the most important, or minimally acceptable, criteria for evaluation be stated. (See box for sample format.) This generic format might be used in an occupational therapy general medical and surgical service, where clients with varied diagnoses are referred for a wide variety of treatment techniques, splinting, or daily living skills training. In addition, several frames of reference for treatment may be considered in this format. Each therapist would be responsible for addressing each of the topic areas in the outline.

This generic format serves only as a foundation or skeleton for providing consistent note-writing among therapists in a facility. The occupational therapists using the format should not delete any of the sections provided but use their professional judgment to select the appropriate measures and information necessary for each client. In other words, for the sake of consistency in documentation, the therapist can add to the outline, but not subtract (or delete) information requested. This guarantees that each note follows a similar format, yet takes into account the individual needs of each patient or diagnosis.

Taking this format strategy a step further, the outline may be detailed and specific. The outline then provides direction for evaluating specific conditions, measurements, functional performance, and criteria for a given patient population or diagnostic group. An example of the use of a specific format might be in an acute head-injury program. In this setting, the note format for the objective section alone might be structured as indicated in the boxed material.

There is no limit to the number of styles that can be developed for any given facility. In addition to providing a consistent style of documentation, each format aids the therapist in accounting for and addressing the criteria, rules, and guidelines of the facility. Overall, the consistency of documentation within the service or facility can be used to address the issues of case management, research, marketing, and legality, as previously discussed.

Detailed Note Format

Objective information

Patient's age: _____ Weight: _____ Height: _____ Handedness: _____

Orientation: _____

Command following: _____

Communication skills: _____

Visual tracking: _____

Field cuts: _____

Peripheral sensation: _____ UE: _____ LE: _____

Range of motion: _____ UE: _____ LE: _____ Head and neck: _____

Motor responses/strength: _____ UE: _____ LE: _____ Head and neck: _____

Bed mobility: _____

Sitting tolerance: _____

Static and dynamic balance: _____ Sitting: _____ Standing: _____

Endurance: _____

Feeding skills: _____

Implementing a Documentation Format

Documentation formats must be developed and followed with some diligence on the part of the occupational therapist. It may take some time to become accustomed to evaluating patients and documenting results in such a structured way, but it is hoped that the reader can now see the advantages of providing structure and consistency in note writing. The following suggestions should facilitate the implementation of a structured note format.

Example of a Generic Note Format

Occupational Therapy Initial Note

Referring information
    Medical history
Subjective information
    Patient's complaints
    Patient's understanding of diagnosis
Objective information
    Evaluation results (ROM, strength, orientation)
    Daily living skills assessment (dressing, bathing, eating)
Assessment
    Patient's functional limitations
    Patient's expected benefit from rehabilitation
    Problem list
Plan
    Patient's goals
    Treatment plan

First, once a format or outline has been established, print it on 5 × 7–inch index cards so therapists will be able to carry and refer to it conveniently throughout the day.

Second, after a format has been established, experiment with it for 2 to 3 weeks and then reevaluate it. Therapists may find that certain topic areas of the outline are redundant, seldom used, or unnecessary. In addition, some other topic areas may be needed.

Third, remember that the outline provides only a skeleton for the note. If additional tests are needed for a patient, they should be added to the appropriate section of the note. Never delete necessary information.

Fourth, sometimes therapists will evaluate a specified topic area and find the patient had no limitations. At that point, instead of deleting the topic area, the therapist should state that the patient demonstrated no limitations. (*e.g.*, Dressing skills: no limitations, independent; UE sensation: no deficits for light touch; Visual fields: no impairment, normal).

Fifth, it is extremely important that therapists learn to report findings in concise, brief, telegraphic phrases. The use of narrative sentences will quickly produce long, cumbersome notes. For example, the subjective statement "the patient reports that he experiences increased pain in his low back with sustained sitting activities" could be more briefly stated as "sustained sitting increases low back pain.") The outline itself will decrease narrative statements, as each heading calls for a statement or measure (*e.g.*, Sitting tolerance: decreased to 10–15 minutes with report of low back pain).

Finally, lists or tables should be used whenever possible to eliminate narrative sections of the note. For example

Grip strength:	R = 150 lb normal = 156 lb	
	L = 125 lb normal = 130 lb	
2-point pinch strength:	R = 15 lb	L = 14 lb
Lateral pinch strength:	R = 20 lb	L = 19 lb

References

1. Commission on Accreditation of Rehabilitation Facilities: Standards Manual for Organizations Serving People with Disabilities. Tuscon, 1986
2. Health Care Financing Administration: Medicare program: Comprehensive outpatient rehabilitation facility services, rules and regulations. Part IV, final rule. Fed Register 47(241): Dec 15, 1982
3. Joint Commission on Accreditation of Hospitals: Accreditation Manuals for Hospitals. Chicago, 1986
4. Weed L: Medical Records, Medical Evaluation and Patient Care. Chicago, Year Book Medical Publishers, 1970

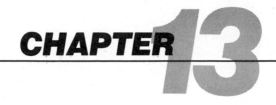

Uniform Reporting   *Sandra J. Malone*

In 1977, PL 95-142 — the Medicare and Medicaid Fraud and Abuse Amendments stipulated that uniform reporting of costs and services be instituted in hospitals certified as medicare providers. Although the law specified only hospitals, its intent was to include all providers, including home health agencies, skilled nursing, and intermediate care facilities. The purpose of this law was to ensure some degree of comparability in the information received from providers in different areas of the country. Medicare and Medicaid officials found that costs reported for the same or similar procedures varied as much as tenfold.

To develop guidelines for uniform reporting of services, the Health Care Financing Administration (HCFA) developed a manual entitled *The System for Uniform Hospital Reporting*. However, within the different branches of the federal government, there was controversy over what this system should do. Because it is directly related to the cost of services, some agencies felt a relative value unit system (RVU) should be used for all services to determine fair costs, whereas others viewed the RVU approach as a form of price fixing. This issue, coupled with the political emphasis on deregulation, has created a holding pattern on the decision related to the use of an RVU system in the reporting of services at this time.

Anticipating the development of a system for uniform reporting, the American Occupational Therapy Association (AOTA) developed a proposal for a national occupational therapy product output reporting system. This proposal, completed in January 1979, is entitled "Occupational Therapy Product Output Reporting System and Uniform Terminology for Reporting Occupational Therapy Services" (see Appendices D and E). This proposal is a valuable tool for any therapist contemplating the development of a uniform terminology for occupational therapy recording.

Impact of Uniform Reporting

Benefits

All occupational therapy services collect data on patient attendance, treatment schedules, fees for treatment, type of treatment given, and so forth. However, not all services collect the same data in the same manner; therefore, we are unable to compare or combine information collected in more than one or two settings. As health dollars become scarce, and as we are asked to describe the impact or outcomes of our intervention's, having comparable data becomes critical.

The benefits of using uniform reporting systems fall

under five general categories important to any occupational therapy service: standards, reimbursement, management, research, and promotion.

Standards

As we develop standards for the treatment of specific disabilities, we must also document the types of evaluation and treatment procedures used. The number of in-hospital days per illness is constantly decreasing owing to attempts to cut costs, and occupational therapy plans of treatment must be modified in order to be implemented over shorter periods of time. Through the development of standards and a uniform way of reporting services, occupational therapists should be able to respond to the following kinds of questions:

What is the average number of occupational therapy treatments needed for a stroke patient to achieve independence in ADL activities?

How many treatment hours would be required if your case load were to increase by 200 stroke patients next year?

If the average number of in-hospital days following stroke were limited to four, what would an occupational therapy plan of treatment include and what would be the expected outcomes?

Reimbursement

Occupational therapy treatment is covered by a variety of third-party payers, each of which uses guidelines to determine the specific type of occupational therapy covered. In order for us to propose guidelines or modifications to existing guidelines for coverage, we must be able to show that a particular type of treatment is in fact common or the "norm" for a particular disability or problem. The use of standard terminology in clinical reporting systems should help to avoid disparity in the types of coverage for occupational therapy services in different areas of the country.

Management

A uniform clinical reporting system can make program planning and management much easier. If the terminology used to describe services is compatible with practice standards, the service manager should be able to project the number of staff needed, the number of treatment hours per week or month, budgetary needs compatible with patient load, and the amount of income that will be generated. A uniform reporting system can serve as a base from which patient care and administrative audits and peer review activities can be conducted. This information can also be extremely important when planning the expansion of services or when developing new services.

Research

More clinical research is needed in occupational therapy. The true test of the validity of any research is the reproducibility of the results. Can someone in another setting get the same results? As our treatment and terminology become standardized, the foundation for clinical research grows.

Promotion

Throughout national, state, and local efforts to promote occupational therapy, we have talked about what occupational therapy is. Through the use of standard terminology and definitions and a uniform way of reporting service, we can now promote what occupational therapists do. Occupational therapy intervention in California should not be unlike what it is in Florida or Michigan. As a profession, we want to have an impact in the public and political arena and on the health care system.

Disadvantages

Whenever a new system or a new approach to handling existing functions is considered, there are advantages and disadvantages. Although the advantages of a uniform reporting system with standard terminology outweigh the disadvantages, such a system does impose more regulation, routinization, and structure on the clinical operation. Some occupational therapists may perceive this as infringement on their professional judgment prerogatives if there is not a thorough review and understanding of the terminology and definitions. Record-keeping procedures will also become more rigid.

A Model Uniform Reporting System

In 1977, the Maryland State Department of Health and Mental Hygiene (MSDHMH) instituted a centralized, computerized system of uniform data collection to be utilized by occupational therapists employed in MSDHMH programs and facilities. During the year prior to the institution of this system, numerous meetings were held with occupational therapists, administrators, program directors, representatives from county health departments, the Maryland Center for Health Statistics, and the state Division of Reimbursements. These meetings focused on the review of existing local statistical recording, identification of common information needs, review of other external systems, review of federal and private data requirements for reimbursement of occupational therapy services, and exploration of data capabilities of the Maryland Center for Health Statistics.

The initial form design incorporated information from the Prince George's County Health Department Rehabilitation Reporting System (Maryland) and the Washington State Hospital Commission Accounting and Reporting Manual (System of Accounts, Occupational Therapy, revised 1976). In 1980, modifications were based on the AOTA report, "Uniform Terminology System for Reporting Occupational Therapy Services."

The MSDHMH occupational therapy data system in its present state of development is patient-centered, meaning a unique record of service is developed about each individual served by the occupational therapy program. Generally, the individual patient is identified by his or her assigned facility number. No other specific identifiers are entered on the computer tape, although a few facilities may stamp the data form with the patient addressograph if the form is to be inserted in the medical record, as it often is to augment occupational therapy evaluation summaries and progress notes and to identify each date service was rendered.

Additionally, the system is designed to produce fiscal and management data through the inclusion of program and project information as part of the basic data set. For example, specific subdivisions of a facility's population (a geographic division, a specific school, a specific budgeted program) can be identified for program planning or fiscal management purposes.

In selecting the system's basic data set, primary consideration was given to the perceived needs of the data users. Experience has verified the usefulness of most of the included elements, although data generated on delivery sites (school, home, kidney dialysis unit, ward, clinic) and by referral sources (physician, family, Division of Vocational Rehabilitation) are of limited use.

The information generated on types of conditions served (for example, arthritis, cerebral palsy, manic depressive syndrome) is currently under review. Although the selected condition identifiers are fairly consistent with similar data generated nationally by AOTA, the trend locally is toward use of the International Classification of Disease. Another approach is to identify the problems addressed (for example, visual impairment, decreased range of motion, poor work habits) as a mechanism for determining the kinds of services being offered to a given population. The best approach to this issue should become clearer with experience.

Figure 13-1 pictures the front of the direct service data form with a case history. Figure 13-2 is the back of the form identifying the coding to be used in completing the front. Definitions for the assessment and treatment

procedures used in the MSDHMH model are contained in Appendix D.

Case History

The patient's identification number is entered in the upper left-hand portion of the form. The patient is male (1) and white (1) and being seen in the outpatient program (03). The first three numbers (123) under primary provider identify the facility from which the services are rendered; the last two numbers (01) identify the therapist—S. Malone, OTR. The patient's birth date is entered—January 1, 1940. His primary condition is renal failure (53). The primary delivery site of service is the operational base occupational therapy clinic (01). The patient's admission status to the service is "new admission" (01), and his status at the termination of service was due to discharge (05). The referral source was his private physician (01), and the county where he resides is Allegany (01).

On January 12, 1981, this patient was initially seen in occupational therapy for an evaluation (005) which took an hour to perform (4 units @ 15 minutes per unit). The evaluation results were documented (945). This documentation required 30 minutes (2 units). The therapist performing those services signs his or her full name and designation. On the 15th, this patient was seen again; his program consisted of body mechanics–energy conservation (051) and self care–survival skills (024). Treatment time was 1 hour (2 units per service). The therapist documented the treatment, which required 30 minutes. The therapist, having signed her full name for the initial visit, can now use her initials for subsequent entries for the rest of the month. Refer to Figure 13-2, the back of the direct service form, and identify the services recorded for January 18, 23, and 28. ☐

A separate form is completed for each patient seen in occupational therapy on a monthly basis. At the end of each month, the service sends all forms to the MSDHMH central office to be keypunched into the computer (Maryland Center for Health Statistics). The forms are then returned to the service, where, in most cases, they are entered into the patient's medical record. In many facilities, copies of the completed monthly data form and other supplementary information are sent to the patient's health insurance company or other third-party payer for reimbursement purposes. Along with the returned forms, each service receives a variety of reports generated from the month's data.

The primary report consists of a listing of all patients by identification number followed by the number of services received and the number of units required to provide those services, for example:

Patient Identification	Total Services	Total Units
RM0006514	9	20

Figures 13-3 and 13-4 are samples of other reports that can be generated monthly. Refer to Figure 13-2 to decode the information.

The quarterly reports contain information that is not needed monthly but is needed more frequently than annually. Figures 13-5, 13-6, and 13-7 are samples of quarterly reports. Fluctuations in service and predictable occurrences can be identified through the comparison of monthly and quarterly reports. Quarterly information can also be used to augment grant reporting.

Alpha codes are being used at many facilities to identify the expected time frame for reaching certain treatment outcomes. Upon completion of the initial assessment and the development of the treatment plan, a particular alpha code is recorded on the form indicating, for example, that the patient will be independent in all dressing, grooming, and personal hygiene activities in 2 weeks or after ten treatment sessions. This use of the alpha codes could prove to be a new management tool.

Annual reports for either the fiscal year or the calendar year can consist of any combination of information collected on the data form. Special reports, such as a listing of all assessment and treatment procedures given to a specific patient population by therapists, can be generated on an annual basis. This type of report can be used to develop expected levels of staff performance or to compare the actual treatment given with departmental or practice standards. Raw data from monthly, quarterly, or annual reports can also be converted into

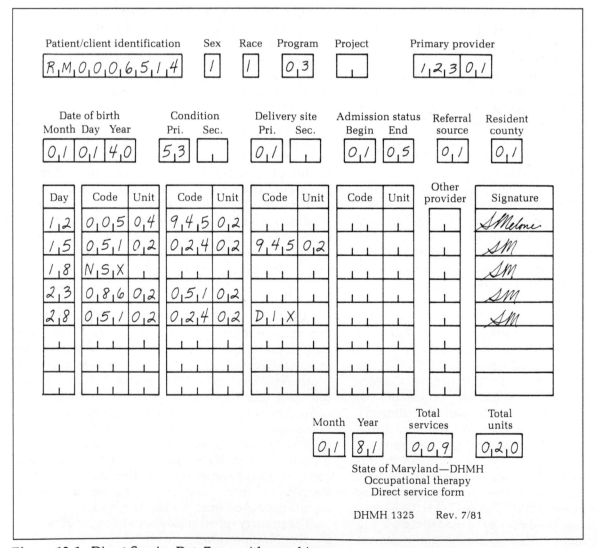

Figure 13-1. Direct Service DataForm with case history

Assessment

001 Screening
002 Patient Related
    Consultation
005 Evaluation
006 Reevaluation
007 Rescreening

Treatment Procedure

Self Care
021 Feeding Skills
022 Grooming/Hygiene
023 Dressing
024 Survival Skills

Cognition
041 Orientation
042 Concept./Comprehen.

Body Mechanics
051 Energy Conserv.
052 Join Protect.
053 Positioning

Therapeutic Adapt.
066 Orthotics
067 Prosthetics
069 Wheelchair
070 Asst./Adapt. Equip.

Psychologic
081 Self Ident./
    Self Concept.
082 Coping Skills

Work
086 Home Management
087 Student/Learner
    Skills
088 Pre-vocational
089 Vocational

090 Infant Stimulation

Play/Leisure
201 Skill/Interest
    Explor.
202 Skill Development
203 Community Resource
    Util.

Sensorimotor
226 Motor
228 Sensory Integration

Social/Interpersonal
251 Diadic Interac.
    Skills
252 Group Interact.
    Skills

800 Other
801 Other
802 Other

915 Patient/Client
    Support Inst.
930 Concurrent Charge
940 Patient/Client
    Related Conf.
945 Documentation
960 Travel
965 Planning
970 Telephone

County of Residence

01 Allegany
02 Anne Arundel
03 Baltimore
04 Calvert
05 Caroline
06 Carroll
07 Cecil
08 Charles
09 Dorchester
10 Frederick
11 Garrett
12 Harford
13 Howard
14 Kent
15 Montgomery
16 Prince George's
17 Queen Anne's
18 St. Mary's
19 Somerset
20 Talbot
21 Washington
22 Wicomico
23 Worcester
30 Baltimore City
40 District of Columbia
41 West Virginia
42 Virginia
43 Delaware
44 Pennsylvania
50 Out of State (other
    than above)
60 Foreign Country
70 Maryland Co. Unknown
90 Unknown

Program
03 Outpatient
04 Inpatient
05 Chronic Obstructive
    Airway Disease
06 Renal Dialysis
07 Mental Retardation
08 Long Term Care
12 Day Care Center
16 Child Health
17 School Health
20 Crippled Children
25 Adult Health
28 Home Health
33 Geriatric Services
96 Other
97 Other
98 Other

Sex

1. Male
2. Female

Race

1. White
2. Black
3. Spanish Surname
4. Oriental
5. American Indian
6. Other

Delivery Site

01 Operational Base
    Clinic
03 Home
04 Community
05 Long Term Care
    Facility
06 School—Public
07 Day Treatment/Care
    Center
08 Kidney Dialysis Unit
10 Ward/Cottage
11 School—Private
12 Other
13 Other

Referral Source

01 Private M.D.
02 Agency Professional
03 Long Term Care Fac.
04 Hospital (other)
05 Community Agency
06 Family or Self
07 Board of Education
08 Other
09 Child Devel. Center
10 Child Health Clinic
11 Diagnostic & Refer-
    ral Clinic
12 Exceptional Child
13 Neurological Clinic
14 Orthopedic Clinic
15 School Health
    Clinic
50 Therapist Initiated
51 Home Health Agency
52 Div. of Vocational
    Rehabilitation
60 Health Department
    (General)
61 Other
62 Other

Admission Status

01 New
02 Continuing
03 Readmission
04 Discontinued
05 Discharged
06 Other

Local Use

A.D.X. New
R.A.X. Readmission
R.R.X. Re-referred
D.I.X. Discharged
D.E.X. Deceased
P.C.X. Program Change
L.O.X. Leave of
    Absence
T.D.X. Temporarily
    Discontinued
N.S.X. No Show
C.D.X. Cancelled
R.E.X. Resumed
M.B.X. Maximum Benefit
O.B.X. Other
O.C.X. Other
O.D.X. Other
O.E.X. Other

Condition

01 Amputee
02 Arthritis
03 Brain Injury
04 Cardiovascular
05 Cerebral Palsy
06 C.V.A.
07 Degenerative Musculoskeletal
08 Developmental Delay
11 Mental Retardation
12 Minimal Brain Dysfunction
13 Orthopedic
14 Perceptual Motor
15 Progressive Neurological
17 Pulmonary
18 Paraplegia
21 Other Neurological
50 Visual Impairment
51 Emotional Problem
52 Hand Surgery
53 Renal Failure
54 Quadriplegia
55 Auditory Loss
56 Burn
57 Medical-Surgical Misc.
59 Malignancy
60 Multiple Anomaly
61 Organic Brain Syndrome
62 Alcoholism
67 Affective Disorder, Bipolar, mixed
68 Affective Disorder, Bipolar, raise
69 Affect. Disorder, Bipolar, depressed
72 Prim. deg. dement., senile onset
73 Dementia assoc. with alcohol
74 Maj. depress., recurrent melancholia
76 Personality Disorder
77 Schizoaffective disorder
78 Conduct disord., undersoc'd non-aggr.
79 Conduct disorder, undersoc'd aggr.
80 Pressure Ulcer
81 Stasis Ulcer
82 General Debilitation
83 Aphasia
84 Other
85 Other
86 Seizure disorder
87 Schiz., disorganized
88 Schiz., catatonic
89 Schiz., paranoid
90 Schiz., undiff.
91 Schiz., residual
92 Substance use disorder
93 Other
94 Att'n deficit disorder
95 Depression
96 Neurosis
97 Character disorder
98 Depressive neurosis

Figure 13-2. Coding for Direct Service DataForm

Occupational Therapy January 1981
Facility 000
Service Codes (1)

Code	Frequency	Percent	Units	Percent
005	11	5.67	46	14.56
007	3	1.55	12	3.80
009	3	1.55	7	2.22
021	1	0.52	1	0.32
022	1	0.52	1	0.32
023	6	3.09	10	3.16
024	7	3.61	17	5.38
042	1	0.52	1	0.32
053	1	0.52	1	0.32
066	6	3.09	13	4.11
070	1	0.52	1	0.32
086	2	1.03	6	1.90
087	34	17.53	42	13.29
090	3	1.55	6	1.90
201	2	1.03	2	0.63
202	4	2.06	8	2.53
226	19	9.79	27	8.54
228	12	6.19	13	4.11
502	1	0.52	0	0.00
915	5	2.58	6	1.90
940	16	8.25	20	6.33
945	21	10.82	33	10.44
960	32	16.49	41	12.97
970	2	1.03	2	0.63
Total	194		316	

Figure 13-3. Sample monthly report. Prepared by the Maryland Center for Health Statistics, March 1981.
Interpretation Notes
This report lists *all* the *Assessment* and *Treatment Procedures* employed by the reporting facility for the specified time frame; *e.g.,* this facility reported six orthotic services (code 066). These represented 3.09% of all services rendered and accounted for 13 units of time or 4.11% of all direct service time.

Occupational Therapy Report January 1981
Facility 000

Program[1]	Patients[2]	Services[3]	Units[4]
07	1	1	1
12	9	39	43
16	9	29	64
17	14	43	61
20	2	8	11
25	1	2	4
28	12	70	132
ALL	48	192	316

	ADMISSION STATUS[5]	
	BEGINNING	ENDING
1	14	0
2	34	43
3	0	0
4	0	2
5	0	3
6	0	0

Figure 13-4. Sample monthly report. Prepared by the Maryland Center for Health Statistics, March 1981.
Interpretation Notes
(1) *Program* refers to Chart of Accounts (*e.g.,* outpatients, renal dialysis, home health).
(2) *Patients* refers to total number of patients seen during specified time frame in that particular program.
(3) *Services* indicates total number of services (*e.g.,* screening, self-care, prevocational).
(4) *Units* indicates total time spent by program — 1 unit = 15 minutes
(5) *Status* refers to admission status both at the beginning and end of the month. During this month for this facility, 14 patients were newly admitted to the Occupational Therapy service, 34 were continued from the previous month, 43 were carried over to February, 2 were discontinued, and 3 were discharged.

July 1981 Quarter 7/81–9/81		Facility 000			
Program	Project	Condition[1]	Patients	Services	Units
033	0	2	3	19	36
033	0	3	1	2	5
004	0	5	6	48	79
→ 004	0	6	8	111	182
004	0	8	15	80	372
003	0	11	5	55	75
003	0	14	2	4	11
003	0	21	2	7	12
→ 003	1	60	1	1	1
Program Totals			43	327	773

Figure 13-5. Sample quarterly report. Prepared by the Maryland Center for Health Statistics, December 1981.

Interpretation Notes

(1) Condition—a listing of all conditions seen by the Occupational Therapy service during the specified time frame, *e.g.*, during this quarter, eight patients were treated with a primary condition identified as cerebrovascular accident (CVA #6). These patients received 111 services for 182—15-min. units of service. All CVA patients were inpatients. Note that a project number (1) was used to indicate that the one patient, with the condition of "Multiple Anomaly" (60), was seen under a federally funded grant program.

graphic displays as in Figures 13-8 and 13-9. Graphs and charts are often used to break the monotony of long narrative reports and enable large amounts of information to be shown quickly. Graphic display of data is frequently used in the development of reports for accreditation and certification reviews such as "Medicare and the Joint Commission on Accreditation of Hospitals."

The MSDHMH data system has had its growing pains, with many more expected before the system reaches maturity. The system does, however, offer some

Figure 13-6. Sample quarterly report. Prepared by the Maryland Center for Health Statistics, December 1981.

Interpretation Notes

(1) The use of alpha codes (alphabet letters) was integrated into the system as a mechanism for offering flexibility to local providers in retrieving data elements unique to their facility. Local providers have used alpha codes to track patients who did not keep scheduled appointments (*i.e.*, NSX—no shows) and to identify specific dates patient/client was admitted, discharged, or discontinued to/from the service.

Because this system does not include number of visits, only units of time, the SPX has been designated for identifying the number of patient visits.

Some of the alpha codes are not listed on the back of the data form because they were developed at the facility and are intended for their internal use only.

Occupational Therapy Quarter 7/81–9/81 Facility 000 Local Use Codes[1]				
Code	Frequency	Percent	Units	Percent
ADX	3	0.46	0	0.00
CBX	1	0.15	0	0.00
CDX	3	0.46	0	0.00
DIX	4	0.61	0	0.00
NSX	80	12.27	0	0.00
OBX	380	58.28	0	0.00
OCX	32	4.91	0	0.00
ODX	4	0.61	0	0.00
SPX	144	22.09	261	100.00
TDX	1	0.15	0	0.00
Total	652		261	

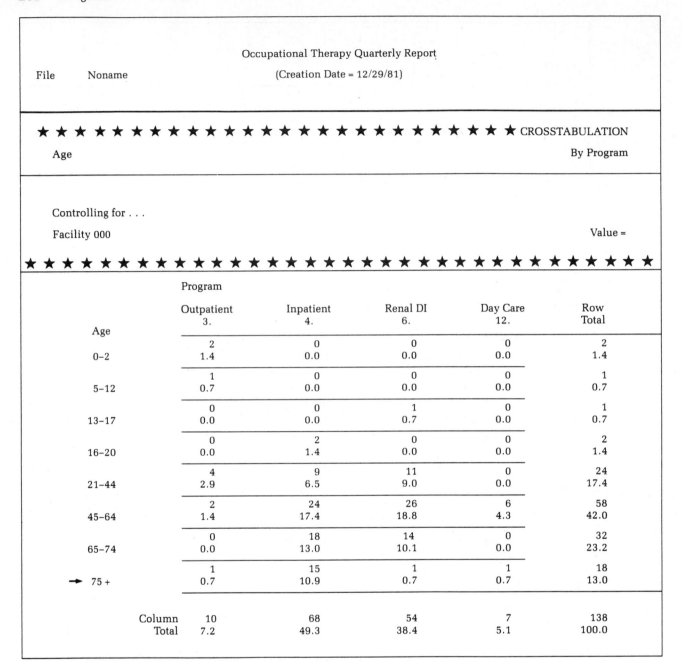

Occupational Therapy Quarterly Report

File   Noname   (Creation Date = 12/29/81)

★ CROSSTABULATION

Age   By Program

Controlling for . . .

Facility 000   Value =

★ ★

Age	Program Outpatient 3.	Inpatient 4.	Renal DI 6.	Day Care 12.	Row Total
0–2	2 1.4	0 0.0	0 0.0	0 0.0	2 1.4
5–12	1 0.7	0 0.0	0 0.0	0 0.0	1 0.7
13–17	0 0.0	0 0.0	1 0.7	0 0.0	1 0.7
16–20	0 0.0	2 1.4	0 0.0	0 0.0	2 1.4
21–44	4 2.9	9 6.5	11 9.0	0 0.0	24 17.4
45–64	2 1.4	24 17.4	26 18.8	6 4.3	58 42.0
65–74	0 0.0	18 13.0	14 10.1	0 0.0	32 23.2
➔ 75 +	1 0.7	15 10.9	1 0.7	1 0.7	18 13.0
Column Total	10 7.2	68 49.3	54 38.4	7 5.1	138 100.0

Figure 13-7. Sample quarterly report.

Interpretation Notes

This table is a cross tabulation of age breakdowns by program and by total. For example, 18 patients were older than 75 years, representing 13% of all patients served. Sixty-eight or 49.3% of all patients were seen on an inpatient basis.

unique features which were unavailable just a few years ago:

Information can be pulled out and presented in a variety of ways: by patient, therapist, program, project, diagnosis, or treatment procedure.

Large amounts of data can be analyzed for program and planning purposes.

The occupational therapy manager is provided with a mechanism for identifying trends and therefore predicting occurrences.

Research on the clinical level can be facilitated.

The next major change in the MSDHMH Occupational Therapy data system will be its incorporation into the states' Hospital Management Information System (HMIS). Occupational therapy managers in state-oper-

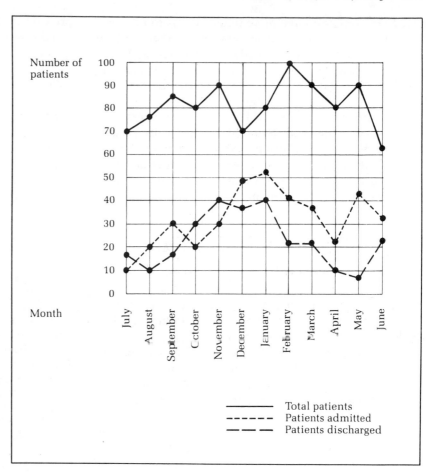

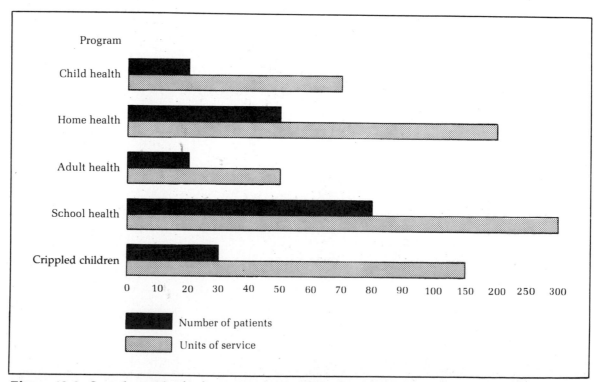

Figure 13-8. Sample graph of information derived from the system of facility Y, July 1980 to June 1981, shows rates of admission/discharge to occupational therapy and total monthly census.

Figure 13-9. Sample graph of information derived from the system of facility B, July 1980 to June 1981, shows total number of patients served by program and units of service.

ated facilities will have more timely access to information and will be able to create new reports that combine occupational therapy information with other service information. Reports could also be generated on a weekly or daily basis. The ability to create special reports will be limited only by the knowledge and ability of the occupational therapy staff. The HMIS system will operate on an IBM computer with terminals located within major departments in each facility. With the variety of computer software programs available and under development, occupational therapy data can be combined in ways rarely possible with manual systems.

Implications for the Future

In developing a uniform reporting system, it must be recognized that changes will be needed in format, content, and the types of reports generated. Current and future changes in federal and state reporting requirements (for instance, Titles IX and XX) all point to the need to maintain a flexible outlook. Concepts on the desirability of reporting in visits, units, or actual time spent per service are changing. The development of similar and potentially compatible uniform reporting systems throughout the country encourages innovations worthy of replication. The terminology used to describe our services needs to be reviewed and updated as technology and research are introduced into the health care system and new sources for the reimbursement for occupational therapy are obtained. Utilizing a unified approach to data collection would not stifle creativity but could prevent unnecessary repetition of errors, and the data generated would be more generally understood.

The importance of uniform terminology and data collection cannot be understated. With third-party encumbrances through reimbursement practices tied to quantifiable delivery of services, it is very important that we, as occupational therapists and as administrator/managers, speak in the same terms and same elements to properly identify and define the scope of our practice. Uniform reporting of occupational therapy data is no longer of the future but rather the future for our profession.

Bibliography

International Classification of Diseases: Manual of the International Statistical Classification of Diseases, Injuries, and Causes of Death, 9th ed., revised. Geneva, World Health Organization, 1977

Prince George's County Health Department Rehabilitation Admission & Forms Service. Cheverly, MD, 1977

The System for Uniform Hospital Reporting: Draft Report—Health Care Financing Administration [for Public Comment]. Washington, DC, 1978

Uniform Terminology System for Reporting Occupational Therapy Services: Commission on Practice Task Force Report. Rockville, MD, American Occupational Therapy Association, 1979

Washington State Hospital Commission Accounting & Reporting Manual: System of Accounts, Occupational Therapy, revised. 1976

CHAPTER 14

Quality Assurance *Patricia C. Ostrow*

Patient well-being and the quality of health care are assumed by most to be interrelated. Few people are aware, however, that the viability of the occupational therapy profession is also tied to the quality-of-care issue. This chapter will look at major factors and issues related to quality of health care to see how they influence patient outcomes and professional growth. An overview such as this also lays the foundation for study of specific quality assurance methodologies, detailed elsewhere, such as monitoring and problem-focused quality assurance, and provides a guide to good quality assurance study topics.[5,11]

Quality Assurance—Improving the Outcomes of Health Care

Accreditation of schools, certification of therapists, licensure, and standards for service delivery—are these enough to ensure that a health care practitioner will provide quality care? Some practitioners believe they are, but many assert that a crucial, and often neglected, element in the quest for quality is a process for clinicians to assess actual service delivery and health care outcomes, be they intermediate or long-range. Quality assurance fills this need. It is a method of studying health care to improve its impact.

Assessing and improving the quality of services are essential components of health care and should be a part of the treatment process itself. Each therapist carries that responsibility for her or his clients. It is as important as evaluating the individual patient before selecting treatment goals. Occupational therapy is committed to outcome-oriented quality review studies; they are specifically mentioned in the *Standards of Practice* approved by the Representative Assembly of the American Occupational Therapy Association in the Spring of 1978. Quality assurance is also included in the Association's *Essentials and Guidelines* for educational programs for occupational therapists and occupational therapy assistants. Therapists should know how to develop and implement quality assurance, while assistants need to know how to collect data for quality assurance purposes.

The evaluation of health care for aggregates of patients with similar problems provides invaluable information to guide a therapist's pursuit of optimal benefits for each client. If, for example, 75% of the patients given activities of daily living (ADL) training do not successfully use the skills they learned in the hospital, then the treatment approach for individual clients needs modification.

In the past, as health care costs became a major social

concern, quality assurance was required by law — health care processes and outcomes became the focus of systematic data collection. Legislators, consumers, and health care practitioners realized that they must find ways to reduce costs and improve quality. The goals were to eliminate unnecessary or ineffective services and to provide feedback information that would enhance professional growth and refine administrative processes.

Because Congress required it, utilization review came into being. It was conducted to measure the necessity for a service, the efficiency of a service, and whether care was given at the least expensive level commensurate with patient needs (for instance, nursing home *vs.* acute care). Lengths of hospital stays were averaged for various diagnostic conditions and patterns of hospital utilization analyzed. Stroke care may be twice as long in one facility as in another. Why? Were the outcomes significantly different? Were the patients significantly different so that one group had more secondary complications? These are the questions for which answers are sought in order to identify underutilization or overutilization.

Quality assurance was another type of data collection that became popular in the years between 1970 and 1987 because it was required by Congress. Quality assurance programs identified problems in health care service delivery and remedied them. Achievable benefits *not* achieved are the focus of quality assurance. Utilization review was initially a separate function from quality assurance. Now, both are frequently considered to be part of a quality assurance program.

The basic steps in quality assurance are directly comparable to the steps a therapist follows to resolve a patient's problems:

Stage 1: *Identify* the significant characteristics of quality care, particularly looking at achievement of patient benefits and satisfaction and any areas where significant problems in service delivery occur (comparable to the initial interview of the patient to identify problems)

Stage 2: *Measure* significant aspects of quality care to confirm and clarify any problems (comparable to specific patient assessments, such as of ADL skills or range of motion, which describe the degree of handicap)

Stage 3: *Improvement planning* to brainstorm and select a cost-effective correction to any quality problems found in Stage 2 (comparable to the treatment plan)

Stage 4: *Improvement action* to improve the problems (parallel to providing treatment)

Stage 5: *Reassessment* to monitor if improvement action was effective; if not, go back to Stage 3 (similar to the predischarge assessment to see if the patient treatment plan was effective)

Quality of Care Defined

The quest for quality in health care services is begun by understanding the meaning of quality. Avedis Donabedian, a well-known theorist in health care, has classified the elements of quality care into structure, process, and outcome. He defined the terms as follows:

Structure — the properties of the resources used to provide care, such as physical facilities, equipment, and qualified personnel and the manner in which these resources are organized

Process — the treatment management activities of health care professionals, such as clinical assessment, treatment, and preventive care, as well as documentation and other related activities

Outcome — the results, to a significant degree, of process and structure in terms of improved health, restored or improved physical and social functioning, and patient satisfaction[2]

A few examples may clarify his terms. One would assess the *structure* of an occupational therapy department by asking questions about the adequacy of space for the number of patients treated, proper certification and licensure of therapists, and the potential hazards equipment may present. *Process* could be evaluated by asking if there was a complete evaluation of the patients' abilities and disabilities as well as patients' goals before a treatment plan was developed, whether the treatment followed the accepted format, and so forth. *Outcome* could be assessed by measuring health care benefits in an aggregate of patients with the same problem or diagnosis. There are numerous intermediate outcomes during a hospital stay, as well as discharge outcomes and long-range outcomes to consider.

As a result of this classification system, polarized opinions have developed about the merits of process or outcome elements in quality assurance studies. Donabedian believes that both are necessary for quality care assessment.[3] From a cost-effective point of view, it seems logical to look at outcomes first. If they do not meet the therapists' standards, then the treatment processes judged to be related to the below-par outcomes must be examined.

Peer Review

As early as 1933, it was agreed that quality of care assessment must rest on the judgment of peers.[7] *Peer review* is a term with a rich variety of connotations. It is used as an umbrella covering all forms of quality review, which include peer judgments, whether or not the standards for determination of quality are written out before the assessment in an explicit, objective, measurable form. (*Quality assurance* refers to later methodologies that rely on objective and measurable standards.)

Enlarging the Concept

The concept of quality health care was enlarged in 1967 beyond the processes performed by recognized leaders to emphasize ". . . diagnosis and therapy, both preventative and curative, based on the best knowledge available from science and humanities; and which eventuates in the least morbidity and mortality in the population."[9] In this quote, equal emphasis was given to treatment processes and beneficial outcomes. Scientific data as the basis for treatment is an important addition to the understanding of quality. Quality care is that based on the best knowledge available. A department providing such care would not only keep abreast of developing theories and treatment techniques but would also systematically review the accumulated knowledge regarding *outcomes relevant to each treatment process* they use.

Another definition of quality, offered in 1975, shows the interplay between technical knowledge or skill and the "art of care," or the ability of the health care practitioner to relate to the client and his or her needs: "Quality of health care is equal to technical care plus the art of care . . ."[3] The art of care here includes patient satisfaction with the milieu, the treatment, communication, and the provider–patient relationship.

Balancing Risks and Benefits

A book by Donabedian, published in 1980, is devoted to the definition of quality. He begins his discourse by posing the following: quality of care is ". . . that kind of care which is expected to maximize . . . patient welfare after one has taken account of the balance of gains and losses (health benefits and risks) that attend the process of care in all its parts."[3] The quantity of health care and its monetary costs are inextricably related to quality. Access to care, sufficient care to achieve results, and inefficient and unnecessary care all become important, assessable elements of quality. Providing care when there is no expectation of benefit reduces the welfare of both the individual and society itself, because it is an improper use of resources. It deprives the client of time and money, and it robs society of the opportunity to provide care to others who may benefit.

Donabedian suggests that the cost of care should be added to the risk as ". . . an unwanted consequence of the provision of care . . ."[3] Considering health care costs in this fashion, he says, allows a more efficient balancing of expected benefits and losses when planning treatment or assessing quality.

Donabedian's description of quality is expanded when he considers how health goals and treatment interventions will be selected. One method is "absolutist": the health care practitioners, as the experts, decide on appropriate health goals and the methods to achieve them. It is a technological decision based on the state of the science and the skill of the professional in applying the science. An "individualistic" alternative for selecting the health goals and treatment plan argues that the client must help select the objectives of care and, by placing his or her values on the benefits and risks of alternate strategies of treatment, share in management decisions. Many clients prefer that these choices be made by the relevant health care practitioner. In that case, the professional is responsible for ascertaining the values of the client. The impact on the client of health care costs thus becomes a necessary consideration in management decisions. Finally, there is a "societal" approach to selection of treatment management decisions. Quality of care in that case could be assessed on the basis of societal health rather than individual welfare. ". . . Quality is the degree to which preventable deaths, preventable functional impairment, and preventable suffering within a defined population are minimized over time."[4]

Efficacy, Effectiveness, and Efficiency

Finally, the understanding of quality can be fully rounded out with three terms: efficacy, effectiveness, and efficiency. John W. Williamson, professor in Health Services Administration at Johns Hopkins University, calls these the ". . . classic evaluation indicators . . . [they] may well provide the foundation for a more successful approach to developing future quality assurance systems."[12] His definitions for these terms are as follows:

Efficacy: The extent to which a health care intervention can be shown to be beneficial under optimal conditions of care (such as clinical research).
Effectiveness: The extent to which benefits achievable under optimal conditions of care are actually achieved in clinical practice.
Efficiency: The proportion of total cost (for instance, money, scarce resources, and time) that can be related to actual benefits achieved.[12]

He suggests these definitions because earlier ones have overlapped in meaning and caused confusion. He proposes that quality assurance, as an evaluation study, is a measure of effectiveness; and clinical research, a measure of efficacy. Too often, hazy thinking on these ideas ruins the intent of a quality assurance study when a cause-and-effect problem (efficacy) will be tackled instead of an effectiveness measure.

Williamson's concept of efficiency echoes Donabedian's concern with cost of care. His definition of efficacy expands the idea of technical knowledge beyond that of the practitioner to the state of the science itself and thus broadens the source of standards for outcomes of care, combining peer judgments with the literature of the field, particularly the scientific data on the cause-and-effect relationship between treatment and outcome. Quality assurance is the interface between clinical research and clinical practice. Williamson and others note the lack of efficacy data, that is, knowledge in the health care field about the causal relationships between treatment variables and patient status.[1,13] In the absence of efficacy data, one can use the consensus of professionals expressed in explicit measurable standards. For Williamson, the assessment of quality care begins with a simple question: In an optimal clinical situation, treatment will accomplish specified results for a particular health problem; are we meeting that achievable goal in this facility?

Application of the Concept of Quality to Health Care

Understanding the issues and factors related to optimal quality in health care assists the professional in two ways:

1. It suggests the areas on which to focus continual review of care for correctable problems.
2. It sets forth standards against which to assess care.

Applying the idea that cost is one of the risks or losses a practitioner must balance against potential improvements, one approaches current pressures to improve therapists' productivity in a new light. Increasing the number of patients treated without monitoring the outcome raises the likelihood that outcomes will suffer. The therapist should balance productivity drives with his or her knowledge of expected treatment benefits as revealed in research or, in the absence of research, as based on the consensus of professionals. Quality assurance studies can aid the clinician in efficiency drives by demonstrating that the expected results are still being achieved. Quality assurance studies are a necessary corollary to productivity and efficiency.

A therapist should consider costs when planning treatment. Many practitioners provide services completely unaware of the total bill for the patient. "Insurance pays for it," is a usual attitude, but insurance runs out. A policy can be depleted in a serious illness. Societal costs must also be taken into account. Achieving the treatment goal in the most efficient manner is the responsibility of the professional and an excellent quality assurance topic, which can increase therapist productivity in a positive way.

The profession cannot ignore the seriousness of the financial issue. Health care costs have reached crisis proportions: "The nation spent $425 billion on health care in 1985, an amount equal to 10.7 percent of gross national product, the highest share in U.S. history," according to the Department of Health and Human Services.[10] These figures are far ahead of inflationary trends. With escalating health expenses seen as draining the economy, third-party carriers seek to curb utilization of health services. They want to avoid reimbursement for services if the outcomes are questionable or insignificant—or if the treatments are held to be unnecessary. Hysterectomies, tonsillectomies, intermittent positive pressure breathing, and diversional activities are examples of services that have been under scrutiny from third-party carriers.

To improve the quality of care, it is the responsibility of the profession at the national, state, and individual levels to maintain access to occupational therapy services for those patients who significantly benefit from them. Access can be impeded not only by the patient's limited finances, but also by limitations in coverage by health insurance programs such as Medicare, Medicaid, Blue Cross, and Blue Shield.

Documentation is an essential weapon in the battle for adequate coverage of occupational therapy. Consider the likelihood of reimbursement, at $50 per hour, for treatment described in this way: "Three home visits by the occupational therapist for Mrs. Jones. Potholders were made to improve manual dexterity." Payment for such treatment is likely to be denied. However, if the therapist says, "Patient participated in an activity providing resistance to finger and thumb flexors to strengthen grasp in both hands. When grasp improves, independent dressing will be achievable," then reimbursement is more likely. The clarity of documentation and the likelihood of coverage would be further served if the therapist noted why this patient was a good candidate for muscle strengthening and how soon results were expected. If the therapist cannot succinctly identify these factors, it is questionable if the patient *should* be making potholders with the therapist at $50 per hour.

Quality assurance studies are of value to help therapists become aware of the outcomes related to a service program. Do stroke patients, for example, achieve the expected improved dexterity and strength while making potholders? That could be assessed in a quality assurance study.

Reimbursement decisions are not always made on a case-by-case assessment unless it is an area under special scrutiny; therefore, the generally held opinion of third-party payers and physicians about occupational therapy becomes crucial to insurance coverage. Quality assurance studies reported within the health care facility and in national professional journals build understanding of the positive impact of occupational therapy services and of the professional commitment to quality care. As the health dollar shrinks, reimbursement and utilization will be influenced by the profession's ability to show that significant patient outcomes are achieved.

Summary

Many aspects of quality, its assessment, and its improvement have been considered. In the earlier part of the 20th century, quality was thought to be most easily achieved by imitating experts. Standard treatment processes used by recognized leaders and teachers were the guide to quality. A new dimension was later added: beneficial outcomes. The knowledge and skill of the provider and the state of the science (as reflected in research & theory), as well as the rapport between provider and client, were recognized as valuable elements of quality. Two names stand out in the quality assurance field: Donabedian and Williamson. Donabedian defined quality care as management reflecting consideration of, and proper balance in, health risks and health benefits.[3] Underutilization, overutilization, access to care, management style, and health care costs become critical factors. Williamson synthesized his concept of quality into three elements: efficacy, effectiveness, and efficiency. The foregoing chapter and the factors related to quality care reveal a wide and varied range of elements essential to optimal health care. Familiarity with these factors and skill in conducting quality assurance studies provide therapists with useful tools to improve the beneficial impact of occupational therapy, enhance their own professional development, and increase appropriate utilization and reimbursement of their services. Step-by-step guides for conducting a quality assurance study are available for both beginners and those with experience.[8,11] In addition, instructional materials have been developed for quality assurance documentation and monitoring.[5,6]

Information about the outcome of treatment for aggregates of patients with similar problems, as measured in quality assurance studies, is probably one of the best ways for a clinician to guide therapeutic efforts that overcome specific handicaps. Quality assurance also provides data that will stimulate the therapist's own selective reach for new information relevant to an improved treatment program.

The three elements of excellence — efficacy, effectiveness, and efficiency — summarize the issues in quality care. They are essential if health care professionals are to meet society's needs for improved health as well as society's demand for reduced health care expenditures. Clearly, outcome-oriented quality assurance studies should be an integral part of every clinician's activities.

References.

1. Brook RH: Quality of Care Assessment: A Comparison of Five Methods of Peer Review, p 21. DHEW Publication No. HRA-74-3100, Library of Congress Card No. 73–699243, July 1973
2. Donabedian A: A Guide to Medical Care Administration, vol 2. Medical Care Appraisal — Quality and Utilization, pp 2–3. New York (now Washington, DC), American Public Health Association, 1969
3. Donabedian A: The Definition of Quality and Approaches to Its Assessment, pp 5–6, 10, 28, and 119. Ann Arbor, MI, Health Administration Press, 1980
4. Ellwood PM, O'Donoghue P, McClure W, Holley R, Carlson RJ, Hoogberg E: Assuring the Quality of Health Care. Instudy, Minneapolis, 1974
5. Joe BE, Ostrow PC: Quality Assurance Monitoring in Occupational Therapy. Rockville, MD, American Occupational Therapy Association, 1987
6. Kuntavanish A: Occupational Therapy Documentation: A System to Capture Outcome Data for Quality Assurance and Program Promotion. Rockville, MD, American Occupational Therapy Association, 1987
7. Lee RI, Jones LW: The Fundamentals of Good Medical Care, p 302. Publications of the Committee on the Costs of Medical Care, No. 22. Chicago, Chicago University Press, 1933
8. Ostrow PC, Joe BE: Quality Assurance Primer. Rockville, MD, American Occupational Therapy Association, 1982
9. Payne BC: Continued evolution of a system of medical care appraisal. JAMA 201:128, 1967
10. Rich S: Health-Care Spending's Share of GNP Reaches a New High, The Washington Post, Section A, July 30, 1986
11. Williamson JW, Ostrow PC, Braswell HR: Health Accounting for Quality Assurance: A Manual for Assessing and Improving Outcomes of Care. Rockville, MD, American Occupational Therapy Association, 1981
12. Williamson JW: Assessing and Improving Health Care Outcomes. pp 9–10. Cambridge, MA, Ballinger Publishing, 1978
13. Williamson JW: Improving Medical Practice and Health Care: A Bibliographic Guide to Information Management in Quality Assurance and Continuing Education. p 9. Cambridge, MA, Ballinger Publishing, 1977

The Occupational Therapy Process — Tools of Practice

CHAPTER 15

Assessment and Evaluation — An Overview*

Helen D. Smith and Elizabeth G. Tiffany

In 1971, Gillette referred to evaluation as a professional responsibility. She defined the functions of the evaluation process[5] as (1) determining the baseline for objectives and providing the foundation for a treatment program, (2) identifying which problems can and cannot be remediated by occupational therapy, (3) giving some indication of the potential for change, (4) enlisting the cooperation of the client in beginning to assess his or her capabilities and dreams, and (5) helping the client begin a course of action designed to master some of the difficulties he or she has previously tried to master alone.

Evaluation also serves the purpose of keeping the therapist's work current, for it is a spiral, building process. Each treatment session should be assessed, and each target area should be reviewed in order to determine the effectiveness of the activity process and to revise the objectives as they are mastered or found to be unreachable. Treatment

should not persist in a straight line. It is the system of evaluation that is built into the treatment process that ultimately determines the effectiveness of treatment.[5]

In occupational therapy, evaluation is a process of collecting and organizing the relevant information about a client so that the therapist will be able to plan and implement a meaningful, effective program of treatment. Several steps are involved:

1. *The collection of data.* This includes the selection and use of tools and methods by which information is obtained. The frame of reference for treatment will determine the kinds of data that will be sought. The participation of the client in this process is critical to the success of the program.

2. *The organization of the data* into a meaningful, dynamic description of the client's strengths and weaknesses with a focus on those areas in which occupational therapy can be of help. The client, the therapist, and others should be able to understand this description readily.

3. *The setting of treatment objectives.* This involves the use of clinical judgment and predictive assumptions on the part of the therapist. Objectives must be based on the accumulated data, including the client's goals, the therapist's knowledge about the

---

* The terms *evaluation* and *assessment* have both been used with regard to procedures used in fact-finding preparatory to and during treatment. In general, the term *assessment* refers to the sum of the results of the *evaluation* procedures used. Assessment yields a composite picture of the patient's functioning. Evaluation refers to the data gathered from specific procedures.

clinical pathology, and the treatment frame of reference.

4. *Commitment to continuing evaluation* as the occupational therapy plan is carried out. The original objectives and treatment plan need constant reassessment. Changes in the occupational therapy plan are dependent on the results of ongoing re-evaluation.

The evaluation process thus represents an organized and systematic way of determining a client's needs. It is essential to objective setting, treatment planning, and assessing the effectivenesss of the implementation of the treatment plan. Careful evaluation and re-evaluation in occupational therapy also adds significant information to the total treatment program of the team as an aid in setting overall goals and in monitoring the effectiveness of interventions such as medication or physical therapy.

It is important to recognize that any fair and valid assessment of a client must be based on several sources, yielding a multidimensional picture of the client's status. It should focus on those data that are pertinent to the occupational therapy process. Any assessment procedure, moreover, includes a clear analysis of the context for treatment, the therapist's skills and resources, and the activities that could be used in treatment.

Types of Evaluation

Evaluation procedures take many forms. There are specific tests for specific functions (*e.g.,* manual muscle testing). There are more complex or comprehensive assessments comprising data from several tests or procedures. Successful evaluation is dependent on the ability of the therapist to gain the trust of the client so that a cooperative effort can take place. The therapist must observe and record data accurately and must make use of a wide range of appropriate information sources pertinent to the treatment process.

Medical Records

The medical record provides valuable information about the client, and it gives indications for precautions that must be considered when planning and carrying out treatment. Data gleaned from the medical record add to the baseline information necessary for effective treatment planning.

The past and present medical history, written by the physician, gives the therapist information on the client's health status, former medical problems, present medical or physical findings, diagnoses, precautions, and prognosis. Daily notes by physicians and nurses list medications and treatments being given, as well as the patient's responses. Reports and evaluations from other specialties (x-ray, dietary, social service, psychiatry, psychology, physical or speech therapy, vocational and/or rehabilitation counseling) are also included. With information from medical records as background, the therapist is ready to move on to the next step in the evaluation process.

Observation

A key to successful evaluation lies in the therapist's skills in observation. The ability to see and to listen well must be accompanied by the ability to sort through the mass of perceptual and conceptual data that may be presented, and to focus on what is relevant to the process.

Human beings communicate information about themselves in a great many ways. There is oral communication—the choice of words and sentences, their meanings, and the quality of tone and inflection with which the words are said. There are the paralinguistic and nonverbal behaviors that accompany oral communication—facial expression, gestures, posture, and body movements. Attention to nonverbal communication is especially important to the occupational therapist, inasmuch as a large part of the occupational therapy process is doing, not talking. Nonverbal expressions in human beings are established earlier in life than verbal ones, and they rely on older neurophysiologic structures.[4] A third mode of communication is the written form. It can be assumed that the written work has been more carefully considered and censored and thus is less spontaneous than the spoken, although this is not necessarily true. What an individual writes about himself or herself may be useful as a representation of a desired or ideal self. The organization and form of the handwriting and its placement on the page have been considered clues to personality, feelings, and cognitive functioning at the time of the writing. Closely related to writing are other forms of psychomotor projection through which communication takes place—the behaviors connected with the use of media and the choice of clothing, colors, and objects. Over a longer period of time, an individual communicates much information by the total effect of behavior, especially small, unconscious, and automatic behaviors, in a variety of circumstances.

The communication process between the client and the therapist lays a foundation for rapport and trust. The client needs to feel that communications have been heard and understood by someone who has not only some empathy, but also some knowledge and skill. The therapist's confidence in his or her abilities and in the profession may be crucial in setting the tone for all future transactions with the client. Four filters affect interactions between people, and they are significant in their potential for distorting the observation process[3]:

Perceptual—how sensory stimuli (color of clothing, perfume) affect the way the other person is perceived

Conceptual—the knowledge base brought to the interaction

Role—the way each person perceives the role he or she is to play in the interaction

Self-esteem—the way each person feels about himself or herself

It is useful for the therapist to consider these filters and the ways in which they might affect objectivity in observation.

The occupational therapist is in a position to observe the patient or client in a variety of structured and unstructured situations. The interview, formal testing procedures, and planned activities represent structured opportunities for observation. These usually involve some elements of prediction or expectation on the part of the therapist, and they will be discussed in the next sections.

The therapist's opportunities to see and interact with clients in situations that are less planned will vary with the setting. If it is possible for the therapist to interact informally and spontaneously with patients in situations where role differentiation may be less clear, information may be available that otherwise might be difficult to obtain. For example, different perspectives on values, interests, and functional levels may be gained by seeing the patient in the local snack shop, in the elevator, or at recreational activities. It is desirable to build some opportunities for informal contact into the evaluation process whenever possible.

Interview

There are occasions when a health professional may wish to interview a client formally or informally. Probably the most important occasion is the initial interview, undertaken as part of the process of evaluation. The initial interview serves several vital purposes. It provides for: (1) collection of information about the client to help develop objectives and a plan for treatment and (2) establishment of understanding on the part of the client about the role of the therapist and purposes of the occupational therapy process, as well as (3) an opportunity for the client to discuss his or her situation and to think about plans for change.

In the *The Helping Interview,*[2] Benjamin refers to important *external and internal factors* that need careful consideration in preparing for an interview. The external factors are such things as the room in which the interview is to take place and the extent to which the place will be private, free of interruptions and other distractions. Internal factors are the attitudes, knowledge, and feelings that the therapist brings to the interview. It is important for the therapist to be clear about the purpose of the interview, to know the kinds of information specifically desired, to be self-trusting, and to be honest.

Allen, in a paper presented at the American Occupational Therapy Association Annual Conference in October 1976,[1] points out there are two requirements for the therapist to be able to conduct a successful interview with a patient: a solid knowledge base and skills in active listening. These requirements are not simple. They necessitate study, preparation, and practice. The solid knowledge base must underlie the therapist's selection of questions or areas to be covered in the interview. It is important that the interview reflect what the therapist knows and that it cover areas that will be relevant to occupational therapy. Active listening means that the interviewer plays a deeply involved role that demonstrates genuine respect for the patient or client.

Benjamin[2] delineates three parts to an interview: initiation, development, and closing. In the initiation phase, the therapist explains the purpose of the interview and his or her role in relation to the person interviewed and begins to establish mutual trust and understanding. It is during the initiation phase that the interviewer should define the parameters of the interview—the amount of time it should take, the kind of material to be discussed, and the uses to be made of the information.

During the development phase, the interviewer seeks information and explores issues with the person interviewed. The occupational therapist doing an initial interview as an evaluation procedure should bring some form of outline or a list of planned questions to the interview to be certain that information vital to the setting of objectives and to treatment planning will be covered. The kinds of questions the occupational therapist may ask should allow the patient to respond with more than a simple "yes" or "no." The occupational therapist needs to have skill in asking one question at a time, tolerating silence, listening carefully, observing both verbal and nonverbal responses, restating or clarifying questions when needed, and encouraging the client to continue or to stay on the track.

Clues marking the end of the interview are either the end of the time defined at the beginning or the end of the list of questions or issues to be explored. It is important for both the therapist and the client to know that the interview is coming to a close. No new material should be brought up at this point. It is best to plan another time and place to discuss new material. Summarizing the material that has been discussed may be a useful way to terminate the interview as well as to double-check on the accuracy of the information gained.

The therapist will need to make notes unless he or she has both an unusual memory and time to record the interview later. The purpose of writing notes or using a tape recorder should be explained to the client at the beginning of the interview. The client should also be told that he or she may read the notes or listen to the tape and that their sole purpose is to provide valid guidelines for the occupational therapy process.

Sometimes it is useful to have clients answer a simple questionnaire before coming to the interview. The use of a questionnaire has some advantages. It may save time in situations where setting aside 30 to 45 minutes for personal interviewing of each client initially is not feasible. It can provide information about the client's ability to read and to respond in an organized fashion in writing. The disadvantage is that some of the richness of detail and interaction will be lost. A written questionnaire can never completely replace a face-to-face interview.

The kinds of information that are best gained through an interview may vary somewhat according to the client population and the general context for treatment. In general, the occupational therapist may learn about education; work experience; leisure interests and pursuits; the way patients' balance their work, sleep, and play and manage time; the quality and extent of their care for their own personal needs (grooming, nutrition, laundry, housekeeping, hygiene); their families or significant people in households; friends or other family members who are supportive; the communities in which they live; their values and familiar objects; their own assessment of their current situations and problems; their personal goals; and current housing situations, including potential architectural barriers.

Knowledge about whether the patient's level of skill has been high enough to accomplish tasks and to fulfill expected social roles successfully provides important clues to the kinds of experiences that should be provided in occupational therapy. The importance of collecting information about this history has been outlined by Moorehead:

> In gathering the occupational history, the investigator is concerned with discovering how and under what conditions the individual patient has learned to approach tasks and role expectations as he does; and whether he was ever more competent than he now appears. Can the therapist expect that the patient will be able to improve his role skills, and if so, how much? In other words, the investigator asks what a patient's particular life style is in terms of occupational function, so that therapy can be structured for him to build upon his experiences for improved function.[7]

A terminal interview, undertaken just before the client leaves treatment, serves other important functions. It gives the client and therapist an opportunity to look together at what has taken place and to identify some of the things that have been learned in the process. Often, the occupational therapy experience may be significant in helping the patient plan how to balance activities at home. For example, the client has learned which activities provide exercise or energy conservation and which are integrative and provide energy release. A final interview helps to reinforce this learning.

Inventories and Checklists

An adjunct to the interview is the checklist, in which the client is asked to respond on paper to questions regarding interests, hobbies, and desires. Janice Matsutsuyu developed the Interest Checklist.[6] This list has served as a prototype for many others. Another useful inventory is the Activities Configuration,[8] developed by Sandra Watanabe and used to identify the qualitative aspects of how a person uses time to meet his or her needs.

Object History

One useful way of learning about a client's values and the cultural system to which he or she belongs is the object history. It is a flexible evaluation tool, and it may be incorporated into the formal interview or used in informal conversation. Written object histories may also be solicited. It may be done individually or in a group. The object history often helps in establishing rapport between the people participating by permitting them to explore their respective backgrounds and experiences. It may also provide some important clues about the beginnings of the patient's pathology. The object history simply asks the client to try to remember something that was important or that he or she valued at earlier periods of life and to explain why it was important or valued. For example, a young man recalled a bush in front of his house where he went to hide as a child whenever he was scolded. From this statement, one can learn that the world of nature may represent refuge to him. Another person recalled an erector set with which he felt he could build anything mechanical in the whole world. Thus one can learn that mechanical things represent pleasure in accomplishment for him. A young woman recalled a stereo set to which she used to dance. From this, one can learn that social dancing once was important to her. Through the exploration of important nonhuman objects, the therapist may learn both the kinds of things that might be integrative to the client and the ability that the client has had in the past to use the nonhuman world to meet emotional needs.

Summary

Over the years, occupational therapists have tended to develop tests and batteries of tests, check lists, and rating scales as the need arose. These tests helped them to evaluate the needs of their own clients within their own contexts. In recent years, a need for reliable, standardized tools has become evident. Occupational therapists have found that they need to identify and employ their tools that are in general use as part of the arduous process of establishing their legitimacy. At the same time, when occupational therapists use tools for which there are standard protocols and which require additional training or certification (*e.g.*, Sensory Integration and Praxis Tests), it is essential for them to make sure that they are fully qualified to use them.

Evaluation of the client's physical or psychological condition is indicated when a suspected or obvious problem exists. Therapeutic procedures chosen depend on the patient's diagnosis, medical reports, lifestyle, interests, and needs. Observations made by the therapist, checklists previously prepared by the client, and information gained in interviews also suggest the best directions for treatment planning. Evaluation of special areas such as perceptual–motor function, activities of daily living, and/or prevocational evaluation may also be indicated. The remainder of this Unit deals with specific evaluation procedures utilized by occupational therapists in problem identification.

References

1. Allen C: The Performance Status Examination. Presented at the American Occupational Therapy Association Annual Conference, San Francisco, October 1976
2. Benjamin A: The Helping Interview. Boston, Houghton Mifflin, 1974
3. Fidler GS: Talk given at Medical College of Georgia, Augusta, Georgia, 1976
4. Freedman A, Kaplan H, Saddock B: Modern Synopsis of Comprehensive Textbook of Psychiatry/II. p 146. Baltimore, Williams & Wilkins, 1976
5. Gillette N: Occupational therapy and mental health. In Willard HS, Spackman CS (eds.): Occupational Therapy, ed. 4, p 79. Philadelphia, JB Lippincott, 1971
6. Matsutsuyu J: The interest checklist. Am J Occup Ther 23:323, 1969
7. Moorehead L: The occupational history. Am J Occup Ther 23:331, 1969
8. Watanabe S: Activities Configuration. 1968 Regional Institute on the Evaluation Process, Final Report RSA-123-T-68. New York, American Occupational Therapy Association, 1968

Bibliography

American Psychological Association: Standards for Educational and Psychological Tests and Manuals. Washington, DC, 1966

Garrett A: Interviewing: Its Principles and Methods. New York, Family Service Association of America, 1972

Hemphill BJ (ed.): The Evaluative Process in Psychiatric Occupational Therapy. Thorofare, NJ, Charles B Slack, 1982

Hurff J: A play skills inventory. In Reilly M (ed.): Play as Exploratory Learning. Beverly Hills, Sage Publications, 1974

Knox S: A play scale. In Reilly M (ed.): Play as Exploratory Learning. Beverly Hills, Sage Publications, 1974

Llorens L: Projective techniques in occupational therapy. Am J Occup Ther 21:266, 1967

Takata N: The play history. Am J Occup Ther 23:314, 1969

CHAPTER 16

Assessment and Evaluation — Specific Evaluation Procedures

SECTION *1*
Psychological, Psychiatric, and Cognitive Evaluations *Elizabeth G. Tiffany*

Procedures have been developed in occupational therapy to assess psychological, psychiatric, and cognitive functioning. They supplement and specify, in occupational therapy terms, the data gathered by other members of the treatment team. The primary use of these procedures has been in the context of psychiatric treatment, but there are indications for their use in the wider range of primary disabilities because occupational therapy seeks to assess clients in terms of their total functioning. In choosing an assessment procedure, the occupational therapist must be clear about the nature of the data to be collected in terms of the frame of reference for treatment and the ways in which the specific data will relate to the subsequent therapeutic management of the client.

Specific occupational therapy assessment procedures are listed in Table 16-1 (see Section 2 of this chapter). General categories include *projective tests*, such as

the Azima Battery,[2] the Comprehensive Assessment Process,[5] the Goodman Battery,[6] and the Shoemyen Battery[7]; *cognitive assessment*, such as the Allen Cognitive Level Test[1]; and *batteries of tests*, which combine performance tasks, interviews, and checklists, such as the Bay Area Functional Performance Evaluation,[3] the Kohlman Evaluation of Living Skills,[5] and the Comprehensive Occupational Therapy Evaluation.[4]

Projective tests used in occupational therapy exploit the rich potential of tapping into unconscious processes through the use of materials, supplies, and structures that permit free expression. These procedures have proven extremely useful in treatment settings that function on a psychoanalytic basis. Their use outside a psychoanalytically oriented treatment setting should be carefully and deliberately understood or avoided. The potential for free association and symbolic expression is high, but in short-term treatment contexts, the possibility of working productively with the material elicited is limited; and there may be results that are counterproductive for the client.

Tests geared to assessing specific functional areas can be valuable if the material elicited can be considered pivotal to the development of a treatment plan. This is the case in the Allen Cognitive Level Test, an assessment procedure developed to provide data to underlie the development of a therapeutic program based on clear knowledge of the client's cognitive functioning.

Comprehensive batteries have been developed to assess a client's total functional level. Because the data yielded in such batteries are extensive and frequently encompass a range of areas, their usefulness may be optimal in those situations where the treatment program is extensive and where occupational therapy is in a position to provide data that will support a number of different services.

References

1. Allen C: ACL in Occupational Therapy for Psychiatric Diseases: Measurement and Management of Cognitive Disabilities. Boston, Little Brown, 1985
2. Azima FJ: Diseases of the Nervous System. Monograph Suppl. 22, 1961, and in Hemphill BJ (ed): The Evaluative Process in Occupational Therapy. Thorofare, NJ, Slack, 1982
3. Bay Area Functional Performance Evaluation. Palo Alto, Consulting Psychologists Press, 1980
4. Brayman S: The comprehensive occupational therapy evaluation. In Hemphill BJ (ed): The Evaluative Process in Occupational Therapy. Thorofare, NJ, Slack, 1982
5. Ehrenberg F: Comprehensive Assessment Process. In Hemphill BJ (ed): The Evaluative Process in Occupational Therapy. Thorofare, NJ, Slack, 1982
6. Evaskus MG: Goodman Battery. In Hemphill BJ (ed): The Evaluative Process in Occupational Therapy. Thorofare, NJ, Slack, 1982
7. Shoemyen C: Occupational therapy orientation and evaluation: A study of procedure and media. Am J Occup Ther 24:276, 1970

SECTION 2

Motor, Sensory, Perceptual, and Physical Capacities Evaluations *Helen D. Smith*

The following evaluations are done before the patient's first treatment to determine his or her assets and limitations. The results are used to establish patient goals, to develop an effective treatment program, and to determine the functional capabilities of the patient in self-care, leisure, and work skills. The initial test results become the baseline with which subsequent test results (during treatment and at discharge) will be compared to ascertain the patient's progress or lack of progress.

Manual Muscle Testing

Manual muscle testing (MMT) determines the strength of a muscle through manual evaluation (Fig. 16-1). Rating is done by having the patient or client move the involved part through its full range of motion against gravity and then against gravity plus resistance. When the patient or client cannot perform the motion against gravity, the part is positioned to eliminate gravity, and then the muscle power is re-evaluated. Manual muscle testing should not be used when spasticity is present, because the increased tone invalidates the results.

Procedure

1. Explain the procedure to the patient.
2. Check the noninvolved extremity for muscle strength and use as a norm.
3. Check the patient's active and passive range of motion (ROM) before beginning MMT of the involved extremity.
4. Position patient so that the muscle will be tested against gravity (start in Fair position).
5. Stabilize the joint above the one being tested to prevent substitution of incorrect muscles.
6. Have the patient perform the motion and observe the performance. If the patient cannot move the part through the full ROM against gravity, reposition to eliminate gravity.
7. Palpate muscle performing the motion to be sure it is contracting.
8. Apply resistance into the opposite motion of the one being performed. (Resistance should be applied in the middle of the ROM.)
9. Grade the muscle strength.
10. Enter the results of each test, and sign and date the form.

(List continues on page 220)

CLINICAL RECORD—MANUAL MUSCLE EVALUATION

Name _____

Age _____

Diagnosis_____

LEFT   RIGHT

				ACTION	PRIME MOVERS	INNERVATION	SP. C. LEVEL				
			N E C K					N E C K			
				Flexion	STERNOCLEIDOMASTOID	Spinal Accessory.	C 2-3				
				Extension	EXTENSOR GROUP	Spinal Accessory.	C 1-8				
			T R U N K	Flexion	RECTUS ABDOMINUS		T 5-12	T R U N K			
				Rotation	EXTERNAL OBLIQUE		T 5-12				
					INTERNAL OBLIQUE		T 5-12				
				Extension	Thoracic	Post. Rami Spinal Nerves					
					Lumbar						
				Pelvic Elevation	QUADRATUS LUMBORUM		T 12 L 1-3				
			H I P	Flexion	ILIOPSOAS	Femoral	L 2-4	H I P			
					SARTORIUS	Femoral	L 2-4				
				Extension	GLUTEUS MAXIMUS	Inf. Gluteal	L 5 S 1-2				
				Abduction	GLUTEUS MEDIUS	Superior Gluteal	L 4-5 S 1				
					TENSOR FASCIA LATAE	Superior Gluteal	L 4-5 S 1				
				Adduction		Obturator	L 2-4				
				External Rotation			L 3 S 3				
				Internal Rotation			L 4 S 1				
			K N E E	Flexion	BICEPS FEMORIS	Sciatic	L 5 S 1-2	K N E E			
					SEMITENDINOSUS SEMIMEMBRANOSUS	Tibial	L 5 S 1-3				
				Extension	QUADRICEPS	Femoral	L 2-4				
			A N K L E	Inversion	ANTERIOR TIBIALIS	Deep Peroneal	L 5 S 1-2	A N K L E			
					POSTERIOR TIBIALIS	Tibial	L 4-5 S 1-2				
				Eversion	PERONEUS LONGUS	Sup. Peroneal	L 4-5 S 1				
					PERONEUS BREVIS	Sup. Peroneal	L 4-5 S 1				
				Plantar Flexion	GASTROCNEMIUS	Tibial	S 1-2				
					SOLEUS	Tibial	S 1-2				
			T O E S	Flexion	DIGITORUM LONGUS	Tibial	L 5 S 1-2	T O E S			
					DIGITORUM BREVIS	Tibial	L 5 S 1-2				
				Extension	DIGITORUM LONGUS & BREVIS	Deep Peroneal	L 4-5 S 1				
			H A L L U X	Flexion	HALLUCIS LONGUS	Tibial	L 5 S 1-2	H A L L U X			
					HALLUCIS BREVIS	Tibial	L 5 S 1-2				
				Extension	HALLUCIS LONGUS	Deep Peroneal	L 4-5 S 1-2				

KEY:
5	N	NORMAL	Complete range of motion against gravity with full resistance
4	G	GOOD	Complete range of motion against gravity with some resistance
3	F	FAIR	Complete range of motion against gravity
2	P	POOR	Complete range of motion with gravity eliminated
1	T	TRACE	Evidence of slight contractility. No joint motion
0	0	ZERO	No evidence of contractility

Figure 16-1. Manual muscle evaluation form. Printed with permission of Moss Rehabilitation Hospital, Department of Physical Therapy, Philadelphia, PA.

CLINICAL RECORD—MANUAL MUSCLE EVALUATION (Cont.)

Name _____ Age _____ Diagnosis_____

								LEFT / RIGHT		

LEFT ... **RIGHT**

LEFT				ACTION	PRIME MOVERS	INNERVATION	SP. C. LEVEL		RIGHT		
						Examiner's Initials					
						Date					
				Elevation	UPPER TRAPEZIUS	Spinal Accessory	C 3-4	S C A P U L A			
			S C A P U L A	Adduction	MID TRAPEZIUS	Spinal Accessory	C 3-4				
					RHOMBOIDS	Dorsal Scapular	C 4-5				
				Abduction	SERRATUS ANTERIOR	Long Thoracic	C 5-7				
				Depression	LOWER TRAPEZIUS	Spinal Accessory	C 3-4				
				Flexion	ANTERIOR DELTOID	Axillary	C 5-6				
				Abduction	MIDDLE DELTOID	Axillary	C 5-6				
			S H O U L D E R	Horizontal Adduction	PECTORALIS MAJOR Clavicular	Ant. Thoracic	C 5-8	S H O U L D E R			
					Sternal		C 5 T 1				
				Extension	LATISSIMUS DORSI	Thoracodorsal	C 5-8				
				Horizontal Abduction	POST. DELTOID	Axillary	C 5-6				
				External Rotation			C 5-6				
				Internal Rotation			C 5-8				
				Flexion	BICEPS	Musculocutaneous	C 5-6				
			E L B O W		BRACHIALIS	Musculocutaneous	C 5-6	E L B O W			
					BRACHIORADIALIS	Radial	C 6				
				Extension	TRICEPS	Radial	C 5-8				
			FORE ARM	Supination	SUPINATOR	Radial	C 6	FORE ARM			
				Pronation	PRONATOR TERES	Median	C 6				
			W R I S T	Flexion	CARPI RADIALIS	Median	C 6	W R I S T			
					CARPI ULNARIS	Ulnar	C 8				
				Extension	CARPI RADIALIS L. & BREV.	Radial	C 6-7				
					CARPI ULNARIS	Radial	C 7				
				Flexion MP joint	LUMBRICALES 1.2	Median	C 7-8				
					3.4	Ulnar	C 8				
				Prox. IP joint	DIG. SUBLIMUS	Median	C 7 T 1				
			F I N G E R S	Dist. IP joint	DIG. PROFUNDUS 1.2	Median	C 8 T 1	F I N G E R S			
					3.4	Ulnar	C 8 T 1				
				Extension	DIG. EXT. COMMUNIS	Radial	C 6				
				Adduction	INTEROSSEI	Ulnar	C 8 T 1				
				Abduction	INTEROSSEI	Ulnar	C 8 T 1				
				Abduction, digit 4	DIGITI QUINTI	Ulnar	C 8				
				Opposition, digit 4	OPPONENS DIGITI QUINTI	Ulnar	C 8				
				Flexion MP joint	POLL. BREV.	Median	C 6-8				
				IP joint	POLL. L.	Median	C 8 T 1				
				Extension MP joint	POLL. BREV.	Radial	C 7				
			T H U M B	IP joint	POLL. L.	Radial	C 7	T H U M B			
				Adduction	ADDUCTOR POLLICIS	Ulnar	C 8				
				Abduction	POLL. L.	Radial	C 7				
					POLL. BREV.	Median	C 6-7				
				Opposition	OPPONENS POLLICIS	Median	C 6-8 T 1				

11. In order to maintain reliability and accuracy, the same therapist should repeat this test on the client at the same time of day.

Grading Scale*

N   Normal: Complete ROM against gravity with full resistance

G   Good: Complete ROM against gravity with moderate resistance

G- Good minus: Complete ROM against gravity with less than moderate resistance

F+ Fair plus: Complete ROM against gravity with minimal resistance

F   Fair: Complete ROM against gravity

P+ Poor plus: Complete ROM with gravity eliminated, takes minimal resistance

P   Poor: Complete ROM with gravity eliminated

P- Poor minus: Less than complete ROM with gravity eliminated

T   Trace: Evidence of contractility on palpation; no joint motion

0   Zero: No evidence of contractility.

Joint Range of Motion — Goniometry

To discuss joint movement, it is necessary to understand the terminology used to describe these motions.

Terminology

Anatomic position. The body in an upright, standing position, face forward, upper extremities at the side, forearms supinated, and palms facing forward

Flexion. A decrease in the angle of a joint as it is being moved

Extension. A return from flexion

Hyperextension. A movement beyond extension and past anatomic position

Abduction. A movement away from the midline of the body

Adduction. A movement toward the midline of the body and a return from abduction

Internal rotation. A rotation toward the midline

External rotation. A rotation away from the midline

Supination. With elbow positioned at 90°, the palm is turned up

Pronation. With elbow positioned at 90°, the palm is turned down

Ulnar deviation. In anatomic position, a movement at the wrist toward the midline

Radial deviation. In anatomic position, a movement at the wrist away from the midline

Circumduction. A combination of movements: flexion, abduction, hyperextension, adduction, and extension

Inversion. Turning the sole of the foot toward the midline

Eversion. Turning the sole of the foot away from the midline

Joint range of motion (ROM) is measured in both upper and lower extremities to determine the existing freedom of motion at a joint. This is done either passively (part moved by an outside force) or actively (part moved by muscle contraction, *i.e.,* muscle power.) The causes of decreased ROM can be spasticity, joint disease, injury, muscle weakness, pain, edema, or bone block. A difference between active and passive ROM in the same joint usually indicates muscle weakness.

Types of Motion

Passive motion is movement performed by an outside force. No muscle contraction can be seen or palpated. *Active motion* is movement performed independently by the individual.

Measurement Tool

The goniometer (Fig. 16-2) is the tool most frequently used to measure joint motion. Other methods used, either alone or in conjunction with the goniometer, are a ruler to measure distance (used especially in hand evaluation); photographs of the client performing the motion(s); outline drawings—for example, tracing the fingers while in abduction; and hand prints made by inking the hands on a stamp pad and pressing them on paper.

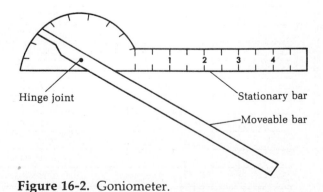

Figure 16-2. Goniometer.

---

* See Figure 16-1 on page 218 for sample form for manual muscle testing.

Procedure—180° Scale

1. Explain the procedure to the patient.
2. Check the noninvolved extremity for active and passive ROM. If no decreased motion is observed, it is permissible to record as "within normal limits" (WNL).
3. When measuring the involved extremity, use anatomic position as the starting position when possible. The starting position is recorded as 0°. Some exceptions to starting in anatomic position are shoulder internal and external rotation and forearm supination and pronation.
4. Demonstrate the desired motion to the patient.
5. Prevent substitution by positioning and stabilizing the joint proximal to the joint being measured.
6. Apply the goniometer to the lateral side of the joint. Some exceptions are forearm supination and hip rotation.
7. Align the axis of the goniometer with the joint axis.
8. Align the stationary bar parallel to the long axis of the stationary bone.
9. Align the movable bar parallel to the long axis of the movable bone
10. Have the patient perform the desired motion. Place the goniometer. Measure both the starting position and the maximum end range; this indicates the arc through which the part moves, thus measuring the freedom of motion at the joint. To determine passive ROM, carefully move the joint through its maximum passive range.
11. Record both the active and the passive degrees of motion on a ROM form (Figs. 16-3 and 16-4). For example, 0° to 95° indicates a limitation in flexion; 35° to 95° indicates a limitation in both flexion and extension.
12. Indicate if any pain, swelling, or spasticity is present.
13. Sign and date ROM form.
14. To maintain reliability and accuracy, the same therapist should measure the client using the same method at the same time of day.

Sensory Testing

Sensory testing is performed when the therapist suspects a sensory problem. A patient or client with neurological disease or damage should always be tested for sensory loss. The following areas are usually examined: tactile sense, temperature, proprioception (position sense), and stereognosis.

General Procedure

1. Explain the procedure to the patient. Ask for feedback to be sure instructions are understood. Give instructions when patient's eyes are not occluded.
2. Occlude the client's vision with a shield such as a file folder, screen, or cut-out box.
3. Sit opposite the patient.
4. Test the nonaffected area first to be sure the patient understands your instructions.
5. Apply stimuli from distal to proximal, both dorsal and ventral surfaces in an unpredictable pattern.
6. Ask patient if he or she was touched. (If aphasic, the patient can nod head.)
7. Enter test results on specified form, date, and sign.

Specific Procedures

1. *Light touch:* Lightly touch the patient's skin with cotton, camel's hair brush, or fingertip or use the Weinstein–Semmes monofilaments.
2. *Deep touch:* Firmly touch the patient's skin with cotton swab or fingertip.
3. *Temperature:* Touch the patient's skin with test tubes of hot and cold water. (Wipe test tubes of excess water.)
4. *Pain:* Touch the patient's skin with large safety pin or opened paper clip for sharp or dull response.
5. *Tactile localization:* Touch the patient's skin with fingertip and ask patient to place his or her finger on the spot touched.
6. *Two-point discrimination:* Touch the patient's skin with two points applied simultaneously. Decrease the distance between the points until the stimulus is felt as one point. Occasionally, touch patient's skin with one point. A two-point aesthesiometer is used to apply the stimulus.
7. *Proprioceptive or position sense* (awareness of position in space: Hold the extremity being tested at bony prominences to avoid excess tactile input and move the specific joint into position. Ask the patient either to imitate the position with the other extremity or to describe the position.
8. *Kinesthesia or movement sense:* Hold the extremity being tested at bony prominences to avoid excess tactile input. Move the joint being tested either up or down. Ask the patient if the part was moved up or down.
9. *Stereognosis* (ability to recognize the shape of familiar objects by touch): Familiar objects of various sizes, shapes, and weights are placed individually into the palm of the client, who is to indicate what object was placed in the hand. If the object cannot be manipulated, the therapist manipulates the object, making sure contact is made with the fingers and thumb. If the client cannot communicate verbally, an alternative is to have him/her point to a duplicate object. Familiar objects such as

(Text continues on page 226)

Joint Range of Motion: Upper Extremity

Patient:		Age:		Diagnosis:		

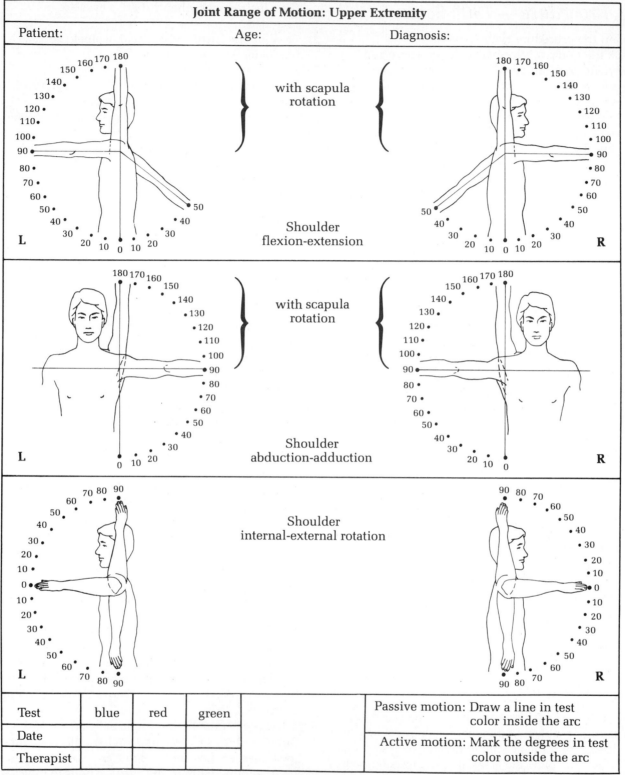

Test	blue	red	green		Passive motion: Draw a line in test color inside the arc
Date					Active motion: Mark the degrees in test color outside the arc
Therapist					

Figure 16-3. Form for measurement of joint range of motion, upper extremity. Redrawn and printed with the permission of Moss Rehabilitation Hospital, Department of Physical Therapy, Philadelphia, PA.

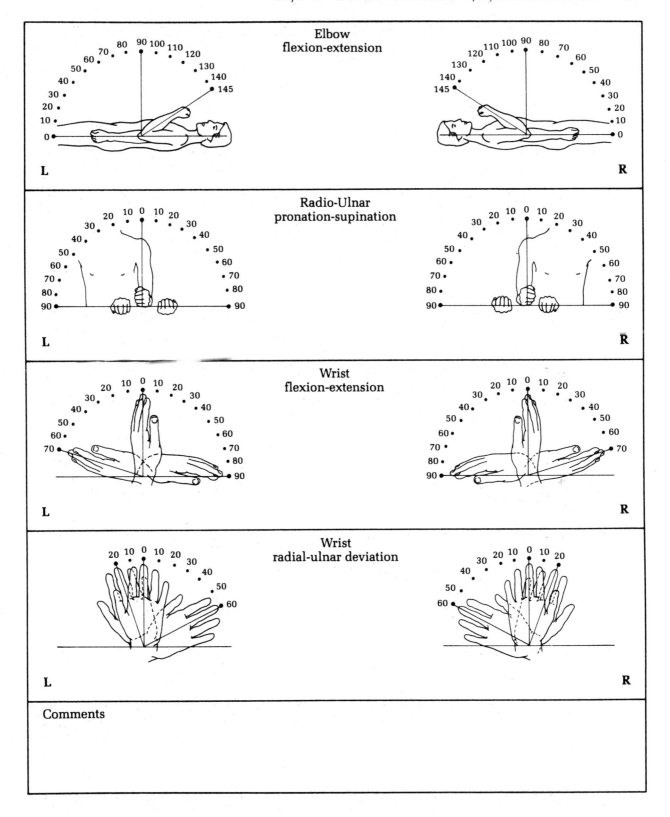

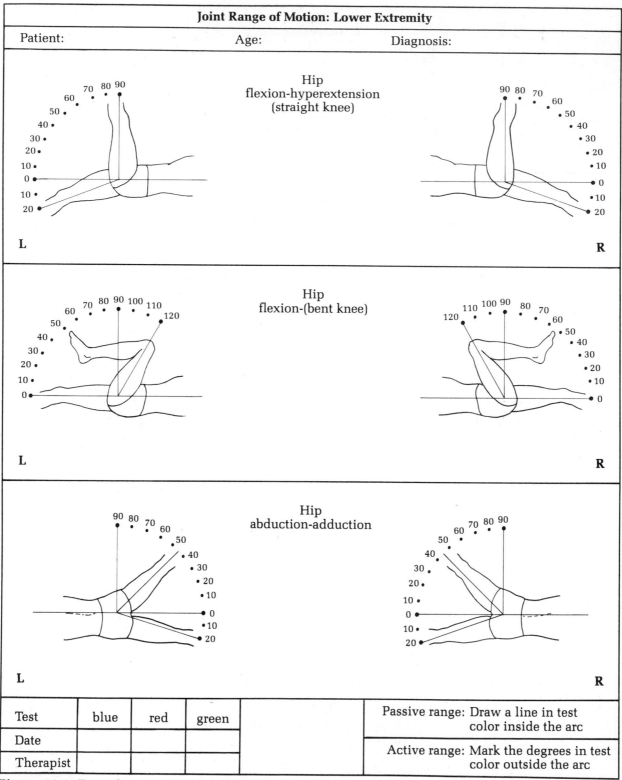

Test	blue	red	green		Passive range: Draw a line in test
Date					color inside the arc
Therapist					Active range: Mark the degrees in test color outside the arc

Figure 16-4. Form for measurement of joint range of motion, lower extremity. Redrawn and printed with the permission of Moss Rehabilitation Hospital, Department of Physical Therapy, Philadelphia, PA.

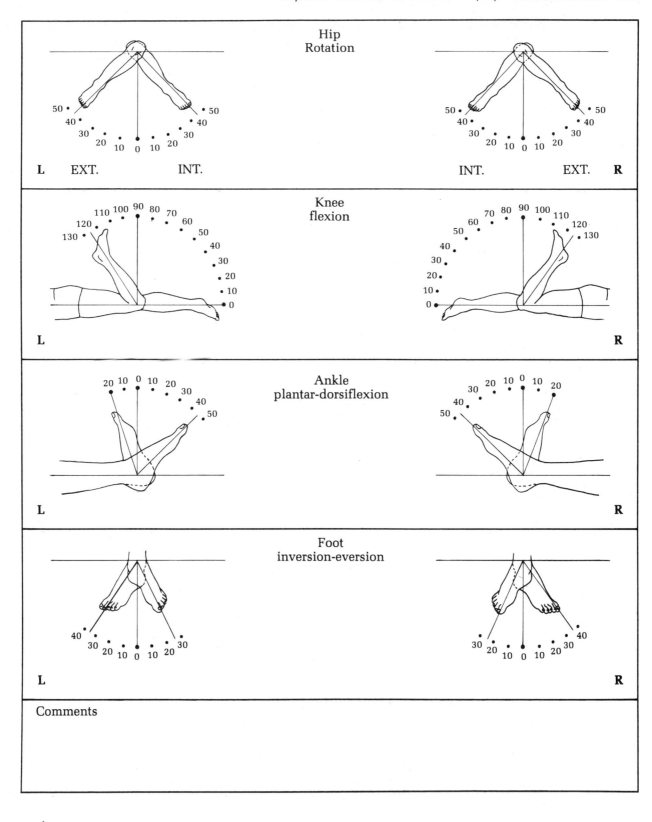

Comments

a coin, key, pencil, or safety pin are examples of objects that are frequently used.

Sample Rating Scale

Intact—A quick, correct response
Impaired—An incorrect or delayed response
Absent—No response

Coordination

Coordination is the working together of muscles or groups of muscles to perform a task. Both gross and fine coordination should be evaluated by the therapist. The tests listed in Table 16-1 under the heading Manual Dexterity and Motor Function Tests are recommended. All are standardized, and most have reliability and validity information. When these tests are not available, a task such as tossing and catching a bean bag or ball or playing a board game will assist the therapist in judging the patient's coordination.

Cognition

Cognition is the mental process by which knowledge is acquired; it is the ability to think and reason. Following disease or injury in which impairment of cognitive functioning is suspected, the following abilities should be evaluated:
1. To follow simple or complex instructions
2. To carry over learned skills from one day to the next
3. To attend to a task (attention span)
4. To follow numerous steps in a process
5. To understand cause and effect
6. To problem solve
7. To concentrate
8. To perform in a logical sequence
9. To organize parts into a meaningful whole
10. To interpret signs and symbols
11. To read
12. To compute

This list of cognitive abilities is not complete. Therapists use a wide range of tests, from short mental-status tests to lengthy and detailed tests. Some of these are standardized, but many have been developed by therapists for use in their work settings.

Hand and Pinch Strength Testing

Hand strength is measured by the patient gripping a dynamometer. The dial is calibrated in either pounds or kilograms, and the indicator will stay at the highest reading until reset manually. An added feature in some dynamometers is an adjustable hand grip.

Pinch strength is measured on a pinch gauge. The dial is calibrated in pounds, and it measures finger prehension force. A quick reading of the dial must be made if the indicator does not stay at the highest reading point. Both the dynamometer and the pinch gauge can be purchased through suppliers of rehabilitation equipment.

It is recommended that standardized positioning and instructions be used for testing, as recommended by Mathiowetz and associates in their 1984 study of grip and pinch strength reliability and validity.[8] A pinch gauge and a Jamar dynamometer were used. The authors used the American Society of Hand Therapists' recommendations for standardized positioning and established procedures and instructions for each test of strength (grip strength, palmar pinch, lateral pinch, and two-point tip pinch). The authors believe that the high inter-rater and test–retest reliability were achieved by using standardized instructions and positioning (see Appendix I).

Endurance Testing

The patient or client is often tested for the ability to reach or maintain the energy output necessary to perform an activity. This is especially important in activities of daily living, homemaker retraining, and work-related activities. The amount of work and the time required to do the work are carefully noted, and work output and time are carefully increased according to the tolerance of the client until either the desired level is reached or the client reaches his or her maximum.

The Physical Capacities Evaluation*

In writing a summary of physical capacities, one should summarize the client's ability, endurance, speed, safety, and strength in all activities tested. The activities that the client was unable to perform should be listed, and it can be stated why he or she was unable to perform each activity. The length of time the test took, the frequency of rest periods, the appliances used, the amount of pain or discomfort, and the client's overall work endurance should also be stated. The client's emotional reactions,

(Text continues on page 239)

---

* This evaluation procedure is based on the physical capacities requirements of the *Dictionary of Occupational Titles* (DOT), US Department of Labor. Developed and reprinted with the permission of Susan L. Smith, Professional Occupational Therapy Services, Inc., Metairie, LA.

Table 16-1. *Sampling of Tests Used in Evaluation**

Name	Type	Description	Features	Source
Manual Dexterity and Motor Function Tests				
Jebsen–Taylor Hand Function Test[7]	Individual test to evaluate functional capabilities	Seven subtests measure major aspects of hand function often used in activities of daily living. Equipment needed: stopwatch	Standardized tasks, objective measurements taken with stopwatch. Norms (360 normal subjects) included. Easy to administer. Test equipment and material are either made or easily available. Subtests are writing, card turning, picking up small objects, simulated feeding, stacking checkers, picking up large light objects, picking up large heavy objects. Time: 12–15 min. Age: child–adult	Jebsen R, et al, Arch Phys Med Rehab 50:311, 1969 Sand P, Am J Occup Ther 28:87, 1974
Purdue Pegboard	Individual test to aid selection of employees for industrial jobs requiring manipulative dexterity	Measures both gross movements of arms, hands, and fingers and fingertip dexterity Equipment: stopwatch	Two operations: rapid placing of pins in pegboard and assembly of pins, washers, and collars. Norms for male industrial applicants, veterans, college students, female college students, and industrial applicants Time: 12–15 min. Has face validity, low acceptable reliability	Science Research Associates, 259 East Erie St, Chicago, IL 60611
Minnesota Rate of Manipulation Test	Individual test of manual dexterity	Designed to measure dexterity of individuals grade 7 to adult	Five operations resulting in five scores: placing, turning, displacing, 1-hand turning and placing, and 2-hand turning and placing. Form board used—wells and round disks Time: 30–50 min.	American Guidance Service, Publishers Bldg. Circle Pines, MN 55014.

(continued)

Table 16-1. *(continued)*

Manual Dexterity and Motor Function Tests (continued)

Name	Type	Description	Features	Source
The Lincoln–Oseretsky Motor Development Scale (Revised Oseretsky Tests of Motor Proficiency)	Scale of motor development. Individual test for hand and arm movements measuring speed, dexterity, coordination, and rhythm	First published in Russian, 1923. Portuguese adaptation, 1943. English translation, 1946. Sloan adaptation, 1948 Items sample variety of motor performances	Items arranged in order of difficulty. Instructions concise, scoring is specific. Correlations of each item score with age and tentative percentile norms. Separate and combined scores given for sexes. Validated in relation to changes with age	CH Stoelting Co, 424 N Hohman Ave, Chicago, IL 60624
Pennsylvania Bi-Manual Work Sample	Individual test of bimanual dexterity: finger dexterity of both hands, gross movements of both arms, eye–hand coordination, and indication of use of both hands	Selection of a bolt with one hand and a nut with the other, assembling the two objects and placing in a receiving hole. Norms given for age, sex, blind, and partially blind	First part—assembly of 100 nuts and bolts. Second part—disassembly of nuts and bolts. Two scores—one for each operation Time: 10 min assembly and 5 min disassembly. Reliable. Validity not indicated	Educational Test Bureau, American Guidance Service, Publishers Bldg, Circle Pines, MN 55014
Crawford Small Parts Dexterity Test	Individual measure of fine eye–hand coordination and manipulation of small hand tools	10-inch-square board. Round wells for parts to be manipulated (*i.e.*, pins, collars, and screws); a metal plate containing 42 unthreaded and 42 threaded holes; two metal trays beneath the plate to receive the pins and screws Tools: Tweezers and small screwdriver	*Part I*—Examinee picks up pin with tweezers, inserts in small hole in metal plate, and places collar over it using preferred hand. *Part II*—Examinee picks up screw, starts it in threaded hole with the fingers, then screws through metal plate with screwdriver, using both hands in operation. Six practice trials. Scored by time required Time: *Part I*—5 min *Part II*—10 min High reliability Face validity	Psychological Corporation, 304 East 45th St, New York, NY 10017

Test	Purpose	Description	Comments	Source
Box and Block Test	Individual test of manual dexterity	Test has been used to measure gross manual dexterity and as a prevocational test for handicapped people. Test is timed. Subjects pick up one block at a time and place in second compartment. Equipment: Stopwatch, boxes; 150 colored wooden cubes, 1-inch square[8]	Normative data for adults, adults with neuromuscular involvement, and normal children 7–9 years old. Standardized instructions; reliability and validity data included	Mathiowetz V, et al, Am J Occup Ther 39:386, 1985

Developmental Tests

Test	Purpose	Description	Comments	Source
Bayley Scales of Infant Development	Individual scales of infant development	A three-part evaluation of a child's development in relation to other children of the same age. Scales include mental, motor, and behavior ratings.	Well standardized. No data on validity of motor scale or predictive validity of mental scale. Reliability is satisfactory. Time: 45–90 min Age: 2–30 mo	Psychological Corporation, 304 East 45th St, New York, NY 10017
Brazelton Behavioral Assessment Scale	Individual score of infant interactive behavior	Evaluates the neonate's reaction to stimuli and responses to the environment	Best performance is scored. Photographs of testing procedures are included. Time: 20–30 min. Research in progress on test reliability and validity	JB Lippincott, East Washington Square, Philadelphia, PA 19105 Four training films: Educational Development Corp, 8 Mifflin Place, Cambridge, MA 02138
Brigance Screen	Individual and group screening test for kindergarten and first grade	Adapted from and cross-referenced to readiness section of the Brigance Inventory of Basic Skills and Inventory of Early Development. Identifies children needing referrals to special services and those needing further assessment; for program planning	Small group screening, individual screening added 2 or 3 min to the time. Cost for manual $19.95; pads of 30 forms 25 cents per child. Scoring—one scale, 100 points. Rank words to score. Time: 10–12 min	Curriculum Associates, 5 Esquire Rd., N., Billerica, MA 01862

(continued)

Table 16-1. *(continued)*

Name	Type	Description	Features	Source
Developmental Tests (continued)				
Callier–Azusa Scale (1975)	Individual developmental scale for assessment of deaf, blind, and multihandicapped children	Designed to be used in a classroom, this scale is divided into five subscales: motor development, perceptual development, daily living skills, language development, and socialization. Subscales are made up of sequential steps describing developmental milestones.	Examples of behavior are provided for many items. (Behaviors were observed on deaf–blind children.) Lists criteria Observation to extend over a 2-week period Reliability information available from author	Robert Stillman, PhD, Callier Center for Communication Disorders, University of Texas/Dallas, 1966 Inwood Rd, Dallas, TX 75235
Denver Developmental Screening Test	Individual formalized observations of normal developmental behavior of infants and children	A screening tool for detecting infants and children with developmental delays. Areas evaluated: gross motor, fine motor, language, and personal–social development	Standardized on children age 2 wk – 6.4 yr in Denver. High percentage came from professional families. Inexpensive, quick, easy to use. Uses common items. Manual and scoring guide are clear. Reliability and validity vary with age groups	Ladoca Project and Publishing Foundation, E 51st Av & Lincoln St, Denver, CO 80216
Developmental Screening 0–5 Years	Individual screening inventory of abnormal development	History and observation ratings in five areas: adaptive, gross motor, fine motor, language, and personal–social (Selected items used from the Gesell Developmental Schedules)	Age: 1 yr – 18 mo. No reliability data available Testing time: 5–30 min	Knobloch H, et al, Pediatrics 38:1095, 1966
The Gesell Developmental Tests	Individual scale of developmental levels	Scale of behavioral observations by age level (5–10 yrs) of the mental growth of the child to aid in determining school readiness	Qualitative measure of motor development, adaptive behavior, and personal–social behavior. Present functional level evaluated Time: 20–30 min	Programs for Education, Box 85, Lumberville, PA 18933

Sensory Integration Tests

Test	Purpose	Description	Comments	Source
Developmental Test of Visual–Motor Integration (Berry K)	Used to detect problems in visual–motor integration in children	Subject is presented with 24 geometric forms arranged in order of increasing difficulty, which are copied into a test booklet	Standardized test that can be group administered. Emphasis is on preschool group. Directions are clear. Separate age norms for each sex. Two forms: ages 2–15 (long form), ages 2–8 (short form). Reliability and validity information does not appear complete. Time: 10 min	Follett Educational Corporation, 1010 W Washington Blvd, Chicago, IL 60607
Marianne Frostig Developmental Test of Visual Perception	Individual and group test measuring visual perception	Five subtests of visual perception: eye–motor coordination, figure-ground, constancy of shape, position in space, and spatial relations	Five areas relate to preschool and early elementary academic performance. Group administration possible. Norms for ages 3–8 yr. Reliability appears adequate. Validity information does not appear to be complete. Time: Individual, 30–45 min; group, 40–60 min	Consulting Psychologists Press, 577 College Ave, Palo Alto, CA 94306
The Imitation of Gestures: A Technique for Studying the Body Schema and Praxis of Children 3 to 6 Years of Age	Individual test of perceptual–motor function	Berges J, Lezine I: Clin Develop Med No. 18. Spastic Society Medical Education and Information Unit. London, W Heinemann Medical Books, 1965		Medical Market Research, 227 South 6th St, Philadelphia, PA 19105
Perceptual Forms Test	Individual and group testing for perceptual and readiness evaluation and training	Two parts: perceptual forms test and incomplete forms in which subject is required to complete partial drawings. Visual–motor coordination is required. Used to identify children who might have problems in school achievement	Geometric forms are copied. Templates are used. Formal scoring on the perceptual form test but not on the incomplete forms. Age: 5–8 yr. Reliability and validity information not complete	Winter Haven Lions Research Foundation, PO Box 111, Winter Haven, FL 33880

(continued)

Table 16-1. *(continued)*

Name	Type	Description	Features	Source
Sensory Integration Tests (continued)				
The Purdue Perceptual Motor Survey	Individual test of perceptual motor abilities	Identifies children with perceptual–motor problems that could interfere with learning of academic skills. Eleven subtests: rhythmic writing, walking board, jumping, identification of body parts, imitation of movements, obstacle course, chalkboard, Kraus–Weber, angels-in-the-snow, ocular pursuits, developmental drawing	Test based on theory. Easy to administer, and instructions and scoring keys are adequate. Reliability and validity information are said to be good. Age: 6–10 yr. Time: 20 min	Charles E Merill Publishing, 1300 Alum Creek Dr, Columbus, OH 43216
Sensory Integration and Praxis Tests				
Figure–Ground Perception Motor Accuracy Postrotary Nystagmus Space Visualization Postural Praxis Finger Identification Graphesthesia Standing and Walking Balance Design Copying Bilateral Motor Coordination Manual Form Perception Localization of Tactile Stimuli Praxis on Verbal Command Constructional Praxis Sequential Praxis Oral Praxis		No specific information available at time of publication	Tests undergoing revision	Western Psychological Services, 12031 Wilshire Blvd, Los Angeles, CA 90025
Illinois Test of Psycholinguistic Abilities (ITPA)	Individual test of cognitive functioning	A test of language perception and short-term memory abilities to assist in diagnosing learning problems	Visual and auditory channels are used for input. Vocal and motor channels are used for output. Norms on children from slightly above average homes, age 2–10 yr. Reliability said to be moderate Time: 45–50 min	University of Illinois Press, Urbana, IL 61801

Intelligence Tests

Test			
Goodenough–Harris Drawing Test	Individual or group test of conceptual and intellectual maturity	Tests accuracy of observation and development of conceptual thinking. The subject draws a picture of a man, woman, and a self-portrait.	A simple nonverbal test. Norms were established on children age 5–15 yr from four major geographical areas representative of various occupations. Reliability and validity information are said to be adequate. Time: 10–15 min Age: 3–15 yr	Harcourt Brace Jovanovich, 757 3rd Ave, New York, NY 10017
Peabody Picture Vocabulary	Individual test of verbal intelligence	Untimed test that estimates verbal intelligence by measuring hearing vocabulary. Subject chooses one of four pictures after hearing a word.	No reading required. Standardized age range 2.5–18 yr. Content and item validity are good, and reliability is said to be adequate.	American Guidance Service, Publishers Bldg, Circle Pines, MN 55014

Psychological Tests

Test			
Adaptive Behavior Scales	Individual scale assessing adaptive behavior of the mentally retarded and emotionally maladjusted individual	Evaluation of subject's effectiveness to cope with environmental demands. Twenty-four areas of social and personal behavior are covered.	Easy to administer but hand scoring is complex. Norms based on institutionalized retardates beginning at age 3. Has face validity but no data on reliability. Time: Children, 20–25 min; adults, 25–30 min	American Association on Mental Deficiency, 5201 Connecticut Ave NW, Washington, DC 20015
Vineland Social Maturity Scale	Individual performance scale of social maturity	Behavioral observations of self-help, self-direction, locomotion, occupation, communication, and social relations. Provides an evaluation of subject's social competency	Useful tool for evaluating mentally retarded individual. Includes 117 items Age: birth to maturity Time: 20–30 min	Educational Test Bureau, American Guidance Service, Publishers Bldg, Circle Pines, MN 55014

(continued)

Table 16-1. *(continued)*

Psychological Tests (continued)

Name	Type	Description	Features	Source
Bender-Gestalt Test	Individual or group projective evaluation of personality dynamics	Measures nonverbal gestalt functioning in perceptual–motor area. The subject copies designs.	Evaluates perceptual–motor functioning, neurologic impairment, and maladjustment. Scoring system quantified and objective. Most validity research done on scoring system. No data on reliability Time: 10 min Age: 4 yr and over	American Orthopsychiatric Association, 1790 Broadway, New York, NY 10019
Minnesota Multiphasic Personality Inventory (MMPI)	Individual and group nonprojective test measuring psychopathology	Assesses the type and degree of emotional dysfunction in adults	Spanish edition is available. Normative and reliability data have not been changed since 1951. Time: Individual, 30–90 min; group, 40–90 min for complete form and 40–75 min for short version	The Psychological Corporation, 304 East 45th St, New York, NY 10017
Nurses' Observation Scale for Inpatient Evaluation (NOSIE)	Nonprojective individual rating scale measuring behavioral status and change	Highly sensitive ward behavior scale that assesses subject's status and change over time	Seven scores: competence, social interest, personal neatness, irritability, manifest psychosis, and retardation. Easy to use. Norms based on adult male schizophrenics age 55–69. Validity and reliability appear to be adequate. Time: 3–5 min	Behavioral Arts Center, 90 Calla Ave, Floral Park, New York, NY 11001
Activity configuration	Pencil and paper schedule with clear legend	Client lists hourly activities for a typical week with personal assessments of the nature of the activity (recreation, social, work, etc), autonomy, pleasure, and adequacy. Especially useful with clients who are depressed	Administration should be accompanied by discussion. Promotes consideration of personal priorities, time management	Watanabe S: AOTA 1968 Regional Institute on the Eval. Process. Final Report RSA 123-T-68 NY, 1968, pp 46–47

Adolescent Role Assessment	Interview—individual or group administration	Semistructured dialogue with specific rating criteria to assess quality of childhood play, family interactions, chores, school skills, work attitudes, and fantasy	Specific questions to be explored with specific rating criteria so that role expectations may be consistent with values and skills	Black M. Am J Occup Ther 30:73, 1976
Allen Cognitive Level (ACL)	Individual cognitive performance	Measures cognitive level through performance of prescribed tasks	Clearly delineated administration. Provides baseline for establishment of task expectations and ongoing monitoring of treatment effectiveness	Allen C. UCLA Med Ctr, Los Angeles
Azima Battery	Projective battery	Assesses mood organization, organization of drives, ego organization, and object relations through client's performance in drawing, finger painting, use of clay and plastic media	Classic psychoanalytically based assessment, first presented in 1961 / Valuable in treatment planning detecting change, prognosis, effects of drug administration / Heuristic considerations with regard to research, use in family therapy (comparative batteries)	Azima FJ: Diseases of the Nervous System, Monograph Suppl. 22, 1961, and in Hemphill BJ (ed) The Evaluative Process in Occupational Therapy. Thorofare NJ, Slack, 1982
Bay Area Functional Performance Evaluation (BAFPE)	Evaluation Battery	Assesses functional performance in ADL with psychiatric clients / Two subtests—Task Oriented Assessment (TOA) and Social Interaction Scale (SIS) / Use of interview, structured and projective tasks, observation	Clear directions for assessment of ADL, motor skills, sensory motor function, sensation, endurance, cognition, appearance / Rating scale and directions, research implications, and video tape available	Consulting Psychologists Press, 577 College Ave, Palo Alto, CA 94306

(continued)

Table 16-1. *(continued)*

Psychological Tests (continued)

Name	Type	Description	Features	Source
Comprehensive Assessment Process	Projective assessment process; includes structured interviews and group activities	Administration of initial interview and follow-up interviews, ADL questionnaire, group activity sessions, to yield observations of grooming, levels of awareness, orientation, affect, motor level, self-esteem, attendance, self-direction, task investment, independence, concentration, following instructions, problem solving, decision making, frustration tolerance, work tolerance, planning, workmanship, leadership, and more	Designed to evaluate overall client behaviors as basis for individualized plans in short-term, acute-care psychiatric treatment facilities Indications for further research	Ehrenberg F, in Hemphill, BJ (ed): The Evaluative Process in Occupational Therapy. Thorofare NJ, Slack, 1982
Comprehensive Occupational Therapy Evaluation (COTE)	Evaluation scale	Assesses 25 identified behaviors in three areas: (1) general, (2) interpersonal, and (3) task Provides guide to observation, interview, tasks, and recording methods	For use in adult acute psychiatric setting to enhance observation and reduce subjectivity in reporting, facilitate team communication; enables therapist to report a large volume of comprehensive and pertinent information quickly, in consistent format with defined terminology Grid with space for daily recording for 16 days	Brayman SF, Kirby T, in Hemphill BJ (ed): The Evaluative Process in Occupational Therapy. Thorofare NJ, Slack, 1982
Goodman Battery	Projective battery	Evaluates cognitive and affective ego assets and deficits affecting function. Tasks presented represent decreasing structure—copying to freehand drawing to clay task	Very specific instructions retest environment, timing, and so forth Rating scales Further research implications	Evaskus MG, in Hemphill, BJ (ed): The Evaluative Process in Occupational Therapy. Thorofare NJ, Slack, 1982

Assessment	Method	Description	Comments	Reference
Interest CheckList	Interview with pencil and paper; checklist	Eighty activities listed with space for client to check interest level (casual, strong, no) Gives indications of client's experience and interests	Administration should be accompanied by discussion Classic checklist, much adapted and widely used	Matsutsuyu J, Am J Occup Ther 3:327, 1969
Kohlman Evaluation of Living Skills (KELS)	Structured interview with tasks	Assesses psychiatric clients' skills in self-care, safety and health, money management, transportation and telephone, work, and leisure	Clear directions for observation, recording, and implications for community living and/or further treatment Protocol Videotape available	Health Sciences Learning Resources Center T 281 SB-56, Univ of Washington, Seattle, WA 98195
Lifestyle Performance Profile	Individual interview	Assesses performance skills and skill levels as determined by age, culture, and biology in the areas of self-care and maintenance; self-needs—extrinsic gratification; service to others	Data gathered yields information to aid description of skill deficits and strengths, sociocultural expectations for performance, lifestyle performance balance, nature of family, sociocultural, economic, and environmental resources or barriers, sensorimotor, cognitive, psychological, and social skill deficits/strengths, individual characteristics, and interests that shape response	Fidler GS, in Hemphill, BJ (ed): The Evaluative Process in Occupational Therapy. Thorofare NJ, Slack, 1982
Schroeder Block S-I Evaluation	Comprehensive assessment tools	Assesses S-I in adult psychiatric clients using specific testing procedures and observation	Definite procedures, observations, scoring, work sheets, and summary sheets required Research implications	Schroeder CV, Block MP, Campbell ET, Stowell M: Adult Psychiatric S-I Eval. San Diego VA SBC Research Assoc, La Jolla, CA 1979
Shoemeyen Battery	Projective battery (one to four clients)	Uses four activities: mosaic tile, clay figure, fingerpainting, sculpture—media and interview—discussion to gain information about attitudes, mood, cognitive and social skills, dexterity, attention, suggestibility, independence, and creativity	Information gained to aid in team treatment planning—to promote relatively natural therapist–client relationship and collaborative planning and implementation of treatment	Shoemeyen C, and in Hemphill BJ (ed.): The Evaluative Process in Occupational Therapy. Thorofare NJ, Slack, 1982 Shands Teaching Hospital, U of Florida, Gainesville, FL

(continued)

Table 16-1. *(continued)*

Name	Type	Description	Features	Source
Stress Tools				
Holmes–Rahe Life Change Index	Individual evaluation of number of major life changes in past year	Self-assessment of stress level produced by major life changes	Age: adult	Holmes TH, Rahe RH, J Psychosomat Res 11:213, 1967
Type A Behavior Scale	Individual evaluation of number of Type A behavior traits in personality	Self-assessment of stress level produced by Type A behavior traits	Age: adult	AIM for Health, PO Box 182, Hanover St Sta, Boston, MA 02113 in study guide for slide–tape program "Stress"
Stress Audit Questionnaire	Individual evaluation of patterns of stressors	Self-assessment of stress level produced by social and environmental stressors	Age: adult	Miller LH, Ross R, Cohen SI, Bostonia Magazine, 56:4, 5, 39–54, 1982
Other				
Parachek Geriatric Rating Scale	Geriatric rating scale	Designed to help in planning treatment programs for the geriatric patient. Areas rated: physical capabilities, self-care skills, social-inter-action skills	Items arranged and rated in developmental sequence. Treatment manual attached Time: 3–5 min once a month	Greenroom Publishing, 8512 East Virginia, Scottsdale, AZ 85257

* Table developed from Buros OK (ed): The Third–Eighth *Mental Measurement Yearbooks*. Highland Park, NJ, Gryphon Press, 1949–1978.

including his or her emotional tolerance, ability to follow directions, appearance, and cooperativeness are also important. An example of a physical capacities evaluation form is presented in the displayed material.

Standardized Tests

Standardized tests of hand function, motor ability, intelligence, learning disability, development, sensorimotor ability, and personality have been incorporated into Table 16-1. Most information was obtained from Buros in *Mental Measurement Yearbooks,*[1-6] with additional material from sources indicated in the table. The tests mentioned are referred to in various chapters of this book. This table is not intended to be a complete listing of all tests used by occupational therapists. See Appendix I for the Hierarchy of Competencies Relating to the Use of Standardized Instruments and Evaluation Techniques by Occupational Therapists.

References

1. Buros OK (ed): The Eighth Mental Measurement Yearbook. Highland Park, NJ, Gryphon Press, 1978
2. Buros OK (ed): The Seventh Mental Measurement Yearbook. Highland Park, NJ, Gryphon Press, 1972
3. Buros OK (ed): The Sixth Mental Measurement Yearbook. Highland Park, NJ, Gryphon Press, 1965
4. Buros OK (ed): The Fifth Mental Measurement Yearbook. Highland Park, NJ, Gryphon Press, 1959
5. Buros OK (ed): The Fourth Mental Measurement Yearbook. Highland Park, NJ, Gryphon Press, 1953
6. Buros OK (ed): The Third Mental Measurement Yearbook. Highland Park, NJ, Gryphon Press, 1949
7. Jebsen R, Taylor N, Triegchmann R, et al: An objective and standardized test of hand function. Arch Phys Med Rehabil 50:311, 1969
8. Mathiowetz V, Weber K, Volland G, Kashman N: Reliability and validity of grip and pinch strength evaluations. J Hand Surg 9A:222, 1984

(Text continues on page 244)

PHYSICAL CAPACITIES EVALUATION

Administrator's Guide for Physical Capacities Evaluation

Performance Rating:
    Within Normal Range (W.N.R.)
    Fair
    Poor
    Unable
    Not appropriate (N.A.)

"Comment" space to be used only for:
    Reason unable to perform
    Other significant performance

Use of exercise mats:
    "Kneeling" and/or "Crawling" if client's knees are tender
    "Reclining" if floor too hard

Standard of comparison:
    "Walking": Army Regulation—66 seconds per 100 yards
    "Climbing" (stairs): Average time between 3 and 5 seconds each way

---

Walking:
  Request:
    1. To walk as ordinarily 100 yd. on rubber tiled flooring.
        A. Performance:
            a. Type of gait:
            b. Appliances used:
            c. Endurance:
            d. Safety:

    2. The client's estimate of distance and length of time he is able to walk.
        A. Estimate:
            a. Distance inside:
            b. Distance outside:
            c. Time inside:
            d. Time outside:

Comment: _____

_____

_____

PHYSICAL CAPACITIES EVALUATION (*continued*)

Running
Request:
  1. To run 30 yds on rubber tiled flooring.
      A. Performance:
          a. Endurance:
          b. Type of gait:
          c. Safety:

Comment: _____

_____

Jumping:
Request:
  1. To jump from a 19 in. & 30 in. high platform onto rubber tiled flooring landing on both feet.
      A. Performance:
          a. Balance: 19": _____ 30": _____
          b. Ability: 19": _____ 30": _____
          c. Safety: 19": _____ 30": _____

Comment: _____

_____

Climbing
Request:
  1. Ramp (8′ × 12° textured brick tile surface): To walk up and down five consecutive times.
      A. Performance:
          a. Gait:
          b. Endurance:
          c. Use of handrail:
          d. Use of appliance:

  2. Stairs: (10 steps, 7 in. rise, steel and stone tread) to walk up and down once.
      A. Performance:
          a. Safety:
          b. Endurance:
          c. Speed:
          d. Use of handrail:
          e. Use of appliances:
          f. Foot-over-foot: Foot-by-foot:

  3. Curbs: (9 in. and 14 in. high) To climb and descend curbs once.
      A. Performance in reference to public transportation:

          a. Ability: 8" _____ 14" _____
          b. Use of appliances:
          c. Safety:

  4. Straight ladder (8 rungs, 10 ft. high): to climb up and down five consecutive times.
      A. Performance:
          a. Foot-over-foot: Foot by foot:
          b. Hand-over-hand   Hand on rail:
              Hand-by-hand:
          c. Balance:
          d. Safety:

  5. Step Ladder. (6 ft. 10 in. rise):   To climb up and down once carrying a 10 lb. paint pail in one hand.
      A. Performance:
          a. Foot-over-foot: Foot-by-foot:
          b. Balance:
          c. Safety:

Comments: _____

_____

PHYSICAL CAPACITIES EVALUATION (*continued*)

Crouching:
Request:
1. To work in a squatting position for 3 minutes placing 1½ lb. cans (4″ × 8″) from the floor to a 19″ high shelf.
   A. Performance:
      a. Ability to carry out task:
      b. Ability to assume position:
      c. Ability to regain standing:
      d. Balance:
      e. Endurance:

Comments: _____

_____

Lifting:
Request:
1. Left Hand—To lift maximum weight from floor to a waist-high surface five consecutive times.
   A. Performance:
      a. Number of lb.:
      b. Ability:
      c. Balance:
      d. Endurance:

2. Right Hand—Same as left
   A. Performance:
      a. Number of lb.:
      b. Ability:
      c. Endurance:
      d. Balance:

3. Both hands—To lift maximum in weighted box from floor to a waist high surface five consecutive times.
   A. Performance:
      a. Ability:
      b. Balance:
      c. Endurance:
      d. Number of lbs.:

Comments: _____

_____

Carrying:
Request:
1. To bilaterally carry maximum weight in weighted boxes 25 yd. while walking on rubber tiled flooring.
   A. Performance:
      a. Number of lb.:
      b. Ability:
      c. Endurance:
      d. Balance:

Comments: _____

_____

Handling:
Administrator's estimate of the maximum weight the testee is able to handle comfortably.
1. Estimate:

Comments: _____

_____

Pushing: Push—Pull
Request:
1. To push a wheelbarrow (heavy duty with inflated rubber tire) for 25 yd. on rubber tiled flooring with maximum load.
   A. Performance:
      a. Ability:
      b. Endurance:
      c. Balance on turning:

PHYSICAL CAPACITIES EVALUATION (*continued*)

2. To alternately push and pull bilaterally to arm's length the maximum in a weighted box on a waist high rough wooden surface, ten times, both from standing and sitting positions.
   A. Performance:
      a. Number of lb. _____   Standing: Sitting:
      b. Ability:

Comments: _____

_____

Pulling:
Request:
1. To pull in a hand-over-hand fashion the maximum weight on a single pulley (¾ in. cotton rope) ten consecutive times.
   A. Performance:
      a. Number of lb.:
      b. Ability:
      c. Endurance:
      d. Balance:

Comments: _____

_____

Stooping:
Request:
1. To perform in 3 min. standing and stooping repeatedly while placing 5 lb. cans (4 in. × 8 in.) from the floor to a 48 in. high shelf.
   A. Performance:
      a. Ability:
      b. Endurance:
      c. Ability to grasp—   Right hand: Left hand:

Comments: _____

_____

Reaching:
Request:
1. Overhead—from a standing position to bimanually reach a 10 lb. box from an overhead shelf; return it to position. To reach with separate hands small objects from the same shelf.
   A. Performance:
      a. Ability: 10 lb.:   Right: Left:
      b. Range of motion
      c. Balance:
      d. Coordination: Grasp:

2. Forward: Standing—To reach forward and pick up a 10 lb. box from a table with both hands.
   A. Performance:
      a. Balance: Both: Right: Left:
      b. Coordination: Both:
      c. Grasp: Right: Left:
      d. Range of motion: Both: Right: Left:

3. Forward: Sitting—To reach forward for a small object on the table with separate hands, both directly and across the body.
   A. Performance:
      a. Balance: Both: Right: Left:
      b. Coordination: Both:
      c. Grasp: Right: Left:
      d. Range of motion: Both: Right: Left:

4. Low: Standing—To pick up small objects on floor from front position with both hands. To pick up same object on right and left sides with separate hands both directly and across body.
   A. Performance:
      a. Balance: Both: Right: Left:
      b. Coordination: Both:
      c. Grasp: Right: Left:
      d. Range of motion: Both: Right: Left:

PHYSICAL CAPACITIES EVALUATION (*continued*)

5. Sitting—To reach directly for small object on floor with separate hands at the right, left, and front positions.
   A. Performance:
      a. Balance: Right: F. Right: F. Left:
      B. Range of motion:
      c. Grasp: Right: Left: F. Right: F. Left:

Comments: _____

_____

Kneeling:
Request:
   1. To assume a kneeling position on a rubber tiled floor and maintain it for a 1 min. period.
      A. Performance:
         a. Ability to assume position:
         b. Ability to regain standing:
         c. Balance:
         d. Endurance:

Comments: _____

_____

Crawling:
Request:
   1. To crawl on rubber tiled flooring 8 ft. forward and then backward with head and shoulders down.
      A. Performance:
         a. Type crawl: 4-point: 3-point: Other:
         b. Speed:
         c. Agility:

Comments: _____

_____

Reclining:
Request:
   1. To assume a backlying position on rubber tiled flooring. When in position.
      A. Performance:
         a. Ability to assume position:
         b. Ability to regain standing:
         c. Ability to turn: Right: Left: Face:
         d. Comfort on: Right: Left: Face: Back:

Comments: _____

_____

Turning:
Request:
   1. To lift maximum weight in box from the floor, to turn trunk only and place it to the right at waist level and back to floor. Repeat for left side.
      A. Performance:
         a. Ability to: Right: Left:
         b. Balance: Right: Left:
         c. Endurance:

Comments: _____

_____

Balancing:
Request:
   1. To one-leg stand on individual legs for 30 sec. each.
      A. Performance:
         a. Ability: Right: _____ Left: _____
         b. Endurance: Right: _____ Left: _____
         c. Leg dominance: Right: _____ Left: _____

Comment: _____

_____

PHYSICAL CAPACITIES EVALUATION (*continued*)

Sitting:
With what ability is the client able to get in and out of a straight-backed chair? For an estimated period how long could he sit comfortably and with what type posture?
1. Ability to sit:
2. Ability to rise:
3. Estimated time:
4. Type of posture:

Comment: _____

_____

Standing:
What type of posture and stance does the client exhibit? Client's estimate of time he can stand.
1. Posture:
2. Stance:
3. Estimate of time:

Comment: _____

_____

Hand Grasp:
As measured with a dynamometer, the strength of the client's hand grasp.
1. Broad grasp: Right: _____   Left: _____
2. Tight grasp: Right: _____   Left: _____
3. Hand dominance: Right: _____   Left: _____

Comment: _____

_____

Bibliography

Specific Procedures

Abreu BC (ed): Physical Disabilities Manual. New York, Raven Press, 1981

Daniels L, Williams M, Worthingham C: Muscle Testing Techniques of Manual Examination. Philadelphia, WB Saunders, 1980

Joint Motion: Method of Measuring and Recording. Chicago, American Academy of Orthopaedic Surgeons, 1965

Kellor M, Frost J, Silberberg N, et al: Hand strength and dexterity: Norms for clincial use, age and sex comparisons. Am J Occup Ther 25:77, 1971

Moberg E: Emergency Surgery of the Hand. London, ES Livingston, 1967

Pedretti LW: Occupational Therapy: Practice Skills for Physical Dysfunction. St Louis, CV Mosby, 1985

Trombly CA (ed): Occupational Therapy for Physical Dysfunction, 2nd ed. Baltimore, Williams & Wilkins, 1983

Weiss MW, Flatt AE: A pilot study of 198 normal children: Pinch strength and hand size in the growing hand. Am J Occup Ther 25:10, 1971

Werner JL, Omer GE: A procedure evaluating cutaneous pressure sensation of the hand. Am J Occup Ther 24:347, 1970

General

Ayres AJ: Interrelationships among perceptual-motor functions in children. Am J Occup Ther 20:68, 1966

Bell E, Jurek K, Wilson T: Hand skill measurement, a gauge for treatment. Am J Occup Ther 30:80, 1976

Brayman S: Measuring device for joint motion of the hand. Am J Occup Ther 25:173, 1971

Brazelton TB: Neonatal Behavioral Assessment Scale. Philadelphia, JB Lippincott, 1973

Brown M, Diller L, Fordyce W, et al: Rehabilitation indicators: Their nature and uses for assessment. In Bolton B, Cook D (eds): Rehabilitation Client Assessment. Baltimore, University Park Press, 1980

Denhoff E, et al: Developmental and predictive characteristics of items from the Meeting Street School Screening Test. Develop Med Child Neurol 10:220, 1969

DeVore GL, Hamilton G: Volume measuring of the severely injured hand. Am J Occup Ther 22:16, 1968

Erhardt RP, Beatty PA, Hertsgaard DM: A developmental prehension assessment for handicapped children. Am J Occup Ther 35:237, 1981

Fiorentino M: Reflex Testing Methods for Evaluating C.N.S. Development, 2nd ed. Springfield, IL, Charles C Thomas, 1965

Hasselkus BR, Safrit MJ: Measurement in occupational therapy. Am J Occup Ther 30:429, 1976

Hurt SP: Considerations in muscle function and their application to disability evaluation and treatment—joint measurement. Am J Occup Ther 1:209, 1947; 1:281, 1947; 2:13, 1948

Kendall HO, Kendall FP, Wadsworth GE: Muscles, Testing and Function. Baltimore, Williams & Wilkins, 1971

Llorens L: An evaluation procedure for children 6–10 years of age. Am J Occup Ther 21:64, 1967

MacBain K, Hill R: A functional assessment for juvenile rheumatoid arthritis. Am J Occup Ther 26:326, 1973

McNary H: Keynote address—A look at occupational therapy. Am J Occup Ther 12:203, 1958

Milani–Comparetti A, Gidoni E: Routine developmental examination in normal and retarded children. Develop Med Child Neurol 9:631, 1967

Sand P, et al: Hand function in children with myelomenigocele. Am J Occup Ther 28:87, 1974

Sand P, et al: Hand function measurement with educable mental retardates. Am J Occup Ther 27:138, 1973

Skerik SK, et al: Functional evaluation of congenital hand anomalies, Part 1. Am J Occup Ther 25:98, 1971

Smith HB: Smith hand function evaluation. Am J Occup Ther 27:244, 1973

Stratton M: Behavioral assessment scale of oral functions in feeding. Am J Occup Ther 35:719, 1981

Turner A (ed): The Practice of Occupational Therapy. London, Churchill Livingstone, 1981

Von Prince K, Butler B: Measuring sensory functions of the hand in peripheral nerve injuries. Am J Occup Ther 21:385, 1967

Weiss MW, Flatt AE: Functional evaluation of the congenitally anamalous hand, Part 2. Am J Occup Ther 25:139, 1971

Zimmerman M: The functional motion test as an evaluation tool for patients with lower motor neuron disturbances. Am J Occup Ther 23:49, 1969

CHAPTER 17

Activities of Daily Living

SECTION **1**

Assessment and Evaluation – Life Work Tasks

Maude H. Malick and Bonnie Sherry Almasy

Activities of Daily Living

The concept of activities of daily living (ADL) has always encompassed eating, dressing, and personal hygiene activities that are basic to an individual's independence. The loss of independence in these basic activities has a traumatic effect on body image and may also affect persons associated with the patient. However, careful assessment, goal setting, planning, and training programs can be geared for accomplishment of short- and long-term goals that aim at self-sufficiency for a patient who is temporarily or permanently disabled. Dependency in self-care is often the first sign of depression or the major cause of depression. Therefore, early recognition of patient needs and ADL training are essential, especially in acute-care settings. Conversely, a chronically disabled person who can be independent in self-care activities requires far less custodial care and thus can be cared for in a more independent unit in a community setting.

The traditional program of ADL has been an integral part of all occupational therapy programs no matter what the setting, disability, or age group. Assessment and training can take place in the home, school, acute-care hospital, rehabilitation center, special school institution, long-term care agency, or nursing home. Many tests are availabe for self-care assessment, with simple grading forms providing ready reference to the nursing and health team. Cognition and judgment should enter into the assessment process. Merely accomplishing a task does not constitute competency. In many cases, simple self-help devices are useful, but they should not be used unless essential. Devices such as built-up handles, attachments to faucet handles, reachers, overhead rings, and mats to anchor plates and tableware are very simple aids that can make a great difference in independence. Simple energy-saving techniques and planning can also change dependence to independence. In all cases, safety should be a prime concern.

ADL, in its broadest sense, encompasses indepen-

Table 17-1. *Health/Disability Scale Determining Illness and Dependency or Health and Independence*

	Internal Limitations (Basic Survival)	*External Obstacles/Adaptations* (Role Identification)
Bodily functions	Self-care	Household tasks
Mobility in space	Mobility	Use of transportation
Communication	Speech, hearing, vision	Aids, equipment, and devices
Social	Appropriateness and self-presentation	Social competence in confronting and using support systems
Cognitive	Orientation and problem solving	Management of personal affairs
Emotional	Tolerance of psychological stress, orientation to goals, phobias, anxiety, depression	Acting out behaviors, motivation

dence in the home, at work, and in the community. In this sense, the individual should be assessed regarding ability to make judgments; function in a community setting; communicate with others; carry out acceptable social behavior; and manage his or her own lifestyle financially, socially, vocationally, and avocationally.

A grant to develop "Rehabilitation Indicators: A Method for Enhancing Accountability" was awarded to the New York University Medical Center, Institute of Rehabilitation Medicine, in 1976, with Diller, Fordyce, and Jacobs as codirectors. An ADL Task Force, chaired by Carl Granger, MD, developed and explored levels of ADL performance indicating the scope of skills assessed under activities of daily living. As a result of this task force meeting and others throughout the country, rehabilitation indicators (RI), which describe a client's behavior and environment, were developed. Four types of RIs have been developed: status, activity pattern, skill, and environment. Phrases have been written to describe what clients actually do, what clients demonstrate they can do, and what clients plan to do.*

A health/disability scale, used to delineate the aspects of ADL function, is given in Table 17-1. In many cases, substitution using strengths in one area to compensate for deficits in another area can be effective. For example, speech and communication skills can supplement writing skills.

Klein and Bell have developed an ADL scale using behavioral measurements to evaluate patient self-care skills. This scale is an objective and valid measure of ADL, and it has been shown to have a high degree of inter-rater reliability. Based on an activity analysis of self-care skills, the scale mirrors the typical breakdown of self-care activities that would be used in occupational therapy evaluation and treatment. Each activity is broken down into separate behavioral segments, and each is rated separately. (Fig. 17-1). The choice for rating is a

simple yes or no: clients receive either full score for performance without human assistance, or they receive no points for any amount of dependence, excluding the independent use of adaptive equipment. This relieves the rater of having to make subjective judgments as to the amount of assistance required. The problem areas can be quickly identified. A treatment plan can easily be developed from the items that are negatively scored. The positive items then constitute an accumulation of skills that is reaching toward total independence. The client receives a score in each of six areas of self-care: dressing, bathing/hygiene, elimination, mobility, eating, and emergency telephone communication (Fig. 17-2). All of the self-care items rated in the scale are applicable to all persons, able bodied or disabled. It is also applicable to children, although not yet standardized to age levels. Having many steps that are components of one overall behavior allows relatively slow but steady progress to be identified and plotted. This gives the client, occupational therapist, and team members a sense of accomplishment.

The statistical reliability of this test was determined using independent ratings by pairs of experienced occupational therapists and rehabilitation nurses. Each pair independently rated patients at the same point in time, and their scores were compared. There was a 92% agreement between pairs of raters for all items on all patients. This high reliability is due largely to the dichotomous ("independent" or "dependent") rating and to the careful analysis and breakdown of each activity.

Validity measurements reflect the functional abilities actually existing with each client. To measure validity, clients were contacted following discharge from a rehabilitation center. By means of a structured interview, a determination was made of the number of hours attendant care was received per week. The correlation coefficient between the Klein–Bell score at discharge and hours per week of attendant care is -0.86 ($p < 0.01$). This consistent relationship indicates that the lower the score on the Klein–Bell ADL Scale, the greater the amount of assistance required.

---

* Further information can be obtained from Margaret Brown, Project Coordinator, NY University Medical Center, Institute of Rehabilitation Medicine, 400 E 34th St, New York, NY 10016.

Pullover Shirt

29. Reach shirt to top of head (2)						
30. Pull head through neck hole (2)						
31. Put R hand through R armhole (2)						
32. Put R elbow into sleeve (2)						
33. Put L hand through L armhole (2)						
34. Put L elbow into sleeve (2)						
35. Pull shirt down over trunk (2)						

Shorts/Pants

23. Reach shorts to foot (2)					
24. Get R leg into R leghole (2)					
25. Get L leg into L leghole (2)					
26. Pull pants up to waist (2)					
27. Zip zipper (2)					
28. Fix fastener (2)					

Figure 17-1. Sample items taken from the Klein–Bell ADL scale.

This scale gives the user a reliable and valid measure of patient performance that assists in meeting many clinical, administrative, research, and educational needs. Other assessment and training techniques described by Lawton in 1963[2] are valid today as when they were written.

Home Management Skills in Occupational Therapy

Homemakers constitute the largest group among the disabled. With current figures exceeding 10 million, it is essential both socially and economically that the rehabilitation process be used to help the individual re-establish his or her place in family, home, and community. Physical rehabilitation services encompass those techniques that are instrumental in developing physical re-

sidual capabilities, whether by training or re-education, with emphasis on modifications of performance or task completion. The occupational therapist introduces a set of tools that can be used to develop a comprehensive home management rehabilitation program.

It is essential in any program to incorporate methods for coping with the individual's physical, personal, and social needs while promoting self-integration as well as integration into family and society.

The rehabilitation process must include provisions for the personal and social needs, goals, and resources of each potential homemaker. According to Switzer:

Homemaking activities—whether carried out by men, women or children—contribute to the welfare and stability of the family and to its economic productiveness and well-being. Homemaking itself is a composite of physical tasks, managerial functions, spirit, emotional climate that holds the family or personality together and fosters devel-

Figure 17-2. A section of the Klein–Bell ADL Scale. The graph depicts scores for a 56-year-old ▶ woman who sustained a right internal capsule cerebrovascular accident with resulting left hemiparesis. Two weeks later, she underwent her initial ADL evaluation. Nine days after that evaluation, she sustained a second CVA, this time in the left hemisphere, with resulting right hemiparesis and dysarthria. The scores shown represent only her initial and final evaluations. Her ADL score decreased after the second CVA; however, she steadily improved and was discharged to her home with a companion/attendant. (An instructional videotape with scales and manual for scoring is available from: Distribution, Health Sciences Learning Resources Center, T-245 Health Science Building SB-56, University of Washington, Seattle, WA 98195.)

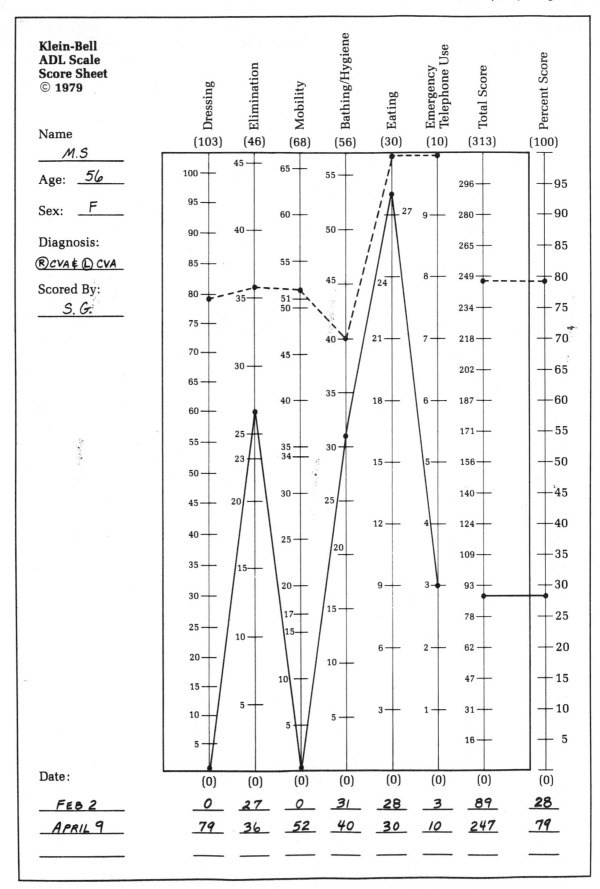

**Klein-Bell
ADL Scale
Score Sheet
© 1979**

Name

_M.S_

Age: _56_

Sex: _F_

Diagnosis:

Ⓡ CVA & Ⓛ CVA

Scored By:

_S.G._

	Dressing (103)	Elimination (46)	Mobility (68)	Bathing/Hygiene (56)	Eating (30)	Emergency Telephone Use (10)	Total Score (313)	Percent Score (100)
Date:	(0)	(0)	(0)	(0)	(0)	(0)	(0)	(0)
FEB 2	0	27	0	31	28	3	89	28
APRIL 9	79	36	52	40	30	10	247	79

opment. Damage to this process at any point weakens its total capacity to function. Where possible, the damage must be repaired; where this is not possible, other measures must be taken. Perhaps the environment can be changed so that the function can continue; perhaps the other areas of the complex must be brought to greater prominence and use; perhaps the very depths of personality must be touched and a new role learned.[4]

The Rehabilitation Act of 1973 and the Social Services Act of 1974 emphasize the pertinence and urgency of developing comprehensive programs for enabling the homebound individual to realize his or her potential. Homemaking is now a viable occupation and should be considered as such when funding is necessary for implementing the rehabilitation process. Schwab says disabled homemakers with a recent rehabilitation experience exhibit positive changes in self-perception in relation to household tasks.[3] The self-respect and self-confidence derived from this experience can transfer to other activities, which may make the individual more productive, even in terms of competitive employment.

The 1978 amendments to the Rehabilitation Act of 1973 established Title VII, "Comprehensive Services for Independent Living." The Independent Living (IL) Center programming is administered by the state vocational rehabilitation agencies. They provide the following:

1. A grant program for IL centers
2. An IL program for older blind persons
3. A protection and advocacy program to guard the rights of severely disabled persons.

Home management programs traditionally have encompassed the teaching and assessment of basic work skills. These programs include the utilization of work-simplification techniques to promote time and energy conservation while concurrently providing therapeutic exercise, teaching the use of prosthetic or orthotic equipment, promoting psychological gains through satisfactory performance, and assisting constructive planning for home adjustment.

Physical or mental disability necessitates many changes. Because of accident or illness, the homemaker may have to cope with changes that are out of his or her realm of control, and he or she may be unable to set realistic goals freely. It is the therapist's role to assist the homemaker in using management skills to bring about the change in an orderly way. This involves the homemaker's adapting to alternatives and finding outside resources in the family. Although functioning may be limited in one area, resources can be channeled in new directions. Tasks do not need to be limited to one member of the family. All family resources must be considered when faced with decision making.

Sometimes, the disabled homemaker is so distraught by the changes that he/she may bypass an essential step in the decision-making process and therefore must be given guidance. The process involved in decision making is relatively simple. It is as follows:

1. State the problem.
2. Seek and explore alternatives.
3. Discuss possible solutions.
4. Choose one alternative.
5. Accept the responsiblity for the decision made.

The working through of this process provides the family with a better communication system, which in turn leads to greater satisfaction with the ultimate decision.[1]

Today's home management programs have grown and expanded in many new and exciting directions, all aimed toward the goal of producing home managers who are functioning to their capacity in all areas. Among the most important areas of concentration is the fulfillment of nutritional needs. This includes basic food preparation skills, with emphasis on planning, purchasing, and serving nutritious meals that meet all dietary needs. Assistance with financial management and information on budgeting, spending, and saving can be incorporated into the basic program. Selection, care, and adaptation of clothing is yet another facet of the program that can make the handicapped homemaker a more effective and efficient home manager. Child care can consume a good portion of the homemaker's day. With instruction on purchasing functional equipment and clothing, as well as in techniques for the feeding, dressing, and bathing of children, the handicapped homemaker can resume many tasks that previously were allocated to other family members or to hired help.

Current home management training programs are the keystone in the structure of rehabilitation that enables the disabled person to build a new life with an emphasis on ability, not disability.

Recording and Scoring of Function in ADL and Homemaking

Because the entire rehabilitation process is directed toward change in the total patient profile—change in attitude, ability, activity, awareness, and aptitude for the program—it is necessary to record changes and use these records in upgrading the client's program. It is essential to establish a scale of performance and a code for noting the levels of performance before an evaluation begins. There are potentially as many scales and codes as there are therapists, and experimentation may be necessary to find one that is flexible and functional in various treatment settings. However, all therapists in a department should use the same recording system, or patients functioning at the same level may receive dif-

HARMARVILLE REHABILITATION CENTER, INC.
OCCUPATIONAL THERAPY DEPARTMENT

NAME _____

ADMITTED _____

DISCONTINUED _____

DATE:						
Feed Self						
Cut Meat						
Liquids						
Light Hygiene/Grooming						
Bathing Face						
Upper Torso						
Lower Torso						
Dressing-Undershirt/Bra						
Shirt						
Underpants/pants						
Socks/Jobst/Ted Hose						
Shoes						
Prosthesis/Orthosis						
Transfer-Bed ⇌ W/C						
W/C ⇌ Commode						
W/C ⇌ Tub						

Pt. Dresses in Bed _____ W/C _____

Edge of Bed _____

Equipment

Splint _____ Day _____ Night _____

Lapboard _____ Armboard _____

Other

Comments/Set-up

CODES

0 - Not applicable or not tested.

1 - Patient is dependent in all aspects of activities.

2 - Patient is able to perform less than 50% of the activity requiring physical assistance or constant direct supervision.

3 - Patient is able to perform 50% or more of the activity; may require some assistance and/or direct supervision for all aspects of activity.

4 - Patient is able to perform all physical aspects of the activity but requires supervision or minimal assistance to perform safely.

5 - Patient is able to perform all aspects of the activity independently with or without adaptive equipment.

Figure 17-3. Activities of daily living evaluation and scale used by the Harmarville Rehabilitation Center, Pittsburgh, Pennsylvania. (reproduced with permission).

fering reports from various therapists, which can be confusing, especially when reporting to other treatment departments. Several ADL and homemaking charts with codes are included as examples (Figs. 17-3 – 17-5).

In order to note a change, a baseline (*i.e.,* a point of reference from the initial evaluation) is needed. It is from this baseline that the program develops. The information obtained from the initial evaluation should be used in setting the goal toward which the therapist and patient will be working. The general levels of function-

HOMEMAKING EVALUATION AND TREATMENT

Name: Age: Date Referred:

Address: Visual Difficulty:

Disability:

Mobility Status:_____independent_____W/C_____cane_____crutches_____walker

Dominant Hand: R   L Limitations:

Goal: Special Diet:

Discharge Plans:

Household members and ages:
1.
2.
3.
4.
5.

Available help within or outside of family:

Description of home or apartment: _____floors_____stairs_____rooms

Are bath facilities functional? _____kitchen facilities functional? _____

(X) Patient formerly responsible for:

( ) Patient wants to return to doing:

( ) ( ) Food preparation
( ) ( ) Serving and cleaning
( ) ( ) Washing dishes
( ) ( ) Grocery shopping
( ) ( ) Meal planning
( ) ( ) Budgeting
( ) ( ) Child care
( ) ( ) Bed making
( ) ( ) Laundry—facilities in home _____
( ) ( ) Ironing
( ) ( ) Cleaning
( ) ( ) Sewing

SKETCH PROBLEM AREA

Special problems:

Special interests:

Patient's attitude toward homemaking:

Family's attitude toward patient's role as homemaker and toward family help:

Figure 17-4. Homemaking Evaluation and Treatment form, and the code (facing page) that is used for the "Goal" entry of the homemaking evaluation. A goal is established after the patient has been interviewed and observed working in the area. At the time of discharge from the area, it is determined whether he or she has reached the set goal. (From the Harmarville Rehabilitation Center, Pittsburgh, Pennsylvania [reproduced with permission])

ing, tolerance, and attitude are determined. Once a program is established, it is of paramount importance to note daily changes and periodic differences in levels of improvement. These are easily coded and marked on the scales. A progress chart frequently provides some motivation for the patient as a visual and concrete indication that he or she is improving.

Daily reports often take the form of short notes that include the activity performed; level of success; tolerance; attitude; pertinent observations, including physical limitations such as cognitive, perceptual, visual, and hearing deficits; use of adapted or standard equipment; ability to solve problems, read, and follow directions; mental reliability (*e.g.,* disorientation or hallucination); and general method of approaching the activity (*e.g.,* precise or careless). Positive or negative changes noted on the chart indicate a need for program adaptation. Retraining may be indicated, or the program may need to be accelerated. It often is helpful for the family to see the coded scales when the therapist explains alterations in the program, as carryover is generally greater when the family is aware of the exact level of functioning that can and should be expected.

Not all information relating to progress or condition can be included on a checklist based on observations or testing because many factors not amenable to coding and scaling will influence the patient's performance. These should not be neglected. Each chart should include space for impressions and subjective observations. Records should be accurate and concise, but they should contain all pertinent information. The treatment goals should be noted. In most cases, the physician will make referrals indicating general treatment procedures.

The final report, usually a discharge summary, should include the results of the initial evaluation, the treatment procedures, the results of the final evaluation, the final level of functioning, the achievement of goals, prognosis, and recommendations for maximal carryover upon discharge. This final report often goes to the sponsoring agency and to agencies that may be working with the patient in an outpatient or home setting.

Case Study

Susan A. is an agile, spirited, 82-year-old widow. She had been living alone in a high-rise building for the elderly not far from the business district of a small mill town in Pennsylvania. Although she has had two strokes, the most recent 1½ years ago, and has a

CODE

A	Independent Homemaker—Patient appears capable of all homemaking activities without assistance or supervision.
B	Independent Light Homemaker—Patient appears capable of all light homemaking activities without assistance or supervision.
C	Good Partial Homemaker—Patient appears capable of most light homemaking activities independently. May require assistance with some heavier or very complex tasks.
D	Partial Homemaker—Patient appears capable of some light homemaking activities independently or with minimal assistance with heavy or complex activities. May be limited in performing certain activities by physical inadequacy.
E	Partial Homemaker with Assistance—Patient appears capable of many light homemaking activities but requires assistance in at least one aspect of most of these activities. May be limited by tolerance or mental ability.
F	Partial Homemaker with Supervision—Patient appears to require general supervision while performing most homemaking activities but physically performs well.
G	Simple Partial Homemaker—Patient appears capable of simple, repetitive homemaking activities without supervision or assistance. May need to be set up at an activity but able to follow through.
H	Simple Partial Homemaker with Supervision—Patient appears to require supervision to perform even simple repetitive tasks.
I	Not Feasible—Patient did not appear capable of working on a homemaking evaluation at the time as a result of either physical or mental insufficiency.
J	Incomplete—Homemaking evaluation had been initiated but not completed because of medical problems, early discharge, or referral to another program.
K	Refused—Patient was referred to the homemaking area for an evaluation but refused to attend the program.

HOUSEHOLD ACTIVITIES PERFORMANCE EVALUATION

MEAL PREPARATION ACTIVITIES	Perf.	Place	Time	Perf.	Place	Time	Perf.	Place	Time	Perf.	Place	Time	Perf.	Place	Time	COMMENTS Equip. & Devices
DATE																
1. Turn on water																
2. Turn on stove																
3. Pour hot liquid																
4. Open package																
5. Open jars																
6. Use can openers																
7. Use refrigerator																
8. Bend to low cupboards																
9. Reach high cupboards																
10. Peel vegetables																
11. Use sharp tools																
12. Measures																
13. Use oven																
14. Use range																
15. Stir against resistance																
16. Use electric mixer																
17. Cut with shears																
18. Read directions																
19. Follow directions																
MEAL SERVICE																
1. Set and clear table																
2. Carry items to table																
3. Wash dishes																
4. Dry dishes																
5. Clean area																
6. Wring out dishcloth																
CLEANING ACTIVITIES																
1. Retrieve objects from floor																
2. Wipe up spills																
3. Make bed																
4. Use dust mop																
5. Vacuum																
6. Use dust pan																
7. Clean bathtub																
8. Sweep with broom																
9. Dust high surfaces																
10. Dust low surfaces																
11. Clean refrigerator																

Figure 17-5. Household activities evaluation form from Harmarville Rehabilitation Center, Pittsburgh, Pennsylvania (reproduced with permission).

HOUSEHOLD ACTIVITIES PERFORMANCE EVALUATION (*continued*)

LAUNDRY ACTIVITIES	Perf.	Place	Time	Perf.	Place	Time	Perf.	Place	Time	Perf.	Place	Time	Perf.	Place	Time	
1. Sort clothes																
2. Wash lingerie																
3. Iron																
4. Fold clothes																
5. Set up board																
6. Use washing machine																
SEWING ACTIVITIES																
1. Thread needle																
2. Make a knot																
3. Sew buttons																
4. Use machine																
5. Diversional activity																
MARKETING ACTIVITIES																
1. Make out list																
2. Put groceries away																
CHILD CARE ACTIVITIES																
1. Bathe																
2. Dress																
3. Feed																

CODES

Performance
X—unnecessary
A—independent
B—with assistance
C—impossible
D—training needed

Place
W—wheelchair
O—ambulatory
Ө—ambulatory with
      assistive devices

Time
N—within normal limits
X—excessive

history of heart trouble, she has returned to independent living following a 6-week stay at a comprehensive rehabilitation center.

Susan tells her story:

I was always a busy lady, active with my family and at church. My husband was hurt badly in a mill accident just after we were married. We had to live some way, so I turned our house into a guest home. My whole life was spent making people comfortable and happy. It wasn't easy. I've had heart trouble for about 30 years now, and then I got a stroke on my left side about 18 years ago. My daughter died of rheumatic heart disease. She left a wonderful husband and two sons. The boys still see me often and send money if I need it.

After my husband died, about 10 years back, I sold the house and moved into this apartment near my sisters. The place is really nice—we have elevators, a laundry room, even grab bars in the bathroom for us old folks.

Just over a year ago, I fell down getting out of bed. By crawling across the floor, I finally got to the phone for help. An ambulance took me to the hospital. It was another stroke, on the left side again. I could shrug my shoulder but couldn't move my hand at all. Two people had to help me to let me walk. For the first time I was really afraid. There was no one who could take care of me, and I surely couldn't do much for myself. Although I could feed myself a little, I couldn't fix my hair or put on my bra, panties, or slacks. Couldn't tie my shoes either. Housework was unthinkable with one hand. I thought they'd make me go to some home for old people. Just to get better and go back to my apartment was all I wanted.

My doctor thought I could make some progress at a rehabilitation center. I'm sure glad I went. They had special groups for discussion about strokes. I got to talk to a lot of people who were in the same shape as I was.

They gave me therapy on my arm and showed me how to walk with a cane. A lady from occupational therapy worked with me and showed me how to dress and feed myself. I got my hair cut on beauty shop day so I could take care of it myself.

The occupational therapist showed me how to cook my favorite meals with one hand, even how to peel potatoes. I was supposed to be on a 2-gram-sodium diet,

---

HARMARVILLE REHABILITATION CENTER, INC.
OCCUPATIONAL THERAPY DEPARTMENT

NAME __Susan A__

ADMITTED __1-8-87__

DISCONTINUED _____

DATE:	1/8/87	1/15	1/29	2/5		
Feed self	4	4	5	5		
Cut meat	3	3	4	5		
Liquids	5	5	5	5		
Light hygiene/Grooming	4	5	5	5		
Bathing face	4	5	5	5		
Upper torso	4	5	5	5		
Lower torso	3	4	5	5		
Dressing-undershirt/(bra)	2	3	3	5		
Shirt	3	4	5	5		
Underpants/pants	4	4	5	5		
(Socks)/Jobst/Ted hose	3	4	5	5		
Shoes	4	5	5	5		
Prosthesis/Orthosis	NA	NA	NA	NA		
Transfer-Bed ⇌ W/C	4	4	5	5		
W/C ⇌ Commode	3	4	4	5		
W/C ⇌ Tub	3	4	4	5		

Pt. Dresses in bed _____ W/C _____

Edge of bed __x__

Equipment

Splint _____ Day _____ Night _____

Lapboard _____ Armboard _____

Other

Comments/Set-up

CODES
0 - Not applicable/Not tested
1 - Dependent
2 - Maximum assistance
3 - Moderate assistance
4 - Supervision/Minimal assistance
5 - Independent

Figure 17-6. Sample form for case study from Harmarville Rehabilitation Center, Pittsburgh, Pennsylvania (reproduced with permission).

but I had never followed it because I didn't know what it was. At homemaking they showed me how to eat what I like and still stay on my diet. I learned lots of tricks, too, so I wouldn't get so tired doing my work. I used to think it was lazy to sit to work, but it's just plain smart. We went grocery shopping too. My sisters thought it was too hard for me to walk and push a cart too, but I did it.

The therapists got me in pretty good shape at the rehabilitation center, but I was still a little leery about going home by myself. Oh, I wanted to—but with my stroke, wasn't sure I could. My sisters wanted me to move in with them, but at my age it's better to live by yourself.

The rehabilitation center had an apartment right in the building. I didn't want to stay there; my doctor had other ideas. I think he thought I couldn't do it—I showed him. I stayed there just like I was at home by myself. I washed and dressed myself, took my pills, made the bed, cooked my meals, did my exercises, and had my social worker in for tea. I thought I could do it, but it sure gave me confidence to know for sure. It gave me a real big lift—I was ready to go home.

My sisters insisted that I get Meals-on-Wheels. I did for a few weeks, but the food wasn't so hot. I started cooking on my own again. The spikeboard I made in occupational therapy was a big help.

After I was home for a few weeks, the occupational therapist came to see me. She brought the long-handled sponge and long shoehorn I had asked for. She showed me how to arrange things in the kitchen to make it easier for me to reach. I showed her how I fixed my calendar so I don't get mixed up about when to take my pills. I learned how to get in the tub at the center so I bought those stick-on flowers so I don't slip. I think the therapist was surprised at how well I was doing. Guess I surprised myself too.

Six months later, Susan was evaluated on an outpatient visit. She was gaining function in her left hand. Ambulation status was independent. She reported participating in apartment activities and utilizing Adult Services for transporation to visit and shop. Figure 17-6 shows Susan's chart; box shows the discharge summary.   □

References

1. Gross I, Crandall EW: Management for Modern Families. New York, Appleton–Century–Crofts, 1963
2. Lawton EB: Activities of Daily Living for Physical Rehabilitation. New York, McGraw–Hill, 1963
3. Schwab LO: Self Perception of Physically Disabled Homemakers. Ed.D. thesis, University of Nebraska, 1966
4. Switzer MW: Foreword. In Rehabilitation of Physically Handicapped in Homemaking Activities. Proceedings of a Workshop, Highland Park, IL, 1963. US Department of Health, Education and Welfare

Bibliography

Abreu BC: Physical disabilities Manual. New York, Raven, 1981

After A Stroke: Patient and Family Guide. Pittsburgh, Harmarville Rehabilitation Center, 1981

Bertelsen J: Small Group Homes for the Handicapped and Disabled: An Annotated Bibliography. US Department of Housing and Urban Development, 1977

Bowe F: Rehabilitating America: Toward Independence for Disabled and Elderly People. New York, Harper & Row, 1980

Davis WM: Aids to Make You Able, 2nd ed. Chicago, IL, Fred Sammons, 1979

Diffrient N, Tilley AR, Bardagiy JC: Humanscale 1/2/3. Designer: Henry Dreyfuss Associates. Cambridge, MA. MIT Press, 1974

El-Ghatit Z, Melvin JL, Poole MA: Training apartment in community for spinal cord injured patients: A model. Arch. Phys Med Rehab 61:90, 1980

Frieden L: Independent Living models. Rehab Lit July–August:169, 1980

Frieden L, Richards L, Cole J, Bailey D: A glossary for independent living. ILRU Sourcebook: A Technical Assistance Manual on Independent Living. Houston: TIRR (Institute for Rehabilitation and Research), 1979. Vol 41, July–August, 1980

Frith GH: The use of professionals in achieving independent living for severely handicapped persons. Rehab Lit 42:18, 1981

Garee B: Ideas for Making Your Home Accessible. Bloomington, IL, Accent Special Publishers, 1979

Discharge Summary

GOAL: Good partial homemaker. This goal was achieved.

Mrs. A's program included:

1. Vegetable preparation—used spikeboard safely and appropriately
2. Food preparation—successfully read and followed directions, opened packages, used range, oven, and refrigerator while ambulating
3. Dishwashing—worked with no apparent difficulty from standing position
4. Bedmaking—balance and tolerance appeared good. Worked neatly and efficiently.
5. Vacuuming—difficulty was noted when patient attempted to move furniture.
6. Laundry—effectively used coin-operated facilities.
7. Received instruction in work simplification techniques and management principles.
8. Received instruction on 2-g-sodium diet and meal planning.
9. Completed 48-hour apartment living experience with excellent results.

Appreciation is extended to Nancy Annunziato, M.S., OTR/L of the Harmarville Rehabilitation Center for her contributions.

Harkness SP, Groom JN Jr: Building Without Barriers for the Disabled. The Architect Collaborative Inc., Whitney Library of Design, Cambridge, MA, 1976

Harmarville Rehabilitation Center, Inc.: Handicapped Homemaker Follow-Up Study, 1972, PO Box 11460, Guys Run Road, Pittsburgh, PA 15238

Jay P: Help Yourselves; A Handbook for Hemiplegics and Their Families, 4th ed. UK, Jan. Henry Pubs., 1985

Klein RM, Bell BJ: Self care skills: Behavioral measurement with the Klein–Bell ADL Scale. Arch. Phys Med Rehab (In press)

Kliment SA: Into the Mainstream: A Syllabus for a Barrier-Free Environment. Prepared under a grant to the American Institute of Architects by the Rehabilitation Services Administration of the Department of Health, Education, and Welfare, Washington, DC, 1975

Klinger JL: Self Help Manual for Arthritic Patients. New York, The Arthritis Foundation, 1974

Klinger JL, Friedman FH, Sullivan RA: Mealtime Manual for the Aged and Handicapped. New York, Simon and Schuster, 1970

Lifchez R, Winslow B: Design for Independent Living: The Environment and Physically Disabled People. Los Angeles, U of California Press, 1981

Malick M: Manual on Dynamic Hand Splinting. Pittsburgh, Harmarville Rehabilitation Center, 1974

Malick M: Manual on Static Hand Splinting. Pittsburgh, Harmarville Rehabilitation Center, 1972

Morgan M: Beyond disability: A broader definition of architectural barriers. A/A Journal 65:50, 1976

National Center for Health Statistics: Use of Special Aids, United States, 1977. Hyattsville, MD, US Dept of Health and Human Services, 1980

Nichols P, Hamilton EA: Rehabilitation Medicine: The Management of Physical Disabilities. London, Butterworths, 1976

Palmer ML, Toms JE: Manual for Functional Training. Philadelphia, FA Davis, 1980

Pan E, Backer TE, Vash CL (eds): Annual review of rehabilitation, vol 1. New York, Springer, 1980

Parmenter TR: Vocational Training for Independent Living. New York, World Rehabilitation Fund, 1980

Pflueger SS: Independent Living. Washington Institute for Research Utilization, 1977

Power PW, Dell Orto AE: Role of the Family in the Rehabilitation of the Physically Disabled. Baltimore, University Park Press, 1980

Rusk HA: Rehabilitation Medicine, 4th ed. St Louis, C V Mosby, 1977

Sargent JV: An Easier Way—Handbook for the Elderly and Handicapped. Ames, Iowa State University Press, 1981

Simkins J: The Value of Independent Living. New York, World Rehabilitation Fund, 1979

Smith BC, Fry R: Instructional Materials in Independent Living. Menomonie, WI, Stout Vocational Rehabilitation Institute, 1978

Walker JM: A Guide to Organizations, Agencies and Federal Programs for Handicapped Americans. Washington, DC, Handicapped American Reports, 1979

Wilshere ER: Equipment for the Disabled: Hoists, Walking Aids. Oxford, UK, Oxford Regional Health Authority, 1980

Yost AC: The rehabilitation home economist. J Home Econ 72:50, 1980

SECTION 2
Activities of Daily Living and Homemaking *Maude H. Malick*

Numerous techniques for training in the activities of daily living (ADL) have been explored and devised, but the primary component for success is the patient's motivation. The patient must understand what his or her needs and deficits are and the purpose and goal of the training. The patient will then be more cooperative and more willing to follow through with personal care. The therapist and patient must assess abilities and determine together which accomplishments are best done supine in bed, in a chair or wheelchair, at the edge of the bed, or standing.

Often, simple assistive devices such as grab bars, trapeze bars, or sliding boards can aid in gross positioning. An overhead trapeze bar or a looped rope attached to the foot of the bed can permit a patient to pull himself

or herself up to a sitting position and comfortably transfer with or without a sliding board to a wheelchair. Once trunk balance can be maintained, a patient may proceed with self-care activities in a chair.

In any disability group, it is important that the patient reach maximum physical strength, balance, and coordination through a structured exercise and activity program. The occupational therapist should work closely with the physical therapist in developing maximum muscle and joint function so that the patient can be trained to use the maximum of his/her abilities and to substitute for any deficits. It is equally important for the occupational therapist to communicate with nursing and with the patient's family regarding proper techniques to ensure carryover of ADL training.

Activities of daily living are of primary concern when priorities must be set. Muriel Zimmerman states there is a direct corollary in planning physical therapy and occupational therapy activities. Mat exercises, for instance, precede and coincide with sitting up in bed and transferring from the bed to the wheelchair. However, the needs and interests of the individual patient should always be considered. Independent eating may be started as soon as a patient can sit comfortably in bed or in a wheelchair, and in some instances, it may be started while the patient is being tilted on a tilt-bed or tilt-board.[8] After the initial evaluation, the patient is scheduled for training sessions in activities in which he is deficient and which are deemed suitable. He may merely need a few practice periods, with or without special guidance or equipment, or he may need carefully planned and supervised methods of procedure, such as sequence of performance, and the placement of the body or the hands, with repeated practice.[7]

In all self-care and dressing procedures, there are some basic considerations that should be employed:

1. The bed, chair, or wheelchair should be positioned properly. All pieces of clothing and self-care items should be placed properly. Visual and perceptual skills should be considered when determining placement of articles.

2. Patients should be encouraged to do tasks independently as much as possible. The patient's own ingenuity is an important factor.

3. Little or no adaptive equipment should be used unless it is absolutely necessary and then primarily for safety or to reduce consumption of energy and time.

4. All safety precautions should be observed, especially when the patient's stability is in question. The wheelchair should be locked at all times while transferring and during dressing and self-care procedures.

5. Cognitive and perceptual skills are major factors contributing to the patient's independence in dressing and self-care skills. Orientation, attention span, judgment, and the ability to plan and solve problems are a few cognitive skills that should be assessed and addressed during ADL.

Physical disability may be increased by pain, edema, and loss of sensation. The therapist must instruct the patient in proper positioning of the arm and leg to prevent injury from burns or trauma. The treatment plan must include training for perceptual, visual, sensory, and cognitive loss as well as for physical dysfunction.

Independence without assistive devices is most desirable, but many patients cannot manage without some special equipment. Assistive devices, when wisely selected and designed, can provide independence and often increase safety, speed, and acceptance. ADL training can be started with an assistive device and later discontinued, as physical gains are made. Perhaps one of the simplest devices is a built-up handle for an eating utensil or a c-cuff with a spoon fitting into a pocket (Fig. 17-7). When wrist strength and stability are insufficient, a simple dorsal or volar splint can be used (Fig. 17-7).

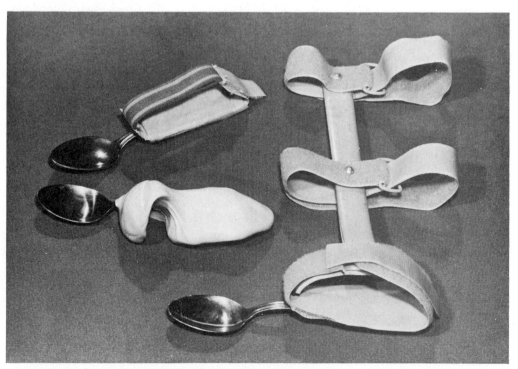

Figure 17-7. Assistive devices for holding eating utensils.

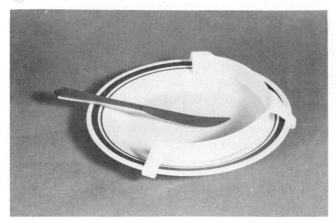

Figure 17-8. Plate guard and rocker knife to aid in feeding.

These are most frequently used with the quadriplegic, multiple sclerosis, or Guillain–Barré patient. A plate guard and rocker knife are frequently used to increase independence in self-feeding for hemiplegic patients or patients who must use one-handed techniques (Fig. 17-8).

The following techniques are used at Harmarville Rehabilitation Center in patient and family education. They are further described in their *Learning and Living* book series.[2]

ADL for the Hemiplegic Patient

Feeding

Depending on the sensory and motor functioning of the affected upper extremity, the hemiplegic patient may be instructed either in one-handed techniques or in using the affected extremity as a stabilizer or as an active assist during feeding. A rocker knife allows the individual to cut food with one hand.

Dressing

Shirts, robes, dresses, and coats should be loose fitting with the opening down the full length of the front of the garment.

Method A. Position the unbuttoned garmet on lap with the front label of the shirt facing up, the collar closest to the waist, and the arm hole for the involved arm centered between legs.
1. Lift involved arm and place it into the arm hole.
2. Lean forward so that the involved arm falls completely into the sleeve.
3. Pull the arm hole well up above the elbow.
4. Push the remainder of the shirt under involved arm and bring it around the back.
5. Pull shirt onto involved shoulder.

6. Reach back and slip uninvolved arm into the arm hole.
7. Adjust the shirt for comfort.
8. Line up the front edges and start buttoning from the bottom, working upward.

Method B. This method tends to be more effective for patients with perceptual deficits.
1. Complete steps 1–3 of Method A.
2. Leave the shirt positioned on lap with the front facing upward.
3. Place uninvolved arm into the arm hole and push completely into the sleeve.
4. Gather the back of the shirt up to the collar.
5. Lean forward while lifting the shirt up and over head.
6. Pull the shirt down in back and around the chest and adjust for comfort.
7. Line up the front edges and start buttoning the shirt working from the bottom, up.
8. Remove shirt from unaffected shoulder and arm before removing from affected arm.

Note: For long-sleeved shirts, cuffs may be buttoned before putting on the shirt. If hands do not fit through the buttoned cuff, sew the buttons on with elastic thread.

Lower extremity underwear and pants usually should be donned while sitting in the wheelchair, chair, or edge of bed.

Method A: For the patient getting dressed in wheelchair, chair or edge of bed.
1. Cross the involved leg over the uninvolved leg. Balance is best maintained if the involved leg is brought to a point directly in front of the midline of the body.
2. Lean forward and place the underwear over the involved foot and onto the leg. The involved arm may be positioned either on the arm rest of the chair or the knee or, if there is increased tone, the involved arm can hang to the side, allowing protraction of the scapula and elbow extension.
3. Uncross the leg.
4. Place the uninvolved foot through the leg hole of the underwear. Pull underwear up over knees.
5. Repeat steps 1–4 for donning pants.
6. Before standing, socks and shoes and/or brace should be donned to increase lower-extremity stability.
7. Stand to pull up pants. Place affected arm in pants pocket to prevent garment from dropping to floor. When standing, the patient should have the weight equally on both lower extremities. The therapist should be standing on the hemiplegic side of the patient.
8. Remove pants from uninvolved leg first.

Method B. For the patient who dresses in the bed (Patients who are dependent in transfers, sitting, and standing balance).
1. Put clothing on involved leg first.
2. Bend involved leg at the knee and hip using the uninvolved hand. Slip on the pant leg, then put uninvolved leg into the other pant leg.
3. Work over the hips either by rolling side to side (roll toward involved side first) or by pulling over the hips with both knees bent. The therapist may need to stabilize the involved leg while the patient pulls the garment over the hips.

Slips and dresses (for women) *and undershirt and pullover shirts* are donned as follows:
1. Position clothing on lap with neck of garment at the knees and the back of garment on top.
2. Gather the back up into hand until the arm hole for the involved arm becomes visible and is located between knees.
3. Lift involved arm up and place it through the arm hole. Lean forward, sliding arm between legs into the arm hole.
4. Pull the entire sleeve up above elbow
5. Put the uninvolved arm through sleeve.
6. Lean forward and pull shirt over head.

Socks are donned as follows:
1. Cross involved leg over uninvolved leg.
2. Use the thumb and finger of uninvolved hand to open the sock.
3. Lean forward with the involved arm either hanging at side or bearing weight with the forearm on the involved leg, if the involved arm is unable to assist with this activity.
4. Place the sock over toes and pull it onto foot.

The recommended style for *brassieres* is a front-opening style which may be easiest to use. Bras can be adapted with Velcro to become front-opening.
Method for back-opening style:
1. Anchor bra strap with thumb of involved hand, pull opening around to front.
2. Hook bra in front at the waist, remove thumb of involved hand from bra strap, and slip fastener around to the back.
3. Place involved arm through the shoulder strap and then place the uninvolved arm through the other strap. Adjust bra.

Shoes and short leg braces (Ankle Foot Orthosis: AFO's) are donned as follows:
1. If patient is dependent in maintaining sitting balance, apply the brace while in bed.
2. Sit in a chair if balance is fair, or sit on the edge of the bed if balance is good.

3. Cross the involved leg over the uninvolved leg. Balance is best maintained if the uninvolved leg is brought to a point directly in front of the midline of the body.
4. Make sure the laces on the shoe are loose, then hold the shoe underneath the heel. Place it over toes and pull it onto heel. (If a short leg brace is attached to the shoe, slip the shoe over toes with the brace behind the leg.)
5. Uncross legs and place uninvolved hand over the involved hand on top of involved knee and push firmly downward. A long-handled shoehorn in the heel of the shoe may make the process easier.
6. Buckle, tie, or fasten the shoe. Use one-handed shoe tie if vision, perception, and coordination of uninvolved hand is intact.
7. Uncross the legs, and put sock and shoe on uninvolved foot.

Hygiene and Grooming

Safety is the main concern during bathing and hygiene and needs to be considered at all times when recommending equipment. Bath stools with suction cups ensure safer transfers, as do stools which are not covered with vinyl. (Vinyl-covered seats tend to stick to the patient's bare skin and therefore make further physical demands on the patient and caregiver.) The recommended equipment is:
1. Electric razor for safety
2. Long-handled bath sponge or soap on a rope
3. Bathtub bench, seats, or chair inside tub for safe transfers
4. Hand-held shower hose for bathing
5. Bedside commode chair for easy accessibility
6. Nail file secured to table with masking tape.

To wash uninvolved arm, place soapy washcloth on uninvolved leg and rub arm up and down on it. Suction hand brushes can enable patients to brush dentures using one hand.

ADL for the Paraplegic Patient
Dressing

ADL training and independence in ADL with the paraplegic patient depend on the patient's level of balance, which is relative to level of the spinal cord lesion.

For donning *shirts, jackets, or dresses* that open completely down the front:
1. Balance body by putting palms of hands on mattress on either side of body.
2. If balance is poor, sit with back supported and legs extended (long sit).

For donning *lower extremity underwear and pants*:

1. Use long-sit position or sit in bed and pull knees into a flexed position. (One leg can be pulled into a flexed position at a time, depending on balance.) If poor balance is noted, use dressing stick and ranging strap to assist with flexing lower extremity.
2. Hold the top of the trousers and flip the pants down to feet.
3. Work pant legs over feet and pull up to the hips. If balance is poor, patient may require use of reacher.
4. Roll from hip to hip in a semireclining position and pull up the garment.

For donning *slips and skirts*:

1. Sit with back supported and legs extended or sit in bed, slip garment over head, and let it drop to waist.
2. Roll from hip to hip in a semireclining position and pull the garment down over the hips and thighs.

For donning *socks*:

1. Socks with tight elastic bands should be avoided.
2. Socks should fit smoothly because any wrinkles may cause pressure areas.

For donning *shoes*, pull one knee at a time into flexed position with hands while in sitting or long sitting on bed, and, supporting leg with upper arms, slip on shoe.

Hygiene and Grooming

The recommended equipment is:

1. A hand-held shower
2. Long-handled bath brushes for ease in reaching all parts of the body
3. Soap on a rope
4. For catheter and bowel training, a bowel training chair is useful if patient has shower or a raised toilet seat with a cutout side
5. Tub bench

ADL for the Quadriplegic Patient

Dressing

The amount of independence and the following suggestions depend on the level of the lesion.

1. Zippers and Velcro fastenings facilitate dressing.
2. Blouses and shirts should be long.
3. Garments should be loose fitting.
4. Loops can be sewn onto pants for arms to fit through.
5. A loop strap can be used to lasso the lower extremity.
6. Dressing sticks can be modified with loops.
7. Tenodesis splints can be used.

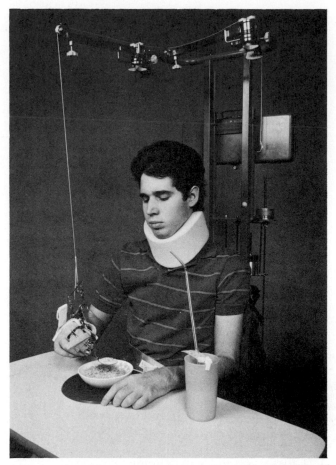

Figure 17-9. Upper extremity supported in deltoid aid and use of tenodesis splints to increase independence in feeding.

Feeding

1. Tenodesis splints can be used (Fig. 17-9).
2. Deltoid aids or mobile arm supports (MAS) can be used for patients with weak shoulder musculature (Fig. 17-9).
3. Plateguards, Dycem pads, long plastic straws, and built-up handles can be used to increase independence in feeding.
4. C-cuffs and/or universal cuffs can be used.

Grooming

Few adaptive devices are required if using tenodesis splints. A cigarette holder or a robot smoker for safety and a mouth stick for turning pages, painting, typing, writing, and dialing the telephone can be easily made if needed. Other aids include:

1. Shower/commode chair or bathtub bench. To overcome severe lower extremity spasm, flex patient's hips and knees when transferring

2. Sliding boards to transfer to shower, commode chair, or tub bench
3. Depending on the level of the lesion, catheterization can be performed with tenodesis splints
4. Bowel training chair

Powered wheelchairs and mobile carts have been perfected and are available. The telephone companies have many options in communication aids for the disabled; these may vary depending on the region of the country in which the patient lives.

ADL for the Head-Injured Patient

Because of the various degrees of cognitive deficits seen in head-injured patients, thorough assessment of the level of cognition is necessary when establishing realistic ADL goals. In order to maximize cognitive skills, the occupational therapist, along with the nursing staff and the family, must provide consistency to achieve successful results. A few of the cognitive areas that should be assessed are: orientation, attention/concentration, initiation/perseveration, impulsivity/judgment, planning, problem solving, and carryover.

Dressing and Hygiene

For patients with hemiplegia as well as head injury refer to ADL training for the hemiplegic patient (page 260). Suggestions are:
1. Before each ADL session begins, orient the patient to person, place, and time if appropriate. A calendar in the room and familiar photos will be helpful.
2. Provide the appropriate amount of structure. For example, if the patient is able, allow him or her decision-making responsibilities by allowing a choice of clothing. If patient is confused or agitated, talk slowly and firmly.
3. Perform dressing and hygiene each day with the same sequence. For example, wash face, brush teeth, and then comb hair.
4. Be aware of the amount of verbal commands you provide so that you do not overwhelm the patient with directions or information.
5. Lists are often helpful for the patient to aid in planning and memory. Lists also provide consistency between nursing and occupational therapy.

Feeding

Due to cognitive deficits, head-injured patients may be unable to initiate, concentrate, or plan while eating.

Again, structure, consistency, and a quiet environment will aid in increasing the patient's level of independence. Some suggestions include:
1. Provide reality orientation if necessary.
2. Assistive devices may be required.

Bathing

1. Bedside commode chair may aid in accessibility.
2. Bathtub seat and grab bars may aid in safety and in independence.

ADL for Patients with Limited Range of Motion

These patients may include those with arthritis, multiple sclerosis, multiple traumatic injury, fractured hip, or chronic low back pain. Generally, there are no standard procedures for ADL for patients with limited ROM; however, the following adaptations may prove helpful:

Dressing

1. Larger clothing
2. Adapted styles of clothing; for example, use of Velcro fasteners
3. Long shoehorn
4. Reachers
5. Sock aids
6. Elastic shoelaces
7. Loops sewn on clothing to facilitate use of hook on a handle

Feeding

1. Built-up handles
2. Elongated handles
3. Long plastic straw
4. Feeding aid

Hygiene and Grooming

1. Hand-held shower
2. Reachers to hold washcloth, powder puff, and so forth
3. Long-handled combs, toothbrush
4. Spray-type deodorant

Homemaking

Home management training can be implemented in treatment plans to improve functional wheelchair mobility or functional ambulation, upper extremity strength and coordination, upper extremity sensory awareness, compensatory techniques for visual or perceptual deficits, and cognitive skills such as following directions and judgment. Home management training is individualized for each patient, depending on capabilities and limitations. However, these considerations can be followed.

Energy Conservation Techniques

The introduction of basic energy conservation techniques is of prime importance to patients with any disability. All patients who participate in managing the home may benefit from home management training. These may include the housewife, husband, bachelor, widow/widower, or young adult living at home. The homemaker must be made aware of new demands and of limitations placed on his or her energy. For example, the use of a wheelchair or assistive ambulation device requires an extra expenditure of energy. Cardiac problems or arthritis may necessitate stopping or altering some activities. Adaptive equipment can often reduce the amount of energy exerted to perform functional activities.

One of the most difficult areas is helping the patient feel comfortable with and accepting of the new rate and method of work. Many individuals become frustrated with their initial attempts at activity, and frustration, fear, and anxiety can drain energy faster than the actual performance of some tasks. Efforts should be made to provide an atomosphere for training and evaluation that is pleasant and conducive to learning and that allows for maximal performance.

Decision making is an integral part of work simplification. The decisions made may indicate role reversal, hiring help, compromise of priority, or modifications in the home. Many homemakers see work simplification techniques as the lazy way to work, and they are uncomfortable with accepting new methods, products, or equipment. The homemaker should first question the reason for doing each task. *Is it necessary?* Many tasks or at least portions of tasks can be eliminated. *Is the homemaker the one best suited to do this task?* Many family members may be capable of assuming the responsibility. The homemaker may, in turn, assume activities more appropriate to his/her present abilities. It is important to consider *when* a task must be completed in relation to other planned activities. It may be necessary to alternate the tasks of a passive nature with more active tasks. Discussion of *how* a task should be completed will provide an opportunity to introduce convenience foods and appropriate small appliances or assistive devices. Many individuals are concerned with excessive cost but, in terms of the cost of time and energy

saved, the homemaker cannot afford to limit herself/himself to old methods or equipment. *Rehabilitation Monograph VIII*[6] offers assistance in developing an improved method in work simplification techniques and principles:

1. Use both hands to work, in opposite and symmetrical motions.
2. Lay out work areas within normal reach. Arrange supplies in a semicircle within normal reach.
3. Slide—do not lift and carry. Use a pushcart to transport equipment.
4. Have a place to do each job so that supplies and equipment may always be kept ready for immediate use.
5. Select equipment that may be used for more than one job; eliminate unnecessary motions. Use recipes that emphasize the "one-bowl" method.
6. Avoid holding—use utensils with a flat base, suction cups, rubber mats, or electric mixers to free both hands.
7. Let gravity work—a laundry chute.
8. Pre-position tools.
9. Store the most commonly used items as the most accessible. Avoid bending and reaching for supplies.
10. Locate machine control and switches within easy reach.
11. Sit to work whenever possible.
12. Select workplace height appropriate for the worker and for the job.

There is no standard height, because body proportions differ.[6]

Incoordination

Incoordination can be caused by a variety of diseases or conditions such as Parkinson's disease, multiple sclerosis, cerebral palsy, cerebral vascular disease, and traumatic head injury. Regardless of the specific cause, it is often necessary and desirable to attempt to use the affected extremity to develop coordination. Homemaking tasks may provide a productive form of exercise. Simple cooking tasks allow the patient to increase coordination by opening containers and holding utensils.

Before introducing specific techniques, it is especially important to allay any of the patient's fears that could aggravate the coordination problem or hinder safe functioning. Also, fatigue can influence the degree of spasticity or incoordination.

Emphasis should be placed on activities that the patient can complete easily and safely. Families should be made aware of all limitations as well as abilities. Self-help catalogs have many gadgets for the individual with the use of only one hand. Although some equipment may be necessary for independent functioning, it should be stressed that most homemaking activities can be completed with nothing more than the proper technique.

A spikeboard, two stainless steel nails on a board, becomes a second hand to stabilize everything from potatoes to cupcakes to meat. A Dycem mat can be used to hold bowls, pans, or plates. Packages or jars can be stabilized for easy opening by placing them between the knees. One-hand-grip scissors are helpful in opening many types of packages. Each person should be allowed to experiment with various techniques and pieces of equipment to encourage the problem-solving methods at home.

The Arthritic Patient

The arthritic homemaker may find it crucial to conserve energy and protect his/her joints from undue stress. Some homemaking tasks provide good exercise and actually may be beneficial. All activities must be monitored with regard to the joint stress produced, the amount of time required in one position, and the contribution to general fatigue. It is important to emphasize the following:

1. Practice energy conservation techniques. All these will apply to the arthritic homemaker.
2. Sit when possible but not for long periods of time.
3. Use fingers in extension whenever possible; for example, in dishwashing and dusting.
4. Use larger joints whenever possible to distribute weight. For example, carry handbag over shoulder instead of in clasped hands.
5. Avoid movements which encourage ulnar deviation.

The arthritic homemaker will be well aware of his/her limitations. A few items of adaptive equipment chosen in the treatment program may eliminate the need for restriction of activity. The *Self-Help Manual for Arthritic Patients* from the Arthritis Foundation[4] answers many questions on equipment needs and specific task techniques.

Because of the progression of arthritis, the homemaker may have psychological problems such as grief, denial, or depression. The therapist may be instrumental in easing these problems as well as in easing pain and increasing function in the affected joints.

The Quadriplegic Patient

The quadriplegic patient must be provided with knowledge and skills to organize and manage his/her daily home management activities effectively. Introduced in the early stages of rehabilitation, basic management skills can help allay the feelings of total helplessness. The therapist can provide the patient with opportunities

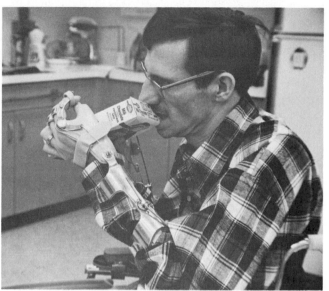

Figure 17-10. Teeth and tenodesis splints work together effectively to open packages.

to develop problem-solving skills that may carry over into other areas of the patient's activities. Financial management, childrearing, diet instruction, and meal planning are initial tasks that can be accomplished to provide positive reinforcement and increase motivation. With the use of telephone and typing skills, manually or by mouth (using mouthstick), it is possible to assume tasks such as ordering groceries and paying bills. It is important that families be involved, especially when role reversals or modifications are indicated.

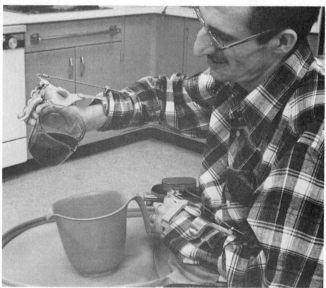

Figure 17-11. A lightweight measuring cup, bowl with handle, and vinyl lap tray promote independence for the quadriplegic patient with natural or mechanical tenodesis functioning.

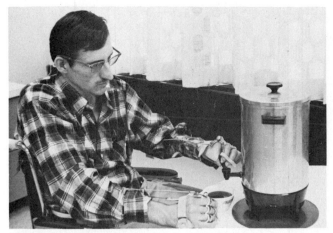

Figure 17-12. Urn stabilized with rubber mat provides hot water for instant cereals, soups, and beverages.

For those quadriplegics (generally C5 lesions and below) who will be assuming some or most homemaking tasks, special attention should be given to equipment selection and utilization of work simplification techniques (Figs. 17-10 and 17-11). The use of such appliances as an electric skillet, can opener, coffee urn, or microwave oven can provide a great degree of independence (Fig. 17-12). *Mealtime Manual for the Aged and Handicapped*[5] offers specific suggestions for the use and selection of adapted equipment and appliances. Because of the patient's loss of sensation, safety should be a prime consideration, especially in the use of heat or sharp objects. The patient must also develop an understanding of the amount of time required to perform simple home management skills. In this way, the patient will be able to plan and organize daily schedules efficiently.

Home Visits and Home Modification

The subject of home modification can be approached when both the patient and the family exhibit signs of acceptance of the disability and an understanding of the permanence of the situation. There are several ways to determine the need for home modifications. One is by receiving information, floor plans, and measurements from the family, the other by making a home visit. The therapist will determine the need for a home visit on the basis of the reliability of the family in providing accurate information and measurements, the patient's level of functioning, and the general description of the home environment.

When a home visit is indicated, it may be advantageous to include the patient. Questions can be answered and fears quelled. Home visits also help the family to prepare emotionally for the patient to return home after hospitalization or rehabilitation.

The occupational therapist and other members of the rehabilitation team such as the physical therapist may participate in the evaluation. The following areas should be considered:

1. Entranceways (concrete versus gravel, slope, steps)
2. Width of doorways
3. Floor coverings (ambulation and wheelchair propulsion are more difficult on carpeting) and door sills
4. Furniture placement (important for transfers)
5. Location of light switches, telephone, and radio. A cordless telephone offers convenience and safety for the handicapped.
6. Safety in the bathroom. Is equipment needed, such as grab bars or elevated seats?
7. Size of bedroom and accessibility of closets and storage areas
8. Size of kitchen and accessibility of appliances and cupboards
9. Accessibility of laundry facilities
10. Installation of a fire extinguisher and smoke detector

After the information has been obtained, the occupational therapist determines the necessary home modifications. Most people are unable to remodel extensively and some, those who rent houses or apartments, find it impossible to make any structural changes. Ingenuity and perseverance are needed and can make even the most unlikely places accessible. Much has been written concerning home modifications with special emphasis on the kitchen and bathroom. Special requirements have been established for wheelchair functioning, proper work heights, and storage areas (Fig. 17-13). Each of the three common types of kitchen—U-shaped, L-shaped, and aisle—has advantages and disadvantages; these depend on the homemaker, the disability, and the family situation. Figure 17-14 is a sketch of sample bathroom facilities.

Dietary Considerations

The incorporation of nutrition principles is an essential part of any home management rehabilitation program. Nutritional needs are established and prescribed by the physician or dietician, but home management rehabilitation provides a natural area for testing, training, and explaining dietary plans. The American Dietetic Association offers many audiovisual aids, posters, and pamphlets that are helpful in teaching nutrition. Increasing nutritional awareness is vital for the cardiac, diabetic, or malnourished patient. The patient must realize that, depending on one's level of activity or wheelchair use

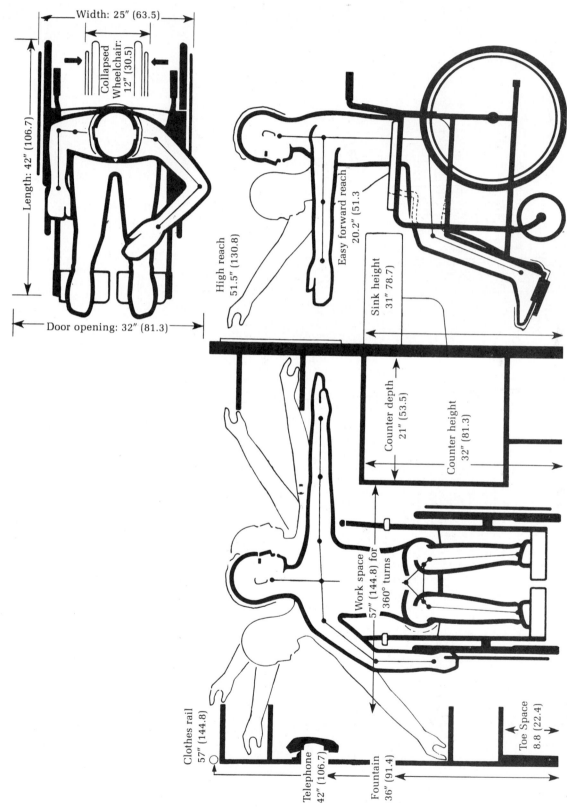

Figure 17-13. Basic measurements and proportions can be utilized when planning home modifications. (Measurements are given in inches and centimeters.) (Adapted from Diffrient N, Tilley AR, Bardagey J: *Humanscale 1/2/3*. Designer: Henry Dreyfuss Associates. Cambridge, MA, MIT Press, 1974.)

Width: 25" (63.5)

Collapsed Wheelchair: 12" (30.5)

Length: 42" (106.7)

Door opening: 32" (81.3)

High reach 51.5" (130.8)

Easy forward reach 20.2" (51.3)

Sink height 31" 78.7)

Counter depth 21" (53.5)

Counter height 32" (81.3)

Work space 57" (144.8) for 360° turns

Clothes rail 57" (144.8)

Telephone 42" (106.7)

Fountain 36" (91.4)

Toe Space 8.8 (22.4)

267

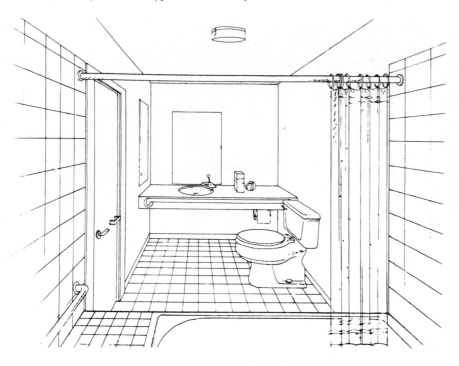

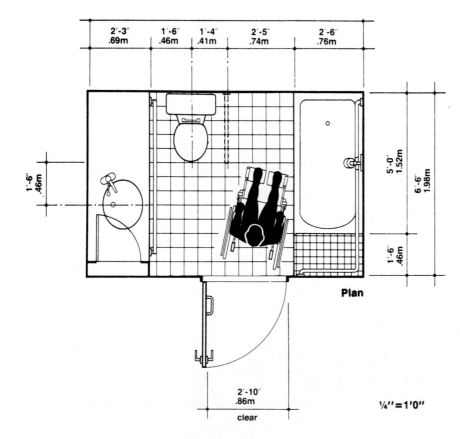

Plan

¼" = 1'0"

Figure 17-14. Two views of a bathroom suitable for use by most disabled persons. (Courtesy of Harkness SP, Groom JN, Jr: *Building Without Barriers for the Disabled.* The Architect Collaborative Inc, Whitney Library of Design, Cambridge, MA, 1976.)

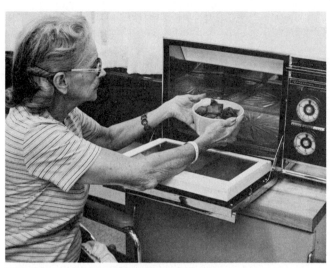

Figure 17-15. Fast no-mess cooking in a microwave oven can encourage those who live alone or are on modified diets to prepare meals that meet their nutritional needs.

there may be an increase or a decrease in caloric needs for the day.

Many patients, due to either premorbid lifestyle or long periods of inactivity during hospitalization, have exceeded their normal weight. Excess weight severely limits a handicapped homemaker in reaching his or her potential. Transfers are more difficult, dressing problems are increased, and more energy is required to ambulate or perform other physical activity. General tolerance and endurance are reduced. Prostheses, if used, often do not fit correctly.

Introduction of new food preparation methods may be helpful. For example, teach broiling instead of frying, or introduce new products such as sugar substitutes. Emphasis should be placed on planning foods that are not only relatively easy to prepare but also are nutritious (Fig. 17-15). There are many diabetic cookbooks to recommend to patients and their families.

Basic nutrition principles are essential, not only for the homemaker, but also for the family. Often, it is necessary to emphasize the manner in which the patient's dietary restrictions can be coordinated with family food planning. The use of food stamps or other government-sponsored assistance programs (*e.g.*, Meals on Wheels) should be explained and the homemaker referred to the appropriate agency.

Financial Management

Evaluation of the patient's ability to manage finances is necessary if the patient will be performing this role after discharge. For many patients who have suffered trauma to the brain, either from cerebral vascular accident or head injury, simple mathematics is difficult. Due to per-

ceptual problems, the patient may be unable to differentiate a quarter from a dime. The therapist may evaluate the patient's ability to sort and count money, figure the correct amount of change, and pay bills. The patient and family must be made aware of any problem areas, so that role changes can be made prior to discharge.

Training Apartment

In addition to basic home management activities, a training apartment provides an essential setting for an important portion of the evaluation process. According to the procedures and policies established for the use of the Harmarville Rehabilitation Center apartment,[3] the purposes of a trial stay in the apartment are:
1. To evaluate patient and family capabilities in a homelike situation. Apartment use must be indicated therapeutically.
2. To evaluate physical and emotional needs of a patient and family
3. To reinforce and follow through on patient care procedures in preparation for discharge and document the level of performance of patient or family in a protected but independent area

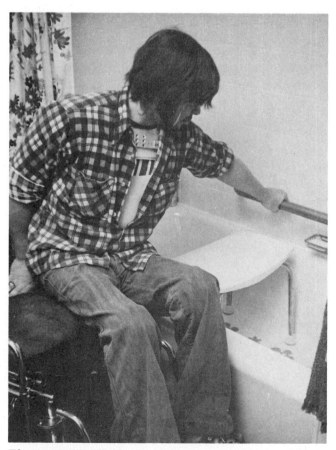

Figure 17-16. The homemaking apartment provides an opportunity for the patient to care for himself, thus preparing him for independent living.

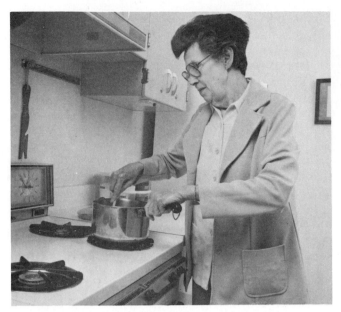

Figure 17-17. The homemaking apartment provides an opportunity for the patient to practice skills that will be needed after discharge.

In addition to being an education tool, an apartment stay can provide a means for increasing the confidence of the patient and family. On a daily basis, the apartment lends itself to use as a training area for activities of daily living, for transfer training, and for the evaluation of large-scale homemaking tasks (Figs. 17-16 and 17-17).

Community Reentrance Skills

Community reentrance skills include mobility (wheelchair, ambulation, transfers), ADL, cognitive, vocational, social, and home management skills. The purpose of community reentrance groups is to evaluate and train the patient to function in typical community settings such as grocery stores, restaurants, and parks. Patients participating in community reentrance groups develop an awareness of social and physical barriers in the community as well as gain knowledge of their capabilities and their limitations. Community reentrance groups can lead to a smoother adjustment after discharge from rehabilitation centers by providing opportunities to practice skills and discover new ones.

Accessibility

Federal and state governments and public and nonprofit groups are becoming involved in breaking the barriers that are keeping the disabled from using public buildings, housing, theaters, stores, recreational facilities, restaurants, and public transportation. In the early 1960s, the President's Committee on Employment for the Handicapped, with the Easter Seal Society for Crippled Children and Adults, led a campaign that made the public aware of this discrimination. Enactment of the Architectural Barriers Act of 1968[8] ensured that certain federally funded buildings and facilities would be designed to be accessible and usable by the physically handicapped. Federal legislation has established standards, which were revised in 1976, for providing accessibility as prescribed by the American National Standards Institute (ANSI). The Architectural and Transportation Barriers Compliance Board was created by the Rehabilitation Act of 1973. By 1974, every state and the District of Columbia had required the elimination of architectural barriers in public buildings either through legislation, building codes, or executive directives.[1]

The International Symbol of Access, officially in use since 1969, has been of assistance to millions throughout the world in the location, identification, and use of facilities designed for the disabled. The symbol signifies barrier-free facilities: ramped entry ways; restrooms with wide stalls and grab bars; 30-inch wide doorways; ground-level entry; telephone, drinking fountains, and elevator controls within reach; or reserved and enlarged parking spaces near accessible entries. The display of this symbol also educates the public to the problems of accessibility faced by the disabled person. The symbol has increased general awareness, and it acts as a catalyst for the elimination of environmental barriers.

References

1. Further Action Needed to Make All Public Buildings Accessible to the Physically Handicapped. Report to Congress by Comptroller General of the United States, July 1975
2. Learning and Living After Your Stroke, pp 83–90. Pittsburgh, Harmarville Rehabilitation Center, July, 1983
3. Handicapped Homemaker Follow-up Study. Pittsburgh, Harmarville Rehabilitation Center, 1972
4. Klinger JL: Self-Help Manual for Arthritic Patients. New York, Arthritis Foundation, 1974
5. Klinger JL, Friedman FH, Sullivan RA: Mealtime Manual for the Aged and Handicapped. New York, Simon & Schuster, 1970
6. Rusk HA: A Manual for Training the Disabled Homemaker, pp. 49–50. Rehabilitation Monograph VIII. New York, Institute of Rehabilitation Medicine, 1970
7. Zimmerman ME: Activities of daily living. In Willard HS, Spackman CS (eds): Occupational Therapy, 4th ed. pp 217–256. Philadelphia, JB Lippincott, 1971
8. Zimmerman ME: Homemaking training units for rehabilitation centers. Am J Occup Ther 20:226, 1966

Bibliography

Accent on Living Buyer's Guide: Your Number One Source of Information on Products for the Disabled. Bloomington, IL, Cheever Publisher, 1986–87

Access in the 80's: Problems and Solutions. Worchester, MA, Massachusetts Easter Seal Society, 27 Harvard St, Worchester, MA 01608

American Automobile Association: The Handicapped Driver's Mobility Guide. Falls Church, VA, The Association, 1981

American National Standard Specifications for Making Buildings and Facilities Accessible to and Usable by Physically Handicapped People. New York, American National Standards Institute, 1980

Anderson H: The Disabled Homemaker. Springfield, IL, Charles C Thomas, 1981

Architectural Barriers Removal: Resource Guide. Office for Handicapped Individuals and Architectural and Transportation Barriers Compliance Board, 1979

Architectural and Transportation Barrier Compliance Board: Resource Guide to Literature on Barrier-Free Environments, with Selected Annotations. 2nd ed. Washington, DC, The Board, 1980

Baum B, Hall K: Relationship between constructional praxis and dressing in the head injured adult. Am J Occup Ther 35:438, 1981

Cary JR: How to Create Interiors for the Disabled: A Guidebook for Family and Friend. New York, Pan Theon, 1978

Carver V, Rodda M: Disability and the Environment. New York, Schocken, 1978

Chasin J, Saltman J: Wheelchair in the Kitchen: A Guide to Easier Living for the Handicapped Homemaker. Paralyzed Veterans of America, 1978

Chollet D: A cost-benefit analysis of accessibility. Washington, DC, US Department of Housing and Urban Development, 1979

Gallender CN, Gallender D: Dietary Problems and Diets for the Handicapped. Springfield, IL, Charles C Thomas, 1979

Guthrie JL, Crist K, Dienicki D, Walls R: Homemaker rehabilitation in the age of accountability. Rehab Lit 49:90, 1981

Jay P: Help Yourselves: A Guide for Hemiplegics and Their Families, 4th ed. Ian Henry, UK, 1985

Jellinek, Hollis et al Functional abilities and distress levels in brain injured patients at long-term follow-up. Arch Phys Med Rehab 63:160, 1982

Jones M: Accessibility Standards. Springfield, IL, Capital Development Board, 1978

Kernaleguen A: Clothing Designs for the Handicapped. Edmonton, University of Alberta, 1978

I Can Do It! Cookbook for People with very Special Needs. Newport Beach, CA, K&H Publishing, 1979

Kottke F, Stillwell GK, Lehman J: Krusen's Handbook of Physical Medicine And Rehabilitation, 3rd ed. Philadelphia, WB Saunders, 1982

Learning and Living: After Your Spinal Cord Injury. Pittsburgh, Harmarville Rehabilitation Center, May 1983

Malick M: Manual on Dynamic Hand Splinting with Thermoplastic Material. Pittsburgh, Harmarville Rehabilitation Center, 1974

Malick M: Manual on Static Hand Splinting, Pittsburgh, Harmarville Rehabilitation Center, 1972

Mealtimes for Severely and Profoundly Handicapped Persons: New Concepts and Attitudes. Baltimore, University Park Press, 1980

Mondale K. Standardization and the handicapped. Bromma, Sweden, International Committee on Technical Aids, Housing and Transport (Information Center: Box 303, S-161 26, Bromma, Sweden), 1980

Morgan M: Beyond disability: A broader definition of architectural barriers. Am Inst Architects J 65:50, 1986

Panikoff L: Recovery trends of functional skills in the head injured adult. Am J Occup Ther 37: 735, 1983

Resource Manual of Canadian Information Services for the Physically Disabled, 2nd ed. Toronto: Canadian Rehabilitation Council for the Disabled, 1980

Roessler RT: Training independent living specialists. J Rehab 47:36, 1981

Sorensen RJ: Design for Accessibility. New York, McGraw-Hill, 1979

Steinfeld E, Schroeder S, Duncan J: Access to the Built Environment: A Review of the Literature. Washington, DC, US Dept of Housing and Urban Development, 1979

Step-by-Step Pictorial Cookbook. St Louis, Ralston Purina, 1979

Strebel MB: Adaptations and Techniques for the Disabled Homemaker, 5th ed. Minneapolis, Sister Kenny Institute, 1978

Svensson E: Rebuilding: A Few Examples of how Accessibility Can Be Improved in Public Buildings. Bromma, Sweden, ICTS Information Center, 1980

Appreciation is extended to Nancy Annunziato, M.S., OTR/L and Bonnie Sherry Almasy of the Harmarville Rehabilitation Center for their contributions.

CHAPTER 18

Occupational Therapy for the Workplace

Work Assessments and Programming *Karen Jacobs*

Joshua attends preschool.
Ariel is an occupational therapist.
Matthew is a retiree who seriously collects coins.
Laela is a homemaker who volunteers twice a week at a local hospital gift shop.

What these four individuals have in common is that they are all workers. "Work refers to skill and performance in participating in socially purposeful and productive activities."[54] These human occupations—that is, student, homemaker, hobbyist, and volunteer—regardless of whether they are reimbursed, are not limited to adults but relevant throughout the life span (school age to retiree) and can be applied to a broad range of individuals; for example, school-aged children with emotional or physical disabilities, adults in rehabilitation facilities, industrial-injured individuals in a work capacity evaluation center, and disenfranchised older adults.

Two important elements constitute the concept of work: (1) work behavior and (2) work skills, aptitudes, and physical capacities. Work behaviors, which have been more familiarly called "prevocational readiness," are the antecedents to specific work (job) skill development; that is, those behaviors that are necessary for successful participation in a job or independent living. They include, but are not limited to, cooperative behavior, attention span, decision making, motivation, attendance, acceptance of supervision, appropriate appearance, punctuality, responsibility, organization, and productivity.

Work skills, aptitudes, and physical capacities, frequently referred to as "vocational skills," are required to perform the tasks of an actual job. More specifically, work skills are capabilities that the individual has learned or has the potential to learn, such as typing, welding, drafting, soldering, and cooking. Work aptitudes are abilities that are, to one degree or another, possessed by nearly all individuals. Some work aptitudes are coordination, dexterity, and intelligence.

Physical capacities are factors such as the ability to lift heavy objects, to bend, to kneel, and to sit or stand for long periods.

History

"Work is at the heart of the philosophy and practice of occupational therapy. In its broadest sense, work, as productive activity, is the concern in almost all therapy."[25] Indeed, the area of work parallels our profession's development, even though it has been an on-again/off-again romance. (Refer to Chap. 2 for a historical review.)

Occupational therapy (OT) "has been linked to vocational education and rehabilitation through legislation in response to war-generated needs and social change. The initial legislative thrust came in the World War I era. Soldiers were the first to receive vocational education and rehabilitation, then civilians. The second thrust came during World War II, when medical services became available.

In the beginning, emphasis was placed on those people who could be returned to employment quickly. As the need for workers decreased, the social value of work was replaced by a social value of a humane response to disability itself: Everyone deserved a chance to work. Finally society decided that everyone also deserved to live as independently as possible."[32a] The accompanying box lists important legislation that has affected work-related practice.

The 1980s have heralded in the reawakening of interest in work-related practice, as evidenced by the appearance of this topic in various forums: the American Occupational Therapy Association (AOTA) publication, in 1980, of an official position paper entitled "The Role of Occupational Therapy in the Vocational Rehabilitation Process"; the development of 5-day advanced training workshops for therapists entitled "Planning and Implementing Vocational Readiness in Occupational Therapy (PIVOT)"; the publication of *Work Hardening Guidelines*; the May 1985 publication of an entire issue of the *American Journal of Occupational Therapy* (AJOT) devoted to work evaluation; an increased number of presentations at the national conference on this subject; and the establishment of the Work Programs Special Interest Section within the AOTA. In general, there has been an increase in the number of professional articles, textbooks, conferences, and workshops on this subject.[15,25] The climate of the nation's economy, with accelerating health care costs, has offered occupational therapy the perfect marketplace to reestablish work practice, particularly outside the medical model. However, despite these advances, Harvey–Krefting, a Canadian occupational therapist, recognizes that there are still major concerns for this area of practice due to the difficulties in defining an area of practice that is so diverse and so ill-defined (particularly in the area of standardized vocabulary), the lack of formulated models of practice, and the absence of standardized instruments.[19] In addition, regulatory agencies such as the Commission on Accreditation of Rehabilitation Facilities (CARF) are

---

Significant Legislation Related to Work

Year   Description of Legislation

1916   National Defense Act
Improved military efficiency and enabled soldiers to become more competitive in civilian life. The focus was educational, but no agency was established to carry out the directives.

1917   PL 64-347: Smith–Hughes Act (Vocational Education Act)
Created the Federal Board for Vocational Education (FBVE)

1918   PL 65-178: Smith–Sears Act (Soldiers Rehabilitation Act)
Enlarged the role of FBVE to provide programs for disabled veterans who were unable to succeed at gainful employment

1920   PL 66-236: Smith–Fess Act (Civilian Rehabilitation Act)
Initiated rehabilitation for the general public. Provided funds for vocational guidance and training, occupational adjustment, protheses, and placement services. Occupational therapy was reimbursed if it was part of medical treatment. No reimbursement for psychiatric or developmentally disabled persons

Year   Description of Legislation

1921   PL 67-47: Veterans Bureau Act
Established the Veterans Bureau as an independent agency with a director responsible to the President

1933   PL 73-2: Veterans Administration Act
Recognized the Veterans Bureau and designated this federal agency as the Veterans Administration

1935   PL 74-271: Social Security Act
Established unemployment compensation, old-age insurance, child health and welfare services, crippled children services, and public assistance for the aged, blind, and dependent children

1943   PL 78-16: Welsh–Clark Act (World War II Disabled Veterans Rehabilitation Act)

Significant Legislation Related to Work *(continued)*

Year   Description of Legislation

Provided vocational rehabilitation for disabled veterans of World War II

1943   PL 78-113: Barden–LaFollette Act (Vocational Rehabilitation Act)

Changed the original provisions of PL 66-236. Physically disabled, blind, developmentally delayed, and psychiatrically disabled were added to those served. Office of Vocational Rehabilitation (OVR) established. New emphasis on activities of daily living (ADL) and adaptation. Removed ceiling on appropriation

1944   PL 78-346: Servicemen's Readjustment Act (GI Bill)

Provided for the education and training (tuition and subsistence) of individuals whose education or career had been interrupted by military service

1945   PL 79-176: Joint Congressional Resolution for a National Employ the Physically Handicapped (NEPH) Week

Established an annually observed NEPH week. In 1954, Truman changed it to President's Committee on Employment of the Physically Handicapped; in 1962, Kennedy changed it to President's Committee on Employment of the Handicapped

1954   PL 83-565: Hill–Burton Act (Vocational Rehabilitation Act Amendments)

Greater financial support, research and demonstration grants, professional preparation grants, state agency expansion and improvement grants, and grants to expand rehabilitation facilities. Many occupational therapists received this money for training and education

1965   Vocational Rehabilitation Act Amendments of 1965

Increased services for several types of disabled and socially handicapped persons. Construction money made available for rehabilitation centers and workshops

1968   PL 90-480: Architectural Barriers Act

Led the way to changes in access for disabled persons

1970   PL 91-517: Developmental Disabilities Services and Facilities Construction Act

States were given broad responsibility for planning and implementing a comprehensive program of services to developmentally delayed, epileptic, cerebral palsied, and other neurologically impaired individuals

1973   PL 93-112: Rehabilitation Act

Expanded services to the more severely disabled. Also provided for affirmative action in employ-

Year   Description of Legislation

ment (Section 503) and nondiscrimination in facilities (Section 504) by federal contractors and grantees

1975   PL 94-142: Education For All Handicapped Children Act

Provided educational assistance to all handicapped children in the "least restrictive environment." Occupational therapists included as "related personnel"

1978   PL 95-602: Amendments to the Rehabilitation Act of 1973

Expansion of rehabilitation to include independent living. Established the National Institute of Handicapped Research. Provided employer incentives for training and hiring disabled individuals

1983   PL 98-199: Education of the Handicapped Act Amendments of 1983

Established better transition from school to work

1984   PL 88-210: Carl D. Perkins Vocational Act

Authorized federal grants to states to assist them in (1) extending, improving, and maintaining existing programs of vocational education; (2) developing new programs; (3) providing part-time employment for youths who need earnings to continue their vocational training on a full-time basis; and (4) assisting persons of all ages (secondary, postsecondary, and adult levels) to enter the labor market, upgrade their skills, or learn new ones. Provides funding for the following grant programs: Adult Training and Retraining, Career Guidance and Counseling, High Technology Training, Title II Basic Grants, Consumer and Homemaking Education, and Community-Based Organizations (CBO) programs

1986   PL 99-357: Carl D. Perkins Vocational Education Act Amendment

A technical amendment to rectify a problem with state allocation of funds, particularly for the Consumer and Homemaking Education program

1986   PL 99-457: Education of the Handicapped Act Amendments

Provides a significant increase in federal funds to encourage states to provide special education and related services to preschoolers ages 3 through 5 years. Federal funds for this age group will be terminated if this is not initiated by school year 1990–91. Also included is a mandate for a new comprehensive, interagency program to provide early intervention to infants and toddlers with handicaps, ages birth through 2 years.

dictating the role of occupational therapists. For example, present CARF standards do not allow an OTR without a Master's degree to be a director of a work program or to be called a vocational specialist.[12,42] These standards allow OTRs with baccalaureate degrees to be hired as vocational evaluators or work-adjustment specialists only if other criteria have been met.

At present, there are many sources for employment in work practice, and the settings appear to be expanding: workshops, schools, and educational facilities; hospitals and institutions; rehabilitation centers; community agencies; nursing homes and residential centers; home health; clinics; correctional facilities and prisons; job sites and industry; and private practice.[45] If occupational therapy is to play an important role in these settings, we will need to respond to the concerns previously described.

The Work Process

A review of the literature reveals the following as some of the occupational therapy functions that relate to work[1,21-23]:

1. Initial screening
2. Interest assessment
3. Support in exploration or identification of possible work objectives
4. Evaluation of motor, perceptual, and cognitive abilities
5. Evaluation of work skills and tolerances
6. Evaluation of work habits and interpersonal skills
7. Evaluation of work-related capabilities, such as transportation, communication, and self-care
8. Work-hardening programs
9. Work adjustment and habit/behavior programs
10. Independent living skills programs
11. Work placement programs
12. Job analysis and work environment evaluation
13. Task and environmental adaptation
14. Follow-up care

From this list, it is possible to group the functions of occupational therapists, related to work practice, into four sequential categories that may be viewed as similar to the vocational rehabilitation process: *assessment, planning, treatment/programming,* and *termination/follow-up care.*[46] Within this process, the therapist will have the opportunity to work with a broad array of personnel. In the rehabilitation field, these individuals may include rehabilitation counselors, work evaluators, work adjustment specialists, employment or vocational counselors, job placement specialists, and rehabilitation nurses. Some additional personnel are teachers, administrators, employers, physicians, physical therapists, and other ancillary services.[61]

Assessment
General Overview

Assessment is a term which has been often misused as a synonym for *evaluation.* In actuality, assessment is much more encompassing and includes evaluation as one of its three phases (1) intake interview, (2) general medical examination, and (3) evaluation.

A variety of processes are used by occupational therapists in assessment:

1. Review of medical, educational, and vocational records
2. Interviews with the individual, the family, employer, teachers, and others
3. Observation
4. Inventories and checklists
5. Standardized and nonstandardized evaluations[47]

Specifically, work assessment uses these processes in an attempt " . . . to predict current and future employment potential by evaluating mental, emotional and physical abilities along with limitations and tolerances. It focuses on the identification of a person's strengths and weaknesses in relation to general employability factors and specific vocational skills."[46] Also important is the assessment of the individual's occupational interests and ancillary (indirect) job needs; that is, mobility skills.

The following discussion briefly reviews observation, inventories, and checklists and then focuses on standardized and nonstandardized evaluations.

Observation

As occupational therapists, we are trained to hone our observation skills. Applying these skills in the assessment process represents the key to developing an accurate performance profile of the individual.[32] (Refer to Chap. 15 for more information.)

Inventories and Checklists

There are many inventories and checklists that can be used to gain insight into the individual's interests, desires, and possible work objectives. The OTR may use the Activity Configuration,[60] the Interest Checklist,[36] the Vocational Behavior Checklist,[59] the Reading-Free Vocational Interest Inventory,[4] and Assessing Your Work Values.[10]

The *Reading-Free Vocational Interest Inventory* provides a series of 55 rows of line drawings arranged in groups of three depicting various unskilled, semiskilled, and skilled tasks (Fig. 18-1). The evaluee is instructed to select one picture from each row of three. After all the

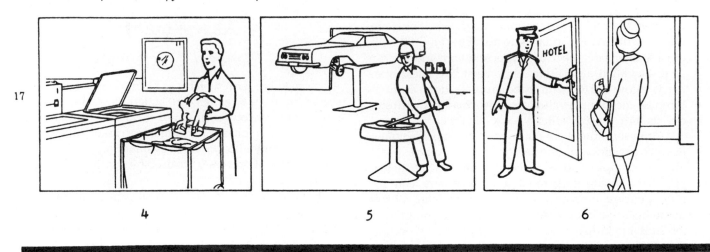

17   4   5   6

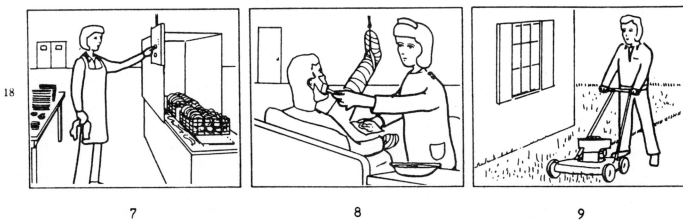

18   7   8   9

Figure 18-1. An example of the Reading-Free Vocational Interest Inventory: M F devised by Ralph L. Becker. The evaluee is instructed to circle the picture in each row that he likes best to ascertain his work interests. The complete inventory contains 55 rows of pictures of people working at various jobs. (Becker RL: Reading-Free Vocational Interest Inventory: M F. Columbus, Ohio, Elbern Publications, 1981)

rows are completed, a profile is calculated based on percentiles of interest within the eleven interest areas (*e.g.,* automotive, animal care, laundry service) presented. Reading comprehension is not a variable of this inventory.

Assessing Your Work Values was developed as a checklist for women who want to plan, begin, change, or advance in their careers and is used to help clarify the individual's motivations for working. Figure 18-2 provides examples of three of the 13 work values the individual may find important.

Additional inventories and checklists can be found in Figure 18-8, under the category of volitional subsystem, which is part of Kielhofner's "model of the person as an open system."[28]

Evaluation

CARF composed the following list as a guide for work evaluation:

Physical and psychomotor capacities

Intellectual capacities; emotional stability; interests, attitudes and knowledge of occupational information; personal, social, and work histories; aptitudes

Achievements (*e.g.,* vocational, educational)

Work skills and work tolerances

Work habits (punctuality, attendance, concentration, organization, and interpersonal skills)

Work-related capabilities (*e.g.,* mobility, communication skills, hygiene, homemaking, money management)

Job-seeking skills

Potential to benefit from further services that are specifically identified

Employment objectives, which may involve either competitive or noncompetitive employment or programs in industry options

Individuals' ability to learn about themselves as a result of information obtained and furnished through the evaluation experience

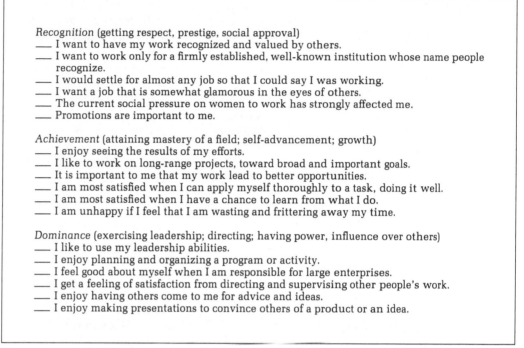

Recognition (getting respect, prestige, social approval)
___ I want to have my work recognized and valued by others.
___ I want to work only for a firmly established, well-known institution whose name people recognize.
___ I would settle for almost any job so that I could say I was working.
___ I want a job that is somewhat glamorous in the eyes of others.
___ The current social pressure on women to work has strongly affected me.
___ Promotions are important to me.

Achievement (attaining mastery of a field; self-advancement; growth)
___ I enjoy seeing the results of my efforts.
___ I like to work on long-range projects, toward broad and important goals.
___ It is important to me that my work lead to better opportunities.
___ I am most satisfied when I can apply myself thoroughly to a task, doing it well.
___ I am most satisfied when I have a chance to learn from what I do.
___ I am unhappy if I feel that I am wasting and frittering away my time.

Dominance (exercising leadership; directing; having power, influence over others)
___ I like to use my leadership abilities.
___ I enjoy planning and organizing a program or activity.
___ I feel good about myself when I am responsible for large enterprises.
___ I get a feeling of satisfaction from directing and supervising other people's work.
___ I enjoy having others come to me for advice and ideas.
___ I enjoy making presentations to convince others of a product or an idea.

Figure 18-2. Examples of a checklist based on 13 work values, such as recognition, achievement, and money, which is used to clarify a person's motivation for working. The evaluee is instructed to check one statement within each value category that is important to him or her. (Catalyst: What to Do With the Rest of Your Life. New York, Simon & Schuster, 1980.)

Assessment of the most effective mode of understanding and responding to various types of instruction Identification of the need for tool and job site modification or adaptive equipment that may enhance the individual's employability.[12]

This listing, although also composed of some secondary treatment goals, is consistent with occupational therapists' education, skill, and experience. In actuality, many of the evaluations commonly used in OT practice to evaluate strength, endurance, coordination, dexterity, activities of daily living, and interpersonal skills can be considered part of work evaluation.[53]

Types of Work Evaluation

Botterbusch categorizes work evaluations within one of the following four techniques:
1. On-the-job evaluations
2. Situational assessment
3. Psychological tests
4. Work samples[7,8]

There is an inverse relationship between the closeness of the technique to real work as viewed by the client and the overall cost of the technique. Botterbusch notes:

. . . tests . . . are the cheapest way of obtaining information about a client. Job site evaluation requires a heavy staff investment in terms of the amount of time needed to develop the initial job site and to maintain a client on the site. Situation assessment requires the existence of a workshop, production contracts, and staff for supervision. If "homemade" work sample techniques are used, they require staff time to develop as well as money and time to construct; commercial work sample systems can cost up to $20,000 for the initial purchase. All work samples eventually require replacement parts and many require expendable supplies. Tests have the advantages of: 1. being cheaper to buy, 2. usually being group administered, and 3. often having separate answer sheets which reduce the expense of expendable supplies.[8]

This can be visualized as in Figure 18-3.

Most often, combinations of these techniques are the most effective way to appraise an individual's work potential and future performance in job training and employment.[61]However, not all the evaluation techniques are used by the OTR or are appropriate for every individual. For example, a school-aged person with no work experience is referred for an evaluation with the purpose of ascertaining occupational interests, whereas another individual who has work experience but has been fired from a series of jobs is referred for the purpose of

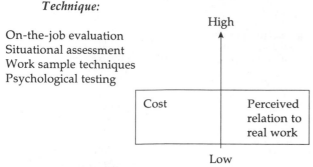

Technique:

On-the-job evaluation
Situational assessment
Work sample techniques
Psychological testing

Figure 18-3. A model that demonstrates the inverse relationship between the closeness to real work as viewed by the client of a work-evaluation technique and the overall cost of the technique.

evaluating behaviors in order to find out which are causing job instability.

On-the-Job Evaluations

On-the-job evaluations "are situations in which the client is assessed in one or more of a variety of real work situations including job site situations in industry, trial training evaluation in a training program, and simulated job stations within the facility."[7] The OT evaluation may include ascertaining the individual's ability to perform and tolerate physical activities of the job such as sitting, kneeling, reaching, carrying, and lifting. Figure 18-4 is an example of a physical capacities evaluation.

Situational Assessment

The method of situational assessment involves placing an individual in a controlled, artificial work environment, where the person can be observed and variables systematically altered. This technique is most often used in more elemental kinds of work, such as unskilled assembly.[33]

Psychological Tests

These include an almost endless variety of paper-and-pencil and apparatus techniques for measuring general intelligence, achievement, abilities, and related characteristics of an individual and are typically administered by psychologists.[7,8,47] Table 18-1 lists some of the most commonly used psychological tests.

Work Samples

Work sampling is the primary technique of work evaluation and has evolved " . . . to meet the growing demand for vocational and special services to a variety of disability groups in traditional rehabilitation settings,

clinics and public schools."[37] A work sample is " . . . well defined work activity involving tasks, materials, and tools which are identical or similar to those in an actual job or cluster of jobs. It is used to access an individual's vocational aptitude, worker characteristics and vocational interests."[49] Work samples have the advantage of resembling actual work, providing an opportunity to observe work behaviors and physical functioning and a variety of work areas.[7] There are four types of work samples according to their degree of correspondence with actual jobs: actual job samples, simulated job samples, cluster trait samples, and single trait samples.[7]

The TOWER, Vocational Evaluation System (Singer), some of the work samples in the Valpar Component Work Sample Series (VCWS) (*i.e.,* VCWS No. 16, Drafting), and the Jewish Employment and Vocational Services (JEVS) Work Samples are commercially avail-

Table 18-1. *Psychological Tests Frequently Used in Work Assessment*

Category	Name
Achievement batteries & reading tests	Adult Basic Learning Examination
	California Achievement Tests
	Gray Oral Reading Test
	Nelson–Denny Reading Test
	Peabody Individual Achievement Test
	Tests of Adult Basic Education
Personality	Minnesota Multiphasic Personality Inventory
	Draw-a-Person Test
	House–Tree–Person Test
Intelligence	Wechsler Adult Intelligence Scale
	Peabody Picture Vocabulary Test
Vocational aptitudes	General Aptitude Test Battery
	Non-Reading Aptitude Test Battery
	Purdue Pegboard
	Crawford Small Parts Dexterity Test
	Stromberg Dexterity Test
Vocational interests	Strong Vocational Interest Blank
	Geist Picture Interest Inventory
	Minnesota Importance Questionnaire
	Kuder Occupational Interest Survey
	Wide Range Interest–Opinion Test

PHYSICAL CAPACITIES EVALUATION

Name: _____   Date: _____

	NORMS	N	G	F	P	O	LIMITS	COMMENTS
1. Sitting								
Standing								
Walking								
Stooping								
Kneeling								
Crouching								
Crawling								
2. Climbing								
Balancing								
3. Lifting (Unilateral)								
Lifting (Bilateral)								
Carrying								
Pushing								
Pulling								
4. Reaching								
Handling								
Fingering								
Feeling								
Placing								
5. Talking								
Hearing								
6. Seeing								
a. Acuity								
b. Depth perception								
c. Field of vision								
d. Accommodation								
e. Color vision								

FUNCTIONAL TOLERANCES

1. Standing								
2. Sitting								
3. General mobility								
4. Fine work								
5. Rapid work								
6. Repetitive work								
7. Sequential work								
a. Short cycle								
b. Long cycle								
8. Stamina								

Norms are based on D.O.T. Standards

KEY: O—Unable to perform, or impractical
P—Performed with assistance, improvement needed
F—Performed without assistance, but improvement needed to be adequate
G—Adequate for practical performance even though affected by disability
N—Performance not affected by disability

Figure 18-4. Sample form for a physical capacities evaluation. Norms are completed by the therapists depending on the task selected; form is from the Delaware Curative Workshop, Wilmington, Delaware (reproduced with permission.)

able *actual job samples;* that is, they are samples of work that have been taken in their entirety from an employment setting and brought to a testing environment for the purpose of evaluating an individual's interest and aptitude. Some of the jobs represented are pipe fitting, refrigeration, electronic assembly, baking and cooking, and cosmetology.

A *simulated job sample* is a representation of the common critical factors of a job. It differs from an actual job sample in that not all factors affecting the job are replicated, for example, environmental stress.[61] Figure 18-5 portrays a simulated job sample of grill work for a fast-food restaurant that has been constructed in a special-needs high school and used with its learning-disabled students. Another simulated job sample is the Baltimore Therapeutic Equipment (BTE) Work Simulator (Fig. 18-6). It is composed of an adjustable shaft that accommodates a variety of tools that simulate jobs (*e.g.,* shoveling) and can be adjusted to different angles and heights and a computer console that displays the

amount of resistance programmed by the therapist. After the completion of an activity, there can be a printout of data such as the amount of time spent on the activity and the force exerted on the tool.[2,5]

The Work Evaluation Systems Technology (WEST) and some of the work samples composing the Valpar Component Work Sample Series (VCWS) (*e.g.,* VCWS No. 4, Upper Extremity Range of Motion) are examples of a *cluster trait sample* because they assess a number of traits inherent in a job or various jobs, such as strength, endurance, range of motion, speed, and dexterity.

The Purdue Pegboard, the Minnesota Rate of Manipulation, the Crawford Small Parts Dexterity Test, the O'Conner Dexterity Tests, the Pennsylvania BiManual Work Sample, the Bennett Hand-Tool Dexterity Test, and the Stromberg Dexterity Test are examples of *single trait samples,* which assess a single worker trait, in this case, dexterity.[53,61] These tests are occasionally included under psychological tests of vocational aptitudes.

There are many standardized and standard work

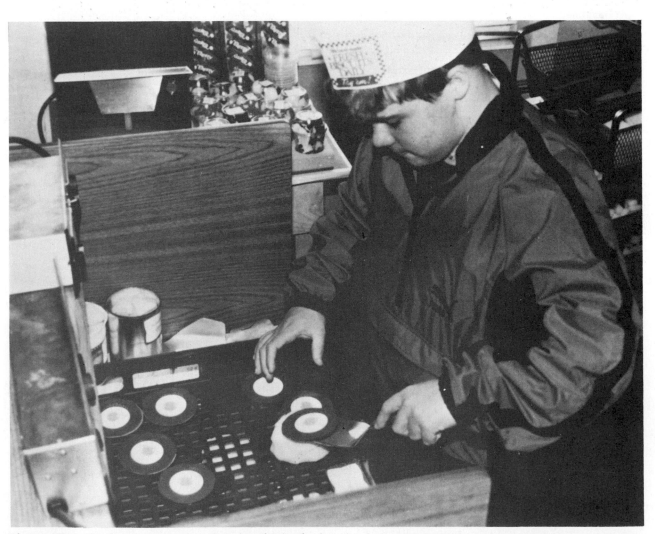

Figure 18-5. Student working in a simulated job of a fast-food restaurant. Job simulation such as this can be used in both evaluation and treatment.

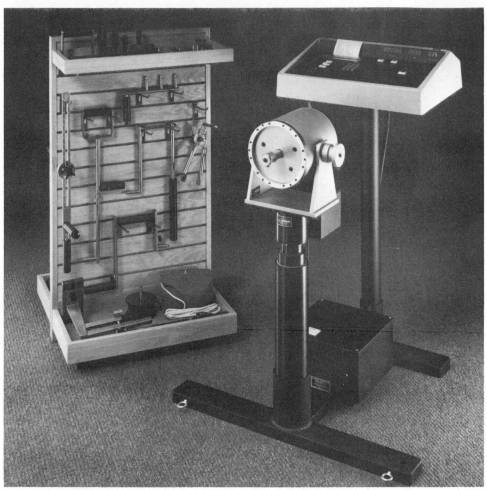

Figure 18-6. Baltimore Therapeutic Equipment (BTE) Work Simulator with attachments; the simulator is used in both evaluation and treatment. (Photography courtesy of Baltimore Therapeutic Equipment Co, Hanover, Maryland)

samples. Because of the high cost of many commerically available work samples, design of work samples by the therapist for a particular population is often appropriate. An example of a therapist-designed work sample system is the Jacobs Prevocational Skills Assessment (JPSA), developed for a learning-disabled adolescent population at the Learning Prep School in West Newton, MA. This 15-task battery relies heavily on observational skills to provide a profile of an individual's skills and behaviors. Table 18-2 is the recording device for the JPSA, which in actuality is an activity analysis of each work sample. Examples of the tasks include quality control, carpentry assembly, office work, and food preparation.[25]

There are a number of additional commercially available work evaluation systems. Many of these are used completely or in part by occupational therapists as well as by other professionals such as work evaluators. Table 18-3 gives a description of 14 systems. The McCarron–Dial System, Valpar, and TOWER will be reviewed in more detail.

Commercial Systems

Botterbusch has authored a monograph through the Materials Development Center, Stout Vocational Rehabilitation Institute, Menomonie, WI entitled *A Comparison of Commercial Vocational Evaluation Systems,* which is one of the best resources on this subject.[7]

McCarron–Dial System

The McCarron–Dial System (MDS) was developed in 1973 by Lawrence T. McCarron and Jack G. Dial to determine the "prevocational, vocational and residential functioning levels of disabled individuals," with revision and expansion of the norm base to include the general population.[37] The system is at present targeted for the learning disabled, emotionally disturbed, mentally retarded, cerebral palsied, closed head-injured, socially handicapped, or culturally disadvantaged persons with adaptations for use with the visually and hearing impaired. MDS is based on a neuropsychological theo-

(Text continues on page 287)

Table 18-2. *The Jacobs Prevocational Skills Assessment (JPSA)*

Tasks	Fine Motor Coordination	Eye-Hand Coordination	Motor Planning	Figure–Ground	Sorting	Classification/Sequencing	Decision Making	Problem Solving	Organizational Skills
1. Quality control	✓			✓	✓		✓		✓
2. Filing A	✓				✓	✓	✓	✓	✓
B	✓			✓	✓	✓	✓	✓	✓
C	✓				✓	✓	✓	✓	✓
3. Carpentry assembly	✓	✓	✓	✓			✓	✓	
4. Classification	✓					✓	✓	✓	
5. Office work A	✓	✓	✓			✓	✓	✓	✓
B	✓	✓	✓			✓		✓	✓
C	✓	✓	✓			✓		✓	✓
6. Telephone directory A	✓	✓		✓		✓			✓
B	✓	✓							✓
7. Factory work	✓	✓	✓	✓			✓	✓	
8. Environmental mobility A	✓	✓	✓	✓				✓	✓
B								✓	✓
9. Money concepts A									
B									
C	✓			✓			✓	✓	
D	✓			✓			✓	✓	✓
10. Functional banking A	✓	✓		✓			✓		
B	✓	✓		✓			✓		
11. Time concept A									
B				✓					
C									
12. Work attitudes A				✓		✓	✓		✓
B							✓	✓	
13. Body scheme	✓							✓	✓
14. Leather assembly	✓	✓	✓	✓		✓			✓
15. Food preparation	✓	✓	✓			✓	✓		

From Jacobs K: *Occupational Therapy: Work-Related Programs and Assessments.* Boston, Little, Brown, 1985.

Use of Tools	Ability to Follow Directions			Conceptual Skills	Task Focus	Behavioral Observations
	Visual	Written	Verbal			
			✓		✓	
		✓		✓	✓	
		✓		✓	✓	
		✓		✓	✓	
✓					✓	
			✓		✓	
✓					✓	
	✓		✓		✓	
		✓		✓	✓	
			✓		✓	
			✓	✓	✓	
			✓		✓	
			✓		✓	
		✓			✓	
			✓	✓	✓	
			✓	✓	✓	
			✓	✓	✓	
		✓	✓	✓	✓	
✓			✓	✓	✓	
			✓	✓	✓	
			✓	✓	✓	
			✓		✓	
			✓		✓	
			✓		✓	
	✓		✓		✓	
✓	✓				✓	
✓	✓				✓	

Table 18-3. *Commercially Available Vocational Rehabilitation Evaluation Systems*

Name	Developer/ Sponsor	Target Population	Work Samples	Scoring and Reporting	Reliability	Address for Information	Cost as of February 1987
Coats	Prep, Inc	Manpower, secondary education, rehabilitation	27 independent samples consisting of job matching, employability attitudes, living skills	Emphasis on quality, standardized reporting forms	Student norms on work samples, data in manuals. Construct validity through factor analysis	Prep, Inc, 1007 Whitehead Rd Ext, Trenton, NJ 08638	Sample 1 ... $ 825 Sample 2 ... $1340 Sample 3 ... $1045 Sample 4 ... $1200 Sample 5 ... $1295 Sample 6 ... $1400 Sample 7 ... $1025 Sample 8 ... $ 495 Sample 9 ... $ 940 Sample 10 ... $1235 Sample 11 ... $1020 Sample 12 ... $1355 Sample 13 ... $ 480 Sample 14 ... $1965 Sample 15 ... $ 910 Sample 16 ... $1190 Sample 17 ... $ 550 Sample 18 ... $ 725 Sample 19 ... $ 480 Sample 20 ... $ 875 Sample 21 ... $1795 Sample 22 ... $ 620 Sample 23 ... $1550 Sample 24 ... $2350 Sample 25 ... $4250 Sample 26 ... $2065 Sample 27 ... $3300
Career Evaluation Systems (Career Hester)	Goodwill Industries of Chicago, Dr. Edward Hester	All intelligence levels, physically disabled	39 test scores	Emphasis on time to completion or number of responses, computer-generated scores, standardized reporting forms	Test scores are integrated by computer to produce a vocational ability profile	Career Evaluation Systems, Inc, 7788 Milwaukee Ave, Niles, IL 60648	$9,000
Jewish Employment and Vocational Services (JEVS)	US Dept of Labor	Initially disadvantaged and handicapped	28 samples arranged according to Dictionary of Occupational Titles 10 worker trait groups and 12 work groups	Time and quality given equal weight. Standardized reporting forms. Little reading required	Norms based on 1100 clients; no data on reliability or recent data on validity	Vocational Research Institute, 2100 Arch St, Philadelphia, PA 19103	$9,980
McCarron–Dial System (MDS)	McCarron and Dial	Neuropsychologically disabled and mentally retarded, mentally ill, learning disabled, normal	Instruments arranged according to five factors	Emphasis on quality, specific time limits, standardized reporting forms	Norms based on several groups of disabled clients, reliability in high 0.80s–low 0.90s	McCarron–Dial Systems, PO Box 45628, Dallas, TX 75245	$1525
Micro-TOWER	ICD Rehabilitation and Research Center	General rehabilitation population	13 samples arranged according to five groups of general aptitude factors	Emphasis on quality, specific time limits for each work sample, standardized reporting forms. Group-administered	19 different norm groups, high reliability	Micro-TOWER ICD Rehabilitation & Research Center, 340 E 24th St, New York, NY 10010	Based on number of tests; approximately $1000 per/set or $10,000 for set of 10

Name	Target population	Samples	Scoring	Norms/Reliability	Source	Cost
Talent Assessment Programs (TAP)	Age 14 and up, mental level above trainable, nonreading	10 independent samples	Emphasis on time, standardized reporting forms. Computer program for job titles based on assessment	Seven different norm groups, reliability of 0.85 coefficient of stability. No data available on validity	Talent Assessment Inc, PO Box 5087, Jacksonville, FL 33247-5087	$5,360
Testing, Orientation, and Work Evaluation in Rehabilitation (TOWER)	Physically and emotionally disabled	110 samples arranged according to 14 training areas	Time and quality given equal weight, standardized reporting forms	Norms based on clients, no data available on reliability and validity	ICD Rehabilitation & Research Center, 340 E 24th St, New York, NY 10010	No hardware; $200 for TOWER manual. Two weeks training on an overview of work evaluations: tools, techniques, and materials available
Valpar Component Work Sample (VCWS)	General population, industrially injured workers	19 independent samples	Weighted combination of time and errors, separate reporting form for each sample	Six different norm groups, time–motion norms, reliability in the 0.80–0.99 range	Valpar International Corp, PO Box 5767, Tucson, AZ 85703-5767	VCWS No. 1 . . . $1095 VCWS No. 2 . . . $ 985 VCWS No. 3 . . . $ 975 VCWS No. 4 . . . $1075 VCWS No. 5 . . . $1950 VCWS No. 6 . . . $1095 VCWS No. 7 . . . $1240 VCWS No. 8 . . . $1525 VCWS No. 9 . . . $1425 VCWS No. 10 . . $1485 VCWS No. 11 . . $1240 VCWS No. 12 . . $1240 VCWS No. 13 . . $1185 VCWS No. 14 . . $2295 VCWS No. 15 . . $1195 VCWS No. 16 . . $1095 VCWS No. 17 . . $2995 VCWS No. 18 . . $3625 VCWS No. 19 . . $2995
VIEWS	Mild to severely mentally handicapped, moderate and severely learning disabled	16 samples arranged according to four worker skill groups	Time and errors given equal weight, standardized reporting forms	Norms based on 452 mentally retarded, no data available on reliability	Vocational Research Institute, 2100 Arch St, Philadelphia, PA 19103	$9,950 for basic system, $11,610 for expanded system
VITAS	Educationally and culturally disadvantaged	22 samples arranged according to worker trait groups	Time and errors given equal weight, standardized reporting forms	Norms based on 600 CETA clients, no data available on reliability	Vocational Research Institute, 2100 Arch St, Philadelphia, PA 19103	$9,950 for basic system, $11,610 for expanded system
Vocational Evaluation System (VES; Singer)	Wide range of rehabilitation, education, and manpower populations	27 independent samples	Time and errors given equal weight, standardized reporting forms	Norms based on clients, employed workers, time–motion norms. Significant test–retest reliability 0.61 and 0.71	New Concepts, Corp, 1802 N Division St, Morris, IL 60450	$698–3,439 per work station; majority in $1,700–2500 range

(continued)

Table 18-3. *Continued*

Name	Developer/ Sponsor	Target Population	Work Samples	Scoring and Reporting	Reliability	Address for Information	Cost as of February 1987
Vocational Skills Assessment	Brodhead–Garrett Co	12 yr to adult handicapped and disadvantaged	18 samples in Phase 1, seven samples in Phase 2, seven samples in Phase 3	Time and quality given equal weight	No data available on norm base or reliability	Brodhead–Garrett Co, 4560 E 71st St, Cleveland, OH 44105-5685	Phase I . . . $6500 Phase II . . . Basic Tools: hardware $2800; software $375 Sheltered Employment: hardware $10,000; software $375 Building Maintenance: hardware $4,000; software $375 Health: hardware $7600; software $375 Agri-Business: hardware $550; software $375 Clerical Sales: hardware $3600; software $375 Construction Trades: hardware $2900; software $375 Phase III . . . Hardware range $350–4400; software all $375
Work Skill Development Package (WSD)	Attainment Co	Severely mentally disabled	20 samples, arranged in three groups	Time and accuracy given equal weight, standardized reporting forms	No data on reliability. Validity correlations between scores and supervisor's ratings: 0.86 and 0.92	Attainment Co, PO Box 103, Oregon, WI 53575	$2995
WREST	Jastak Associates	Severely mentally and physically disabled	Ten independent samples	Emphasis on time, standardized form for reporting quality score	Norms based on three major groups, characteristics well defined; test–retest coefficients in 0.80s–0.90s	Jastak Assoc, 1526 Gilpin, Wilmington, DE 19806	$1,409

Updated from Reynolds–Lynch K: Vocational assessment: The field in general. In Kirkland M, Robertson S (eds): *Planning and Implementing Vocational Readiness in Occupational Therapy.* Rockville, Maryland, American Occupational Therapy Association, 1985.

Table 18-4. *McCarron–Dial System Factors, Definitions, Instruments, and Supplementary Measures*

Factor	Factor Definition	Instruments
Verbal–Spatial–Cognitive	Language learning ability, achievement, memory	Wechsler Adult Intelligence Scale (WAIS or WAIS-R) or Wechsler Intelligence Scale for Children (WISC or WISC-R)*
		Peabody Picture Vocabulary TEST (PPVT or PPVT-R)
		Perceptual Memory Test (PMT)[†]
		Wide Range Achievement Test (WRAT)[†]
		Peabody Individual Achievement Test (PIAT)
		Woodcock–Johnson Psychoeducational Battery[†]
		Booklet Category Test[†]
Sensory	Perceiving and experiencing the environment	Bender Visual Motor Gestalt Test (BVMGT)
		Haptic Visual Discrimination Test (HVDT)
		Haptic Memory Matching Test (HMMT)[§]
Motor	Muscle strength, speed and accuracy of movement, balance and coordination	McCarron Assessment of Neuromuscular Development (MAND)[‡]
Emotional	Response to interpersonal and environmental stress	Observational Emotional Inventory (OEI or OEI-R)
		Emotional Behavioral Checklist (EBC)[†]
Integration–Coping	Adaptive Behavior	Behavior Rating Scale (BRS)
		Street Survival Skills Questionnaire (SSSQ)
		Survey of Functional Adaptive Behaviors (SFAB)[†]

* Used in educational evaluation of individuals under the age of 16 years

† Supplementary tests or procedures

‡ Used in clinical neuropsychological evaluation

§ Used instead of the HVDT for evaluating the blind

From the McCarron–Dial Systems Manual.

retical framework to assess five factors: verbal–spatial–cognitive, sensory, motor, emotional, and integration–coping/adaptive behavior. The basic system consists of six widely accepted assessment instruments in combination with performance and behavioral observation. Table 18-4 contains a summary of MDS factors, definitions, and instruments. The system provides flexibility based on the needs of the individual or the setting, with the ability to add or substitute other instruments.

The evaluation process begins with a preliminary screening through interview and referral information. Administration of assessment instruments (work samples) starts with factor one and proceeds through factor five. Both a formal testing setting and a period of placement in a work or classroom setting are utilized. The formal testing can be completed in approximately 3 hours, and the systematic observation in a work or classroom setting can last for up to 5 days.

The basic MDS is packed in three kits, each the size of a large briefcase, with the only expendable items being various answer sheets, behavioral observation, and report forms. Some tasks are timed, with the em-

phasis in scoring on the quality and quantity of performance. The reporting format includes the various scores profiled for each of the five factors, strengths and weaknesses, programming priorities, and programming recommendations.

The McCarron–Dial system requires a commitment to pursue training as a prerequisite for purchase of the system, with each basic training workshop taking 3 days. (See Table 18-3 for further information.)

Valpar Component Work Sample Series

Valpar International Corporation has devised a diverse product line in vocational evaluation which includes self-reporting interviews, microcomputer evaluation and screening assessment (MESA and MESA-SF2), a computer-based job-search program (which provides both a national job data base and training bank program and the capability to build your own local job data base and training bank), computerized self-reporting (Comport), the self-reporting Physical Functioning Questionnaire, and work samples, as well as the Valpar National

Training Institute. It is important to note that occupational therapists are among the target audiences for their products. For the purpose of this section, only the Valpar work samples will be described.

The various Valpar tools have been designed, according to their literature, to meet " . . .the vocational evaluation needs of the population continuum"; this includes the nonhandicapped through the profoundly handicapped or disabled.[49] However, Valpar work samples have been used extensively with industrially injured workers.

At present, there are 19 Valpar Component Work Samples (VCWS), which involve a worker trait and work factor approach utilizing task analysis:

1. Small tools (mechanical)
2. Size discrimination
3. Numerical sorting
4. Upper extremity range of motion
5. Clerical comprehension and aptitude
6. Independent problem solving
7. Multilevel sorting
8. Simulated assembly
9. Whole-body range of motion
10. Trilevel measurement
11. Eye – hand – foot coordination
12. Soldering and inspection
13. Money handling
14. Integrated peer performance
15. Electrical circuitry and print reading
16. Drafting
17. Prevocational readiness battery
18. Conceptual understanding through blind evaluation (CUBE)
19. Dynamic physical capacities.[58]

The work samples are intended for use as individual components, are packaged separately, and have minimal expendable materials. Although the company offers suggestions for use, the order and number of samples given to an individual is left to the therapist's discretion.

The work samples most frequently used by occupational therapists are the VCWS No. 1, Small Tools (Mechanical); VCWS No. 8, Simulated Assembly; VCWS No. 9, Whole-Body Range of Motion; and VCWS No. 19, Dynamic Physical Capacities* (Figure 18-7). The VCWS No. 19 is used particularly in work evaluation/work-hardening programs. It is composed of 28 individual tasks similar to those of a shipping and receiving clerk or parts-order clerk (*i.e,.* lifting, climbing and balancing, and stooping). These tasks measure the physical demands factor of the Worker Qualifications Profile of the Dictionary of Occupational Titles.[46]

Scoring emphasizes quality and time. These scores can be converted to Methods Times Motion (MTM), an industrial standard, and to percentiles with one or more of the eight norm groups.[7,29] A five-point scale is used to rate individuals on each of 17 worker behavior characteristics, such as ability to work alone, ability to respond to change, ability to communicate, and ability to make decisions. Norms are available for various groups. Reliability coefficients are generally high, and descriptions of different types of validity are provided in each manual.

Training is not required as a condition of purchase, although it is available. Valpar International Corporation provides support to their customers, including a support line (800-528-7070), four regional training offices, newsletters called the "Valparspective," and a yearly Valpar National Training Institute, which offers courses and workshops on the use of their products. (See Table 18-3 for additional information.)

In general, the work samples are appealing to the evaluee and are easy to administer and score.

TOWER

Work sampling began in 1936 with the development of the TOWER system by the New York Institute for Crippled and Disabled (ICD, which is now known as the International Center for the Disabled). TOWER has served as a model over the years. It is an acronym for "Testing, Orientation, and Work Evaluation in Rehabilitation." Originally developed for use with the physically disabled, it is now used with all types of disabled individuals, including the emotionally disabled.

The system is composed of 110 work samples arranged in 14 occupational areas: clerical, drafting, drawing, electronics assembly, jewelry manufacturing, leather goods, machine shop, lettering, mail clerk, optical mechanics, pantograph engraving, sewing machine operating, welding, and workshop assembly. Each of the 14 areas is independent, with selection of areas at the therapist's discretion. Within each area, the work samples are arranged in order of complexity. For example, the work sample jewelry manufacturing is composed of the following tasks, from simple to complex: use of saw, use of needle files, use of electric drill press, piercing and filing metals, use of pliers, use of torch in soldering, and making earring and brooch pin.*

A list of hardware and equipment needs, purposes, and procedures can be obtained from the ICD publication of the system's manual and a separate book, *TOWER.* The use of a realistic work setting and atmo-

---

* Mowbray–Swallow, D, personal communication, 1987.

---

* Rosenberg, B (Director of Vocational Rehabilitation Services, ICD, and one of the originators of the TOWER), personal communication, 1987.

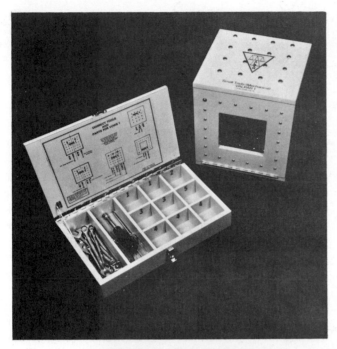

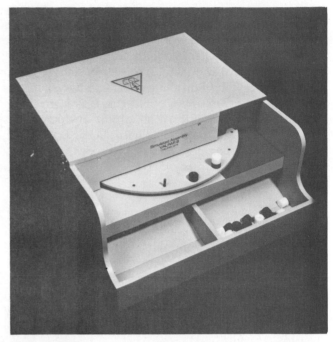

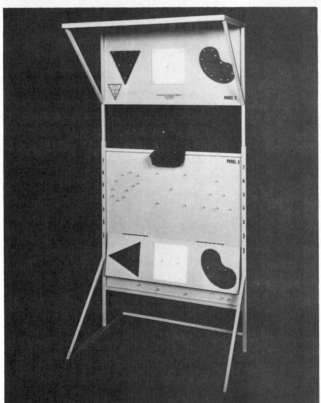

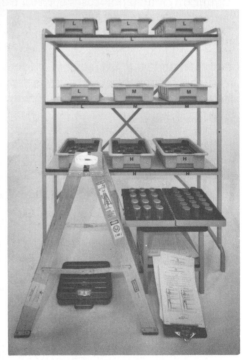

Figure 18-7. Valpar Component Work Samples: A. No. 1 = small tools (mechanical). B. No. 8 = simulated assembly. C. No. 9 = whole body range of motion. D. No. 19 = dynamic physical capacities. (Photographs courtesy of Valpar International Corp, Tucson, Arizona.)

sphere is recommended when administering the samples. Completion of the entire system by an average evaluee takes 3 weeks; however, most samples are usually not administered to each individual.

Time and work quality are given equal weight in scoring, with scoring on a five-point scale. Work factors and work behaviors are recognized by ICD as an essential part of the TOWER. Although the evaluator rates these different factors and behaviors in the final report, they have not been described or incorporated formally into the TOWER manual.[7,29,47] (See Table 18-3 for additional information.)

Selecting An Evaluation

One finds the state of the art of work evaluation being consistently refined and improved. External forces such as reduction in funding have forced decreases in the amount of time spent in evaluation and the amount spent for tools while increasing the need to obtain a large amount of data in a short time. This is particularly significant in litigation cases such as worker's compensation.

Many of the well-known commercially available work evaluation systems and work samples have been computerized and are able to perform job-matching with the *Dictionary of Occupational Titles* (DOT) in a matter of minutes.[55] (See References in Section 2 of this chapter.)

The selection of an evaluation or evaluations must be based on the characteristics of the target population in relation to the factors of cost, time, effectiveness, and use of manpower. The following listing is presented as a guide to the selection of appropriate evaluations:

1. Investigate the range and types of jobs available in the local catchment area; determine the relevance of the evaluation to local jobs and training programs.
2. Analyze your client population, considering their assets and deficits.
3. Review commercially available systems, either by visiting other facilities that have them or by borrowing them for a period of time. The Materials Development Center[8] (MDC) has many audiovisual materials reviewing vocational evaluation that may aid in decision making.
4. Carefully review the evaluation manual, its answer sheet, and other parts to answer the following: What is its purpose? What is the reading level? Are the instructions and procedures clearly presented? How much does it cost? How much time does it take to administer and score? Is training necessary? How much space is needed? For what population was the evaluation designed? Does the evaluation have reliability, validity, and established norms? Read the review of the evaluation in the *Handbook of Measurement and Evaluation in Rehabilitation*[6] for a critical overview.
5. Investigate the resources you already have available within your facility or a neighboring facility.
6. Consider whether you need to purchase an evaluaion. Can you borrow it or develop your own from existing subcontract work, in-house jobs, or other sources?

Conceptual Framework for Evaluation Selection

A review of the literature indicates the need to base practice on a clear conceptual framework. Although various schemata have been developed, such as Clark's model of human development through occupation,[11] Mosey's three frames of reference,[40,41] and Kielhofner's "paradigm of the future,"[28] which is based on general systems theory, Creighton states that "no recent attempt has been made to identify the specific implications of various theoretical orientations for specialized areas of occupational therapy practice, such as vocational rehabilitation."[14] In her article, Creighton selected Mosey's three frames of reference as one theoretical perspective on which to base planning, assessment, and treatment in the area of work practice.

Thompson has followed Kielhofner's model of the person as an open system to organize the classification of various work assessment tools.[27,53] Figure 18-8 lists the different instruments within the three subsystems: volitional, habituation, and performance. Kielhofner describes the human being as a dynamic system composed of these three subsystems that interact and influence each other. The volitional subsystem, at the top, comprises values, interests, motivation, and personal causation. The habituation subsystem, viewed as below the volitional subsystem, is composed of roles and habits. The performance subsystem (formerly called production) is at the base and comprises aptitudes and skills (*e.g.,* sensory, motor, perceptual, cognitive, and social).

Planning

Following the assessment, ideally the therapist *and* the individual should plan programming priorities and establish short- and long-term goals. In this planning stage, there are many factors that should be taken into account, particularly if the work program is just being established within the OT department. Some factors include: (1) What are the individual's interests? (2) What are his or her aspirations and interests regarding future employment? (3) Are the individual's job goals realistic? (4) What is the extent of the individual's job experience? (5) What type of work is available to the individual, particularly in his or her local community? Does the individual have the necessary skills to perform this kind of work? (6) What resources are available to you at your

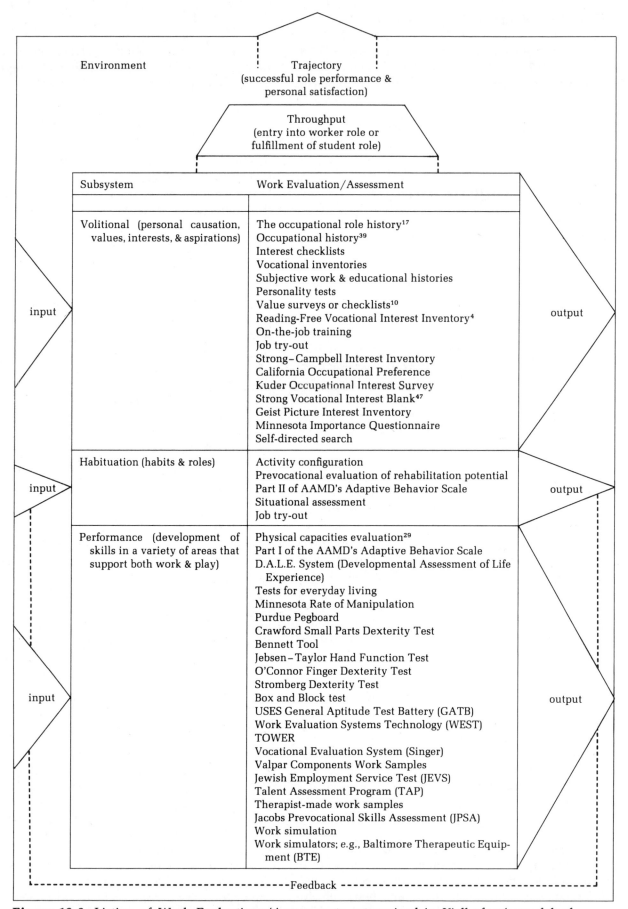

Figure 18-8. Listing of Work Evaluations/Assessments categorized in Kielhofner's model of human occupation. (In Kielhofner G: A model of human occupation, Part 3. Benign and vicious cycles. *Am J Occup Ther* 34:731, 1980).

facility and in the community for use as simulated job experiences? (7) What kind of budget do you have for developing and operating this program? (8) Do you have access to equipment and supplies that may relate to programming? (9) How much physical space will you have for the program? and (10) Do you have the support of the administration and staff of your facility?[25]

Programming

Traditionally, the occupational therapist has been faced with individuals of various ages who are unsuccessful at work, unable to work for a variety of reasons, or have never had the opportunity to acquire work behaviors and work skills. Such persons may include a nurse with a chronic back injury who now perceives herself as unable ever to return to work; the older adult who has been replaced by high technology, feels disenfranchised, and has become severely depressed; the institutionalized developmentally disabled adolescent who has never been exposed to appropriate work behaviors; the homemaker, who, after severe head trauma due to a car accident, has limited cognitive and physical functioning; and the upper-extremity amputee from a recent industrial accident.

Functionally, these individuals' dysfunctions can be viewed in two major categories: a lack of work behaviors or work skills, and neurophysiologic impairments. The importance of work behaviors is emphasized by the fact that most unemployed workers are unable to obtain jobs or have lost their jobs because of problems with interpersonal relationships; that is, trouble getting along with co-workers and supervisors, rather than inadequate work skills, aptitudes, or physical capacities.[16,25,35] In addition, "limited concentration, distractibility, or psychological pressures that limit tolerance for specific activities might preclude employment even though job skills are present."[30]

Types of Programming

The outcomes from assessment may be one of the following types of programming:
1. Direct competitive job placement
2. On-the-job training
3. Educational training
4. Remediation
5. Rehabilitation workshop employment

As previously identified, some of the functions of OT related to work programming include: support in exploring or identifying possible work objectives, work hardening, work adjustment/habit and behavior programs, independent living skills programs, work placement, job analysis and work environment evaluation, and task and environmental adaptation. Some of the functions provided by the occupational therapist within each type of programming will be described.

Direct Competitive Job Placement

The individual has been deemed work ready. Although many consumers believe that we "get people jobs," the OTR rarely does formal job placement. However, she or he can play an active role in the decision-making process through assisting in career exploration and identification of work objectives, ascertaining when the individual is ready for competitive employment, what type of job is feasible and the extent, if any, of adaptations, work simplification, and modifications that need to be made at the job site. Familiarity with references such as the *Dictionary of Occupational Titles,*[55] the *Guide For Occupational Exploration,*[56] and "Selected Characteristics of Occupations Defined" in the *Dictionary of Occupational Titles*[57] can aid in the process (see References in Section 2). Job analysis is also a useful tool that the OTR can use in assessing the individual's work site needs.

For those OTRs working in industry, the roles may include the aforementioned, with the addition of becoming a researcher/practitioner working to prevent initial work-related injury.[3] Many injuries that could be prevented " . . . are caused by the use of poorly designed tools and work stations and improper work performance movements."[3] Bear–Lehman and McCormick, hand therapists/occupational therapists, remark that OTRs " . . . can be influential in injury prevention by work with local safety and industrial groups to develop educational programs and to investigate injuries."[3]

Another evolving population for the OTR's services is the disenfranchised worker or "the new poor." These are individuals who are unemployed due to modernization, lack of current skills, or sagging markets. The OTR can be part of a consortium effort by providing retraining techniques, job analysis, and occupational exploration.[50]

On-The-Job Training (OJT)

The individual is placed on the job where training is provided at the work site. The individual placed in an OJT situation, has good basic work behaviors and the potential to be successful on the job; however, there is a need for a period of formal training. Institutions, hospitals, and schools are good sources for OJT situations, since they provide ready access to jobs in departments such as housekeeping, dietary, maintenance, secretarial, and accounting. The occupational therapist may have the opportunity to train and supervise these OJT individuals or to play an active role as a member of their rehabilitation team. The Learning Prep School in Massachusetts provides an example of the role of the therapist in OJT, where frequently the OTR or COTA will work at a job site.

Educational Training

For some individuals, success on a job may be predicated on the need to receive vocational or academic training prior to job placement; for example, a work/study program in a secondary school or a vocational technical program. The implementation of Public Law 94-142, Education of the Handicapped Act, has made OT a well-recognized profession within the educational arena. (See the box, Significant Legislation Related to Work.)

Career Theories

The work of a child is play, and as this child enters school, his or her role is being a student, and studying is

Table 18-5. *Three Theories of Career Development*

Ginzberg and Associates *Stage/Characteristics*	*Super* *Stage/Characteristics*	*Havighurst* *Stage/Characteristics*
Fantasy Period Below age 11: Choices are governed by wish to engage in exciting adult activities.	**Growth Stage** Ages 4–10—Fantasy: Needs are dominant; role playing is important. Ages 11–12—Interests: Likes determine aspirations.	**Stage I** Ages 5–10—Identification with a Worker: Individual identifies with significant people; concept of working is incorporated into egoideal.
Tentative Period Ages 11–12—Interest: Choices are governed by likes/dislikes. Ages 13–14—Capacity: Individual begins to consider own abilities objectively. Ages 15–16—Value: Individual attempts to clarify goals. Age 17—Transition: Individual is suspenseful about future.	Ages 13–14—Capacity: Abilities are given more weight. **Exploration Stage** Ages 15–17—Tentative: Variety of factors are considered, choices tried out. Ages 18–21—Transition: Reality is given more weight: individual attempts to implement self-concept. Ages 22–24—Trial: Beginning job is tried out as life work.	**Stage II** Ages 10–15—Acquiring the Basic Habits of Industry; Individual learns to organize time and energy, put work ahead of play. **Stage III** Ages 15–25—Acquiring Identity as a Worker in the Occupational Structure: Individual chooses and prepares for occupation, gets work experience.
Realistic Period Age 17—Young Adulthood (stages not closely correlated with chronological age)— Exploration: Individual obtains information about various vocations. Crystallization: Individual assesses all factors influencing choice and commits self. Specification: Individual considers field of specialization, particular career objectives.	**Establishment Stage** Ages 25–30—Trial: Changes may be necessary before life work is found. Ages 31–44—Stabilization: Career pattern becomes clear; individual attempts to make secure place in work. **Maintenance Stage** Ages 45–64: Concern is to hold place in world of work. **Decline Stage** Ages 65–70—Deceleration: Pace or nature of work changes to fit declining capacities. Age 71 on—Retirement: Occupation ceases.	**Stage IV** Ages 25–40—Becoming a Productive Person: Individual masters skills and moves up ladder in occupation. **Stage V** Ages 40–70—Maintaining a Productive Society: Individual emphasizes societal aspects of worker's role. **Stage VI** Age 70 on—Contemplating a Productive and Responsible Life: Individual withdraws from worker role and reviews/accepts productivity.

(Adapted from Ginzberg E, Ginsburg SW, Axelrad S et al: Occupational Choice: An Approach to a General Theory, New York, Columbia University Press, 1951; Super DE: The Psychology of Careers. New York, Harper & Row, 1957; Havighurst RJ: Youth in exploration and man in emergence. In Borow H (ed): Man in a World of Work. Boston, Houghton Mifflin, 1964; Creighton C: Theories of career development. In Kirkland M, Robertson S (eds): Planning and Implementing Vocational Readiness in Occupational Therapy. Rockville, MD; American Occupational Therapy Association 1985)

Composite List of Play-Leisure and Household Activities that Promote Vocational Development

1. Construction sets: erector sets, Tinkertoys, Lego sets
2. Toy cars and trucks
3. Doll play
4. Household odds and ends
5. Toy tools
6. Handcrafts
7. Collections
8. Dress up
9. Cops and robbers
10. Doctor–nurse–patient
11. Space fantasy games
12. Other dramatic play
13. Races
14. Contests
15. Model building
16. Photography
17. Playing cards
18. Sketching
19. Drawing and coloring books
20. Painting
21. Scrabble
22. Dramatics
23. Musical instruments
24. Creative writing
25. Inventions
26. Experiments
27. Videogames and computer play
28. Soccer
29. Basketball
30. Baseball and softball
31. Aerobic exercises and dancing
32. Care for pets
33. Care for younger siblings
34. Help with housework
35. Clean own room
36. Make own bed
37. Wash and dry dishes; help load dishwasher
38. Remove trash
39. Help with yardwork
40. Set dinner table
41. Prepare simple foods
42. Run errands for parents
43. Do chores for neighbors and teachers

(Adapted from Goldstein B, and Oldham J: *Children and Work: a Study of Socialization.* New Brunswick, NJ, Transaction Books, 1979; and Shannon P: Occupational choice: decision-making play. In Reilly M (ed): *Play as Exploratory Learning: Studies in Curiosity Behavior.* Beverly Hills, Sage Publications, 1974; Stephens LC, Clark PN: Schoolwork tasks and prevocational development. In Clark PN, Allen AS: *Occupational Therapy for Children.* St Louis, CV Mosby, 1985)

the work. An understanding of career theories may be beneficial to the therapist developing work programming for children and adolescents.

There are five widely accepted theories of career development, which were originated by psychologists and sociologists and have been adopted by practitioners: (1) trait-and-factor,[44] (2) sociologic,[9,38] (3) psychodynamic,[48] (4) developmental,[18,20,52] and (5) systems.[31,43] An understanding of these theories may assist in the development of appropriate OT work programming.

Developmental theories are currently applied in OT educational programs as well as in schools for counseling and career education. Developmental theory views career development as a gradual process within human growth that takes place over the life span in predictable stages.[13] Ginzberg and co-workers,[18] Super,[52] and Havighurst,[20] although developmental theorists, have different beliefs about how and why development occurs (Table 18-5).

Work is a dynamic process, where programming must begin at a young age with the introduction of career awareness and exploration of work capabilities and interests. Although this awareness and exploration must be reinforced with normal children, it is particularly critical for programming to be presented developmentally and initiated at an early age for special-needs children. The rationale supporting this is that: (1) these children have " . . . fewer opportunities for free play experiences with other children,"[51] (2) they typically have little or no exposure to the world of work; and (3) they are thought to have limited career expectations by parents and society.[25] In addition, too often people around these children tend to "do for" them or to assign others tasks that the children could accomplish if expectations were not based on time, tolerance, or temperament.[51] It is important that "training materials and work performance requirements should increasingly approximate actual industrial demands and that training should move from the school to the actual work site as soon as possible."[31]

The creation of simulated business enterprises, such as a fast-food restaurant (Fig. 18-5), supermarket, cookie company, or library, can create a milieu of a work environment within the confines of a classroom. Academic training and the reinforcement of work behaviors and skills can be incorporated into this setting through a collaborative effort of the OTR and the teacher. For example, simple arithmetic problems can be designed around the purchase of a week's groceries or a hamburger and French fries while practicing appropriate interpersonal skills. The accompanying box, devised by Stephens and Clark, is a composite list of play–leisure and household activities that promote readiness for work and may be incorporated into the classroom activities.[51]

Work programs particularly targeted to special-needs students should include the following options, which can be visualized in a hierarchy: regular vocational education, adapted vocational education, special vocational education, individual vocational training, and prevocational evaluation services.[24]

Regular Vocational Education

In regular vocational education, specific vocational and academic programming is provided to the student. Training is dependent on the individual's age, strengths and weaknesses, interests, motivation, and goals. The occupational therapist may work directly with the student in vocational classes, provide individual or group therapy or both, or act as a consultant to the faculty.

Adapted Vocational Education

Regular vocational programs may be modified to meet the needs of the special students. Occupational therapists may act as direct consultants to the vocational teacher by providing adaptive devices, work simplification techniques, or task analysis or work directly with the student in class to implement these recommendations. In addition, individual or group treatment or both may be provided by the OTR.

Special Vocational Education

For those students whose impairment is so severe as to preclude success in a regular vocational program, a self-contained special education class or placement in a facility specializing in the student's needs is a valuable option. Programming is usually focused on the development of work behaviors and skills that may be utilized in entry-level semiskilled jobs or vocational training programs. Rehabilitation workshops may be used for training. Once again, the role of the OTR or COTA may be one of consultant to the classroom teacher in developing appropriate tasks that facilitate work behavior and skill development or one of direct programming with the student. Direct treatment is typically in the form of group activities relating to work; for example, role playing the job of a grocery bagger or babysitter.

Individual Vocational Training

Programming may also be tailored to meet the individual needs of each student, because the level of functioning may vary greatly. Some students may be capable of performing rudimentary academic, work-related tasks and self-care activities, whereas another student who is severely and profoundly disabled may require constant supervision and intensive individual and group training. Programs may be offered in a variety of settings, such as school, community, work/study, or OJT. The

OTR can assist in planning goals for the student, perform job analysis, and provide direct and consultative care. Occupational therapy programming usually requires that the tasks be performed in highly structured environments under close supervision. Some commonly used work tasks may be categorized as independent living activities; for example, sweeping, mopping, dusting, folding clothes, washing dishes, setting tables, and handling and moving materials.

Prevocational Evaluation Services

Prevocational evaluation services are "designed to provide vocational assessment to students whose disability precludes the use of the regular education sequence."[24] These services are usually provided by facilities under contract with the school, such as rehabilitation workshops and private vocational assessment centers. Subcontract activities are often used in programming: collating, packaging and labeling, envelope stuffing and stamping, and assembly.

Remedial Services

When the individual has been identified through the assessment process as having medical, psychological, social, or physical limitations, remediation is needed. Kester states that "some conditions are temporary and do not prevent return to previous employment, even before remediation is completed. Other disabilities that are more permanent in nature might not preclude return to work if adaptive devices or environmental changes could compensate for the personal limitation. A third category involves the permanent . . . disability that is severe enough to prevent return to previous employment . . ." or even the exposure to work in the first place.[30] *Direct treatment* is typically utilized for the first two categories and *work adjustment* services for the latter one.

Direct Occupational Therapy Treatment

For the individual with a physical or medical disability, the OTR has at his or her command an almost limitless number of activities to use in treatment. Depending on the facility and its philosophy, treatment may involve support in exploring or identifying possible work objectives, independent living skills training, and prevention education training. Some modalities used are work simulations or work samples and crafts such as woodworking or leatherworking. Work hardening is a frequently used approach to treatment (see Section 2 of this chapter).

Often, success in treatment is predicated on the individual's motivation to succeed with established treatment goals as well as on addressing the psychosocial ramifications of the disability. The individual's involvement in planning the treatment goals, along with use of treatment activities of interest to them (which often can be tasks from their work), may be the best course of action. The OT department at the Liberty Mutual Medical Service Center in Boston uses various work samples, such as a multiwork station that resembles a two-story house under construction and a cross-section of a truck cab, which involve common job tasks for their industrially injured clients, as treatment modalities. In addition, they use a very popular modality, the work simulator, as a treatment method.[5,25]

For the individual with psychosocial disabilities, the variety of treatment modalities is almost limitless, too, although there may be specific safety precautions that eliminate some of the options. Some additional variables may need to be considered in designing programs. For example, these individuals often have difficulty making transitions and tend to decompensate when adapting to change, usually because of their fear of failure. Also, inconsistencies in their behavior and work performance can be due to medication, including changes in what is administered or its inconsistent use or disuse.[25] Activities that provide the opportunity for group interaction are highly recommended. The designing of a business enterprise that allows for grading jobs in various levels of difficulty has met with much success; for example, the establishment of a greeting card company whose jobs might include stamping precut designs on paper, folding paper, wrapping and packaging, inventory, and bookkeeping.

Work Adjustment

"Work adjustment is an educational/training process involving individual and group work, and work-related activities, to assist individuals in understanding the meaning, value and demands of work; to modify or develop attitudes, personal characteristics, and work behaviors; and to attain a functional level of vocational development."[37] Emphasis in work adjustment services should be centered on the following objectives:
1. Development of work tolerance
2. Motivation to do productive work
3. Development of self-reliance
4. Acceptance of supervision
5. Relating effectively to co-workers
6. Development of safety habits
7. Punctuality
8. Development of concentration, accuracy, and speed on the job[34]

Occupational therapists use some or a combination of the following techniques in work adjustment: individual or group therapy, planned work experience, modeling and imitation learning, behavior modification, and individual and group classroom instruction.

Rehabilitation Workshop Employment

Rehabilitation workshop employment offers assessment, training, employment, and other rehabilitative services in a controlled and protective setting that allows the individual to work at his or her own capacity and often to receive remuneration.[26] These facilities are typically privately operated and serve either the developmentally or the emotionally disabled. Although often generically called "sheltered workshop," there are actually four categories under this model: transitional workshops, sheltered workshops, work activity centers, and avocational or day adult activity centers.[26]

Occupational therapists and certified occupational therapy assistants may be employed in rehabilitation workshops in full- and part-time capacities and as consultants. Typically, they work as consultants to the rehabilitation staff and directly with individuals to develop work behaviors and skills. Common activities used with clients are activities of daily living, subcontract piece work, and work simulations. In addition, the OTR may utilize job analysis, work simplification, and adaptation techniques.

Termination/Follow-Up Care

For some individuals, the vocational rehabilitation (work) process is finite and can be terminated after programming goals are attained. For others, this may be a life-long process or one that is entered into periodically, with follow-up care provided.

Case Study

J., age 59, was seen over a period of 4 months in OT at a local vocational rehabilitation center. J. had been an assembly-line worker at a local factory for 40 years, since his graduation from high school. When the factory was sold, the new owner modernized the factory, replacing J.'s job with high technology. Shortly thereafter, J. was laid off and went on unemployment. For 3 months, he diligently looked for employment similar to his past job, to find that all jobs of a similar nature had been replaced by high technology. During this period of job searching, J. became depressed and developed carpal tunnel syndrome in his left (nondominant) hand. After seeing his family doctor for his physical complaints, he was referred to the local vocational rehabilitation center. At the center, the vocational rehabilitation counselor coordinated J.'s assessment process. The occupational therapist was included in J.'s rehabilitation team. As part of the assessment process, the occupational therapist reviewed J.'s records and had the opportunity to interview his family (wife and son). An interest inventory was provided to explore and identify interests, desires, and possible work objectives. He was given the following three Valpar Components Work Samples: VCWS No. 1, Small Tools (mechanical); VCWS No. 8, Simulated Assembly; and VCWS No. 19, Dynamic Physical Capacities; and a partial sensorimotor evaluation.

J. was cooperative and pleasant during the evaluation sessions. The interest inventory indicated that J. enjoyed many activities that involved fine-motor skills, use of tools, reading, and spectator sports.

J.'s confidence increased and his depression decreased as he was able to complete the work samples with an above-average speed, no errors, and a quality of average and above and was able to lift the required weight and perform the physical tasks required at each strength level. The only potentially limiting factor was revealed in the sensorimotor testing: paresthesia and some pain involving the first three fingers of his left hand, forearm, and wrist. Sensation was slightly diminished along the median nerve distribution. No edema was noted. J. noted that his discomfort usually increased in the evening.

Evaluation results were shared with J.'s vocational rehabilitation team. It was felt that J. became aware of his capabilities through the evaluation process. From the support of the vocational rehabilitation team, he was able to make the transition from feeling disenfranchised to developing the confidence to make a commitment to learning a new job which required his already developed work behaviors, physical capacities, and aptitudes. It was recommended that J. could benefit from OJT, which could be provided at a local air conditioning repair company. The job placement specialist would assist J. with the formal training period at this job. Follow-up care would be provided if needed.

A prescription for a neutral-position splint was obtained from J.'s physician, and the OTR constructed a splint to be worn in the evenings.   ☐

References

1. Ad Hoc Committee of the Commission on Practice: The role of occupational therapy in the vocational rehabilitation process: official position paper. Am J Occup Ther 34:881, 1980
2. Baltimore Therapeutic Equipment Co., 1201 Bernard Dr, Baltimore, MD, 21223, 1987
3. Bear–Lehman J, McCormick E: The expanding role of occupational therapy in the treatment of industrial head injuries. Occup Ther Health Care 2:79, 1985–86
4. Becker RL: Reading-Free Vocational Interest Inventory: MF Columbus, Elbern Publications, 1981
5. Bettencourt CM, Carlstrom P, Brown SH, et al: Using work simulation to treat adults with back injuries. Am J Occup Ther 40:12, 1986
6. Bolton B (ed): Handbook of Measurement and Evaluation in Rehabilitation. Baltimore, University Park Press, 1976
7. Botterbusch KF: A Comparison of Commercial Vocational Evaluation Systems, 2nd ed. Menomonie, WI, Materials Development Center, Stout Vocational Rehabilitation Institute, University of Wisconsin–Stout, 1982
8. Botterbusch KF: Psychological Testing in Vocational Evaluation. Menomonie, WI, Materials Development Center, Stout Vocational Rehabilitation Institute, University of Wisconsin–Stout, 1978
9. Caplow T: The Sociology of Work. Minneapolis, University of Minnesota Press, 1954
10. Catalyst: What to Do With the Rest of Your Life. New York, Simon & Schuster, 1980
11. Clark PN: Human development through occupation: Theoretical frameworks in contemporary occupational therapy practice, part 1. Am J Occup Ther 33:505, 1979
12. Commission On Accreditation of Rehabilitation Facilities: 1987 Edition of The Standards Manual For Organizations Serving People With Disabilities. Tucson, Commission On Accreditation of Rehabilitation Facilities, 1987
13. Creighton CC: Career development theory. In Kirkland M, Robertson S (eds): Planning and Implementing Vocational Readiness in Occupational Therapy. Rockville, MD, American Occupational Therapy Association, 1985
14. Creighton C: Three frames of reference in work-related occupational therapy programs. Am J Occup Ther 39:331, 1985
15. Cromwell F (ed): Work-Related Programs in Occupational Therapy: Occupational Therapy in Health Care. New York, Haworth Press, 1985–86
16. Distefano Jr MK, Pryer MW: Vocational evaluation and successful placement of psychiatric clients in a vocational rehabilitation program. Am J Occup Ther 24:205, 1970
17. Florey LL, Michelman SM: Occupational role history: a screening tool for psychiatric patients. Am J Occup Ther 36:301, 1982
18. Ginzberg E, Ginzberg SW, Axelrad S, et al: Occupational Choice: An Approach to a General Theory. New York, Columbia University Press, 1951
19. Harvey–Krefting L: From another perspective: an overview of the theme. Occup Ther Health Care 2:3, 1985
20. Havighurst RJ: Youth in exploration and man in emergence. In Borow H (ed): Man in a World of Work. Boston, Houghton Mifflin, 1964
21. Hightower–Vandamm M: Nationally speaking: The role of occupational therapy in vocational evaluation, part 1. Am J Occup Ther 35:563, 1981
22. Hightower–Vandamm M: Nationally speaking: The role of occupational therapy in vocational evaluation, part 2. Am J Occup Ther 35:631, 1981
23. Holmes D: The role of the occupational therapist–work evaluator. Am J Occup Ther 39:308, 1985
24. Howard R: Vocational Education of Handicapped Youth—State of the Art. Washington, DC, National Association of State Boards of Education, 1979
25. Jacobs K: Occupational Therapy: Work-Related Programs and Assessments. Boston, Little, Brown, 1985
26. Jacobs K, Mazonson N, Pepicelli K, et al: Work center: A school-based program for vocational preparation of spe-

cial needs children and adolescents. Occup Ther Health Care 2:47, 1985–86

27. Kielhofner G: A model of human occupation 3: Benign and vicious cycles. Am J Occup Ther 34:731, 1980
28. Keilhofner G: Health Through Occupation: Theory and Practice in Occupational Therapy. Philadelphia, Davis, 1983
29. Kester, D: Prevocational evaluation. In Hopkins H, Smith H (eds): Willard and Spackman's Occupational Therapy, 6th ed. Philadelphia, JB Lippincott, 1983
30. Kester D: Prevocational training. In Hopkins H, Smith H (eds): Willard and Spackman's Occupational Therapy, 6th ed. Philadelphia, JB Lippincott, 1983
31. Kiernan WE, Petzy V: A systems approach to career and vocational education programs for special needs students: Grades 7–12. In Lynch KP, Kiernan WE, Stark JA (eds): Prevocational and Vocational Education for Special Needs Youth: A Blueprint for the 1980s. Baltimore, Paul H Brookes Publishing, 1982
32. Kirkland M, Robertson S: An overview of tests and measurements. In Kirkland M, Robertson S (eds): Planning and Implementing Vocational Readiness in Occupational Therapy. Rockville, MD, American Occupational Therapy Association, 1985
32a. Kirkland M, Robertson S: The evolution of work-related theory in occupational therapy. In Kirkland M, Robertson S (eds): Planning and Implementing Vocational Readiness in Occupational Therapy. Rockville, MD, American Occupational Therapy Association, 1985
33. Marshall E: Notes on Situtional Assessment. Loma Linda, Dept. of Occupational Therapy, School of Allied Health Professions, Loma Linda University, July 1983
34. Materials Development Center: Work Adjustment Program: An Overview (slide/tape). Menomonie, WI, Materials Development Center, University of Wisconsin–Stout, 1984
35. Materials Development Center: Vocational Evaluation: An Overview (slide/tape), Menomonie, WI, Materials Development Center, University of Wisconsin–Stout, 1980
36. Matsutsuyu J: The interest checklist. Am J Occup Ther 23:323, 1969
37. McCarron L, Dial JG: McCarron–Dial Evaluation System: A Systematic Approach to Vocational, Educational and Neuropsychological Assessment. Dallas, McCarron–Dial, 1986
38. Miller DC, Form WH: Industrial Sociology. New York, Harper & Row, 1951
39. Moorehead L: The occupational history. Am J Occup Ther 23:329, 1969
40. Mosey AC: Occupational Therapy: Configuration of a Profession. New York, Raven, 1981
41. Mosey AC: Three Frames of Reference for Mental Health. Thorofare, NJ, Slack, 1970
42. Occupational Therapy Benefits From CARF Changes. Occup Ther News 41:1, 1987
43. Osipow SH: Theories of Career Development. New York, Appleton–Century–Crofts, 1973
44. Parsons F: Choosing a Vocation. Boston, Houghton Mifflin, 1909
45. Reed K, Sanderson SR: Concepts of Occupational Therapy. Baltimore, Williams & Wilkins, 1980

46. Reynolds–Lynch K: Prevocational and vocational assessment in occupational therapy. In Kirkland M, Robertson S (eds): Planning and Implementing Vocational Readiness in Occupational Therapy. Rockville, MD, American Occupational Therapy Association, 1985
47. Reynolds–Lynch K: Vocational assessment: The field in general. In Kirkland M, Robertson S (eds): Planning and Implementing Vocational Readiness in Occupational Therapy. Rockville, MD, American Occupational Therapy Association,1985
48. Roe A: Early determinants of vocational choice. J Counseling Psychol 4:216, 1957
49. Rosenberg B: The work sample approach to vocational evaluation. In Hardy RE, Cull JG (eds): Vocational Evaluation for Rehabilitation Services. Springfield, Charles C Thomas, 1973
50. Small LM: Disenfranchised worker strategies. Occup Ther News 40(11):28, 1986
51. Stephens LC, Clark PN: Schoolwork tasks and prevocational development. In Clark PN, Allen AS (eds): Occupational Therapy for Children. St Louis, CV Mosby, 1985
52. Super DE: The Psychology of Careers. New York, Harper & Row, 1957
53. Thompson G: Work-related assessment in occupational therapy: An overview. Work Programs Special Interest Sect Newslett 1:1, 1987
54. Uniform Terminology For Reporting Occupational Therapy Services. Rockville, MD, American Association of Occupational Therapy, 1979
55. US Department of Labor: Dictionary of Occupational Titles, 4th ed. Washington, DC, US Government Printing Office, 1977
56. US Department of Labor: Guide for Occupational Exploration. Washington, DC, US Government Printing Office, 1979
57. US Department of Labor: Selected Characteristics of Occupations Defined in the Dictionary of Occupational Titles. Washington, DC, US Government Printing Office, 1981
58. Valpar International Corporation: Valpar International Corporation Brochure. Tucson, Valpar International Corporation, 1986
59. Walls RT, Zane T, Werner TJ: The Vocational Behavior Checklist. Dunbar, West Virginia University, West Virginia Research & Training Center, 1978
60. Watanabe S: Activities Configuration. 1968 Regional Institute on the Evaluation Process, Final Report RSA-123-T-68. New York, American Occupational Therapy Association, 1968
61. Wright GN: Total Rehabilitation. Boston, Little, Brown, 1980

Bibliography

Bailey D: Vocational theories and work habits related to childhood development. Am J Occup Ther 25:298, 1971
Brolin DE: Vocational Preparation of Retarded Citizens. Columbus, Charles E Merrill, 1976
Cromwell FS: Occupational Therapist's Manual for Basic Assessment—Primary Prevocational Evaluation. Altadena, Fair Oakes Printing, 1976

Cromwell FS: A procedure for prevocational evaluation. Am J Occup Ther 13:1, 1959

Ethridge DA: Prevocational assessment of rehabilitation potential of psychiatric patients. Am J Occup Ther 22:161, 1968

Fidler GS: A second look at work as a primary force in rehabilitation and treatment. Am J Occup Ther 20:72, 1966

Granofsky J: A Manual for Occupational Therapists on Prevocational Exploration. Dubuque, WC Brown, 1959

Maurer PA: Antecedents of work behavior. Am J Occup Ther 25:295, 1971

Wegg LS: Eleanor Clarke Slagle Lecture: The essentials of work evaluation. Am J Occup Ther 14:65, 1960

Woodside HH: Occupational therapy—a historical perspective: the development of occupational therapy 1910–1929. Am J Occup Ther 25:226, 1971

SECTION 2

Occupational Therapy in Industrial Rehabilitation   *Sallie E. Taylor*

Historical Overview

The current relationship between occupational therapy (OT) and the world of work has arisen from a tradition that goes back to the very roots of our profession. Some periods in the practice of OT may be more definitely identified with the work role of patients than others, yet there has remained within the profession a small group of therapists who have retained a practice emphasizing the building or rebuilding of skills and tolerances necessary to enable patients to enter or to return to the labor market. The serious student of history is referred to the several references listed at the end of this chapter that detail the occupational therapy legacy of "work" and of "workplace" focus in the field of rehabilitation.

Conditions that Created the Market

Following a period of economic "stagflation" in the early to mid 1980s, corporations in America needed new strategies for holding their positions in the marketplace. Companies that had always been able to increase prices to achieve acceptable profit found themselves in danger of pricing themselves out of business. As an alternative method of retaining adequate profit to stay viable in the marketplace, management turned to cost reduction.

In the mid 1980s, payments connected with on-the-job injuries ran into the millions of dollars per year, representing a substantial cost to business. These costs had always been considered an inevitable expense of doing business. However, the possibility of decreasing the financial outlay for workers' compensation payments, medical and rehabilitation treatment, compensation for "pain and suffering," as well as other fees associated with litigation, was attractive to industry. Costs incurred in connection with on-the-job injuries were a natural target for closer control.

Conditions that Created the Opportunity for Occupational Therapy

While corporations were desperately seeking ways to cut the cost of production, three other significant phenomena were occurring that put into place the elements necessary to launch many occupational therapists into a different application of their skills.

In 1983, the national health insurance, Medicare, shifted from a fee-for-service to a prospective payment system for hospital services provided to individuals who receive Medicare coverage. Occupational therapy, which, as a profession had followed the medical model of service delivery since the 1920s, was primarily situated within the hospital structure. As hospital administrators redirected management practices to minimize operational costs under the new payment system, many hospital-based OT departments were either reduced or eliminated. Suddenly, there were a number of occupational therapists available to move into a new area. In addition, the pressure on hospital-based OT departments caused by Medicare cutbacks provided the incentive for OT department directors and hospital administrators to consider new options and more nontraditional practice opportunities.

A significant influence on occupational therapists' stepping forward to reclaim a position in industrial rehabilitation was occurring simultaneously. A psychologist with Master's level training in vocational rehabilitation, Dr. Leonard Matheson, initiated a series of workshops on a national basis on work tolerance screening and work hardening. He described his highly successful program of returning workers to the job. Although his workshops were open to anyone, Matheson urged occupational therapists, especially, to apply their professional skills to the needs of modern industry.

The response to Matheson's appeal from occupational therapists was, initially, slow and cautious. The effects of Medicare cutbacks, however, continued to pinch the profession.

Carolyn Baum, OTR, FAOTA, American Occupational Therapy Association (AOTA) President in 1982 and 1983, was simultaneously advocating the exploration of new opportunities for OT. She strongly supported its re-entry into the work place.

By 1984, occupational therapists were ready to learn from Matheson. Assisted by Linda Dempster Niemeyer, OTR, Matheson provided leadership that was critically needed at that time by occupational therapists. With his instruction, occupational therapists learned to maximize their opportunity to build work-focused programs.

The Transition

With the encouragement of Matheson, Baum, and others, occupational therapists began to envision this new application of their skills. The transition from the medical model of practice to work-focused service delivery occurred smoothly for most therapists. Skills previously used to guide patients from dependence to independence in the school, hospital, or community were easily translated to guiding clients into functional independence in the job setting.

Interfacing with Business

Communication

Occupational therapy practice in an industrial rehabilitation framework demands that the practitioner communicate in nomenclature familiar in business and industry. The "language" of this market has been established by the United States Department of Labor and differs from the medical terminology in which occupational therapists have been schooled. The occupational therapist becomes "bilingual" in a very real sense. Information regarding a client's performance during evaluation or treatment may be reported to the referring physician in one way and to insurance carriers, attorneys, Social Security administrative law judges and employers in different phraseology in order to provide the clearest meaning to the reader.

Reference Works

The United States Department of Labor has compiled several documents that provide excellent references for the therapist who wishes to develop his or her "second language" in work-related practice. The first of these is *The Dictionary of Occupational Titles* (DOT). The DOT and its companion publications, *The DOT Supplement* and *The Classification of Jobs According to Worker Trait*

Factors (COJ), provide information about the more than 20,000 jobs which exist in the United States economy.

The DOT and the DOT Supplement contain the following useful information:
1. An alphabetical listing of all occupational job titles
2. A brief description and job title for most jobs encountered in the United States labor market
3. An occupational listing of titles arranged by industry
4. An analysis of requirements placed on a worker who performs the job

The COJ is a document which is used in tandem with the DOT and the Supplement. A full range of worker trait factors is cross-referenced in these documents for each job title listed in the DOT and the DOT Supplement. Worker trait factors include the following:
1. Environmental conditions surrounding the worker, such as extremes of heat or cold, noise, fumes, and hazards
2. General educational level or training required to perform the job proficiently
3. Aptitudes generally needed for successful job performance, such as intelligence, form perception, and manual dexterity
4. Interests and temperaments commonly found in individuals who successfully perform the job, such as adaptability to accepting responsibility or to performing repetitive work
5. Physical demands of the job, such as seeing, hearing, feeling, handling, lifting, carrying, and climbing

One of the most useful sections of the COJ is the "Physical Demands" classification section. One of the first criteria for determining a client's ability to do a job is his or her ability to lift the amount of weight which is ordinarily handled in a given job. For this reason, all jobs are classified, initially, by the primary "strength" requirements needed for successful performance of each job (see the box, Classification of Work Levels). The strength components include ability to lift, carry, push, and pull. Consideration is given to the frequency with which the client's strength is employed. The COJ provides the work level at which a given job is generally performed. This is important information for the therapist in setting up a job simulation.

Referral Sources

Referrals to the work performance program may be initiated by any of a number of people. Referrals are generally made by one who is seeking definitive information about a client's capabilities and limitations. Often, the physician will make the referral. Other times, the workers' compensation insurance carrier or the carrier's case manager or the managing rehabilitation nurse or

---

Classification of Work Levels

1. *Sedentary work* requires a maximum lift of 10 lb, infrequently, and occasional lift or carry of papers, small tools, or file folders. Sedentary work may require occasional walking or standing.
2. *Light work* requires a maximum lift of 20 lb with frequent lifting or carrying of up to 10-lb objects. If a great deal of walking, standing, or pushing and pulling of arm or leg controls is required by the job, the job will be classified at the light level even though the lifting requirements do not exceed 10 lb.
3. *Medium work* requires a maximum lift of up to 50 lb with frequent lifting and carrying of weights up to 25 lb.
4. *Heavy work* requires a maximum lift of 100 lb with frequent lifting or carrying of objects weighing up to 50 lb.
5. *Very heavy work* requires lifting objects greater than 100 lb with frequent lifting or carrying of objects weighing 50 lb or more.

---

specialist will initiate work performance program entry. Either the plaintiff's or the defendant's attorney may request work performance evaluation or treatment in personal injury or workers' compensation cases. Rehabilitation counselors often request information obtained from a work-hardening program regarding a client's potential to perform a certain job for which he or she may be trained under the sponsorship of vocational rehabilitation services. Educational institutions may refer students to work performance programs for this same reason. Occasionally, a client will be referred directly from his employer or present himself or herself for referral.

Range of Services Provided

Whether the industrial rehabilitation program deals primarily with clients with psychosocial or with physical problems, many of the program services may be the same. Work-focused programming offers a variety of service components for the occupational therapist. The two program areas that have provided the bulk of practice for most therapists to date have been functional capacity evaluation and work-hardening therapy. Before discussing these two program concepts, several other services merit review.

Pre-Employment Evaluations

Pre-employment evaluations may be provided by the occupational therapist. These usually consist of the test-ing of prospective employees in areas which are critically important to job performance. Materials handling or lifting and carrying specific weights required in the job, for example, may be evaluated in a test setting, and the results may be considered in reviewing the prospective employee's qualifications for the job. This service is usually purchased by a company in an effort to reduce the risk of injury by ensuring that individuals hired are indeed physically able to perform the high-risk job components.

Prevocational Evaluation

Prevocational evaluation and treatment programs help clients achieve a level of mastery of self-care or general work skills prior to determining job placement. School-based OT programs, head-trauma centers, pain management units, and rehabilitation centers provide a first step toward the long-term goal of entry or re-entry into the work force.

Prevention or Wellness Programs

Many companies offer their employees short training programs to assist them in coping with the emotional stresses of today's fast-paced lifestyle. The objective is to equip the employee with skills needed to avoid lost time from work because of job or personal problems. Among the more popular training programs provided by occupational therapists are materials handling and body mechanics training, stress management, relaxation, development of leisure skills, and energy-saving techniques for home or work management.

Job Modification

Business and industry are increasingly cognizant of the importance of safe, efficient placement or location of job components in the design of a job in the prevention of occupational injuries. The occupational therapist may recommend job or equipment modifications to reduce the physical or psychological stress imposed on the worker. Sometimes, adjustment of the height of the work surface, the distance or angle of reach, or the seating arrangement can make a significant difference in the stress imposed on the worker by the task he or she must perform.

Expert Witness Testimony

Increasingly, occupational therapists are engaged to provide expert witness testimony in a court of law. The therapist may be hired by either the plaintiff's or the defendant's attorney. When the therapist is engaged by the plaintiff's attorney, the primary interest will often be in the client's limitations and the negative effects of an injury. When the therapist is engaged by the defendent's attorney, the primary interest will usually be in the plaintiff's functional capabilities.

In either case, the occupational therapist's testimony is usually based on a functional capacity evaluation (FCE) administered to the plaintiff. The FCE must be conducted and documented in the same way for either situation, regardless of the focus the attorney will give the reported findings. The therapist must remain, in either case, as objective and unbiased as possible, or the credibility of the testimony will be damaged.

Functional Capacity Evaluation

The FCE or work performance assessment (WPA), as it is sometimes called, stands alone as a one-time evaluation. The FCE measures a client's performance against given criteria and predicts his or her potential to engage in work. The criteria against which measurements are made may be job-specific, as in the case of an injured worker who may eventually return to his job. Alternately, the measurements may be made using the general physical demands of work criteria as defined by the United States Department of Labor to identify a general work level in which the client may be expected to function successfully.

Reasons for Referral

Functional capacity evaluations may be requested from a variety of sources. A physician may request an FCE to obtain data on which to base a client's disability rating. An insurance carrier may require data on which to base the settlement of a workers' compensation claim. An attorney in personal injury litigation may seek a clear definition of a client's ability to function normally. A rehabilitation counselor may require physical performance parameters in order to develop an individualized employment plan (IEP) with a client.

Preparing for the Evaluation

Preparation for assessment begins several days in advance of the actual evaluation. The therapist must arrange for review of medical records, including the records of any therapy the client has received relative to his reason for entering the industrial rehabilitation program. Before the first measure is taken, it is important for the therapist to be acquainted with three things from the client's perspective:

1. What the client perceives has happened to him or her
2. What the client recognizes has been done about it
3. What the client expects will happen in the future with regard to recovery and return to work

This information may be obtained by telephone contact with the client or by a questionnaire mailed in advance of the appointment. Use of a mailed questionnaire in advance of a work performance evaluation is highly desirable because it allows the client to respond thoughtfully to queries in his own home without feeling rushed. This permits the client to consider the questions carefully, to refer to his records, and to note names and dosages of present medications directly from the labeled container. Generally, educational and work histories will be more extensive if the client prepares them in advance of the appointment.

When the client arrives for the initial visit, information may be obtained from the receptionist regarding the client's manner and any physical limitations exhibited as he or she enters the evaluation center. Any assistance required by the client during the registration process is noted by the receptionist and related to the evaluating therapist.

The Four-Step Evaluation Process

An interview, which can be accomplished in 15 to 30 minutes if a completed questionnaire has arrived with the client, allows the therapist and the client to initiate their working relationship. In addition to obtaining subjective information from the client, the therapist begins the objective evaluation by observing the client's sitting tolerance for the duration of the subjective interview.

With subjective reporting by the client covered well, the evaluation moves into a second phase, or a period of specific and direct measurement. The basic measures of muscle strength, joint range of motion, sensibility, coordination, balance, and functional mobility are performed and recorded.

After the client's limitations and abilities have been established by direct measure, the client enters the third section of the evaluation, performance on standardized tests. A number of standardized tests are employed at this point. Tests such as dynometric grip strength, the Minnesota Rate of Manipulation Tests, the Jebson–Taylor Test of Hand Coordination, and any combination of the many standardized instruments now on the market provide useful information and normative data for comparison. Standardized tests are useful evaluation instruments for one time only or for test–retest application.

Finally, the FCE has a work sample or simulated job task component that is individualized for each client. When the client's job is specified, the therapist selects those factors essential to the job but which, based on the information concerning the nature and extent of injury in the medical record, the therapist deems likely to challenge the client's ability to perform. These functions of the job are set up as nearly as the therapist can manage, to require the same motion, pace, and resistance required on the job.

When there is no specific job targeted for the client, a generic evaluation may be conducted. The client is started out at a level slightly less than that in which the therapist estimates the client's performance will fall. This is accomplished by first taking an objective measure of the client's lifting achievement on the day of the test. Simulated job tasks can be selected just under the client's best performance of full range of motion under load. The therapist then rather quickly advances the client through the United States Department of Labor classifications of work levels. Tests that give a good idea of the client's cognitive as well as physical function are included in this component of the total evaluation.

Evaluation Findings

Upon the conclusion of functional capacity testing, the therapist will have obtained considerable data regarding the limits of the client's functional performance for the day of testing. Many tests will have been performed to the client's point of maximum strength or endurance. Other tests will have provided comparison data that allow the therapist to compare the client's performance with that of a normal group.

Following review of the data collected in the work performance assessment, the therapist is able to identify the client's strengths and weaknesses for job performance as the job is known to him or her. The therapist can identify the factors that are impeding the client's return to his or her job at the time of testing. These are called "primary limiting factors for the job." The therapist can also determine the extent to which the limitations prevent the client's performing the job.

Calling upon professional experience, the therapist will be able to make an estimation regarding which of the limiting factors may yet be responsive to remediation, adapted devices, or adapted environments. The therapist will also identify which skills the client has to offer in the labor market.

In discussion with the client, and then in a written report to referral sources, the therapist will recommend a course of action appropriate for the client from the perspective of preparing to enter or re-enter the work force. The recommended procedures may be incorporated into the client's treatment plan if he or she is to continue in a period of work-hardening therapy. In this case, the therapist also estimates the length of time work-hardening therapy may be expected to last.

Work-Hardening Therapy

Work-hardening therapy has provided a large portion of the practice of occupational therapists engaged in industrial rehabilitation programs. Work hardening may be defined as *the therapeutic technique that moves the worker from a submaximal level of performance to a level of performance adequate for entry or re-entry into the work force.* It is the carefully planned and guided, graded process of maximizing an individual's performance in relation to a work goal. The program is governed by the physiological principles of gradually increasing strength, endurance, and tolerance for activity.

The Evaluation

The key to successful treatment in work-hardening therapy, as in other OT treatment, is well-executed evaluation. A strong evaluation procedure provides the therapist with data upon which to construct a strong treatment plan. Therefore, an FCE will be the first step in work-hardening treatment.

Generic versus Job-Specific Treatment

Work hardening may be generic in nature, meaning that, in general, it provides the client with challenges at a level of physical and cognitive demand determined by US Department of Labor criteria. Generic work-hardening programs are appropriate for clients who have not yet selected or targeted a specific vocational or job goal. Most often, however, work hardening is job-specific; that is, the client and the therapist know the job for which the client is preparing. In many cases, as with a client who has been injured on the job, the employer to whom the client will return is also known. Detailed requirements for that job may be known to the client and to the therapist. Job elements that challenge the client's physical or cognitive abilities are the focus of the job-specific work-hardening program.

Program Entry

Entry into work hardening occurs in one of two modes. The client may enter a program immediately following an injury. Many times, however, clients are referred to work-hardening programs some time after the injury has occurred. In general, it is preferable for work-hardening therapy to closely follow the completion of the acute phase of rehabilitation. Work hardening, then, becomes a progressive step in the total rehabilitation process. When little time is allowed to elapse between the injury and enrollment in an aggressive rehabilitation program focused on return to work, few changes in life roles for the client or for family members are likely to occur.

Treatment Process

Regardless of the client's mode or chronologic point of entry into a work-hardening program, the treatment consists of graded activity to increase the client's strength and tolerance for tasks required on the job.

Exercise, activity, and simulated work tasks are fundamental to the treatment protocol. The therapy program is carefully designed to require the client to move in the same planes and distances and to use the same muscle groups required by the job. The therapist also designs tasks that require the client to lift and carry materials of the same size and weight for the same distances as the job demands.

Psychosocial Considerations

Although the physical effects of the injury may appear to be the primary focus of a work-hardening treatment program, the psychosocial needs of the client will not be underestimated by the prudent therapist. Although these will not be explored here, the following are some of the issues the injured worker finds himself or herself facing during work-hardening therapy:

1. Fear of reinjury if he returns to the same job
2. Concerns regarding supervisory response to his return to the job. Although employers must take back a worker who has been injured on the job, if the employee–supervisor relationship was cool before the injury, the client may expect an even cooler reception upon return to the job.
3. Concerns from peers regarding the client's competence to perform job duties adequately, to carry his or her fair share of the work load, and, perhaps more importantly, to avoid injury to them
4. Diminished financial settlement if he or she returns to work
5. Concerns regarding the permanence of the job if he or she does go back to work. In recent years, many companies have changed ownership, with resultant layoff of both long- and short-term employees. Other companies, unable to hold market position, have simply gone out of business. As a result, some clients feel they must calculate whether they will "come out better" with the maximum worker's compensation settlement they can obtain or whether they will be able to support their family better on unemployment benefits.
6. Concerns regarding change in the role assignments within the family structure if the client shifts from a "patient" to a "worker" role

Although the client may give fleeting thought to these issues upon entry into a work-hardening program, initially, the focus of the program is primarily biomechanical. As the client shows improvement in physical function and becomes aware that he or she may, in fact, achieve return to work status, these psychosocial issues play a more dominant role in the total treatment process. The work-hardening staff must provide the client with sensitive assistance in working through these common concerns.

Disposition

When the client has demonstrated proficiency in accomplishing the job requirements for an 8-hour day over a 3- to 5-day period, he or she may be released to return to the physician for final disposition. At this point, it is appropriate for the therapist to recommend to the physician that the client return to full duty without restrictions if the work-hardening therapy performance has demonstrated his or her ability to do so.

However, not all work-hardening clients are successful in meeting return-to-work requirements. When this is the case, the therapist may recommend a return to restricted work. The therapist will specify to the physician the limitations or restrictions that will allow the client to perform in his or her maximum job capacity. If return to former or modified work is deemed to be impractical, a referral to a vocational rehabilitation counselor will very likely be appropriate. The aim is to assist the client in retaining gainful employment at his or her maximal functional level in the work force.

The Client's Job Performance

One of the most difficult yet interesting challenges for the occupational therapist in industrial rehabilitation is the issue of performance inconsistency. There is a somewhat frequent demonstration of inconsistent performance by the client in the industrial rehabilitation setting. During the course of the evaluation and treatment processes, the therapist must be sensitive to *any* inconsistencies in the client's performance. The client who is unable to move shoulders higher than 90° in abduction during direct measure or in simulated work tasks but, who abducts the shoulder to place his cap on his head when it is time to go home, is demonstrating an inconsistency in performance. The client who clings to the banister during direct testing of stair climbing but, walks downstairs without holding hand rails at the end of the evaluation or the simulated work day, is demonstrating a performance inconsistency. The client who cannot bend forward on direct testing but does so to obtain a soft drink from the soda machine is performing inconsistently. These inconsistencies often represent the client's effort to impress staff with greater than actual impairment. This misrepresentation may be called "symptom magnification" or "exaggerated pain or impairment behavior." Inconsistencies must be documented in the evaluation or progress report.

When inconsistencies are noted, the client should be confronted by the therapist in a supportive way and provided with a retest opportunity. It is hoped that in the retest situation, the client will "discover" an expanded capacity compared with the previous performance. In the case where inconsistencies of performance are called to the attention of a client and retest shows no change, the events are also recorded in the industrial rehabilitation record and are reported to referral and payment sources.

Litigation

Because the question of financial settlement is often pending when clients enter an industrial rehabilitation program, many clients are not totally committed to attaining or to demonstrating complete recovery from their injuries. It is extremely important for the therapist to be sensitive to the implications of pending litigation. Some of the implications are:

1. The client may put forth less than maximum effort in the FCE or work-hardening program. This will very likely reveal itself in observed or measured inconsistencies in performance during the testing or treatment period.
2. The client's motivational level for return to work may be very low.
3. The client is sensitive to the fact that all documentation of performance in the industrial rehabilitation program will be reviewed by parties involved in the litigation.

The Impairment Rating

Since the client seen in industrial rehabilitation is frequently ultimately rated by a physician for the effect of the injury, a word about that rating procedure is of interest to the occupational therapist.

Impairment determination is the purview of the physician in the United States. It is a statement of the client's physical or psychiatric impairment, made by a physician, based on the injuries the client has received. Traditionally, the impairment determination or impairment rating has been based entirely on the individual's loss of functional use of a body part. Until the advent of work-hardening therapy in the early 1980s, little or no consideration was given to the extent to which the client's job was affected by his injury, nor was it necessary to determine whether the job was affected at all by the injury. Monetary settlements, sometimes of vast sums, were made on the basis of the existence of an injured body part. This medical assessment for economic adjustment almost totally ignored the client's abilities.

With the establishment of industrial rehabilitation programs, however, came the possibility of observing an injured worker in a simulated work setting. Many physicians now rely heavily on data obtained from an FCE or from a course of work-hardening therapy to make a final impairment rating. This allows the physician and other parties involved, including insurance carriers, attorneys, and the client, to consider the client's

strengths and assets for job performance, as well as the limitations or disabilities.

Vocational Rehabilitation and Vocational Evaluation

Sometimes, an experienced worker's ability to perform his or her job adequately is permanently affected by accident or disease to the extent that he or she is unable to return to the previous work. The inability to meet job demands may be immediately obvious, as in the case of a barge deckhand whose leg is traumatically amputated in a motorcycle accident and who would be unsafe walking or hopping on a string of river barges in choppy water. The construction worker whose back is broken in a fall, resulting in partial paralysis of both lower extremities, provides another example. With other clients, limiting factors that prevent return to previous work may not show up until the FCE or even until a period of work hardening has been accomplished and the client's functional limitation consistently interferes with the performance of simulated job tasks. When the occupational therapist makes the judgment that the client will be unable to return to the original or modified work, a referral to a vocational rehabilitation counselor or to a vocational evaluator is appropriate. Members of these two professions may be, at this time, more highly qualified than occupational therapists in the artful matching of the client's transferrable skills with opportunities for employment.

The role of worker is an important life role for the client. The client's livelihood, and often that of his or her family, are dependent on work. He or she deserves the expertise of the trained vocational evaluator or rehabilitation counselor in making a major job change. Although workshops, college credit course work, and continuing education courses will enhance the occupational therapist's skills in the identification of a client's transferrable or marketable skills, this function requires more specialized training than occupational therapists routinely receive at this time.

The Therapists' Roles

The OTR or COTA will be able to more accurately guide the client in the work tasks that simulate the most critical components of the client's job when he or she sees it performed by one of the client's peers.

The COTA may perform functions beyond treatment provision in the work-focused program. Progress notes prepared and signed by the COTA are cosigned by the OTR and distributed to physicians and insurance carriers. The OTR or COTA, then, may be contacted by these outside agents for additional information or for clarification of some point in the progress note. The

COTA can provide information effectively and thus represents the program to the public in a professional manner.

The summary note, which documents the discharge status of a work-hardening client, usually contains data from rather extensive final evaluations. A synthesis of the data is prepared, and a prognosis for the client's successful entry or re-entry into the work place is projected in the discharge summary. It is, therefore, prudent for the OTR to prepare the discharge summary. Even so, he or she will find the COTA's observations and input extremely valuable for this final report.

Curriculum Considerations

New areas of professional practice are opening with implications for the curricula which prepare occupational therapists for registry and occupational therapy assistants for certification. As the practice of industrial rehabilitation flourishes, faculty at both of these teachings levels must review their course content to ensure that, at a minimum, the following topics are covered to some extent:

1. Consideration of the life role of worker for all patients
2. Evaluation of lower as well as upper extremity function
3. General descriptors for functional ambulation
4. Methods of materials handling or body mechanics
5. Orientation to pain management therapy
6. Orientation to workers' compensation procedures and practices
7. Orientation to United States Department of Labor terminology related to job analysis and performance
8. Orientation to standardized tests which evaluate functional, job-oriented performance

Although fieldwork placement in a work-hardening program may be interesting to the student who has identified industrial rehabilitation as her or his primary job interest, she or he will find that field experience in other areas of adult treatment will be invaluable in the work-focused setting. A therapist who has worked with orthopedic patients will have an understanding of the healing of both tissue and bone. A therapist who has worked in acute-care rehabilitation or with cancer patients will rarely be fooled by a client attempting to feign pain. Experience in a psychosocial setting serves to better prepare the new therapist for dealing with the myriad psychosocial ramifications of an industrial injury.

A Look Toward the Future

At the time of this writing, work-hardening therapy has captured both health care and corporate dollars. It is a growth industry. Members of the various health care professions are competing with each other to carve as large a place as possible for themselves and their professions in the control of this popular new service. Yet some therapists are committing their skills and talents to a broader area. They are identifying and addressing the scope of the needs in the area of industrial rehabilitation. These therapists have not limited their practice to FCEs and work-hardening therapy. Rather, they have viewed work hardening as the entree into a new "product line" for occupational therapists to be found under the broader umbrella of industrial rehabilitation.

Is work hardening, or industrial rehabilitation for that matter, a viable "product line" for occupational therapists, or are therapists momentarily distracted from the "real work" of occupational therapy? These are important questions. They are the same questions, however, that occupational therapists must ask themselves about each of their service areas, on a regular basis. Health care services are provided in a rapidly changing social and economic environment. A service that fails to address a societal need is doomed to failure. It is wise, therefore, for the occupational therapist to review the range of services offered on at least an annual basis and to make appropriate adjustments for the market in which the services will be delivered. If occupational therapists will do this, the appearance of their programs will reflect some change from year to year. It is unlikely, however, that occupational therapists will soon give up their position again in work-focused program provision.

Bibliography

Acquiaviva JD: Federal law and access to rehabilitation services. In Kirkland M, Robertson, SC (eds): Planning and Implementing Vocational Readiness in Occupational Therapy. Rockville, MD, American Occupational Therapy Association, 1985

Cantor SG: Occupational therapy and occupational medicine—a merger. Am J Occup Ther 33:631, 1979

Cromwell FS: Work-related programming in occupational therapy: its roots, course and prognosis. Occup Ther Health Care 2:9, 1985–86

Dictionary of Occupational Titles, 4th ed. Washington, DC, US Department of Labor, 1982

Dictionary of Occupational Titles (Supplement), 4th ed. Washington, DC, US Department of Labor, 1984

Ellsworth P, Davy J, Mitcham M, et al: The role of occupational therapy in the vocational rehabilitation process: Official position paper. Am J Occup Ther 34:881, 1980

Field TF, Field JE: The Classification of Jobs According to Worker Trait Factors, ed. rev. Athens, VDARE Service Bureau, 1984

Holmes D: The role of the occupational therapist–work evaluator. Am J Occup Ther 39:308, 1985

Jacobs K: Occupational Therapy: Work-Related Programs and Assessments. Boston, Little, Brown, 1985

Kester DL: Prevocational and vocational assessment. In Hopkins HL, Smith HD (eds): Willard and Spackman's Occupational Therapy, 6th ed. Philadelphia, JB Lippincott, 1983

Kirkland M, Robertson SC (eds): The evolution of work-related theory in occupational therapy. In Kirkland M, Robertson SC (eds): Planning and Implementing Vocational Readiness in Occupational Therapy. Rockville, MD, American Occupational Therapy Association, 1985

Macdonald EM (ed): Occupational Therapy in Rehabilitation, 4th ed. Baltimore, Williams & Wilkins, 1976

Matheson LN: Work Capacity Evaluation. Anaheim, ERIC, 1986

Taylor SE, Blaine JM: Work hardening: A bridge to return to work. In Fry R (ed): Second National Forum on Issues in Vocational Assessment: The Issues Papers. Menomonie, WI, Materials Development Center, Stout Vocational Rehabilitation Institute, University of Wisconsin–Stout, 1986

West WL: The role of occupational therapy in work adjustment. In Jones M, Kandel D (eds): Work Adjustment as a Function of Occupational Therapy. Dubuque, WC Brown, 1962

CHAPTER 19

Upper Extremity Orthotics   *Maude H. Malick*

Great strides have been made in the construction of orthotics for the upper extremities using plastic materials as a result of the NASA (National Aeronautics and Space Administration) programs. Reliability of dynamic splinting also has increased as a result of the greater sophistication in electronics and external power sources. This is true not only in the United States, but also in Europe, South Africa, and Australia. Since low-temperature plastic materials are remoldable, splints can be easily constructed or adjusted while the patient waits. Many splints can be custom designed, constructed, fitted, and applied within an hour. Temporary progressive splinting can be fabricated with minimal effort. Orthotic principles applicable to the low-temperature materials are the same as those applying to the metal or high-temperature materials. Low-temperature materials require more contour or reinforcement when rigidity is required.

A series of polycaprolactone materials, such as Polyform, Polyflex II, Ezeform, Ultra Form, and Ultra Form 294, Kay-Splint, and Aquaplast, are effective low-temperature materials. These materials can be handled easily if the molding temperature requirements are strictly adhered to. Static and dynamic splints can be constructed readily but should be considered only for 3 to 6 months of use. Laminated plastic, high-temperature materials, and metal are indicated if splint (orthotic) requirements dictate longer wear. Where moving parts such as metal joints, hinges, and telescopic units are needed in the wrist-driven orthosis, they should be constructed and assembled by a qualified orthotist. A good example of this is the Engen telescopic reciprocal wrist orthosis which, in a modular fashion, utilizes laminated plastic, metal, and rods to make an effective orthosis for the quadriplegic patient.

When evaluating the orthotic requirements of the patient, careful analysis should be made of the upper extremity to evaluate what stability is lacking and what motion is needed to perform functional tasks. Range-of-motion tests and functional motion tests should be used to evaluate strength, range, coordination, and sensory deficiencies, noting whether and where spasticity is present. When orthotic devices are indicated, it is important to do the following:

1. Fully explain the upper extremity evaluation to the patient and involve the patient in the design and selection of the orthosis.
2. Fabricate the orthosis so that it will be well fitted, designed, and constructed.
3. Begin use of the splint early in the treatment program and then discard the splint if it is no longer useful.

The therapist must always consider the psychological aspects of splinting. Patient acceptance may vary, but ease of acceptance can be greatly influenced by proper explanation of its necessity. The orthosis should meet functional requirements and be cosmetically acceptable. Comfort, stability, and value of the orthosis are probably the greatest factors in patient acceptance.

Initially, the splint should be worn only under the therapist's supervision for short periods to be sure no pressure areas exist. Straps must be adequate and secure so that the orthosis retains its correct position. Distal slippage, with its accompanying misfit, is the greatest cause of pressure areas.

Most ADL are performed more usefully when the forearm and hand are in the best functional position. An orthosis provides the proper position, supports weakened muscles, and stabilizes joints. In most cases, the dominant hand, when affected, is splinted, but if both upper extremities are affected, bilateral orthoses may be considered. When shoulder and elbow function are impaired, consideration should be given to the flail arm splint (FAS), overhead slings, and balanced forearm orthosis (mobile arm supports) to provide support to and position the upper extremity and hand in the most functional position.

The FAS (Fig. 19-1) is basically the skeleton of the upper limb prosthesis. It fits around the flail upper extremity and enables the patient to position the elbow in one of five positions, which in turn increases the functional range of the extremity. By protracting the unaffected scapula, the patient can operate various terminal devices, thereby increasing his functional capability. The FAS is modular, and this allows for variations in its construction to compensate for less extensive or recovering lesions. The patient should be trained to put on and take off the orthosis and instructed about its proper fit and mechanics. Many simple assistive devices can be quickly constructed with the low-temperature plastics for temporary use before those of a permanent nature are considered.

Orthotics of the Hand

The terms *"orthotics"* and *"splinting"* are often used interchangeably, especially in reference to the upper extremity. With the availability of low-temperature plastics, the occupational therapist can readily make nearly any splint to meet the requirements of patients. Since occupational therapists outnumber orthotists 19.7:1, the responsibility for upper extremity splinting largely falls to the occupational therapist.

The occupational therapist must assess or evaluate both the patient's affected hand and the unaffected hand in order to determine the specific purpose of the splint and the parts to be splinted. The purpose determines whether the splint should be static or dynamic, as well as the regimen in which it is to be used. All splints are a part of an overall patient management program.

Static splints may be protective, supportive, or corrective in their design. A static splint may be indicated to protect weak muscles from being stretched by providing the force to counteract a strong muscle group and in this way provide a functional balance while healing is taking place. The splint can support the hand, joint, or arch as a substitute for weak muscles, as in the case of arthritis. Corrective splinting can specifically position or force an involved joint or bone into correct or near-correct alignment. Static splints have no movable parts and wherever possible should hold the involved forearm and hand in a functional position.

All splints must be taken off at intervals and be a part of a maintenance exercise program. The splint and the patient's hand should be washed and dried and the hand carefully replaced in the splint in the correct position. The therapist must always be aware of swelling or edema. Edema can be due to constriction by the splint or its strap. Prolonged static splinting can cause joint immobility. The patient should be encouraged to use the

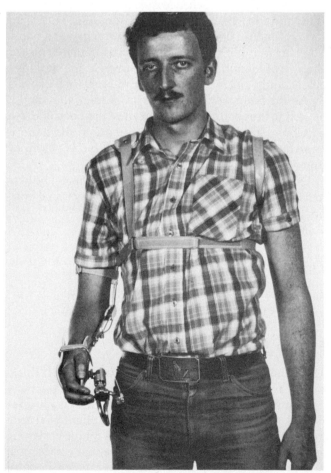

Figure 19-1. Full flail arm splint with shoulder girdle, elbow lock, and forearm support with terminal device.

splinted extremity as much as possible to maintain muscle tone and joint mobility. No splint should immobilize more joints in the hand than are specifically indicated by the evaluations.

All splints should be neat and constructed with careful craftsmanship. They should be lightweight, durable, cosmetically acceptable, washable, and carefully designed to avoid loss of the special properties of the thermoplastic material.

Choice of Splinting Materials

There is a wide variety of splinting materials available, the various properties of which must be understood in order to use them properly. They can be classified in four groups:
1. High-temperature materials
2. Moderate-temperature materials
3. Low-temperature materials
4. No-heat, or layered, materials

All materials except the layered materials come in sheets of various thicknesses.

In general, high-temperature materials are best cut flat with hand or power tools such as a jigsaw; they should be formed on a plaster positive mold to avoid burning the patient. Low-temperature and layered materials may be cut with scissors; they do not require a mold and can be molded directly on a patient. Application of the various materials is dependent on their thickness and rigidity and the design of the splint. The less rigid materials will require more area and contour for support.

High-temperature materials include Nyloplex, Copolymar, Royalite, and Kydex. A splint of this type is shown in Figure 19-2. A moderate-temperature material is high-impact vinyl. Low-temperature materials include Orthoplast, Polyform, Polyflex II, Ezeform, Ultra-Form, UltraForm 294, San-Splint, Kay-Splint, SOS Plastazote, and Aquaplast. An example of no-heat or layered material is plaster of paris bandage. In general, low-temperature plastic materials are used for temporary progressive splinting and the high-temperature plastic materials for long-term splints.

Construction of the splint requires not only a thorough knowledge of the properties of the materials but also the imagination of the occupational therapist. Patterns and models are guidelines only and should be modified to meet each patient's special requirements. Static splints should never be used longer than is physiologically indicated and should never be used if a dynamic splint would be equally effective. Splints should immobilize only the intended joints, leaving all the adjacent joints free to move. Static splints can do the following:
1. Prevent unwanted motion
2. Relieve pain
3. Prevent deformity and contractures
4. Substitute for weak or lost muscle function
5. Maintain a functional position for bone, muscle, tendon, or ligaments during healing

Physiologic Considerations

It is essential that each occupational therapist understand the bony skeleton, joint locations, and muscle insertions and functions of the forearm, wrist, and hand. The versatility of motion in the hand depends on the amount of motion in every joint above it; the shoulder, elbow, and wrist must be stable and functional in order to use the hand. Without shoulder motion, the hand is limited to the arc of motion in front of the body allowed by elbow motion. Without elbow motion, the hand is limited to the small arc in which the hand is placed by the wrist.

No matter what splint is used, the hand must be kept in a functional position (Fig. 19-3). The functional position of the hand is as follows:
1. Wrist in 30° dorsiflexion
2. Normal transverse arch
3. Thumb in abduction and opposition with the pads of the four other fingers
4. Metacarpal and proximal interphalangeal joints in 45° flexion

Palmar Creases

The palmar surface of the hand is covered with thick, tough, and not very pliable skin. This lack of pliability accounts for a system of palmar creases, which allow for flexion and motion. These creases differ slightly on each individual and should act as guidelines for the designing and fitting of each splint. The distal palmar crease must not be impinged upon if full metacarpophalangeal (MCP) flexion is required. Likewise, the thenar crease must not be impinged upon if opposition is required.

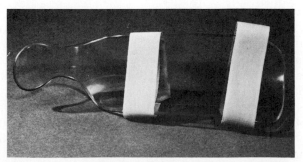

Figure 19-2. A simple palmar wrist cock-up splint made of Nyloplex provides an aesthetically appealing rigid wrist support. Nyloplex is a high-temperature plastic that must be formed over a plaster mold.

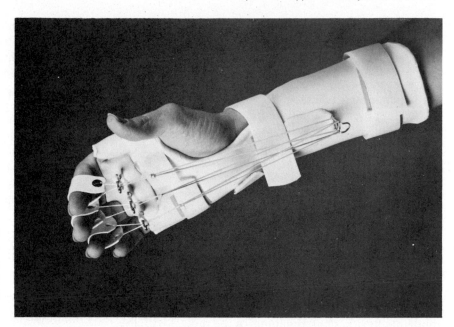

Figure 19-3. Palmar splint used to maintain wrist and metacarpophalangeal joints in functional position while low-profile dynamic outrigger is used to achieve flexion of proximal interphalangeal joints.

The wrist creases indicate the best location for a splint strap to stabilize the splint and prevent it from sliding forward.

Arches of the Hand

The palm of the hand is concave from side to side and also in its length. This shape is formed by three arches (Fig. 19-4), which are of prime consideration when constructing a splint.

Transverse Arch

The distal transverse arch is also called the metacarpal transverse arch. When the hand is at rest, the arch is slightly oblique. This arch is deepened when the hand is used functionally. The mobility of the fourth and fifth metacarpal within the arch contributes directly to the dexterity of all the fingers. If this metcarpal mobility is constricted, the functional motion of the fingers is directly impaired. Therefore, the ability of the arch to deepen should always be considered when designing a splint. There should be freedom and some excursion if a palmar bar or support is designed into a splint.

The proper functioning of the thumb depends on the integrity of the transverse arch also. If the arch is depressed, the hand becomes flat, and the thumb is unable to oppose the fingers. This opposition is possible only when there is some cupping of the palm, and when the curve of this arch can be increased voluntarily. Any weakness or damage to this arch will impair the strength, mobility, and precision of the motion of the thumb.

Longitudinal Arch

The longitudinal arch follows the long lines of the phalanges and metacarpal and carpal bones at a slightly oblique angle and primarily involves the third finger. The mobility of the phalanges (fingers) directly affects the efficiency of the hand grasp.

Figure 19-4. The three arches of the hand are of primary importance to function: (*1*) transverse arch; (*2*) longitudinal arch; and (*3*) proximal transverse arch. All can be identified easily by the creases of the hand.

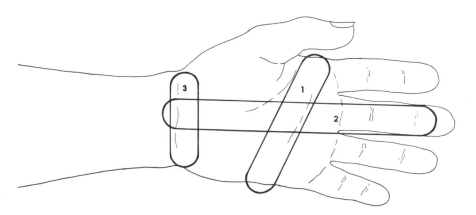

Proximal Transverse Arch

The proximal transverse (or carpal) arch is located at the wrist and is troughlike. It is formed by the annular ligaments and the carpal bones. It is this arch that provides the mechanical advantage to the tendons of the finger flexors by providing the fulcrum.

The "Ball" and Functional Position

The "ball" is the result of the combination of the three arches. It is located directly over the metacarpals which the three arches form. Often, the ball is the best pivotal position of support for the hand in a splint. It can be noted when grasping an object. The splint must conform to this ball if it is to fit properly and allow normal function.

When the hand is in the position of function, it maintains its arches, slight dorsiflexion of the wrist, and moderate flexion of all the joints of the fingers with the thumb in opposition. This position is maintained primarily by two key sets of joints: the wrist for the hand and the metacarpophalangeal joints for the fingers.

Requirements of a
Well-Designed Splint

A well-designed and fitted splint should be individually constructed to support, re-establish, or facilitate normal coordinate movement, preserve normal physiological status of muscles, and prevent deformities. The splint should provide the patient with as functional a hand as possible for performing as many activities as possible. This is best done when the splint conforms to the following characteristics:
1. Maintains normal arches
2. Retains the normal axis of motion
3. Permits balanced function of unaffected muscles
4. Provides the most practical prehension pattern
5. Allows maximal mobility with optimal stability
6. Frees the palmar surface of hand and digits for greatest sensory perception

Precautions Regarding Pressure Areas

Pressure areas can be created in splinting by the force placed on hand areas for correct positioning. Certain areas are prone to pressure, including:
1. Dorsum metacarpophalangeal joints (with a dorsal splint)
2. Palmar (volar) surface of metacarpophalangeal joint of thumb and index finger (with C-bar of opponens cuff)
3. Palmar (volar) surface of distal joints of fingers (with palmar resting-pan splints, especially with flexion contractures)
4. Dorsal surface of the first phalanx of each finger (with lumbrical bar)
5. Head of ulna (with the wrist strap of the dorsal opponens splint or the forearm section bar of the long opponens splint)
6. Metacarpal joint of the thumb just distal to the head of the radius (with the opponens bar)
7. The center of the palm (with the palmar (volar) surface of a wrist cock-up, especially when there is wrist flexion contracture)

Pressure areas can be avoided by correct splint designs that include the following features:
1. Following the contours of the normal hand and forearm
2. Placing minimal stretch on joints or muscles in deformed positions over a longer period rather than striving for immediate correction
3. Increasing the splint surface area to distribute pressure and using padding

General precautions include the following:
1. Design and modify splints individually to meet the needs and changes in each patient's extremity. The splint should be viewed systematically and re-evaluated according to need, fit, and purpose.
2. Have the patient wear the splint intermittently. The length of time is determined by the physician or therapist and usually is not more than 10 to 12 hours daily. Splints should be worn only as long as they are performing a function.
3. Avoid tight encircling straps to prevent constrictions. There should be no blanched areas where circulation is decreased.
4. Avoid pressure areas over bony prominences.
5. Avoid making too short a forearm section because this will provide inadequate leverage. Conversely, too long a forearm section will impinge on the elbow joint and limit flexion. A good general rule is for the forearm section to be two-thirds the length of the forearm. The splint should be checked when the patient is seated.
6. Fit the palmar piece over the metacarpal transverse arch accurately and allow the metacarpal joints to flex to a right angle.
7. Contour the sides of finger, thumb, and platform splints to follow the natural curve of the digits. Metacarpal and proximal interphalangeal joints should be flexed to about 15° to 45°. Avoid positions which would lead to hyperextension of finger joints. The thumb should be held in a functional position of 45° abduction and opposition.

Dynamic Splints

Purpose of Dynamic Splinting

Dynamic splinting is the application of a force on a moving part that remains nearly constant as the part moves. Often, it is called active splinting; this refers to the specific and directional mobility that the splint gives the joints by providing forces that substitute for absent muscle power. This joint mobility decreases adhesions, maintains joint function, and prevents ankylosis.

Dynamic splints must be designed and constructed carefully to provide specific traction with good directional control. Outriggers, which must be placed accurately and secured firmly to the body of the splint, often can be used (Fig. 19-5). The stability and maintenance of splint position on the hand are of prime importance.

A large percentage of patients requiring dynamic splinting are seen in acute-care hospitals following surgery or trauma to the forearm and hand and subsequently are seen as outpatients and in rehabilitation centers. Dynamic splints frequently are used to substitute for absent muscle power, to prevent contractures or impending contractures, to maintain balance, to promote rest, or to mobilize specific joints.

Splints may be required for the following reasons:

1. Skeletal substitution
   a. To aid in fracture alignment
   b. To support bones and joints having pathology
2. Muscle balance
   a. For paralyzed muscles
   b. For divided tendons or muscles
3. Joint motion
   a. To preserve joint motion
   b. To increase joint motion
4. Rest
   a. To promote wound healing of newly repaired structures
   b. To treat infection
   c. To relieve pain

The patient should be under close supervision of the physician and the occupational therapist. He or she should be encouraged to maintain and restore joint motion, to follow the exercise program, and to have the splint checked and adjusted regularly. The therapist must maintain an accurate joint measurement progress record.

Medical Principles

Good general medical principles must be considered in dynamic splinting. These principles include:

1. Moving muscles must be given an opposing, balancing force in order to maintain joint mobility and freely gliding tendons. A corrective force, often in the form of a finger cuff and rubber band, is necessary.
2. Movement prevents joint limitation, muscular atrophy, and deformity such as ankylosis.
3. Joints never should be immobilized needlessly.
4. Where there are injuries on the *flexor* surface, the wrist and fingers should be placed in flexion.
5. Where there are injuries in the *extensor* surface, the wrist and fingers should be placed in a neutral (resting) position.
6. Whenever possible, the position of function should be maintained prior to the application of any dynamic unit.
7. The hand should be elevated in the presence of edema, since edema causes fibrosis and prevents function. The edema should be reduced as quickly as possible so that early motion can be encouraged and the movement in the uninvolved parts of the hand maintained.
8. Straps that constrict venous return should not be used. Excessive tension of circular straps causes edema and increases the danger of ischemic contractures.

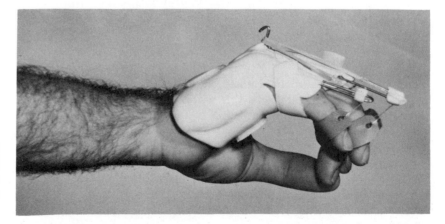

Figure 19-5. Hand-based dorsal splint that holds the metacarpophalangeal joints blocked in flexion. Low-profile dynamic outrigger is used to achieve proximal interphalangeal extension.

Static Base of the Dynamic Splint

The static base of the dynamic splint is of primary importance, as this base is the secured (anchored) foundation upon which all the support and moving parts rely. The static base of the splint does the following:

1. Provides foundation for proper (functional) alignment of joints
2. Provides a foundation to which the outrigger is attached with its traction components
3. Provides the foundation for a hinge joint
4. Aids in the relaxation of any spastic muscle
5. Allows tissues to adapt to their new position
6. Protects a newly repaired structure
7. Provides the support for proximal parts to allow increased function in distal joints or uninvolved parts
8. Aids in the positioning for edema control

Immobilization leads to joint stiffness; this must be remembered when constructing the static base of a splint.

Forces

Dynamic splinting should provide constant force over a long period of time rather than strong, short-term pressure. It operates according to a principle similar to that an orthodontist uses in straightening teeth. Active motion can be encouraged, for the pumping effect of muscle contraction helps relieve edema and increases joint range of motion. Eight hours of light, steady tension are more successful than vigorous passive exercise for 20 minutes, especially where contractures are present. Progressive alteration to a static splint can draw out a contracture, and active dynamic splinting can aid in maintaining the correction.

Active dynamic splinting has a physiological effect as well, for when the muscles are moving they pump away stagnant fluids that wash out the toxins, and the tendons keep gliding and the joints keep moving. Thus, the formation of adhesions is prevented, and the good mobility of joints can be maintained.

Directional Pull

Generally, the force to be applied should be at right angles to the axis of the bone. When applying flexion traction to the fingers, the direction of the pull is of paramount importance. The pull on the fingers must not draw them straight down to the palm of the hand but rather aim them obliquely at the scaphoid bone or the base of the third metacarpal. In normal opening of the hands, fingers abduct; in normal closing of the hand, fingers adduct, moving in an oblique arc of motion (Fig. 19-6).

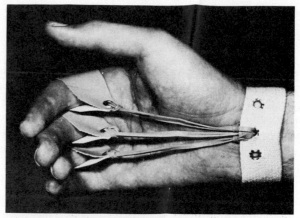

Figure 19-6. Dynamic flexion cuff demonstrating the correct line of pull.

All the fingers except the middle one (which may flex straight down) cross the palm obliquely from 10° to 30°. The same line of pull or of direction should be maintained when finger traction is used. If the splint is incorrectly designed, with the finger pulled straight down in flexion, a serious ulnar deviation will appear when the patient tries to extend the fingers. If bone callus has formed, the deformity may need surgical intervention.

Exercise Program

Dynamic splints are used to maintain forces and position, as well as to be a part of a graduated exercise and activity program. The combination of good dynamic splinting and an exercise program aids in hand rehabilitation.

The exercise and activity program aids in the excursion of the joint and is good for maintaining the tone of the skin and improving the circulation to the injured part. A patient also can gain confidence by seeing to what degree the hand can be moved safely. Exercises are best performed by the patient following instructions from the therapist so as not to go beyond the point of pain.

When there is lack of sensation, one must be extremely careful to avoid pressure or increase resistance too rapidly in a traction program. Applying heat prior to the exercise program is often a great help in relaxation and in facilitating movement.

Instructions for the Patient

A patient should understand the purpose of the splint, its accurate positioning, and exactly what motion or movement or range is being sought. The therapist should explain the functional anatomy of the hand to the patient. The therapist could demonstrate his or her own hand movement and range of motion so that the patient can understand the regimen more clearly and have confidence in it. The patient can use the unaffected hand to explore normal ranges of motion.

Careful instructions in the use of the dynamic splint are absolutely necessary, and written instructions are imperative when a splint is given to the patient on an outpatient basis. The patient should be seen at least once a week to measure the range of motion of hand joints. Adjustments must be made as gains are achieved in the mobilization of joints and as muscle power increases. The regimen is successful when there is improvement, little or no pain, and minimal edema. One must be careful in the follow-up program to make sure that the hand does not begin to shift back into its old or nonfunctional position as soon as the dynamic splint has been removed.

Bibliography

Anderson MH: Upper Extremities Orthotics. Springfield, IL, Charles C Thomas, 1979

Barr, NR: The Hand: Principles and Techniques of Simple Splint Making in Rehabilitation. London, Butterworths, 1975

Bunch WH, Keagy RD: Principles of Orthotic Treatment. St. Louis, CV Mosby, 1976

Cailliet R: Hand Pain and Impairment. Philadelphia, FA Davis, 1982

Fess E, Gerrle K, Strickland J: Hand Splinting: Principles and Methods. St. Louis, CV Mosby, 1981

Hunter JM: Rehabilitation of the Hand. St Louis, CV Mosby, 1984

Johnson MK: The Hand Atlas. Springfield, IL, Charles C Thomas, 1975

Malick MH: Manual on Dynamic Hand Splinting. Pittsburgh, Harmarville Rehabilitation Center, 1974

Malick MH: Manual on Management of Specific Hand Problems. Pittsburgh, Harmarville Rehabilitation Center, 1984

Malick MH: Manual on Static Hand Splinting. Pittsburgh, Harmarville Rehabilitation Center, 1972

Redford JB, Orthotics, Etc. 2nd ed. Baltimore, Williams & Wilkins, 1985

Robertson E: Rehabilitation of Arm Amputees and Limb Deficient Children. London, Bailliere–Tindall, 1978

Robinson C: Brachial plexus lesions II: Functional splintage. Br Occup Ther 49:331–334, 1986

Wolfort FG: Acute Hand Injuries: A Multispecialty Approach. Boston, Little, Brown, 1980

Wynn–Parry CB: Rehabilitation of the Hand, 4th rev. ed. London, Butterworths, 1981

Appreciation is extended to Cathryn J. Robinson, Dip COT, OTR/L of the Harmarville Rehabilitation Center for her contribution.

CHAPTER 20

Interpersonal Relationships in Occupational Therapy *Elizabeth G. Tiffany*

Conscious Use of Self

The occupational therapist is only one of the many people to whom the client is exposed when he or she becomes involved in treatment. Within the complexity of this situation, the interactions between the therapist and the client may be critical to the desired processes of growth and change. The therapist's conscious use of self is one of the important tools of the therapeutic process.

Although the therapist's role is usually defined by the context, it may not always be entirely clear to the client. It is therefore vital that the therapist be clear about his or her role. In the occupational therapy process, the therapist's use of self means bringing together knowledge, skills, caring, and basic personality strengths to help the client overcome difficulties and maximize abilities. A therapist is a helper. The kind of helper may vary. The therapist may help by teaching, giving support, fabricating adaptive devices, aiding in communication, engineering opportunities for growth, confronting problems, clarifying, reinforcing progress, or promoting plans for the future. In the therapeutic context, the therapist may be friendly but never the client's "friend," "buddy," or close confidante. This

means that the therapist especially must monitor the influence of personal needs and feelings. If, for example, a therapist has a strong need to prove that occupational therapy will cure a client, there is a risk of feeling angry if the client rejects the help offered or feeling disappointed if the client fails to respond. The reaction, in either case, would be a distortion and ultimately not helpful to the client. Because the maintenance of objectivity within the relationship is important, it is helpful and often necessary for the therapist to have another professional with whom to discuss feelings and events as they arise.

People with psychiatric problems may have great difficulty in developing healthy and health-promoting relationships with other people. Often, the relationships they have experienced either just before becoming ill or throughout longer periods of their lives have been negative. The precedents for human relationships may be fraught with distortions. There may be unrealistic positive or negative expectations of authority figures. Other human beings may be perceived as lacking constancy or predictability or as being threatening or hurtful. On the other hand, the emotional needs of the client may be so powerful as to cloak the reality of the situation in a cloud of wish-fulfillment. Frank has referred to the problems of avoidance, selective inattention, and self-fulfilling prophecy on the part of the client.[1] Fear of being hurt or of an unknown new mode of behavior may prevent the client's correction of a pathologic self-image. It is the task of the therapist to break through these problems and to develop with the client a new, different set of transactions, ones that will "confirm healthy expectations and disappoint pathological ones."

Initially, it is necessary to gain some measure of the client's trust. Trust is a feeling that is based on the perception of the therapist's ability and caring. Trust potentiates motivation: a client who trusts the therapist will be more easily motivated to participate in the occupational therapy process than one who does not feel trust. The issues of trust and motivation are important throughout the entire time the therapist and client are involved with one another.

How are trust and motivation developed? In the therapeutic context, there may be many factors. Apart from the direct interpersonal experiences of the therapist and client, there may be the distant uninvolved appraisal the client may make of the therapist based on observations of the transactions between the therapist and other clients or other staff members. There may be the halo effect of the encouragement to be involved in occupational therapy from the client's physician, other staff members, or other clients. The client may have made a simple, uncritical assumption (based on wish-fulfillment) that if the therapist is on the staff, the therapist must know how to help.

It is, however, in the direct interpersonal transactions between the therapist and the client that true and effective trust is established and reinforced. It is first necessary for the therapist to communicate empathy for the client's feelings and respect for the client as a human being. Such communication may be very simple, like a nod, or asking the client how he or she wishes to be called rather than automatically using a first name, nickname, or a formal name.[2] Communication must be clear and consistent throughout the total process. This is not always easy. For example, the silent, nonverbal client who may be depressed and despairing may show a strong wish to avoid involvement. The client who may be acting out feelings with hostile language or behavior may seem to be trying to put the therapist off. Such behavior may make it difficult for the therapist to communicate empathy and respect, yet it is these people who most need to feel they are cared for and valued in spite of the strange or threatening behaviors they show. Unless they feel valued, it is not really worth the effort for them to invest in making changes. The therapist, too, must be able to recognize the pain that underlies their behavior in order to wish to invest in making a change

process possible. Sometimes, this means sitting silently with a client; sometimes, it means confronting behavior or setting clear limits in a way that indicates an expectation that change is possible. It always means maintaining a clear contact with reality and being willing to communicate that reality to the client, who needs to know that the therapist can be counted on to point out what is real.

The therapist's own self-confidence and self-knowledge are critical to the development of a truly therapeutic relationship. It is the therapist's knowledge base, combined with the therapist's personal trust in his or her own skills, that make it possible for the therapist to have the confidence necessary to instill confidence in the client. What the therapist knows about the disease or deficit, about the client, and about the kinds of interventions occupational therapy can make will determine the effectiveness of what is communicated about the program. If the client experiences the program as effective, this will promote trust and motivation.

There are a number of fears that often inhibit a client's willingness to participate in occupational therapy. Many of the ordinary things that are part of normal living, such as sometimes expressing anger, or receiving anger expressed by someone else, or making a mistake, may be perceived by the client as extremely risky. In the therapeutic relationship, an important contribution may be made when the therapist who is trusted expresses or receives anger without becoming upset or makes a mistake and is able to admit it.

There are certain other issues that may emerge in the course of a therapeutic relationship in occupational therapy. Among these are dependency, control, and transference. The ultimate goal of the program is to facilitate the client's ability to function as successfully as possible. This means recognizing the issues when they arise, often naming them with the client, and planning strategies for dealing with them. The frame of reference within which the therapist is working will determine the way in which issues are perceived and the kinds of strategies that may be used.

At all stages in the course of the therapeutic relationship, initiation, implementation, and termination, it is important to remember that the relationship is a dynamic one involving both therapist and client. Their concepts of themselves and others, as well as their values and biases, will affect the quality and extent of their commitment to a program of change. In this way, an authentic, acting, feeling self on the part of the therapist lends strength to the relationship.

References

1. Frank J: The therapeutic use of self. Am J Occup Ther 12:215, 1958
2. Purtillo R: Health Professional/Patient Interaction. Philadelphia, WB Saunders, 1978

SECTION *2*

The Group Process in
Occupational Therapy

Groups form the context for much of the treatment that takes place in occupational therapy. Some group occupational therapy is deliberate, with the formation of a group specifically to accomplish stated goals. Some occupational therapy takes place in groups because it is expedient or necessary where staff limitations prevent extensive one-to-one treatment. In either case, when working with clients in a group, the occupational therapist has a powerful therapeutic tool in the dynamics of the group itself. For this reason, an understanding of the theoretical and practical issues relating to groups is important.

A group has been defined as "associations between two or more persons who are in some kind of interdependent relationship with one another."[8] Because the individuals are in a situation of interdependence, they are necessarily going to become organized around levels of interaction. It is the organization and the interaction that evolve in a group which provide the valuable tools for learning about clients, for fine-tuning a plan of treatment, and for implementing that plan.

Group process has been the subject of serious study since the 1950s. In the time since groups were first studied, groups have been examined, and group dynamics approaches explored, from a variety of theoretical perspectives in order to understand the behavior of individuals within the group context. It has become clear that there are predictable patterns to group behavior and to the evolution of groups. It also has become clear that an individual's behavior within a group can provide useful evaluative information that can add to the value of treatment implementation. The management of the group has emerged as a means to further therapeutic goals for the individuals who are part of that group.

Any consideration of the group as a context for treatment requires attention to a number of points, regardless of the frame of reference or theoretical perspective: the *size* and *structure* of the group, the *goals* of the group, the criteria for *membership*, the nature of the group's *leadership*, the *roles* of the group members, and the *norms* that the group has developed.

The ideal *size* for a group is difficult to identify without first identifying the group's purpose and goals. For example, a group of diabetic patients, in which the primary goals relate to emotional and social support, would probably be smaller than a similar group whose primary goal was education. The smaller the group, the greater the possibility for individual participation and

personal interaction. This is an important key to the determination of the number of members desirable in a treatment group. An upper limit of 12 to 15 members is suggested if group interaction is to be observed and group process used consciously as a part of treatment. For much of the treatment in occupational therapy, groups would be smaller.

The *structure* of the group refers to the way the relationships within the group are organized. The group may be structured so that there is a designated or elected leader or so that there are officers with clear responsibilities (*e.g.,* president, secretary, treasurer). The therapist may be the leader, a consultant, or purely a resource person and observer, depending on the structure of the group. The structure may be rigidly or loosely defined but in any case defines and regulates the behavior of the group members and provides for group stability and predictability.[9]

The *goals* of groups in occupational therapy are sometimes, although not always, well defined. There are groups established to meet clearly specified goals of providing support, education, and socialization for individuals who share the experience of living with a given disability or problem, such as hemiplegia, diabetes, amputation, or heart disease. There are groups that have a clear goal of helping individuals in the process of change or growth, such as groups for substance abusers or people with anxiety disorders or depression. Other groups may be formed with the development of interpersonal skills as a primary goal. Fidler proposed the task-oriented group as a context for treatment in which individuals would be able to use the group in exploring and practicing interpersonal relationships.[5]

The criteria for *membership* in a group are usually defined by the group's goals. If the group is established for clients with a given disability or set of problems, membership criteria are clear. Other criteria that might be used include age, sex, geographic area, individual treatment goals, and developmental level of functioning. Occupational therapists have found it useful, in some contexts, to identify the level of adaptive skill development in the area of group interaction, as it can be assessed in individual clients, and then to structure occupational therapy groups to match the clients' abilities to function. This approach is based on the work of Mosey,[7] who proposed that adaptive skills, consisting of sets of subskills, must be acquired sequentially in the process of development. Membership in treatment groups based on developmental adaptive skill levels facilitates progress toward therapeutic goals. Mosey defined group interaction skill as "the ability to be a productive member of a variety of primary groups."[7] Sequentially, the individual levels, defined developmentally, are that the individual would be able to participate in (l) a parallel group; (2) a project group; (3) an egocentric cooperative group; (4) a co-operative group; and finally (5) a mature group. Each of these levels of group interaction has been defined in terms of the degrees and quality of the inter-actions among the members and the nature of the leadership.

The *leadership* of the group in occupational therapy often is vested in the therapist at the beginning, but, as mentioned before, the structure will determine the exact nature of the therapist's relationship to the group. It is important to recognize that, in groups, leadership is a *quality* that is not necessarily demonstrated by the desig-nated leader. One may observe leadership emerging from various members of the group at different times during the group's life.

On the basis of the work of Bales[1] and of Benne and Sheats,[3] the *roles* that individual members may assume within a group can be defined in three major categories: *task* roles, *group maintenance* roles, and *individualistic* roles. Task roles are those roles which are involved pri-marily in accomplishing the group's stated agenda, with getting the job done. Maintenance roles are concerned with the comfort and effectiveness of the group through encouraging, harmonizing, and compromising. Individ-ualistic roles are ones which bring personal agendas to the group, such as seeking special help or recognition and using the group for personal reasons.

Lewin has suggested that an additional role exists in most groups, that of *gatekeeper*.[6] The gatekeeper is pow-erful in that it is this person who can affect the structure of the group and the criteria for membership. For the health professional, it is important, if not critical, to identify the gatekeeper if access to an existing group is to be attempted.[9] Roles can be fluid, and members may find themselves assuming different roles at different times.

As groups meet, they develop *norms* which exceed those implicit in the stated criteria for membership. Norms are standards of behavior and action that tend to be developed around such issues as language, dress, approaches to problem solving, expressions of feelings, and degrees of tolerance for deviant behavior. The norms that emerge within a group exert powerful pres-sure on its members; any consideration of individual behavior within a group must take into account the ef-fect of the group's norms.[8]

A number of group theorists[4] have proposed that groups go through a series of predictable *developmental stages*. Understanding groups as developing entities

with lives of their own is useful for the therapist who is working with clients in groups.

Tuckman outlined four stages: (1) *forming*, the time when group members first come together, get to know one another, and define what the group is to do; (2) *storming*, the time when the group may begin to deal with its tasks, a time of conflict over leadership and role issues, when subgroups may be formed and sides drawn representing different points of view; (3) *norming*, the time when the conflicts and disagreements are resolved and the group is free to develop norms and standards and to find ways to work together cohesively and coop-eratively; and (4) *performing*, the time when the group actually is doing the task it set out to do.[10] Schutz sug-gested that group development may be conceptualized around three sets of issues, which emerge in sequence as groups meet and work together.[9] The issues are basic human interpersonal needs, and the character of the group at any given time will reflect the needs of the individuals who are its members. The first issue is that of *inclusion*, each individual's need to feel truly a member of the group on an informal, interpersonal, and subtle basis. The second issue is *control*, with a focus on indi-vidual issues of authority, dependence, and autonomy. The third issue is *affection*, when the members of a group are bonded into a cohesive whole. As a group termi-nates, Schutz hypothesized that it may go through the same stages but in *reverse order*. Bales proposed that groups go through three stages, similar to but not the same in emphasis as the previous theorists: (1) an *orien-tation* stage, focusing on definition of the group's pur-poses; (2) an *evaluation* stage, focusing on emotional issues; and (3) a *control* stage, during which decisions about the group's work are made.[2]

The parallels among the group development theories are striking. It is important to note that these theories offer guideposts to the therapist in understand-ing what may be occurring in a group at any given time. It should be further noted that not all groups, at all times, go through the sequential steps. Individual members or other circumstances may move a group's interactions back and forth between the characteristic stages.

It is beyond the purview of this section to elaborate further on the theoretical perspectives for understand-ing groups. It is hoped that the therapist who works within the context of groups will think through and investigate further the potential of this important tool of practice.

References

1. Bales RF: A set of categories for the analysis of small group interaction. Am Sociol Rev 15:257, 1950
2. Bales RF: The equilibrium problem in small groups. In Hare AP, Borgatta EF, Bales RF (eds): Small Groups. New York, Alfred E Knopf, 1955

3. Benne KD, Sheats P: Functional roles of group members. J Social Issues, Vol IV, 1948
4. Bion WR: Experiences in Groups. New York, Basic Books, 1959
5. Fidler GS: The task oriented group as a context for treatment. Am J Occup Ther 23:1, 1969
6. Lewin K: Group decision and social change. In Maccoby EE, Newcomb TM, Hartley EL (eds): Readings in Social Psychology, 3rd ed. New York, Holt, Rinehart and Winston, 1958

7. Mosey AC: Recapitulation of ontogenesis. Am J Occup Ther 22:426–438, 1968
8. Sampson EE, Marthas M: Group Process for the Health Professions. New York, John Wiley and Sons, 1981
9. Schutz W: FIRA: A Three-Dimensional Theory of Interpersonal Behavior. New York, Holt, Rinehart and Winston, 1960
10. Tuckman B: Developmental sequence in small groups. Psychol Bull 63:384, 1965

SECTION 3

Leisure Counseling

As change takes place in an individual in the occupational therapy process, it is hoped that he or she will experience a sense of greater control over living. The use of the time that can be called "leisure" may be an issue for a variety of reasons, and it is an issue that could and should be addressed in occupational therapy. For the child who has been disabled since birth, the world of play may be limited to times when there are individuals around to play with him or her. For the young person who, in adolescence, becomes paralyzed by a spinal cord injury, a previously cherished world of physical activities may seem to be closed. For the depressed adult, the whole idea of leisure or play may feel like a cruel fantasy. For the elderly who may no longer have the physical vitality or intellectual acuity they once had, the possibilities for recreation become limited.

These situations represent challenges for the occupational therapist. There are a number of approaches that a therapist should consider, including external measures, such as adapting equipment, teaching compensatory functions, and providing activities which can be carried out as hobbies. Some therapists also make a point of exploring and keeping an inventory of recreational resources and resource people. In this way, the therapist is prepared to offer advice, encouragement, and even, at times, referral. Occupational therapists, as a matter of course, need to assess the background, interests, skills, and values of their clients. The message inherent in the kind of information yielded by these assessments is one to which the therapist should pay careful attention. The critical balance of the client's growing sense of efficacy, his values with regard to the uses of time, and his sense of purpose become part of the picture of the individual. For some clients, deeper issues may need to be addressed before they are ready to seek the pleasure of play, or before they have the confidence to try something new. For example, the amputee needs time to mourn his loss. The disabled child needs reassurance about undertaking activities that are new and demanding. The occupational therapist has an important role and an important opportunity to contribute to the skills and attitudes that will support the development of healthy leisure habits. But it is a role that, in most instances, must be shared with others: the patient's friends or family and other members of the professional team, such as a psychologist or social worker, recreational therapist, or nurse.

Possibilities exist in many communities for structured pursuit of such activities as swimming, horseback riding, and skiing by disabled individuals. There are social clubs, art centers, dramatic groups, and evening classes where a wide range of subjects are taught. Interests in cooking, horticulture, or computer science can be pursued in a structured fashion within regular community settings. Occupational therapists in some areas have undertaken the development of specialized leisure groups.

It is in the development of interests that the client can pursue at home, alone or with family or friends, that occupational therapists may be able to make the most important contribution. The list of such activities is as extensive and creative as the therapist, the client, and others who are involved can make it. Plants, musical instruments, cooking, photography, table games, puzzles, handcrafts—the possibilities are too numerous to list. The important point is, the occupational therapist can provide opportunities for activities to be tried, valued, or discarded and may be able to direct the client to the resources for further development.

It is critical for the occupational therapist to be sensitive in doing leisure counseling. Because the occupational therapist has the tools to evaluate and to support the development of competence, he or she has the special responsibility to help the client to internalize his or her own sense of the worthwhileness of the pursuit of leisure activity.

CHAPTER 21

Stress Management *Maureen E. Neistadt*

Stress is the collection of physical and emotional changes that are felt in response to a challenge or threat. These changes produce a certain amount of wear and tear on the body over time.

Stress affects health. Too little stress can lead to boredom, malaise, and, in extreme cases, confusion and disorientation. Too much stress can lead to or exacerbate illness and disability, causing a decrease in functional abilities. Stress management programs, by relieving anxiety, can promote wellness and help people to function optimally. Consequently, occupational therapists offer structured stress management programs for many clients, particularly those with cardiac, mental health, and pain problems.[12,24,35,36,44,51,53] Many occupational therapists also practice stress management techniques themselves to help them cope with work-related pressures and demands. This chapter looks at the elements of an effective stress management program: an examination of common stressors; the neurophysiologic effects of the stress response; conceptual model for stress management techniques; and guidelines for choice among these techniques.

Common Stressors

Any agent or circumstance capable of triggering our stress reactions is called a *stressor*.[47,48] It is important to be aware of the many and varied stressors so that when we or our clients feel too stressed or tense, we can accurately identify the causes of those feelings. Knowing the sources of stress can help us predict and control the amount of stress in our lives.[1,32,34,37,47,48]

The potential stressors that are encountered in everyday lives fall into three major categories: external physical, internal physical, and social environmental. Some of these stressors can cause direct biological trauma and illness in addition to triggering stress reactions.

External Physical Stressors

External physical stressors include noise, crowding, poor lighting, inadequate ventilation, and environmental pollutants. Research has shown that excessive or continuous noise (90 decibels or higher) at home or at work can cause high blood pressure and hearing loss.[41,42] Crowding can make people irritable and aggressive. Poor lighting or ventilation has been reported to cause eye irritation, headaches, nausea, and drowsiness in workers.[39,40] Environmental pollutants have been correlated with a wide range of health problems. Short-term exposure to many of the chemicals in the craft, ceramic, and woodworking supplies used in some occupational therapy clinics can cause health problems ranging from headaches to respiratory distress, and longer-term exposure can cause more serious health problems.[31,45] Daily exposure to external physical stressors makes a baseline coping demand on our nervous systems, and additional stressors make demands on a nervous system already engaged in responding to larger environmental stressors.

Internal Physical Stressors

The internal, neurobiologic environment also affects stress responses. Patterns of neurologic organization—expressed in individual biorhythms, relative brain hemispheric lateralizations, and different personalities—partially determine susceptibility to stress. Also, ingested chemicals can affect the nervous system's reaction to potential stressors.

Blood levels of enzymes, hormones, and other body chemicals fluctuate daily in conjunction with circadian rhythms or biorhythms. These are normal cycles of change in metabolism that occur daily and are indicated by fluctuations in body temperature, pulse and breathing rates, blood chemistry assays, and sleep patterns.[11] Changes in work schedules or normal sleep patterns can disrupt circadian cycles and deplete one's ability to cope with stressors. Nurses are an example of persons who work a variety of shifts that change frequently or abruptly and thus may experience the greatest disruptions of biorhythms.[10] Such schedule irregularities have been correlated with a high number of stress-related errors on the job.[22]

Left-handedness, or motor dominance of the right hemisphere, has been correlated with a statistically higher incidence of dyslexia, headaches, allergies, and autoimmune diseases. There is speculation that this pattern of cerebral organization may result in a compromised immunologic system, which would make people more susceptible to environmental stressors.[15,16]

Overvigilance of the right hemisphere has been linked to excessive timidity and fearfulness or depression in some people. Research has suggested that inability to screen out extraneous nonverbal stimuli can result in a neurologically overwhelmed person who is extremely susceptible to stressors.[20,21,27]

Individual patterns of brain organization express themselves in behavioral styles or personalities. Kabosa, Hilker, and Maddi[26] have identified three personality factors that distinguish stress-prone and stress-resistant people. The latter see change as a challenge, feel they have control over their environments, and have a sense of commitment and purpose about their lives. Stress-prone people, in contrast, see change as a threat, feel helpless to control their environments, and have a sense of alienation about their lives.

Friedman and Rosenman[14] have identified a stress-prone, or type A, personality as hard-driving, achievement-oriented, hostile, and highly sensitive to time pressures. A type A personality might be seen as a reaction formation to the stress-prone feelings identified by Kabosa, Hilker, and Maddi. This behavior pattern has been correlated with an increased risk of heart disease.

Certain chemicals that most people ingest regularly can interfere with the nervous system's ability to cope with other stressors. For example, caffeine and nicotine, as sympathetomimetics, produce many of the same physiologic reactions seen during a stress response and so sap the nervous system of the energy needed to cope with other stressors. As little as 250 mg of caffeine can cause headache, tremors, nervousness, insomnia, and irritability.[37] One 5-oz cup of coffee contains from 110–150 mg of caffeine; one 5-oz cup of tea contains from 9–50 mg of caffeine, depending on the preparation method and length of brewing time.[54] Caffeine can be found not only in coffee and tea, but also in colas, cocoa, baked goods, frozen dairy products, soft candy, gelatins, puddings, and some nonprescription drugs.

Central nervous system depressants like alcohol or diazepam (Valium) inhibit the ability of the nervous system to react constructively to stressors. Abuse of these and other drugs can cause somatic symptoms, disrupt social relationships and increase levels of stress.

Social Environmental Stressors

Social environments can also be a source of stressors. Major life changes that alter social roles and relationships—marriage, divorce, a job change, a serious illness, or the death of a loved one—can increase susceptibility to stress, especially when several of these changes occur within a brief period of time. Studies have shown that for some people, multiple major life changes within a year's time correlate with a higher risk of injury or illness.[23,38] Other studies have shown that middle-aged widowers have a significantly higher mortality rate than do married men of the same age and that separated and divorced women have an increased mortality rate for some diseases.[6,19] The link between major stressors and illness appears to be the immunologic system. For instance Kiecolt–Glaser and her colleagues have found bioassay evidence of depressed immunologic function in medical students during examination periods. This has been correlated with an increased incidence of infectious diseases such as colds during the same period.[33]

Minor changes or day-to-day aggravations can also act as stressors. Lazarus has identified three minor "hassles" rated as most annoying by adults aged 18 to 64 years of age: misplacing or losing things, being concerned about physical appearance, and having too many things to do.[29] Other common annoyances listed by survey subjects included economic pressures, household chores, and crime. These petty vexations can have a cumulative effect and are magnified during periods of major life changes. Major life changes, in addition to their immediate impact, can create a ripple effect of continuing minor hassles.

Changes in social roles caused by major life changes necessitate changes in daily activities. A divorce, for example, may force both partners to assume chores and financial obligations that had previously been shared. The duration, frequency, intensity, and context of these relatively minor hassles influences how potent they are as stressors. Clusters of stressful events have been correlated with an increased incidence of accidents and job-related errors.[50]

The lack of an active social network of family and friends contributes to stress responses and decreases life expectancies by denying people emotional support and nurturing. Without a network, a person lacks an important source of practical information and assistance. A social network can provide information about employment opportunities and medical care, for instance, and assistance in matters such as grocery shopping and small loans.[4,46] One's sense of involvement with his or her network may be as important as the existence of that network. One study found that feelings of isolation, even in the presence of a social network, contributed to higher cancer incidence and mortality rates in women.[33]

Some people are *stress carriers*. People who fail to clearly communicate their expectations or a plan of action and then get angry at others for not doing things the "right" way can provoke stress reactions. Stress carriers often question in a manner that puts people on the defensive and give nonconstructive criticism that undermines the recepient's self confidence.

Stress Response

Occupational therapy clients are particularly prone to some of the stressors mentioned above. Illness and disability are major life changes in and of themselves. In addition, they can cause social role changes and generate a host of minor aggravating changes in daily activities. Hospital routines can be extremely disruptive to some clients' biorhythms. Changes in appearance or behavior can leave a client constantly fearful of rejection. The larger society that our clients hope to join is not always socially and physically accessible to them.

On the other side of the therapeutic relationship, therapists have to deal with some trying job-related stressors that can easily lead to burnout, chronic fatigue, and irritability caused by too much stress. Time pressures are intense in many settings, with demands for direct treatment, documentation, interdepartmental and intradepartmental communication, and continuing education being made constantly and simultaneously. Since the establishment of the Medicare prospective payment system and similar cost-containment proce-

dures from other insurers, many clinics are experiencing drastic changes in the types of caseload and in client/staff ratios. Inadequate space is an issue in most occupational therapy clinics, and the constant client need for empathy can be emotionally draining.

Stressors do not automatically trigger stress responses in everyone. Response to any potential stressor is a matter of interpretation. A minor change in routine may be upsetting to one person but insignificant to another. Our bodies respond to potential stressors only when we interpret those events as significant. When we do respond, our pysiologic reactions are the same, regardless of whether the stressor is viewed as positive or negative. For instance, whether a move to a new house or apartment is viewed as devastating or exciting, our bodies would need to organize a stress response to deal with the demands of relocation. The emotional labels we attach to stressors influence our ability to work through the stages of our stress response.

General Adaptation Response

Selye describes the body's stress reaction as the general adaptation response.[47,48] This response occurs in three stages: the alarm reaction, the adaptive or resistive stage, and the exhaustion phase. Not everyone experiences all three stages; the exhaustion phase is reached only if the person either gets stuck in the alarm stage or goes through the alarm and adaptive stages too often.

Alarm Reaction

The alarm reaction is the fight, fright, or flight response that prepares a person to meet a challenge or threat. During this stage, the cerebral cortex activates the reticular activating system to generally alert the organism. The cortex also activates the sympathetic nervous and endocrine systems by way of the hypothalamus. The sympathetic system releases epinephrine from its nerve endings to effect increases in heart rate, blood pressure, sweating, muscle tone, and cell metabolism. Blood vessels just under the skin constrict, and digestion is slowed. The endocrine system releases hormones from the adrenal and thyroid glands that increase the body's supply of glucose and help cells accelerate their metabolism. In addition, the hypothalamus triggers the release of beta-endorphins from the pituitary. Beta-endorphins are endogenous opiate proteins that elevate mood and decrease pain perception. They have also been linked to suppression of the immunologic system.[49] Figure 21-1 provides more details about this stage.

Adaptive or Resistive Stage

In the adaptive or resistive stage, the body returns to its pre-excited state and recovers from the physiologic

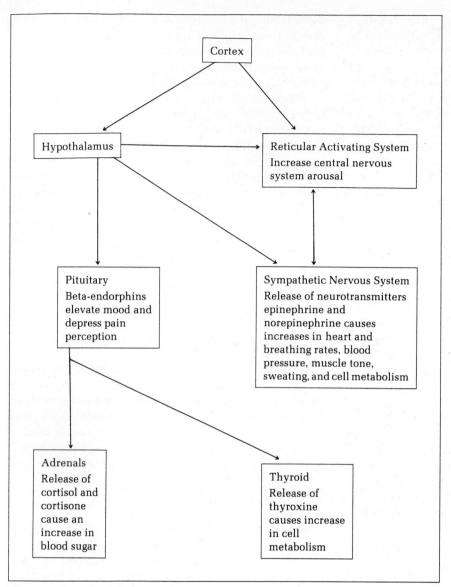

Figure 21-1. Stimulation pathways of the alarm stage.

strains of the alarm stage. Stress-prone or overstressed people, who may interpret even normal events as negative stressors, are often unable to reach this particular stage. They get stuck in the alarm reaction until their bodies enter the exhaustion stage. People who are able to transit to the adaptive stage may also reach the exhaustion phase if there are too many stressors in their lives.

Exhaustion Phase

The exhaustion phase is a reaction to the constant high metabolic demands of the alarm stage. During this phase, the person no longer has the neurophysiologic ability to respond to stressors effectively.

Chronic Stress

The constant physiologic demands of chronic stress have been linked to many diseases and disorders. A continual state of stress-linked alertness can deplete the neurotransmitters used to record and store new information, thus making it difficult to learn. Constantly elevated blood pressure can lead to hypertension, which is a risk factor for stroke. Increased muscle tension can result in headaches and low back pain. Changes in circulation can aggravate heart disease, Raynaud's disease, and diabetes; changes in the digestive process can affect ulcers.[34,37] Some people experience ventricular fibrillation in response to stressful situations of interpersonal conflict, threat of or actual marital separation, bereavement, business failure, or public humiliation.[43] Uncorrected ventricular fibrillation can lead to heart failure and death within minutes.

Stress Management Techniques

Stress management techniques have been developed to help avoid chronic stress and its detrimental effects. These techniques are all learned behaviors that interrupt the nervous system's stress reactions. Different techniques influence nervous system processing at different levels. Some techniques, like imagery and time management, use cortical strategies either to change the interpretation of stressors or to avoid them altogether. Biofeedback facilitates control of the stress response by giving the cortex sensory feedback that would not normally be registered consciously. Benson has theorized that meditation stimulates the anterior hypothalamus, which controls the parasympathetic nervous system.[3] Stimulation of the parasympathetic system offsets the stress responses of the sympathetic system. Quiet, dark environments decrease the stimulation of the reticular activating system and can consequently calm stress-induced vigilance. Progressive relaxation techniques[25] provide an outlet for release of sympathetic nervous system–induced increases in muscle tone.

Specific Techniques

Table 21-1 lists some common stress management techniques according to the level of the nervous system on which they have their greatest impact.

A brief description of the various techniques and hints for teaching them follow. Many excellent resources that describe these techniques in more detail are available.[1–3,8,18,25,32,34,37,52,55] Biofeedback is discussed in more detail in the following chapter.

Aerobic Exercise

Aerobic exercise involves slow, repetitive, rhythmic contractions of the large muscles of the legs and arms. Examples include walking, running, bicycling, and swimming. This type of exercise is called "aerobic" (in the presence of oxygen) because muscles use aerobic metabolism to get energy for this type of movement. In aerobic metabolism, muscles use oxygen to break carbohydrates down into carbon dioxide and water, and adenosine triphosphate (ATP), an energy-releasing compound. The muscle demand for oxygen inherent in this cycle forces the body to increase the efficiency of its systems for oxygen supply (pulmonary system), oxygen delivery (cardiovascular system), and oxygen utilization (musculoskeletal system). Consequently, if aerobic exercise is done regularly, breathing capacity improves and the heart muscle becomes stronger, resulting in increased stroke volume and a decreased heart rate. In addition, circulation improves, blood pressure decreases, and overall muscle strength increases.[2,8] These physiologic changes also stimulate alterations in brain biochemistry that can increase deep sleep and improve mood.[7,30]

Aerobic exercise, then, can have an immediate stress

Table 21-1. *Stress Management Techniques*

Nervous System Level / Stress Function	Stress Management Techniques	Client Skills Needed	Environmental Resources Needed
Cortex (interpretation of events, control of emotional reactions, planning of behavior)	Autogenic training, biofeedback, communication skills, mental imagery, time management, verbalization	Abstract thinking, concentration, delay gratification, sequencing	Cost of equipment (biofeedback), time and quiet*
Hypothalamus (autonomic nervous system and endocrine system control)	Deep breathing Laughter, meditation	Concentration, concrete thinking Concentration, delay gratification	Time and quiet*
Reticular activating system (alertness levels)	Aerobic exercise, dark and quiet room, vestibular stimulation	Concentration, sensorimotor skill	Rocking chair (vestibular stimulation), equipment (exercise), time, quiet, and space*
Peripheral nervous system (sensory input and motor output)	Aerobic exercise Progressive relaxation exercises	Concentration, sensorimotor skill	Equipment (exercise), Time*

* Relevant to all techniques in category

management effect by allowing someone to work off built-up tensions. If done regularly, aerobic exercise can make a person more stress-resistant by improving overall health and mood. Anyone planning to start an aerobic exercise program should first see his or her physician for a complete checkup; all exercise programs should begin gradually and work slowly toward increased difficulty to avoid injuries. Specific guidelines for setting up individualized aerobic exercise programs are available from other sources.[2,8]

Autogenic Training

Autogenic training is a meditative process that uses autosuggestion or self-hypnosis and mental imagery to achieve relaxation. Autosuggestions typically involve imagining sensations of physical heaviness and warmth to achieve muscle relaxation and vasodilation, respectively. Imagining oneself in settings where one would feel warm, comfortable, and heavy can facilitate these autosuggestions.

There are six steps in autogenic training: (1) assuming a mental stance of open passivity, (2) physical relaxation of muscles, (3) induction of feelings of warmth, (4) cardiac regulation and respiratory control, (5) inducing a sense of warmth in the abdominal region, and (6) cooldown. Learning this process requires daily practice over many months. Only those who have been specifically trained in this technique should consider teaching it.[34,37]

Biofeedback

Biofeedback refers to a collection of devices and techniques that increase a person's awareness of subtle changes in body functions like heart rate and muscle tension. Biofeedback training is a process of learning to use information from those devices and techniques to control body functions.

Biofeedback training helps people to change their characteristic bodily responses to stressors. Through biofeedback training, one can learn to modify the autonomic nervous system's response to stressors and decrease the detrimental health effects of prolonged stress. Features of biofeedback are discussed in the next chapter.

Communication Skills

Many stressful situations are caused by misunderstandings that result from unclear communication between people. Practicing effective communication skills like clarifying expectations, defining needs honestly, and providing tactful and constructive feedback, can decrease the number of stressful misunderstandings. It is also helpful to examine troublesome interpersonal exchanges from the perspective of transactional analysis, a psychological theory and method of diagramming social interactions that helps identify individuals' hidden agendas. Information from such an analysis can be used to change our behaviors or to modify our reactions to the behavior of others. Further details are provided in other sources.[5,18]

Deep Breathing

Deep, or diaphragmatic, breathing involves slowly inhaling and exhaling to slow down our general pace and work off tension in the shoulders, trunk, and abdomen. Since this technique involves quiet concentration on a rhythmic body function, it is also a form of meditation.

The process begins with focusing on one's normal breathing in a quiet and comfortable place. This is followed by a period of deep inhalation and slow exhalation. During inhalation, the abdominal muscles should be relaxed. During exhalation, the abdominal muscles should be contracted. It is often helpful to rest a hand lightly on the abdomen during this process; during inhalation, the abdomen should puff up; during exhalation, the abdomen should flatten. Just a few minutes of this can be very relaxing.

This technique is relatively easy to learn, requires no equipment, and can be done anywhere so long as the person is able to ignore outside distractions. It is a quick and easy way to relax at any time of the day.

Laughter

The healing power of humor has received increasing attention from health care professionals over the past few years. Some writers have suggested that laughter may stimulate the release of endorphins, our brain's endogenous opiates, thereby helping to alleviate pain and stress.[9] It is important for therapists to remember that therapy does not have to be solemnly serious to be effective.

Meditation

Meditation involves focusing one's attention on a rhythmic, repetitive word, phrase, or sensation (e.g., breathing, heart rate) in order to achieve relaxation. Benson has suggested that this mental process blocks the stress response of the sympathetic nervous system by activating the anterior hypothalamus, which controls the parasympathetic nervous system. This technique requires considerable mental discipline and can take many months to learn.[3,34,37]

Mental Imagery

Mental imagery techniques use both passive and active daydreaming to interrupt habitual stress patterns. Passive techniques can offer temporary escape from a stressful situation, giving the nervous systems a reprieve. Imagining oneself in a calm and pleasant setting like a deserted beach or forest is an example of passive techniques.

More active methods of imagery can change stress patterns by expanding the perspective from which stressful situations are viewed or by exploring alternative ways of responding. The blow-up technique, for instance, involves imagining all the worst possible, most exaggerated consequences of a problem. After that exercise, the original problem looks quite harmless and mild in comparison to our overblown speculations. Mental role plays of difficult interpersonal interactions allow the practice of different behavior patterns in response to stressful situations.[55]

Progressive Relaxation Exercises

Jacobsen's progressive relaxation exercises involve systematically tensing and relaxing all muscle groups in the body, one group at a time, from head to foot. This teaches the difference between muscle tension and muscle relaxation by exaggerating the contrast between the two tone states. The learning sequence for this technique is: (1) systematic tensing and relaxing of muscle groups to verbal cues, (2) systematic relaxing of muscle groups to verbal cues, (3) relaxation of muscle groups by autosuggestion. This technique requires mental discipline and daily practice and can take months to master.[25] The first step in the learning sequence can be used to provide temporary relief from excess muscle tension but is not recommended for clients with upper-motor-neuron lesions and spasticity.

Time Management

Time management techniques include realistically scheduling and organizing time, setting priorities about task accomplishment, making lists, setting limits, and accepting the fact that everything cannot be done at once. Changing schedules or daily routines to avoid stressful situations is also a form of time management.[28]

Verbalization

Talking to friends and acquaintances about stressors can help us to ventilate pent-up feelings and to find new solutions to old problems. Friends can offer different perspectives, new suggestions, and support, all of which are helpful in extricating ourselves from feeling stuck with a problem situation.

Vestibular Stimulation

Slow, rhythmic rocking or rotary motions of the head produce mild vestibular stimulation and can have a calming influence on the nervous system. These motions are part of both rocking in a rocking chair and aerobic exercise. The physiologic mechanism for the relaxing effect of these motions may be reticular activating system activation of the parasympathetic nervous system.[13]

General Guidelines for Choice of Technique

Self-Assessment

Guided self-assessment of individual stressors and stress reactions is the first step in designing an appropriate stress management program. The guiding can be done by another person or by structured forms that an individual can fill out. Many occupational therapists use the Holmes–Rahe Life Change Index,[23] or variations on it, the type A behavior scale,[17] or the "pie of life" exercise (Fig. 21-2) to assess stressors. Other forms are available to help people assess their physical, emotional, and behavioral stress responses.[1,34,55] Care should be taken to interpret scores on formal stress scales as only gross, relative indications of stress levels and behavior patterns. On the Holmes–Rahe scale, for instance, the statistical correlation between higher scores and the risk of illness or injury, although positive, is relatively weak. If scores on these instruments are taken too literally, those scores can become self-fulfilling prophecies. A list of the categories of stressors mentioned earlier might be a more useful, less restrictive and less suggestive way to structure a person's self-assessment. The pie of life is a very useful way for someone to look at both their time management strategies and the work/play balance in their daily activities.

General Factors

Some stressors can be avoided; others cannot. Some general factors to consider in suggesting stress management techniques for clients or deciding on such techniques for oneself include:

Learning style (concrete *versus* abstract)
Level of financial and interpersonal resources
Life style and daily routine and
The amount of time available to learn a new technique

For example, if a cardiac client does not have the finances to purchase a biofeedback unit for home use, it would not be useful for an occupational therapist to spend the client's hospitalization time teaching him or her to use such a unit for stress control. Meditation takes many months to learn properly and could not be taught within a short hospital stay. Deep breathing techniques, on the other hand, are relatively easy to learn, require no outside equipment, and can generally be taught fairly quickly.

Purpose: To give you a graphic representation of your patterns of time use.

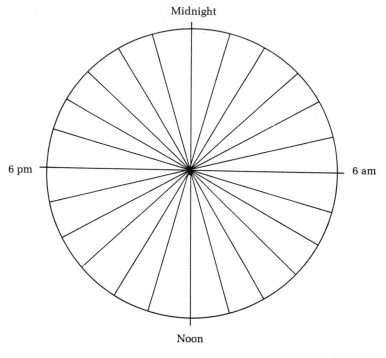

Directions: Use two charts—one for a typical weekday and one for a typical weekend day. On each chart, fill in each hour with what you do during that time.

Analysis:

Rest and Relaxation	Responsibilities
How many hours do you spend sleeping? _____ How many hours do you spend resting? _____	How many hours do you spend fulfulling responsibilities to others? (Job, childcare, homemaking, meetings, etc.) _____
How many hours do you spend relaxing, doing something just because you enjoy it? _____	How many hours do you spend on self-maintainance tasks? (Dressing, grooming, meals, chores, etc.) _____
Total: _____	Total: _____

Do the totals from these two columns match? What changes might you make in your life to achieve a more satisfactory work/play balance?

Figure 21-2. Pie of life.

Effective stress management programs can be part of individual or group therapy sessions and are particularly helpful for clients with stress-related illnesses or with high stress levels that seriously impede their functional progress. Though not all clients will need formal stress management training, it is important to remember that all clients are in stressful situations by virtue of their illness or disability. All clients will, therefore, be tense and anxious to a certain degree. Occupational therapists need to keep this in mind and to do their best to help their clients relax during any treatment session. Explaining procedures and making clients partners in the treatment process will go a long way toward relieving their stress and helping them to achieve their maximal functional potential.

References

1. Aronson S, Maschia M: Stress Management Workbook. New York, Appleton–Century–Croft, 1981

2. Batten J: The Complete Jogger. New York, Harcourt Brace Jovanovich, 1977

3. Benson H: The Relaxation Response. New York, Avon, 1975

4. Berkman LF: Social network analysis and coronary heart disease. Adv Cardiol 29:37, 1982

5. Berne E: Games People Play. New York, Grove Press, 1964

6. Bower B: Social isolation: Female cancer risk? Sci News 129:166, 1986

7. Carr DB, Bullen BA, Skrinar GS, et al: Physical conditioning facilitates the exercise-induced secretion of beta-endorphin and beta-lipoprotein in women. N Engl J Med 305:560, 1981

8. Cooper K: The Aerobics Way. New York, Bantam, 1977

9. Cousins N: Anatomy of an Illness as Perceived by the Patient. New York, Bantam Books, 1979

10. Czeisler CA, Moore–Ede MC, Coleman RH: Rotating shift work schedules that disrupt sleep are improved by applying circadian principles. Science 217:460, 1982

11. Dale A: Biorhythym. New York. Pocket Books, 1976

12. Ericson LL: Occupational therapy in a cardiac teaching program. Occup Ther Forum II(35):1, 1986

13. Farber S: Sensorimotor Evaluation and Treatment Procedures for Allied Health Professionals, 2nd ed. Indianapolis, Indiana University–Purdue University at Indianapolis Medical Center, 1974

14. Friedman M, Rosenman RH: Type A Behavior and Your Heart. New York, Alfred E. Knopf, 1974

15. Geschwind N, Behan P: Left-handedness: association with immune disease, migraine, and developmental learning disorder. Proc Natl Acad Sci USA 79:5097, 1982

16. Geschwind N, Galaburda A: Cerebral lateralization: Biological mechanisms, associations, and pathology: I. A hypothesis and program for research. Arch Neurol 42:428, 1985

17. Glazer HI: Type A Behavior Pattern. EHE Stresscontrol Systems, Inc. (available in ref. 47)

18. Harris TA: I'm OK, You're OK. New York. Avon, 1969

19. Helsing KJ, Szklo M, Comstock GW: Factors associated with mortality after widowhood. Public health 71:802, 1981

20. Herbert W: Depression: Too much vigilance? Sci News 124:84, 1983

21. Herbert W: Sources of temperament: Bashful at birth? Sci News 121:36, 1982

22. Hilts P: The clock within. Science 80 1:61, Dec 1980

23. Holmes TH, Rahe RH: The social readjustment rating scale. J Psychosomat Res 11:213,1967

24. Jackson J, Kylan C: Occupational therapy for the spinal pain patient. Physical Disabilities Special Interest Sect Newslett 4(4):1, 1981

25. Jacobsen E: Progressive Relaxation. Chicago, University of Chicago Press, 1938

26. Kabosa SC, Hilker RR, Maddi SR: Who stays healthy under stress? J Occup Med 21:595, 1979

27. Kagan J: The Nature of the Child. New York, Basic Books, 1984

28. Lakein A: How to Get Control of Your Time and Life. New York, Signet, 1973

29. Lazarus R: Little hassles can be hazardous to your health. Psychol Today 15:58, July 1981

30. McCann IL, Holmes DS: Influence of aerobic exercise on depression. J Personality Social Psychol 46:1142, 1984

31. McCann M: Artist Beware. New York, Watson–Guptill, 1979

32. McQuade W, Aikman A: Stress. New York, Bantum, 1975

33. Miller JA: Immunity and crises, large and small. Sci News 129:340, 1986

34. Miller LH, Ross R, Cohen SI: Stress: What can be done? Bostonia Magazine 56:4, 1982

35. Mueller S, Suto M: Starting a stress management programme. Mental Health Special Interest Sect Newslett 6(2):1, 1983

36. Neistadt ME: An occupational therapy program for adults with developmental disabilities. Am J Occup Ther 41:433, 1987

37. Pelletier K: Mind as Healer, Mind as Slayer. New York, Delta Press, 1977

38. Rahe RH: Life change events and mental illness: An overview. J Hum Stress 5:2, Sept 1979

39. Raloff J: Basement parking and high rise CO_2. Sci News 120:316, 1981

40. Raloff J: Building Illness. Sci News 120:316, 1981

41. Raloff J: Noise can be hazardous to your health. Sci News 121:377, 1982

42. Raloff J: Occupational noise—the subtle pollutant. Sci News 121:347, 1982

43. Reich P, DeSilva RA, Lowin B, Murawski BJ: Acute psychological disturbances preceeding life threatening ventricular arrhythmias. JAMA 246:233, 1981

44. Sanborn, CP: Chronic pain management: Occupational therapy role. Physical Disabilities Special Interest Sect Newslett 4(4):1, 1981

45. Science News: Beware the supplies of arts and crafts. Sci News 119:325, 1981

46. Science News: Social ties and length of life. Sci News. 118:392, 1980

47. Selye H: Stress Without Distress. New York, Signet, 1974

48. Selye H: The Stress of Life. New York, McGraw–Hill, 1978

49. Shavit Y, Terman GW, Martin FC, et al: Stress, opioid peptides, the immune system, and cancer. J Immunol 135(2 Suppl):834s, 1985

50. Sheehan DV, O'Donnell J, Fritzgerald A, et al: Psychosocial predictors of accident/error rates in nursing studies: a prospective study. Int J Psychiatr Med 11:125, 1981–82

51. Simari J: Cardiac rehabilitation. In Logigian MK (ed): Adult Rehabilitation: A Team Approach for Therapists. Boston, Little, Brown, 1982

52. Trombly CA: Biofeedback as an adjunct to therapy. In Trombly CA (ed): Occupational Therapy for Physical Dysfunction, 2nd ed. Baltimore, Williams & Wilkins, 1983

53. Trombly CA: Cardiac rehabilitation. In Trombly CA (ed): Occupational Therapy for Physical Dysfunction, 2nd ed. Baltimore, Williams & Wilkins, 1983

54. Union Hospital: Caffeine and your health. What's News, p 2, Mar 4, 1982

55. Wall N, Neistadt ME: Stress: A Study Guide to Accompany the Slide–Tape Program "Stress." Boston, AIM for Health, 1982

CHAPTER 22

Computer Technology in Occupational Therapy *Renee L. Okoye*

Computer applications in the field of occupational therapy seem to have evolved from two major, and distinct sources. Although computer use is now much more widespread throughout the field, the main thrust for implementation still rests in these two major areas. The forerunner and initial impetus came from the structured use of video games in clinical applications.[3] The impetus for use of the computer in administrative areas seems to have emerged from the development of the personal home computer. Systems originally used at home by educators, chiefs of service, and other occupational therapy administrators were eventually brought into the clinical arena and embraced as tools for management to ease tedious but necessary paper-shuffling details.

Thus, two distinct applications began to emerge in the use of the computer. Administrative support functions emerged through expanded use of data-management software packages. Clinical support functions emerged through expanded use of drill-and-practice software packages. Unfortunately, the computer systems and software packages were not readily interchangeable: for the most part, computer systems and software applications suitable for administrative functions were not amenable to clinical applications, and the converse was also true. At present, the ideal system that can serve both necessary functions has yet to be designed.

Packages for data management allow the administrator to store and retrieve patient data in an integrated manner. The flexibility of design built into data-management packages allows the occupational therapist to focus on the specific types of information that are particularly important to them. It allows retrieval, sorting, and coding of the data so that justification for items such as hiring of additional staff, training programs for staff in particular areas of need, and requests for additional pieces of equipment can be supported.

Packages used for drill and practice allow the clinician to apply specific intervention in an integrated fashion. Rehearsal of deficient skills can be accomplished easily within the developmental framework determined by program selection. In addition, the unparalleled consistency of visual, motor, and auditory feedback inherent in most computer programs is said to result in more efficient mastery of the deficient skills.[6]

These two general areas of applications, which parallel the development of the computer as a tool in education, have now broadened to impact on almost every aspect of occupational therapy. This chapter will review use of the computer as a tool for the support of our administrative functions as occupational therapists and then present uses of the computer as a tool for support of our clinical functions.

Administrative Support

Word Processing

Word processing is perhaps the most common of all computerized administrative support functions. Computer software that performs this function differs from its business machine counterparts in several ways. Ease of use is an asset. Most well-written word processing packages are easy to use and require little or no memory of complicated codes by the user. Most prompts are on the screen or can be accessed on a "help" screen with only a keystroke. Integrated software packages allow the user to merge documents created by the word processor with data stored in other formats. For example, mail merge letters, notes, or memos can easily be sent to selected people whose file have been stored in a compatible data-management format. By using the mail merge capabilities of a word processor, it is possible to notify affiliating students, vendors, patient relatives, and others of upcoming changes in staff or services at a facility without investing hours of manpower.

Data Management

Data-management packages offer the administrator the option of designing an electronic filing system that organizes forms, charts, and indexes in a manner suitable for individual departmental needs. Integrated data-management packages typically offer file management, report generation, word processing, and access to the disk-operating system, so that files can be easily manipulated.

A *file manager* forms the data base or basic platform of information from which other aspects of data management are derived. The file manager allows the user to design the filing format he or she prefers. Although any number of files can be constructed for special use, the skilled administrator will usually design one master file that contains most of the basic information commonly needed for day-to-day clinical operations. Data will then be manipulated based on the sorting of this basic information. The generation of reports and the siphoning off of other smaller files will be based on selected items from the master file. Once the data are filed, the system can retrieve specific items and group, match, or chart similar items so that area needs, trends, or patterns of utilization can easily be seen.

Putting this information into a usable format is the responsibility of the *report generator*. Questions regarding how many, how much, and how often can be quickly formatted to reflect departmental statistics and patterns of operation. The report generator can be used to highlight aspects of clinical involvement important to the day-to-day operation of the department. For example, the report generator could be used to sort through files to show differences among the clinical treatments required by right- versus left hemiplegic patients. The number of treatments required, the types of treatment required, the amount of time required per treatment, and the type of patient supervision required during each treatment could be used to adjust the caseload of therapists, depending on how many left hemiplegics are being carried.

Another routine but very useful application of a report generator is the listing of supplies and equipment available for specific types of treatment intervention. Reports can be generated frequently to keep the staff up to date on which programs are available and what types of skills can be remediated with each program. The file should include fields for the title, publisher, suggested mental age, a rank ordering of skills needed to use the program, and any special instructions needed to run the program. The file can be consulted frequently for suggestions of computer activities available for upgrading, downgrading, or parallel movement in a particular level of skill development during treatment.

Spreadsheets are used to manage numerical data by organizing displays into rows and columns. Common administrative uses of spreadsheets are in billing and in the preparation of annual budgets. Some of the more enjoyable functions of a spreadsheet are automatic calculations, copying of intricate formulas, and the ability to move rows, columns, and blocks of cells at a keystroke. Spreadsheets are also helpful in locating outstanding items such as deficit or past-due accounts, back-ordered items, or significant differences between expenses and designated supporting funds.

Record Keeping and Scheduling

Record-keeping processes such as scheduling, treatment documentation, individualized educational plan (IEP) generation, and intake and exit summaries can be greatly enhanced yet simplified and expedited through use of the computer. Although dedicated packages exist for many of these functions, creative use of an integrated data-management system can provide a less costly alternative. In addition, when treatment documentation and IEPs are maintained through integrated data-management programs, the data are readily available for generating reports and for research purposes.

An example of *treatment documentation* maintained through a file-management function of an integrated data-management package is shown in the box. The files are maintained on the computer screen and are regularly printed out by the department secretary. The routine data, such as the diagnosis, date of birth, physician, and frequency of treatments, are copied onto the

---

Occupational Therapy
Treatment Record

LAST: _____ FIRST: _____ DATE: _____
    (Name)

DIAGNOSIS: _____   D.O.B.: _____

PHYSICIAN: _____   Fx of Tx: ____

Tx METHOD:_____

OBJECTIVE: _____

SPECIFIC GOALS: _____

                            _____

                            _____

EQUIPMENT USED:_____

Duration of Tx: _____

Response to Tx:

Comments:

Therapist:

---

form by the computer, so that only 1 or 2 minutes of the therapist's time is needed to enter the specific details of an average treatment session. Criteria-referenced statements are used as often as possible in the "response" field. Differences form the basis of progress reports and treatment summaries. The data fields on the treatment record shown were designed to hold information selected by the staff of the department so that annual statistics could be easily retrieved. Given the fields defined, the following types of information could be formatted into a report: (1) age range of patients treated, (2) frequency of diagnostic groups treated, (3) frequency of use of particular treatment methods, (4) most commonly pursued treatment objectives, (5) equipment usage, and (6) duration and frequency of treatments for major diagnostic groups. Another report that could be generated with the data is a justification for budgetary requests for replacement of equipment frequently used, purchase of needed equipment, or additional staff educational leave. The data could also be used to support research on correlations between diagnostic categories and methods of treatment, treatment media, duration or course of treatment, and so forth.

Although software packages are available for the generation of IEPs, the variety of selections among objectives, methods, and materials generally are not appropriate for occupational therapy services. An alternative strategy for computerized generation of IEPs is to (1) use a full-function word processor or file-management system to specify the objectives, methods, materials, and criteria used within the department on one extensive form and then (2) complete and print out only those fields that apply to the patient whose IEP is being written.

In the accompanying example, the therapist enters only the variables in the desired fields (see box). The word processor converts the variables into the designated phrases and criteria as indicated. To prepare a criteria-referenced objective relating to Johnny S's ability to dress himself, the therapist would enter "Johnny S. A.1.,1A, $x\%=2$, $y\%=4$, a)" on screen H. The word processor would dutifully write: "Johnny S shall be able to take off tops in 2 out of 4 trials with minimal assistance."

Research

Another example of administrative support available through computer applications is use of the system for *management of research data*. Given a file formatted with fields to hold background information, a statistical package can be used to analyze and chart the data. By

---

H. Activities of Daily Living

The student shall be able to:

A. Dressing

1. Take off _____
   in $x\% =$ ____ out of $y\% =$ ____ with ____

2. Put on _____
   in $x\% =$ ____ out of $y\% =$ ____ with ____

3. Wash/dry _____
   in $x\% =$ ____ out of $y\% =$ ____ with ____

B. Feeding

1. Manipulate utensil with food to mouth
   in $x\% =$ ____ out of $y\% =$ ____ trials

2. Separate food in $x\% =$ ____ out of $y\% =$ ____ trials

3. Manipulate cup to mouth
   in $x\% =$ ____ out of $y\% =$ ____ trials

Listing of variables

1A tops	2A upper torso
1B bottoms	2B lower torso
1C shoes	2C face
1D coat	

a) with minimal assistance
b) with moderate assistance
c) with physical set-up only

NTM Pilot-Simulated Feeding (Dominant/Nondominant Upper Extremity)

(a) Students	(b) Diagnosis	(c) Sim. Feed Pretest Dominant	(d) Sim. Feed Posttest #1 Dominant	(e) Differ- ence (c − d)	(f) % Change (e/c)	(g) Sim. Feed Pretest Nondominant	(h) Sim. Feed Posttest #1 Nondominant	(i) Differ- ence (g − h)	(j) % Change (i/g)
Group #1									
Laura M.	Spas. Quad.	24	24	0	0	120	103	17	.14
Oscar M.	Spas. Hemi.	30	10	20	.67	113	44	69	.61
Maria B.	Spas. Quad.	32	22	12	.38	37	24	13	.35
Tammy A.	Spas. Quad.	19	14	5	.26	34	12	22	.65
Averages		26.25	18	9.25	.33	76	46	30	.44
Group #2									
Rachel W.	M.C.D.	30	17	13	.43	36	38	−2	−.06
Thomas W.	M.C.D.	19	16	3	.16	50	25	25	.50
Christopher H.	M.C.D.	15	11	4	.27	14	11	3	.21
Christopher O	M.C.D.	59	20	39	.66	32	20	12	.38
Averages		31	16	15	.38	33	24	10	.26
Group #3									
Matthew M.	Hypotonia	28	26	2	.07	40	38	2	.05
Kevin H.	M.C.D.	18	15	3	.17	16	14	2	.13
Jason L.	Spas. Quad.	38	21	17	.45	96	77	19	.20
Jennifer O.	Spas. Hemi.	29	18	11	.38	216	65	151	.70
Nicholas L.	Cereb. Atax.	33	41	−8	−.24	78	64	14	.18
Averages		29	26	5	.16	89	39	37.60	.14

Figure 22-1. Example of a spreadsheet.

highlighting comparisons among various fields in the format, relational inferences and differences may be observed that would otherwise be difficult to define. The data can be formatted into columnar reports, graphs, and charts that convey meaning far more effectively than would lengthy descriptions. Use of the computer as a tool to assist with research aids in the initial organization and compilation of the data, the process of sorting and grouping similar items for comparison, and the statistical analysis of the data. Figures 22-1 to 22-3 demon-

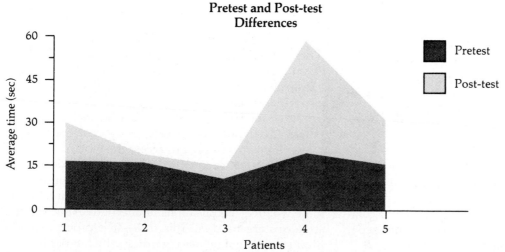

Figure 22-2. Example of a filled line graph, showing the same results as those in the spreadsheet (see Fig. 22-1).

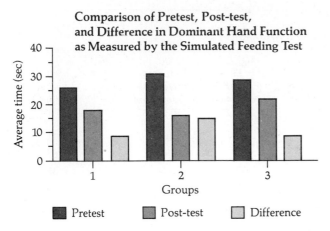

Figure 22-3. A bar graph showing in pictorial form the information summarized in the spreadsheet (Fig. 22-1).

strate ways of presenting the results of a research project.[4] The spreadsheet in Figure 22-1 shows the results in tabular form. Figure 22-2, a filled line graph, shows the results that are charted in the spreadsheet in columns "(c)" and "(d)" of group 2. The bar graph in Figure 22-3 shows in pictorial terms the information summarized by the group averages in the spreadsheet. Use of a spreadsheet, report generation, and graphing capabilities of a computer system enhance the finished presentation by giving it an aura of professionalism and credibility.

The administrative support functions enhanced through computer applications in occupational therapy thus are myriad. An oversimplified but somewhat appropriate comment would be that whenever an occupational therapist becomes involved in processes requiring excessive paper shuffling, it would be worthwhile to consider whether a computer might be a more efficient tool for the task.

Clinical Support

Although the medium is a new one, the primary method of factoring out the potential of a computer application for use as a therapeutic activity is very traditional. Skilled use of an activity analysis is essential for unlocking the abilities of an occupational therapist in the use of computerized activities in the clinical arena.

Task Analysis

The process of task or activity analysis is a basis for use of any medium, including the computer, in occupational therapy. However, due to the multifaceted possibilities of this modality, both the tools and the media of computer-assisted treatment need to be considered separately.

The tools of this activity are the physical components of the computer system, commonly referred to as

hardware—the keyboard, printers, disk drives, joysticks, drawing tablets, and so forth. Each physical component may require separate consideration regarding its suitability for inclusion in a particular treatment program, depending on the nature of the disability and the unique abilities of each patient. Ease in accessing the tools of the computerized activity is another important consideration. Analysis of the physical and mental requirements for handling each peripheral device is also necessary to determine which tools can be used by the patient independently, which ones will require additional supportive equipment, which will require mental assistance with direct supervision of the therapist, and which will require simple modifications. The process of task analysis will also help to highlight those tools that look attractive but are inappropriate for patient use.

The medium or vehicle for computerized activities is the software itself. Separate processes of evaluating the medium in terms of the content and format of the screen presentation will determine which programs are appropriate for a select patient population and the sequence in which the programs should be presented for maximum therapeutic benefit. Aspects such as the clarity of screen format, rate of program flow, specific perceptual motor/sensory integrative skills required, and the developmental level of their presentation need to be considered.

The activity analysis of a computerized task should stimulate thinking about the many physical and mental skills required to use the computer as a tool. The physical demands of the task in terms of postural alignment, range of motion, and the like need to be viewed equally with academic, attentional, and perceptual motor requirements of the task. A wide array of perceptual-motor and sensorimotor skills need to be assessed, because most computerized activities require simultaneous integration of these skills. The ability to coordinate the integration of multiple sensory subsystems is a prerequisite for most computerized activities. Academic competencies, particularly in the areas of reading and mathematics, also need to be noted, because software is written at so many different educational levels. Attentional skills, compliance, and the ability to prioritize, follow instructions, and maintain an organizational set also need to be assessed.

Three major steps are involved in an analysis of computerized activities: (1) broadly categorizing the physical requirements needed to access the tools, (2) broadly categorizing the cognitive requirements needed to access the medium, and (3) comparing these requirements with the abilities and limitations of the patient to determine whether modifications or alternative intervention strategies are needed. This three-step process should produce clear guidelines regarding which types of tools and media would be appropriate for the patient. Software programs should be selected with these guidelines in mind. The extent to which any aspect of the task limits application of the medium to a given patient depends to a large extent on the software and peripheral devices selected. For example, producing a greeting card with the "Print Shop" can be accomplished with minimal academic abilities, muscle power, range of motion, and coordination, whereas producing a document with a word processor is an entirely different matter. The activity analysis form (see box) demonstrates one way of broadly analyzing and categorizing both the physical and the perceptual requirements for a computerized activity.

Access

Review of the activity analysis gives rise to three issues commonly overlooked when planning clinical application of computerized activities. The first factor is that of access, the ability of the patient to approach and engage the keyboard, disk drive, and printer. Since access is largely a function of range of motion, muscle power, and coordination, only two distinct populations seem to have major difficulties: the high-level quadriplegic patient lacks the muscle power and the range of motion, whereas the severely multiply-handicapped patient

---

Activity Analysis

Part One: Analysis of Ability to Access the Tools

Given specific pieces of hardware . . .

Yes No

A. Physical Orientation

*If "no," what adjustments might be needed in placement of keyboard, monitor, or patient's base of support? ** (common solutions)*

1. Are the components aligned for ease of pt. use?
(use a computer stand)
2. Is the patient seated properly?
(use an adjustable-height table or get pt. out of the w/c and into a seat with feet touching the floor)

3. Are there postural deviations?
in the frontal plane?
(vary the position of the keyboard and/or monitor)
in trunkal alignment?
(provide pelvic or thoracic support)
in head/neck orientation?
(use biofeedback software for training head alignment)

B. Physical Requirements
1. Can the patient reach the tools?
(use slings, feeder arms, a breakaway keyboard, or switching devices)
2. Is the patient's finger function adequate?
(use dowels or pencils with a universal cuff)
3. Is the patient's coordination adequate?
(use an expanded keyboard, or an adaptive firmware card)

Part Two: Analysis of Ability to Access the Medium

Given a specific type of software . . .

Yes No

A. Attentive functions

*If no, which clinical problems limit success? What alternative programs, instructional methods, tools, or media might be used? ** (common solutions)*

Can the patient:
1. Maintain adequate attention to the task?
(use software with limited number of processes . . . use software with ↑ audio reinforcers)
2. Sequence the steps required?
(use software with less-detailed processes)
3. Perform the problem-solving operations required?

(Chart continues on following page)

Activity Analysis   *(continued)*

Part Two: Analysis of Ability to Access the Medium *(continued)*

Given a specific type of software . . .

                                                        Yes   No

B. Visual Functions

Does the patient have the:
1. Visual-associative language concepts   (use software with more-concrete, less-stylized
   required?   graphics)
2. Visual-discriminative skills required?   (use software with a less cluttered screen format)
3. Visuospatial skills required?   (use developmentally lower-level software for this
                                                   task)

4. Oculomotor skills required?   (use software with slower speed options)

C. Sensory–Integrative Functions

Does the patient have the ability to
integrate the:
1. Kinesthetic cues required?   (use software with slower speed options)
2. Simultaneous tactile–proprioceptive   (add textural cues to the joystick and fire button or
   cues?   tactile dots to the corners of the keys)
3. Bilateral motor integration   (use a joystick with suction feet or center stick fire
                                                   button)
4. Optic–kinetic skills required?   (use a Koala pad for training, substitute use of a
                                                   keyboard joystick)
D. Fine Motor Functions

Does the patient have the:
1. Unilateral fine motor skills required?   (use a splint to position fingers and/or wrist)
2. Isolated finger function required?   (use an expanded keyboard)
3. Bilateral hand function   (use keylocks for toggle functions)

---

lacks the coordination. Many other patient populations can access the computer without additional technological support with traditional methods of intervention commonly used by occupational therapists to compensate for loss of muscle power and range of motion. For example, standard clinical equipment such as suspension slings, forearm orthoses, splints, inclined table tops, and adjustable-height tables can be used to overcome many of the physical barriers to use of the computer by the physical disabled.

Positioning

Positioning the equipment for optimal use is the second issue commonly overlooked during the planning stages. The computer systems with lightweight, portable, and separate components seem to be the most useful in clinical applications, because separate portable monitors, disk drives, and keyboards can be positioned for easy access. Separate components reduce the amount of extraneous equipment needed for the majority of patients and thus the clutter in the computer area.

Simultaneity

The third and final issue raised in the activity analysis is that of simultaneity—the ability to sort, prioritize, and integrate multiple sensory cues. For the psychiatric, brain-injured, learning disabled, and developmentally delayed patient, the cognitive requirements of a given program may be exasperating and limiting. The computer medium is able to provide neither the variety nor the nuances of orienting cues available from a therapist. Instead, the patient must deduce what behavior is desired entirely by attending to the screen presentation. Fortunately, however, as frustrating as this may be, the medium can usually provide an extremely desirable type of consistent feedback which may be difficult to duplicate in other media. Computerized activities can also be extremely engaging, providing their own intrinsic motivators and rewards.

The activity analysis correctly indicates that the process of software selection requires a well-thought-out approach to ensure that the programs offered to the patient will be both developmentally appropriate and geared to the specific treatment objectives.

Software

The selection and use of software to achieve therapeutic goals is a clinical skill that can be readily mastered given background information, time, and practice. The ability to develop skill in this area is also dependent to some degree on familarity with the processes of task analysis and the ability to apply those processes to computerized activities.

Software that is appropriate for use in occupational therapy applications is not always easy to locate. This may be due to the types of software generally available *versus* the types of software that meet the needs of our particular clinical orientation. Therapists seem to be using one of three strategies for acquiring software for clinical application: (1) selecting software from the array that is widely available from all fields, (2) selecting software developed for rehabilitation fields that share some of our views of patient needs (*i.e.*, neuropsychology and special education), and (3) developing software written specifically to meet patient needs as viewed from the perspective of occupational therapy. Since the occupational therapy perspective is distinct in its holistic view of the patient from a developmental, neurobehavioral, and neuromuscular frame of reference, it would seem unlikely that another profession would be able to develop software that would meet our clinical needs. It would seem more likely that occupational therapists, out of necessity, would begin to develop their own software to reflect their specific contributions to patient treatment.

Although a wide variety of software is available, selecting software amendable to clinical applications in occupational therapy is no easy matter. Given divergent patient populations with equally divergent treatment objectives to be met, selecting appropriate software for each population requires diligence and perseverence. Nevertheless, certain programming features tend to make software more amenable to clinical applications. These features include simplicity in screen format, multiple levels of difficulty, variable timing options, and record-keeping facilities.

Types

Some of the more common types of software can be described as follows:

Drill and Practice

Software that helps the learner rehearse skills that have already been taught is called drill-and-practice software. This type of software can be used clinically for rehearsing competencies such as visual discrimination, typing, bookkeeping, reaction time, sequencing, ordering, and other attentive functions.

Tutorials

Software that is designed to teach a specific competency is a tutorial. The hallmark of a tutorial is that it can branch upward (to advance) or downward (to retard) program presentation to match the needs of the learner. This type of software can be used clinically to teach vocational and daily living skills such as typing, basic banking transactions, reading a utility bill, and budgeting as well as preacademic and para-academic competencies.

Interactive Video

Software designed to interact with a video playback system is called interactive video. This type of software can be used clinically with adults having psychiatric and developmental disabilities, as well as with children having psychosocial and learning disorders. It is particularly suitable to group applications and is generally used to simulate social learning experiences.

Educational Games

Software can be designed to teach basic educational competencies through a game format. Educational games can be used with both children and adults, depending on the program format. Common clinical applications include improving skills such as map reading, visual discrimination, visual association, coding, problem solving, and spatial relations.

Motor Games

Software has been designed to improve medium and fine motor skills through game playing. The hallmark of motor games is the use of a joystick, trac ball, biofeedback leads, or similar peripheral devices for input to the computer. Motor games can be used clinically to provide a wide range of teaching, training, and testing activities. Directionality, bilaterality, hand turning, isolated finger function, visual pursuit, and reciprocal upper-extremity movements are some of the skills that are amenable to intervention through the use of motor games.

Action-Consequence

This software is designed exclusively to teach attending behaviors to the cognitively young. The hallmark of action-consequence software is the tendency for it to use the computer as a switch or timing device that provides auditory and visual reinforcement for specified motor behaviors. This type of software can be used in clinics involved with early intervention, child psychiatry, and severely brain-injured populations.

Evaluation

Evaluating software for clinical application requires the ability to set aside preconceived notions of the needs of any one particular patient group in order to extract the broadest possible application from each piece of software. After the software has been fully evaluated, a determination of whether and how it can be used in the clinic can be made.

There are many formats available for software evaluation, most of which have been borrowed from fields of educational technology.[2] However, due to the wide variety of applications possible within the field of occupational therapy, it would be advantageous for the clinician to consider applications broader than those currently focused on in a particular area of practice. When the broader view is applied, one piece of software can be

---

Software Evaluation for Computer Applications in Clinical Practice

A. Name of Program _____
   Game or level available _____
B. What is the primary intended use of this program? _____
C. What is the primary targeted population for this program? _____
D. List the specific primary clinical problems that may be remediated through use of this program.
1. Cognitive disorders of attention, sequencing/organization of thought, memory, and problem-solving skills.

   _____   _____

2. Visual-processing disorders of visual discrimination, visual association, and visuo-spatial skills.

   _____   _____

3. Sensory–integrative disorders of kinesthetic, visuomotor, and somatosensory skills.

   _____   _____

4. Movement disorders of unilateral, bilateral, or reciprocal hand function and fine motor or medium motor coordination skills.

   _____   _____

E. List specific secondary clinical problems that may be remediated by use of this program.
1. ADL disorders of dressing, eating, communication, ambulation, hygiene, and grooming.

   _____   _____

2. Para- and/or pre-academic disorders or impairments of reading, writing, and mathematics concepts.

   _____   _____

3. Prevocational and/or independent living skills.

   _____   _____

F. List the specific functional skills that are inherent in successful use of this program.*
1. Check the level of competence that is required: Low   Moderate   High

   a. Cognitive skills   _____
   b. Reading skills   _____
   c. Computational or decoding skills   _____
   d. Motor skills   _____
2. Which of these functional skills may be improved through use of this program?

   _____   _____

3. Which of these inherent functional skills may not be "taught" through use of this program?

   _____

4. If the intended patient population does not have the specific functional skills that are required for this program, are there alternative methods/media/tools available to provide the necessary instruction?

             yes _____ no _____

   (If no, perhaps it might be best to consider using a different program for treatment of the clinical problems that have been identified as amenable to computer applications.)
G. List one or two preparatory activities that might precede the computer-assisted instruction.

   _____   _____

H. List one or two follow-through activities that might provide appropriate rehearsal of skills learned during computer-assisted instruction.

   _____   _____

   * An "ideal" sort of program for clinical application would allow for a wide range of competence, and drill and practice in skill areas that have been targeted for remediation through use of this program.

used as a therapeutic medium in a variety of settings. For example, "Print Shop" can be used in the remediation of spatial relations with the cerebral palsied and learning disabled child, in prevocational exploration with the developmentally delayed adolescent, and in cognitive remediation with the brain-injured adult. When this broader view is maintained, the therapist utilizes clinical skills to vary the task so that the medium becomes appropriate for a wider range of treatment applications. A software evaluation (see box) is included as an example of ways in which this broader view can be maintained when evaluating specific pieces of software.

The process of software evaluation is crucial to appropriate application of both tools and media in clinical practice. After this process is completed, the clinician will be better able to discern which aspects of the medium should be changed to make it suitable for application with a particular patient. Use of alternative methods of presentation can be considered, as well as use of alternative peripheral devices.

Hardware

Hardware used in clinical applications may be divided into two categories, the components of the computer system (*e.g.*, keyboard, disk drives) and peripheral devices. Any type of computer system may be used in clinical practice as long as it supports the clinical functions needed. Unfortunately, at the present, no one system seems to be able to handle the diversified needs of patients being served through computer applications, nor do the computers used for administrative support functions handle a wide variety of clinical applications. They may be suitable for prevocational and business applications but are not adequately supported for motor re-education, biofeedback, daily living skills, or applications for the developmentally delayed. On the other hand, computers used for motor re-education and biofeedback are not designed to handle the large business functions of a typical occupational therapy department. At present, most departments seem to have compromised by choosing a computer system designed primarily for either business or educational purposes but which can be adapted to meet the needs of the physically handicapped through the use of peripheral devices. Any computer system used for clinical applications should be selected on the basis of how well it meets the needs of the patient population most commonly treated in a given clinic. However, because no one system is truly adequate in multipurpose clinical applications at this time, the clinician involved in computer applications will have to compromise to some extent.

System Features

The hardware features most commonly seen as desirable are:

1. A breakaway keyboard: a lightweight portable keyboard that is separate from the disk drive and monitor. This feature allows independent access to the keyboard by many disabled users, since it allows the user to position the keyboard on a lapboard or other accessible work area. The breakaway keyboard is commonly available both in the business computer systems and in those designed for home, hobby, and game enthusiasts. However, most systems with breakaway keyboards are only beginning to support the peripheral accessing devices needed for the high-level quadriplegic or severely uncoordinated patient.

2. A hard disk. Using hard rather than floppy disks for storage increases the speed and storage capacity of the computer system. It also eliminates the need to manipulate floppy disks, which is difficult for the handicapped user. Hard disks are optional equipment but are available for most computer systems.

3. Function keys. When the system is to be used for prevocational applications, having a keyboard with function keys is essential in retraining the conceptual processes associated with business software and toggle functions. Use of function keys is a design feature that is not built into all computers.

An adaptive firmware card functions somewhere between hardware and software because it is packaged as a card that is installed into the circuit board of a computer. An adaptive firmware card is a "transparent" interfacing device with multiple applications for the handicapped user. For example, it can be used to slow down commercial software so that it can be used by severely disabled persons. It also allows use of a wide variety of switches and other input devices as opposed to the keyboard by the severely disabled.

Accessibility of disk drives and printers can be achieved by selection of special features at the time of purchase, by careful layout of the computer work station, or by use of adapted equipment to steady the disks or paper for insertion and removal from their holders. Assorted peripheral devices can be used to increase the accessibility of computers for handicapped users. However, the occupational therapists' most frequently considered option for a peripheral device continues to be the home-made variety. Devices that are fabricated of thermoplastic materials, ranging from individually designed mouthsticks to splints, slings, and pointers, are more readily available, more universally appropriate, and less expensive than their commercial counterparts.

Peripheral Devices

A broad assortment of accessing devices is available for the severely handicapped or users with special needs. However, direct keyboard access is generally preferable in most instances due to speed and availability of a wider range of software. Peripheral accessing devices include expanded keyboards, switches, the mouse, joysticks, graphic tablets, touch screens, light pens, and puff and sip controls. Commonly used devices, their functions, and vendors are listed in Table 22-1.

Another sort of peripheral device, which is not used for access in the strictest sense of the term, is the mini-computer used for biofeedback. These minicomputers translate data available in analog form (such as skin temperature, heart rate, and localized EMG) into digital information, which then serves as input for the host computer system. This sort of peripheral device is used in muscle re-education programs, cardiac rehabilitation, stress reduction clinics, and the like.

Being able to match hardware, software, and peripheral devices to a specific patient need requires creative problem-solving skills. Unraveling the details of the tools and media needed to accomplish desired treatment objectives can be likened to solving a puzzle. Although the puzzle can have many possible solutions, each alternative will have the potential to drastically improve the quality of a life.

Common Clinical Applications

Computer-assisted treatment (CATx) applications have been implemented in almost every area of occupational therapy practice. In most instances, this has resulted in an expansion of the scope of practice. Through the use of CATx, both the means and the methods to extend services to underserved areas of practice (*e.g.*, prevocational exploration, early intervention, activities of daily living) became a practical reality. The following section will list some of the more common areas where CATx is being implemented in clinical practice and briefly indicate how the tools and the media are being applied.

Table 22-1. *Peripheral Devices and Their Function*

Devices	Function	Vendor
Accessing Devices		

Switches:
  Single
  Dual
  Multiple
	Allows those with severely limited range of motion/muscle power/coordination to access computers, telephones, communication aids, environmental control systems	TASH
		70 Gibson Drive
		Unit 1
		Markham, Ontario, Canada L3R 2Z3
		(416) 475-2212

Expanded keyboards	Allows those with severe limitation to input directly to the computer keyboard	Prentke Romich 8769 Twp. Rd. 513 Shreve, Ohio 44676-9421 (216) 567-2906
Softkey	Allows direct access to the computer keyboard via touch-sensitive pad	Softkey Systems, Inc. 4737 Hibiscus Ave Edina, MN 55435 (612) 926-4905
Keyguards	Prevents unintentional hitting of keys	Preston Corp. 60 Page Rd Clifton, NJ 07012 (201) 777-2700 Unicom 297 Elmwood Ave Providence, RI 02907 Don Johnson Developmental Equipment 981 Winnetka Terrace Lake Zurich, IL 60047 (312) 438-3476
Voice input module	Allows direct access to the keyboard through voice activation	MCE, Inc 157 S. Kalamazoo Mall Kalamazoo, MI 49007 (800) 421-4157

(continued)

Table 22-1. *Peripheral Devices and Their Function*   (continued)

Devices	Function	Vendor
Pediatric Training Devices		
Activity board	Highly versatile switch-activated aid to teaching cognitive functions to the young, moderately involved preschooler or older, limited child	TASH (see above)
Training aids	Switch-activated toys designed to teach action–consequence to severely and multiply handicapped child	Linda J. Burkhart 8315 Potomac Ave College Park, MD 20740
Koala pad	Koala Painter and Koala Bear can be used to teach sequencing, unilateral fine motor skills, and visuomotor coordination skills	Local computer stores and larger toy stores
Chalk pad	Programmable touch pad used with overlays for the cognitively young and preschoolers	Dunamis 2856 Buford Highway Duluth, GA 30136
Miscellaneous Devices		
Firmware card	Used to slow rate of program flow and allow use of Morse code and other special modes. Enables physically disabled and slow users to benefit from standard software that is commercially available	Adaptive Peripherals 4535 Bagley Ave N Seattle, WA 98103 (206) 633-2610
Light pens	Used by young or brain-injured users as an alternative to keyboarding with specially designed software	Tech Sketch, Inc 26 Just Road Fairfield, NJ 07006 (201) 227-7724
Touch screen	Overlay device applied to screen for direct input by touch (finger)	Sunburst 39 Washington Avenue Pleasantville, NY 10570

Pediatrics

Use of computer applications has been spurred through close association with the fields of special education and speech pathology. Careful application of software developed for special education populations and accessing devices used as communication aids have improved our understanding of which children occupational therapy can best serve through CATx.

Early Intervention

Therapists in early intervention treatment facilities often use computer applications with the cognitively young to improve motor and attentive skills. In some instances, computer systems are being used as sophisticated switching devices to activate toys, train sets, or audiovisual presentations while collecting data about frequency of response, response delay time, and so forth.[5] Computers are being used with the severely developmentally delayed to improve orienting reactions, attending behaviors, and motor skills in response to multisensory or selective-sensory stimulation.[7] Therapists are using this medium to improve head righting, maintained visual regard, and postural alignment, as well as unilateral and bilateral medium-motor skills. CATx can be used as a motivator to encourage exploratory motor behavior with paretic extremities. The early stimulation of cognitive strategies of gaming and action–consequence can be achieved with the severely involved infant through the use of CATx.

An important feature to look for when considering software for this population is screen presentations that include objects common to the life experience of the cognitively young rather than stylized or "cutesy" pictures that are learned through acculturation. This concept should also be expanded to include sound effects. One research project, "Babies on Line," featured a screen format of a scoop of ice cream to motivate one multiply handicapped, cognitively young child to roll over and reach out toward the computer keyboard. The screen presentation of a favorite toy was used to encourage repeated reaching and grasping by another child.[1]

Preschool

Therapists involved with preschool facilities often use CATx to present structured tasks for remediation of developmental apraxia and visual–perceptual disorders. Peripheral input devices, keyboard modifications, and voice synthesizers are commonly used to introduce this medium to preschoolers. Remediation of sensory–integrative disorders of body scheme, body concept, directionality, and reciprocal upper-extremity function can be incorporated into CATx through careful selection of programs designed to link movement with multisensory screen presentations. Learning to use a joystick with low-level motor games fosters development of bilaterality, reciprocal use of the upper extremities, and basic motor planning skills. Programs using peripheral graphic devices such as a Koala pad or light pen are commonly used to help remediate visual-associative and visual-discriminative disorders in the developmentally delayed preschooler who is at risk for learning disabilities. Use of peripheral graphic devices presents a unique medium for remediation of optic-kinetic/visuomotor integrative functions and paves the way for later use of a pencil as a tool.

Software features to look for with preschoolers include: (1) simple, rather than cluttered, screen presentation and (2) graphics that are self-explanatory and tend to prompt an automatic correct response without lengthy instruction.

Physically Handicapped

Therapists treating physically handicapped children are often involved with teaching mastery over the physical environment through use of the computer as a tool in the classroom. With this population, the occupational therapist is primarily involved in using CATx for solving problems of physical manipulation and remediating perceptual motor deficits. Home-made accessing devices, expanded keyboards, switches, and touch screens are commonly used to resolve problems of access with this population. Software is available for treatment of visual, motor, and auditory sequencing deficits from special education sources. However, the occupational therapist will generally need to alter the presentation or focus of the programs garnered from these sources due to professional differences in perspective and treatment objectives. Programs for rehearsal of visual discriminatory skills of shape, closure, and figure–ground are readily available to the clinician using a computer as a tool in the clinic.

Learning Disabled

Therapists involved with learning disabled children who have multiple sensory–integrative deficits are able to improve the quality of treatment by using multisensory computer presentations to assist in the integration of body scheme, praxis, and visuomotor skills. Many clinicians find it helpful to use motor games in the remediation of visuospatial disorders with this population. However, programs that separate the cognitive aspects of spatial relations, such as position in space, space visualization, and movement, through use of the keyboard are also helpful in the remediation of visuospatial disorders. Specific types of attentional deficits such as ordering, sequencing, and simultaneity can be remediated through careful selection of software.

Software features for the physically handicapped and learning disabled child should offer: (1) simple rather than "busy" screen presentations, (2) multiple levels of play within the program that offer increases in timing or sequencing or increasingly refined use of discriminatory skills, and (3) developmental progression of skill acquisition.

Psychosocial Applications

The use of computer applications in psychiatry has become much more sophisticated since the days of its infancy in the use of video games in treatment.

Behavior Disorders

Therapists involved with patients having behavior disorders are able to use the computer as a tool in behavior management. Studies have been conducted using the computer as a reinforcer of positive behavior in token economy wards with teens.[3] Alternatively, computers have been used as a tool to reinforce compliant behaviors in autistic populations by selecting programs that render all keys "dead" except for desired input sequences. To some extent, limit setting and reinforcement of compliant behaviors are inherent in computer use, in that when program instructions are not followed, the results provide negative reinforcement. This aspect of working with computers can be heightened by the therapist through the deliberate selection of software that provides on-screen instruction to use only certain keys or certain sequences.

Plan to look for teacher options when selecting software for the behavior-disordered. This is a feature that allows the therapist to modify the program content, the number of trials presented, the duration of each trial, and the frequency of positive reinforcers.

Small Group Therapy

Therapists involved with small groups of patients having psychosocial disorders have been using computerized video games as a tool for several years. Computer applications have expanded to the use of video disk technology and other computer simulations to aid interactional skills and ego functions within the group setting. The use of learning development software is now emerging in adolescent psychiatry to assist in identification and treatment of perceptual–motor deficits and problem-solving difficulties within small groups.

Software that requires cooperative effort is a helpful feature when working with group dynamics. This type of software is available in game format and in life-task simulations. The software is strategically designed to require multiple cooperative inputs to achieve the desired goal.

Reality Testing

Therapists involved with patients having disorders of reality testing have begun to use some of the nonhuman aspects of computer applications to their advantage. Computer programs can be selected for their unlimited tolerance for incorrect responses and their inability to be socially manipulated by erratic or provocative behavior. Use of a computer system to provide consistent, valid feedback about performance has been used to reinforce ego functions and to provide a concrete platform from which to build relational skills.

Personality Disorders

Therapists involved with patients having personality disorders, particularly those involving substance abuse and criminal behavior, have been able to make extensive use of educational and prevocational computer applications. In institutionalized treatment settings, CATx can be valuable in identifying underlying perceptual disorders, areas of academic difficulties, and specific vocational aptitudes. It also provides a fashionable alternative medium for remediation of deficits. CATx has also been used as a structured medium to increase the accountability of patients who require contract setting and other modifiers to limit negative behaviors. Strategies such as scheduling computer access time and defining ratios of game to educational applications or creative to structured tasks can help reinforce greater sensitivity to interpersonal behaviors until adequate internal controls have developed.

Simple spreadsheets can be used to reinforce behavioral contracts by having the patient construct a personal chart of target behaviors. Charting frequency, duration, and formulas resulting in increased time on-line can then be used to reinforce behavior management strategies.

Adult Physical Disabilities

Therapists who treat the physically handicapped adult have applied CATx extensively in many areas of their practice. Depending on the severity of the disability, the adult may require several different types of computers throughout the various stages of rehabilitation. Initially,

motor re-education or attention training may be required. Biofeedback, motor games, and programs for cognitive rehabilitation are available. For the high-level quadriplegic or severely involved adult patient, solutions to problems of environmental control will usually involve a computerized system. Furthermore, CATx can be used to help clarify discharge plans relating to vocational concerns and the capacity for return to independent living within the community.

Cognitive Rehabilitation

Therapists working with patients in need of cognitive rehabilitation have tended to rely heavily on programs developed by neuropsychologists to assist in the remediation of attentive and visual–perceptual disorders. Although these programs sought to achieve objectives that were similar in style to those commonly sought by occupational therapists, they were not conceptually equivalent in terms of task analysis or results.

A few therapists, in the spirit of true pioneers, have ventured into the software development arena by developing programs that bear our distinct professional characteristics. CATx for the remediation of motor and visuomotor skills with the brain-injured patient has been accomplished primarily through the skillful analysis of motor games. Both the tools and the media must be carefully reviewed to achieve treatment objectives in terms of bilaterality, unilateral fine motor skills, grasp, dexterity, motor sequencing, visual pursuit, conjugate gaze, and so forth. Peripheral devices such as modified joysticks, trac balls, mice, graphic tablets, switches, and adaptive firmware cards have been among the tools used. Therapists working in long-term facilities have been able to rehearse the cognitive aspects of safety, shopping, budgeting, and other skills with patients who will be returning to the community through use of software developed to teach daily living skills.

Features to look for when selecting software for cognitive rehabilitation depend somewhat on the specific focus of treatment in this broadly defined area of practice. However, software should: (1) offer a progression of levels for remediaton of skills within a developmental framework, (2) offer a progression of levels for simultaneous integration of skills to be remediated within a developmental framework, and (3) offer tasks clearly related to meaningful life tasks that are being rehearsed through other media in occupational therapy.

Environmental Control

Therapists working with patients needing environmental control have historically used technological advances to further the independence of their patients. At present, computerized systems for environmental control are available for most major brands of computers. However, the scope of practice for occupational therapists in this area has now expanded to include vocational applications for the severely handicapped adult. Major issues in this area involve system configuration and the resolution of problems of positioning, set-up, and access of all the components of the computer. Extensive use is initially made of peripheral devices and their fittings to promote a measure of environmental independence. Prevocational aspects of CATx raise further issues of system and software compatability for those programs commonly used in business and the ability of the patient to access these.

Biofeedback

Therapists working with patients needing biofeedback are no longer tied to large, complex industrial computers. Portable, personal configurations are being used to aid in motor re-education and stress reduction and to perform monitoring functions in cardiac rehabilitation. In addition, the scope of practice has expanded to include computerized work simulators capable of giving feedback about muscle power and range as patients perform activities designed to simulate their specific job tasks.

Software features to look for include: (1) user-friendly features such as ease of use, (2) simple screen formats for patient interpretation, and (3) inherent positive reinforcement such as competition with a pre-set baseline or game format.

Motor Re-education

Therapists working with patients in need of motor re-education are able to exploit several aspects of hardware and peripheral design to their advantage. Reciprocal upper-extremity functions can be rehearsed through use of joysticks. Joystick adaptations that are readily available include suction feet, a variety of handles to promote alternative types of grasp, and a variety of fire button positions to accommodate right- or left-handed approaches to motor functions. Optic-kinetic integration can be finely tuned through use of motor games that promote the subordination of kinesthetic awareness while providing sensory feedback about movement through visual modalities. Separation of finger function can be achieved through use of the keyboard, a number pad, a mouse, or other peripheral device. Both muscle power and range of motion can be improved by increasing the thresholds for biofeedback games and through use of work simulators.

Prevocational Applications

The use of CATx has broadened the ability of the occupational therapist to assess and prepare the disabled for vocational training programs. Available software ranges from vocational interest and aptitude instruments to training for a variety of jobs that require paper or data handling. Software packages that provide an inventory of vocational interests are available from almost every major publisher of educational materials. Use of these packages allows the occupational therapist to borrow from the expertise of other professionals rather than limiting the patient to the prevocational experience of the clinician alone. Detailed interest inventories provide job descriptions and work simulations for a variety of professions so that the patient can get a preview of the academic requirements of the job as well as some of the ramifications of the profession being considered. Objective skill assessments can also be provided through CATx so that a degree of vocational steering can be achieved at a prevocational level. Therapists can also initiate training for data entry and data management with the multiply-handicapped and physically disabled in preparation for computer-based cottage industry or sheltered work experiences.

In prevocational practice, heavy reliance has been placed on use of educational software for review of basic academic competencies. Business software and simplified modifications intended for home use have been used to teach concepts relevant to business applications. Software selection should again be based on developmental constraints, and the program should move from simple to more complex processes appropriate to the background of each patient. Use of software for drill and practice can be very effective in prevocational applications.

Summary

Computer applications in the field of occupational therapy represent a broadly expanding sphere of influence. Computer technology is beginning to impinge on almost every aspect of practice. From the administrative support available through use of word processors, spreadsheets, and data management packages to the technical aspects of clinical application, our profession is moving ahead to incorporate advanced technology.

However, certain negative consequences of computer applications are also beginning to be expressed. Among these are: (1) territorial rivalry from other professions that is beginning to limit the use of computers within our profession to those objectives that are clearly within our sphere of licensed practice; (2) the lack of software designed to meet our professional treatment objectives, which limits our ability to serve our patients through this medium; and (3) the lack of research documentation for the use of CATx which limits clinicians in all areas of occupational therapy practice. It also limits the ability of administrators to justify hardware and software expenditures. At the same time, many very positive influences are beginning to emerge from use of computer applications in occupational therapy. Among them are: (1) increased efficiency in administrative functions, which provides more time for administrators and clinicians to be involved with patient care rather than paperwork; (2) increased professional visibility and credibility, which results as occupational therapists are seen as being technologically competent in the computer age; and (3) expansion of the scope of occupational therapy practice through use of computer applications to offer a broader spectrum of services to the disabled.

References

1. Aprin S: Babies on line. Presented at the National Conference on the Use of Microcomputers in Special Education, Hartford, Connecticut, March 1983

2. Humphrey M: Evaluating educational software. Creative Computing, October 1981
3. Lynch WJ: The contribution of video games to computer assisted cognitive training. Presented at the Annual Convention of the American Psychological Association, August 1983
4. Okoye R, Malden J: Use of neurotransmitter modulation to facilitate sensory integration. Neurol Rep 10:4, 1986
5. Rosenberg S: A microcomputer playstation for severely handicapped children. Presented at Closing the Gap Annual Conference, October 1986
6. Taber F: Microcomputers in Special Education. Reston, VA, ERIC Clearinghouse on Handicapped and Gifted Children, 1983
7. Wright C, Momura M: From Toys to Computers: Access for the Physically Disabled Child. San Jose, Wright 1985

CHAPTER 23

Biofeedback* *Abby Abildness*

In its present state, biofeedback employs simple devices to detect signs of physiological activity. These tools have been used for acquiring evaluative information in medical and biological research for many years. Now, biofeedback is used, not only to diagnose disease, but also to provide information to the patient about his or her own state and to enable the patient to alter that state by using cortical control.

The use of biofeedback for self-control has developed in the behavioral sciences over the past 20 years. This has excited and challenged a wide variety of health care professionals. Through awareness of the patient's psychophysiological status, patients and therapists can learn together to manipulate the patient's internal environment to promote changes in maladaptive behavioral responses. The exciting implication is that the therapist – patient relationship changes from the professional's imposing treatment on the patient to the therapist's facilitating the patient's ability to change internal psychophysiology. Such change can reduce the need for medications, which can have harmful side-effects, decrease the need for adaptive equipment, and reduce environmental stress.

Overall, feedback has an impact not only on preventive and restorative comprehensive health care alternatives, but, through its emphasis on self-control, on medicine's philosophical and psychophysiological concept of human beings.

The Biofeedback Process

Electronic feedback on physiological events is given to patients in the form of visual or auditory signals. Biofeedback machines have transducers that detect heart rate, blood pressure, muscle tension, peripheral blood flow, skin temperature, sweat gland activity, and brain wave rhythms. Machines detect much more subtle changes than can be perceived otherwise and thus give feedback on minute biological changes. The feedback process' consists of five operations (Fig. 23-1):

1. Detection and amplification of bioelectric potentials that are otherwise undetected
2. Conversion of bioelectric signals to auditory and

---

* Material in this chapter is intended to inform therapists about the potential of biofeedback, not train them in the use of biofeedback machines. Other educational resources should be studied to develop expertise in the use of the technology. The American Occupational Therapy Association has produced a biofeedback strategies training package, including text and six videotapes authored by Abby Abildness, that is available for purchase or rental.

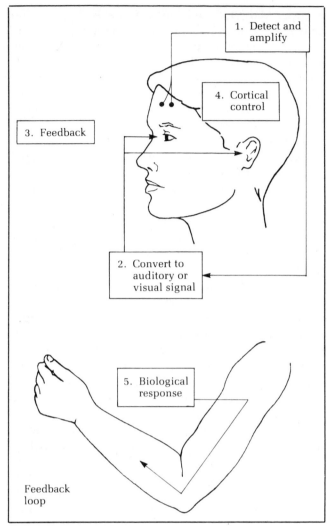

Figure 23-1. Five operations in the biofeedback process.

visual signals that are understandable to the individual
3. Instantaneous feedback on the status of, and changes in, the biological state
4. Triggered cortical awareness of biological status, enabling an individual to learn volitional control of the biological state
5. Biological response, with continuous feedback as an operant reinforcer to enable skilled execution of a biological response; for instance, a motor response

It is critical for accurate learning that the feedback be continuous, instantaneous, and directly proportional to the biological change. The instrument's feedback becomes the reinforcer, stimulating learning that is "shaped" by the therapist to obtain the desired behavioral outcome.

Biofeedback is not intended as a treatment in itself but as an adjunct to traditional occupational therapy procedures. It enhances the possibilities for restoring health by providing information needed by the patient to gain control of biological events previously thought to be uncontrollable.

The Feedback Concept in Occupational Therapy

The effectiveness of biofeedback is determined by its integration into a therapist's total treatment framework. Individuals can readily use biofeedback sensory aids to learn to change physiological or psychological arousal, but unless the learned skill is applied to functional daily life, it is useless. Biofeedback should be one of a variety of means used to achieve goals.

Biofeedback offers crucial advantages in the early stages of treatment, because it focuses on cortical remediation of psychophysiological ills. Its unique asset is its capacity to register the psychological and physiological aspects of disordered functioning simultaneously. Biofeedback demonstrates to patients their ability to control physiology. It also provides direct information about the symptom to be changed. Finally, it monitors physiological changes during treatment. The overall treatment advantages, documented by multiple sources, include:
1. Reduced training time: patients achieve desired goals more rapidly when biofeedback is used
2. Cost-effectiveness: therapist time and hospitalizations are shortened
3. Enhanced initiation of motion or emotion that could not otherwise be elicited
4. Objective evaluative data for documenting treatment progress or effectiveness
5. Improved client self-image as a result of increasing responsibility in self-managing treatment
6. Longer-lasting effects, owing to development of cortical awareness and control

Biofeedback in Continuous Activity Analysis

Biofeedback technology offers invaluable adjunctive, objective, evaluative information for analysis of activities and their therapeutic effects. Continuous monitoring of specific biological parameters during prescribed functional activities will demonstrate the degree of appropriateness of each. Some examples of monitoring include:
1. *Electromyography* (EMG) monitoring of the triceps during reaching, grasp, and release activities in different planes to determine the strength, endurance, and appropriate relaxation of contraction
2. *Galvanic skin response* (GSR) or sweat response monitoring of psychiatric clients involved in

individual or group activities to determine stress or relaxation effects
3. *Heart rate* monitoring during exercise for cardiac patients to determine the actual limits of physical demand provided by the activity

A procedural approach devised by Wolf and associates[4] to assess treatment goals is known as *concurrent assessment of muscle activity* (CAMA). CAMA uses muscle biofeedback to inform clinicians about muscle activity as the patient responds to therapeutic intervention. By implementing CAMA, the therapist can receive quantified documentation about muscle behavior during treatment and modify the treatment approach to elicit a more desirable response. This is more precise information than muscle palpation or observation of movement. It allows direct data acquisition to demonstrate treatment efficacy and thus helps justify reimbursement for clinical services.

Dual-channel EMG recordings are done during the application of neuromuscular facilitation or inhibition techniques. The immediate and accurate information on EMG activity enables therapists to make more appropriate and efficient modifications during treatment sessions. CAMA enhances patient responses to therapeutic interventions. Its method helps the occupational therapy community in the necessary transformation from appreciated art to acknowledged science.

However, therapists must remember that biofeedback alerts patients to the strength of their psychophysiological behavior but not to the nature of the reaction. Therapists should use other clinical skills to explore the meaning and clinical significance of the behavioral response and its therapeutic application.

Major Biofeedback Applications in Physical Dysfunction

Biofeedback in Neuromuscular Re-education

Traditional neurodevelopmental rehabilitation procedures are aimed at providing appropriate proprioceptive input for the patient. EMG biofeedback can detect any latent motor unit potentials in seemingly paralyzed muscles. This information is relayed to the patient through the intact auditory and visual systems rather than the neurologically impaired proprioceptors. Biofeedback thus enhances the neurodevelopmental treatment process by providing information about motor responses too slight to be sensed by the patient or therapist otherwise.

When upper or lower motor neurons are injured, electrical impulses from the brain to the muscle are interrupted, and the muscle may become paralyzed. However, as Marinacci and Horande have shown, a few active motor units may remain in the muscle even if it appears to be totally paralyzed.[9] The patient and therapist may not detect the potential for recruiting other motor units and regaining some functional control, but the EMG biofeedback machine detects and amplifies these electrical potentials either to enable the patient to learn to elicit a motor act or as feedback for accurate execution.

Normal learned motor responses occur through proprioceptive feedback of muscle tension and position, indicating how movement was performed. Biofeedback technology can provide information on exact tension changes, but coordinated motor control requires position feedback, which must come from the client's and therapist's observation of the limb performing a functional task.

Spasticity or hypertonicity may also develop owing to diminished proprioceptive information concerning muscular tension, causing a loss of the inhibiting or modulating influences of the brain on the lower motor neurons. In the case of excessive tension, biofeedback provides information regarding exact tension levels, enabling the patient to learn to relax the tension.

The ability to substitute for absent, impaired, or faulty kinesthetic feedback is the most important advantage of EMG biofeedback as an adjunct in neuromuscular re-education. At first, patients rely heavily on feedback display representations of actual motor activity, but as the ability to initiate and terminate contraction develops, they become less dependent on electronic cues and more reliant on associated internal sensory cues and visual observation of limb changes.

Cerebrovascular Accident

In rehabilitation, EMG biofeedback has gained a firm place in the treatment of upper motor neuron lesions, particularly in retraining extensor muscles and inducing relaxation of spastic muscles of stroke patients. Most neuromuscular biofeedback research has been done with stroke patients 2 to 5 years after injury to ensure that the findings do not represent spontaneous recovery. After standard rehabilitation attempts had maximized motion, biofeedback greatly increased strength and volitional control, even in muscles previously thought to be paralyzed. A representative study compared biofeedback with standard physical therapy and showed biofeedback to excel in strengthening the anterior tibialis muscle and in reducing the need for short leg braces in most cases.[1]

Hand and forearm extensor paralysis combined with flexor spasticity requires dual-channel EMG feedback to combine inhibition training of flexors with neuromotor facilitation training of weak hand and forearm extensors.

Spinal Cord Injury

Biofeedback training facilitates development of full motor potential at, or sometimes below, the identified cord lesion. It is believed that spinal shock impairs the brain's ability to detect minimal proprioceptive signals. Biofeedback externally and artificially provides the necessary feedback to facilitate motor activity otherwise undetected and may functionally lower the cord lesion.

The techniques of Bernard Bruckner at the University of Miami in Florida lead the field in training spinal cord-injured patients to take the focus off the limb and put it on the neurosignal combinations.[4] Prior to training, it must be determined that motor signals are not simply reflex firing in the cord itself. There must be neural tissue in the spinal cord available for operant learning. There need not be observable limb movement, but some trace of neurosignal operating from the brain and travelling through the cord past the point of injury must be found. EMG training then teaches recruitment of motor neurons to produce a motor signal to travel to the muscle site. Combining this training with resistive activities, occupational therapists have more potential muscle action with which to work. Initial treatment focuses on hand-to-mouth functions and progresses to finger grasp and release, working proximally to distally.

Dramatic results are also being found with quadriplegic patients who suffer from orthostatic hypotension. Direct blood-pressure monitoring enables them to learn to raise and maintain their blood pressure cognitively to a sufficient degree to prevent fainting.

Cerebral Palsy

Biofeedback efforts in cerebral palsy are aimed at regaining motor control in characteristic disorders of posture, gait, and involuntary athetoid movements. Harris and his associates identify athetoid movements as faulty kinesthetic monitoring.[5] Accurate simultaneous biofeedback of opposing muscles encourages coordinated motor control. Suger and co-workers[12] train hemiplegic children to achieve a symmetric gait by providing auditory feedback from a load-sensitive insole inserted in the shoe on the hemiparetic side and encouraging them to increase the weight-bearing load by increasing the feedback signals from the machine. This addition to the functional ambulation treatment program is a great advantage for children who do not understand what they are doing wrong. They simply learn to make the feedback signal happen. The feedback helps them calibrate the proprioceptive sensory information they normally receive, thereby improving motor control. Proper learned behavior becomes a habit and is followed through outside the treatment setting. This method reduces the need for manual stretching of the calf, night splints, and surgical intervention.

Special head-control caps are also being used for teaching postural control. These provide tape recorder feedback when the patient sits erect, with the sound diminishing in proportion to the slouch. A variety of feedback transducers are gaining wider use in cerebral palsy and other musculoskeletal disturbances. These include electrogoniometers and pressure-sensitive and position-sensing devices.

Peripheral Nerve Injury

Feedback from isolated muscles can be used to prevent substitution problems and to encourage peripheral nerve regeneration following disease or crushing. Force position and joint-angle monitors help increase range of motion by improving the instrument's feedback response. This improves the specific coordinated control of patients with neural, musculotendinous, and articular limitations.

Guillain–Barré Syndrome

Recent promising Guillain–Barré case studies show biofeedback to enhance activities of daily living (ADL) training even after more traditional therapies have been discontinued. Marked benefits for wrist and finger musculature are reported.[6] EMG biofeedback enhances natural recovery in neuromuscular disorders not only by providing activities that utilize recovering muscles appropriately on an individual, specific basis but also by providing direct information concerning muscle use. Electrical feedback serves the dual purpose of reinforcing only correct motor behaviors and of motivating the patient because correct effort is immediately rewarded and improvements are seen. ADL training involving strength of gross and fine finger movements uses feedback to improve specific strengthening during eating and dressing.

Rehabilitation Engineering Feedback Tools for Activity Analysis and Training

Instrumentation adaptations may be among the most important contributions of occupational therapists to the field of biofeedback. Electrokinesiologic devices have already been developed at Emory University and at Boston University.[3,13] These include electrogoniometers for elbow, wrist, and finger joints and pressure feedback devices for grasp and prehension strengthening. Each of these devices has calibrated threshold settings that allow setting of multiple strength or range-of-motion goals during prescribed activities. The devices are useful for evaluating range and strength changes, as well as the therapeutic value of functional tasks. A bioconverter has been reported to provide more motivating feedback to children.[2] It can send EMG signals through any household appliance or electrical toy, thus increasing the child's attention span and perseverance in performing accurate motor tasks in order to see electrical toys move.

Microcomputer-based wearable devices are being used to assess treatment effects as well as to improve transfer of skills training. These devices can provide a profile of a patient's selected behaviors in the home during daily activities that may be more difficult or contribute to poor behavior patterns. For example, Rubow and Swift developed a wearable biofeedback device that provides a Parkinson's patient with information about speech intensity outside the clinic.[11] The feedback allows the patient to focus on maintaining adequate loudness once the basic behaviors have been learned in the clinic. As the patient develops a habit of speaking with adequate vocal intensity, he or she becomes independent of the wearable aid.

Other occupational therapy evaluative and treatment tools could lend themselves to feedback adaptations. It simply requires a creative therapist who understands the feedback concept and its therapeutic use. The therapist can explain the type of feedback required to a biomedical engineer or electronic technician, who can devise simple adaptations at minimal cost.

Heart Rate

Heart rate biofeedback is one of the most widely researched areas. Because heart rate responses are such sensitive indicators of stress and anxiety, and because nervous regulation of heart beat is relatively simple heart rate has been easy to control through conditioning. Cardiac arrhythmias are the predominant category for clinical treatment. The direct relationship between nerve stimulation and heart rate lends itself to modification by higher cerebral control limited chiefly by the integrity of nerve connections. The strength of biofeedback applicability to certain pathological conditions of heart-beat conduction by way of neural involvement can positively relieve any emotional overlay aggravating the conditions.

Blood Pressure

Because of the psychogenic nature of blood pressure variability, biofeedback treatment is part of a program dealing with underlying stresses. Biofeedback can help patients recognize the role of emotion in precipitating their illness; it can also help them identify harmful emotion-arousing situations or conditions. It facilitates control over overt activities associated with emotional arousal and autonomic responses.

Temperature Self-Regulation (With Raynaud's Disease)

Initial temperature clinical applications were applied to Raynaud's disease, in which paroxysms of cutaneous vasospasm cause reduced blood flow. Peripheral constriction causes pain, skin discoloration, and ulcers and can lead to gangrene of the digits. Skin temperature, a measure of peripheral vascular activity, can be internally raised by vasodilation and relax sympathetic activity. Control is recognized when the treatment is effective during the coldest months of the year and is maintained over seasonal variation. Maintenance and generalization of the learned behavior change (temperature control) must be programmed by continued logging of vasospastic attacks. Learned control must be practiced frequently for short periods to prevent or terminate episodic symptoms.

Temperature training is being expanded to encompass inflammatory arthritis, wound healing, tumorous growth reduction, diabetic peripheral neuropathies, and renal blood flow problems. Trained vasodilation and vasoconstriction alter blood flow to specific regions.

Breathing (with Bronchial Asthma)

Biofeedback relaxation training can increase peak respiratory flow rates in asthmatic children.[8] A counterconditioning desensitization approach reduces the frequency, duration, and severity of attacks as patients learn bronchodilation as an antagonistic approach to bronchoconstriction. Children develop a sense of self-confidence in controlling mild attacks, which lessens the fear and apprehension believed to induce natural asthmatic attacks.

Biofeedback with Psychosomatic and Psychopathologic Disorders

Biofeedback counterconditioning strategies are designed to bring mastery of psychobiologic stress by developing awareness of certain stress indices (muscle tension, increased blood pressure, increased sweating) and learning to inhibit them. Awareness of the ability to change or control stress reactions internally, rather than be controlled by them, increases the patients' potential to be healed. For example, the patient with bronchial asthma who senses the beginning signs of an attack can intervene and stop or minimize the attack, rather than fear its onset and so heighten its effects.

General Stress Management

Many epidemiological studies initially investigating psychoses and psychosomatic symptoms have shown that conditions producing psychological stress greatly increase the risk of adverse consequences, such as psychiatric hospitalizations, stomach lesions, diabetes, hypertension, and many other medical complaints.[10] Stress is usually accompanied by a generalized arousal of the neuromuscular, autonomic, and central nervous systems. Once stimulated, people with psychosomatic or psychiatric symptoms will experience maladaptive, heightened arousal more frequently and for longer periods of time and have difficulty returning to prestress levels. Specific physiological patterns of arousal to stress may vary. One person may show greater cardiovascular changes, while another may have gastrointestinal or neuromuscular alterations. Therefore, a stress profile must be taken using various biofeedback machines as part of a complete medical and behavioral analysis. This will provide information about the physiological systems that should be altered to promote healthful responses to stress.

Feedback dermography is used to measure generalized arousal mechanisms. It monitors skin conductance characteristics by detecting the direct current potential between two electrodes on the skin's surface. Physiologically, current is primarily mediated by sweat gland activity and activated by sympathetic nervous system stimulation. During evaluation or treatment, the dermograph feedback magnitude will reflect the intensity and nature of anxiety-provoking topics discussed or events experienced.

Patients having stress-related disorders typically demonstrate multiple symptoms and initially need generalized relaxation training. Lowering physiological arousal to provide relief of psychiatric symptoms is based on Jacobson's premise that anxiety is incompatible with relaxation and that controlled relaxation is sufficient to provide relief from physical or emotional stress.[7] Trainees are taught to enter a state of relaxation, or cultivated low arousal, characterized by parasympathetic dominance and antagonistic to the pattern of physiological arousal exhibited in stress-related disorders. This results in reduction in skin resistance and a redistribution of the blood supply to the body periphery, with resulting lowered blood pressure. Therefore, learning to relax can bring internal responses under control, adding many health benefits.

These responses are readily controlled in the clinic; far more difficult is the task of controlling them during daily life. Therefore, therapists must wean a patient from the machines by turning them off for short periods and then for longer periods until the patient can maintain control unassisted. Therapists also need to teach the skills matched with activities directly related to the patient's condition and lifestyle stresses. By first using feedback machines reflecting generalized emotional responses and progressing to those measuring specific functions, such as heart rate or isolated muscle tension, patients are taught control over generalized arousal and then isolated physiological functions applied to real-life stressors. Patients perform self-monitoring and document for themselves symptom changes. Instrument feedback facilitates awareness of tension levels and how to monitor and inhibit them cortically. This enhances simple relaxation strategies by enabling patients to realize their progress and to decide which techniques are most effective.

Specific Psychotherapeutic Applications

Biofeedback can help many patients modify specific responses or response patterns associated with a mental disorder. It is most suitable for patients and disorders in which physiological processes can be identified as relevant. Biofeedback methods can help patients achieve physical and mental relaxation through reduction of muscle tension or calming of other physiological processes. Biofeedback can also help sensitize individuals to their own bodily responses and the associations of those responses with cognitive processes and behaviors, thereby facilitating more adaptive responses.

Feedback treatment methods have distinct positive rewards because they actively involve the patient in the therapeutic process and provide him or her an opportunity for successful self-control. Biofeedback can readily lead to a sense of mastery because it incorporates graded practice, gradual improvement, and an objective index of success.

Neurosis

Neurosis, in physiological terms, is a form of neuromuscular hypertension complicated by pathological habit formation. Excessive tension begins to control the individual as he or she loses an internal locus of control. As an adjunct to insight therapy, biofeedback promotes self-awareness as patients learn their physiological response to stress and learn more appropriate responses. As they learn to relax, mental tension is relieved. Reasoning becomes clearer and verbalizations more coherent. Confidence gained in the ability to control oneself increases independence, which decreases reliance on external substances such as medications.

Phobia

Electrodermal feedback has been used as a physiological measure of the autonomic components of phobic responses to identify the specific fear. This enhances accuracy in the development of a stress hierarchy, or graded stress situations, for patients not in touch with their emotions. Feedback alerts patients when relaxation is achieved in each progressive stress situation and helps them determine when they may move to the next level.

Drug Addiction (Substance Abuse)

Biofeedback is a nonpharmacological intervention used to reduce the anxiety and tension associated with detoxification. Sources of anxiety can be withdrawal symptoms in recovery programs as well as environmental or emotional situations that promote drinking or drug-taking behaviors.

Biofeedback is used to offer an alternative to anxiety-relieving addictive substances. Many addicts cannot tolerate withdrawal from the substance without some type of alternative. They feel unable to overcome powerful drives to use substances that fill an emotional void. Biofeedback and relaxation alternatives help addicts gain control of their psychophysiological arousal, thus decreasing the need for the substance. Biofeedback can be preferable for anxiety reduction because it has functional specificity and does not need to subdue the entire central nervous system.

Pain

Biofeedback deals directly with muscle or vascular tension resulting in pain. Biofeedback develops awareness of tension levels, as well as their triggering stimuli, thereby enabling patients to recognize early pain and abate it before it becomes incapacitating. Pain applications most frequently discussed include migraine headaches, bruxism, low-back syndrome, cancer, and spasticity pain associated with neurological disorders.

Biofeedback relaxation strategies are effective in increasing activity levels, decreasing use of pain medication and improving levels of pain and mood. The best results are found when patients are taught coping skills in the form of relaxation methods and behavioral cognitive techniques that are applied to the home or work environment. With functional backache symptomatic of muscle spasms, cocontraction relaxation procedures are a useful behavioral technique for assessment and treatment. Simple acquisition of resting-level relaxation procedures is less beneficial for excessive spasms unless it can be applied to functional daily tasks.

Treatment methods should be matched to the patient's lifestyle needs and goals based on a thorough behavioral analysis of the problem. Because it is difficult to return patients to a prepain level of functioning, treatment should be oriented toward helping them live as normally and productively as possible while preventing the development of chronic pain.

The Occupational Therapist's Role in Biofeedback Training

The therapist should plan and monitor treatment with biofeedback, viewing it as one tool for accomplishing the treatment goals. The therapist acts as coach and educator and teaches the patient to interact and derive meaning from the biofeedback. Changes are observed in physiological activity as the patient develops the ability to alter feedback displays, and verbal cues are provided to encourage the development of cortical awareness of physiological change. The therapist must be aware of other aspects of the patient's homeostasis being affected by changes in the monitored system.

Since biofeedback strategies do not specifically address a person's maladaptive appraisals and behaviors in the natural environment, the therapist must guide the patient in translating learned internal control skills into real-life behavioral adaptations. If environmental modifications have already been made, they may no longer be necessary once internal control is achieved. Observing internal control on biofeedback displays is a reinforcer in itself, yet a greater motivational challenge is to be able to achieve more gratifying personal activity goals.

Therapists train patients to modify physiological behaviors by shaping responses with the aid of visual or auditory cues proportional to the magnitude of that activity. Treatment success or failure is contingent on the patient's motivation and ability to modify internal physiological responses and motor behaviors and to transfer the training into meaningful functional consequences. Treatment success repeatedly is found to be linked to training during functional life tasks. This fact emphasizes the need for this electrical tool to be used by the occupational therapist within the total treatment perspective.

Occupational therapists are becoming increasingly conscious of a need to treat patients from a holistic perspective. This takes into account treatment of the total person, including attention to physical, psychological, spiritual, and environmental needs. Biofeedback and its concomitant behavioral strategies lend themselves well to this perspective. The biofeedback equipment simultaneously records a composite of psychophysiological behavioral responses. The behavioral strategies, particularly those dealing with stress-related disorders, can guide patients through the use of meditation into recreating silences in the inner world of contemplation, which results in true psychophysiologic peace and inner healing. Some therapists employ yoga or meditative prayer techniques. The therapist's ultimate goal in biofeedback treatment is to call upon the resources of the cortical mind and use it as healer. A thorough understanding of the patient's beliefs and needs will best ensure successful treatment.

References

1. Basmajian JV, Kukulka CG, Narayan MG, Takebe K: Biofeedback treatment of foot drop after stroke compared

with standard rehabilitation technique: Effects on voluntary control and strength. Arch Phys Med Rehab 56:231, 1975

2. Brown DM, Basmajian JV: Bioconverter for upper extremity rehabilitation. Am J Phys Med 57:233, 1978
3. Brown DM, Dibaucher GA, Basmajian JV: Feedback goniometers for hand rehabilitation. Am J Occup Ther 33:458, 1979
4. Goldsmith MF: Computerized biofeedback training aids in spinal cord injury rehabilitation. JAMA 253:1097, 1985
5. Harris FA, Spelman FA, Hyner JW: Electronic sensory aids as treatment for cerebral-palsied children: Inaproprioception II. Phys Ther 54:354, 1974
6. Ince LP, Leon MS: Biofeedback treatment of upper extremity dysfunction in Guillian–Barré syndrome. Arch Phys Med Rehab 67:30, 1986
7. Jacobson E: Progressive Relaxation. Chicago, University of Chicago Press, 1942
8. Kotses H, Glaus KO, Crawford PL, et al: Operant reduction of frontalis EMG activity in the treatment of asthma in children. J Psychosom Res 20:453, 1976
9. Marinacci A, Horande M: Electromyogram in neuromuscular re-education. Bull Los Angeles Neurol Soc 25:57, 1960
10. Miller NE: Biofeedback and visceral learning. Annu Rev Psychol 29:373, 1978
11. Rubow R, Swift E: A microcomputer based wearable biofeedback device to improve transfer of treatment in parkinsonian dysarthria. J Speech Hear Disorders 50:178, 1985
12. Suger BR, Caudry DJ, Scholes JR: Biofeedback therapy to achieve symmetrical gain in hemiplegic cerebral palsy children. Arch Phys Med Rehab 62:364, 1981
13. Trombly CA, Cole JM: Electromyographic study of four hand muscles during selected activities. Am J Occup Ther 33:440, 1979
14. Wolf SL, Edwards DI, Shutter LA: Concurrent assessment of muscle activity (CAMA): A procedural approach to assess treatment goals. Phys Ther 66:218, 1986

CHAPTER 24

Human Sexuality *Marianne Rozycka Dahl*

The role of sexuality in the health of an individual has been increasingly recognized as a legitimate aspect of rehabilitation. Also, health professionals are becoming more aware of their responsibility to deal directly with the sexual health of their clients as part of activities of daily living (ADL) training.[1,3,7]

The subject of human sexuality encompasses a complex and subtle blend of the biological, psychological, social, and interpersonal aspects of being either a man or a woman. Some physiological functions and anatomical structures distinguish male from female. Family responsibilities and other life roles are influenced by sex. Clothing and the way it is worn reflect sexuality. Even the choice of friends and leisure-time activities may be affected by one's sex. Religious beliefs and socioeconomic and ethnic influences also have an impact on a person's sexual attitudes and knowledge.

Sexuality and sexual function are not synonymous. Sexual function refers to the physiological reaction to psychic or physical stimulation. Masters and Johnson's human sexual response cycle facilitates an understanding of the anatomic and physiologic changes that occur during sexual functioning.[5] In men, the response cycle can involve erection, increased blood pressure, sweating, ejaculation, and a sensation of climax, with subsequent reduction of tension (Table 24-1). In women, the response cycle can involve vaginal moistening, increased blood pressure, sweating, a flush, and sensations of climax (Table 24-2).

Sexual functioning may occur alone or with another person. Some people elect to abstain, whereas others may masturbate or engage in intercourse.

Acute or chronic illness impacts numerous areas of a person's life and may disrupt sexuality, including sexual functioning. Specific disabilities or illnesses may affect sexual functioning in different ways. For example, anatomy or physiology may be affected, so that sexual function is impaired directly. Weakness, easy fatigability, pain, or limited range of motion can markedly disrupt sexual function.

Many people, including health professionals, find it difficult to deal directly with explicit sexuality. It is important, however, that the occupational therapist foster a recognition of the fact that all persons have sexuality, and to initiate discussion of this aspect of life. By recognizing the sexual components of medical, social, psychological, and vocational aspects of physical disability, the occupational therapist becomes better prepared to assist the disabled person with sexual adaptation.

Suggestions regarding sexual adaptation depend on knowledge of a patient's or client's values, medical condition, medications, psychological well-being, and so-

Table 24-1. Male Sexual Response Cycle

	Able-Bodied Male	Disabled Male
Penis	Erects	Erects ±
Skin of scrotum	Tenses	Tenses ±
Testes	Elevate in scrotum	Elevate in scrotum ±
Emission	Yes	No ±
Ejaculation	Yes	No ±
Nipples	Erect	Erect
Muscles	Tense, spasms	Tense, spasms
Breathing rate	Increases	Increases
Pulse	Increases	Increases
Blood pressure	Increases	Increases
Skin of trunk, neck, face	Sex flush	Sex flush

Adapted from Cole T. by Glass DD: Sexuality and the spinal cord injured patient. In Oaks WW, Melchiode GA, Fisher I (eds): *Sex and the Life Cycle*, p 187. New York, Grune & Stratton, 1976. Reprinted with permission.

Table 24-2. Female Sexual Response Cycle

	Able-Bodied Female	Disabled Female
Wall of vagina	Moistens	±
Clitoris	Swells	Swells ±
Labia	Swell and open	Swell ±
Uterus	Contracts	±
Inner ⅔ of vagina	Expands	±
Outer ⅓ of vagina	Contracts	±
Nipples	Erect	Erect
Muscles	Tense, spasms	Tense, spasms
Breasts	Swell	Swell
Breathing	Increases	Increases
Pulse	Increases	Increases
Blood pressure	Increases	Increases
Skin of trunk, neck, face	Sex flush	Sex flush

Adapted from Cole T. by Glass DD: Sexuality and the spinal cord injured patient. In Oaks WW, Melchiode GA, Fisher I (eds): *Sex and the Life Cycle*, p 187. New York, Grune & Stratton, 1976. Reprinted with permission.

Table 24-3. Implications of Certain Disabilities/Dysfunction for Sexuality

Disability/ Dysfunction	Impact on Sexuality	Considerations
Cardiovascular	Decreased sexual activity due to fear Elevated blood pressure and heart rate Angina with exertion or stress	Monitor heart rate and grade sexual activity so body can deal with this physiologic exercise Use positions that are enjoyable and least taxing Do not have sex after a heavy meal or alcoholic beverages Include spouse/partner in discussions about sexual activity Take physician-prescribed medications before sex
Endocrine		
Gonadal disorders	Infertility Inability to ejaculate Impotence Amenorrhea	Hormone replacement therapy Psychological counseling
Diabetes mellitus	Varying impotence Retrograde ejaculation Absence of orgasm in female	Improved metabolic control through diet and/or insulin Suggestions for noncoital sexual activity Surgical implantation of penile prosthetic devices
Disorders of the thyroid	Decreased libido Dysmenorrhea Impaired fertility Weakness Fatigability	Reversible with re-establishment of metabolic control

(continued)

Table 24-3. *(continued)*

Disability/ Dysfunction	Impact on Sexuality	Considerations
Neurologic		
Cerebrovascular accident	Fear of another stroke	Inconclusive information regarding risks of sex
	Combination of mechanical difficulties (from decreased strength, coordination, or maneuverability), cognitive/emotional factors, paralysis, pain, spasticity, communication difficulty	Identify areas of intact sensation and focus lovemaking stimulation on those areas
		Define effective positions for sexual activity that use residual strength and coordination
	Drug side-effects	Use pillows to compensate for weak musculature
		Side-effects can be minimized with medical management and counseling
Epilepsy	Drug side-effects	Sexual behavior and sexual functioning usually normal
	Anxiety regarding seizure during sexual activity	
Multiple sclerosis	Episodic sexual dysfunction involving erection, ejaculation, decreased libido, orgasm, lack of vaginal lubrication	Plan sexual activity during levels of high energy
		Use vaginal lubricant to allow easy penetration
	Impaired sensation and muscle tone	Define positions for effective coitus
	Easy fatigability	Intervals of remission and exacerbation may result in varying styles of sexual activity
Cerebral palsy	Increased spasm/athetoid movement from arousal	Positioning for comfort and effectiveness
	Spasticity may make coitus painful or difficult	Medication or positioning to decrease spasticity
	Libido unimpaired	
	Genital sensation unimpaired	
Spinal Cord Injury	Capabilities vary regarding erection, ejaculation, orgasm, fertility, mechanical ability to engage in coitus or self-stimulation, and sexual satisfaction	Open, honest, sensitive counseling essential
		Common sense accurate individualized information using known facts and psychosocial characteristics of each situation
		May include catheter care, coital positioning, hygiene, and nongenital sex options
Amputation	Upper extremity dexterity difficulty	Positioning changes
	Lower extremity balance problems	Pain-relief methods such as biofeedback, medication, psychotherapy, TENS
	Pain or phantom sensation	
	Distorted body image	Time, rehabilitative therapy aimed toward independence and counseling as necessary to re-establish self-esteem.
Arthritis	Diminished sexual energy and responsiveness due to fatigue, pain, malaise, joint deformity	Analgesic effects of sexual intimacy may last for hours
	Inhibited libido due to corticosteroids	Plan sex activity when pain is least (midday)
		Coordinate medication effects and sex
		Use massage, heat during foreplay
		Incorporate energy- and joint-conservation techniques such as waterbed, support pillows, adaptive positioning for coitus
		Abstinence from coitus may need to be recommended in some situations (predisposition to fractures, delayed healing, and for several weeks after hip replacement)

Kolodny RC, Masters WH, Johnson VE: Textbook of Sexual Medicine. Boston, Little, Brown, 1966 cial situation. These suggestions should focus on education, attitudinal support, referral to appropriate diagnostic services or intensive sexuality counseling services as needed, and specific information to assist with functional problems (Table 24-3). Specific adaptations may involve ways of participating in nongenital sexual activity or various positions for coitus that minimize

pain. Information that considers the person's bladder function may be essential. For example, for persons with bladder impairment, it is recommended that the bladder be emptied prior to intercourse, whereas persons with a catheter may be advised to double back the catheter tubing over the penis to permit intercourse.[2,6]

A therapist who wishes to counsel a client regarding

Table 24-4.   *Suggestions for the Occupational Therapist in Dealing with Sexuality-Related Issues*

Issue	*Suggested Approach*
Healthy sexuality is a part of total rehabilitation, and all team members are responsible for helping the client achieve a better state of health.	Initiate discussion and endorse sexuality. Be aware of physiological mechanisms of sex. Recognize that it is difficult for many people to deal directly with explicit sexuality. Know when to refer a client to an appropriate team member for specific information or counseling.
Rehabilitation facilities are designed to promote constant interaction, sometimes with loss of privacy, but some activities require privacy for learning to occur.	Be sensitive to privacy needs. Don't overreact to human sexual behavior should it occur (*e.g.,* erection during ADL training). When appropriate, recommend opportunity for aloneness (*e.g.,* hospital pass for home visit).
Learning of social sexual skill should be expected and encouraged, just as people are expected to learn other ADL. Sexuality is a natural part of life, and awareness of sexuality belongs in the rehabilitation process.	Encourage sexual awareness and responsibility as part of ADL. Teach skills in attractive dressing and grooming techniques, including application of cosmetics, aftershave, and so forth. Teach skills in relating to others as appropriate to the client's need and lifestyle (*e.g.,* role-play slow dancing with a client with loss of coordination who plans to attend school dance on weekend with his girlfriend).
Methods of expressing sexuality can be developed by problem solving rather than punishment. Ignoring or reprimanding a disabled person for testing a self-image of a whole person may communicate that he/she is incompetent and "not okay."	Avoid overreacting to behavior with sexual content. Objectively share information with team members so that the behavior can be understood. Deal with the client as you would like to be dealt with. Encourage the client to discuss feelings with appropriate team members.
Sexuality is an early concern of many disabled people; acknowledging feelings will endorse honesty and responsibility. Denying our own sexual feelings could inhibit them in our clients.	Deal with personal aspects of therapy openly and sincerely. Be aware of your effect on a client, especially during dressing or bathing training. Acknowledge your client's effect on you. Realize that nonverbal communication can give the client input as to his/her own sexuality.
Some people are shy and need "permission" to speak freely about sexuality. The disabled person will appreciate sensitivity and concern. When sexuality is discussed, new disability may be avoided.	Recognize that we are all sexual beings. Be aware of the possibility of sexual response for the disabled. Anticipate sexual concerns and be prepared either to deal directly with them or to refer the person to another for help. Take the responsibility of becoming comfortable with your own sexuality.

Adapted from Cole TM: Program in Human Sexuality. University of Minnesota Medical Center, Minneapolis (unpublished material).

explicit sexuality should develop an increased understanding of his/her own attitudes and sexuality and become comfortable discussing these topics. All therapists should develop an ability to respond appropriately to clinical situations that reflect sexuality. Table 24-4 suggests an approach for the occupational therapist in dealing with sexuality-related issues and problems.

References

1. Conine JA, Evans JH: Sexual reactivation of chronically ill and disabled adults. J Allied Health 11:251, 1982

2. Heslinga K, Schellen AMCM, Verkuyl A: Not Made of Stone: The Sexual Problems of Handicapped People. Springfield, IL, Charles C Thomas, 1974

3. Isaacson J, Delgado HE: Sex counseling for those with spinal cord injuries. Soc Casework 55:622, 1974

4. Kolodny RC, Masters WH, Johnson VE: Textbook of Sexual Medicine. Boston, Little, Brown, 1979

5. Masters WH, Johnson VE: Human Sexual Response. Boston, Little, Brown, 1966

6. Mooney TO, Cole TM, Chilgren RA: Sexual options for paraplegics and quadriplegics. Boston, Little, Brown, 1975

7. Sidman JM: Sexual functioning and the physically disabled adult. Am J Occup Ther 31:81, 1977

Implementation of the Occupational Therapy Process in Specific Areas of Practice

CHAPTER 25

Psychiatry and Mental Health

SECTION *1*

Sharan L. Schwartzberg

Introduction   *and Elizabeth G. Tiffany*

Different objects present themselves to consciousness as constituents of different spheres of reality.
Peter L. Berger and Thomas Luckmann[1]

The term *mental health* covers a broad spectrum of concerns that have been of primary interest to occupational therapists since occupational therapy began. In all parts of life, the mental health of the individual is a vital component of adaptation. What, then, of "mental illness," or of the shades of emotional, cognitive, and psychomotor problems in adaptation that become the focus of psychiatric intervention?

If we look for definitions, perhaps the most effective one today is a functional one. People who, through the centuries, have been called mentally ill, psychiatrically disabled, or maladjusted have been those who have lacked the ability to organize their thoughts, feelings, attitudes, and actions in a way that would permit them to function within society for either a brief or extended period of time. Such a broad definition seems necessary. The phrase "ability to organize" covers a wide range of etiologies, including physiologic, toxic, psychologic, and social. Such a definition permits consideration of the severe psychological pathologies that sometimes accompany physical illness or trauma and require special attention if rehabilitation is to be effective. It does not exclude the possibility that the mentally retarded or the neurologically impaired may have components of psychiatric disability. The phrase "within society" recognizes that the environments and social systems in which people live are varied and that what constitutes healthy behavior in one may be seen as highly undesirable, perverted, or ill in another. We find that, at the outer edges of our definition, the distinctions between "mental" and "physical," "individual" and "societal," tend to blur.

Occupational therapy, like medicine, is concerned

with the restoration or maintenance of function in people who are ill or otherwise disabled. Like medicine, occupational therapy must always reflect and act upon the knowledge of the time. What is known and understood about people and their functioning dictates what is perceived as possible. Like medicine, occupational therapy will always be bound to some degree by the values of the time and the place in which it provides service. Occupational therapy, like medicine, is practiced by people, individuals who bring to their profession their own strengths and weaknesses, value systems, needs, and unique ways of perceiving, thinking, feeling, and acting. These factors explain some of the differences one finds in occupational therapy practice, especially in psychiatric settings. They also compel us to define clearly and in detail the premises of psychiatric occupational therapy practice.

It is an illusion to proclaim any definition of occupational therapy practice in mental health as universal. Since the late 1960s, vast changes have occurred in the field. For example, the 1963 edition of this textbook, now only historical material, included this statement: "Without a transference and countertransference problem arising in the relationships with the patient, no real therapeutic practice will be achieved."[2] More than 20 years later, we know that intrapsychic exploration can be toxic for many individuals, that it can promote unnecessary regression in occupational functioning, and, further, that some occupational therapists consider it outside the profession's domain. By 1971, the time of this book's fourth edition, state hospitals were being deinstitutionalized. In developing a community mental health center's partial-hospitalization program, psychodynamic theory became secondary to knowledge of social systems theory.

This chapter is an effort to synopsize current occupational therapy process in psychiatry and mental health.

It no doubt contains some biases and is at times skewed toward hospital care because of trends in practice and the authors' educational beliefs and experiences. Further, the practice area is explained primarily from the perspective of a clinical reasoning process. No attempts will be made to detail specialized frames of reference or techniques used in evaluation and treatment. Finally, underlying this presentation is the premise that each patient is an individual whose unique set of interacting biological, psychological, social, and behavioral circumstances require selective application of occupational therapy processes.

The chapter is divided into six sections. Section 2 examines the historical roots of psychiatric occupational therapy in the societal changes of this country. Each decade is reviewed as psychiatric occupational therapy adapts, develops, and institutes changes. Section 3 explains the basic principles of psychiatric occupational therapy practice. After an examination of the roles and functions and theoretical foundations of practice, the generic tools of practice are overviewed in the Section 4. Section 5 explains the generic processes of practice in some detail. Emphasis is given to evaluation because of its complex nature and critical role. Section 6 attempts to summarize and highlight issues and trends in occupational therapy in mental health and psychiatry in the near future.

References

1. Berger PL, Luckmann T: The social construction of reality: A treatise in the sociology of knowledge, p 21. Garden City, NY, Anchor Books, 1967
2. Dundon HD: Psychiatric occupational therapy. In Willard HS, Spackman CS (eds): Occupational Therapy, 3rd ed, p 64. Philadelphia, JB Lippincott, 1963

SECTION 2
Historical Roots *Elizabeth G. Tiffany*

On close perusal of the history of psychiatric occupational therapy, it is evident that there are threads of thought that are woven into the fabric of the profession as a whole. These constant strands are what have given the profession its consistent uniqueness through the years. Competence, mastery, self-image, motivation, total function, adaptation, integration, satisfaction — these are some of the key words that appear throughout the literature of occupational therapy.

Holistic Approach

A thoughtful look at the meanings of these key words reveals a fundamental belief that has permeated the history of occupational therapy: the belief that human beings are whole, that mind and body are intricately linked, and that anything that impinges on or influences one must affect the other. Dunton, one of the founders of occupational therapy, said in 1922, "The primary objects to be obtained by occupational therapy may be divided into two groups, mental and physical, although it is impossible to divorce these functions."[14] To work toward the restoration of function in their physically disabled clients, occupational therapists have relied on psychological involvement in the *meanings* attached to the *doing* process. To work toward restoration of function in their mentally ill clients, occupational therapists have used movement, doing, touching, and sensing; that is, physical factors. In working with all kinds of clients, occupational therapists have been concerned with stress, anxiety, tension, and learning, all of which have long been known to have both emotional and physical components.

Moral Treatment

It is generally thought that the principles of "moral treatment" formed the base for modern psychiatric practice and for the specific concern with the uses of activity for treatment as we know it in occupational therapy. What are the tenets of moral treatment which, in the late eighteenth century, were so great a departure from the existing beliefs and practices with regard to the mentally ill? Moral treatment was based on the belief that mental illness occurred as the result of physical and psychological, not mystical, factors. Environmental stresses were recognized as major causes. Therefore, attention to a patient's environment or milieu was a primary concern, and institutions for the mentally ill gave attention to providing pleasant surroundings, kind and consistent treatment, and opportunities for patients to be productive. There was a belief that, no matter how ill or bizarre the patient appeared, there were still healthy parts to his or her personality; therefore, treatment should include ways for the patient to develop self-esteem.

The institution to which the mentally ill were sent became their community. At a time when cultural and social systems were homogeneous and communication and transportation methods were limited, the establishment of a fairly uniform institutional community was possible. Patients were committed to institutional care for long periods of time, in some instances for life. Moral treatment sought to develop in the institutional community a sense of family living. The milieu was one of daily routines, with chores and responsibilities shared by staff and patients for the good of all. Staff members provided role models for the patients. When staff members and patients came from the same kinds of cultural and ethnic backgrounds, as they often did during this period, such a milieu could be quite successful.

Because the work ethic was dominant in society, work prevailed as a major means for the individual to experience satisfaction and purpose in life. "The patient is now one of our best workers, and in other respects improves much . . . I had the most rational conversation with him that I had ever had . . . It was truly pleasing to discover such rationality."[12] So wrote Isaac Bonsall, who in 1817 became the first superintendent of the Friends Asylum in Frankford, located in Philadelphia. Bonsall was describing the effect of occupation on a severely disturbed patient.

Development of Psychiatric Occupational Therapy
Emergence of the Profession

Occupational therapy developed into an identified profession during the years after World War I (see Chapter 2). At that time, Dr. Adolf Meyer and Eleanor Clarke Slagle developed the use of carefully planned goals and methods for promoting health through the use of activities. It was in the 1920s that Meyer restated the principles of moral treatment and gave a context and philosophy for the development of the profession of occupational therapy.[36] At the same time, Slagle began training occupational "therapeutists." She divided rehabilitation efforts into three distinct groups: those directed toward patients who in all likelihood would continue their lives within the institution, those directed toward return to the community, and those directed toward prevention through the use of a prehospital work clinic. The approaches of Meyer and Slagle to the use of activities and relationships, examined in the light of today's knowledge and practice, were remarkably modern — they emphasized developmental needs and had a sense of the importance of preparing the individual patient to function within society.[51,52]

In the 1920s, behaviorism dominated psychology, while psychoanalytical theory dominated psychiatry. The pioneers in occupational therapy, however, focused on the patient's outer reality and functional behavior. In the institutional setting, the patient was involved in work assignments. These assignments seemed effective in promoting adjustment.

William Rush Dunton, Jr., the psychiatrist whose commitment to and belief in the principles of occupational therapy were a cornerstone of the profession, wrote several books and articles on the subject. In *Prescribing Occupational Therapy*, published in 1928, he systematically categorized activities and kinds of patients. He thoughtfully delineated principles for matching activities with the needs of patients in a way that could be therapeutic. He classified activities in terms of their demands for attention, repetition, physical or intellectual effort, social factors, and criteria for rest, surprise, or creativity. He simplified the categories of mental disorders and suggested the kinds of activities that could be most desirable and most therapeutic with each category. He also described the importance of the therapist's approach and attitude for each:

For the manic — steady, quieting activity to reduce motor restlessness and train concentration; sedative activity, rhythmic and repetitive, with little variety.

For the depressed — stimulating activity, although the therapist may need to give a preliminary course of stereotyped activity. The activity should have the potential for replacing the patient's preoccupations with depressive ideation. The therapist must use tact and be sensitive.

For the demented (dementia praecox or schizophrenia) — re-education activities to train better habits of thought and action. Social activities that would place the individual into simple, structured work with others — activities which demand constant attention to overcome daydreaming and activities to emphasize reality contact.

For the paranoid — activities which would create or stimulate interest in concrete things such as caring for goldfish or canaries or working in hospital industries.

For the psychoneurotic — activities to reduce egocentricity and to allow sublimation of repressed conflicts.[14]

In Dunton's work, we see a major attempt to analyze activities, to categorize patient needs, and to suggest therapeutic approaches. He considered the core of the occupational therapy process to be making the correct matches among these elements.

Other proponents of the clear, deliberate application of activities to meet specific patient needs were Louis J. Haas and L. Cody Marsh. Haas' publications, *Practical Occupational Therapy* and *Occupational Therapy for the Mentally and Nervously Ill*, contain interesting detailed descriptions of crafts projects in addition to theoretical formulations about the use of crafts.[24,25] Haas stated emphatically that "being busy is not necessarily therapeutic."

Marsh, in a speech at the Sixteenth Annual Conference of the American Occupational Therapy Association (AOTA), defined the uses of carefully matched work assignments as therapy.[30]

Aides to the Psychiatrist

In the 1930s and 1940s, psychiatric occupational therapists clearly identified themselves as aides to the psychiatrist in treating the mentally ill. The occupational therapist's activities included music, psychodrama, bibliotherapy, recreation, work, and arts and crafts. In effect, occupational therapy was concerned with the whole person and his or her total life of work and play within the institutional setting.

At the same time that occupational therapy developed as a profession, there began a search for theoretical concepts that would provide frames of reference for treatment. Therapists began to be dissatisfied with basing their practice purely on intuitive and empirical success. Occupational therapists saw their roles as closely aligned with the psychiatrist responsible for patients. The situation in which they worked involved a written prescription from the psychiatrist or physician before the occupational therapist could initiate treatment. The prescription gave basic information about the patient, including special precautions, and requested that the occupational therapist provide specified services. The occupational therapist's areas of service to the psychiatrist included: (1) diagnostic aid (through observation of the patient's behavior and performance in occupational therapy), (2) facilitating the patient's adjustment to the hospital environment, (3) supplementing shock therapy, (4) supplementing psychoanalytic therapy, and (5) habit training.[52]

Psychoanalytical Bases

The theoretical base for occupational therapy as a true intervention and treatment modality within a psychoanalytical frame of reference was specified by William C. Menninger. His six categories of the functions of activities as treatment are: (1) as an outlet for aggression and hostility, (2) to provide opportunities for advantageous identifications, (3) as atonement for guilt, (4) as a means of obtaining love, (5) to provide opportunities to act out fantasies, and (6) to allow for an experience of creative work.[35] The occupational therapist working within this context needed basic knowledge of the principles of psychoanalytical psychiatry, especially of defense mechanisms, as well as sensitivity to the potentials of given activities for fulfilling the functions listed.

Although intuition, common sense, and empirical success provided the only guidelines for selecting activities, it is evident from the literature of the time that there were tendencies to seek a more scientific base and to define occupational therapy professionally.

Electric and insulin shock therapies were being employed. These presented special challenges to the occupational therapist. The psychiatric casualties of World War II provided the impetus for the development of programs under the Veterans Administration. One is struck by the number of articles written by physicians in collaboration with occupational therapists during this period.

Training Programs for Aides

Obviously, for the number of patients hospitalized, there were never enough trained therapists, especially as training programs grew longer and more academic. The professional occupational therapist, in many instances, became a program planner and a supervisor of aides, particularly in the large hospitals. It became a major concern of professional therapists to find ways to transmit theoretical knowledge to untrained staff members and to facilitate the communication of treatment goals and methods. In the large hospitals, psychiatrically trained physicians were also in short supply. Although the psychiatrist's written prescription could serve an important purpose, effective communication of this kind often was more an ideal than a reality.

Radical Changes of the 1950s

Psychosurgery

At the beginning of the 1950s, in addition to shock therapies, psychosurgery in the form of the prefrontal lobotomy was added to the list of medical attempts to cure the mentally ill or at least to provide symptomatic relief. Occupational therapists had to find ways to work effectively with the lobotomized patient, which was often discouraging. Psychosurgery, although initially considered promising, was to be a short-lived form of treatment.

Activity Analysis

Psychodynamic principles for treatment and activity analysis were explored in greater depth in the 1950s. The occupational therapist began to look at the patient's behavior and symptoms in terms of "externalized or internalized aggression, projection, withdrawal and regression." Gail Fidler, in an article in the *American Journal of Occupational Therapy* in 1948, presented an outline of activity analysis through which the materials, tools, actions, and interpersonal relationship potentials of activities could be explored.[17] Professional occupational therapists attempted to match activities with patient needs based on this kind of thinking.

Case Study

TIME: 1949

PLACE: An occupational therapy shop in a private psychiatric hospital

The occupational therapist enters her office, a screened-off area in the back of the bright, pleasantly decorated large room known as the "OT Shop." (A sign, carefully painted in old English script, hangs outside the door to designate this fact.) She stops for a moment to smooth her starched white uniform and notes that she will soon have to have her hair cut or fasten it up. On her desk lies a copy of *Discovering Ourselves* by Strecker and Appel,[47] an old book, but one she finds stimulating and helpful, not only in understanding her patients, but also in understanding herself.

Her patients have just left, and the day is about over. There were ten in this last group, men from the locked ward. An attendant brought them down to her shop and stayed with them for the hour they were there. She thinks, with satisfaction, how much better it is in this bright new area than it was in the dingy basement shop next to the boiler room. It was more than the change that felt good—it was the idea that the hospital superintendent seemed to appreciate and support occupational therapy. Until the shop was moved 2 months ago, she had needed to take supplies to the men on the ward. It seems so much better to get them out of that atmosphere. Here, she could give them so many more things. There are floor looms, where patients can beat out their hostility on rugs, and there is a bicycle jigsaw and a workbench. Good masculine activities. And, of course, the radio, so they could have music. The only drawback is that the men can come only when they're on good behavior. That's a problem she's been thinking a lot about. She was planning to get together with the ward personnel to see if there would be some way to put a punching bag or something right on the ward for the men to use whenever they began to feel upset.

Now, however, her mind is focused on one patient. He is new in the hospital and she had already received a written prescription for occupational therapy from his physician. She thumbs through a pile of cards on her desk until she finds his prescription. The card reads:

NAME: John Jones   AGE: 31
DIAGNOSIS: Schizophrenia, paranoid type

O.T. PRESCRIPTION: Activities to divert attention from hallucinations, improve reality testing and attention span, increase socialization

---

PRECAUTIONS: Patient has auditory hallucinations. May become assaultive. Currently being treated with insulin coma therapy. Observe for insulin reactions.

PHYSICIAN: *M. Brown, M.D.*

WARD: 5B

John Jones had come to OT that day. He seemed mild-mannered and polite but a little vague in his thinking, probably because he'd had an insulin treatment earlier. That was the problem with the patients who were getting insulin or electric shock therapy; they sometimes seemed to forget everything or be really out of touch. John Jones had picked copper tooling to do. This had seemed a good choice to the occupational therapist because it would require some planning and attention; its actions involved hard pressure but also controlling, and it was masculine. He already was planning to use it as a gift. He had chosen a picture of two sheep, with a little lamb standing between them. When he started to work on it, he seemed able to follow the directions all right. He said that the little lamb reminded him of himself, in between his mother and his wife. The occupational therapist jots down a note to mention that to his physician. She also decides to set aside time to read John Jones' chart before he comes to the shop tomorrow.

The occupational therapist then opens a cabinet and takes down rolls of brightly colored crepe paper, some construction paper, paste, and a box of blunt-pointed scissors. She places these items on a cart, ready to take to the women's locked ward first thing in the morning. They would need an early start to make the decorations for the party that evening.

One more thing, before she could call it a day. She picks up the telephone and calls the lady in charge of the hospital auxiliary. She needs to check a few more details about the OT sale next week.

"Sometimes," she thinks, "I really do feel like a jack-of-all-trades, but I like what I'm doing and I feel sure that the activities I give my patients help them. They know I'm interested in them and accept them as human beings." She remembers, in a flash, having seen the movie *The Snake Pit* the week before. "Thank goodness it doesn't have to be like that any more," she thinks as she locks up the cabinets and desk, puts on her coat, and leaves. □

Psychopharmacology

The mid-1950s saw a revolution take place in mental hospitals. The introduction of psychopharmacology, the use of tranquilizers and psychic energizers, opened a new world of possibilities. The medicines seemed to reduce most of the gross pathological symptoms and acting-out behaviors that previously had interfered with treatment.

Therapeutic Community

Social psychiatry and anthropology explored new vistas for handling the problem of mental illness. Maxwell Jones' "therapeutic community" in England received attention.[27] The therapeutic milieu, open-door policies, halfway house, family treatment, aftercare services, and volunteer involvement all became possibilities.

Diagnostic Categories

The American Psychiatric Association, in 1952, published the first edition of *Diagnostic and Statistical Manual of Mental Disorders*, the first official manual to describe diagnostic categories of mental problems. These descriptions reflected the view of Adolf Meyer that mental disorders were reactions of the personality to psychological, social, and biological factors.

Social Adaptation

Occupational therapists at this time began to look in greater depth at the social adaptation of their patients and to focus on the meaning and use of activities and their interpersonal components in treatment. Two major events took place in psychiatric occupational therapy. One was a book; the other was a study that culminated in a book. In 1954, *Introduction to Psychiatric Occupational Therapy* was written by Gail S. Fidler, OTR, and Jay W. Fidler, M.D. This book represented professional occupational therapy as the use of productive activities as treatment in a collaborative effort between the occupational therapist and the psychotherapist. It suggested the concept of the occupational therapy area as a laboratory in which the patient could experiment with new ways of handling emotions and developing living skills. It presented a much refined, psychoanalytically flavored activity analysis process; suggested ways in which groups could be used to facilitate treatment; and encouraged the study of projective techniques. While acknowledging that many occupational therapists were working without psychiatric supervision to the extent described, it encouraged occupational therapists to formulate treatment goals and programs in the most meaningful way on their own and to work toward effective communications with all involved staff. The Fidlers candidly stated, "These views cannot be presented without the realization that occupational therapy is a young field and that there are great potentialities for future development. This is especially emphasized by the fact that the entire field of psychiatry is still in its youth and therefore any of the subsidiary techniques must also be as elementary if not more so." [18]

In 1956, following a 2-year study funded by a grant to the AOTA by the National Institute of Mental Health, a conference of leaders in the field of psychiatric occupational therapy was held at Boiling Springs, Pennsylvania. Under the leadership of Elizabeth P. Ridgway and Gail S. Fidler, the participants explored and questioned many emerging issues of psychiatric occupational therapy practice. These were identified as *use of self, of group and group techniques, and of activities; creation of the therapeutic milieu; development of special treatment goals as a supplement to psychotherapy;* contributions to psychodynamic formulations through the *use of personality, social, and skills evaluations;* and, finally, *bridging the gap between community living and the hospital.*[54] In her introduction to the published proceedings of the conference, Wilma West said, "Several developments and changes in the treatment of psychiatric patients during recent years made this project a timely one. These include an awareness of the reversibility of the process of mental illness, the growth of the team approach and resulting collaboration of all concerned, utilization of group interaction and an increasing emphasis on the total individual and the milieu in which he functions." [54] This is a fair assessment of the state of psychiatric occupational therapy at that time.

Case Study

TIME: 1957

PLACE: OT shop in a large, progressive state institution

Barbara and Jack, OTRs, are seated at the end of a long table near a window in the large, somewhat cluttered OT room. They've just come back from lunch and are working together warping a table loom.

Two copies of the *American Journal of Occupational Therapy* lie on the windowsill.

Barbara comments to Jack, "Did you see the article in the September Journal about the study they made—the one that proved that if the occupational therapist is able to work on developing relationships with the patients, the patients become more active?" [42]

Jack replies, "Nope. But it makes sense, doesn't it? I know that sometimes it looks as if I'm goofing off when I just sit and talk with the guys from Ward B, but they really do seem to want to come to OT, and I think I get further with them . . . you know . . . it's like they trust me more."

"Yes," Barbara says, and adds, "By the way, has Dr. Brown started having team meetings for Ward B? He said he wanted to because soon they want to make it an open ward. He wants to start having ward meetings for all the patients too. He really wants to make sure that everybody's involved in the changes."

Jack recalls, "They're supposed to start next week, at eight o'clock Wednesday morning. That's the time when most of the nurses and attendants are around. I wonder how it will work. Incidentally, since you mentioned the *Journal,* I did look at that article about changes in OT due to tranquilizing drugs.[15] Did you see it? I guess because I'm a recently graduated OT, I'm not so aware of the differences the new drugs are making. I know the things they told us about in school, the kinds of crazy actions we heard about. Well, I just haven't seen them, at least not many of them. What worries me, though, is that half the time I feel as if I'm working with zombies. The article says that a lot of your time and energy used to go into finding ways to channel excess drives, controlling hyperactivity, and so forth. Is that true? I almost think that would make OT more interesting!"

Replying to Jack's comments, Barbara says, "Oh, I don't know about that. It got pretty wild sometimes. Now, in some ways it seems easier, but in other ways it seems harder—like working through a mask. And we've got a whole new set of things to watch for and report. By the way, has Dick complained to you about his eyesight? He was trying to draw the squares on that chessboard he's making and he was having an awful time. Said everything was going blurry on him. Better check it out. Uh-oh, it's one o'clock and the crowd is about to arrive."

They fasten down the pieces of warp with tape, open the supply cabinets, and unlock the OT room doors. Jack says, "See you," and retreats through a back door that leads to the men's shop.

A group of 20 women, in hospital dresses, presses through the door. Two nursing aides accompany the group. As if preprogrammed, they go to the supply cabinets, take out boxes neatly labeled with their names, and seat themselves around the table. Some begin to work on embroidery and some on knitting;

one goes to an upright loom on which a braided rug has been started. Two of the women, apparently new, stand still until the aides talk them into taking seats at the table. Barbara sits down near them and suggests to them that they draw some pictures. She gives them crayons and construction paper. Barbara is uncomfortable. She has been reading, for the second time, the book, *Introduction to Psychiatric Occupational Therapy*.[18] The scene before her seems so very far removed from the exciting ideas about what OT could be. She begins to think about things they could do, especially if the hospital really goes into teams.

She moves about the group of patients, offering help to some, encouraging others, stopping to listen while one complains about a problem in the dining room, occasionally chatting with the whole group about some current event and trying to interest the group in planning an afternoon party to which they would invite their physicians, visitors, or any special friends. The atmosphere is quiet and subdued. It is hard to feel enthusiasm. On another level, Barbara's mind is racing ahead. She's devising a form—one that would list the kinds of information the therapist gets about patients when they do activities—the way they use the materials and the way they relate to the OT and to each other. And she's planning a new method for reporting to the physicians and nurses. And, remembering that the hospital has just hired a volunteer director, she's thinking about ways volunteers can help them in new kinds of activities. She'll have to talk to Jack about all this. ☐

Community Mental Health

The Mental Health Study Act was passed in 1955, establishing the Joint Commission on Mental Illness and Health. The charge of the Commission was to establish priorities and appropriate methods of services for the mentally ill. *Action for Mental Health*, the report of the commission, was published in 1961.[1] This report proposed a concerted attack on mental illness in the following ways: (1) better distribution and community-oriented philosophic reorientation of psychiatrists; (2) increasing participation of lay people at various levels in programs of prevention, treatment, and rehabilitation; (3) shift of emphasis from institutional to community services; and (4) plans for shared federal, state, and local funding of community mental health centers. Thus was launched the community mental health movement.

In 1963, the Community Mental Health Act was passed, mandating the National Institute of Mental Health to establish and fund community mental health centers in local catchment areas with populations from 75,000 to 200,000. This gave impetus to the development of new approaches to treatment. Transactional analysis, gestalt therapy, and milieu therapy came to the fore. Family therapy became a treatment of choice for some individuals, on the interesting premise that the mentally ill person in a family may simply be expressing the symptoms for a whole family's pathology.[41] Behavioral approaches to treatment such as desensitization and operant conditioning techniques, developed by Joseph Wolpe and others, grew rapidly.[56] "Token economies" or behaviorally oriented milieus were developed and seemed promising, particularly in treating the long-term chronically disabled and institutionalized mentally ill, the mentally retarded, and some kinds of childhood psychoses.

Research efforts were intensified in the areas of biochemistry, neurophysiology, and metabolic, including genetic, abnormalities. Psychosomatic illnesses were explored in greater depth. The wholeness of human function and the connections between mind, body, and emotions were proved repeatedly. Each new research finding, it seemed, pointed to new questions and new areas for exploration. Research efforts and techniques were aided by the enormous capabilities introduced by the growth of computer technology.

There was a shift away from emphasis on the long-term, deep methods of treatment by psychoanalysis toward exploring ways in which individuals could be returned to function as rapidly as possible. Partial hospitalization programs opened so that patients could continue their lives in the community and attend treatment programs during the day or evening. Mental health professionals, including occupational therapists, began to visit the homes of their patients and to look into important aspects of work and recreation in the community. In some settings, patients began to be called *clients*, *residents*, or *members*. The atmosphere of psychiatry had taken on a new and optimistic perspective.

Creativity of the 1960s

The worlds in which psychiatric occupational therapists worked were greatly expanded by these changes. The spirit of experimentation, of questioning, and of unrest which characterized society as a whole during the 1960s permeated occupational therapy as well. Knowledge grew, and new techniques were developed for the management of the mentally ill.

The second *Diagnostic and Statistical Manual of Mental Disorders* (DSM-II) of the American Psychiatric Association was published in 1968 and represented an effort to base the classification of mental disorders on the corresponding section of the eighth revision of the *International Classification of Diseases* (ICD-8) that was published at the same time. This edition of the DSM, like the ICD, did not attempt to define the diagnostic categories in terms of a theoretical framework, as the previous one had, but simply gave descriptions of the classifications.

In 1963, the Fidlers wrote a second book, *Occupational Therapy: A Communication Process in Psychiatry*.[19] They emphasized the enormous potential of the occupational therapy process as another vital language for communication, especially in view of its use of the nonverbal and its work regarding object relationships. They identified three major emphases for occupational therapy in psychiatry: (1) *treatment*, directly applied intervention in a pathological process to effect change in the patient, with subcategories defined as *psychoanalytic*, *supportive*, and *directive* (repressive); (2) the *mental health process*, by enhancing the milieu and supporting the healthy parts of the individual; and (3) *rehabilitation*, helping the patient learn to use existing strengths more effectively. This book provided carefully analyzed and synthesized material, especially regarding the meaning of activities and interpersonal transactions in the activity process. Though strongest in its psychoanalytical orientation, it acknowledged as well the changes that were taking place both in psychiatry as a whole and in psychiatric occupational therapy.

The early 1960s were also influenced by the development of instruments for evaluation or assessment of the client. This was a period when there was significant interest in the use of the *Azima Battery*.[10] Gail Fidler also developed a battery, similar to the Azima Battery, through which information about a client's psychodynamics could be obtained.[16] These two batteries, and a number of local modifications of them, used art media and clay. The client's behavior and his or her projections were interpreted to provide meaningful data to aid in treatment planning.

Cognitive – Perceptual – Motor Research

Another very significant development was taking place during the 1960s. A. Jean Ayres was beginning to publish her observations of perceptual motor development and dysfunction in children.[9] Her research, which is still going on, was based on neurophysiology and seemed to point to some areas of major concern to the occupational therapist working in psychiatry. Lorna Jean King, in Arizona, began a daring experiment with chronic schizophrenics and exhaustive research in the literature on perception, neurophysiology, and mental illness. She adapted and applied the theoretical base and some of the techniques developed by Ayres. The results of her work with severely regressed, institutionalized, chronically ill, schizophrenic patients were most encouraging. By the end of the 1960s, it appeared that continued research and application of *sensorimotor-integrative* techniques for certain groups of patients was indeed indicated and contained heuristic value in terms of other, related psychiatric concerns.

Developmental Theory

In psychological and educational circles during this time, there was a growth of interest in the work of Piaget. Developmental theory, especially theories of cognitive development, were being explored generally. Psychiatric occupational therapists began to explore the significance of Piaget's work as it might relate to the occupational therapy process in psychiatry.

Activities Therapists

It should be noted that, with the increased attention to direct services for the mentally ill, there were not enough trained occupational therapists to fill the critical positions in both institutions and community. New activity specialties grew up: therapeutic recreation, art, music, dance, drama, and horticulture. These specialties grew from at least two roots: (1) independently and in a parallel stream of thought with occupational therapy, based on existing knowledge in education and psychology; and (2) as an outgrowth of the training of workers in occupational therapy in the two preceding decades. Each new discipline using activities has sought to develop its own professional identity, its own special areas of practice, and its own research base. Taking as its foundation the same base as occupational therapy, namely that activity can be used for evaluation and for treatment, the new activity specialties presented a challenge to occupational therapy to refine its own theory and practice and to work toward developing viable ways of communicating and cooperating with them.

Funding for a Consultant

Under the Social Rehabilitation Services Grant (#123), the AOTA was funded in 1964 to have a full-time consultant in psychiatric rehabilitation in the National Office. Through the efforts of this consultant, and with the backing of the Association, a number of regional and national institutes were held across the United States. The main foci of these workshops, which were held between 1964 and 1968, were supervision, group process, object relations, and education. In addition to the effects of deepening the knowledge base and strengthening the skills of practicing therapists, there was a concomitant development of a sense of community among them, as they shared in the search for greater professional effectiveness.

The project director for this particular grant was June Mazer. Actually, the project RSA No. 123 had been started in 1958 as a consultancy program in physical dysfunction; at that time, Irene Hollis was director. Mary Alice Coombs joined the project in 1961, and it became a joint physical – psychiatric consultancy. In December 1962, the physical dysfunction phase was concluded. The psychiatric phase continued until 1968. Fourteen regional institutes were held on group process, administration, object relations, and evaluation, and 21 national institutes were held on education and advanced object relations.

Search for a Comprehensive Theory

The Psychiatric Special Interest Group of the Council on Practice of the AOTA became especially active on a nationwide basis during the 1960s. There was a surge of interest in exploring ways to incorporate the expanding approaches and the ever-widening knowledge base into occupational therapy practice. Local special interest groups flourished in many areas and became forums in which practicing therapists studied together, shared their questions and their ideas, and supported each other as they faced the critical issues emerging in psychiatry as a whole. The Psychiatric Special Interest Group, on a national level, participated in a number of special projects.

In 1968, the *American Journal of Occupational Therapy* invited occupational therapists practicing in psychiatry to submit papers describing the application of concepts to practice. The resulting issue of the *Journal* might be considered a landmark, as the authors attempted to define theoretical frames of reference and to describe viable approaches to their use. The words of the introduction to the special section describe the situation of occupational therapy in psychiatry at that time: "It is evident that many therapists are involved in the struggle to formulate and/or apply various theories in their practices, even though none of the submitted papers proposed a truly comprehensive theory of occupational therapy. Each article is accompanied by critical discussions and an author's response. We hope that these will stimulate further critical thinking and discussion. Our dream is that this special section may herald the beginning of a period rich in clinical exploration and research."[34] The four articles and the conference report included in this issue focused attention on the difficulties of developing such a comprehensive theory. The authors identified the work still to be done by describing both their thought and their practice.[13,33,39,49,53]

Following the institutes on object relations in 1967, a small group of therapists met in Albion, Michigan, to attempt to relate "a large number of divergent theories and thoughts to a specific framework that would include all aspects of the organism."[33] The object relations institutes and their culminating seminar attempted to explore in some depth the existing knowledge bases in anthropology, sociology, psychology, neurophysiology, and philosophy, as well as in psychiatry. There seemed to be little doubt that all of these could be significant in contributing to the knowledge base of occupational therapy. This was a most ambitious task, and the problem seemed to be one of providing bridges among all the possibilities. The charge was stated, "A necessary step toward building a body of knowledge specifically related to the kind of experience occupational therapy is able to provide is a frame of reference which utilizes a truly holistic developmental approach."[33]

The climate of optimism, enthusiasm, and investigation characterizing psychiatric occupational therapy at this time was reflected in a number of articles which were published during 1969 and 1970. Mary Reilly and her colleagues and students at the University of Southern California began to make their contributions to the field through the study of the work–play continuum, the patient's real world, and concepts of competence as the keys to the theoretical base of psychiatric occupational therapy.

The "occupational behavior" frame of reference for occupational therapy in psychiatry, as explored and proposed by Reilly, has taken the earliest principles and approaches of occupational therapy, as practiced in "moral treatment" and expressed in 1922 by Adolf Meyer, and examined them in depth and in the light of current psychological and sociological literature. This group proposed that occupational therapy shift its "initial perspective of patients from diagnostic labels to those of occupational roles of worker, student, housewife, retiree, preschooler and even career patient. . . ."[31] Occupational therapists were urged to look into the influences of the experiences found in childhood play.

In 1970, a symposium, "The Skill Continuum from Play through Work," was conducted in Boston under the sponsorship of the United States Department of Health, Education and Welfare's Maternal and Child Health Service. The papers presented were published in the *American Journal of Occupational Therapy* in September 1971.[11,22,26,32,37,48,55] The important message of this orientation was expressed by Matsutsuyu: "It was found that the perspective based on pathology held few guidelines for working knowledge of healthy function. It is not enough to accept the definition of health as the absence of disease."[31] The framework for this thinking had been expressed earlier by Reilly when she said: "Play, in a chronological or longitudinal sense, we believe, is the antecedent preparation area for work. In a cross-sectional sense, we have found it clinically useful to see an adult social-recreation pattern of behavior as a sublatent support to a work pattern. The entire developmental continuum of play and work we designate as occupational behavior."[45]

Case Study

TIME: 1969

PLACE: The OT office in a day program in a mental hospital of medium size

Alice, the occupational therapist, sits at her desk, writing a note. She has just finished working with a group that is planning an issue of the program's newspaper. The clients in the group are Don, a middle-aged man who is just recovering from a depression; Marie, an obese young woman whose obsessive-compulsive tendencies have interfered with her ability to work at her job; and Jim, a 19-year-old man who is suffering from an anxiety neurosis.

"How can I express what seemed to be happening when Jim and Don and Marie were starting to plan the next issue of the newspaper?" she thinks, her pen poised above the paper. "It was as if Don and Marie were Jim's mother and father, and he was their little child. And Jim seemed to fit right into that role. Maybe it's because Don and Marie really have had a lot more experience with the paper. On the other hand, we have seen so much of Jim's dependency in just about every aspect of his life. We've seen it in our evaluations too. This is probably just another expression of that. Putting the paper out could be a good way to help him grow, because he certainly has the basic skills. I'll talk with Don and Marie about letting Jim do the typing first . . . then maybe they'll show him how to do the paste-up, if he's interested."

At this point, there's a knock on the door, and a pleasant-faced woman, the unit's social worker, pokes her head in and says, "They're going to run the videotape of the activity group again, so the group can watch. Maybe you'd better be there for the feedback session."

Alice gets up and goes to the door saying, "You bet. I want to have another look at the way Jim handled the situation. I have a feeling he may want to talk about it. By the way did you want to borrow my Arieti?[8] And sometime could you let me look at your *Freedom to Learn?*"[46] ☐

Consumerism and Prevention in the 1970s

In American society, the early 1970s was a time of some disenchantment. Out of the chaotic and creative flux of the late 1960s, there emerged a public tiredness. The Vietnam War dragged on, draining off money and manpower that more and more Americans began to feel could be better used. Government spending priorities moved further away from the social and health concerns of the 1960s. The economy seemed doomed to increasing inflation as a worldwide problem. Watergate set off widespread questions about trust and accountability, which had ramifications beyond the political arena, touching business, education, and health care delivery systems.

The focus of the consumer movement on greater personal involvement, concern for human rights, and issues of responsibility and accountability led to some important changes in the way mental illness and its treatment were viewed. There was a general increase in public interest in abnormal psychology, nurtured by the use of psychological themes in the media and popular literature and by the development of opportunities to study about it at all educational levels. This interest and knowledge, coupled with a growing concern for clients' rights, led to questions and demands with regard to mental health practices. The lay population, no longer altogether naïve, sought to define health care in terms of its costs, benefits, risks, and hazards. It became increasingly important for all health professionals to justify their services. This meant clearly defining their goals and methods and the populations to be served. Reporting systems needed refinement to be consistent with professional aims and relevant to patients' needs.

A new chaos and creative flux developed in society as a whole. The civil rights movement begun in the 1950s extended into concerns that profoundly affected health care professionals. It aroused consciousness of inequities suffered by many segments of the population. The women's movement mobilized many people to change some of society's most fundamental attitudes and practices. The elderly and the handicapped organized to demand long-overdue rights, opportunities, and concern. Homosexuality no longer was considered an illness in itself, and people with various sexual orientations "came out of the closet." Other taboos were lifted. Death and dying, as part of the continuum of living, became a subject of conversation and study. *Patients' rights* became a major concern. The nation experienced what Alvin Toffler called "future shock."[50] People were increasingly bombarded with facts, new orientations, and the rapid fabrication and just as rapid decline of materials, ideas, and fads. All of this has had enormous significance to occupational therapy, a profession with a commitment to help others to "do for themselves."

Legal Decisions

The US legal system lent support to these developments. In 1971, in a milestone decision, the Alabama courts (Wyatt *vs* Stickney) ruled that an individual who has been involuntarily confined to a mental institution has a right to treatment — as opposed to simply maintenance or incarceration. Minimum standards for institutional staffing and treatment were spelled out.[23] In 1975, a US Supreme Court decision (O'Connor *vs* Donaldson) ruled that "a finding of mental illness alone cannot justify a state's locking a person up against his will and keeping him indefinitely in a simple custodial confinement. . . . In short, a state cannot constitutionally confine without more (than custodial care) a non-dangerous individual who is capable of surviving safely in freedom by himself or with the help of willing and responsible family members or friends."[23] Across the country, states were compelled to look into their laws, policies, and practices regarding institutional management of the mentally ill. There were a number of local changes in laws which reflected three broad themes: (1) access to mental health care; (2) the rights of mental patients to receive or to refuse treatment; and (3) social acceptance of deviance.

Occupational therapy was forced during the late 1960s and early 1970s to look carefully at its uses of work as therapy. For many years, in some of the large public institutions, patients had been assigned to work in the laundry, maintenance shops, farm, and a variety of other areas. Frequently, in these assignments, patients were able to experience the success of developing real proficiency at given tasks and the sense of being contributing, productive members of the institutional community. Unfortunately, the very positive personal effects these work assignments had on some patients, also, within the institutional setting, tended to reinforce their need to stay in the hospital. There was not enough attention, given the total milieu of the institution, and not enough effort put into helping the patients generalize their skills so they could use them in the world outside the institution. To the public, it appeared that patient labor was being seriously exploited.

The question of institutional peonage was brought into the courts. (The case, Nelson Eugene Souder *vs* Peter J. Brennan, Civil Action 482-73, resulted in a law in April 1974 requiring that patients be paid the statutory minimum wage for performing work within the institutional setting. The date when vigorous enforcement was to begin was set as December 1, 1974.) Therefore, the assignment of patients to work without pay in situations that benefited the institution became illegal. The act resulting from the above-mentioned court action required that institutions provide pay for patients' work. Few institutions could afford either this or the necessary staff and paperwork to justify work as therapy. There were some patients, the seriously institutionalized and chronic, who lost in the process their one successful, however rote, activity. And so, a concomitant, and possibly resultant, movement arose to develop more community, business, and industrial contacts so that patients could be given work assignments in the real world with real renumeration. Occupational therapists needed to examine this concept.

New Preventive Models

In 1971, Geraldine Finn presented the Eleanor Clarke Slagle Lecture at the Annual Conference of the AOTA in Cleveland. Her lecture discussed the societal and technological changes during the preceding decades and examined the efforts that had been made at Boston State Hospital to shift occupational therapy services to a prevention model. She identified nine major issues which were part of that process[21]:

1. The function of primary institutions in maintaining the health of the people of a community and the need for occupational therapists to understand the functions, goals, and policies of these primary institutions
2. The planning of appropriate programs and services based on man's need to engage in interaction with the objects of his environment in order to maintain his health throughout his life
3. The need to reinterpret the body of knowledge available within the profession of occupational therapy in order to apply it in the service of keeping people healthy rather than in helping people minimize their disabilities
4. The creation of new associations of our available knowledge in order to respond more accurately to the pressing reality needs of today
5. The establishment of an organizational model which will allow translation of abstract plans about activities, human action and the delivery of health services into concrete actions
6. The presence of risk taking and its ramifications on one's ability to function and persevere when faced with an unfamiliar environment
7. The necessity of reexamining communication patterns to ensure real communications among people
8. The need to create a climate of acceptance for a planned program and the development of the skills needed to assist others in seeing the value of these programs
9. The role of supervision in maintaining the performance and professional growth of the staff members.

The kinds of programs described by Finn included early intervention programs for children, consultation services to teachers, inservice programs on developmental screening, and program planning, outreach programs for the elderly, workshops for mothers and preschool children, inservice programs on perceptual-motor development for mental health workers, development of new models of parent education and counseling and the introduction of knowledge about developmental levels of human performance in a community drug program.[21]

In 1977, President Carter appointed a Commission on Mental Health to study and make recommendations regarding the status of mental health and mental health services in this country. Their findings led to the following statement: "Because of the pluralistic nature of the American Society and cultural order, social problems and social deviances, when applied to mental health issues, must be approached from a cultural relativity frame of reference."[44]

Development of Professionalism

Thus, during the 1970s, the psychiatric occupational therapist was plunged into a new and challenging set of perspectives. In many ways, the occupational therapist was beginning to accept and identify with a peer professional role along with physicians, social workers, psychologists, and nurses. The search for a unifying theory of occupational therapy had disclosed in sharp relief the unique contributions that could be made by the therapist. The occupational therapist as an aide to the physician gave way to the occupational therapist as another professional cooperating with a number of other disciplines in the treatment of the mentally ill, at least in some of the newer and less traditional settings. The contexts for treatment and the constitution of the treatment teams were considerably extended. By 1970, occupational therapists were working in schools, community programs, and homes in addition to the traditional settings. In some of the more traditional settings, nontraditional staffing patterns and new approaches were being explored.

As popular trends in psychiatry gained momentum and prominence, many occupational therapists working in psychiatry saw the value of learning and gaining skills in their use. Transactional analysis, gestalt therapy, meditation, bioenergetics, assertiveness and effectiveness training, and a variety of humanistic and self-actualization group techniques are just a few of the movements that were beginning to offer new avenues for the development of healthier, more productive, and more satisfying lives in the general (normal to mildly neurotic) population. Some occupational therapists, as well as psychologists, social workers, and others, saw in these techniques opportunities for enhancing the treatment of their clients. With various degrees of effectiveness, therapists incorporated these methods into existing treatment techniques. This happened most readily and most often in those settings where the occupational therapist's role was blended with the roles of other members of the treatment team.

Human Development Reference

The work of Anne C. Mosey, Lela Llorens, and others encouraged occupational therapists in several parts of the country to study and articulate the principles of human development as a basic frame of reference for psychiatric occupational therapy. This approach led to further interest in perceptual and cognitive functioning and the concepts of stress and regression.

Societal Changes

The 1970s saw the resurgence of interest in, and attention to, the significance of societal attitudes, values, and life-styles. Community-based programs, partial hospitalization, and home treatment programs have made it essential for occupational therapists to consider the impact of these social changes as well as the impact of their own personal value systems on all aspects of treatment.

Behavior Therapy

In some areas, psychiatric occupational therapists began to experiment and work with behavioral approaches to treatment. Usually working within a team and in a setting where behavior therapy was being used, therapists developed methods of treatment based on schedules of reinforcement, operant conditioning, modeling, shaping, and chaining procedures. For some patients, these techniques proved useful in changing or extinguishing undesirable behavior patterns and in establishing and reinforcing healthy behavior patterns.

Neurophysiological Approach

At the same time, neurophysiological knowledge and neurophysiological approaches to treatment have been gaining momentum; they promise to make a significant impact on psychiatric practice. Refinement and development of the work of Ayres and King have continued. There has been increased attention to the effects of the functions of the reticular activating system. In 1975, Josephine Moore, in her Eleanor Clarke Slagle Lecture at the Annual Conference of the AOTA in Milwaukee, "Behavior, Bias and the Limbic System," spoke eloquently of the need for greater consideration of the influence of basic neurophysiological mechanisms in determining human feelings and actions.[38]

Conceptual Models

The search for clear conceptual models, clear frames of reference, and a unifying theory of occupational therapy continued to preoccupy the profession during the 1970s. The work of several prominent occupational therapists during this period and a special consciousness on the part of the AOTA sought to provide guidelines to practice.

In her book, *Three Frames of Reference for Mental Health*, published in 1970, Mosey discussed three conceptual approaches to psychiatric occupational therapy: (1) psychoanalytic, (2) acquisitional, and (3) developmental. She suggested that each of these frames defines specific aspects of the occupational therapy process.[40] According to Mosey, each frame of reference has postulates regarding the nature of the individual, the characteristics of health and illness, and viable approaches to evaluation and treatment. Clarity with regard to the frame of reference used in treatment is seen as highly desirable. It permits the therapist to work from a specific body of knowledge and encourages consistency among expectations, goal-setting, and approaches to evaluation and treatment.

Mental Health Task Force

In 1975, a special task force comprised of psychiatric occupational therapists was appointed by the AOTA to identify issues of concern in the practice of occupational therapy in mental health and to recommend solutions to the identified problems. The task force surveyed practice in psychiatric occupational therapy and, based on their assessment of the status of occupational therapy in psychiatry, made their recommendations, which were published in the AOTA newspaper in September 1976. The task force reported that "mental health practice lacks standardized clinical techniques and therefore is dependent on a conceptualization of the fundamental value of performance which has never been clearly articulated."[7] The task force went on to make recommendations geared to refining the knowledge base and strengthening the technology of occupational therapy practice. Specific recommendations were made regarding research, graduate education, continuing education, and the definition of occupational therapy practice in psychiatry. Although the work of this task force was addressed to psychiatric occupational therapy practice, it had serious implications for the profession as a whole.

Case Study

TIME: 1977

PLACE: Kitchen area of a community mental health center

Bill (a registered occupational therapist with 5 years of experience in psychiatry) and Rona (an occupational therapy student in the sixth week of her second fieldwork experience) are having a cup of coffee before starting the day. They are in the kitchen, an area partitioned off from a pleasant living room, part of the program's small ADL apartment. Bill and Rona have papers spread out on the table in front of them. They have been discussing the clients.

Rona comments, "I finished checking out Roberta yesterday. It didn't work at all to place her in the group on Monday. She just went into her shell and stayed there. So I decided to work with her on a one-to-one basis for a while. She has a lot of rote skills, old familiar schemes, I guess, at a pretty high level—things like making coffee and setting the table—but when she tries something she never did before, or when there's some special emotional strain, she falls apart unless we give her a lot of structure.

She seems able to handle only about two steps at a time, so you have to stay near. I think it's really important to give her that support. Don't you?"

Bill comments, "She certainly needs to succeed. Just watch that she doesn't get too dependent."

Rona replies, "I know. That's tricky, and I may need help to recognize it if it's happening. I was thinking—you know, her husband is going to stop by for lunch today. I thought I'd have her make something like grilled cheese sandwiches—which I'm sure she can handle—but use ready-mades like potato chips and tomatoes and finish it out with ice cream for dessert. She's coming in at ten o'clock to decide the menu and seems to feel okay about going down the street to buy the food. I just think it's important for her to make the meal, but it can't be too complicated. What do you think?"

Bill says, "Sounds good to me. You're using her integrated skills well and that's probably important, because, while it's neat that her husband is coming, it's bound to be somewhat stressful. You know he's been doing most of the cooking at their house for a couple of years! Good luck."

Bill leaves Rona and goes down a short hall to his office to check his schedule of activities for the day. A 9:30 meeting with the director to review the budget. The meeting will be sticky. Everybody's looking for ways to cut corners and save money. At 10:30, he will work with a small group of clients, both men and women, in the workshop next to the kitchen. They will be doing simple repairs to broken pieces of furniture they have brought in to the center. Most of the work is gluing and clamping, but there are some minor painting and refinishing jobs. Bill has found that this activity is good both as evaluation and as treatment.

In the afternoon, he will be taking Rona with him to the home of one of their clients. Mrs. Smith, the client, is 45 years old. An arthritic condition prevents her from getting out of the house. She is depressed and anxious. An occupational therapy program has been started to see if there are ways she could be helped to handle her basic activities of daily living. The situation is difficult because her family are all hard-working, energetic people, who were used to having Mrs. Smith depend on them but who tended also to resent it silently. And the house is full of architectural barriers.

Somewhere, Bill is going to have to fit in time to read over the AOTA Mental Health Task Force Report again, because there will be a local hearing about it this evening. He had read it once and had felt excited about parts, depressed about other parts, and disturbed about some of the recommendations.

"It could matter a lot, how this gets handled!" he thinks.   □

Evaluation Tools

In 1977, the Mental Health Specialty Section of the AOTA expressed concern about the need for valid and reliable evaluation tools. A series of activities designed to survey the field and to encourage the development and standardization of methods and techniques for evaluation of clients in mental health was launched.

Need for Philosophical Base

In 1978, Lorna Jean King, as the Eleanor Clarke Slagle lecturer, eloquently addressed the need for occupational therapy to have a comprehensive, unifying theory. She suggested that the adaptive process could be considered the unifying principle of occupational therapy. King identified the four unique features of adaptation in the individual human experience as: (1) active participation in adjustment to different conditions or environments; (2) adaptation as called forth by the demands of the environment; (3) adaptation as most efficiently organized subcortically; and (4) the adaptive response as self-reinforcing. She stated that, "I am implying that the essential purpose of occupational therapy is to stimulate and guide the adaptive processes through which an individual may best survive and develop." [29]

A landmark meeting of the AOTA officers, the Representative Assembly, and academic and clinical leaders took place in Scottsdale, Arizona, in the fall of 1978. At this meeting, major issues of education, clinical practice, and research in occupational therapy were discussed, and the status of occupational therapy as a true profession was analyzed. Papers were presented by ten leaders in the field, who thoughtfully and provocatively addressed the history, philosophy, current status, and future of occupational therapy. Resolutions were generated to affirm a philosophical base, to encourage support for research, and to reassess the levels of preparation required for entry into practice. These resolutions and the decisions that ensued had a significant effect on the field of occupational therapy as a whole. The impact was experienced in the field of psychiatry, especially in the momentum that developed around the standardization and dissemination of instruments and methods of evaluation and in an increase in the publication of books and articles. [3,4]

Significance of the 1980s

Publication of DSM-III

In 1980, the American Psychiatric Association published the *Diagnostic and Statistical Manual of Mental Disorders*, Third Edition (DSM-III), a task that had been laboriously and conscientiously undertaken over a period of 6 years by its Task Force on Nomenclature and

Statistics. The DSM-III, while compatible with the Ninth Edition of the *International Classification of Diseases* (ICD), is not identical. It was prepared to reflect the current knowledge in such a way as to be clinically useful and to provide a basis for research and administration. Mental disorder is conceptualized in terms of significant behavior or psychological syndromes or patterns that cause individuals to experience subjective distress or functional disability. An important feature of the DSM-III is its multiaxial system for evaluation. This system recommends consideration of the individual in terms of five different dimensions or *Axes*: (I) clinical syndromes; (II) personality or specific developmental disorders; (III) physical disorders; (IV) severity of psychosocial stressors; and (V) highest level of adaptive functioning during the past year. The developers of the DSM-III state that this revision represents only "one still frame in the ongoing process of attempting to better understand mental disorders." [6]

The major classifications representing the categories within Axis I are: disorders usually first evident in infancy, childhood or adolescence; organic mental disorders; substance use disorders; schizophrenic disorders; paranoid disorders; psychotic disorders not elsewhere classified; affective disorders; anxiety disorders; somatoform disorders; dissociative disorders; psychosexual disorders; factitious disorders; disorders of impulse control not elsewhere classified; and adjustment disorders. Unlike DSM-II, DSM-III does not have a separate category for neurotic disorders but includes them under the affective, anxiety, somatoform, dissociative, and psychosexual classifications. Personality disorders are categorized under Axis II. Psychiatric factors affecting physical condition are categorized under Axis III, and codes are given for conditions that are not attributable to a mental disease but are a focus of attention or treatment.

The significance of the DSM-III to occupational therapists lies in its attempt to take a holistic approach to understanding mental disorders. Certainly, adding the considerations of Axes IV and V (psychosocial stressors and the highest level of adaptive functioning) underscores concerns of special importance to the occupational therapist.

There has always been some controversy over the usefulness of diagnostic labels when one is working with people in a treatment context. The practice raises the issue of depersonalization or of predisposing the professional to perceive a classical picture or fantasy patient rather than a unique human being with a personal gestalt different from that of any other person. On the other hand, a diagnosis represents a compilation of research and experience with large numbers of people over a long period of time and, as such, presents important guidelines for understanding the disease process, methods for treating it, and certain expectations regarding its prognosis. It is a professional responsibility for mental health professionals to recognize both aspects of this issue and to seek the balance in their use of diagnosis that will serve their clients best.

American Psychiatric Association – American Occupational Therapy Task Force

The Commission on Psychiatric Therapies of the American Psychiatric Association began a study of the existent therapies in practice and asked the AOTA to join in the effort to prepare a report. A committee of occupational therapists, chaired by Gail Fidler, addressed the background, practice, and issues of psychiatric occupational therapy in its paper, "Overview of Occupational Therapy," which was submitted to the American Psychiatric Association in May of 1981.[20] This report emphasized the neurobiologic and sociocultural framework for understanding human experience and behavior as underlying the practice of occupational therapy. It stressed the emphasis of occupational therapy on the value of purposeful activity in the development of a person's sense of competence and worth and underscored the "integrative, adaptive qualities of doing, and the significance of doing in the acquisition of age-specific, culturally relevant performance skills."[20] It outlined the psychiatric contexts within which occupational therapy works and emphasized the need for continuing research into the relationship between purposeful activity and neurophysiologic integration.

New Publications

The year 1980 also saw the beginning of a journal, *Occupational Therapy in Mental Health*, providing another medium through which practice and research issues might be shared.[43] The AOTA also began publication of a journal of research for the field as a whole.[5]

New books addressing occupational therapy in mental health have become available, offering a wide range of resources and levels. The thrust toward graduate education has increased the interest in research and the number of articles published in the occupational therapy journals and in the journals of other related professions.

Emerging Approaches

During this period, the study of cognitive function and dysfunction as critical aspects of mental health and mental illness continued under the leadership of Claudia Allen in California. Defining cognitive function as the quality of thought an individual uses in doing a task, Allen suggested that the occupational therapist is in a unique position. Using the knowledge of task analysis and of human cognitive levels, the occupational therapist can evaluate cognitive function and provide specific remediation where dysfunction exists. This is a far more specific and focused approach to occupational therapy in psychiatry than most, and one which presents new directions and new challenges for refining practice.[2]

There is, in the 1980s, increasingly productive research in the biochemical and biogenetic bases of human emotional and cognitive functioning. Health care professionals need to be able to understand and use the knowledge gained from this research. The occupational therapist's skills in the observation of the task behaviors of patients are important in the effective use of medications and other biological treatments.

Another approach, built on the earlier contributions of Mary Reilly and of the founders of occupational therapy, has gained attention. Gary Kielhofner and a large number of other occupational therapists have proposed that occupational therapy can best be developed around a model of human occupation emphasizing a systems frame for viewing balance in human functioning.[28]

Societal Influences on Mental Health

The delivery of health care is related to factors that affect society as a whole. On the one hand, the development of electronic devices, video games, and home computers, as well as the flights of the space shuttles, have captured the popular imagination, suggesting unlimited potential for "progress." But this optimism was countered by economic and political problems—runaway inflation, assassinations, military intervention and takeovers, unemployment, economic dislocations, terrorism by small hit squads and established governments, cutbacks in social services. People were bombarded by the news media. Immediate and vivid coverage of devastating events invited mass empathy, but the feeling that they could do nothing to control world-scale occurrences caused people to retreat into despair or numbness. The threat of nuclear destruction, by accident or conscious act of war, was changing the consciousness of human civilization—in one direction or the other. Some chose to deny for political reasons. Others had no choice but to deny because the threat was too great to comprehend, but they suffered a growing sense of powerlessness in their denial. Broad segments of the western European population, as well as many members of the scientific and medical establishments in the United States, claimed it was pathological to continue such denial and set out to oppose the destruction. All of these factors combined to compromise the mental health of individuals on a broad scale. "Burnout" and stress management became clichés, especially among people working in human services. Self-help and group-help programs designed to aid people in developing and using coping strategies proliferated.

The community mental health movement has often lacked adequate financial support or structural understanding. In most metropolitan areas, thousands of formerly institutionalized individuals are barely existing in the community—the fortunate ones in "good" boarding homes or independent living facilities. Too many of them are literally homeless and are known as "bag ladies" or "vent people," living on the streets, seeking warmth, shelter, and food wherever they can be found.

All of these factors, the positive and the negative, powerfully influence thinking and behavior. To mental health professionals and everyone else, the crisis exists as a danger or an opportunity.

Case Study

TIME: 1982

PLACE: Community mental health center in a large city

Marvin, an OTR, and Carie, a mental health aide, are seated at a table in a large room that is divided into areas by the placement of furniture. There is a work area with a long table and folding chairs and cupboards along the wall; a socialization area with a coffee urn, a couch, some soft chairs and a coffee table; and a library with tables, chairs, and bookshelves half full of paperback books and well-used magazines. Large bright posters are taped to the walls, and there are two bulletin boards on which schedules and notices have been posted. One section of the wall has large windows that look out on the busy street below. Potted plants line the window sill. Several folding chairs face the window.

Marvin and Carie have just said goodby to their group, 20 former state hospital patients, who leave on the center's bus each day at 3:30 p.m. to be delivered to their boarding homes. About six more travel independently by public transportation to their families' homes.

Carie calls Marvin's attention to the chairs at the window. They both sigh. No matter how often they have tried to find substitutes for staring out the window, it seems that there are always a few clients who prefer to withdraw in this way. (But is it really withdrawal? Marvin wonders.) The last activity that afternoon had been a current events discussion group. This is a daily activity, in which clients are encouraged as "homework" to bring in news items to discuss with the group. Marvin and Carie talk about some of the clients.

Carie says, "Mary's too good for this group. She is so much smarter and 'with it' in every way. How come they keep her here?"

Marvin replies, "It's a strange thing—she has tried other programs, but she always goes to pieces. I think she's scared and this group makes her feel superior. She's beginning to sound that way in group therapy. That's why we're doing some special individual treatment sessions . . . It's old Joe I'm worried about."

"Yeah!" says Carie. "Now he's bragging about getting some money from his buddy who plays the casinos—and some slick guy wants to sell him a car! I don't think he even knows how to drive." Marvin grunts and frowns. He had done some evaluations with Joe, and it was evident that it would take intensive work to help him to develop even basic living skills like money management and the ability to recognize when he needs to ask for assistance.

Carie gets up to straighten the room and prepare supplies for the next day's activities. Marvin picks up a pen and poises it over a blank paper. There are so many clients and such a limited staff! Staff burnout has become a real problem, and they were trying to find ways to reorganize themselves to deal with it. Marvin was hoping to convince his administrator to add a position for a COTA to replace the mental health aide who just left. He decides to put the request in writing. There is no point in going home, because there is a supper meeting of the local community board to discuss plans for getting support for further program development. Marvin knows that the big issue is to decide whether to mount a fund-raising campaign or to cut back further on the existing program. A good movie would be in order after this meeting! □

Economic, political, and social change and the phenomenal development of knowledge and technology have continued. Mental health professionals, occupational therapists among them, have moved in three significant directions as the 1980s draw to a close: the development of private practices; increased encouragement of graduate study, both for the credentials involved and in a genuine quest for greater understanding; and research into the roots of our treatment claims.

Case Study

TIME: 1987

PLACE: The campus of a large university

Anita skips down the stone steps of the university library. She is pleased that she has finally been able to find and borrow the Luria book which was listed as supplemental reading for her graduate course in neuropsychology. At the foot of the steps, she is greeted by Hiroki, a fellow student, and an old friend, an occupational therapist with whom she used to work.

"I see you got it! Good!" he says. "At last . . ." says Anita, "This course has really raised my curiosity. I wish I had taken it before, when I was working in the state hospital." Hiroki nods. "So do I," he says. They sit down on a bench. "What are you doing now?" he asks. Anita says, "Well, I've taken the big leap and have gone into private practice, mostly seeing people in their homes. I'm also doing some consultation. It works out well with my graduate work, in terms of time, anyway. It's not easy, but sometimes it's really exciting. There's certainly a big need. Are you still at the community mental health center?" Hiroki nods. "We are still very, very busy. You know, we're hoping to receive a grant for more extensive liaison services with the state hospital. If we get it, the center will set up a halfway house on the grounds of the hospital and we'll need a lot more staff. Think you'd be interested?" "Hmmm — maybe — but not right away. I'm working on the research proposal for my thesis. Come to think of it, you might be able to help. I want to study the validity of the community readiness activities we use. I think occupational therapists are in a position to exert a lot more influence on the discharge process, but we need to be able to demonstrate better that we can evaluate whether a patient is ready to move out. I'm afraid that community readiness activities in an institutional setting sometimes are a lot different from the real thing outside. I hope that I can tease out ways of identifying the critical elements so we can do a better job." "Wow! It sounds like your state hospital experience, the private practice, and this course are all coming together. Sometimes, the criteria used for sending patients out are the pits — not as clear as they could be. We are working on the whole idea of using the community itself more. We are also beginning to use computer games and programs as treatment. The clients love them: they provide immediate feedback. Why don't you come over and spend a day with us? You could probably help us and maybe we can help you." "Great!" says Anita, "Listen; could we plan on it next week? I've got to run now, but I'll see you in class tomorrow."

Hiroki bids Anita goodby and sits for a minute watching the sharp lines of sunshine and shadows on a rock by the campus walk. His mind is on one of his clients, a young woman who comes to the center because she has been all but paralyzed by fear and depression since her separation from her husband. The center's team has set goals for her, which include helping her to regain control of her life in terms of developing job skills. Hiroki knows that for her, this means providing her with activities which will permit her to feel successful, competent and whole; ones that can move her, in small increments as she is ready, into the interpersonal challenges of her life. They'd already started with the computer. . . . □

References

1. Action for Mental Health: Joint Commission on Mental Illness and Mental Health. New York, John Wiley & Sons, 1961
2. Allen C: Occupational Therapy for Psychiatric Diseases: Measurement and Management of Cognitive Disabilities. Boston, Little, Brown, 1985
3. American Occupational Therapy Association: Occupational Therapy 2001 A.D. Rockville, MD, American Occupational Therapy Association, 1979
4. American Occupational Therapy Association Representative Assembly: Proceedings. Am J Occup Ther 33:785, 1979
5. American Occupational Therapy Foundation: Journal of Research. Rockville, MD, American Occupational Therapy Foundation, 1981
6. American Psychiatric Association: Diagnostic and Statistical Manual of Mental Disorders, Edition III (DSM-III). Washington, DC, American Psychiatric Association, 1980
7. A Report of the American Occupational Therapy Association Mental Health Task Force. Occup Ther Newspaper 30, 1976
8. Arieti S: The Intrapsychic Self. New York, Basic Books, 1967
9. Ayres, AJ: The development of body scheme in children. Am J Occup Ther 15:3, 1961
10. Azima FJ: The Azima Battery. In Mazer J (ed): Materials from the 1968 Regional Institutes Sponsored by the American Occupational Therapy Association on the Evaluation Process. Final Report RSA-123-T-68. New York, American Occupational Therapy Association, 1968
11. Bailey D: Vocational theories and work habits related to childhood development. Am J Occup Ther 25:298, 1971
12. Bonsall II; quoted in Van Atta K: An Account of the Events Surrounding the Origin of the Friends Hospital, p 24. Philadelphia, Williams Brothers Printing, 1976
13. Diasio K: Psychiatric occupational therapy: Search for a conceptual framework in the light of psychoanalytic ego psychology and learning theory. Am J Occup Ther 22:400, 1968
14. Dunton WR: Prescribing Occupational Therapy. Springfield, IL, Charles C Thomas, 1928
15. Elkins HK, Van Vlack NM: Changes in occupational therapy due to the tranquilizing drugs. Am J Occup Ther 11:269, 1957
16. Fidler GS: Diagnostic battery, scoring and summary. In Mazer J (ed): Materials from the 1968 Regional Institutes Sponsored by the American Occupational Therapy Association on the Evaluation Process. Final Report RSA-123-T-68. New York, American Occupational Therapy Association, 1968
17. Fidler GS: Psychological evaluation of occupational therapy activities. Am J Occup Ther 2:284, 1948

18. Fidler GS, Fidler JW: Introduction to Psychiatric Occupational Therapy, p 170. New York, Harper & Row, 1954

19. Fidler GS, Fidler JW: Occupational Therapy: A Communication Process in Psychiatry. New York, Macmillan, 1963

20. Fidler GS, Shapiro D, Falk–Kessler J, et al: Overview of Occupational Therapy. Report submitted to American Psychiatric Association Commission on Psychiatric Therapies, 1981

21. Finn G: The occupational therapist in prevention programs. Am J Occup Ther 26:65, 1972

22. Florey L: An approach to play and play development. Am J Occup Ther 25:275, 1971

23. Goldstein MJ, Baker BL, Jamison KR: Abnormal Psychology: Experiences, Origins and Interventions, pp 616–622. Boston, Little, Brown, 1980

24. Haas LJ: Occupational Therapy for the Mentally and Nervously Ill. Milwaukee, Bruce Publishing, 1925

25. Haas LJ: Practical Occupational Therapy. Milwaukee, Bruce Publishing, 1944

26. Johnson J: Considerations of work as therapy in the rehabilitation process. Am J Occup Ther 25:303, 1971

27. Jones M: The Therapeutic Community. New York, Basic Books, 1953

28. Kielhofner G, Burke J: A model of human occupation I: Framework and content. Am J Occup Ther 34:572, 1980

29. King LJ: Toward a science of adaptive responses. Am J Occup Ther 32:429, 1978

30. Marsh LC: Shall we apply industrial psychiatry to psychiatry? Occup Ther Rehab 12:1, 1932

31. Matsutsuyu J: Occupational behavior: A perspective on work and play. Am J Occup Ther 25:292, 1971

32. Mauer P: Antecedents of work behavior. Am J Occup Ther 25:294, 1971

33. Mazer J: Toward an integrated theory of occupational therapy. Am J Occup Ther 22:451, 1968

34. Mazer J, Mosey AC: Introduction to special section: Theories of psychiatric occupational therapy. Am J Occup Ther 22:398, 1968

35. Menninger WC: Psychiatric hospital therapy designed to meet unconscious needs. Am J Psychiatr 93:347, 1936

36. Meyer A: The philosophy of occupational therapy. Arch Occup Ther 1(5):1, 1922

37. Michelman S: The importance of creative play. Am J Occup Ther 25:285, 1971

38. Moore J: Behavior, bias and the limbic system. Am J Occup Ther 30:11, 1976

39. Mosey AC: Recapitulation of ontogenesis. Am J Occup Ther 22:426, 1968

40. Mosey AC: Three Frames of Reference for Mental Health. Thorofare, NJ, Charles B Slack, 1970

41. Nagy I, Framo J: Intensive Family Therapy. New York, Harper & Row, 1965

42. Niswander GD, Haslerud GM, Dixey E: The effect of the professional activity of the occupational therapist on the behavior of acute mental patients. Am J Occup Ther 11:273, 1957

43. Occupational Therapy in Mental Health: A Journal of Psychosocial Practice and Research. New York, Haworth Press, 1980

44. President's Commission on Mental Health: Task Panel Reports, Vol 3, appendix. Washington, DC, US Government Printing Office, 1978

45. Reilly M: The educational process. Am J Occup Ther 23:302, 1969

46. Rogers C: Freedom to Learn. Columbus, Charles E Merrill, 1969

47. Strecker EA, Appel KE: Discovering Ourselves, 2nd ed. New York, Macmillan, 1948

48. Takata N: The play milieu. Am J Occup Ther 25:281, 1971

49. Tempone V, Smith A: Psychiatric occupational therapy within a learning theory context. Am J Occup Ther 22:415, 1968

50. Toffler A: Future Shock. New York, Random House, 1970

51. Slagle EC: Training aides for mental patients. Arch Occup Ther 1:14, 1922

52. Wade B: Occupational therapy for patients with mental disease. In Willard HS, Spackman CS (eds): Principles of Occupational Therapy, 1st ed, pp 99–109. Philadelphia, JB Lippincott, 1947

53. Watanabe S: Four concepts basic to the occupational therapy process. Am J Occup Ther 22:439, 1968

54. West W (ed): Changing Concepts and Practices in Psychiatric Occupational Therapy. New York, American Occupational Therapy Association, 1959

55. White RW: The urge towards competence. Am J Occup Ther 25:271, 1971

56. Wolpe J: Psychotherapy by Reciprocal Inhibition. Palo Alto, Stanford University Press, 1958

SECTION 3

Principles of Psychiatric Occupational Therapy Practice *Sharan L. Schwartzberg*

Roles and Functions

Psychosocial principles and therapeutic processes are applied today in all areas of occupational therapy and are an essential component of entry-level curriculums. The specific purpose of occupational therapy practice in psychosocial dysfunction is "to improve people's capacity for and involvement in healthy occupations."[4] Practitioners in psychiatric and mental health occupational therapy have a primary interest in the psychosocial aspects of practice.

Added to their basic professional education, psychiatric occupational therapists have specialized knowledge and refined intervention skills concerning mental health problems. Several therapists further narrow their practice by limiting it to an age group, setting, role, or therapeutic model. Therapist preparation for such highly specialized roles is beyond basic professional education. The educational routes include graduate education, continuing education, and supervised clinical experience.

Evolution of Roles

The occupational therapist's role in mental health practice has changed over time, largely as the result of new knowledge concerning mental illness, of developments within the profession, and of social, political, and economic forces. All affect both the kinds of services delivered and the types of settings in which therapists work.

Psychosocial occupational therapy is particularly influenced by the role of women in defining the profession. Psychiatry as a branch of medicine, a male-dominated profession, also has considerable impact on the roles occupational therapists assume. Both the role of women and the forces of medicine and economics are evident in the evolution and role of group work in occupational therapy.[10] Howe and Schwartzberg, in their analysis of this subject, point out that the "occupational therapy collective," popular in the profession's early years, had both an economic and a therapeutic rationale. This occurred at a time when patient labor became a necessity as hospitals changed from charity to paying institutions. Predominantly women—and probably because of this social background—occupational therapists were also comfortable directing a collective of individuals in ordinary daily tasks under the supervision of male physicians.[10]

Raising questions about the role of women and the forces of medicine is important in understanding the unique changes and purposes of occupational therapy as a mental health discipline. An equally important concern is the role of economics in shaping practice.

Currently, payment systems have reduced the length of the hospital stay. Efforts to avoid duplication of services, control costs, and provide effective time-limited services are paramount, forcing occupational therapists to focus their energies on functional evaluation and management as primary roles in acute care. As a result, therapists must aggressively shift to differentiated roles in community-based programs, private practice, and alternative modes of health care delivery such as health maintenance organizations, independent practice associations, and home health. In addition to the influence of changing reimbursement patterns, with current social changes and the knowledge explosion, occupational therapists' roles must respond to newly identified target populations, including, among others, primary roles in adolescent treatment, adult day care, stress management and prevention programs in industry, and services for the elderly and young adult chronic patient.

Internal and External Influences

As previously highlighted, the roles and functions of occupational therapists are influenced by several factors internal and external to the profession. These variables significantly affect the degree of autonomy therapists have in their work. This subject, although relevant to the whole profession, is especially important in understanding identity problems and the diversity in mental health practice.

When occupational therapists act as verbal psychotherapists rather than enable individuals to function and adapt through the use of purposeful activities, professional identity and autonomy are lost. Furthermore, as is common with other psychiatric treatment modalities, the research knowledge base in psychosocial occupational therapy is notably incomplete. Although this situation appears to be improving, the gains will be lost if occupational therapists negate the profession's mission by failure to be explicit about the philosophical, conceptual, and empirical bases of their practice. Paradoxically, absence of knowledge of research in the other fields of psychiatry and mental health is also problematic. Such information can help to validate the occupational therapist's unique value and shape research and policies concerning the profession.

Research on occupational therapy education, clinical reasoning, and therapist values helps explain role definition problems and differences among therapists. For example, significant differences in the knowledge and perceived value of theory was found between therapists with different amounts of education and experience.[7,20] The degree of conceptual consistency and practice of beliefs also differs between therapists educated at the undergraduate and graduate levels.[3]

Interestingly, a study on mental health evaluations in occupational therapy revealed a discrepancy between the evaluations used in practice and those taught in occupational therapy educational programs. Further, it was found that existing occupational therapy evaluations were not being used in practice.[8] Finally, Barris' research on role variations in psychosocial occupational therapy suggests a relationship between role practices and therapist ideology and that the work setting acts as a variable in shaping practice.[1] This notion appears further supported by Barris' later study of clinical reasoning in psychosocial occupational therapy. As part of this investigation, she found the focus of psychosocial occupational therapy evaluations to be related to the treatment population, hospital setting, time frame, and tradition within the occupational therapy department.[2]

Contemporary Practice

There is no one universal model of occupational therapy practice in mental health. Therapists assume a variety of roles and employ a wide range of modalities.

Current Roles and Functions

Practice includes direct service roles in patient care and indirect service roles in administration, supervision, education, training, consultation, and research. The duties assigned to these roles vary depending on the goals, priorities, and resources of a given setting. Also probably related to role functions are a therapist's education, experience, theoretical orientation, and areas of expertise.

The AOTA's 1985 manpower report lends insight into current trends in practice.[17] In general, there is a declining proportion of occupational therapists who work with mixed age groups and an increased proportion working with the elderly and with patients under 20 years of age. The 1986 Member Data Survey results also show that an increasing percentage of occupational therapists in mental health are working with individuals over 65 years of age. However, there is a slight increase in the proportion of these therapists working with mixed ages and a decline in those working with patients

18 years and under. In descending order, based on 1986 data, the top seven primary health problems of patients most frequently seen by registered occupational therapists who work primarily with mental health patients are: (1) mental retardation, (2) schizophrenic disorders, (3) affective disorders, (4) organic mental disorders, (5) adjustment disorders, (6) alcohol/substance use disorders, and (7) personality disorders (Table 25-1). The 1982 data are also detailed in the table for comparison.

Table 25-1. *Profile of Occupational Therapy in Mental Health*

	Percent	
Primary Work Setting	*1986*	*1982*
College, 2-year	0.3	0.2
College/university, 4-year	1.3	1.3
Community mental health center	6.4	8.1
Correctional institution	0.3	0.4
Day care program	2.3	2.0
Halfway house	0	
Health maintenance organization (includes preferred provider organization/independent physicians association)	0.1	0.1
Home health agency	0.2	0.2
Hospice	0	
General hospital—rehab. unit only	0.8	
General hospital—all other	21.5	
Pediatric hospital	0.4	0.7
Psychiatric hospital	30.3	25.0
General hospital—all	22.3	21.2
Outpatient clinic (free-standing)	1.1	1.4
Physician's office	0.1	
Private industry	0.2	0.1
Private practice	2.0	1.0
Public health agency	0.4	0.3
Rehabilitation center or hospital	1.4	1.0
Research facility	0.1	0.3
Residential care facility, group home, or independent living center	9.4	12.2
Retirement or senior center	0.2	
School system (includes private schools)	10.1	15.9
Sheltered workshop	1.2	1.8
Skilled nursing facility or intermediate care facility	5.8	1.7
Vocational or prevocational program	0.8	
Voluntary agency (*e.g.,* Easter Seal/UCP)	0.4	0.4
Others	2.4	4.3

(Note: the bracket spanning "General hospital—all other", "Pediatric hospital", and "Psychiatric hospital" is labeled "either short- or long-term".)

(continued)

Table 25-1. *Profile of Occupational Therapy in Mental Health* (continued)

Age Range of Patients	Percent 1986	Percent 1982
Infant (under 1 year)	0.1	0.3
Preschool (1–4 years)	1.7	2.7
Primary school (5–12 years)	5.1	7.6
Secondary school (13–18 years)	6.2	4.8
Two or more of the above	8.6	14.1
19–64 years	49.5	50.8
65–74 years	2.9	
75–84 years	3.2	
85+ years	1.1	
65+ years	7.2	1.6
Mixed ages	21.5	18.2

Primary Health Problems of Patients	Percent 1986	Percent 1982
Adjustment disorders	5.7	
Affective disorders	17.9	
Alcohol/substance use disorders	5.1	5.0
Anxiety disorders	1.4	
Autism		1.0
Behavior disorders		10.1
Mental retardation	27.8	37.5
Neuroses		8.1
Organic mental disorders (includes dementias, Alzheimer's and organic brain syndromes)	7.2	
Personality disorders	3.7	5.7
Psychoses		32.4
Schizophrenic disorders	27.3	
Other psychotic disorders	1.1	
Other mental health disorders	2.7	

Note: According to 1986 data, 22.1% of OTRs and 39.4% of COTAs are working in mental health (as defined by the primary health problems of their patients). For 1982 data, the percentages are 27.0 and 38.9, respectively. The data detailed are based on the OTR groups.

Source: American Occupational Therapy Association, Research Information and Evaluation Division, 1982 and 1986 Member Data Surveys.

Standards of Practice

Psychiatric occupational therapy practice is guided by the profession's philosophical base and governed by professionally agreed upon ethics and standards (see Appendices B and C). Therapists must also comply with federal and state regulations when providing services. Also relevant to mental health practice are policies concerning entry-level role delineations for the registered occupational therapist and the certified occupational therapy assistant[6] and differences in their roles and functions in activities programs and long-term care.[18]

Practice Settings

Several types of psychiatric and mental health settings exist. Three models of care are suggested as examples of inpatient psychiatry: the general hospital, the private psychiatric hospital, and the state public hospital.[19] The public–private arrangement and Veterans Administration system can be added. These models help to explain inpatient practice settings and larger systems of outpatient care.

Variables that may distinguish the previous structures include: (1) staff hierarchy (*e.g.*, team concept, medical model of care); (2) principal form of treatment (*e.g.*, individual treatment plan and therapeutic milieu, therapeutic community); (3) fiscal system (*e.g.*, not-for-profit, private for-profit investor-owned, state- or government-supported); (4) institutional purpose and affiliations (*e.g.*, direct service, research and training, a business that provides health care); (5) source of referral; (6) source of payment and admission policies concerning compensation; (7) involuntary capacity; (8) length of stay; and (9) geographic source of patients and nature of physical setting.[19] For example, unlike the private psychiatric hospital, the state hospital is required by law to provide psychiatric care to all individuals regardless of their circumstances. Psychiatry in a general hospital has the unique role of providing acute care in close proximity to medical care and in the community setting, as well as of offering services to medical and surgical patients through psychiatric consultation–liaison services. In addition to clinics for outpatient services and private practices, community-based services include public and private day programs, halfway houses, and night programs for general and specialized psychiatric services.

The location of occupational therapy services in mental health is most realistically portrayed by a profile of practice (Table 25-1). As one would expect, practice is concentrated in hospital and community settings that provide services for severely disabling conditions such as schizophrenia rather than in outpatient office-based supportive psychotherapy for the "worried well." In fact, for more than half the mental health occupational therapists, 1986 data show that a hospital is the primary work setting. This represents a growth in hospital-based practice since 1982, which may be coupled with a projected need for services in outpatient community settings.

Despite the array of settings and practitioners that deliver psychiatric care, many people lack needed mental health services. In fact "only 20 percent of the estimated 47 million Americans who suffer from a mental disorder in a given six-month period actually receive psychiatric care, according to a recent survey by the National Institute of Mental Health."[5] It is likely this statistic reflects in part the large number of chronically mentally ill individuals who are underserved and require occupational therapy intervention for multiple handicaps.

Theoretical Foundations of Practice

The theoretical foundation of occupational therapy is composed of many theories. Mosey describes the scientific bases of practice: "selected theories from the biological sciences, psychology, sociology, the arts, and medicine and theories generated through the practice of occupational therapy form the theoretical foundation of occupational therapy."[15] On the basis of scientific reasoning, a healthy profession's theoretical foundation is never complete; theories are continuously developed, refined, and verified or refuted as a result of empirical research. The thoretical bases of occupational therapy and its specialties are undoubtedly incomplete. Naturally, with this deficiency, there is no one universally accepted conceptual model that explains occupational therapy practice in mental health and psychiatry.

Conceptual Models

With supporting research, certain theories are more strongly accepted by the profession than others and are more comfortably incorporated into conceptual models of practice. For a variety of reasons, including those outlined, several models are used in clinical practice.

Definition, Purpose, and Types

A conceptual model is an abstract representation of practice. As explained by Reed, a model of practice consists of a frame of reference and an organized system of assumptions, concepts, goals, assessment instruments, intervention strategies, deductions, and intervention principles.[16] Its overall purpose is to assist therapists to make sound judgments concerning methods of evaluation and intervention.

Two general types of conceptual models exist in the psychosocial area, which in psychiatry Lazare labels the *categorical* and *individualistic* approaches.[12] The latter is consistent with the occupational therapy profession's Meyerian historical roots and philosophical assumptions. It also, in my opinion, best explains psychiatric occupational therapy.

A simple explanation of the individualistic approach is contained in an occupational therapy belief: the body, mind, and environment of an individual are inseparable.[15] Similarly, Lazare points out that pathologic be-

havior is not caused solely by a person's biology, psychology, conduct, or social system: "Each provides a different level of explanation. At the same time, there are interactions between the systems that must be attended to."[11] Conversely, in the categorical approach, disease is viewed as unidimensional and diagnostic categories are not seen as abstract concepts.[11]

Overview of Categorical Models and Contributions

Because occupational therapists do not directly treat symptoms of a mental disorder, their models of practice are never truly categorical. However, approaches that fit with categorical models include: developmental, neurodevelopmental, and sensorimotor; analytical; behavioral; and cognitive. (For further discussion of these concepts see Chapter 3.)

In simple terms, a common characteristic of categorical approaches is that function and dysfunction are determined by assessing an individual according to a fixed schedule of expectations. Using a developmental frame of reference, for example, an occupational therapist may ask, does this person have age-appropriate skills and behaviors to function in the environment? That is, at ages 15, 16, or 17 — the teen years — one would expect a certain level of functioning and capability, whereas at mid-life, there are other expectations. If highly specialized or narrow definitions of function or adaptation are used, the therapist may consider only the neurological, sensorimotor, or analytic stages of development when evaluating a person.

Another feature of a frame of reference concerns the process of change. Expecting individuals to change their ways of relating because of insights gained from interpretations of motives, in a task-oriented group is an example from the categorical perspective. There is an assumption that maladaptive styles of interaction can be changed when unconscious conflicts are identified and explored. As an illustration, a patient may be skilled in a craft yet repeatedly seek the therapist's help. The patient also complains of receiving inadequate supervision at work and desperately wants praise from family members. With group and self-analysis, the patient may come to see that this behavior is motivated by an unfulfilled wish for parental approval. In the behavioral frames, task adaptation and environmental modification, reinforcement techniques, role modeling, and sequentially organized learning activities are some methods used to help patients.

Overview of Individualistic Models and Contributions

The individualistic models used in the psychosocial area include the occupational behavior or human occupation model (see Chapter 8-Section 4), the biopsychosocial model,[13,14] and the ecological systems model.[9] The contribution of these models is reflected in this chapter's content and emphasis.

Changing Assumptions and Concepts

Lazare cautions about the hazards of the categorical approach. Problems with such explanations include viewing all diagnostic categories as equally valid and ignoring other theoretical perspectives. Yet Lazare also believes that one needs to be scientific and clinically relevant, to be able to move between categorical and individualistic approaches. He further observes that the more multiple the etiology, the more individual a disease will be.[12]

Psychiatric occupational therapy evaluation and intervention are in part concerned with a person's component skills. Since technology and concrete approaches have appeal for several reasons, there is a temptation to focus on these specifics and to avoid practice and research concerning general occupational performance areas. This was seen in the past when therapists focused exclusively on psychodynamics. The current wave of enthusiasm for cognitive and sensorimotor techniques poses a danger, if other domains such as life satisfaction and work, play, and self-care are ignored.

There are considerable historical and empirical reasons to support individualistic approaches in psychosocial occupational therapy. It appears the profession nevertheless will continue to struggle with the value of maintaining its comprehensive, integrative approach to helping.

References

1. Barris R: Toward an image of one's own: Sources of variation in the role of occupational therapists in psychosocial practice. Occup Ther J Res 4:3, 1984
2. Barris R: Clinical reasoning in psychosocial occupational therapy. Presented at the Annual Conference, American Occupational Therapy Association, Minneapolis, April 1986
3. Barris R, Kielhofner G: Generating and using knowledge in occupational therapy: Implications for professional education. Occup Ther J Res 5:113, 1985
4. Barris R, Kielhofner G, Watts JH: Psychosocial Occupational Therapy Practice in a Pluralistic Arena, p 309. Laurel, MD, RAMSCO, 1983
5. Carey J: Bleak days for psychiatry: A search for answers. US News & World Report, p 74, February 25, 1985
6. Entry-Level OTR and COTA Role Delineation. Rockville, MD, American Occupational Therapy Association, 1981
7. Fox JV: Occupational therapy theory development: Knowledge and values held by recent graduates. Occup Ther J Res 1:79, 1981
8. Hemphill BJ: Mental health evaluations used in occupational therapy. Am J Occup Ther 34:721, 1980
9. Howe MC, Briggs AK: Ecological systems model for occupational therapy. Am J Occup Ther 36:322, 1982
10. Howe MC, Schwartzberg SL: A Functional Approach to Group Work in Occupational Therapy. Philadelphia, JB Lippincott, 1986
11. Lazare A: A multidimensional approach to psychopathology. In: Outpatient Psychiatry Diagnosis and Treatment, p 9. Baltimore, Williams & Wilkins, 1979
12. Lazare A: Two paradigms of the mind: A 3000 year old debate in medicine and psychiatry. Boston, Harvard Medical School course: Inpatient Psychiatry: Practice and Politics, March 1986
13. Mosey AC: A model for occupational therapy. Occup Ther Mental Health 1:11, 1980
14. Mosey AC: An alternative: The biopsychosocial model. Am J Occup Ther 28:137, 1974
15. Mosey AC: Occupational Therapy: Configuration of a Profession, p 71. New York, Raven Press, 1981
16. Reed KL: Models of Practice in Occupational Therapy. Baltimore, Williams & Wilkins, 1984
17. Report of the Ad Hoc Commission on Occupational Therapy Manpower: Occupational Therapy Manpower: A Plan for Progress, pp 56–57. Rockville, MD, American Occupational Therapy Association, 1985
18. Rogers JC, AOTA Commission on Practice: Roles and functions of occupational therapy in long-term care: Occupational therapy and activity programs. Am J Occup Ther 37:807, 1983
19. Sederer LI, Katz B, Manschreck TC: Inpatient psychiatry: Perspectives from the general, the private, and the state hospital. Gen Hosp Psychiatr 6:180, 1984
20. Van Duesen J: Relationship of occupational therapists' education and experience to perceived value of theory development. Occup Ther J Res 5:223, 1985

SECTION 4

Generic Tools *Sharan L. Schwartzberg*

Psychiatric occupational therapy consistently involves four tools: (1) therapeutic use of self, (2) purposeful activity, (3) activity analysis, and (4) activity adaptation. Although these are general to the profession, this section emphasizes their application in mental health practice. A profile of these generic tools is offered. Detailed descriptions of their restricted use to achieve goals in specific occupational performance areas and component skills can be found in more specialized literature.

Therapeutic Use of Self

The therapist's use of self is critical to engaging the patient in occupational therapy. Although the patient–therapist relationship is not the central focus of occupational therapy, it is used as a therapeutic device in helping emotionally troubled individuals. Three ingredients are essential to establishing a therapeutic relationship: (1) understanding, (2) neutrality, sometimes called empathy, and (3) caring.[20] As Siegel explains these principles, the therapist accepts the patient as he or she is. In addition, the therapist is tolerant and interested in the patient's painful affects. Finally, the therapist is able to communicate to the patient what the patient expects from the therapist. By remaining neutral but engaged, the therapist encourages the patient to interact.[20]

Conscious Use of Self

On the basis of the previous definition, one may ask if a therapeutic relationship is like a paid friendship. To qualify as therapy, however, the therapist must do more than be tolerant and empathic. Therapists must also manage their own subjective responses or countertransference problems.

Self-Awareness

Both patients and therapists have personalities. It is the clinician's first job to understand his or her own vulnerabilities, biases, and wishes. This understanding is instrumental to therapist neutrality and objectivity.

Monitoring Objective Observations and Subjective Responses

Objective observations are behavioral descriptions of perceived external characteristics. Subjective observations are descriptions of internal visions, feelings, and thoughts, which are based on an individual's needs, past experiences, and assigned meanings. An example of an objective observation is: the patient was silent during the community outing to the Museum of Fine Arts. A subjective observation of the same incident might be: the patient's withdrawal from the group caused me to feel angry and confrontational.

Therefore, observations include objective and subjective perceptions. Both frames of reference are brought to the therapeutic relationship. Objective perceptions permit systematic analysis and reporting; subjective perceptions are useful for understanding how the therapist or others might be reacting to a patient. Responses based on subjective perceptions, however, might not be in the best interest of the patient. For example, unconscious anger may cause a therapist to be overly protective and to passively encourage the patient's nonparticipation in activities. To identify a subjective response, the therapist may ask questions such as: Is my reaction to this situation or person exaggerated? Am I attempting to fulfill my own unmet needs?

Establishing and Modulating a Therapeutic Relationship

A therapeutic relationship is a developmental process. The therapist needs to determine how much support and gratification are necessary to sustain the patient's health and well-being. This varies depending on the nature and phase of a therapeutic relationship. Trust is preliminary to any therapeutic relationship. Concerns related to termination of therapy vary. In more long-term and intense relationships, feelings of anger, sadness, and loss may be particularly acute during periods of separation and at termination. Anxiety concerning the future is common in short-term therapeutic relationships. In addition, each patient's unique history and set of problems requires that the therapist respond on an individual basis.

Facilitating Self-Initiated Communication and Action

Patient involvement in the doing process is key to occupational therapy. To encourage patient-initiated communication and action, the therapist behaves in ways that make the patient feel cared for, understood, and masterful. For example, the patient is involved as much as possible in setting goals for therapy. A noncritical atmosphere with realistic expectations also seems to inspire adaptive action. Pleasant physical surroundings and challenges within the patient's capabilities appear to foster feelings of self-respect and competence.

Impasses to the Therapeutic Relationship

Noninvolvement of the Patient

Patients are uninvolved in the therapeutic relationship for several reasons. One may ask: what is motivating the noninvolvement? To answer this question requires hypotheses or explanations from the biological, psychological, social, and behavioral domains. An approach to this reasoning process is given in Section 5, under Evaluation.

Countertransference Difficulties

Both the patient and the therapist bring thoughts, feelings, and unconscious reactions to the therapeutic relationship. There are bound to be problems in the therapeutic process when therapists are unaware of their own perceptions and unconscious impulses. For example, as Maltsberger explains, patients with a borderline personality disorder make us hate them—they need to be hated; they need to feel victimized and rejected. In order to acknowledge countertransference impulses, which are mostly unconscious, he suggests that therapists be aware of their own feelings such a nervousness or anxiety.[14]

Purposeful Activity

Purposeful activities are goal-directed tasks that characteristically involve active participation of the doer, with attention directed at the task rather than at the processes required for task accomplishment.[2,16] The use of purposeful activities as a therapeutic modality is a very significant feature of the profession. As Fine comments

> . . . the over-riding focus on actual engagement in a task or activity distinguishes occupational therapy from the verbal psychiatric therapies. Its concerns for the full spectrum of human performance (work, play and self-care); for the relationships and balance among these in coping and adaptation; and for the prerequisites and components of performance, distinguishes occupational therapy theory and practice from that of other activity disciplines whose specialties are based upon the application of a single modality.[7]

Purposeful activity involves a human and a nonhuman environment, process, and, often, materials and a product. Each of these elements will be briefly discussed from the vantage point of mental health practice.

The Human Environment

Occupational therapists work with patients in dyads and groups and on an individual basis. In fact, in Duncombe and Howe's survey of occupational therapy practice, they found that all respondents working in community mental health centers and psychiatric hospitals used groups.[5]

Individual and Dyads

Although the group format is well suited for goals such as those related to socialization and life tasks, at times it is more appropriate to meet with patients in dyads or on a one-to-one basis. Those patients who are easily distracted, require limited stimulation, or need constant supervision and structure do better with individual therapy. Some patients are unable to tolerate working with others, lack the prerequisite skills for participating in a group task, or simply do not have the therapeutic need for a group. Finally, certain interviews, assessments, and teaching–learning processes require one-to-one or dyadic formats.

Group

Occupational therapists use a variety of group formats in mental health. Howe and Schwartzberg propose a model for group work in occupational therapy based on the profession's long-standing interest in groups as a therapeutic tool.[9] The Howe and Schwartzberg model is a functional approach to group work that relies primarily on the use of purposeful, self-initiated action for the fulfillment of individual member and group goals. Duncombe and Howe's profile of occupational therapy group practice, a survey view, includes the following categories: exercise groups, cooking groups, activities of daily living groups, task groups, arts and crafts groups, self-expression groups, feeling-oriented discussion groups, reality-oriented discussion groups, sensorimotor and sensory-integration groups, and education groups. Interestingly, two-thirds of the activities of daily living groups were organized for adult patients with psychosocial dysfunctions. They focused on predischarge living skills and preparation for independent community living, primarily to increase task skills and share information. Overall, 76% of the groups reported were small (fewer than ten members), and all therapists reported that their groups had more than one goal.[5]

Recently, attention has once more been given to studying the unique value of occupational therapy group work with psychiatric patients. Examples of such research include DeCarlo and Mann's study of the effectiveness of verbal *versus* activity groups in treatment of interpersonal communication deficits as a psychiatric day treatment center[4] and Schwartzberg, Howe, and McDermott's comparative investigation of three group treatment formats for facilitating social interaction in a psychiatric acute-care inpatient setting.[19]

The Nonhuman Environment

The nonhuman environment is a critical tool in psychiatric occupational therapy. It includes all nonhuman objects surrounding the patient, such as materials for projects or tasks, decorations, and functional objects such as furniture, tools, and machines. The external physical and emotional atmosphere is also considered part of the nonhuman environment.

During the profession's birth and in the recent past, a significant number of occupational therapy articles addressed concerns about the effects of environment on the deterioration of occupational skills and behaviors.[8,18] Recently, emphasis is being given to incorporating environmental concepts into the profession's theoretical base.[3] There is also renewed interest in empirical studies that examine the relationship between environment and psychiatric occupational therapy. An example of such research is Dunning's 1972 investigation of psychiatric outpatients and their home environments.[6]

Based on her recent analysis of studies on psychiatric ward atmospheres, Kannegieter observes that "research suggests that patients and staff be matched to behavioral settings that facilitate types of behavior compatible with the patient's response modes, and that patients be placed on wards or in occupational therapy settings with other patients who respond with similar response modes and with staff displaying congruent characteristics."[10] Kohler's study of the effect of activity environment on emotionally disturbed children supports the previous conclusion that settings should be matched with patients' ways of responding. This investigator found that the subjects in a room without distractions were more attentive than those in a room with distractions. Furthermore, the children involved in a structured activity were found to be less distractible than the children involved in an unstructured activity.[12]

Mehrabian's study of "environmental load," the information rate of an environment,[15] is important to psychosocial occupational therapy. It offers a broad explanation of the impact of nonhuman environments on psychiatric patients. In addition, because medical–surgical patients are at risk for problems related to environmental load, the concept reinforces our work with activity environments in psychiatric consultation–liaison services. Mehrabian believes that an individual's reaction to an environment creates either approach or avoidance behaviors. Thus, an environment can be designed to elicit a set of responses based on the wish to approach or avoid. The load level is the amount of perceived information in the environment. It is considered a high load if a person perceives the environment as unpredictable, if it makes him feel uncertain. If the environment is low load, it is experienced as common and certain; that is, it contains a low rate of information per unit of time.

Mehrabian explains that for the newly admitted psychiatric patient, excessive environmental loads can increase anxiety and discomfort. Conversely, the long-term patient needs variety and opportunities for rewarding interactions. Mehrabian also proposes that predischarge hospital activities be at a load level typical of the patient's expected community living environment, which, he points out, is the rationale behind halfway houses. Thus to avoid a repetition of preadmission anxieties or stresses, it is advisable that the patient be able to cope with the demands of community living prior to discharge.

It would therefore be advisable to create a relatively predictable, routine, and structured environment for occupational therapy in acute-care settings. As much as possible, therapists may want to provide patients with familiar objects, activity situations, and interactions. To encourage initiative and participation among long-term patients, occupational therapists should provide a tolerable amount of complexity or novelty in the environment and schedule of activities. As one may well imagine, if patients feel that a room is overcrowded with people or things, they will want to avoid that situation. Thus, occupational therapists must monitor and adapt the load levels in their own treatment environments and may also offer advice and consultation concerning environmental loads in the overall institution and program milieu.

Materials, Process, and Product

It is apparent that behavior is influenced by both the human and the nonhuman aspects of purposeful activities. By observing behavior and reactions to a variety of tasks, we gain knowledge about an individual's biological, psychological, social, and behavioral makeup and level of occupational functioning. In relation to a patient's mental disorder, psychiatric occupational therapy also involves selective application of purposeful activities to specific problems in performance areas and performance component skills. This sytematic approach requires knowledge of typical and atypical responses associated with various materials, processes, and end products of occupational therapy.

To offer an example: it is well accepted that long-term institutionalization in an understimulating environment puts elderly individuals at a higher risk for mental problems associated with sensory deprivation. Because of this knowledge, occupational therapists are well advised to consider the environmental load when evaluating and planning treatment for institutionalized geropsychiatric patients. In acknowledging this factor, Paire and Karney conducted a study of the effects of a sensory stimulation program on hospitalized geropsychiatric patients. As one might have expected, they found that the sensory stimulation treatment was effective for increasing patients' interests in group activities and in improving their personal hygiene.[17] However, sensory stimulation was less effective for improving reality orientation than had been expected.

Activity Analysis

The psychiatric occupational therapist uses activity analysis to understand the component demands and meanings of activities. Activity analysis helps answer questions such as: Why does a patient with multiple substance abuse regularly attend cooking group and avoid work-oriented groups? Several levels of explanation may be offered. The patient, forced to abstain from alcohol and nonprescription drugs, might be attempting to fulfill his or her oral dependency needs through eating. In addition, work groups may require interaction that the patient is attempting to avoid. The patient may be experiencing memory and learning problems because of an alcoholism-related cognitive deterioration. Because of such difficulties, work issues may be a particular source of anxiety for the patient. Given the variety of possibilities, multidimensional-integrative activity analysis is extremely useful.

Multidimensional-Integrative Analysis

In analyzing an activity, it is preferable to examine demands at the behavioral, psychological, social, and biological levels. The interactions among these components also deserve attention. In summary, the therapist asks three major questions: (1) What are the human and nonhuman qualities of an activity? (2) What skills and abilities are required to perform the activity successfully? and (3) Can these elements be modified for the purposes of intervention?

The Human Environment: Patient–Therapist Relationship

The qualities of a patient–therapist relationship are central to activity analysis. Patient-to-patient relationship requirements for performance of an activity should also be considered.

When analyzing demands in the biological domain, the therapist is often concerned with biological stimulus conditions. The therapist may ask, for example, is the relatedness required in an activity stressful to human organisms, or does it evoke feelings of safety? From the psychological perspective, one may consider symbolic meanings and transference potential in the activity relationship. More simply, individuals react through past experiences. Activities may require a type or frequency of interaction that resembles the past. An activity can recall certain thoughts, memories, or feelings, and these reactions may confuse the patient, cause some discomfort, or even be pleasurable. It is therefore critical to analyze things such as the degrees of trust, intimacy, independence, and dependence necessary to perform an activity.

It is also important to understand the sociocultural meanings attached to the human relationship aspects of an activity. This can be done by studying a patient's culture and social networks. For example, an Ultra-Orthodox Jewish woman, who is, by custom, expected to take care of her husband and children, would find it difficult to accept help from younger patients and therapists or from men in an occupational therapy activity group.

Finally, from the behavioral domain, the therapist attempts to identify dyadic and group human–object relationship skills required to accomplish a task. Mosey's progression of developmental groups[16] is a very useful framework for analyzing group interaction skills required in a task-oriented group. She identifies five levels of group interaction skill: (1) parallel, (2) project, (3) egocentric-cooperative, (4) cooperative, and (5) mature. As one moves up the developmental continuum, an increasing degree of member skill in group task and maintenance functions is required.

The Nonhuman Environment: Materials, Process, and Product

In one study, it was found that chronic psychiatric patients in a day treatment program had different feelings about three activities commonly used in occupational therapy. The activities studied were a craft activity, a sensory awareness activity, and a cooking activity. Of the three, the cooking activity was rated the highest on the evaluation factor — the measure of positive or negative feelings. However, in regard to power or action factors, no differences were found. The researchers speculated that the cooking activity might be most valued because it fulfilled the patients' oral needs, was concrete, and had an understandable purpose.[13]

The previous example demonstrates the need to analyze the nonhuman material, process, and product components of an activity. One level of this analysis addresses the sociocultural and psychological meanings of these environmental elements. Questions are raised about social, cultural, and developmental reference group definitions. Opportunities for sublimation and self-expression are analyzed. Task demands are also examined from behavioral and biological perspectives. From the behavioral frame of reference, one inquires about the skills prerequisite to activity completion. In considering the biological factors, attention is paid to demands on the physical human systems and to the functional level required of those systems.

Activity Adaptation

Occupational therapy intervention in mental health involves modifications of the therapeutic relationship and doing process. Since activity adaptation is essentially generic to the profession, it is briefly discussed in this chapter.

Therapist as Teacher, Resource Person, Counselor, or Role Model

The patient–therapist relationship is adapted to meet a patient's particular therapeutic and developmental needs. For example, one would expect limit setting and role modeling to be an important aspect of therapeutic relationships with emotionally troubled adolescents. The treatment setting and differences between OTR and COTA role definitions also influence the type of relationships established with patients. Usually, the needs of patients in community rehabilitation programs require therapists to act in the role of teacher and role model rather than emphasize the counseling aspects of the relationship. To summarize, the therapist may act as teacher, resource person, counselor, or role model.

Modifications in the Doing Process: Task, Social, and Nonhuman Environment

Because task performance involves skills that are related, there are risks in viewing each of the human subsystems in isolation. The concept of attention span is a good example of this problem. What regulates attention span? One can find cognitive, sensorimotor, social, and psychological explanations in occupational therapy. With a measureable description of attention span, it would be easier to adapt activities for intervention purposes.

In modifying the doing process, psychiatric occupational therapists consider the task, social, and nonhuman environment. An interesting example of this process is Allen's neurobehavioral approach to task adaptation. As Allen explains, in this cognitive model of psychiatric occupational therapy, "the same motor actions and sensory cues that specify the cognitive levels are used to specify task equivalence. This specification makes it possible to provide an activity that is within a patient's range of ability."[1] She further notes that the criteria for task equivalence involve analysis of *task demands*, *task directions*, and *individual differences* based on past experiences and preferences.[1]

Eliciting an Adaptive Response

King describes how the adaptive response is facilitated by active participation, elicited by environmental demands organized below the conscious level, which of itself is self-reinforcing.[11] In so doing, occupational therapists in mental health are structuring activities to meet particular goals. These goals are based on an evaluation process, which is described in section 5 of this chapter.

Graded Structured Activities

Since activities can require a continuum of abilities, their structure can be graded to various levels of complexity. Finally, given the wide range of purposeful activities appropriate to occupational therapy in mental health, practitioners can be selective about the modalities they use.

References

1. Allen CK: Occupational Therapy for Psychiatric Diseases: Measurement and Management of Cognitive Disabilities, pp 81–83. Boston, Little, Brown, 1985
2. American Occupational Therapy Association: Purposeful activities. Am J Occup Ther 37:805, 1983
3. Barris R: Environmental interactions: An extension of the model of occupation. Am J Occup Ther 36:637, 1982
4. DeCarlo JJ, Mann WC: The effectiveness of verbal versus activity groups in improving self-perceptions of interpersonal communication skills. Am J Occup Ther 39:20, 1985
5. Duncombe LW, Howe MC: Group work in occupational therapy: A survey of practice. Am J Occup Ther 39:163, 1985
6. Dunning H: Environmental occupational therapy. Am J Occup Ther 26:292, 1972
7. Fine SB: Occupational therapy: The role of rehabilitation and purposeful activity in mental health practice, p 5. White Paper, Executive Board of the American Occupational Therapy Association, 1983
8. Gray M: Effects of hospitalization on work-play behavior. Am J Occup Ther 26:180, 1972
9. Howe MC, Schwartzberg SL: A Functional Approach to Group Work in Occupational Therapy. Philadelphia, JB Lippincott, 1986
10. Kannegieter RB: Environmental interactions in psychiatric occupational therapy: Some inferences. Am J Occup Ther 34:720, 1980
11. King LJ: 1978 Eleanor Clarke Slagle Lecture: Toward a science of adaptive responses. Am J Occup Ther 32:429, 1978
12. Kohler ES: The effect of activity/environment on emotionally disturbed children. Am J Occup Ther 34:446, 1980
13. Kremer ERH, Nelson DL, Duncombe LW: Effects of selected activities on affective meaning in psychiatric patients. Am J Occup Ther 38:522, 1984
14. Maltsberger JT: Hospital treatment of borderline patients: Problems of suicide. Presented at the 37th Institute on

Hospital and Community Psychiatry, American Psychiatric Association, Montreal, October 1985

15. Mehrabian A: Public Places and Private Spaces: The Psychology of Work, Play, and Living Environments. New York, Basic Books, 1976
16. Mosey AC: Occupational Therapy: Configuration of a Profession. New York, Raven Press, 1981
17. Paire JA, Karney RJ: The effectiveness of sensory stimulation for geropsychiatric inpatients. Am J Occup Ther 38:505, 1984

18. Parent LH: Effects of low-stimulus environment on behavior. Am J Occup Ther 32:19, 1978
19. Schwartzberg SL, Howe MC, McDermott A: A comparison of three treatment group formats for facilitating social interaction. Occup Ther Mental Health 2:1, 1983
20. Siegel A: Prerequisites for engagement in psychotherapy: Implications for the therapist. Cambridge, MA, Mount Auburn Hospital Psychiatry Grand Rounds, April 1986

SECTION 5

Generic Processes *Sharan L. Schwartzberg*

Evaluation

The primary purposes of evaluation are to identify areas of function and dysfunction in occupational behavior and to engage the patient in a therapeutic process that will ultimately improve his or her level of adaptation and life satisfaction. *Occupational behavior* is generally defined as the human sphere of routine activities or occupations of daily living.

According to Barris, Kielhofner, and Watts, "healthy occupational behavior represents a balance between inner needs and external requirements. When either or both are not met, disorder is present."[6] Hence, occupational behavior dysfunction occurs when individuals are unable to satisfy their urge to explore and master the environment through daily occupations or when individuals are unable to meet the requirements of the external environment.[6]

Generating and Testing Clinical Hypotheses

Lazare's hypothesis-generation and -testing approach[18] is applied here as a framework to explain the processes involved in occupational therapy evaluation. The approach first requires that a manageable list of hypothesized partial formulations be developed on the basis of current psychiatric knowledge. Lazare organizes his hypotheses into four categories: biologic, psychodynamic, sociocultural, and behavioral (Table 25-2).

Next, the clinician repeatedly carries out a three-step mental process of hypothesis generation and testing. The operations are as follows:

1. From multiple sources, the clinician collects early critical negative and positive data pertaining to the partial formulations.
2. On the basis of data collected, hypotheses are generated, confirmed, and refuted.

3. Methods are employed to elicit further data that will lead to the generation of new hypotheses and the confirmation or refutation of old ones.

It was assumed, in selecting this approach to clinical formulation, that contemporary occupational therapy

Table 25-2. *Lazare's Hypothesized Partial Formulations*

Conceptual Framework	Explanatory Factors
Biologic	Syndromes or biologic conditions
Psychodynamic	Personality style
	Stress or precipitating event and psychological meaning
	Unresolved grief
	Developmental crisis
	Ego functioning and related psychodynamic issues
Sociocultural	Nature and social impact of stressful life events
	Social resources
	Reference group's definition of and response to mental illness
	Meaning of symbolic communication
Behavioral	Specific antecedent events
	Stimulus conditions
	Reinforcements
	Behavioral and skill deficits
	Areas of effective functioning and skill assets

Summarized from Lazare A: Hypothesis testing in the clinical interview. In: Lazare A (ed): *Outpatient Psychiatry Diagnosis and Treatment*, pp. 131–140. Baltimore, Williams & Wilkins, 1979.

practice is derived from multidimensional-integrative conceptual models. Although this view may be questioned, and the models may be scientifically incomplete, it appears to have validity in light of the current literature and consensus in fields of psychosocial practice.

Furthermore, it is assumed and emphasized that

1. The type of occupational therapy evaluation selected and the meaning assigned to the data collected must be made explicit through a stated conceptual model.
2. The outcomes of an evaluation imply the treatment goals and therapeutic modalities to be chosen.
3. The patient must be involved as fully as possible in the evaluation and treatment planning process.
4. Problems in the conduct of activities of daily living, the domain of occupational therapy, may result in part from psychological, social, or behavioral variables or be associated with the disease process itself.
5. Occupational behavior dysfunction may actually precipitate an individual's mental disorder.[6]
6. The patient's mental disorder or order may be inseparable from dysfunction or function in areas of occupational performance and performance component skills.[6]

Hypothesized Partial Formulations

The following partial formulations are suggested for generating hypotheses about the patient's occupational behavior dysfunction. Lazare originally identified the conditions or factors mentioned below as useful concepts for understanding psychiatric outpatients[6] (see Table 25-2). The "Skills and Performance Areas"[3] are discussed later in this section and are listed in Appendix F.

First, the patient's occupational behavior dysfunction can be understood in part as resulting from a *syndrome or biologic condition*[18] that affects skills and performance areas. Syndromes and biologic conditions include clinical psychiatric syndromes, personality disorders, and nonmental medical disorders (Axes I, II, and III of DSM-III).[19] Lazare emphasizes that, although the syndromal diagnoses in DSM-III are systematically considered in biologic hypotheses about the patient's problem, the previous conditions may have nonbiologic explanations.[19] Nevertheless, since problems in occupational functioning may be associated with the disease process itself, biologic hypotheses should be considered when evaluating every patient. This is particularly important because the occupational therapist's direct observations of occupational behavior yield critical information about the patient's level of adaptive functioning. For example, because somatic treatments are often useful in management of biologic disorders, by monitoring symptoms and the side-effects of medication during

task performance, the therapist establishes a baseline for evaluating change.[1,27] On a psychiatric inpatient unit, this type of occupational therapy consultation is vital. It can assist the psychiatrist in determining an appropriate diagnosis and plan for somatic therapy. In addition, by also screening for functional skills and residual disabilities, such clinical data acknowledges psychodynamic, sociocultural, and behavioral variables influencing a patient's level of functioning. Finally, a biologic hypothesis should be considered since there is a neurobehavioral approach to occupational therapy treatment of schizophrenia.

Second, the patient's occupational behavior dysfunction can be understood in part on the basis of *psychodynamic factors*[18] that affect skills and performance areas. These explanatory factors may include manifestations of personality style; the stress or precipitating event and its psychological meaning, unresolved grief, a developmental crisis, and ego functioning and related psychodynamic issues.[18]

The occupational therapist has many opportunities to observe a patient's natural psychological response to the human and nonhuman environment. Psychodynamic patterns can easily be identified through examination of an individual's response to the range of activities, materials, and processes employed. Strategies used for coping with a variety of task situations (structured, unstructured, and semistructured) can further the clinician's understanding of the patient's personality style and emotional vulnerabilities.[27] For example, does the patient quit a project when near success? Regardless of repeated errors, is the patient unwilling to accept help in learning a new activity? Does the patient always blame himself or herself, the therapist, or other patients for difficulties in the task? Does the patient avoid interaction by choosing solitary, complex, and detailed projects? Is the patient attempting to resolve a developmental crisis; for example, children leaving home, by continuously looking to help others engage in activities?

Third, the patient's occupational behavior dysfunction can be understood in part in terms of *sociocultural factors*[18] that affect skills and performance areas. In evaluating a patient, the social and cultural factors to consider include the nature and social impact of stressful life events, such as stress leading to role change or role loss and its effect on the patient and his or her social system; the extent, nature, and accessibility of social support — the social resources that facilitate movement toward goals; the definition and response to breakdown in the person's sociocultural groupings; and the meaning of symbolic communication, such as symptoms serving as messages.[18]

Through observation of the patient in occupational therapy, especially in groups, the therapist can learn about an individual's value system and temporal management of various social roles and capacity to use social supports.[27] The premorbid and current activity patterns should also be compared in investigating sociocultural hypotheses. The therapist likewise secures data about the patient's values and the preferences of significant others concerning how time should be occupied.

This assessment provides valuable information about the loss of valued social and occupational roles, changes in available personal, nonhuman, and social supports, and the meaning of occupational behavior problems from the perspectives of the patient and individuals in his or her social system. For example, a family may assume homemaking duties for the identified patient who values that role and can perform it well. Thereby, the family system promotes a social condition that maintains the patient's occupational behavior dysfunction.

Changes in the external environment are bound to occur when individuals are removed from their immediate social settings and roles. In fact, for some individuals, psychiatric hospitalization itself may precipitate occupational behavior dysfunction. Patients are commonly impaired by consequences such as loss of employment or a shift in family role distribution. This is especially acute when their primary gratification and status are derived from a former occupational role.

Fourth, the patient's occupational behavior dysfunction can be understood in part by an analysis of *behavioral factors*[18] that affect skills and performance areas. An individual's behavior may be considered disordered and thus causally related to specific antecedent events, determined by sociocultural and biologic stimulus conditions, or resulting from reinforcing consequences of the behaviors. Occupational behavior dysfunction may also result because of a deficit of behaviors or a lack of requisite skills for effective functioning. The patient's behavior can be further understood by an analysis of the areas of effective functioning.[18]

The occupational therapist's knowledge of activity analysis is particularly important in considering behavioral hypotheses. By observing the patient's actual performance of life tasks, one can glean general information about assets and deficits in skills and performance areas. However, the therapist should first determine the skills necessary for adaptive functioning. Several questions may be addressed. What skills are necessary for this individual to meet external environmental demands and mastery needs? How might the home, community, program, or hospital environment be contributing to skill loss or atrophy? In addition, are there conditions that might be stimulating or reinforcing disordered occupational behavior? What are the conditions that reinforce functional occupational behavior?

Knowledge of the behavioral domain helps to identify whether the patient has the prerequisite skills and performance necessary for a type of therapy. For example, insight-oriented therapy would be a poor choice if the patient is cognitively impaired by innate or primary skill deficits in orientation, conceptualization, or cognitive integration. Behavioral data also help isolate motivating factors. Particular skills can be further evaluated and perhaps learned. By understanding behavioral conditions, one can more easily speculate about the major aims of therapy: (1) there-and-then re-experience, (2) here-and-now experience, or (3) adaptation of the biological, physical, intellectual, or social–emotional environments.

Collect Early Critical Data

The AOTA "Uniform Occupational Therapy Evaluation Checklist"[3] (see Appendix F) is suggested as a format for collecting critical data related to the partial formulations. As Rogers observes, "the Checklist forces the therapist to examine occupational performance from a panoramic view rather than microscopically. In so doing, it fosters the search for information that might suggest hypotheses the therapist might not otherwise have entertained."[25]

In using the checklist, the occupational therapist will need to select methods of evaluation that may include record review, interview, observation, and the administration of specific data collection procedures. The checklist partially includes the following global categories, which are further detailed in the document along with other categories. As this is a fixed data-collection schedule, whether the data confirm or disprove a hypothesis, the therapist must report about all major categories. All the terms are defined in the AOTA "Uniform Terminology for Reporting Occupational Therapy Services"[4] (see Appendix D).

I. Demographic Information
  A. Personal information
  B. Referral related information
  C. Personal history
II. Skills and Performance Areas
  A. Independent living/daily living skills and performance
    1. Physical daily living skills
    2. Psychologic/emotional daily living skills
    3. Work
    4. Play/leisure
  B. Sensorimotor Skills and Performance Components
    1. Neuromuscular
    2. Sensory integration
  C. Cognitive Skills and Performance Components
    1. Orientation
    2. Conceptualization/comprehension
    3. Cognitive integration
  D. Psychosocial Skills and Performance Components
    1. Self-management
    2. Dyadic interaction
    3. Group interaction

Generate, Confirm, and Refute Hypotheses

Once the critical data have been collected, the partial hypotheses are reviewed and confirmed or refuted on the basis of the data. Those hypotheses that seem most probable and relevant are subjected to further testing. A hypothesis certainly deserves further investigation, for example, if, on the basis of theory and research, one would expect to find such a pattern.

Elicit Further Specific Data to Confirm or Refute Hypotheses Under Consideration and Possibly Generate New Ones

The therapist needs to continue data collection until no new relevant information is being generated.[25] There is no one universal standardized tool to gather sufficient data for a multidimensional-integrative case analysis and formulation. Several occupational therapy evaluation tools and methods of data collection are required.

Methods of Data Collection

The evaluation data base in occupational therapy is usually derived from several sources. Data collection methods may include any of the following in various combinations:

1. Review of referrral, screening, and record information
2. Informal, semistructured, or structured interviews
3. Unstructured observation of task performance
4. Structured observation of task performance with standarized or nonstandardized rating scales
5. Written questionnaires or self-report inventories with open-ended questions, fixed categories, standardized administration and scoring, or nonstandardized formats
6. Standardized or nonstandardized tests

Models of integrative evaluation protocols for preliminary data gathering can be found in the literature.[10,12,14,27] An initial protocol is chosen or devised according to the treatment setting and patient population.

Specific instruments also need to be selected or designed on the basis of hypotheses generated for testing to make final biologic, psychodynamic, sociocultural, and behavioral inferences. A partial list of evaluation tools organized by conceptual categories is given in Table 25-3. Several sources, including this textbook, contain comprehensive reviews of tools that may be used for data collection in generating and testing hypotheses.[6,9,15,16,21,24]

Appropriate selection, administration, and interpretation of an evaluation demands considerable experience and expertise, especially when protocols need to be created for particular environments and populations. In order to be successful as an evaluator, the beginning therapist most certainly will require supervision by and consultation with senior colleagues in occupational therapy.

Program Development

As a result of screening and evaluation, the therapist determines if a patient is in need of occupational therapy services. It is generally accepted that occupational therapy can serve the following several purposes: (1) fulfillment of ordinary health needs, (2) prevention of occupational behavior dysfunction, (3) change processes of development or restoration, (4) maintenance of functioning, or (5) management of disabling behaviors.[20] Like any health profession, with additional research and discoveries, the purposes of occupational therapy in mental health will also be further clarified and refined.

In developing a program, the therapist first establishes a treatment plan. The occupational therapy plan outlines long-term goals, short-term goals, therapeutic methods and media, and the treatment environments to be used. Also included are methods for evaluating progress, the frequency of service, procedures for termination, and discharge plans.

The treatment plan is often devised in cooperation with other health team members. In some settings, occupational therapy services are determined by a unit director or prescribed by the patient's attending psychiatrist. For example, services such as evaluation and treatment, on a hospital inpatient unit require a formal medical referral if they are to be eligible for insurance coverage.[26]

As one can see, program development is not only based on the needs of patients. Economics, staff politics, and technological resources also play a role in the amount and type of intervention delivered. Because coverage for occupational therapy services is not uniform and unlimited in the United States, third-party payment criteria for reimbursement must be considered in program development, administration, and documentation.[23] An occupational therapy program is further influenced by external accreditation requirements, professional standards, and policies in the immediate setting.

Setting Goals with the Patient

Ideally, goals are formulated on the basis of hypotheses confirmed during the evaluation process. This requires the patient's participation and consensus. As was mentioned earlier, in the very first contact, the therapist attempts to establish a therapeutic climate for such mutual goal setting. In fact, there is mounting evidence to suggest that a patient's understanding of the therapeutic purposes of occupational therapy can influence his or her participation and satisfaction.[11,22]

When the patient is unable to engage in a dialogue

Table 25-3. *Conceptual Frameworks and Evaluation Tools**

	Title	Source
Biologic	Allen Cognitive Level (ACL) Test and Lower Cognitive Level (LCL) Test	Allen CK: Assessment procedures. In Allen CK: *Occupational Therapy for Psychiatric Diseases: Measurement and Management of Cognitive Disabilities*, pp. 105–129. Boston, Little, Brown, 1985
	Person Symbol	King LJ: The person symbol as an assessment tool. In Hemphill BJ (ed): *The Evaluative Process in Psychiatric Occupational Therapy*, pp. 169–194. Thorofare, NJ, Charles B Slack, 1982
	Schroeder Block Campbell Adult Psychiatric Sensory Integration Evaluation (SBC)	Schroeder CV, Block MP, Trottier EC, et al: The adult psychiatric sensory integration evaluation. *Ibid.*, pp 227–253
	Southern California Sensory Integration Tests (for children)	Ayres AJ: Southern California Sensory Integration Test Manual. Los Angeles. Western Psychological Services, 1974
Psychodynamic	Azima Battery	Azima FJ: The Azima battery: An overview. In Hemphill *op. cit.*, pp. 57–61
	BH Battery	Hemphill BJ: The BH battery. *Ibid.*, pp 127–138
	Diagnostic Test Battery	Andores L, Dreyfus E, Bloesch M: Diagnostic test battery for occupational therapy. Am J Occup Ther 19:53, 1965
	Fidler Diagnostic Battery	Fidler GS: Diagnostic battery, scoring and summary. In Mazer J (ed): *Materials From the 1968 Regional Institutes.* Sponsored by the American Occupational Therapy Association on the Evaluation Process. Final Report RSA Grant 123-T-68. New York, American Occupational Therapy Association, 1968
	Goodman Battery	Evaskus MG: The Goodman battery. In Hemphill, *op. cit.*, pp 85–125
	Magazine Picture Collage	Buck RE, Provancher MA: Magazine picture collage as an evaluation technique. Am J Occup Ther 26:36, 1972 Lerner C: The magazine picture collage. In Hemphill, *op. cit.*, pp 139–154
	Shoemyen Battery	Shoemyen CW: The Shoemyen battery. *Ibid.*, pp 63–83
Sociocultural	Activity Configuration	Mosey AC: *Activities Therapy*, pp 101–102. New York, Raven Press, 1973
	Adolescent Role Assessment	Black M: The adolescent role assessment. In Hemphill, *op. cit.*, pp 49–53
	Assessment of Occupational Functioning (AOF)	Watts JH, Kielhofner G, Bauer DF, et al: The assessment of occupational functioning: A screening tool for usein long-term care. Am J Occup Ther 40:231, 1986
	Interest checklist	Matsutsuyu JS: The interest checklist. Am J Occup Ther 23:323, 1969
	Occupational history	Moorhead L: The occupational history. Am J Occup Ther 23:329, 1969
	Occupational performance history interview	Henry A, Kielhofner G, et al: *The Occupational Performance History Interview: Preliminary Version.* Rockville, MD, American Occupational Therapy Association, 1985

(continued)

Table 25-3. *Conceptual Frameworks and Evaluation Tools* *(continued)*

	Title	*Source*
	Occupational role history	Florey LL, Michelman SM: Occupational role history: A screening tool for psychiatric occupational therapy. Am J Occup Ther 36:301, 1982
Behavioral	Bay Area Functional Performance Evaluation (BAFPE)	Bloomer J, Williams S: The Bay Area functional performance evaluation. In Hemphill, *op. cit.*, pp 255–308
	Comprehensive Evaluation of Basic Living Skills (CEBLS)	Casanova JS, Ferber J: Comprehensive evaluation of basic living skills. Am J Occup Ther 30:101, 1976
	Comprehensive Occupational Therapy Evaluation (COTE)	Brayman SJ, Kirby T: The comprehensive occupational therapy evaluation. In Hemphill, *op. cit.*, pp 211–226
	Kohlman Evaluation of Living Skills (KELS)	McGourty LK: *Kohlman Evaluation of Living Skills.* Seattle, Health Sciences Learning Resources Center, University of Washington, 1979
	Mosey Skills Surveys and Interview Guides	Mosey AC: Evaluation. In Mosey, *op. cit.*, pp 83–103
	Parachek Geriatric Rating Scale	Parachek J, King LJ: *Parachek Geriatric Rating Scale.* Scottsdale, AZ, Greenroom Publishing Company, 1976

* Although tools may elicit data useful for more than one framework, categories reflect predominant features of the tools listed.

about these concerns, the therapist must adapt the interview process. This may occur, for example, if a patient is cognitively impaired and unable to make decisions about the future. Also, patients with acute distress may feel overwhelmed with emotions or be distrustful of others, and it is common to find patients who are unmotivated to change their occupational behavior. This may occur for complex biologic, psychological, and social reasons or because the patient lacks the skills necessary for change.

The general types of occupational therapy goals in mental health include *treatment, maintenance, rehabilitation, and prevention.* Programs usually have more than one goal. Each type will be discussed briefly.

Stated in measureable terms, occupational therapy *treatment* goals are the expected outcomes of intervention for an individual's occupational behavior dysfunction. Treatment goals include aims to restore functioning to a premorbid level or to target areas for new learning. The goals are established for skills and performance areas affected by biologic, psychodynamic, sociocultural, or behavioral factors. A goal may be specific and restricted to performance component skills or global and related to occupational performance areas. However, since there is usually a relationship between skill deficits and performance area dysfunctions, considerable overlap exists between restricted and global treatment goals.

Goals for *maintenance* of functioning are often established through general activity program aims. In order to foster a healthy milieu, the therapist plans and structures activities to provide opportunities for normal human gratifications such as those found in exercise, recreation, self-care, and other activities of daily living. As part of the discharge planning process, goals to prevent future occupational behavior dysfunction may also be established. These goals often involve the use of community resources and interactions with future environments such as the family, school, and workplace.

Finally, *rehabilitation* goals are central to any occupational therapy program. Rehabilitation does not, however, aim to change the individual. Rather, its general purpose is to adapt or change the physical, social, and emotional environment so that a person may function as well as possible.

Whether rehabilitation is a primary or secondary goal depends on several factors. The patient's resources, intervention setting, and time interval in the intervention process are a few of these variables. For example, central objectives of a short-term psychiatric hospitalization are containment and emotional distance from overwhelming affects.[28] In addition to the use of medicine, an occupational therapy rehabilitation program is a common form of management used to achieve these conditions. In contrast, rehabilitation goals are often more ambitious in long-term hospital and outpatient programs.

Determining Methods and Developing a Plan

Intervention methods are determined on the basis of the goals established. A plan is thereby developed that indicates the personnel, intervention media, procedures, and environment to be used for program implementation. In developing a plan, the therapist must address the following questions:

1. What is therapeutic about the methods selected?
2. What outcomes are expected and why are they expected? Therefore, is there theoretical or empirical support for use of these methods?
3. Are the methods appropriate to the nature and priorities of the patient, intervention setting, and problems identified?
4. Are there qualified staff and ample nonhuman resources to implement the intended program?

Program Implementation and Evaluation

A program is implemented once the problem areas, long-term goals, short-term goals, therapeutic methods, and program rationale are established. Program changes are made in tandem with the patient's progress. The patient's performance and program are periodically re-evaluated. The former is documented within a time frame appropriate to the setting's requirements in the patient's record.

Team Collaboration

The occupational therapist collaborates with several mental health professionals. In direct service, the therapist may work jointly with other team members for general management or specific treatment of patients' clinical conditions. An additional, primary yet auxiliary role for the occupational therapist is observation and evaluation of medication effects and side-effects. Therapists also give and receive supervision and consultation at a level commensurate with their education, training, and experience. All direct and indirect service roles include information sharing through oral and written communications.

Roles of Mental Health Professionals

A variety of professionals and paraprofessionals are educated to work as specialists in the area of mental health (Table 25-4)[7,29,31] Their educational backgrounds range from the postdoctoral level to no formal education other than inservice education in the work setting. Al-

Table 25-4. *Mental Health Service Providers*

Discipline	Generic Team Role	Minimum Education
Art, music, and dance therapy	Facilitate communication and awareness through creative modality	Master's degree
Nursing	Milieu and nursing care	Psychiatric nurse clinical specialist: Master's degree; Nursing generalist: associate degree, diploma, baccalaureate degree
Occupational therapy	Functional assessment and activities to promote occupational functioning and adaptation	Baccalaureate degree
Paraprofessional counseling	Maintain therapeutic milieu	No standard education
Psychiatry	Medical care	Doctorate in medicine and psychiatric residency
Psychology	Psychologic testing and assessment	Doctorate in clinical psychology
Recreational and activity therapy	General social, recreational, and activity programs	Baccalaureate degree
Social work	Family work; identify social resources and community referrals	Baccalaureate degree

though there is some variation according to the setting, generic roles exist for each of the formal disciplines. Role blurring and a lack of clear role definition are more common in nontraditional settings and for paraprofessional staff with no standard education or training in a mental health field.

Supervision and Consultation

The complex intrapersonal and interpersonal nature of a therapeutic relationship requires delicate supervision. Regular supervisory sessions with a senior therapist offer the neophyte therapist an opportunity to reflect and to organize plans of action. Unlike a personal therapy, which is solely for the therapist's gain, supervision is a professional growth process aimed primarily to benefit the patient or fulfill the institution's aims. The supervisor also has direct responsibility for evaluating and instructing the supervisee's work. Therapists with advanced clinical training and experience usually voluntarily seek out individual supervision or peer supervision groups.

Occupational therapists act as consultants for patients, other professionals, programs, and institutions. In a consultation, the therapist offers his or her expert opinion regarding the matter in question. The person or individuals in receipt of this service are consultees. They are free to follow through on the recommendation or can choose to reject the advice. Consultation does not impose the obligations found in formal supervision.

Role of Somatic Therapies, Types, and Side-Effects

Somatic therapies play an important role in contemporary treatment of major mental disorders. These biologic interventions primarily include pharmacotherapies and electroconvulsive therapy (see box). Apart from their negative side-effects, somatic therapies may benefit patients by shortening the duration of acute phases of an illness, decreasing the frequency of episodes, helping engagement in interpersonal therapies, and lessening or shortening periods of hospitalization. Antipsychotic agents, in particular, are praised for drastically reducing periods of hospitalization for patients with schizophrenia as well as helping prevent relapse and rehospitalization.

Although it is the psychiatrist's role to prescribe

Somatic Therapies Commonly Used in Psychiatry

Pharmacotherapies

Antipsychotic Agents ("Major Tranquilizers," Neuroleptics)
Common trade names: Thorazine, Vesprin, Mellaril, Serentil, Prolixin, Trilafon, Stelazine, Taractan, Navane, Loxitane, Haldol, Moban, Serpasil

Major value: Management of acute psychotic symptoms; particularly useful in treatment of schizophrenia and mania

Limitations: Many patients with chronic schizophrenia do not respond well. Drug of choice depends on history of response (or failure) in patient or family and side-effects. Compliance is a problem because of unpleasant side-effects. Risk of acute, long-lasting, and potentially irreversible side-effects in form of neurological disorders of the extrapyramidal motor system (*e.g.*, dystonias, akathisias, parkinsonism with acute administration, and tardive dyskinesia after prolonged use)

Potential side-effects: Sedation, dry mouth, blurred vision, constipation, urinary hesitation, restlessness, muscle spasms, rigidity, sluggishness, tremor, itching, sun sensitivity, weight gain, bone-marrow suppression

Antimanic Agents (Lithium Salts)
Common name: lithium carbonate

Major value: Management and prophylactic effectiveness for patients with bipolar manic–depressive illness and recurrent depressive disorders

Limitations: Clinical actions may be delayed for a week or more; this may necessitate hospitalization and use of antipsychotic agent for the very disturbed patient (*i.e.*, in acute severe mania). Requires close medical supervision because of relatively narrow margin of safety; very low risk of later lithium-induced renal damage when monitored carefully

Potential side-effects: Nausea, vomiting, diarrhea, metallic taste, tremor, awkwardness, unsteadiness, thirst, urinary frequency, skin rashes
Note. Tegretol is a good second choice for mania.

Antidepressant Agents
Common trade names: Monoamine oxidase (MAO) inhibitors: Parnate, Nardil. Tricyclic antidepressants: Elavil, Norpramine, Pertofrane, Adapin, Sinequan, Tofranil, Aventyl, Vivactil. Second-generation antidepressants: Desyrel. Experimental antidepressants: Xanax, Tegretol

Major value: Alleviation of serious depression in major depression and depressive episodes of bipolar disorder

Limitations: Unpleasant side-effects, relatively toxic, potentially lethal, and used in a population at high suicidal risk. MAO inhibitors not widely prescribed because of potential toxic effects (*e.g.*, hypertensive crisis); tricyclics are first choice

Potential side-effects: Sedation, dry mouth, blurred vision, urinary hesitation, constipation, skin rashes, agitation, excitement

(Text continues on following page)

Somatic Therapies Commonly Used in Psychiatry   *(continued)*

Antianxiety Agents ("Minor Tranquilizers," Anxiolytics)

Common trade names: Xanax, Tranxene, Librium, Valium, Ativan, Serax. For sleep: Dalmane, Restoril, Halcion

Major value: Antianxiety and sedative effects

Limitations: Increasing doses required due to tolerance; can produce psychological dependence and physical addiction. Severely dangerous withdrawal syndromes. Toxic and potentially lethal when taken acutely in high doses above the usual daily dose

Potential side-effects: Excessive sedation, unsteadiness, skin rashes; sedation in morning from sleep medications

Disulfiram

Common trade name: Antabuse

Major value: As a component of supportive therapy for alcoholism, this drug helps motivated individuals avoid impulsive drinking by causing unpleasant symptoms when alcohol is ingested (*e.g.*, throbbing headache, nausea, vomiting, respiratory difficulty).

Limitations: The drug cannot cure alcoholism or prevent drinking. It is useful only for patients who want to remain sober, since a person can "safely"

ingest alcohol a few days after the last dose. Severe alcohol–Antabuse reactions can result in grave medical consequences (*e.g.*, coma, death).

Potential side-effects: Sedation, a metallic taste, mild gastrointestinal disturbances

Electroconvulsive Therapy (ECT)

Major value: For severely depressed patients who have not responded to an adequate trial of antidepressants or whose medical condition makes use of medications risky. Also highly effective for severely manic patients

Limitations: Without maintenance pharmacotherapy, relapse rate is as high as 50% within 1 year

Potential side-effects: Amnesia, confusion, headache, muscle aches, nausea, adverse reactions to anesthesia

Compiled from: Baldessarini RJ: The use of chemotherapy in outpatient psychiatry. In Lazare A. (ed): *Outpatient Psychiatry: Diagnosis and Treatment,* pp 563–595. Baltimore, Williams & Wilkins, 1979; Glenn M, Taska RJ: Antidepressants and lithium, pp 85–118. In Karasu TB (chair): *The Psychiatric Therapies.* Washington, DC, American Psychiatric Association, 1984; Tomb DA: *Psychiatry for the House Officer,* 2nd ed. Baltimore, Williams & Wilkins, 1984.

these therapies, occupational therapists observe and report about somatically induced changes in occupational behavior and performance. In treatment and discharge planning, the therapist must raise questions about how somatic therapy may limit and enhance a patient's functioning. The following should be considered:

1. What side-effects may one expect as a result of the somatic therapy? How might these side-effects interfere with the patient's occupational functioning?
2. As a result of somatic therapy side-effects, are there any contraindicated activity processes, materials, products, or environments? For example: avoiding activities requiring mental and physical alertness if the patient is excessively sedated from an antianxiety agent, avoiding undue exposure to the sun if the patient is taking an antipsychotic agent, and avoiding very fine work with patients who have blurred vision or tremor.
3. How has the patient's occupational behavior and performance changed as a result of somatic therapy?
4. How should treatment activities and discharge plans be adapted or modified to accommodate

changes in functioning as a result of somatic therapy?
5. What is the patient's capacity to understand the medication he or she is taking, including its side-effects and benefits?

Information Sharing

Multiaxial Classification Systems: DSM-III (Axes I–V) and Occupational Therapy Uniform Terminology

Two information-reporting systems are central to psychosocial occupational therapy practice and research in the United States. One is the *Diagnostic and Statistical Manual of Mental Disorders* (DSM-III),[5] the official classification scheme of the American Psychiatric Association. The other is the Uniform Terminology for Reporting Occupational Therapy Services (see Appendix D), the official occupational therapy services description and definitions of the AOTA. The DSM-III will here be described in some detail because of its particular relevance to mental health services.

In order to achieve a common language from which clinicians and researchers could communicate about mental disorders, the DSM-III contains operationally defined criteria for psychiatric diagnoses. As a multiaxial system of classification, multiple diagnoses are permitted for an individual. To make a diagnosis, a psychiatrist matches information from the patient's clinical history and presentation with criteria from a likely diagnosis. The diagnosis is established when an adequate number of criteria are met.

With the DSM-III, a patient is evaluated on each of the following five axes:

Axis I: The clinical psychiatric syndromes
Axis II: Personality disorders and specific developmental disorders
Axis III: Physical disorders or conditions
Axis IV: Severity of psychosocial stressors
Axis V: Highest level of adaptive functioning in past year

Although only the first three axes are needed for an official diagnosis, full classification includes a code for each of the five axes. Since adaptive functioning is defined as a composite of the individual's social relations, occupational functioning, and use of leisure time, occupational therapists naturally make an important contribution to the psychiatrist's Axis V evaluation.

Documentation — Record-Keeping Methods

For several purposes, as already mentioned, the patient's status and course of occupational therapy intervention are routinely documented in a permanent record. It is advisable to follow the AOTA's *Guidelines for Occupational Therapy Documentation*.[2] (Appendix G) According to these guidelines, and following requirements established by the individual facility, accreditation bodies, and government agencies, each patient's record should include:

1. *Identification and background information*: Name, age, sex, date of admission, treatment diagnosis, and date of onset of current problem; referral source, services requested, and date of referral to occupational therapy; pertinent history that indicates prior levels of function and support systems; secondary problems or pre-existing conditions; and precautions and contraindications
2. *Assessment and reassessment*: Refer to the Uniform Occupational Therapy Checklist for specific skills and performance — tests and evaluations administered and the results; summary and analysis of assessment findings; references to other pertinent reports and information; occupational therapy

problem list; and recommendations for occupational therapy services.
3. *Treatment planning*: Long- and short-term goals; activities and treatment procedures; type, amount, and frequency of treatment; anticipated time needed to achieve goals; and statement of potential functional outcome
4. *Treatment implementation*: Activities, procedures, and modalities used; patient's response to treatment and the progress toward goal attainment as related to the problem list; goal modification when indicated by the response to treatment; change in anticipated time to achieve goals; attendance and participation with treatment plan; statement of reason for patient missing treatment; assistive/adaptive equipment, orthotics, and prosthetics if issued or fabricated and specific instructions for the application and/or use of the item; patient-related conferences and communication; and home programs.
5. *Discontinuation of services*: Summary of assessment and treatment implementation; home programs; follow-up plans; recommendations; and referral(s) to other health care providers and community agencies.

Formats for the psychiatric case record vary; however, the Weed Problem-Oriented Record (POR)[30] is widely applied to psychiatric clinical record keeping. The POR contains four main parts: (1) the *data base* — history, physical examination, and routine laboratory data; (2) the *problem list* — a numbered list of the patient's problems; (3) *initial plans* for each problem; and (4) *progress notes* on each problem.

The progress note itself generally comprises the following elements; hence, it is commonly called a SOAP note:

S = *Subjective data*: What the patient says about problem areas and feelings
O = *Objective data*: Repeatable findings of specific evaluations and tests; objective descriptions of behavior; and treatment done to the patient and results achieved
A = *Assessment*: Professional conclusions about the preceding subjective and objective data; effectiveness of the treatment and any changes needed; and goals
P = *Plan*: Course that will be taken, based on preceding assessment to achieve goals for identified problems: further evaluations, specific treatments or modalities, and recommendations

Record keeping, a formalization of care provided, is particularly important to the legal aspects involved in mental health service delivery. As Gutheil notes, "complex and difficult decisions made on the firing line deserve the protection from liability that scrupulous documentation provides." [13]

Forensic Psychiatry

The whole specialized area where law and psychiatry mix is called forensic psychiatry.[17] Some of the problems dealt with in forensic psychiatry have relevance to the occupational therapist, including professional negligence or malpractice; preparing evaluations for probationary, child custody, and compensation for injury cases; and determining an individual's functional capacity or competency to care for self, others, and property. Certainly, any occupational therapist working in mental health is well advised to become familiar with legal issues concerning patient confidentiality, hospitalization, criminal responsibility, and informed consent.

Borofsky and Levine suggest the following guidelines for mental health professionals conducting "psychological evaluations" in the role of expert witness[8]:
1. Clarify the referring question in a legal referral. Questions that ask for predictions about the future or for cause-and-effect relationships are poor questions to attempt.
2. Use objective, structured interview methods and tests with normative data.
3. Do not write speculations in a report or be conjectural; be short and concise.
4. Meet with the referring attorney prior to giving testimony to find out questions likely to be asked in cross-examination.
5. If asked, state opinions based on "reasonable professional certainty."

Clinical Conditions

Diagnoses are abstract classifications. They help clinicians select appropriate interventions based on empirical trends observed in patients with similar histories, presenting pictures, and responses to therapeutic modalities.

Since individuals are open biopsychosocial systems, problems in occupational functioning can stimulate, exacerbate, or result from a mental disorder. Similarly, several variables influence the course of a disorder and an individual's potential for functioning. Unfortunately, in spite of technological advances in treatment, not all patients will return to their highest level of functioning after an acute episode of mental illness. Although some disorders are transient, others are unremitting or chronic, with persistent residual impairments in functioning and recurrent acute episodes. Other persons may experience recurrent acute exacerbations with either no or increasing residual impairments between episodes.

Following this nonlinear model, treatment and management of the individual with an acute mental disorder requires knowledge of the individual, his or her clinical condition, and social systems. When possible, intervention is first directed at treatment of the primary cause(s) of a disorder. Management of the manifestations of an acute mental disorder concurrently aim to provide relief from acute distress, prevent complications, and assist the patient toward the treatment process.

If the patient's problem is primarily viewed as a biological illness because of data such as genetic history and positive response to medication, as often found with schizophrenic and affective disorders, then somatic modalities are a priority in care. However, a toxic family situation or stresses related to life roles may be the primary problem for other individuals with the same diagnoses. In such cases sociotherapies such as occupational therapy, milieu therapy, and family therapy may play more dominant roles in acute care. In depression, unresolved grief may be a precipitating factor and psychological work a necessity to symptom relief.

In some instances, inpatient medical treatment is absolutely necessary before psychosocial intervention can take place. This may be the case with conditions such as psychophysiological disorders, substance use disorders, eating disorders, and organic mental disorders and for patients who have medical complications from a suicide attempt.

Thus, for psychiatric conditions, acute care usually focuses on crisis stabilization, diagnosis, symptom reduction, medication management, alliance building, and aftercare planning. For severely disabling disorders and life-threatening conditions, at the very least, this care is provided in a hospital setting. Ideally, as soon as it is possible, the staff prepares a patient for long-term or follow-up care in the community. If there are residual impairments in functioning, family education, sheltered living environments, or outpatient training for community living may be necessary, depending on their severity.

Patient Management

Mental disorders are manifest as distressing thoughts, feelings, and behaviors for patients and those who are significant to them. Although these problems can diminish when treatment is successful, many individuals will still require long-term support, therapeutic management, and care. Thus, patient management remains primary to the occupational therapist's role and to that of other mental health providers. With emphasis given to the occupational therapist's interests, the goals and methods for short-term and inpatient management of impairments resulting from several mental disorders are highlighted in the box.

Short-Term Management Goals and Methods

Alcoholism

Problems: Impairment in social or occupational functioning; denial of illness

Goal: Effectively engage in a therapeutic program

Methods: Educate about alcohol—its effects on daily life activities and community treatment resources available

Anorexia Nervosa

Problems: Abnormal eating habits and improper nutrition; inability to identify and verbalize internal states; excessive physical exercise

Goals: Regulated food intake and exercise; engagement in a variety of activities

Methods: Prescribed meals and accompanied eating; opportunities for self-expression and experimentation with novel activities; structured milieu with a balanced routine of daily activities

Borderline Personality Disorder

Problems: Physically self-damaging acts; impulsive and self-destructive behaviors; transient psychotic states; depressive symptomatology; inability to contain feelings, particularly anger; unstable affect; feelings of helplessness; difficulty being alone

Goals: Physical safety; containment; distance from overwhelming feelings

Methods: Clear, prompt, firm, and consistent limits; structure and routine; minimize stress; provide soothing activities; empathic and reliable relationships with staff members

Delirium

Problems: Transient global impairment of cognitive functions (*e.g.*, disturbances in attention, orientation, recent memory, perceptual discrimination, and sleep)

Goals: Determine etiology of delirium: prevent complications (*e.g.*, accidents); relieve distress from acute symptoms; maximize self-esteem and sense of mastery

Methods: A milieu structured to provide an optimal sensory and social environment (*e.g.*, quiet, well-lighted room); order, consistency, and familiarity; instructions given in a repeated, concrete, and slow manner; tasks presented one at a time; interactions orienting and clarifying, warm and yet firm, expression encouraged; participation in unit activities and self-care encouraged as tolerated; unrestrained movement when patient is no danger to self.

Dementia

Problems: Progressive, static, or reversible impairment of cognitive functions that affects social or occupational performance; for example, disturbance of recent and later remote memory; disorientation; impaired judgment and ability to learn new knowledge and skills; often personality change; attention and ability to abstract may be impaired

Goals: Compensate for deficits to support functioning at maximal capacity; minimize debilitation secondary to limited ambulation

Methods: Reduce tension and change in environment; routine, familiar, and structured environment; frequent contact with nonstressful and familiar objects and people; assistive/adaptive equipment and orthotics when needed; range of motion and muscle relaxant activities when indicated

Depression

Problems: Withdrawal; sense of hopelessness and pessimism; loss of interest or pleasure in daily activities; feelings of worthlessness, helplessness and dependency; lack of energy, fatigue; decreased concentration and productivity; self-destructive behavior

Goals: Safety from self-harm; stress reduction; restore sense of competence

Methods: Safety measures to prevent self-harm; empathic relationships; opportunities for socialization and gratification as tolerated; support for and expectation of functioning in activities of daily living; realistic, structured program to re-experience prior sustaining relationships, interests, and activities

Mania

Problems: Distractibility; hyperactivity; impaired judgment; denial; euphoric and irritable moods

Goals: Mood stability and limits on destructive behaviors

Methods: Empathic support; reality test and recognize conflicts; firm, consistent limit setting and restrictions; minimize stimulation; provide activities that are constructive outlets for energy

Psychological Factors Affecting Physical Conditions

Problems: Tension; illness not responding to medical treatment or in chronic phase

Goals: Minimize stress

Methods: Ego support concerning related emotional crisis, conflict, or fear, often in groups; relaxation activities and techniques

(Text continues on following page)

Short-Term Management Goals and Methods *(continued)*

Schizophrenic Disorders

Problems: Danger to self or others; withdrawal; loose associations and illogical thinking: delusions, hallucinations, magical thinking, illusions; inappropriate, flat, or blunted affect; ambivalence; disorganized behavior; deteriorated habits and functioning in self-care, work, leisure, or social relationships

Goals: Safety of patient and others; psychotic symptom reduction; restored sense of self

Methods: Prompt, firm, and strict limits on harmful behaviors; clear limits and realistic expectations and privileges; structure and distance from emotional – social stimulation and stress; reality testing; reality-orientation activities; support; ego-organizing activities and balanced daily routines

Adapted from: Kaplan HI, Sadock BJ: *Modern Synopsis of Psychiatry/IV*, 4th ed. Baltimore, Williams & Wilkins, 1985; Lazare, A (ed): *Outpatient Psychiatry: Diagnosis and Treatment.* Baltimore, Williams & Wilkins, 1979; Sederer LI (ed): *Inpatient Psychiatry: Diagnosis and Treatment,* 2nd ed. Baltimore, Williams & Wilkins, 1986

References

1. Abeles J, Schwartzberg SL: An occupational therapy approach to functional assessment. Boston, Harvard Medical School course: Inpatient Psychiatry: Practice and Politics, March 1986
2. American Occupational Therapy Association: Guidelines for Occupational Therapy Documentation. Rockville, MD, American Occupational Therapy Association, 1986
3. American Occupational Therapy Association: Uniform Occupational Therapy Evaluation Checklist. Am J Occup Ther 35:817, 1981
4. American Occupational Therapy Association: Uniform Terminology for Reporting Occupational Therapy Services. Rockville, MD, American Occupational Therapy Association, 1979
5. American Psychiatric Association: Diagnostic and Statistical Manual of Mental Disorders, Edition Three (DSM-III). Washington, DC, American Psychiatric Association, 1980
6. Barris R, Kielhofner G, Watts JH: Psychosocial Occupational Therapy Practice in a Pluralistic Arena, p 217. Laurel, MD, RAMSCO, 1983
7. Benfer BA: Defining the role and function of the psychiatric nurse as a member of the team. Perspect Psychiatric Care 18:166, 1980
8. Borofsky G, Levine E: The perils and pleasures of being an expert witness. Cambridge, MA, Mount Auburn Hospital Psychiatry Grand Rounds, October 1985
9. Briggs AK, Duncombe LW, Howe MC, et al: Case Simulations in Psychosocial Occupational Therapy. Philadelphia, FA Davis, 1979
10. Ehrenberg F: Comprehensive assessment process: A group evaluation. In Hemphill BJ (ed): The Evaluative Process in Psychiatric Occupational Therapy, pp 155–167. Thorofare, NJ, Charles B Slack, 1982
11. Feder J: Inpatient satisfaction with occupational therapy: One hospital's experience. AOTA Mental Health Spec Interest Sec Newslett 9:2, 1986
12. Fidler GS: The activity laboratory: A structure for observing and assessing perceptual, integrative, and behavioral strategies. In Hemphill BJ (ed): The Evaluative Process in Psychiatric Occupational Therapy, pp 195–207. Thorofare, NJ, Charles B Slack, 1982
13. Gutheil TG: The psychiatric medical report. In Sederer LI (ed): Inpatient Psychiatry: Diagnosis and Treatment, p 316. Baltimore, Williams & Wilkins, 1983
14. Howe MC, Schwartzberg SL: A Functional Approach to Group Work in Occupational Therapy. Philadelphia, JB Lippincott, 1986
15. Jacobs K: Occupational Therapy: Work-Related Programs and Assessments. Boston, Little, Brown, 1985
16. Kaplan HI, Sadock BJ: Modern Synopsis of Psychiatry IV, 4th ed, pp 887–898. Baltimore, Williams & Wilkins, 1985
17. Kaplan K: Short-term assessment: The need and a response. Occup Ther Mental Health 4:29, 1984
18. Lazare A: Hypothesis testing in the clinical interview. In: Outpatient Psychiatry: Diagnosis and Treatment, pp 131–140. Baltimore, Williams & Wilkins, 1979
19. Lazare A, Keller MB, Rubinstein JF, et al: The clinical record: A multidimensional/hypothesis testing/negotiated approach. In Lazare A (ed): Outpatient Psychiatry: Diagnosis and Treatment, pp 238–245. Baltimore, Williams & Wilkins, 1979
20. Mosey AC: Psychosocial Components of Occupational Therapy, pp 9–11. New York, Raven Press, 1986
21. Mosey AC: Three Frames of Reference for Mental Health. Thorofare, NJ, Charles B Slack, 1970
22. Peloquin SM: The development of an occupational therapy interview/therapy set procedure. Am J Occup Ther 37:457, 1983
23. Peters ME: Reimbursement for psychiatric occupational therapy services. Am J Occup Ther 38:307, 1984
24. Reed, KL: Models of Practice in Occupational Therapy. Baltimore, Williams & Wilkins, 1984
25. Rogers JC: Eleanor Clarke Slagle Lecture 1983: Clinical reasoning: The ethics, science, and art. Am J Occup Ther 37:601, 1983
26. Schwartz SC: Reimbursement and psychiatric occupational therapy: Administrative issues. AOTA Mental Health Spec Interest Sec Newslett 9:5, 1986
27. Schwartzberg SL, Abeles J: Occupational therapy. In Sederer LI (ed): Inpatient Psychiatry: Diagnosis and Treat-

ment, 2nd ed, pp 308–323. Baltimore, Williams & Wilkins, 1986

28. Sederer LI: First do no harm: Inpatient psychotherapy of the borderline patient. Cambridge, MA, Mount Auburn Hospital Psychiatry Grand Rounds, November 1985

29. Sienkielewski K: Evolution of inpatient psychiatric nursing. In Stuart GW, Sundeen SJ: Principles and Practice of Psychiatric Nursing, 2nd ed, pp 570–591. St Louis, CV Mosby, 1983

30. Weed LL: Medical Records, Medical Education, and Patient Care. Cleveland, Case Western Reserve University Press, 1969

31. Wilson HS, Kneisl CR: Psychiatric Nursing. Menlo Park, CA, Addison–Wesley, 1979

Appreciation is extended to Janet Abeles, M.Ed., OTR, for her continuing support and solid commentary concerning my work; to Lloyd I. Sederer, M.D., for his enthusiastic response, concrete suggestions, and detailed review of the material on somatic therapies; and finally, to Milt, Teddy, and Harriet for their humor, love, and appreciation of my nature.

SECTION 6

Summary, Trends, and Challenges

Elizabeth G. Tiffany and Sharan L. Schwartzberg

Historically, occupational therapy has been philosophically committed to a view of man that is consistent with the metaphysical concept of embodiment. Embodiment or wholism is that perspective where mind and body are perceived as inextricably connected, integrated as one entity, in contrast to the dualistic perspective where mind and body are perceived as separate and hierarchically related entities (one entity superior to the other).

P.D. Shannon[2]

As theory and practice in psychiatric occupational therapy are traced through the years, a pattern emerges that indicates that the profession has maintained certain consistent awareness and concerns.

Wholeness

The therapist has sought to promote in clients a sense of wholeness, as well as the ability to adapt and to function as fully as possible. To do this, the therapist has tried to maintain a level of awareness and sophistication that keeps pace with growing knowledge and advancing technology and with the expanding consciousness that has characterized both health care and society in general.

Sharrott proposes that the profession's holistic beliefs require that a phenomenological view of people be contained in the theoretical bases of its approaches. Concepts central to this view of human functioning include self-actualization, intrinsic motivation, active participation, and satisfaction of personal and social requirements for productivity. Sharrott concludes that the major theoretical perspectives for occupational therapy in mental health are not holistic, and that the psychoanalytic and developmental perspectives are particularly deficient.[3]

Others caution that practice and education are rapidly moving away from a holistic orientation. As Shannon explains it, "specialization is the demise of a wholistic philosophy."[2] Nevertheless, he believes that by shifting to a philosophy-questioning process, occupational therapy will draw knowledge from the holistic disciplines. Unlike the dualistic groups, who view people as controlled by their environment, these disciplines perceive adaptation as an interactive process between individuals and their environment.

Changes and Development

Allying itself with psychiatry, occupational therapy has been subject to the excitement, dilemmas, and ambiguities that have characterized the development of psychiatric practice. As psychiatry has grown and become more diversified, it has had to become more responsive to and interested in the changes, diversification, and growth that have taken place in the social sciences. Changes in society have been close to revolutionary and have forced psychiatry and all of its related professions and services, including occupational therapy, to develop new alliances and new perspectives.

Broader Concepts

There has been a need to develop broader concepts of health and illness and to accommodate the greater demands for preventive services, in addition to providing for treatment, maintenance, and rehabilitation. The move has been away from institutional care and toward diverse community programs. Creativity and frustration tolerance have been challenged as fiscal constraints make it difficult to accomplish what needs to be done. Psychiatric practice and occupational therapy seem to be in a period of disequilibrium, out of which the development of new levels of understanding and adaptation could grow.

Issues and Trends

To date, the psychiatric occupational therapist has had only embryonic conceptual models and frames of reference to address some of the issues that present themselves. Nevertheless, issues have been there to be addressed. Should we accommodate the new approaches or fads in popular mental health self-help? How do we work with other activities therapy professionals? How can we maintain our commitment and work within the constraints imposed by some standards that are well meaning but seem to be depersonalizing to the client? How do we deal with increasingly complex concerns for accountability and legality? How can we be involved productively in the important developments in biogenetic and biochemical research? How can we relate what we know about human adaptation and activities to these developments? Are we ready to discard some of our long-cherished assumptions if we learn that they are not scientifically accurate?

These are only a few of the issues we need to explore, study, think about, and adapt if we are to grow and act as a true profession. Some of the issues are critical and some even painful. Some of them are truly exciting!

If one were to characterize the trends, directions, and, in fact, major goals of psychiatric occupational therapy in recent years, one would find three important themes. First, with the increasing sense of urgency that emanates from newly acquired knowledge, there has been the need to establish strong scientifically based support for the apparent therapeutic effects of our practice. Second, there have been significant efforts to promote an identity and public visibility for occupational therapy as a distinct profession. Third, there has been a continuing need to examine the models that best represent our bases for practice, whether they are medical, sociological, or biopsychosocial. These concerns are widespread and must be considered not only in practice but in education and research as well. The future appears to promise opportunities and challenges for the occupational therapist who works in mental health. Perhaps the most demanding of the challenges will be to achieve true professionalism in a way that will most effectively serve our ultimate purpose: to be able to help our clients to achieve the highest possible quality of life and function.

The Future: A Postindustrial Society

In the future, occupational therapists will need to help their patients adjust to a postindustrial society. A technologically based society brings about stresses such as lack of work, fear of nuclear holocaust, high-tech isolation, and rapid change. It is likely that our occupation-based tools will be crucial in treating the effects of these psychosocial problems, including an increased incidence of anxiety-related disorders, depression, and substance abuse.[1]

One already sees a rise in adolescent mental health problems. These problems include eating disorders, depression, alcohol and drug abuse, runaway behavior, and suicidal behavior. In addition, therapists are increasingly coming into contact with patients who have psychosocial problems associated with autoimmune deficiency syndrome (AIDS), alcoholism, divorce, incest, sexual abuse, and child abuse.

What about the great numbers of chronic institutionalized expatients who have been discharged to live in the obscurity of boardinghouse rooms, nursing homes, bus stations, and the streets? How can we give them proper care? What about the increase in computer technology and the devaluation of the work ethic? What about the agony of unemployment and its stress on the individual and families? What about the segment of an increasingly aged population that is neither sick nor well but which might be helped to continue to be productive, contributing members of society? Who helps the aged with Alzheimer's disease? And who helps their families adjust and survive emotionally, physically, and financially? As there is more stress on middle-aged and older adults to care for aging parents, how can they be helped through parent–child role reversals? Even though great strides have been made in increasing consciousness of racism, sexism, and the rights of the handicapped, how do we reach or maintain goals of equality in such a quickly changing society?

On the positive side, there are new biological approaches to psychiatric diagnosis of psychotic disorders, such as positron emission tomography (PET) scanning. Geriatric psychiatry is a rapidly advancing field. More attention is also being given to psychiatric disorders in patients who are medically ill or neurologically impaired. The medical psychiatric unit in a general hospital, for patients who are too medically ill for the usual psychiatric unit and at the same time too psychiatrically ill to be managed on a medical unit, is becoming more common. Finally, the unique needs of individuals with chronic mental disabilities are being considered. Occupational therapists can play a vital role in developing alternative approaches to long-term and acute management of disabling conditions in community settings. It is perhaps because of, rather than in spite of, our holistic heritage that occupational therapy practice is compatible with contemporary acute and long-term care in psychiatry and mental health.

The influence of a prospective payment system on psychiatric care in this country remains unclear. It implies that occupational therapy resources will be limited to the acutely ill, hospitalized patient. The question remains whether attitudes will permit ample money to be designated for follow-up care and services for the chronically disabled. Finally, the American Psychiatric Association's edition of its *Diagnostic and Statistical Manual of Mental Disorders*, the DSM-IV, is bound to have a significant influence on the practice of occupational therapy in psychiatry and mental health.

References

1. Schwartzberg SL: Work and play: Process or product? Presented at the Second Annual Northeast Region Occupational Therapy Student Conference, Hamden, CT, February 1983
2. Shannon PD: Statement of philosophy. In: Toward a Philosophical Base for Occupational Therapy Working Papers 1977–1983, pp 27, 30 Rockville, MD, American Occupational Therapy Association, 1984
3. Sharrott GW: An analysis of occupational therapy theoretical approaches for mental health: Are the profession's major treatment approaches truly occupational therapy? Occup Ther Mental Health 5:1, 1986

CHAPTER 26

Mental Retardation *Reba M. Sebelist*

Although this is a nation of skills and opportunities and rights for all, these are not available equally to all citizens. The physically and mentally handicapped have been the recipients of much physical and verbal abuse. As demeaning as physical abuse might be to the mentally retarded person, verbal abuse is much more destructive of human worth. After hearing derogatory designations over the years, individuals begin to refer to themselves in the same manner—a self-perpetuating process of breaking down their sense of worth.

Well-meaning groups have attempted to change the labels from early ones like "idiot" or "imbecile" to "trainable" or "educable." These new, supposedly complimentary, terms are now being fought by organizations such as the National Association for Retarded Citizens (NARC), which changed its name from the National Association for Retarded Children. Throughout this chapter, the retarded are referred to as individuals who have feelings, rights, obligations, and ego needs.

What is Mental Retardation?

In 1973, the American Association on Mental Deficiency (AAMD) stated: "Mental retardation refers to significantly subaverage general intellectual functioning existing concurrently with deficits in adaptive behavior and manifested during the development period."[11]

The mentally retarded do not demonstrate a single area of difficulty but rather manifest an interaction of multiple factors, among which are sociocultural, psychological, and physical influences.

Etiology

The AAMD definition of mental retardation refers to causes acting during the developmental periods of life. Most frequently, a cause is associated with interruption in the sequence of one of three time frames: prenatal, perinatal (neonatal), or postnatal. Each stage may have its own particular etiologic component but may also include a causation crossing all three periods, thus demonstrating the multiplicity of factors involved in mental retardation (Table 26-1). Only a sampling of causations is identified here; more comprehensive information may be found in *Birth Defects Compendium, Atlas of Mental Retardation,* and *Mental Retardation.*[1,4,9]

Table 26-1. *Causation of Mental Retardation and Developmental Period Of Occurrence*

Causation	Prenatal	Perinatal	Postnatal
Infection	X	X	X
Trauma	X	X	X
Genetic disorders	X		
Drugs or intoxication	X	X	X
Prematurity		X	
Low birth weight		X	
Anoxia	X	X	X
Parental age and health	X		
Sensory deprivation		X	X
Cultural deprivation		X	X

Mental Retardation versus *Mental Illness*

Frequently, the public does not comprehend the difference between mental retardation and mental illness. Some very basic differences are indicated in Table 26-2.

Incidence

The people known as mentally retarded comprise approximately 3% of the general population. This represents a very large number of individuals who require aid in meeting particular needs. The greatest number of these individuals demonstrate symptoms at birth or shortly thereafter. The remainder, are mentally retarded as a result of problems occurring after the neonatal period. Within this 3%, there are distinctions based on functioning levels. Those considered profoundly retarded comprise 1.5%, the severely retarded 3.5%, the moderately retarded 6%, and the mildly retarded 89% of the total.[5]

Table 26-2. *Differences Between Mental Retardation and Mental Illness*

Mental Retardation	Mental Illness
Primary defect in intellect	Intellect relatively unimpaired
Usually oriented in time and place	Difficulty with time and place orientation
Not curable, long-term	Often significant cure possible
May not differ in aptitude, interests, and feelings	Cluster of behaviors differing from normal

Historical Perspective

In early times, the mentally retarded were ignored, received little or no care, or were placed in the woods to fend for themselves or die. Life for the average person was short and living arduous; hence it was extremely difficult to support those who required extra care. Contributing to the desertion and persecution of these individuals was the belief that they were possessed by demons.

During the Middle Ages, the role of the court jester was usually filled by a retarded individual. Art from this period shows individuals now recognizable as having Down syndrome as jesters. Frequently, when these individuals remained with their families, they filled the role of "village idiot."

Various religious orders became so distressed with the lack of physical care, the ridicule, and the abuse given the retarded that they built sheltered communities. Unfortunately, with the kindly intended isolation, a sense of hopelessness grew. No change was envisioned. Good care and shelter were provided, but there was little mental stimulation; this in turn caused more regression and deterioration.

In the 1800s, Jean Itard, a physician who worked with the deaf, became involved with a boy about 12 years of age who had been captured in the forest of Aveyron, France. The lad had been considered severely retarded. Believing that intellectual performance and potential could be affected by environmental stimulation and opportunity, Itard began working with sensorimotor techniques to improve the boy's level of functioning. Initially, he worked with Victor (his name for the young man) through the sense of hearing: after occluding visual stimuli, he bombarded Victor with auditory stimuli and required from him an acceptable response. Next, he required discrimination of types of noises, proceeding afterward to verbal clues. When Victor was able to respond to emotions such as anger, sadness, and happiness in vocalizations, Itard proceeded to the sense of touch, followed by the senses of smell and taste. Itard worked with Victor for 5 years, and although gains were made by this previously animalistic "Wild Boy of Aveyron," they were not sufficient for him to fit into the dandified Paris society; Itard felt he had failed.[13] He did indeed fail if we use the goal of fitting into society as a criterion; nonetheless, his greatest contribution was to effect attitudinal change regarding the mentally retarded.

Seguin, a student of Itard, elaborated on Itard's work and developed what he called the "physiological method" of training. After coming to the United States, Seguin became a prime mover in the opening of residential facilities such as Fernald in Massachusetts and Germantown (now Elwyn) in Pennsylvania. His involvement led to the establishment of an organization now known as the American Association on Mental Deficiency (AAMD).

As with most specialty areas, unqualified persons promised cures that they could not effect, since mental retardation is not a curable illness but a condition. Many felt that if the condition could not be cured, time, money, and energy expended were wasted. As a result, these unqualified persons caused a reversal in feelings regarding the potential of the mentally retarded and negated the work of Itard and Seguin, with a resultant return to the sense of hopelessness. This attitude of futility continued with the development of larger residential facilities, mostly in isolated areas. Society was convincing itself that it was meeting the needs of the mentally retarded by assuring them care for their basic physical needs, while showing little concern for their psychosocial and mental needs.

By the end of World War II, emphasis shifted, and programming was demanded by the NARC to meet the needs of all retarded individuals regardless of age, thereby permitting the recognition of the adult population. Organizations such as AAMD had assisted the professionals serving the mentally retarded but did not hold themselves responsible for defining and justifying the service provided. Now, for the first time, professionals were being held accountable for both resultant behavioral changes in clients and the expenditure of funds.

Following lengthy litigation between the Commonwealth of Pennsylvania and parents regarding the availability of educational opportunities for the mentally retarded, a Right to Education Consent Agreement was implemented in 1973.[10] This guarantees educational opportunities for all mentally and physically handicapped persons to the age of 21 years. This was indeed a major accomplishment for the parents, who were supported in the action by the Pennsylvania Association for Retarded Citizens (PARC), an affiliate of NARC. Many other states used this Agreement as a model in legal actions for defining and providing educational and therapeutic programs.

Public Law 94-142, the Education For All Handicapped Children Act, was passed by the federal government in 1975. The major effect of this act on occupational therapy has been that all special education programs were to have physical or occupational therapists available, either on their staffs or as consultants, by September 1977.

A positive change has now been seen in the role of training centers. Funds had not always been available to provide personnel to effect change. Society had been content to have the retarded isolated or institutionalized and to receive mostly custodial care. Professionals had not assumed responsibility for preparing themselves to work with the mentally retarded. Pressure from organizations such as NARC, along with federal and state regulations, have forced accountability by staff. They, in turn, have demanded and are receiving more efficient and appropriate training from colleges, universities, and professional schools, which are producing staff members less hesitant to assume responsibility for education and training.

Methods of Classification

Intelligence Quotient

For many years, the only method used to designate the functioning level of the retarded was the measurement of intellectual skills. The evaluator would use test instruments and issue an IQ score. These scores have both positive and negative aspects, and an inexperienced evaluator can do irreparable damage. The IQ score with a descriptive statement frequently influenced the amount of effort expended on an individual and would remain on the record permanently. Staff members with large case loads would have to set priorities. Little thought was given to motivation, previous program exposure, or plateauing, ignoring the fact that an individual with a low score might be motivated and ready for change and thus might benefit more from therapy than a less motivated person with a higher score. It is not only unfair but also unrealistic and weak programming to base decisions on IQ evaluations only.

On the other hand, a skilled evaluator who looks at the total person, the physical abilities and limitations, verbal or nonverbal communicative state, and so forth, and then chooses an evaluation instrument that is appropriate, can do invaluable work. This type of evaluator elicits responses that produce a higher functioning level and aids the treatment team in developmentally designed programming.

Many states require that a numerical IQ score be given. This information is useful for record keeping, statistics, and research but is not in itself meaningful for the goal-directed team.

Medical Diagnosis or Causation

The World Health Organization (WHO) has been concerned with obtaining uniform information for international sharing. WHO feels this process would clarify communication in addition to encouraging sharing for improvement of international health concerns. In the United States, to implement the request of WHO, the International Classification of Diseases has been utilized by the medical team in an attempt to classify mental retardation according to etiology or causation. Initially, a number from 310 to 315, based on intellectual functioning according to the Revised Stanford–Binet Tests of Intelligence Forms L and M, is assigned: 310 for borderline, 311 for mild, 312 for moderate, 313 for severe, and 314 for profound retardation. The 315 designation is for those who have not been assigned a specific functioning level but who demonstrate behaviors associated with retardation.

Following this number is a fourth digit signifying a clinical subcategory based on etiology: .0 following infection and intoxication; .1 following trauma or physical agent; .2 with disorders of metabolism, growth, or nutrition; .3 associated with gross brain disease (postnatal); .4 associated with diseases and conditions resulting from unknown prenatal influence; .5 with chromosomal abnormality; .6 associated with prematurity; .7 following major psychiatric disorder; .8 with psychosocial (environmental) deprivation; .9 with other (and unspecified) conditions. There may come to be a fifth and sixth digit as a means of further pinpointing causation. Hence, for example, the numerical designation 314.5 indicates that an individual is profoundly retarded as a result of chromosomal abnormality.

The greatest values of this type of classification is the ease of comprehension and utility in research. This system does, however, remove the human element while social agencies and families are attempting through legal maneuverings to give dignity to the mentally retarded.

Information including numerical designations desired by the mental retardation section of the International Classification of Diseases is available in the *Diagnostic and Statistical Manual of Mental Disorders* (DSM-II).[7]

It is desirable to know the etiologic factors, but this information is not essential for program planning. Combining the two classifications provides information regarding the IQ and the etiologic factors but does not indicate what the individual is capable of doing and thus should not be used in isolation as a determinant for training.

Education

A frequently used classification method is one designed for use by educators. Terms such as *life support, dependent, trainable,* and *educable* are assigned. These terms are meaningful to those who use them daily but are relatively useless to others.

The use of case histories to provide relevant information has been frustrating because the focus in the past has been on describing what has been done and includes neither past nor present performance levels of the individual. The use of the educational terms also reinforces in most instances the same lack of information.

Adaptive Behavior Level

The AAMD definition refers to impairment in adaptive behavior in the mentally retarded. As early as 1955,

Sloan and Birch began defining these behaviors.[12] A monograph supplement to the *American Journal of Mental Deficiency* prepared by Heber gives four levels of behavior with three appropriate age groupings. Descriptive paragraphs are given for Levels 1, 2, 3, and 4, with Level 4 referring to maximal ability and vocational adequacy. Useful as this information was, it still was not an adequate system of classification. Thus, it was updated in 1973 with age-level delineation of skills in areas such as activities of daily living, communication, physical, social, self-motivation, and occupation.[11] This method now offers quick reference, with information indicating at what level on the developmental continuum the individual is functioning. It also provides a possible recommendation for setting achievable goals.

In 1974, the AAMD issued a revision of the Adaptive Behavior Scale.[14] This revision has a more comprehensive method of evaluating adaptive behavior and will be discussed more fully under Assessment below.

Composite Classification

Finally, a compilation of information that is meaningful is evolving. From the generic term of mental retardation, it is possible to progress through the use of demonstrable IQ score, etiological factors with indications of possible progressive deteriorating conditions, and educators' designation and conclude with adaptive behavioral levels. A combination of all these factors is not only desirable but essential for designing a program to meet the needs of the individual.

Assessment

As with all aspects of programming for the mentally retarded, assessment must be a combined effort. Some well-staffed centers are implementing a decentralized system of management, which can be an asset for evaluating abilities and limitations. A group of experienced professionals is charged with devising composite evaluative measures affecting the full range of activities existing at the center. This evaluation device is administered either by the professional services staff or by other qualified evaluators working in the unit. The results are shared with all the staff working with the involved individual. Also, the professional services staff meets with the direct-care staff to learn the individual's level of response in the residential unit and with representatives of other program staff to ascertain behaviors, gains, regressions, or plateauing. In addition, the professional service staff observes each individual in a variety of program experiences for on-site evaluation and completion of an all-inclusive assessment.

This sophisticated level of assessment will not be possible in all centers because of size of staff and range of responsibilities. However, a complete goal-oriented training program cannot exist without evaluative measurements, because change cannot be measured if no initial or re-evaluative information is available. However, there continue to be programs in which change is recorded only through periodic subjective progress notes without an initial assessment.

Regardless of the sophistication of the assessment team or the materials used, the most important factor is the relevance of the instruments for measuring the desired results. As the use of a standardized test written in English is unfair to a Spanish-speaking person, so also is use of one for the mentally retarded that is not level-appropriate. After defining the purpose of a specific assessment and the goals to be achieved, the instrument with the greatest potential for determining the functional level of the individual is chosen and administered.

There is a controversy regarding where assessments should be done. Valid arguments can be presented to substantiate the various points of view. Concerns include questions of where the activity is usually done, the discomfort of the individual being evaluated in a strange setting, the distractibility of the individual, and so on. Just as it is true that most people function better in a familiar environment, it follows that the distractions of that same area might affect performance. The professional doing the assessment must consider the location, time of day, and family members present when choosing the optimal setting.

A representative listing of some instruments that have been demonstrated as useful with the mentally retarded follows. Although the list is incomplete, it illustrates the scope of available formal instruments. With most mentally retarded individuals, the number of areas to be assessed is such that one or more program areas may be involved in doing the evaluations that are peculiar to the contribution of their disciplines. A more comprehensive description of each of these instruments and their validity and reliability can be found in *The Eighth Mental Measurement Yearbook*, edited by Buros.[3] With, all screening devices, it is essential to remember that they are only as useful as the skill of the evaluator in comprehending the behaviors of the mentally retarded.

Many occupational therapy departments devise evaluation forms to meet the requirements of their service. The tool can be as simple or as complex as desired but should elicit such information as physical status, mental functioning level, and adaptive behavioral level. Other information obtained is dependent on the age level served, the type of program, and the relationship of the department to other program services. An instrument based on the type described by Currie is most useful.[6] This type evaluates neuromuscular status, perceptual–motor abilities, activities of daily living, and performance abilities.

Intelligence and Developmental Scales

Bayley Scales of Infant Development

Devised for use with infants from 2 to 30 months of age, this instrument has a mental scale, motor scale, and infant behavior record. It does not predict potential abilities but does establish an infant's status in relation to others of the same age. The instrument aids in the recognition and diagnosis of sensory and neurologic defects as well as of emotional distress or disturbance. It is standardized and has good reliability.

Denver Developmental Screening Test

This is a screening device for children from 2 weeks to 6 years of age. Four sections evaluate gross motor, fine motor–adaptive, communication, and personal–social development. The score sheet with its key gives the average age by which each skill should be attained. In addition, the score sheet provides columns for re-evaluation, thus producing a quick composite reference. This is a practical, efficient evaluative tool.

Peabody Picture Vocabulary Test

This instrument was devised for use with persons aged 2½ to 18 years. The individual responds to verbal cues by indicating the correct picture from a choice of four. Negative features of this instrument are that directions are given in English, thus making it invalid for persons who do not speak that language. It does not take colloquialisms into account. A very useful instrument for nonverbal individuals, it requires only pointing to the correct picture. Those with motor involvement can also be evaluated because the test pictures are of a good size and are well-separated on the page. The positive aspects of this test outweigh its negative features.

Stanford–Binet Intelligence Scale (IQ)

This very old instrument was devised for use with individuals aged 2 years or older. The current, third, revision was published in 1960 and combines items from Forms L and M to become the Revised Version Form L-M. This use of the better items is thought to produce a more valid instrument. The instrument relies heavily on verbal ability. It requires the use of six different items from a possible seven for each age level. Although this tool has good validity, it does not adequately evaluate older, severely retarded individuals.

Wechsler Intelligence Scale for Children

A stable general-purpose scale, this instrument was devised for use with individuals from 5 to 15 years of age.

From the composite of 12 subtests, information is accumulated for verbal, performance, and full-scale scores. The division of items in this scale is based on content rather than level of difficulty; some evaluators consider this the reason that the scale is easy to administer and is successful in gaining responses from children. Individually administered, this instrument is valid in measuring current mental functioning.

Illinois Test of Psycholinguistic Abilities

The recommended age range for use of this instrument is 2 to 10 years. In the development of this tool, the purpose was to produce a diagnostic device for analyzing intellectual deficits in the learning disabled and mentally retarded. Nine subtests evaluate communication performance in decoding, association, and encoding; levels of language organization; and channels of input and output of language. Although there are areas needing some revision, this instrument has served the purpose of diagnosing learning difficulties. A practical, valid test, it can be a valuable tool.

Goodenough–Harris Drawing Test

The age range for this test is 3 to 15 years. This updating of the Draw-a-Man test presents an opportunity to use a quick, nonthreatening instrument that frequently evokes useful comments while the individual is completing the task. Of vital importance in the use of this instrument is the *purpose* for its use. As a result of motor difficulties and impaired mental functioning, the retarded individual responds not only as a definite individual but also as one who has obvious aberrance. Recognizing these limitations, the evaluator must know how to administer the test and be skilled in the use of the information it evokes.

Adaptive Behavior Scales

Vineland Social Maturity Scale

This instrument has been widely used, although no true standardization has been done. Interpretations are based on the experience of the developer. An important feature of this instrument is that the information comes from a general population sample. Because of the subjective nature of this test, the relationship between the evaluator and the individual being tested may have either a "halo" or negative effect on scoring. It provides a useful broad evaluation of adaptive behaviors.

Adaptive Behavior Scale

This instrument, published by the American Association on Mental Deficiency in 1969, is composed of two scales, one for ages 3 to 12 and the other for ages 13 and older. The tool was developed for use with the mentally retarded and emotionally maladjusted.

The scale devised for adults (13 years and older) measures behaviors in the areas of independent functioning, physical development, economic activity, language development, number and time concept, occupation-domestic, occupation-general, self-direction, responsibilities, and socialization in Part One. Part Two evaluates factors such as violent and destructive behavior, antisocial behavior, rebellious behavior, untrustworthy behavior, withdrawal, stereotyped behavior, odd mannerisms, inappropriate interpersonal manners, unacceptable vocal habits, self-abusive behavior, hyperactive tendencies, sexually aberrant behavior, and psychological disturbances. Because many of the behaviors listed have more than one item to be evaluated, the final score totals the assigned point values from each item.

This is a broad scale and presents a global view of the individual. The scale is well-constructed and easily administered and has much to offer in the assessment of easily discernible areas for habilitation training.

An updated revision of this scale was published by the AAMD in 1974. This edition tends to be more refined and, with increased data collection, should evidence greater validity and reliability. The Profile Summary makes it possible to study a composite survey of the individual's behavioral changes. Careful use of different colors in plotting scores will produce a meaningful record of the individual over time.

Perceptual Motor Instruments

Marianne Frostig Developmental Test of Visual Perception, Third Edition

The age range recommended for this test is 3 to 8 years. Measuring visual perceptual skills in five areas, the instrument contributes valuable data. The global scores have reasonable reliability.

Although this tool is a good instrument, the value of its use with the mentally retarded is limited to individuals with higher levels of functioning. Low scores are not necessarily an indication to start perceptual training but rather might indicate that the instrument was not the most appropriate one for testing that individual.

The Purdue Perceptual Motor Survey

This tool was designed for use with children 6 to 10 years of age and aids in identification of children lacking perceptual motor abilities necessary for acquiring academic skills. As such, it has potential for use with the "borderline" and "mildly" retarded but is not useful with the severely or profoundly retarded. It is an action or performance survey. Thus, it is easily administered to the individual who cannot read.

Pluralistic Tools

System of Multicultural Pluralistic Assessment (SOMPA)

This relatively new evaluative tool approaches diagnostic determination from a broader framework, viewing the individual from medical, social, and pluralistic aspects. The recommended age range is 5 through 11 years. Scoring is converted to percentiles and is recorded in a profile format.

The logic on which the instrument is based is that all factors influencing development are not equal. Therefore, there is increased emphasis on sociocultural impact on the individual's ability to learn.

This rather revolutionary tool needs further field testing to prove its value to health care professionals in assessment and program determination. Should it substantiate the theory developed by its authors, it will fill a void for those who espouse the total child approach to treatment of individuals with mental retardation.

Habilitation Training

The training of a mentally retarded individual requires the cooperation of many persons filling a variety of roles. The mentally retarded individual, depending on his or her functioning level and comprehension, must be a team member. Lack of desire and motivation or a high degree of resistence could interfere with the success of a well-planned developmentally appropriate training sequence.

The family must be involved in a positive manner and must be given much encouragement and reinforcement in an attempt to allay unwarranted guilt feelings. The family members must be aided in adjusting to the fact that progress will be slow and gains small or minimal, yet they must be demanding and supportive of the retarded individual so that the greatest possible level of achievement is obtained.

The individual may require drugs to aid in control of seizures or aberrant behavior or may use dietary supplements. For example, an individual having causative phenylketonuria (PKU) requires a dietary supplement for maintenance or for prevention of further changes. Although physicians and nurses are busy, most will respond to questioning about the individual's medication record. In turn, the medical representatives have the responsibility of informing other team members of changes in the medicinal regimen, especially if consequences or side-effects that could influence the program are anticipated. Physicians are becoming more aware of the type of contribution the occupational therapist may make in observing drug reactions, but it is the responsibility of occupational therapists to make their skills and contributions clear.

The psychologist and social case worker are vital team members. They frequently can elicit from the individual or the family information important to program development. The skill of these people can be helpful in the evaluation and compilation of program goals and can forge another link in the development of a total program team.

The staff members considered to be giving direct service vary with almost every center; they are the persons who have daily contact with the individual. This group provides a vital source of information, because they see retarded individuals for extended periods of time; they can report on specific needs, the carry-over of learning from therapies, the reaction of the individual to peers and activity, the individual's tolerance for frustrations, and the response to daily living situations.

The interaction of physical therapists, occupational therapists, speech therapists, teachers, recreation therapists, and other concerned persons should occur not only at unit staff meetings but whenever a concern arises. The staff should feel free to discuss problems without having to follow a rigid bureaucratic process; however, the staff does have the responsibility to share information with supervisors so they can be aware of and able to contribute to the program.

Roles of Occupational Therapy

Occupational therapy assists in improving the individual's ability to meet the demands of his or her culture with satisfaction and in a manner that is acceptable to and compatible with that environment. It is essential that the occupational therapist have a knowledge not only of normal growth and development but also of the cultural and social requirements the particular individual must fulfill. For example, those from a ghetto in a large urban area have different demands to meet than do those from the farming heartlands. In addition, there must be an awareness of the differences resulting from their social, cultural, and value systems, since these, too, affect program implementation and cooperation of both the individual and the family.

The diversity of skills possessed by occupational therapists makes it possible for them to fill a variety of roles both in administration and in providing direct service. In a small understaffed center, the occupational therapist may be expected to provide recreational activities in addition to occupational therapy. In other settings, the implementation of an approved work training program may be the occupational therapist's responsibility. As staff is acquired in other disciplines, the occupational therapist is able to relinquish some of these extra duties.

Occasionally, the occupational therapist is placed in an administrative role. One difficulty here might be keeping occupational therapy in its proper perspective as a part of the team. Members of all disciplines must contribute to the team, coordinated by an administrator whose major responsibility is to best use the skills of each team member to serve the mentally retarded individual clients.

Traditional Practice

Initially, there were few available trained staff who understood the needs of the retarded for participation in gainful activity. Little activity was available beyond occasional entertainment. This lack of activity produced fertile ground for regression (even in those with a higher functioning level), self-abuse, public masturbation, fights, broken windows, destroyed furniture, and torn clothing. These negative behaviors reinforced society's attitude that the retarded person could not be taught or benefit from positive experiences.

A few determined staff members would not accept this attitude and began implementing arts and crafts activities on the premise that busy work is better than idle hands. This was a positive step for some individuals, as was evidenced by improved ego strength. Much fine work was produced, but usually little thought was given to the individual's symptoms, interests, or desired goals. A negative feature of the arts and crafts programs was that most were self-funded: individuals had to produce in order to buy supplies, making production the primary function of the activity.

The low institutional housekeeping budgets produced another type of traditional programming — that of the individual's doing much of the work around the institution that was not done by paid help. Properly assigned and supervised work within the institution is a useful therapeutic tool. However, the mentally retarded person was often put to work in areas of need (laundry, grounds, kitchen) for long hours with little or no compensation beyond a pinch of tobacco, a cigar, or a cup of coffee. Days off were unheard of, with the retarded individual frequently doing more physically demanding labor than the paid staff.

This type of abuse led to involvement by labor unions. After much discussion, numerous lawsuits, and negotiations, the pendulum has swung to the other extreme. Individuals may work only if they agree, sign a voluntary consent form, and receive the minimum or prevailing wage, whichever is higher, prorated to the level of performance. This federal regulation may hinder the use of therapeutic work as a part of habilitation, because many refuse to participate in it voluntarily. Also, most live-in centers have not been given funds either to hire the retarded individual or to employ additional staff.[8]

Current Practice

As an example of current practice, the system developed in one state is described. In Pennsylvania, the directors of occupational therapy departments serving the Commonwealth Department of Public Welfare Office of Mental Retardation institutions for the mentally retarded defined major program areas in which occupational therapy has a valid contribution to make toward eliciting behavioral change. The list is not to be considered a complete, all-inclusive one but one that is subject to revision and updating. Each of the areas is discussed more fully later in the chapter but is recorded here for a global view of their thinking. Some areas are evaluation, maintenance, research, resource, and consultancy. The areas listed cannot be considered separate entities, as there are many situations in which their functions overlap. They were difficult to define and are impossible to separate; therefore, staff must be prepared to see needs in one or more program areas, set priorities, and plan the program accordingly.

There also appears to be a variety of function and program types to meet specific needs. The group of directors of occupational therapy had difficulty separating the role responsibilities but have listed them for more clarity of comprehension.

Although these program areas were defined for institutional training, they also are relevant to community centers that provide day care, special education, preschool, and infant stimulation programs.

The Occupational Therapy Program
Assessment/Evaluation

The intent of evaluation is to appraise and assess the functioning levels of the individual. This may be done for program placement within the occupational therapy service or at the request of a member of another discipline. A physician, psychologist, or community agency may ask that evaluation be done in order to determine the readiness of the individual for a program or to determine the individual's current functioning level.

Instruments for screening help to determine the need for further evaluation in specific areas. However, if it has been determined that the individual presents symptoms of physical or mental retardation, then further screening is repetitious and unnecessary. Assessment should then be used to determine the level of function of the individual.

Most therapists use a selected battery of instruments. One caution is that the chosen battery must be appropriate and produce meaningful results. A department may assemble a collection of standardized tests with good reliability and validity that produces results to meet their needs. Others may devise a composite battery of their own, combining materials appropriate for their needs. No one instrument or battery will fill all needs. How extensive the battery should be depends on the function of the center, the age of the individuals served, and the basic goals of the service. For example, it would be meaningless for a preschool program to compile a prevocational interest and skill battery, or for an infant stimulation program to develop a battery on cognitive tasks or refinements of self-care. The type of battery promulgated by Currie[6] is broad enough to cover many age and involvement levels but can be limited to meet specific needs.

Evaluation is not a one-time event. It is an ongoing process to provide current information on level of ability. Within the training process, one must be careful not to teach items used in the test: it is easy to elicit good scores on evaluation yet have poor results in performance if an individual has become test-wise. Evaluation must be done with care and skill.

A major responsibility of the occupational therapist is the preparation of clear, concise, and comprehensive reports. If occupational therapists are to function usefully as evaluators they must produce reports that are understandable, meaningful, and useful. Long reports can be meaningless because they may not be read thoroughly.

Neurodevelopmental Sequence

All individuals follow a similar sequential pattern of development. The mentally retarded persons have had their sequence interrupted in some manner — physical, mental, emotional, or as a result of multiple factors. They will therefore require special training in order to progress along the developmental sequence.

For years, well-meaning and skilled therapists used adaptive support devices such as braces and splints in order to get individuals into the upright position and ambulating. When the individuals did not progress, it was concluded that they were too handicapped, too retarded, or too uncooperative. Little thought was given to developmental sequence.

Frustration on the part of the staff and lack of progress on the part of the individual caused a review of programs of different types and goals. Staff began to question whether the goals were appropriate for the skill level of the individual. Finally, various techniques aimed at developmentally realistic goals evolved, with therapists providing sensory stimuli to the individual to aid the integration process and permit performance of a motor act. Of vital importance is the awareness of normal growth patterns and the proper level and type of sensory input needed to achieve the desired result. For example, a person must have head control before sitting and be able to knee-stand before standing upright.

As in many other areas of dysfunction, there is no one technique to meet all the needs. The occupational therapist must evaluate and, after determining the most appropriate technique, proceed with program implementation. There must be constant contact with specialists from other disciplines so as to achieve the greatest potential function for the individual in this highly specialized treatment process.

The Multiply Handicapped

Many individuals who are designated mentally retarded have multiple handicaps. Some are blind, deaf, nonverbal, or cerebral palsied or have missing or incomplete body parts. Many of these involvements alone would demand much adjustment in life-style and learning; when coupled with mental retardation, the problems are severely compounded. A sensory disturbance may be the only manifestation, but more often it is accompanied by a motor disturbance, which indeed creates a complex training need.

There is much overlapping in this program area. The primary need may be in the neurodevelopmental level or in the area of activities of daily living. The role of the occupational therapist must be to determine the need, set the priority for the service, and implement the indicated program.

The Emotionally Disturbed

This program area encompasses a wide scope of problems ranging from the difficulties of mildly and moderately involved individuals to the persons who demonstrate autistic-like behaviors.

The multiple problems faced by the mildly and moderately retarded do not preclude emotional disturbances. Frequently, these persons are alert enough to recognize their difference, feel society's rejection acutely, and yet strongly want to be a part of that society. Many internalize their feelings and develop physical malfunctions such as ulcers and colitis. Occupational therapy can aid these individuals by providing an outlet for, and encouraging the release of, feelings. The release felt while using the beater on a floor loom or wedging clay is immeasurable, and it also is a positive, acceptable behavior. The results derived from the use of various activities are shared with the program team for use by all those working with the individual.

Programming for those who demonstrate autistic-like behavior must first determine whether the individual is profoundly retarded or is demonstrating such symptoms as a result of extreme emotional distress. The assistance of the total program team is vital in making this decision before goals can be set and programming instituted.

This is an expensive type of programming initially, because it requires a one-to-one relationship, but the results are gratifying to the team. The occupational therapist may be the original worker in the process or may be called upon as a consultant or resource person.

Activities of Daily Living

On rare occasions, inability to learn is the main cause for the individual's not performing self-care activities. More frequently, the mentally retarded person has not been required or permitted to undertake his or her own self-care. The behaviors demonstrated by the retarded in this area are often related to the demands made on them. It is unfair if the individual is given an unpressed, buttonless shirt or blouse and then criticized for sloppy appearance. Likewise, if open zippers are permitted, the therapist is negligent in training for community living. Similarly, there should not be one dress code for the retarded persons and another for the staff. There must be consistency in what is expected or accepted.

Use of cosmetics and hair styling should be realistic and meet reasonable current standards. Proper use of cosmetics is a useful tool in teaching body scheme and image.

Self-feeding for some individuals is a slow process, and often staff have done the feeding. Frequently, small, inexpensive, dishwasher-safe adapted utensils can be made for more independent self-feeding. More involved adaptations may require greater on-site assistance from the occupational therapist and demand the training of other staff members in their use and purpose. Adapted equipment should be kept as simple as possible in construction in order to encourage use by all staff.

Self-care in personal hygiene is a topic frequently avoided by most disciplines. The use of the toilet and toilet tissue and handwashing must be encouraged. Teaching of self-care for menstrual needs is increasing. Unfortunately, little is being done to instruct individuals about or to discuss these bodily functions.

A successful method of teaching self-care in feeding, dressing, and personal hygiene is the process known as *chaining. Forward chaining* means building upon a series of simple steps to develop a more complex series and finally to complete the task. For example, the donning of slacks would progress from having the individual insert his feet into the leg openings, to pulling up the trousers, and finally to fastening them. For some individuals, *backward chaining* is an easier learning process. This involves having the individual first complete the task—buttoning, fastening the clamp, pulling up the zipper—and then expanding to include the pulling up process and finally the insertion of feet into the leg openings.

Each procedure ends with the same result, but the manner used is dependent on the individual's perceptions and physical status. Chaining can be utilized for teaching most activities of self-care through individualized occupational therapy training as well as through sharing the process with the direct-care staff for reinforcement and implementation.

Vocational Exploration

The extent of the role of occupational therapy in this area varies according to the roles taken by members of the other disciplines. It may be that, in one setting, a registered occupational therapist has the responsibility for evaluating potential, planning, and implementing the total program. In a larger, more extensively staffed center, the occupational therapist's role could be that of evaluation through offering work experiences for exploration and determination of readiness for progression to workshop assignment.

It is imperative that the therapist be aware of the individual's feelings toward work and those of his or her culture. To many, the ability to work is a sign of health and usefulness. Unfortunately, many mentally retarded persons feel they do not have any responsibility in this area. The occupational therapist can be of value to the team by attempting to motivate the individual to become involved in a work training experience.

Maintenance

For the want of a better term, the descriptive word "maintenance" is used to designate programming for those who have reached what is probably their maximum level of functioning. The goal is to prevent regression.

The individual with a progressive disorder needs assistance in retaining ability in range of motion, activities of daily living, and cognition for as long as possible. The aid the therapist can give the individual and the family is important. There are few progressive disorders causing mental deterioration among those diagnosed as mentally retarded. However, those that do exist require additional skill and effort from the program team.

The normal aging process and the acquisition of additional physical or neurologic involvements compound the care and responsibility of the program teams. A senile, 80-year-old, mentally retarded individual may demonstrate behaviors similar to those seen throughout his or her lifetime but will probably demonstrate less skill than other 80-year-old senile individuals. This individual requires an evaluation and adjustment of goals by the program team to function at his or her highest level.

Although the term "maintenance" can be interpreted negatively, in this aspect of programming, it is given a positive connotation and is meant to be an area in which therapy is not only desired but strongly indicated.

Research

Unfortunately, few occupational therapists have been involved in research, and those working with the mentally retarded have been just as remiss as those in other specialty areas. Occupational therapists are involved in facilitating change and are attempting to meet current needs; but understaffing, heavy case loads, and required paperwork have frequently been used as excuses for avoiding involvement in research. Research does demand time, but the occupational therapist has the responsibility to share findings with others. Research projects also improve level of skill.

Resource and Consultancy

The increase in numbers of small facilities providing interim care, extended care, and community living arrangements, and the requirement that such centers have a registered occupational therapist as a consultant in order to meet government regulations for funding provides another potential role for the therapist working with the mentally retarded. Agencies such as AAMD and NARC have encouraged the return to community centers of those who can profit from living in such settings. Being closer to the family has been desired by many, but the level of functioning requires more care than the family can provide. In addition, many mentally retarded persons with no families can be placed in a center where they might go to a workshop and return to minimal supervision at night-time. Others who require more skilled care may be placed closer to their families so family members may visit them more easily.

The role of occupational therapy can be that of assisting the staff in providing needed adaptations for self-care, in developing an activity program that is therapeutic, and in aiding the staff to meet the particular needs of the mentally retarded individuals so that they may adjust more easily to a new life-style.

Composite Treatment

The mentally retarded develop acute or chronic physical or emotionally disabling conditions, as does the nonretarded population. Special intervention techniques must be implemented to remediate the secondary condition. The overall concern, however, remains the elicitation of behavioral change in regard to the level of mental retardation.

The following is a sampling of the types of program-

ming occupational therapists may emphasize during five broad age periods of the individual.

During the *preschool period,* it would be essential to assess and then to remediate through early intervention and neurodevelopmental techniques. Second, therapy would include encouraging the development of self-motivation, a skill useful throughout the individual's life. A third program is the use of play.

Early school age treatment would probably include continuation of neurodevelopmental training with appropriate re-evaluation. The child should be placed in a school environment compatible with his or her functioning level. The occupational therapist can assist with adaptive and seating devices to alleviate physical dysfunction. Modalities are also used to aid in cognitive development. Motor behavior evaluation and remediation techniques, as described by Beter and colleagues, would be a valuable tool for use with the early school child.[2] The expansion of living skills is most important at this age level.

Adolescent years might entail continued use of earlier modalities and techniques for evaluation and assessment. In addition, the occupational therapist may be involved in prevocational exploration. Activities of daily living would be expanded and include basic sex education.

For the *adult years,* there would be increased emphasis on community living, including work responsibilities and behaviors and basic finances and budgeting. Dating, sex education, marriage, and homemaking skills may be included in the expansion of daily living skills.

During the *aging years,* it is essential that the occupational therapist differentiate the mental retardation component from that of the normal aging process. One must continually reassess skills in order to maintain the individual's maximum functional level. With improved medical care, the mentally retarded are living longer, thus extending the demands on the therapeutic team.

Advances
Accountability

Families, community agencies, funding sources, and professional organizations are demanding proof of the results of time, energy, and funds expended. Staff no longer can report impressive-looking statistics for attendance at mass activities, numbers of pounds of food served, tons of laundry washed, or gallons of water used. Instead, they are expected to produce behavioral change in individuals, with some exhibiting extreme change that will permit independent living apart from the family unit, whereas in others, seemingly minimal change in self-care is seen that permits more active participation within an institutional community.

Family Contribution

Initially, families were encouraged to institutionalize and forget a retarded member. For those who conformed to this counsel, there was increased guilt and shame, compounded, on the rare occasions that they were permitted to visit, by the lack of recognition on the part of the mentally retarded individual and, in some instances, by lack of interest on the part of the staff. For those who kept the member at home, stress was placed on the total family by a society that did not understand, gaped at, and commented on aberrant behaviors. Fortunately, these types of abuse have lessened, and families are being involved as a total unit in a variety of community treatment activities.

The increased involvement of the family is only one product of family counseling. The family is being given help in adjusting to the needs of any member who is mentally retarded; it is aided in deciding where and when to go for assistance and in comprehending how to ask for and obtain the maximum level of function of the retarded individual. The family also is helped in planning for the care of the individual when the primary family can no longer meet his or her needs.

Medical Advances

Genetic counseling is of immeasurable importance; individuals who have the potential for conceiving an involved child can be informed and counseled. Those known as high-risk mothers because of age, exposure to infection, or possible genetic complications have access to amniocentesis.

Much progress has been made, with an even greater prospect for the future, as a result of prenatal care. Early care during pregnancy will aid in improving the nutrition of both the mother and the baby. Various medical and dietary supplements providing a well-balanced diet will aid in the reduction of premature births, as well as in the prevention of disorders such as hypothyroidism that result from endocrine imbalances.

Some geographic areas are now developing a high-risk registry. Individuals considered to be candidates for extended care are listed in the registry and observed closely, with therapeutic intervention occurring as early as possible. Increased use of tests at birth, such as those for phenylketonuria, will show whether there will be a need for dietary supplements or other special measures for the baby.

Legal Rights and Obligations

The right to an education to the extent of the individual's potential is mandated in Public Law 94-142. Expansion of programs such as infant stimulation may decrease the numbers of those considered retarded as a result of insufficient stimulation during the early, formative years.

In addition, mainstreaming is required in states receiving special federal funds. Mainstreaming is defined as educational programming in the least restrictive environment along a continuum of seven levels—from those who can function in a regular classroom to those homebound or in institutions. Education is defined broadly so that the individual receives service compatible with his or her functioning level.

Other legal issues include voting, securing and maintaining employment, appropriate housing, marriage, and parenthood. With each of these rights come obligations and responsibilities, such as total housing rental and upkeep, taxes, and involvement with the community and family.

Many states, as well as the federal government, have enacted legislation mandating that institutions be phased out and that individuals be placed in community housing. In addition, many strict requirements for housing have been compiled for placement in community living arrangements. For those families and staff involved in locating housing, it is recommended that contact be made with the local treatment agency, the mental health–mental retardation unit serving the area, or the state office of mental retardation. It is essential to comply with the constantly updated standards and to make the transition to community living easier for the individuals and their families.

Combined with legal rights and responsibilities is an awareness of ethical and societal concerns. With expanded freedom and legal rights, the mentally retarded should be afforded societal opportunities but must be expected to conform to the mores of their culture.

Acknowledgment

Sincere appreciation is expressed to my patients, colleagues, and students who have contributed immeasurably to my knowledge over the years. A special acknowledgment to Mrs. Noel Higginson for her typing of the manuscript and to Mrs. Judy Blaisdell for her critiquing and editing skills. To my family, a thank you for their support and encouragement.

References

1. Bergsma D (ed): Birth Defects Compendium, 2nd ed. New York, Alan R Liss, 1979
2. Beter T, Cragin W, Drury F: The Mentally Retarded Child and His Motor Behavior. Springfield, IL, Charles C Thomas, 1972
3. Buros OK (ed): The Eighth Mental Measurement Handbook. Highland Park, IL, Gryphon Press, 1978
4. Chinn P, Drew C, Logan D: Mental Retardation. St Louis, CV Mosby, 1979

5. Copeland M, Ford L, Solon S: Occupational Therapy for Mentally Retarded Children, p 27. Baltimore, University Park Press, 1976
6. Currie C: Evaluating function of mentally retarded children through use of toys and play activities. Am J Occup Ther 23:1, 1969
7. Diagnostic and Statistical Manual of Mental Disorders, 2nd ed. (DSM-II). Washington, DC, American Psychiatric Association, 1968
8. Employment of Patient Workers in Hospitals and Institutions at Subminimum Wages. Washington, DC, US Government Printing Office, 1975
9. Gellis S, Feingold M: Atlas of Mental Retardation Syndromes. Washington, DC, US Government Printing Office, 1968
10. Goldberg I, Lippman L: Right to Education. New York, Teachers College of Columbia University, 1973
11. Grossman HG (ed): Manual on Terminology and Classification in Mental Retardation. Baltimore, Garamond/Pridemark, 1973
12. Heber R (ed): A Manual on Terminology and Classification in Mental Retardation, pp 63–64. Monograph supplement to Am J Mental Deficiency, 2nd ed. Springfield, IL, American Association on Mental Deficiency, 1961
13. Itard J: The Wild Boy of Aveyron. Englewood Cliffs, NJ, Prentice–Hall, 1962
14. Nihira K, Foster R, Shellhaas M, et al: AAMD Adaptive Behavior Scale for Children and Adults, 1974 Revision. Washington, DC, American Association on Mental Deficiency, 1974

Kindred M (ed): The Mentally Retarded Citizen and the Law. New York, The Free Press, 1976
Krajicek MJ, Tearney AI (eds): Detection of Developmental Problems in Children. Baltimore, University Park Press, 1977
Magrab PR (ed): Psychological Management of Pediatric Problems, Vol 1, Early Life Conditions and Chronic Diseases. Baltimore, University Park Press, 1978
Magrab PR (ed): Psychological Management of Pediatric Problems, Vol 2, Sensorineural Conditions and Social Concerns. Baltimore, University Park Press, 1978

Bibliography

Banus BS, Kent EA, Norton Y, et al: The Developmental Therapist, 2nd ed. Thorofare, NJ, Charles B Slack, 1979
Batshaw ML, Perret YM: Children with Handicaps: A Medical Primer. Baltimore, Paul H Brookes, 1981
Breines E: Perception: Its Development and Recapitulation. Leban, NJ, Geri-Rehab, 1981
Clark PN, Allen AS: Occupational Therapy for Children. St Louis, CV Mosby, 1985
Fairchild TN, Parks AL: Mainstreaming the Mentally Retarded Child. Austin, TX, Learning Concepts, 1977
Fiorentino MR: Reflex Testing Methods for Evaluating CNS Development. Springfield, IL, Charles C Thomas, 1972
Houts P, Scott R, Leaser J: Goal Planning with the Mentally Retarded. Hershey, Milton S Hershey Medical Center, Pennsylvania State University, 1973

Recommended Periodicals and Journals

American Association on Mental Deficiency:
    AMERICAN JOURNAL OF MENTAL DEFICIENCY
    MENTAL RETARDATION
American Occupational Therapy Association:
    AMERICAN JOURNAL OF OCCUPATIONAL THERAPY
American Orthopsychiatric Association:
    AMERICAN JOURNAL OF ORTHOPSYCHIATRY
American Physical Therapy Association:
    PHYSICAL THERAPY
American Speech-Language-Hearing Association:
    ASHA
    JOURNAL OF SPEECH AND HEARING DISORDERS
Council for Exceptional Children:
    EXCEPTIONAL CHILDREN
Haworth Press:
    SOCIAL WORK IN HEALTH CARE
Insight Publishing Company, Inc.:
    PEDIATRIC ANNALS
Macmillan Journals Ltd.:
    NURSING TIMES
National Association for Retarded Citizens:
    ACTION TOGETHER/INFORMATION EXCHANGE
National Rehabilitation Association:
    JOURNAL OF REHABILITATION
Perceptual and Motor Skills:
    PERCEPTUAL AND MOTOR SKILLS
Professional Press, Inc.:
    JOURNAL OF LEARNING DISABILITIES
Society for the Experimental Analysis of Behavior
    JOURNAL OF APPLIED BEHAVIOR ANALYSIS

CHAPTER 27

Acute Care *Judy Feinberg*

Occupational therapists working in a general hospital setting need to be knowledgeable about a variety of diagnoses, medical and occupational therapy assessments, treatment approaches, and community resources. The patients seen in this setting are acutely ill. They may have more than one problem, and the process of diagnosis may be just beginning. Therefore, the patients' adjustments to their medical problems may also be just beginning.

Many of the patients found in a general hospital are discussed in other sections of this book, such as those with cerebral vascular accident, arthritis, or spinal cord injuries. This chapter will cover other acute medical conditions and focus on the occupational therapy assessment and treatment procedures in an acute-care setting. The approach of the occupational therapist in this setting differs from that elsewhere because of the nature of the medical problems seen in the acute stages of disease.

Acute-Care Hospitals

General hospitals are the mainstay for medical care of the acutely ill individual. They serve all ages, from birth to death, and serve as the entry point for all types of diagnostic, medical, and surgical problems, including birth defects, trauma, and chronic illnesses. It is important to recognize that a general hospital exists for acute-care problems or for episodic care of chronic conditions.

The length of stay in general, acute-care hospitals is decreasing, and now averages about 7 days. Short-term hospitalizations mean that the therapist often has time only to complete assessments and program planning, with the implementation being done by another therapist, in another center, or in the patient's home. Discharge planning is vital in assuring that all patients receive quality care. It is essential that occupational therapists assess the potential benefits of treatment to a patient, so that recommendations can be made regarding whether the patient should remain hospitalized for a longer period, be discharged home, or be sent to another facility.

The constraints of time and resources in the acute-care situation often require prioritization of patients, as do natural fluctuations in caseloads or unexpected staff absences. Occupational therapists in acute care, therefore, need to develop a philosophy that will allow them to establish a logical prioritization system. One such philosophy of acute care is "the belief that the ability to perform basic self-care is intimately connected with recovery from illness and essential for successful timely discharge."[13] On the basis of this philosophy, Rausch and Melvin[13] classified the types of acute-care patients referred to occupational therapists as one possible method of determining the allocation of both staff and resources:

1. The single-episode or injury population; for example, patients admitted for total hip replacement or hand injury. These patients typically have a short hospitalization with a predictable course of treatment.
2. Patients in the acute phase of long-term rehabilitation, such as those with head trauma, cerebral vascular accident, or spinal cord injury. The length of hospitalization for these patients is more variable, and the patients often have life-threatening medical complications.
3. Chronically ill patients admitted for an acute exacerbation, surgical procedure, or concomitant disease. This group includes persons with diabetes, arthritis, cardiac conditions, neurological diseases, or cancer. This group of patients stays for an unpredictable length of time and may require a period of complete bed rest.
4. Patients admitted for invasive diagnostic testing or regulation of medications. Typical diagnoses in this group are acute back injury, poorly controlled diabetes, or Parkinson's disease. The course of hospitalization for these patients typically is brief and relatively predictable, and it may include activity restrictions.

These categories are not meant to be all-inclusive or restrictive but rather to provide useful guidelines for the acute-care occupational therapist.

Assessment

Assessment of the patient must be completed in a short time to maximize the time for treatment. In many instances, it is not practical to do a complete and specific evaluation of the patient's physical status at the time of initial interview due to time limitations or the condition of the patient. A complete evaluation may be accomplished as part of the overall treatment plan during the course of treatment.

Demographic Information

The demographic factors considered should include personal information: name, address, telephone number, date of birth, age, and sex. The date of admission to the hospital, referral date, date first seen by the occupational therapist, and who referred the patient to occupational therapy should be recorded. The type of insurance coverage is important for both billing and planning for occupational therapy treatment. For example, certain insurance coverage requires prior approval for oc-

cupational therapy services. Other data include the diagnosis being addressed in occupational therapy and additional diagnoses that may affect the patient's life, the date of onset, present problems and symptoms, medications, precautions, complications, and other pertinent medical history. The family situation, including marital status, family members at or near the home, people who are with the patient during the day and night, and the family members who are employed, need documentation. There should be a brief description of the home, including whether it is an urban or rural setting, the type of structure, and the number of stairs to be negotiated by the patient.

Independent Living and Daily Living Skills

During the initial assessment, the self-care status should be documented. It should be noted whether the patient is independent, requires assistance of a person or adaptive equipment, or is dependent in any given task. The areas that should be considered are grooming and hygiene, eating, dressing, leisure activities, functional mobility within the home and in the community, and object manipulation. There is some evidence that professionals and perhaps even patients tend to overestimate the ability to perform daily living activities.[15] Although patients may appear capable of performing certain tasks, therapists should know whether these tasks actually are being performed at home.

Documentation of family involvement is an important aspect of the patient's daily living assessment. The amount and appropriateness of the assistance provided should be noted, as well as how both the patient and the family feel about the assistance. If assistance will be needed following hospitalization, and these needs cannot be satisfied by the family or adaptive equipment, social services should be consulted.

Work

Data should be gathered regarding the patient's former and present occupations. Specific education and training, as well as job requirements and responsibilities, should also be documented. Any potential need for occupational change should be noted by the acute-care therapist; such situations usually necessitate referral for later intervention.

Sensorimotor Skills and Performance Components

If appropriate, reflex integration, range of motion, gross and fine coordination, strength and endurance, sensory awareness, visual and spatial awareness, and body integration should be assessed.

Cognitive Skills and Performance Components

This assessment should include orientation, cognitive integration, and conceptualization. Concentration, attention span, memory, and problem-solving abilities of the patient should be noted.

Psychosocial Skills and Performance Components

Information regarding the patient's self-concept and self-identity, situational coping, and community involvement must be obtained. Self-management and dyadic and group interaction also should be documented.

Therapeutic Adaptation

The use of prosthetic or orthotic devices should be recorded. The occupational therapist should ask and record whether the patient has any adaptive equipment and if it is used regularly. The appropriateness of fit of these devices should be checked, so modifications can be made if indicated.

Patient Goals

The therapist should document the patient's short-term and long-term goals. The therapist should note the patient's understanding of the disability or disease, responses to a brief description of the occupational therapy program, and the attitude of the patient toward the program.

Therapist's Impression

Before treatment goals can be developed, the therapist must take into consideration the potential benefit of treatment, the presumed reliability of the patient's responses, and the motivation of the patient to participate in the occupational therapy program.

Occupational Therapy Program Plan

The treatment plan should state the need for any additional specific evaluations. Treatment objectives, treatment modalities, follow-up or referral considerations, and estimated duration of occupational therapy are components of the plan for patients in an acute-care setting.

Special Treatment Procedures

Intensive Care Unit

It is common for occupational therapists to provide services to patients in intensive care units (ICUs) of general hospitals. To develop an occupational therapy program on a given ICU, the therapist must know the purpose of the unit and work supportively with the physician and nursing teams. Any occupational therapy program represents a coordinated effort that considers the patient's medical needs, nursing procedures, and physical and respiratory therapy programs.

The ICU is an equipment-laden environment that provides constant monitoring of patients' vital signs. It is of the utmost importance that therapists have a thorough knowledge of where invasive lines go, what they do, what problems they can cause, and what precautions they warrant (Table 27-1).[2]

There are three problems that commonly occur in the ICU for which occupational therapy intervention is appropriate: immobility and long-term bed rest, sensory deprivation and stress, and long-term mechanical ventilation. Patients who have been on extended bed rest will have very low endurance, low sitting tolerance, and generalized weakness, effects that can be reversed through therapy. Activities such as bed mobility, transfer training, graded self-care, avocational or stress management activities, and communication activities may be helpful. These activities can be graded in terms of length of treatment time, amount and speed of active movement, level of assistance given, adaptive aids, and position and postural support. Because of the nature of the ICU, close teamwork is necessary to provide the patients with a daily schedule that can balance rest, mobilization, and functional recovery directly and effectively.

The highly technical environment of the ICU may be stressful to the patient. The effects of constant monitoring with complete disruption of daily life routines, together with the fear, depression, and pain of being ill, can lead a patient to a state of generalized disorientation and thought disorganization. Occupational therapy programs in the ICU can alleviate some of the problems of isolation and sensory deprivation by providing gradual application of specific stimuli to increase arousal and awareness. The therapist should orient the patient repeatedly when necessary and use calendars, clocks, and family visits to keep the patient oriented. Activities of daily living programs can help to restore a sense of daily routine and personal independence. Relaxation techniques can be incorporated with reality-orienting programs to provide organized, patterned stimulation and to develop an increased sense of personal control.[1] Individualized activity programs using meaningful tasks can promote cognitive and motor recovery in patients and enhance their motivation to participate in their overall

Table 27-1. *Common Life Support and Monitoring Lines*

Line/Catheter	Location	Purpose	Precautions	Implications
CVP*	Threaded through superior vena cava into right atrium	Monitors right side of the heart filling pressures; used to introduce drugs	Line is sutured in; *do not pull.* Normal CVP is 9–12 mm Hg	Should not restrict ROM at head, shoulder, or scapula. Should not restrict activity.
Arterial pressure (art line)	Usually in radial or femoral artery; can also be in artery in the foot (dorsum pedis)	Used when continuous monitoring of blood pressure is indicated or when frequent blood gas measurements are required	Inserted into artery; looks like an IV but is not. Usually sutured in; *do not pull.* Normal MAP is 70–90 mm Hg; transducer must be at level of patient's heart for accurate reading.	Know patient's normal MAP and monitor with any change in activity. Notify nurse of any change.
Swan–Ganz catheter	Threaded into the superior vena cava into right ventricle. Pulmonary valve catheter tip rests in pulmonary artery	Indirectly monitors function of the left side of the heart; can also obtain CVP and cardiac output readings; used following open heart surgery, trauma, heart failure	Line is sutured in; *do not pull.* Usually, patients with this line are in serious condition. Check activity orders closely. Nurse monitors PAWP.	Specific activity order with specific parameters for each patient's MAP from physician. Watch pulmonary artery pressure wave for damping with activity.
TPN	Most commonly in subclavian vein	Used to administer very high concentration of calories, often following extensive surgery or trauma when oral or NG intake is inadequate	Line is usually sutured in; *do not pull.*	Usually, activity is indicated secondary to high calorie intake; line should not restrict mobility or ROM.
Neurological monitors Examples:		Monitors ICP following surgery or trauma	Head of bed usually limited to no more 30° Normal ICP ≤ 15 mm Hg	Usually on bed rest; check with physician
1. IVC	1. IVC tip rests in the ventricle of the brain			
2. Subarachnoid bolt, Richmond bolt	2. Subarachnoid space—CSF in contact with column of H₂O to measure pressure			
Chest tube	Usually through intercostal or subcostal space into pleural space	Drains fluid from chest cavity and restores normal pressure relationships within pleural space	Usually sutured in; *do not pull.*	Avoid tension, torque, or kinking

* CSF, cerebrospinal fluid. CVP, central venous pressure. ICP, intracranial pressure. IV, intravenous. IVC, intraventricular catheter. MAP, mean arterial pressure. NG, nasogastric. OTR, occupational therapist, registered. PAWP, pulmonary artery wedge pressure. ROM, range of motion. TPN, total parenteral nutrition.

Reproduced in modified form with permission from Affleck AT, Lieberman S, Polon J, Rohrkemper K: Providing occupational therapy in an intensive care unit. Am J Occup Ther 40:325, 1986.

care. Patients should be allowed choices when possible to combat feelings of loss of control.

Mechanical ventilation is commonly used to sustain cardiopulmonary homeostasis in critically ill patients. Communication problems may be reduced with writing tablets or communication boards. The occupational therapist provides meaningful and functional tasks such as stress management activities, activities of daily living, or patient-selected activities during the weaning process. These activities can help reduce or eliminate the patient's experience of air-hunger panic or anticipatory anxiety as mechanical ventilation is decreased. Therapists may help patients to come off the ventilator by providing short sessions of therapy interspersed into their daily schedules. Activity analysis is required to obtain the best match between the task demand and the patient's capacity for mental and physical activity.

Depending on concomitant diagnoses, the therapist may employ selected rehabilitation techniques as appropriate to the physical condition of the patient and the limitations of the ICU setting. Emotional support of the patient and the family is extremely important.

Home Assessment

If the patient, the patient's family, or the therapist foresees problems in the return to the home from the general hospital, the therapist should arrange to do a home assessment before or immediately after the patient's discharge. This may be particularly relevant now that hospital stays are shorter and patients are discharged before attaining full independence. Home assessments are particularly relevant when a patient is returning to his home with a decrease in mobility, either temporary or permanent, imposed by his medical or surgical condition. Ideally, the therapist should arrange for the patient and other members of the household to be present in the home during the assessment. If a home assessment cannot be done due to time constraints or the distance of the home from the hospital, the therapist may review the floor plans with the patient and family in the clinic.

The purpose of the home assessment is to determine whether barriers there will interfere with the patient's performance of daily living tasks. By doing the home assessment before discharge, the therapist can make realistic recommendations to the patient, implement further treatment goals, and arrange for any necessary adaptive equipment to ease the transition from the hospital to the home. A home visit can help the therapist determine whether additional occupational therapy services are needed either as an outpatient, through a home health care agency, or at another facility.

Home assessment should include accessibility of the home itself as well as individual rooms. Manipulation of the environment (*e.g.*, light switches, faucets, telephones, and television) by the patient should be as-

sessed. Safety should be a major consideration; therefore, the therapist should note, for example, the presence of throw rugs where a patient may walk and consider putting hand rails and grab bars in appropriate places. If the disability is new to the patient and family, the therapist should realize that any recommendations for change, either temporary or permanent, may be rejected initially. The patient and family must be ready to accept necessary changes before they will be willing to accept the recommendations of the therapist. Also, few patients will be able to make extensive changes in their living environment; therefore, simple, creative solutions should be made whenever possible. Much has been written regarding home modifications for the handicapped, and this topic is addressed in other areas of this book.

Examples of Treatment Programs

This section will address specific diagnostic categories frequently seen in the acute-care, general hospital setting. Symptomatology will be briefly discussed, and the role of the occupational therapist with each specific category will be presented. Many of the orthopedic and neurological conditions seen by the occupational therapist are covered in other sections of this book.

Cancer

The term "cancer" refers collectively to all malignant tumors. Malignancy implies the ability of the tumor, or neoplasm, to invade and destroy adjacent structures and to spread to distant sites (metastasis). Tumors are classified according to their histogenesis; tumors of mesenchymal origin are called sarcomas, whereas tumors of epithelial origin are called carcinomas. Classification and terminology are important because they convey the specific clinical significance — the likely behavior — of a given neoplasm.[14] The location, rate of growth, spread, and amount of interference with normal function determine the pathological effects of a tumor. Cancer often strikes in middle age, but no age group is unaffected. Although the cause(s) of cancer has not yet been determined, several factors have been identified that favor its development, including heredity, hormonal states, and exposure to carcinogens.

The means of slowing, arresting, or curing the disease include surgery, chemotherapy, and radiation. These can result in amputation, seriously altered ways of functioning, changes in self-image, adjustment of lifestyle, and varying states of well-being. Survival time is increasing as early detection and improved treatment methods allow control of the disease for longer periods of time. For some patients, cancer becomes a chronic disease requiring long-term monitoring and treatment. As in other chronic diseases, rehabilitation can maintain optimum function in the cancer patient and improve the quality of the individual's life.

Rehabilitation

In general, the goals for cancer rehabilitation may be divided into four categories.[7] The *preventive* category includes treatment in anticipation of potential disability to lessen its severity or shorten its duration. In the *restorative* category are programs for the patient who can be expected to return to premorbid status without significant handicap. The *supportive* category is defined by controlled disease or handicap that will persist, where much disability can be eliminated by training or treatment. The last category is *palliative*, where there is increasing disability from progressive disease but where appropriate rehabilitation can prevent complications such as bedsores, contractures, problems of personal hygiene, and emotional deterioration due to inactivity and depression.

Rehabilitation of cancer patients differs from standard rehabilitation in several important ways. The single most important factor is that cancer rehabilitation is an ongoing process that does not wait for the patient to be medically stable. Therapists must develop a philosophy of treatment which enables them to cope with the realities of the situation[3]:

1. Occupational therapy may be started before the long-term results of the patient's medical treatment are known.
2. Patients may be discharged before rehabilitation is complete.
3. Much treatment is done at the bedside, which limits activities.
4. Evaluation is brief and ongoing, rather than complete.
5. Rehabilitation sessions are often interrupted by treatment or diagnostic procedures.
6. Side-effects of treatment may prevent occupational therapy treatment.
7. Rehabilitation may not be foremost in the mind of the patient.

The task of the occupational therapist is to trigger useful coping mechanisms, to teach adaptation and compensation, to help the patient regard problems as challenges, and to foster creativity and flexibility. Interventions may include psychosocial support, physical restoration, training in the use of adaptive equipment, design and construction of orthotic devices, retraining in activities of daily living, teaching of satisfying leisure activities, and family support and teaching. The physical restoration measures necessary to rehabilitate the residual problems of the disease or its treatment follow the usual principles of functional occupational therapy. However, the patient may deteriorate in other areas due to disease progression during or after the rehabilitation therapy.

The psychosocial aspects of the treatment of the patient are as important as the physical restoration measures. Although occupational therapy may be limited and intermittent, if an effective therapeutic relationship is developed between the patient and the therapist early in the disease, it will be easier to reinstitute treatment as new problems occur. With each successive rehospitalization, the patient and family lose more of their hope for recovery. Feelings of helplessness and loss of control appear as patients face increasing dependence on others and relinquishment of their social roles of wage earner, homemaker, or parent. Occupational therapy can be instrumental in reestablishing the patient's area of control by helping him or her identify attainable short-term and long-term goals.

Patients Undergoing Radical Mastectomy

Occupational therapy services for women who have undergone radical mastectomies are designed to help prevent problems of decreased shoulder range of motion (*i.e.*, pain, edema, and weakness), to provide education through discussion, and to demonstrate available adaptive equipment such as bras, prostheses, clothing, and cosmetics to obscure scars. The therapist should explain which activities are contraindicated postoperatively while providing therapeutic activities. Instruction in the principles of work simplification and energy conservation may be helpful.

Surgeons vary in their referral patterns, but physical activity and exercise are usually not initiated until 3 or 4 days after the operation. It is important that therapists consult with the surgeon to establish the specific rehabilitation program and rate of progression for each patient. The specific objectives must take into consideration that patient's premorbid condition and activity level in addition to any postoperative complications such as shoulder–hand syndrome.

In coordination with the social services or rehabilitation psychology departments, psychological support for the individual and her family should be offered to facilitate acceptance of her condition. If appropriate, referral should be made to community agencies such as the Reach for Recovery Program of the American Cancer Society. Following discharge from the hospital, the patient may be seen for review and reinforcement of instructions presented during hospitalization. Outpatient treatment may be done in groups to facilitate mutual support in conjunction with physical rehabilitation.

The Dying Patient

People dying from cancer experience physical isolation, an actual withdrawal by family and medical personnel.

It is not uncommon for patients, their families, and the medical staff to experience feelings of denial, avoidance, and anxiety. The therapist who works with dying patients must be secure in his or her own attitude toward death and dying. The therapist must be able to listen, hear, understand, be sensitive, and be able to respond verbally and nonverbally to spoken and unspoken requests. The ability to recognize when a patient needs you, and the willingness to give the time, regardless of personal or professional schedule, are essential.

Occupational therapy is unique in that the patient's physical, psychosocial, and occupational performance needs are assessed and incorporated into treatment. The occupational therapist can provide meaningful, purposeful activity to help the patient maintain occupational functioning and preserve dignity, self-respect, and self-esteem.[12] The patient should ultimately determine the quality of life and the occupational roles he or she wishes to maintain. Activities that promote a feeling of self-worth and productivity may be used to facilitate the adaptive process. Frequent re-evaluation is necessary due to the continuing deterioration of the patient's condition, so that priority setting and goals may be adjusted accordingly.

Cardiac Disease

Cardiac disease is one of the most common causes of death in the United States, and patients with this diagnosis are frequently treated in general hospitals. Myocardial infarction (MI), at present one of the most common manifestations, causes permanent heart damage, as tissue anoxia from occlusion of the blood supply results in necrosis of muscle fibers in an area of the myocardium. Eventually, this area shrinks and scars. The extent of functional impairment varies with the amount of damage, area of damage, length of time elapsed since the event, and patient cooperation during the acute and convalescent stages. Arrhythmia, valvar damage, thromboembolism, shock, pump failure, and anxiety states may prolong recovery time.

Rehabilitation

The primary goal of the rehabilitation program for individuals with recent acute MI is return to optimal physiological, psychological, social, and emotional status by creating a therapeutic environment that not only promotes healing of the damaged myocardium but also helps to prevent any further insult to the heart. The objectives to be achieved are: (1) providing a systematic approach to the advancement of activities throughout convalescence, (2) active participation by the patient and family in the rehabilitation program, (3) explaining to the patient the disease process and its consequences for lifestyle, and (4) providing emotional and psychological support for the patient and family by all members of the rehabilitation team.

When dealing with an acute medical problem such as MI, it is essential that the occupational therapist consult with the nursing staff and review the medical records to keep current on the patient's status. The occupational therapist must also consult with the physician to determine when the patient's activity level should be reduced, sustained, or upgraded. Therapists who want to specialize in cardiac rehabilitation need to acquire more knowledge of cardiovascular physiology, management of heart disease, electrocardiographic interpretation, and exercise physiology.

The occupational therapist starts the program by completing an assessment, including an interview to obtain information on the patient's prehospital lifestyle, current living situation, household and work responsibilities, and leisure interests. Depending on the facility and the region of the country, one may find different rehabilitation professionals performing the same role in different programs. Thus, the occupational therapist's role may vary widely. He or she may provide one or more of the following components of the program[11]:

1. Progressive activity and exercise, to assess, and help the patient to develop, tolerance for activity
2. Work equivalent activity, to teach the patient about the energy cost of activity and to promote a vocational interest
3. Activities of daily living (ADL) evaluation and training, to assess cardiac response to these activities and to make appropriate recommendations
4. Work simplification training, to promote maximum independence in patients whose cardiac reserve is impaired
5. Patient education about activity and exercise
6. Psychosocial support, to assist the patient in coping with the event and in making life-style changes
7. Leisure counseling, to assist the patient in emotional adjustment and stress management
8. Stress management training

Stages of the Treatment Process

Each stage of the treatment involves four basic areas of daily living: self-care, mobility/ambulation, exercise, and other activities, including recreation. The occupational therapist usually does not see the patient during the period of complete bed rest, which is considered stage one. Stage two, three, and four are defined by energy expenditure, and the patient is advanced from one stage to the next after consultation with the primary physician.

Stage One

An activity chart should be given to the individual during the first contact (see the box). The purpose and stages of the program are explained, and appropriate initial activities are filled in by the therapist. The purpose of an activity chart is to demonstrate visually to the patient, family, and other staff the level of physical activity permitted. The activity program maintains and increases physical tolerance, prevents loss of muscle tone, promotes relaxation, develops interests to replace

---

CARDIAC REHABILITATION PROGRAM ACTIVITY CHART

Name: _____   Room: _____

Admission: _____   Date program started: _____

Doctor: _____

Occupational Therapist: _____

	1 — 1.5 Mets. Stage II	1.6 — 2.0 Mets. + U.E. Tension (Static) Stage III	2.1 — 3.0 Mets. Stage IV
○ Supervision needed ○ Can do without supervision ○ Activity no longer applies			
Self-care	Wash hands and face ○ Feed self in bed ○ Fingernail care ○ Brush teeth ○ Feed self in chair 　with feet elevated ○	Bathe body in bed 　except back and 　legs ○ Shave self (seated, 　electric razor) ○ Comb hair (short) ○ Bathe body except 　back, seated at sink ○ Dress/undress in 　bedclothes ○	Eat in dining room 　in w/c. ○ Dress/undress in 　street clothes ○ Go to beauty parlor 　in w/c. ○ May take shower ○
Mobility	Bedside commode 　with assisted 　transfer ○ Chair rest with feet 　elevated: 　　bid. 20 min. ○ 　　bid. 30 min. 　　tid. 20 min. 　* As tolerated . . . 　　tid. 30 min. ○ 　　tid. 45 min. ○ 　　tid. 60 min. ○	Walk to bathroom 　for toileting ○ Progress to walking 　in room tid ○ Walk in room ad lib ○ Sit in chair ad lib ○	Walk in hall — slow 　pace 44 ft. ○ Walk in hall 44 ft. in 　15 secs. (2 mph.) ○ Walk in hall 55 ft. in 　15 sec. (2.5 mets.) 　(2.5 mph.) Walk in hall 66 ft. in 　15 secs. (3.0 　mets.) (3 mph.) ○
Exercise	Deep breathing 　every hour — 5 　deep breaths ○ Shoulders — 1 arm 　at a time ○ Quad. setting — 1 　leg at a time ○ Hips and knees — 1 　leg at a time ○ Ankles and toes — 1 　leg at a time ○	Quad setting ○ Hips and knees ○ Straight leg raising 　— 1 leg at a time ○	Straight leg raising ○ Trunk side bending ○ Trunk twisting ○

(continued)

CARDIAC REHABILITATION PROGRAM ACTIVITY CHART *(continued)*

Other activities			
Listen to radio		Watch T.V. in bed	
Read light weight		sitting	○
book with book-		Read newspaper	○
stand or otherwise		Yarn activities	○
supported	○	Table games and	
Use of telephone		activities	○
3–5 mins., 2–3		Light craft activities	○
calls/day	○		
Crossword puzzles	○		
Write short letters	○		

Get items out of	
drawers, closet. . . .	○
Observe, participate	○
in recreation pro-	
grams in w/c	
talking, singing,	○
table games	
Sit outside in warm	○
weather, not in hot	
sun	
Stair climbing	○
	○

Reprinted with permission. Hays C: General medicine and surgery In Hopkins H, Smith H (eds): *Willard and Spackman's Occupational Therapy*, 6th ed. p 740. Philadelphia, J B Lippincott, 1983.

previous, more strenuous activities, and aids in long-term rehabilitation and adjustment to convalescence.

Stage Two

At stage two, some of the self-care activities allowed are washing the hands and face, feeding self in bed or in a chair with the feet elevated, fingernail care, and brushing teeth. In the mobility/ambulation area, the patient should be able to use a bedside commode with the cardiac method of transfer and start sitting with the feet elevated in a chair twice a day for 20 minutes. After the patient's condition is stable, sitting time can gradually be lengthened to 60 minutes three times a day. Other activities allowed include listening to the radio, reading a book placed in a bookstand or otherwise supported, reading a newspaper or magazine, using the telephone for 3 to 5 minutes at a time two or three times a day, doing crossword puzzles, and writing short letters. When the patient can tolerate this level of activity, the therapist consults with the physician about advancing to stage three.

Stage Three

During stage three, in the area of self-care, the individual should be able to bathe (except for the back and legs) in bed or seated near a sink, to shave with an electric razor, to comb short hair, and to dress and undress in bedclothes. Regarding mobility/ambulation, a patient should first be able to walk to the bathroom for toileting, progress to walking about the room three times a day, and then progress to walking about the room as desired. Other activities are watching television while in bed and reading a newspaper. Light activities such as yarnwork, table games, or light crafts can also be initiated. When able to tolerate all stage three activities, the patient can progress to stage four with the physician's approval.

Stage Four

During stage four, in the area of self-care, the individual should be independent in eating when seated in a chair and in dressing and undressing in street clothes. The patient may take a shower. The individual should be able to do some activities such as going to the occupational therapy clinic, a hospital beauty or barber shop, or a hospital coffee shop. At this stage, ambulation includes walking in the hall at a slow pace (approximately 2 miles per hour, or 44 feet in 15 seconds). This should be increased gradually until the patient is able to walk in the hall at 3 miles per hour (66 feet in 15 seconds). Other acceptable activities would include taking items out of drawers and the closet; observing and participating in activities such as talking, singing, and light crafts; and sitting outside in warm weather. The individual should be able to begin some stair climbing.

Among the indications for stopping an activity are signs of ischemia or undue fatigue: chest pain, shortness of breath, dizziness, diaphoresis, pallor, cyanosis, and nausea. Another sign for caution is incomplete recovery, indicated by fatigue 1 hour after an activity has been completed. All changes need to be analyzed within the context of the situation or activity. In all cases of distress, consultation with the attending physician is required before initiating or resuming activities. Observations and actions taken are to be noted on the medical record.

Psychosocial Aspects of Care

Consideration of the psychosocial problems is essential when dealing with a patient with MI. This individual goes through the common stages of coping with serious illness, including disbelief, shock, denial, anxiety, anger, depression, and, finally, adjustment and adaptation. Some of the goals of the cardiac rehabilitation program should be to decrease the patient's and family's fears through education and to facilitate understanding of the disease and what can be expected. It is important that the therapist maintain daily contact with the patient to establish rapport and allow maximum opportunity for discussion of the risk factors of MI, the roles of activity, stress management, limitations of activities, relationships, return to work, signs and symptoms of fatigue, and ischemia. Inadequate or ambiguous information about coronary disease and its management, symptoms, prognosis, planned tests and procedures, allowable activities, return to work, and similar factors are a major concern of patients recovering from MI.[16] Discussion of these features before discharge from the hospital is important, since adequate time to discuss problems and receive information often is not available during follow-up outpatient visits. By the time of discharge, the patient and family should have a clear understanding of these factors and should be reassured about a safe return home.

Postdischarge Planning

The hospitalization phase of a cardiac rehabilitation program is just the beginning of the patient's recovery; complete rehabilitation requires that the patient participate in long-term exercise and risk factor modification. Positive life-style changes are paramount.

The occupational therapist may provide a detailed assessment of the patient's job requirements and duties; the physical demands of the job, such as sitting, walking, climbing, and lifting; the mental demands or stress of the job; production rate and output on the job; and the patient's responsibilities for others. The amount of break time allowed and the availability of places to rest should be assessed. The usual method of getting to and from work, the distance and travel time, and the availability of a bus from the parking lot to the building entrance are additional considerations. Other aspects of returning to work that need to be evaluated include the company's attitude toward part-time employment increments until an employee is able to resume full-time employment, the feasibility of a change of job within the company, and the policies of the company regarding sick leave, vacation, and retirement. All possible sources of income, such as sick pay, disability insurance, Social Security, other family members' salaries, and public assistance, should be considered. Planning must take into account the attitude of the patient about returning to the same job, consideration of a job change, and willingness to work. Simulated work evaluations provide objective data on which to develop realistic decisions about the patient's ability to return to work that involves nondynamic effort.[17] On the basis of the information gathered, the therapist supplies the physician and the patient with recommendations about returning to work, vocational

evaluation, retirement, employment opportunities that may be open to the individual, or referral to a vocational rehabilitation service.

Before discharge, a home program should be developed by the occupational therapist and the clinical nurse specialist in cardiology and reviewed by the physician. In some facilities, other team members may be part of the home care team. Although there are some basic premises for preparing home programs, each program must be developed for an individual on a personal basis and must be reviewed with the patient and family before discharge. Telephone contact or a follow-up outpatient visit 1 to 2 weeks after discharge may be useful to answer any questions that may have arisen and to check on the patient's functional progress.

Chronic Obstructive Pulmonary Disease

Chronic obstructive pulmonary disease (COPD) is one of the nation's fastest-growing health care problems, with more than 450,000 new patients seen each year.[4] People with COPD have difficulty moving air in and out of their lungs because their airways are narrowed by spasms, secretions, or loss of elasticity of the lung tissue, which traps air in the lungs. COPD results from emphysema, chronic bronchitis, bronchiectasis, or diseases that cause pulmonary fibrosis or cardiac disease. Symptoms include decreased physical tolerance, shortness of breath, cough with production of sputum, chest pain, hemoptysis, and noisy breathing.

Pulmonary rehabilitation is similar to cardiac rehabilitation in that it requires a coordinated effort by a team of health professionals. The rehabilitation program may be initiated in the hospital but is frequently continued in an outpatient setting because progress may be slow. Rehabilitation of patients with a chronic illness such as COPD is a very gradual process and requires a high level of patient and staff motivation, as well as intensive participation by the family. Patient education is important in addition to the physical, psychological, and vocational aspects of the program.

There are two principal objectives of pulmonary rehabilitation: (1) to control and alleviate as much as possible the symptoms and pathophysiologic complications of respiratory impairment, and (2) to teach the patient how to achieve optimal capability for carrying out his or her activities of daily living. The demonstrated benefits of pulmonary rehabilitation include: (1) reduction in symptoms; (2) reversal of anxiety and depression and improved ego strength; (3) enhanced ability to carry out activities of daily living; (4) increased exercise ability; (5) better quality of life; (6) reduction in the hospital days required; and (7) prolongation of life in many patients.[10]

Four primary objectives for occupational therapists

treating patients admitted to the hospital for COPD are:

1. Evaluating and teaching compensatory skills for loss of physical tolerance, including work simplification and energy conservation, and use of diaphragmatic breathing during ADL
2. Exploration of job responsibilities and vocational evaluation to decrease occupational exposure to dust and toxins
3. Provision of graded activity or exercise programs
4. Psychological support

Because the pathological changes are irreversible, physical training is used to rehabilitate the rest of the patient's body. Consequently, the aim of physical training is to reduce the ventilatory demand of physical exercise and to improve cardiovascular and muscle fitness.[6] Patient education topics include the physiological aspects of smoking and how to quit; the effects of respiratory irritants and infections; environmental controls; taking the pulse; coping with anxiety, fear, and stress; relaxation techniques; principles of exercise; proper nutrition; and taking care of home equipment.

Diabetes Mellitus

Diabetes mellitus is a disorder of the metabolism of insulin. In type I diabetes, there is an insulin deficiency, and most affected persons require insulin injections to survive. Type I diabetes, also referred to as insulin-dependent diabetes mellitus or IDDM, is usually of sudden onset and most commonly appears in childhood and adolescence. Hence, it is sometimes called juvenile or juvenile-onset diabetes. Type II diabetes is characterized by the presence of some insulin in the blood — levels may be normal, elevated, or depressed — to which the response is abnormal. Type II diabetes, or noninsulin-dependent diabetes mellitus (NIDDM), has a gradual onset and may appear at any age, although most commonly in persons over age 40. It often is associated with obesity. Lessening insulin requirements by diet or weight loss or stimulation of insulin production with oral medication may be sufficient to control type II diabetes; however, the administration of insulin may be necessary in some cases.

In diabetes mellitus, a balance must be achieved between available insulin, intake of food, and consumption of energy in activities. Long-standing diabetes may lead to decreased vision from retinal vessel disease, kidney lesions and renal failure, neuropathies, arteriosclerosis, and peripheral vascular disease, resulting in gangrene or even amputation.

There are four potential objectives of occupational therapy in persons with diabetes: (1) providing regulated activity to assist in insulin regulation, (2) providing an environment in which the individual can demonstrate knowledge of diet regulations through meal planning or preparation, (3) evaluating and teaching compensatory skills when the patient has complications that result in visual loss, sensory loss, or amputation, and (4) providing psychological support. The pervasiveness of the treatment regimen can produce feeling of depression, anger, and dependency, and the patient may demonstrate manipulative behaviors. Patients may feel overwhelmed, and the occupational therapist should allow them to make as many choices as possible within the therapy situation to facilitate self-control.

Renal Disease

Chronic renal failure (CRF) is a condition in which the kidneys fail to function as a result of progressive destruction of the nephrons, the functional units of the kidney. Filtration, secretion, and reabsorption take place in the nephrons while the kidney regulates the volume and chemical composition of blood and extracellular fluid. When CRF occurs, the kidney is unable to perform its normal functions. Metabolic end products, such as urea, build up in the bloodstream, producing uremia. The clinical manifestations of uremia vary with the medical condition of the patient and may include gastrointestinal upset, decreased mental concentration, apathy, lethargy, confusion and increased irritability, peripheral neuropathy, dermatological changes, generalized itching of the skin, anemia, weakness, and changes in cardiovascular function.[5]

Medical treatment of chronic renal failure consists of hemodialysis, peritoneal dialysis, or kidney transplantation. Hemodialysis uses a blood circuit to a machine called a hemodialyzer. The most common vascular access is an internal arteriovenous fistula, an anastomosis created surgically between an artery and a vein. The radial artery and cephalic vein in the upper extremity are used most often. When arteries cannot tolerate a hemodialysis vascular access, when the patient prefers another method of treatment, or while the patient is waiting for a permanent hemodialysis vascular access, peritoneal dialysis may be used. This type of dialysis involves the insertion of a catheter into the abdominal cavity, where the peritoneum acts as a semipermeable membrane. Patients may receive a kidney transplant (allograft) from a carefully matched living related donor or from a cadaver.

Patients on peritoneal or hemodialysis may develop disuse atrophy, distal edema, and contractures. Those confined to bed are at risk for decubiti. The occupational therapy program for a renal patient should include:

1. Activities or exercises to increase strength and mobility as well as to increase vascular flow
2. Activities of daily living, including leisure skills for both physiological and psychological reasons
3. Instructions in energy conservation and work

simplification to increase functional status despite low tolerance
4. Psychological support.

The amount of therapy a kidney allograft recipient will require depends to a large extent on the patient's medical condition before the transplant: the patient with recent renal failure will probably have fewer problems than the patient who has been on dialysis for several months or years.

The psychological reactions of renal patients are similar to those of patients with other chronic diseases. Feelings of helplessness and depression are common. Lack of motivation toward rehabilitation may be encountered, particularly when uremia is manifest as decreased mental concentration, apathy, and lethargy. Patients with end-stage renal failure must tolerate considerable life restrictions: dependency on and proximity to the kidney machine and multiple dietary and fluid restrictions. Among patients who have undergone successful kidney transplantation, psychological concerns have included: hesitancy to leave the dependent sick role, the need for more social skills to re-enter society, concerns about re-entering the work force, continued opportunity to vent feelings about prior and current health care providers, the importance of being needed rather than needing, maintenance of hope during periods of allograft rejection, continued need for detailed information about their condition, and the need to escape feelings of uniqueness in terms of both physical and psychological symptoms.[9]

Dysphagia

Swallowing impairment often results from mechanical deficits (from radical neck surgery, laryngectomy, or long-term tracheostomy), from neurological deficits (from acoustic neuroma, brainstem tumor, multiple sclerosis, myasthenia gravis, or other progressive neurological diseases), or from cerebrovascular accidents. A swallowing program should be conducted in close cooperation with the medical, nursing, and dietary staffs; the patient; and the family. The occupational therapist should be knowledgeable about the anatomy and neurophysiology of swallowing, including specific volitional and reflexive components. Mandibular kinesiology should also be reviewed.

In developing a program, the therapist should complete an initial assessment as presented earlier, obtaining a general history, including specific facts related to the swallowing problems. There needs to be an evaluation of the peripheral speech and swallowing mechanisms, including resistance to mouth opening, jaw deviation, tongue lateralization, strength of the tongue on protrusion and retraction, soft-palate elevation and depression, and laryngeal rise. Cortical and reflex coordination of motor function should be assessed by having the patient suck, chew, and swallow. Sensory examination should include testing the cheeks, lips, oropharynx, soft palate, and tongue. The gag reflex should be elicited as part of the assessment.

Prerequisites for Treatment

Before implementing a swallowing program, there are several prerequisites. First, the patient must be mentally alert and able to follow instructions, carry them over from day to day, and concentrate on the task well enough to support a reflex behavior. Second, the physiological potential to swallow must be ascertained. Last, a gag reflex must be present. If a patient has little or no gag reflex unilaterally or bilaterally, a stimulation program needs to be initiated before food is introduced. In addition, tongue mobility and good laryngeal closure should be established through tongue exercises and stimulation to ensure propulsion of food through the mouth to the esophageal opening, as aspiration of foreign material into the lungs is the major cause of morbidity and mortality in patients with swallowing dysfunction.[18] Testing for aspiration may be done by asking a patient to swallow ice chips stained with methylene blue. Aspiration is indicated by choking, coughing, or changes in breath sounds and is confirmed by the appearance of methylene blue dye at the tracheostomy stoma or in the tracheal aspirate. Signs of aspiration do not always occur immediately after swallowing but may be evident some time later.

Treatment Program

A swallowing program has three basic components: (1) exercises to improve strength, coordination, and range of motion; (2) verbal coaching to bring swallowing under volitional control; and (3) graduated feeding. Exercises to strengthen the mechanical swallowing abilities include those for tongue lateralization, tongue elevation, tongue retraction, strengthening the cheeks and lips, chewing, swallowing, and gag reflex. Facilitation with pressure and ice might be used together with the exercises. A swallowing treatment kit consisting of items such as straws, mouth care swabs, suckers, and a button on a string can be helpful in the exercise program. For example, the button on a string may be used to provide resistance to lip closure and thus strengthen the perioral musculature.

When the patient is ready to attempt oral feeding, several factors must be considered in the diet selection, including other methods by which the patient may be receiving nutrition or hydration (*e.g.*, intravenous, nasogastric, or other tube feedings), the evaluation results, and the patient's food preferences. Specific foods are selected to provide maximum sensory feedback to enhance the volitional and reflexive components. The common practice in general hospitals is a dietary progression from clear liquids to thick liquids, purees, and soft solids. Unfortunately, patients with swallowing dysfunction have difficulty with this sequence. Liquids provide poor sensory stimulation and present the greatest difficulty.[18] Pureed or minced foods provide good sensory stimulation within the mouth and are easier to swallow, but may not have an aroma and may taste bitter. Sweet foods decrease saliva, while the casein in milk products thickens mucous secretions thereby decreasing sensation and making control of secretions more difficult. Sour food facilitates swallowing. Bland and unattractive foods should be avoided. Applesauce and various baby foods are examples of foods that may be used in oral feeding training of patients with dysphagia.

While motor deficits are being treated, the therapist should begin to teach the patient to "think swallow." The patient must think about chewing, about holding saliva or food in the mouth, and then about swallowing. This is accomplished by constant verbal coaching. When the patient chokes, he must be taught what went wrong and how to prevent it. The patient must trust the therapist in order to comply with the program. There are numerous emotional ramifications resulting from the inability to eat and the necessity for relearning the process: it is usually an unpleasant experience; it is uncomfortable, even painful; and the patient is often embarrassed because he or she may be sloppy. Dysphagia rehabilitation is a slow process and requires persistence by both the patient and the therapist.

Positioning during the swallowing program is important to decrease the chance of aspiration. The patient should sit in a chair at 90° with the neck slightly flexed. If the therapist is spoon feeding the patient, the utensil should be placed at or below chin level to encourage neck flexion. The food should be placed in the mouth at the point where the patient will get the most sensory feedback from the taste, pressure, and the temperature of the food. Placement of the food on the back of the tongue may be helpful with patients having decreased tongue mobility. There should be pauses between swallows to allow the patient to rest, as swallow efficiency decreases with fatigue; and the therapist should inspect the mouth periodically to make sure all food has been swallowed. Small portions given five or six times a day are preferred to larger portions three times a day. After eating, the patient should continue to sit up for a period of time (1 hour, if tolerated). The therapist should instruct the nursing staff and family in the swallowing program, including ways to advance the diet so as to allow them to continue the program until independence is reached.

Summary

Solutions to the variety of problems that an occupational therapist may encounter in a general hospital are limited only by the therapist's creativity, knowledge, and adaptability. Some additional diagnoses that might be encountered and guidelines for the occupational therapy services appropriate for those diagnoses are listed in Table 27-2. Despite a move toward shorter hos-

Table 27-2. *Acute-Care Problems Encountered and Guidelines for Solving Them*

Diagnosis	Common Problems	Occupational Therapy Services
Parkinson's disease	Muscular weakness	Activities of daily living
	Tremors	Therapeutic activities to increase coordination, range of motion, and muscle strength
	Extreme rigidity	Work simplification
Rheumatic heart disease	Decreased physical tolerance	Work simplification
	Poor cardiac reserve	Energy conservation
		Graded activity program
Scleroderma and other collagen diseases	Excessive fatigue	Therapeutic activities to maintain or increase range of motion and muscle strength
	Limited range of motion	Physical tolerance programs
	Decreased muscle strength	Activities of daily living
		Splinting
		Psychological support
Blood dyscrasias	Excessive fatigue	Work simplification
		Energy conservation
		Graded physical tolerance program

(continued)

Table 27-2. *Acute-Care Problems Encountered and Guidelines for Solving Them* (continued)

Diagnosis	Common Problems	Occupational Therapy Services
Renal insufficiency	Dependency on artificial dialysis Limited energy Variety of neurological manifestations Limited work potential	Hospital and home program to help maintain a balance of fluids and body chemistry by medication, activity, and diet Graded physical tolerance program Vocational (work) evaluation Avocational pursuits Activities of daily living
Hip fracture	Self-care problems, especially reaching, transfers, and lower extremity dressing Household management Nonoperative fracture treated by bedrest or traction	Self-care evaluation and treatment Avocational program Work simplification Physical tolerance program
Hemophilia	Hemorrhage into joints causing limited range of motion	Activities to maintain or increase range of motion Vocational (work) evaluation Static splinting to prevent contracture or deformity Self-care evaluation and treatment
Obesity	Limited reach Poor cardiac reserve Poor self-concept Lack of appropriate work skills	Graded physical activity program Self-care evaluation and treatment Activity assimilation program Vocational (work) evaluation Behavior modification
Low back pain	Pain–medication cycle Inability to carry out life tasks	Work simplification with emphasis on proper methods for lifting and carrying Activity assimilation program Psychological support Behavior modification Vocational (work) evaluation
Thoracic surgery— cardiac	Decreased physical tolerance Unable to carry out home management tasks Employment concerns Fear of surgery	Work simplification Energy conservation Graded activity program Psychological support Vocational (work) evaluation
Psychosomatic illness	Inability to function in daily life tasks	Behavior modification program Psychological intervention Avocational pursuits Energy expenditure programs

Reprinted with permission from Hays C: General medicine and surgery. In Hopkins H, Smith H (eds.): *Willard and Spackman's Occupational Therapy*, 6th ed. pp 751–752. Philadelphia, J B Lippincott, 1983.

pitalizations and alternative health care settings, hospitals have a wide range of resources and are, therefore, in a better position to provide occupational therapy services than are free-standing clinics. According to the results of a 1985 American Occupational Therapy Association survey, since the initiation of Medicare's prospective payment system, there have been significant increases in early referrals to occupational therapy and more ICU referrals so that evaluation and treatment can begin early.[8] There has also been a greater intensity of services; that is, more occupational therapy treatment over a shorter period. The role of the occupational therapist in an acute-care setting is primarily one of assessment, provision of efficient prioritized treatment, and participation in discharge planning, including provision of a home program, recommendations for outpatient therapy, home health referral, or referral to other facilities offering traditional rehabilitation services. To have a good occupational therapy department in an acute-care setting, therapists must not only keep current on medical treatment but must be able to apply their skills in an efficient and cost-effective manner.

References

1. Affleck AT, Bianchi E, Cleckly M, et al: Stress management as a component of occupational therapy in acute care settings. Occup Ther Health Care 1(3):22, 1984
2. Affleck AT, Lieberman S, Polon J, Rohrkemper K: Providing occupational therapy in an intensive care unit. Am J Occup Ther 40:323, 1986
3. Bierenger A: Cancer and impaired independence. In Abreu BC (ed): Physical Disabilities Manual. New York, Raven Press, 1981
4. Brooks JL, Brawner BH: COPD: A new frontier for rehabilitation in the 80s. J Rehab 47(2):32, 1981
5. Chyatte S (ed): Rehabilitation in Chronic Renal Failure. Baltimore, Williams & Wilkins, 1979
6. Degre S, Sobolski J: Controversial aspects of physical training in patients with COPD. Pract Card:37, 1979
7. Dietz JH, Jr: Rehabilitation Oncology. New York, John Wiley and Sons, 1981
8. Gray MS: Occupational therapy use rises under PPS. Hospitals 59(11):60, 1985
9. Gulledge AD, Buszta C, Montague DK: Psychosocial aspects of renal transplantation. Urol Clin North Am 10:327, 1983
10. Hodgkin JE: Pulmonary rehabilitation. In Bayless TM, Brain MC, Cherniack RM: Current Therapy in Internal Medicine–2. Philadelphia, BC Decker, 1987
11. Killeen K: I'm glad you asked. Occup Ther News 40(10):15, 1986
12. Pizzi MA: Occupational therapy in hospice care. Am J Occup Ther 38:252, 1984
13. Rausch G, Melvin JL: A new era in acute care. Am J Occup Ther 40:319, 1986
14. Robbins SL, Angell M: Basic Pathology. Philadelphia, WB Saunders, 1971
15. Spiegel JS, Hirshfield MS, Spiegel TM: Evaluating self-care activities: Comparison of a self-reported questionnaire with an occupational therapist interview. Br J Rheumatol 24:357, 1985
16. Wenger NK: Rehabilitation after myocardial infarction. Comp Ther 11(3):68, 1985
17. Wilke NA, Sheldahl LM: Use of simulated work testing in cardiac rehabilitation: A case report. Am J Occup Ther 39:327, 1985
18. Zimmerman JE, Oder LA: Swallowing dysfunction in acutely ill patients. Phys Ther 61:1755, 1981

Bibliography

Assessment

Cautela JR: Organic Dysfunction Survey Schedules. Champaign, IL, Research Press, 1981
Hays C, Kassimer J, Parkin J: Sample Forms for Occupational Therapy. Rockville, MD, American Occupational Therapy Association, 1980
Kottke FJ, Stillwell GK, Lehmann JF: Krusen's Handbook of Physical Medicine and Rehabilitation, 3rd ed. Philadelphia, WB Saunders, 1982

Cancer

Dudgeon BJ, DeLisa JA, Miller RM: Head and neck cancer: A rehabilitation approach. Am J Occup Ther 34:243, 1980
Grabois M: Physical rehabilitation following mastectomy. Tex Med 74:53, 1982
Maguire P: The psychological impact of cancer. Br J Hosp Med 34:100, 1985
May HJ: Psychosexual sequelae to mastectomy: Implications for therapeutic and rehabilitative intervention. J Rehab 46:29, 1980
Mehls JD: Occupational therapy as a component of cancer rehabilitation. Prog Clin Biol Res 121:231, 1983

Cardiac

Atwood JA, Nielson DH: Scope of cardiac rehabilitation. Phys Ther 65:1812, 1985
Harrington KA, Smith KH, Schumacher M, et al: Cardiac rehabilitation: Evaluation and intervention less than 6 weeks after myocardial infarction. Arch Phys Med Rehab 62:151, 1981

Chronic Obstructive Pulmonary Disease

Gale J, O'Shanick GJ: Psychiatric aspects of respiratory treatment and pulmonary intensive care. Adv Psychosom Med 14:93, 1985
Moser KM, Bokinsky GE, Savage RT, Archibald CJ, Hansen PR: Results of a comprehensive rehabilitation program: Physiologic and functional effects on patients with chronic obstructive pulmonary disease. Arch Intern Med 140:1596, 1980
Moser K, Archibald C: Shortness of Breath: A Guide to Better Living and Breathing: A Manual for Patients, 3rd ed. St Louis, CV Mosby, 1983

Death and Dying

DuBois PM: The Hospice Way of Death. New York, Human Sciences Press, 1980
Kubler–Ross E: On Death and Dying. New York, Macmillan, 1971

Diabetes

Cyrus J: Role of exercise in management of diabetes. J Kent Med Assoc 84(4):159, 1986

Holliman K: Another device for one-handed insulin management. Am J Occup Ther 33:393, 1979

Dysphagia

Gallender D: Eating Handicaps: Illustrated Techniques for Feeding Disorders. Springfield, IL, Charles C Thomas, 1979

Groher ME: Dysphagia: Diagnosis and Management. Boston, Butterworths, 1984

Heimlich HJ: Rehabilitation of swallowing after stroke. Am Otol Rhinol Laryngol 92:357, 1983

General Medicine

Steinberg FU: The Immobilized Patient: Functional Pathology and Management. New York, Plenum Medical Books, 1980

Warfel JH, Schlagenhauff RE: Understanding Neurologic Disease: The Text Book for Therapists. Baltimore, Urban and Schwarzenberg, 1980

General Practice

Baum CM: Occupational therapists put care in the health system. Am J Occup Ther 34:505, 1980

Bell E: The changing faces of practice. Am J Occup Ther 39:637, 1985

Florian V, Sacks D: Reasons for patient referral to occupational therapy units by health care professionals. J Allied Health 14:317, 1985

Hays C: Sample Job Descriptions for Occupational Therapy. Rockville, MD, American Occupational Therapy Association, 1981

Schwartz KB: Balancing objectives of efficient and effective occupational therapy practice. Am J Occup Ther 38:198, 1984

Low Back Pain

Caruso LA, Chan DE: Evaluation and management of the patient with acute back pain. Am J Occup Ther 40:347, 1986

Obesity

Humphrey R: A practical approach to exercise in the treatment of obesity. Obesity Bariatr Med 10:6, 1981

Wise JF, Wise SK: The Overeaters: Eating Styles and Personality. New York, Human Sciences Press, 1979

Parkinson's Disease

Lavigne J: Home Exercises for Patients with Parkinson's Disease. New York, The American Parkinson Disease Association, 1978

Robbins JA, Logemann JA, Kirschner HS: Swallowing and speech production in Parkinson's disease. Ann Neurol 19:283, 1986

Renal Disease

Carney RM, McKevitt PM, Goldberg AP, et al: Psychological effects of exercise training in hemodialysis patients. Nephron 33:179, 1983

Kutner NG, Cardenas DD: Rehabilitation status of chronic renal disease patients undergoing dialysis: Variations by age category. Arch Phys Med Rehab 62:626, 1981

Victor–Gittleman B: The role of the occupational therapist in the rehabilitation of end-stage renal disease patients. Dial Transpl 10:738, 1981

Scleroderma

Melvin JL: Rheumatic Disease: Occupational Therapy and Rehabilitation, 2nd ed. Philadelphia, FA Davis, 1982

Rodnan GP: Progressive systemic sclerosis. In McCarty D (ed): Arthritis and Allied Conditions, 9th ed. Philadelphia, Lea & Febiger, 1979

Appreciation is extended to Carole Hays, MA, OTR, FAOTA, for allowing me to revise her previous work and to Becky Barton, MS, OTR; Marty Torrance, MS, OTR; Lucinda Dale, MS, OTR; Karen Sherman, OTR; and Barbara Shepherd, COTA, for their assistance and sharing of their expertise in acute-care occupational therapy.

CHAPTER 28

Functional Restoration: Preliminary Concepts and Planning *Elinor Anne Spencer*

so much
depends upon

a red wheel
barrow

glazed with rain
water

beside the white
chickens

William Carlos Williams[8]

The outward simplicity and inherent complexity of Williams' poem is analogous to the impact of debilitating disease or injury on an individual's life. Although the poem conveys an initially simple and colorful image, through it surges an underlying current of symbolism that adds meaning and dimension to the words. So, too, the process of functional restoration following a disabling condition embodies the totality of human potential.

Functional restoration is the primary objective of rehabilitation. Assisting a person to build or restore his or her life to its fullest use and satisfaction is a philosophical mandate of occupational therapy. Thus, the occupa-

tional therapist is an essential member of the rehabilitation team.

Traditionally, occupational therapists have directed their efforts toward enabling patients and clients to achieve maximum performance in daily functions regardless of the disease, injury, and resulting dysfunction. Evaluation and treatment methods have developed from a disease orientation based on a medical model. During its growth as a profession, occupational therapy has progressed from an allied medical profession to an allied health profession. Therapeutic intervention is used to prevent further disability, to reverse current disability, or to improve ability. An outgrowth of the disease orientation is a disability orientation; an outgrowth of the health orientation is an ability orientation.

Health care professionals, including occupational therapists, are in the midst of a positive health-oriented movement directed toward assisting individuals to take responsibility for their own health. Occupational therapists have long contributed to the promotion of health through a commitment to habilitation, rehabilitation, and prevention.

Changes in the health care system, described more fully elsewhere in this volume, have resulted in shorter institutional stays for persons needing functional rehabilitation. Programs of acute or initial hospital care, ambulatory or outpatient care, and rehabilitation services in hospitals or rehabilitation centers are often forced to provide minimal initial restorative services for the temporarily or permanently disabled individual due to cutbacks in medical reimbursement. There is an increasing emphasis on home and community programs for continuation of rehabilitation services.

The effects of disability are reflected in psychosocial and physical responses reaching into all areas of an individual's life, often requiring adjustments in life patterns. The extent and quality of adjustment depend on the premorbid context of the individual's life, the prognosis of the functional outcome, and the goals set by the individual, family, and rehabilitation team.

Impact of Trauma and Disease

Trauma and disease that result in physical and mental disabilities can be devastating to a person's life. The onset can be *sudden* or *gradual.* The course can be *nonprogressive* or *progressive.* The manifestations of disability may be *temporary* or *permanent.*

Sudden onset of external trauma is characteristic of spinal cord injury, brain injury, fractures, peripheral nerve injury, and amputation. These injuries are often caused by accidents involving cars, sports, industrial machinery, falls, or weapons and usually affect the young adult or middle-aged population. Although the manifestations may result in permanent limitations, the injuries are generally nonprogressive. Sudden onset also is characteristic of internal trauma from such neurological causes as a cerebrovascular accident (CVA, stroke). The symptom complex may take several hours to develop until the stroke is "completed." After the attack, clinical signs generally do not increase; however, there can be a subsequent CVA.

A gradual or insidious progressive onset is seen in diseases such as multiple sclerosis, Parkinson's disease, arthritis, myasthenia gravis, and amyotrophic lateral sclerosis. These diseases tend to have an inconsistent but progressive pattern of remissions and exacerbations. When in remission, the disease process is quiescent or at rest; when in exacerbation, the disease process is active, and the individual experiences, increased symptoms. The severity of the exacerbation is unpredictable, as is the duration of remissions. During these periods, the person may show marked differences in functional ability. The progressive aspects of a condition may be primary causes of disability. Secondary effects (contractures, decubiti, or weakness) may result from initial deficits caused by the disease or trauma. For example, spasticity may be a primary disability resulting from a CVA, and contracture may be a secondary disability resulting from the spasticity. Whereas impaired sensation may be a primary deficit resulting from a spinal cord lesion, a decubitus ulcer or serious skin breakdown may result from prolonged pressure on the desensitized area, causing a secondary deficit.

With an effective rehabilitation program suited to the individual's needs, persons suffering from temporary disability from orthopedic or neurological conditions can be assisted in returning to independent living. A more complex and challenging situation is the individual suffering permanent or progressive disability. In this case, the long-term functional and psychological implications may not be recognized or accepted by the individual or family in the early stages of recovery. Unanswered questions, unmet needs, and unresolved problems contribute to the development of long-term denial that leads to anger, depression, and rejection of both individual potentials and therapeutic programs.

The immediate or eventual difference between what was and what is may result in confusion, fear, questions, insecurity, feelings of inadequacy, or disequilibrium. A previous level of life adjustment and understanding may be replaced by unknown and unfamiliar or unacceptable conditions or situations. In order to establish a relationship that will help the individual regain self-acceptance, the occupational therapist must determine the psychosocial significance of the patient's medical condition and what its impact will be on his or her life-style.

Disability can have a variety of effects on the educational development of an individual. For example, a student with congenital anomalies or with disabilities resulting from injury or disease may be compelled to use a wheelchair. This student depends on such environmental adaptations as ramps, curb cuts, and wide doorways for access to school, classrooms, and other functional areas, yet even though public schools in rural and urban environments are required to be accessible to wheelchair users, many are not. The occupational therapist can greatly assist the school in enhancing the environment by advising the school on how to meet the needs of the disabled student.

The person suffering a brain injury may have damage to perceptual or intellectual centers in the brain, thus hindering visualization, communication, and retention of information necessary for learning and preventing continuation of academic studies without appropriate adaptation. A student who becomes disabled suddenly may not have developed the ability or interest in pursuing academic goals, although such goals may offer outlets to compensate for the loss of normal physical function and mobility. The student or adult experiencing remissions and exacerbations resulting in fluctuating functional abilities is challenged to maintain a positive attitude toward using and improving those capacities. With the increased interest in and necessity of providing adequate educational opportunities for all students, improved special services are becoming available to the disabled individual.

The economic implications of disability can be devastating for both an individual and the family. Financial assistance is available according to age, extent of financial assets, type of illness or disability, duration, vocational or educational prognosis, governmental benefits, private insurance coverage, and liability coverage. Without financial aid, rehabilitation costs can drain individual or family resources. Possible expenses include outlays for surgery, special treatment, assistive devices, wheelchairs, special home equipment, home modifications, adapted transportation aids, home health care, personal-care attendant, outpatient treatment, follow-up, and adaptation of the employment site.

The premorbid life-style and psychological attitudes can help the individual cope with the struggle to regain continuity in life and to set new goals to achieve physical and emotional satisfaction. The occupational therapist must learn when and how each patient can work through each concern most beneficially.

Functional Implications

The effects of trauma and disease influence the total life experience of the individual. The extent to which adjustments are essential to assure continued success in personal relationships and the achievement of life goals varies with the extent and course of the disease or injury and the resulting dysfunctional manifestations. As the daily patterns of a familiar life-style change, the individual and family are forced to adjust to an unfamiliar and imposed combination of independent and dependent levels of function dictated by the course of the disease or injury. The familiar patterns of personal behaviors and social interactions influence how these challenges are met. An accurate analysis of the biopsychosocial context by the therapist is essential to determine the functional implications of the patient's condition.

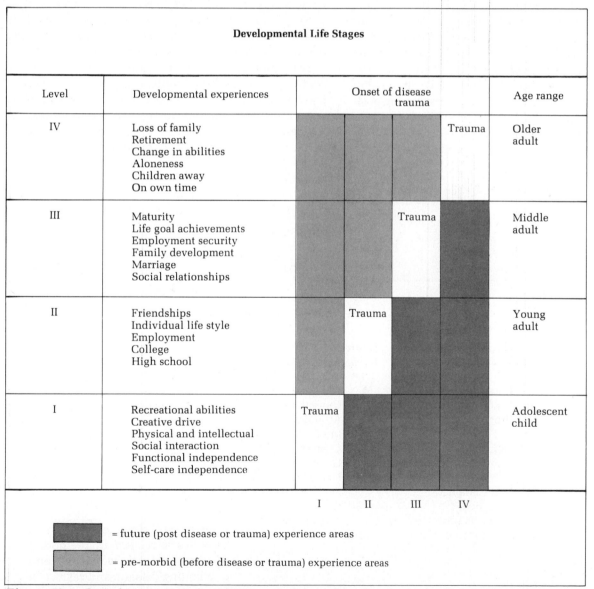

Figure 28-1. Sample experiential activities according to four developmental life stages as related to pre–disease/trauma and post–disease/trauma experience.

Temporary or permanent disability takes on a unique meaning for each individual. Age, developmental stage, previous ability, achievements, life-style, family status, self-concept, interests, and general responsibilities affect attitudes such as understanding, acceptance, motivation, and emotional response (Fig. 28-1). The process of rebuilding or rehabilitating begins with guidelines set by the individual before the trauma or disease. Preceding experiences, abilities, and problems affect the rehabilitation process by enhancing or hindering the accomplishment of goals. Thus, the therapist learns as much as possible about these factors for the individual.

As an example, a child born with a congenital disability experiences early life development with the disability, which becomes part of the body image, a part of him or her as he or she grows. The congenitally disabled adult thus shows a high level of developmental integration because he lacks experiential guidelines to "normal" functioning. In contrast, the adolescent or adult who has experienced life as an able-bodied person knows the implications of loss of function. It appears that the higher the physical, mental, or social achievement the person has reached premorbidly, the greater the challenge in accepting the loss and developing positive alternative goals compatible with the balance of permanent functional deficits and assets. The stage of development and the age of the person can be both advantageous and disadvantageous to necessary adjustments.

Another concept relating to the functional implications of trauma or disease is that of the transitions from *ability* to *disability* and then back to *ability* during rehabilitation. Although the first contact the occupational therapist has with an individual may be after the trauma or disease, the therapist must first consider the previous functional life of the patient. The patient with a sudden imposed disability maintains the self-concept, self-awareness, and responses of an able-bodied individual. Thus, the actual functional limitations and implications may be unrecognized or denied. For the individual suffering remissions and exacerbations of a progressive disease, the self-concept may be more flexible, even tentative or bordering on dependent. The positive trend of rehabilitation is to focus on ability rather than disability and to assist the person who has limitations to become aware of his or her functional potential and to explore these resources in therapeutic programs. It is essential for the therapist to assist the patient in making the transitions. If the individual has suddenly, and possibly unknowingly, made the transition from the ability context to the disability context, therapeutic intervention directs him or her into an integration of both aspects of function into adaptive, ability-oriented performance.

Figure 28-2 illustrates the ability/disability/ability pattern. Areas where changes from premorbid patterns

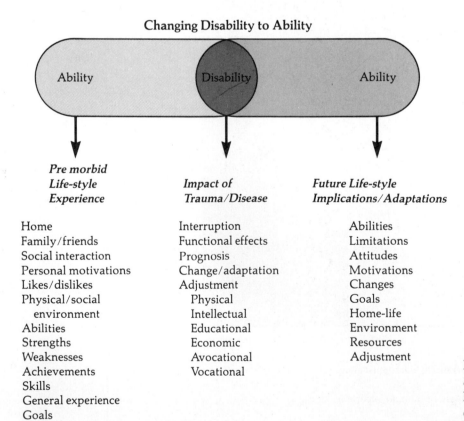

Changing Disability to Ability

Pre morbid Life-style Experience	Impact of Trauma/Disease	Future Life-style Implications/Adaptations
Home	Interruption	Abilities
Family/friends	Functional effects	Limitations
Social interaction	Prognosis	Attitudes
Personal motivations	Change/adaptation	Motivations
Likes/dislikes	Adjustment	Changes
Physical/social environment	Physical	Goals
Abilities	Intellectual	Home-life
Strengths	Educational	Environment
Weaknesses	Economic	Resources
Achievements	Avocational	Adjustment
Skills	Vocational	
General experience		
Goals		
Values		

Figure 28-2. Sample experiential activities *developed* in premorbid lifestyle, *affected* by trauma and debilitating disease, and *adapted* in future lifestyle planning.

may have occurred are listed, as are those affected by trauma and disease and those requiring adaptation for optimum function following formal rehabilitation.

The life experiences listed in Figures 28-1 and 28-2 are global. The functional restoration needed by the individual experiencing limitations from disease or trauma, although specifically related to such special programs as therapeutic activity, activities of daily living, homemaking, avocational pursuits, or vocational pursuits, must be geared toward the context of the individual to be acceptable and appropriate to his or her particular interests, abilities, and goals. Program planning that does not directly involve the patient's input and commitment will not serve the person well upon discharge and thus will not encourage continued rehabilitation. It is crucial to work directly with the patient to remain aware of his or her abilities, activities, and priorities with regard to functional limitations, implications, and potential gains.

Factors Affecting Rehabilitation Process and Outcome

Personal Development

The premorbid level of development in all areas of function provides the person suffering from dysfunction with ways to deal with the effects on his or her present life, which has suddenly come to be made up of unfamiliar events, people, patterns, and procedures. The prognosis is determined in part by the premorbid characteristics the individual has to invest in the process of rehabilitation. As noted earlier, these are crucial resources that can have a positive or a negative effect. A person fortunate enough to have had the resources to develop a strong sense of values and self-esteem, personal independence and achievement, healthy physical activity, and social interaction, with optimum work habits and motivation for productive activity brings a healthy background to the challenge of rehabilitation. On the other hand, a person with poorly conceived or developed skills, poor work habits, and unhealthy attitudes toward personal performance or responsibility brings poorly developed resources to the rehabilitation challenge and process. Negative personal attitudes can combine with negative social attitudes toward illness or disability to thwart the effect of rehabilitation resources. Thus, long-standing personal attitudes and biases can deter the positive gains from a therapeutic program. For example, the fear of the unknown path ahead may be reinforced by a growing dislike of self due to the disability. This can result in denial or rejection of the reality of long-term infirmity or physical limitation. The individual or the family that harbors the belief that disabled persons are "not normal" (*i.e.,* are less intelligent, less socially acceptable, less physically attractive, less functionally capable, and less significant than nondisabled persons) is forced to adjust perspectives in order to accept the reality of long-term disability. Nonacceptance leads to: rejection of therapy as a means of adapting to disability and achieving ability; rejection of association with disabled persons in a therapeutic milieu or within the community; and development of dependency patterns due to decreased self-value and lesser independent function.

Recognizing, accepting, and working through negative personal attitudes with the patient are crucial parts of rehabilitation. Generally, biases necessitate supportive understanding by professionals working with the individual. During the initial interview covering the previous experience of the individual, respect must be given to the personal development of the individual. The value of the therapist will be in the flexibility of attitude available to meet the variety of cultural variables that may be presented by the patient and the family.

Social Interaction

Social interaction is essential for healthy human development, whether a person is gregarious or shy. At some point, a person has need of others. When tragedy occurs, friends and family rally, but the duration of their commitment to the needs of the traumatized person will depend on the nature of the disability, the demands it makes on people, the ability to give and the personality of the individual, and the duration of need. The sequelae of disability (disfigurement; assistive devices; pathological motor patterns; the presence of tremors, drooling, or peculiar voice patterns; or deviations in normal behavioral or intellectual patterns) present a challenge to continuing social contact.

The difficult adjustments experienced by a person in a rehabilitation program may be influenced by personal or social attitudes, concepts, associations, taboos, experiences, or dreams. Words take on a new meaning; personal associations may positively or negatively affect the rehabilitation process. Some examples of varying concepts are as follows:

Recreation—fun, skill, talent, game, leisure, physical, win, group

Therapy—discipline, shame, parent–child, pain, discomfort, fear, anger, help

Paralysis—dumb, inferior, crippled, stupid, useless, unknown, frightening, confining

Disabled—bad, unpleasant, dumb, inconvenient, impatient, unattractive, someone else, child-like

Man—able-bodied, masculine, strong, controlling, manipulating, smart, social

Woman—attractive, weak, subordinate, mother, kind, supporting, loving

Dependent—children, old people, women, undesirable, lazy, reversible, weak, sick, poor

Work—remunerative, masculine, hard, strong, difficult

Leisure—nonremunerative, fun, frivolous, social, relaxing

Well—normal, walking, talking, doing, working, desirable, nondependent, able-bodied, independent, capable

Ill—dependent, lazy, undesirable, controllable, noncontrollable, unmasculine, unproductive

In the social milieu, the disabled person is faced with a new arena of behavior, one in which gains in self-awareness are challenged by a complex environment. Strong self-concepts and self-acceptance are essential for expanding perceptions and reactions to include others and for being able to function effectively within a group. Here, as well as in the nonhuman (object) environment, gains in the ability to function will depend on the type and level of opportunities available. In order to interact with a group, the patient must be able to perform at the level expected by the group; otherwise, the patient will not be included as a significant member.

Role of Occupational Therapy

Occupational therapy practice has been influenced by changing medical concepts and practice with regard to life-support systems; diagnostic accuracy; awareness of and referral to allied medical, health, and therapeutic services; the effect of drugs on human behavior and function; and the technical development of diagnostic, therapeutic, and adaptive equipment.

Occupational therapists and occupational therapy assistants have participated in the growth within therapeutic services by joining team efforts with physicians and other professionals and by developing specific techniques. A rich variety of specific treatment approaches is available to the clinical occupational therapist and assistant. Because the therapeutic approaches and modalities used must be appropriate to a person's needs, specific approaches and techniques are often combined into an eclectic grouping. Methods developed and researched for use with children are being modified for use with adults with similar needs; approaches in psychiatry and physical dysfunction are combined where the clinical signs call for a melding of treatment objectives and techniques. Examples of global approaches that have been adapted for use in a variety of situations are the sensory–integration approaches and the neurophysiological techniques.

Therapeutic perspectives have progressed from localized specific treatment of an injured part to a comprehensive consideration of psychosocial, environmental, educational, and vocational implications. This is particularly emphasized in the rehabilitation programs where a patient may be involved in sensory integration, group treatment, adapted recreation, activities of daily living, work-simulated tasks, and homemaking programs leading to independent living. The traditional concern of the occupational therapist with assisting the individual in functional development within the context of the "whole person" maintains its strong focus in the rehabilitation programs, whether in the hospital, in the ambulatory clinic, or in the community. Specific programs becoming more prevalent are hand rehabilitation, cognitive retraining, development of work capacity, driver training, and independent living readiness.

Principles of Functional Restoration

The rebuilding of a lifestyle demands a creative, realistic, and practical day-to-day adaptive approach to daily living skills, activities, and tolerance. The patient knows the *meaning of ability* in functioning but must learn the *meaning of disability*. The therapist can challenge the patient to become an independently functioning individual, both mentally and physically, and aid him or her in maintaining a balance in all abilities, no matter how well or how poorly developed.

The therapist sets the stage for attitudes regarding the physical setting, the techniques used, the individual, the staff members, and the other patients. By constructing an environment conducive to optimum functional performance, the therapist conveys personal attitudes about the characteristics of the diagnosis, disability, and behaviors demonstrated by the patients. The therapist provides respect, dignity, and reality to the patient during the initial period of fear, stress, confusion, or denial, so that the patient can achieve self-awareness and self-respect as well as understanding of the situation, a sense of support from others, and acceptance of the therapist and the rehabilitation program. The therapist helps the patient achieve integration, reconciliation between predisability life and the life imposed by disability, between the known self and the unknown, new self. In programming for success, the therapist assumes a positive attitude. If the therapist's behavior does not convince the patient that occupational therapy plays a significant role in rehabilitation, the patient may not respond well to the objectives and potentials of functional restoration.

The following principles are basic to functional restoration through occupational therapy:

1. *Correlation of the program* with the medical condition of the patient, general assessment information, motivation level, and stated goals of the patient or client, the family and home situation, other treatment programs and services the individual is receiving, the medical and functional prognoses,

and joint planning for admission, treatment, and discharge

2. *Use of therapeutic relationships* during evaluation and treatment sessions between patient and therapist or assistant, patient and patient, patient and group, patient and family, and treatment team, patient, and family

3. *Use of the environment* to aid in adjustment and adaptation by the patient for functional living, including: (1) adjusting the setting for effective evaluation of functional level, (2) adapting the level of external stimuli for tolerance and interaction, (3) adjusting for successful and satisfying daily living activity, and (4) ensuring self-worth through productive and social activity

4. *Use of therapeutic positioning of the body* for evaluation, treatment, and rest using equipment appropriate for the individual's need and level of function and using the principles of body mechanics

5. *Use of a variety of evaluation techniques* including observation, interviews, standardized tests, and performance tests

6. *Use of purposeful activity* during evaluation and treatment

7. *Use of activity analysis* in the choice of activity for evaluation and treatment and the choice of treatment method as related to the therapeutic value of the selected activity

8. *Correlation of physical treatment procedures* with the person's level of receptivity, the person's behavior, the person's potential

9. *Use of activities of daily living* in evaluation and treatment to provide body awareness and acceptance, daily exercise, and indication of independent-skill level and assistance needed

10. *Use of adaptive devices and equipment* to obtain maximum involvement in functional physical activity, provide independence in daily self-care, and provide self-esteem and self-worth in task completion

11. *Use of work simplification and energy conservation techniques* for motivation, accomplishment, and productivity; maximum achievable independent living functions; and task accomplishment

12. *Use of community resources* for successful community re-entry, continued level of independence post-discharge, social stimulation and benefit, and independence in continuing rehabilitation goals

In the provision of these services, the occupational therapist and occupational therapy assistant must ensure that the recipient can benefit from what is provided. They must provide an opportunity for the patient to improve and to gain functional abilities related to personal daily living requirements and desires. In providing appropriate therapeutic services, the therapist helps the patient learn about the medical aspects of the specific disability and its causes to enable the patient to assume responsibility for the rehabilitation program. The relationship between the therapist and the patient is one in which the therapist lends support, guidance, and opportunity to the patient to achieve independent functions at his or her own speed, ability, and tolerance—not at that of the therapist. The therapist facilitates a qualitative assessment of functional progress by the patient to assist the development of self-concept, self-assessment, and continued awareness of rehabilitation capabilities.

Components of Therapeutic Intervention

Environment

Occupational therapy is based on the belief that people are capable of relating to the human and nonhuman environments in a manner that is self-directed, purposeful, meaningful, and satisfying. Throughout the developmental continuum from birth to death, human beings grow by adapting to the challenges and stresses confronted in daily living. Adaptation is enhanced, thwarted, encouraged, or delayed by the individual's unique abilities to progress through the myriad learning experiences toward integration of sensorimotor and cognitive awareness and function necessary to accomplish meaningful tasks.

The occupational therapist's greatest challenge is to motivate a person toward self-direction and achievement for personal satisfaction. To this end, the occupational therapist organizes the patient's immediate environment to provide opportunities for achievement of independent and productive functions.

In order to reach independence at any level, the disabled person must achieve enough control over the natural and the man-made environments to achieve his or her goals with self-respect and satisfaction. Although there may be limitations that render the individual "handicapped" in specific situations, the extent to which the person with temporary or permanent disability can accomplish his or her goals depends on this control. The following are helpful in gaining self-confidence and strength to cope with the challenges of the environment:

1. Determining what one can do independently
2. Determining what one can do with some assistance
3. Determining what one cannot do without assistance
4. Ability to ask for assistance and get it
5. Knowing whom to ask for assistance
6. Ability to instruct the person giving assistance
7. Ability to adjust to changes imposed by disability (appearance, special equipment, changes in abilities)

8. Development of knowledge of available resources (people, services, equipment, construction)
9. Development of knowledge of rights
10. Development of knowledge and acceptance of physical and mental tolerance

The environment consists of all persons (human environment) and things (nonhuman environment) surrounding an individual. Human performance is greatly affected by environmental influences and the way a person interprets them. The person encumbered by disability and its accompanying emotions may find on re-entry that a previously known environment is now unfamiliar and unknown. Instead of having a safe, familiar, and comforting feeling for the individual, it may have an unfriendly, unsafe, unwelcoming, or even hostile aspect. The environment is continually changing during the recuperation of the disabled person; this phenomenon may represent an overwhelming and continuing challenge and may pose an obstacle to adaptation.

In adapting to the familiar environment with a different body and mind, the individual may be in the situation of having to adjust to the old with decreased adaptive ability and to adjust to the new with even less ability to adapt. However, the recovering patient may actually be more aware of the adaptive challenges of the environment through a sudden slowing down of all physical and mental adjustment mechanisms.

Dunning suggests that occupational therapists are managers of space (to promote stimulation), people (to encourage social interaction), and tasks (to develop skills).[3] In this role, the therapist analyzes the effects of the surroundings on a person in terms of the individual's response. Deficits found during the initial interview and evaluation cue the therapist to changes needed in the environment, either to stimulate or to inhibit the person's behavior or adaptation. The therapist must assist the patient in adjusting to the challenges of the environment by increasing appropriate performance within it.

The occupational therapy program provides the patient with activities in order to create awareness of self in time and space, develop awareness of the environment, and reveal behavior changes and development of abilities. To enhance these awareness areas, the occupational therapist should use the following objectives in planning the treatment program: encourage movement and performance, involve the patient with those nearby and with the environment to provide opportunities, channel abilities, facilitate action, and eliminate barriers to function. Through a program of normal activities in an appropriate environment, the therapist helps the patient establish a new self-image and accept changes in physiology, feelings, and appearance. The therapist also aids the adjustment in preparation to re-enter the home and community and to assume healthy attitudes toward self and family.

Environmental influences can have positive or negative effects on the evaluation and treatment of the person with physical or neurological dysfunction. The following elements can structure the environment for success:

1. *Atmosphere.* The area used for evaluation and treatment should have adequate comfortable space, lighting, and temperature. The therapist initially orients the patient to the meaning of the room, its contents, its location, and its functions and introduces the patient to the other people there. The therapist controls the visual and auditory stimuli in order to relieve any anxiety or confusion.

2. *Sensory bombardment.* Excessive, unexpected sensory impulses (visual, auditory, tactile, proprioceptive, or kinesthetic) can confuse, fatigue, or frighten the patient. Therefore, the therapist controls *all* of the stimuli.

3. By using voice and body in a supportive, nonthreatening way, the therapist becomes a *therapeutic tool.*

4. An acceptable *level of achievement*, commensurate with the patient's interests, is necessary as positive feedback.

5. In some situations, familiar objects may be threatening early in the treatment. Therefore, *unfamiliar activities and exercises* may be better for initial evaluation and treatment.

The occupational therapist assists in providing an optimum living environment. Arrangement of furniture in the room, bed location in relation to the door and to other patients, accessibility of personal items, proximity to the emergency call button, and accessibility and ease of use of the bathroom all contribute to or detract from mental, physical, and emotional well-being. Wherever the patient eats and socializes (own room, cafeteria, or dining room), the facilities should be accessible and should encourage independent functioning; the patient should be placed with compatible persons during meals and for social functions.

In the occupational therapy room, depending on the goals of the treatment program at a given time, the patient should be allowed to work in a secluded area if he or she desires or to work in proximity to others who could have a therapeutic effect.

Family members and friends can have various effects on the patient; some may be encouraging and may stimulate functional recovery, whereas others may be patronizing or pitying and thus may retard progress. The objective of stressing environmental interaction is to assist the patient in adjusting to the return home and in using skills to adapt to the environment for maximum function and minimum stress.

Able-bodied persons tend to limit their perception of

the environment to what they know or where they are rather than notice the conditions to which the disabled person must adapt. In evaluating the needs and the steps to be taken for readaptation, it is important to get a picture of what the patient will be going into. The gradual building of adaptive skills will then aid in the preparation for future environmental changes. Aspects of the environment to be evaluated are: the responsibilities of the patient and others sharing the immediate surroundings; the expectations of the patient for performance and role; others' expectations and roles; housing design; location of living quarters; type of neighborhood; use of private or public transportation; and location of community resources.

Relationships

The relationship between the therapist and the patient is crucial to the patient's reception of the resources available. As the patient is confronted by the need to make myriad adjustments in the initial phases of trauma or disease, the therapist must recognize the impact of evaluation and treatment methods on the patient's level of awareness and acceptance of the debilitating condition and its implications. Essential to the establishment of an effective and functional relationship is awareness by the therapist of his or her personal limitations and biases. The therapist must maintain objectivity toward the patient and not feel personally rejected if the patient balks at program procedures. Working closely with the patient and listening to his or her views of the situation allows the patient adequate self-expression and self-awareness. In the progression of health care from the acute-care facility to outpatient services to postdischarge follow-up visits, the objective of therapeutic involvement is to assist the patient in gaining maximum independence and personal control of all aspects of daily living. This includes being able to maintain and establish effective relationships with family, friends, service providers, and others.

In her distinction between the *sick role* and the *disabled role*, Daniels states that choice of role affects the type and value of health care given to and received by the patient.[2] She describes the patient in the sick role as receiving care focused on noncontinuing or acute illness, with the medical treatment directed by a physician. In this role, the person "acts sick" and responds to the authority of the physician, lacking the knowledge and experience to care for herself or himself.

During the initial acute-care phase of disability, a person may respond to this sick role due to the overwhelming nature of the symptoms and hospitalization. The patient avoids anxiety and uncomfortable feelings of confusion and helplessness by reaching out for protective denial of the implications to use as a crutch or as a retreat from reality. The unwanted reality may be severe

damage to body parts and bodily functions implying undesirable long-term personal and social changes. Vargo states that, in this denial stage, "the individual is not emotionally prepared to accept the reality and the implications of the disability and consequently will deny that such a disability exists."[7]

During this period, the patient attempts to regain old abilities, interests, and habits, if only in fantasy, in a desperate attempt to deny the temporary or permanent loss of them. These fantasies may be repressed in euphoric and cooperative behavior to minimize the anxiety that surfaces in anger or hostility when the patient is challenged to dig into true feelings. As there may be many unfamiliar medical procedures during this time, the patient may slide into the beginning of a habit of dependency, encouraged by the need to fit into an unfamiliar, authoritative medical system. With the prime focus on the person being medical, the disabled person becomes hypersensitive to his or her own thoughts. The patient may try to ward off the fearful recognition that his or her body represents a nonintegrated group of parts no longer totally under control. Fear and confusion may lead to feelings of shame and rejection of the body. This effectively blocks the patient's investment in rehabilitative measures and places the full responsibility for motivation to get well on the shoulders of those serving him or her.

Daniels states that the sick role should not be applied to a disabled person, for this can result in undertreatment (not enough information being provided to the patient regarding the medical condition and treatment), overtreatment (too much or inappropriate care being given), or mistreatment (descisions regarding the medical condition and treatment being made without consulting the patient). To avoid these errors, the health care providers should use the disabled role. Daniels describes this as a continuous process in which the treatment is centered on the patient and the patient's goals, coordinating the care with lifestyle and working through cooperation. In this role, the patient seeks rehabilitation, accepts disability as a personal characteristic, and, through growing knowledge of the disability, takes an authoritative role in his or her own care.

The disabled role is often difficult to follow in a general hospital setting, where care is directed toward acute medical intervention. However, a disabled person hospitalized for acute distress should be allowed to carry out as much self-care as possible, as being treated for the long-term disability rather than for the acute illness constitutes "overtreatment"; "interrupted established routines can injure the self-sufficiency of the disabled person."[2] This advice, of course, refers to the patient who has already been through the process of rehabilitation and has been living in the community as a disabled person.

The hospitalization of the newly disabled patient

may terminate during the denial stage, with the patient unreconciled to the implications of disability and unprepared to leave the sterile protection of the medically oriented environment. In acknowledging the patient's difficulty in accepting alternatives to prior decisions and actions, Heijn and Granger state that the occupational therapist "introduces unfamiliar devices and techniques that substitute for actions that have become difficult or impossible due to functional loss" which may be "direct non-verbal confrontation with existing deficits" necessitating "recognition of the permanence of the impairment."[5]

After the period of autocratic denial of disability and unsuccessful attempts to regain the past, the affected person begins to recognize the facts regarding the condition and passes into a period of bitter mourning where the fantasy of denial can no longer be maintained. Medical changes begin to plateau, and the patient sees that his or her new life does not fit into old patterns. During this depression, the patient may consider suicide or wish for death, become uncooperative toward care, and hurt both family members and those most able to aid him or her in improving the condition.

Heijn and Granger state that "a patient must be able to mourn his losses to see the options in a restricted life."[5] A patient puts limited effort into learning new methods if she or he insists on holding onto past and out-of-reach methods. In adjusting to a new body image, the patient must accept a new or adapted lifestyle and indeed may wish to change it. The strength for these life changes is won by developing a new sense of self-worth by participating in experiences that allow abilities to grow and to be accepted. Although the patient benefits from the support of loved ones, the patient will be the best teacher of how they can accept and adapt to him or her.

Self-worth is developed through trial and result, whether successful or unsuccessful. One's concept of ability is proven through accomplishment of tasks and recognition by oneself and others. When the opportunity to repeat the same successful performance is removed by inability to perform a part or all of the task, one may doubt one's future ability, and the gradual destruction of self-confidence and motivation may begin. Then self-worth must be regained by the acceptance of one's actual ability.

Although the patient may not be aware of what has happened to disrupt normal function or of the implications and potentials of progressive functional restoration, the patient is acutely aware of a *selfness* inside. Although physical abilities may be lacking, the patient focuses on personal signs of achievement. The patient may even hold on to destructive concepts of overjudging and anticipating gains. The therapist must remember that the patient's views are as important as those of the treatment team. Only if the patient's views are known and respected is the therapist able to assist the patient in developing positive ideas about himself or herself.

When the patient is no longer in the hospital, the relationship with the therapist becomes a formal resource to the patient. For example, in the outpatient situation, the patient has returned home and comes to the hospital for specific evaluation or treatment. The patient may be referred to as a client rather than a patient due to this change in the relationship. Responsibility falls on the patient and family for continued connection with the hospital as a resource rather than as a temporary "home." When the patient returns home, he or she is likely to become more cognizant of the importance of rehabilitation objectives previously presented in the confines of the hospital. The individual has the opportunity to integrate hospital gains with the challenges of increased control of his or her own time in the home environment. The occupational therapist may visit the patient in the home to ensure that the social and physical aspects of the environment are conducive to further gains in the person's independent functioning. Here, the therapist becomes an important link in the continuity of care as well as a resource if there are further needs.

Performance

For the disabled individual, reaching previous physical activity levels or potential may seem inconceivable or unachievable; this feeling may reduce motivation to achieve at any level. This patient may be described as "unmotivated" because his or her goals may differ from the rehabilitation goals. The therapist must be sensitive to the patient's physical and mental levels, reactions, and apprehensions with regard to acceptance and tolerance of limitations and changes in ability imposed by the medical condition. The therapist is challenged to assist the patient in developing a "path of achievement" in accordance with medical and personal goals, the current medical condition, and the medical prognosis. Generally, patients need and benefit from assistance in channeling and controlling their energies into appropriate outlets designed to result in realistic, positive feedback regarding their current abilities.

One of the basic practices of occupational therapy is the use of performance as feedback to assist the patient in becoming involved in self-initiated, purposeful activity (Fig. 28-3). Adaptive techniques to assist in the achievement of independent functions (self-care, social interactions, planning and initiating tasks) are often employed. To perform is:

to do

to carry out

to fulfill

to carry to completion

to accomplish.

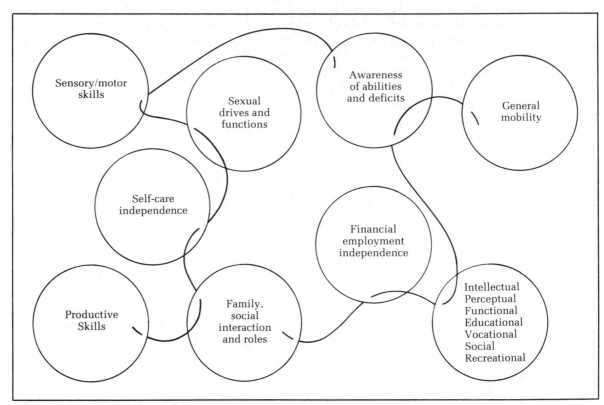

Figure 28-3. For the patient, the experience of and feedback from performance in one area of function can facilitate motivation and accomplishment in another. The timely interrelationship of tasks is connected by the thread of achievement.

In occupational therapy, observation and evaluation of a person in the performance of a task provide the therapist with a picture of the abilities and the limitations the person has in the accomplishment of that task. As a treatment facilitator, performance provides the experience of *doing*, from which the patient can gain an indication of whether he or she is able to accomplish the task and how well he or she can do it. Thus the patient gains feedback for self-awareness. Performance of a specific movement such as repetitive reaching or supination may increase function for use in task completion. To effect a feeling of self-worth, what a person does must be meaningful to him. Since people value the opinions of others, the patient will also derive self-worth when significant persons recognize accomplishments.

Successful performance appropriate to a person's level of functioning facilitates a sense of personal ability. Increasing the demand challenges increased ability which, when gained, provides additional feedback for self-worth. Levels of performance also serve as an indicator of *in*ability and are important for the person's awareness of reality in adjusting to permanent disability. Patients develop self-awareness in the performance of tasks and develop realistic self-concepts and goals through experiencing their own levels of accomplishment.

From the very beginnings, the human being progresses through life experiences and growth in a delicate balance of physical and psychological impressions, reactions, effects, and behaviors. They are interdependent and interchanging and stand in a cause-and-effect relationship to function. The mind and the body work together in providing feedback from function to effect change, adaptation, and improvement in the ability to relate to people, things, and tasks. As the person is motivated to act, the mind designs the task for the body to perform. The nature of performance determines the sensory feedback, which motivates for continuation or for change in the performance. The performer gains an awareness of social and personal acceptance dependent on the quality and appropriateness of the performance.

The Activity Factor

The theory expressed by Mary Reilly, EdD, OTR, "that man, through the use of his hands as they are energized by mind and will can influence the state of his own health,"[6] has long guided the occupational therapist in the use of manual activity for therapeutic purposes. The therapeutic value of the activity depends on its meaning to the person performing it.

Activity provides the patient with information about what he or she is capable of doing. When presented with a situation in which to perform, the patient can deny neither ability nor inability related to a specific task. Although the patient may object to the nature of the activity and reject its importance and significance to rehabilitation, performing it does provide the patient with important gauges for measuring his or her own abilities and attitudes.

A. Jean Ayres suggests that doing the activity is a more meaningful way to improve human functioning than is thinking or talking about the activity. She further suggests that the brain needs information from gravity, movement receptors, muscles, joints, and the skin of the entire body for effective integration:

> The interaction of the sensory and motor systems through all their countless interconnections is what gives meaning to sensation and purposefulness to movement.[1]

Ayers describes purposeful activities as things that begin, continue, and end. In the process of purposeful activity, one follows through to the purpose one wants by doing something *with* something, *to* something, or *for* something.[1]

In the adjustment period after diagnosis of disease or disability, the patient's premorbid attitudes, behaviors, and personality become a part of the rehabilitation process. The drive to regain the premorbid lifestyle may be a strong motivation to the patient in setting goals. Careful and sensitive probing by the therapist into professed interests and proven abilities and self-concepts of the patient helps reveal what the patient was and how he or she views the future.

First gained in the initial contact, this information is reviewed periodically with the patient throughout rehabilitation. Insight into the patient's interests with regard to educational and vocational pursuits, home life, lifestyle, responsibilities, and leisure activities must be gained. Areas to explore include feelings and plans related to family, social contracts, physical and mental potential, life goals for achievement, competitiveness, interest in creative activity, skills, and plans.

The types of activity in which the patient has shown interest may become important in the adjustment to disability. It is important to find out what sort of association and objective the patient had or expects to have with an activity. For example, if one patient is interested in sports, is it in order to compete with skill or ability, to participate socially, to dream of being outstanding, to describe or review, or to enjoy watching a game either in person or on television? If another patient's interest is in music, does this person wish to perform well, to perform adequately, to listen, to be knowledgeable in discussions, or to attend performances? Are the patient's favorite leisure activities socializing with friends at home or at community events, camping with family or friends, traveling, or engaging in such solitary outdoor activities as fishing?

The disabled person may never be able to accept the fact of physical or neurological disability. Mourning a loss, the person goes through periods of denial, hope, delusion, hate, guilt, complacence, sadness, depression, hostility, adjustment, and, sometimes, acceptance. The ability to reason aids in passage through these stages, although the person must deal with the disability emotionally as well as intellectually.

Diagnostic Aspects

Performance in an activity appropriate to the patient's rehabilitation level and goals can show the patient and the therapist what functional level the patient is able or willing to achieve. Regardless of negative feelings about the medical condition, the patient is able to experience specific feelings about the level of achievement. Activity allows myriad opportunities for self-expression. Depending on how it is designed and presented by the therapist, activity provides information regarding quality of performance, level of task completion, skill, talent, insight, strength, tolerance, and ability.

Restorative Aspects

Activity provides a structure for graded improvement in abilities and gives proof of the current level of achievement. It presents reality with regard to what patients are able to do and accomplish. It also aids in bringing them into interaction with people and tasks. The patient is able to learn about himself or herself and to begin to make a functional link with the environment.

As self-awareness and recognition of the realities of dysfunction grow, the patient becomes able to share in the plan for recovery of abilities. Activity provides the patient with the practice of abilities, a sense of continuous accomplishment, a sense of continuity in recovery, and a gradual process of planning. With the development of awareness and an insight into how to begin to plan daily activity, the patient is able to progress with daily feedback concerning performance and to reestablish the link with peers through social interaction. This aids the patient in understanding his or her place in society.

In the process of achieving adaptive behavior through the use of activity, the patient assists in realistic planning through self-staging and gradual accomplishment and begins to adjust to people and to the environment. The patient begins to see herself or himself as a functioning member of society, regains independent functioning, and begins to reach out to family and peers.

In providing adjustment to disability through the use of therapeutic activities, the occupational therapist assists the patient in learning:

1. Physical, mental, and emotional abilities and limitations

2. How to compensate for physical dysfunction
3. The limits of physical and mental tolerance
4. How to compensate for disability by using substitutes for familiar functions
5. How to cope with emotional frustrations caused by lost or decreased function
6. The social, economic, interpersonal, and familial implications of dysfunction
7. How to cope with economic problems caused by long-term disability (cost of hospitalization, expense of continuing treatment and assistive devices and equipment, decrease in job opportunities, and the necessity to be dependent on others in previously independent areas of function)
8. How to adapt to a new functional level of achievement
9. How to use leisure time functionally
10. How to organize, adjust to, and accept a new lifestyle.

In the rehabilitation process, the patient must be encouraged and allowed to function independently at the level of his or her ability in all areas of activity. This approach begins with self-care and ends with vocational independence. If deprived of the experience of doing independently whatever is possible, the patient will lack the opportunity to work through the stages of achieving maximum independence. If a therapist or other team member does the job, he or she encourages dependency. When uninvolved in the treatment plan and implementation, the patient loses commitment to the regaining of self-care skills, self-reliance, identity, and individuality. In assisting the patient to regain these functions, the therapist must put aside his or her own needs and help the patient in the struggle to self-awareness and acceptance.

The patient can do much to make maximum use of remaining physical abilities, adding to them as strength, endurance, and motivation increase. Activity that is specifically and therapeutically directed toward an increase in functional ability can provide important feedback by showing tangible proof that the patient *can* perform. Although the level of performance may not reach the patient's former physical or intellectual competence, incentive can be derived from small gains if the activity is directed properly. As the gains increase, so does the motivation, the willingness to try, and the acceptance. In the early treatment sessions, the patient must be supported in the forms self-expression may take as she or he experiences the feelings described above.

Personal and Environmental Adaptation

Seeing oneself as having less self-worth as a result of disability is a normal reaction to loss. This is confirmed by the social signs of difficulty in acceptance and "for-giveness" of disability such as in attention to making the environment accessible to the physically disabled. Feelings of anger and helplessness against these attitudes can be channeled positively into assisting the community to recognize disabled persons as citizens with equal human rights. Community, state, and national organizations of disabled people provide peer support and channels for action for those interested in becoming involved in changing attitudes.

In considering the impact of disability from a social point of view, it is interesting to note Vargo's comment that, although *disability* is regarded as an observable impairment in the functioning of a body part, a *handicap* is a function of the interaction between individuals and their total environment. A society's political and fiscal priorities will determine whether people will be able to manage in spite of their disabilities. In a totally accessible society, a disabled person is not handicapped; in a society filled with stairs, curbs, visual identifications of locations, and auditory warning signals, handicapping situations confront every disabled person.[7]

A person's attitude toward his or her disability affects others as well. For example, a quadriplegic using a wheelchair can diminish the awareness of the wheelchair and a condescending attitude from others by practicing assertive behavior. An upper-extremity amputee learns to use his prostheses to perform needed and desired functions in public (putting a coin in a machine, mailing a letter, driving a car, or opening a door for others). A woman who has had an arm amputation as a result of cancer will need to overcome her sensitivity regarding both the use of her prosthesis and the feel of it as a part of her body; by doing this, she can engage in social life with her family and friends.

Housing accessibility for the physically disabled person is complex. The home itself may be difficult to get into and out of, regardless of its inhabitants' limitations. It may also have architectural idiosyncrasies that make it difficult for the disabled person to perform daily activities previously done independently.

Checklists to aid in complete evaluation and recommended measurements for access areas (entrance hallways, rooms, and garages) are provided through many resources; some of them are listed in Appendix J.

Wheelchair users should be instructed in how to determine if a building and its functions are accessible or adaptable. Considerations of the accessibility or challenges presented by any building will become a natural part of planning. National accepted standards of accessibility are available on request from the American National Standards Institute. Federal and state laws stipulate accessibility regulations and provide enforcement mechanisms for demanding proper construction of public buildings. These are used both in constructing new buildings and in renovating existing ones to ensure equal access by all persons, regardless of disability.

Community Re-Entry and Functional Recovery

The fact that a person has been a part of a neighborhood, school class, or working team prior to disability entails many adjustments in returning to these familiar friends and formerly comfortable places; residual disabilities may render this person limited in relation to former abilities. How the newly disabled person feels with old friends and in making new friends while using a wheelchair, for example, will depend on the acceptance of the wheelchair as an important part of functioning. The middle-aged man returning to work as a hemiplegic, recovered enough from his stroke to perform somewhat modified tasks with his fellow workers, may have to accept a slower pace of physical performance and intellectual functioning.

A handicap can be imposed on a disabled person by a society that lacks understanding or information regarding what an individual can or cannot do. For example, an employer may focus on the fact that a physical disability exists, rather than on what the person is actually capable of doing in relation to job requirements. Implications for prevocational evaluations and programs are to plan realistic alternatives for the disabled individual leading to employment that can be performed with success and pride.

Referral to Occupational Therapy Services

The *referral* is the basic request for services to be provided to an individual by an occupational therapist. It may be called a "referral," a "consultation," or an "order." The form and concept of the request for services varies among facilities and programs and may range from recommendations regarding a specific problem to a request for complete assessment and treatment program for functional restoration. The frequent lack of specific instructions in the referral request allows the occupational therapist to choose from a variety of individualized approaches and techniques in determining the method of data gathering and treatment provision and coordination with other involved professionals.

Inherent in the role and the value of the work of the occupational therapist and assistant is helping the patient, client, or school-age child return to the community as a functioning individual. In order to do this, it is essential that the occupational therapy contact be directed toward this objective from the very beginning and continue in this way throughout therapeutic programs to the final referral to optimum independent living.

Referrals to occupational therapy are likely to come from physicians, therapists, nurses, psychologists, social workers, counselors, employers, teachers, or administrators. For services within a hospital, rehabilitation center, nursing home, or other medically oriented setting, the referral must come with a physician's signature, as mandated by accrediting and reimbursement parties. Lack of reimbursement mechanisms can result in denial of services regardless of referral or need, resulting in loss of valuable available resources necessary to assist the patient in reaching independent living status. There also are situations in which an occupational therapist can provide direct services and recommendations when a physician is not involved. Such examples can be found in contract consultation services to schools, employers, group homes, and other nonmedical areas. For example, an occupational therapist may be called on to assist in determining architectural modifications to the home or the school for a disabled school-age child or in providing adaptive equipment for residents in a group home or for disabled students in a public school. An employer may consult an occupational therapist for recommendations regarding work station or equipment modifications for safe functioning of a disabled worker. In the community, the services of an occupational therapist may be sought to provide community orientation to barrier-free design and other informational resources for rehabilitation programs and needs, disabilities, and general adaptations for access to community functions.

Assessment Planning and Process

The occupational therapy assessment and treatment components are thoroughly identified in the *Uniform Terminology for Reporting Occupational Therapy Services*, adopted by the American Occupational Therapy Association in 1979 (see Appendix D). Briefly, assessment includes screening, consultation, and evaluation. Evaluation areas include: (1) independent living/daily living skills and performance, (2) sensorimotor skill and performance components, (3) cognitive skill and performance components, (4) psychosocial skill and performance components, (5) therapeutic adaptations, and (6) specialized evaluations (special training required for administration). Occupational therapists use a variety of evaluation procedures to gain an accurate historical and clinical picture of the functional capacities in these areas. Specific approaches vary from setting to setting.

In preparation for the formal functional assessment of a person, the therapist or assistant develops pertinent identifying information regarding the subject. Information gathered includes: the reason for the referral, relevant background of the individual, medical and nonmedical information, the specific information or program requested by the referring party, and the type and location of the referral source. A referral signature is an essential part of the patient's permanent record (see section on documentation). After obtaining this information, the therapist begins a process such as that outlined in the occupational therapy flow sheet (Fig. 28-4). The therapist first reviews the documentation received on the patient and then determines the time available for the assessment, which may be determined by the referring party or reimbursement source. If time is limited, it may determine the extent and type of evaluation tools used. If it is unlimited, the therapist must ensure that the assessment is relevant to the needs of the patient: in no case should the patient go through hours of evaluation which, although providing interesting information, is not appropriate or necessary for determining treatment needs and components or delineating the manifestations of the condition or the prognosis.

In the initial contact, it is good to allow the patient full freedom to express feelings and concerns before beginning the gentle but firm program of evaluation. By getting acquainted with the patient in this manner initially, the therapist is better equipped to elicit cooperation in continuing the evaluation.

Although it is helpful to have an organized evaluation routine, it is frequently necessary to adjust the routine to meet the specific needs of a patient. For example, if a patient is physically fatigued, the therapist can evaluate an aspect of the condition that will not cause additional fatigue. Similarly, if the patient is anxious because of emotional stress and mental fatigue, the therapist should choose an evaluation area and method that will be acceptable, comfortable, and tolerable. For the most accurate results, it is essential to adjust the chronology of the evaluation procedures to the individual's needs while trying to complete the evaluation as quickly and as thoroughly as possible.

Usually, a comprehensive assessment includes enough methods of evaluation to provide the patient with alternatives in performance, thus making the process tolerable and even enjoyable. In creatively adapting the methods to the patient, the therapist can use these different approaches for various lengths of time and in different order: oral questioning in the interviewing approach, timed aspect in the speed test, coordination of the performance test under stress, and the quality of the product in the functional test. Throughout the evaluation, it is essential to derive accurate, factual information. The more the patient understands and becomes involved in the procedure, the more progress will be made.

A coordinated team effort can minimize the time required for the assessment process and maximize the information gained from it. Working out roles among occupational therapy staff and interdisciplinary staff is essential to avoid unnecessary overlap and to provide the most accurate, economical, and effective proce-

dures. The occupational therapy assistant participates under the supervision of the occupational therapist, particularly in the use of standardized tests and evaluations. Specific role delineations with regard to both assessment and treatment provided by the occupational therapist and the occupational therapy assistant are identified in detail in the *Entry-Level OTR and COTA Role Delineation*[4] by the American Occupational Therapy Association (AOTA) (see Appendix H). The therapist and the assistant collaborate in the assessment conclusions.

The occupational therapy assessment includes all results derived from specific evaluation procedures in the areas mentioned. It thus provides a composite picture of a person's functional capacity and behavior. The methods used may be structured, standardized, or nonstandardized. A *structured* instrument or evaluation provides guidelines for the content and process of assessment. For example, the plan of the self-care evaluation is structured to progress from one functional area to another and provides a functional assessment of the degree of independence the individual shows in the areas evaluated. This evaluation may or may not be standardized. Evaluation of homemaking skills and the home environment may fall in this category. A *standardized* assessment provides a measurement against a norm. This type of testing is done according to a specific protocol and may be timed. Examples of this type are coordination tests and perceptual tests. The *nonstandardized* assessment provides significant information that is not compared to norms nor completed according to a specific protocol. Task performance testing is an example of this type of evaluation.

In addition to the methods described above, the therapist uses observation as well as interviews to derive the composite meaning from the assessment process. The four methods are described briefly in the following discussion: observation, interview, structured or standardized evaluation and testing, and nonstandardized assessment of performance.

Observation

The preliminary approach to the patient is observation, which begins with the first contact. Apart from reading the chart or learning about the patient from other team members, observation is not only the first direct contact but is the one from which the initial impression is formed. How the therapist greets the patient, makes introductions, and involves him or her in the surroundings all convey how acceptable she or he is as a person. The therapist must continually be aware of how she or he, the environment, and the tests are affecting the patient. Signs of the mental and physical condition should be observed closely. Observation requires no previous contact with either the chart or with other people and

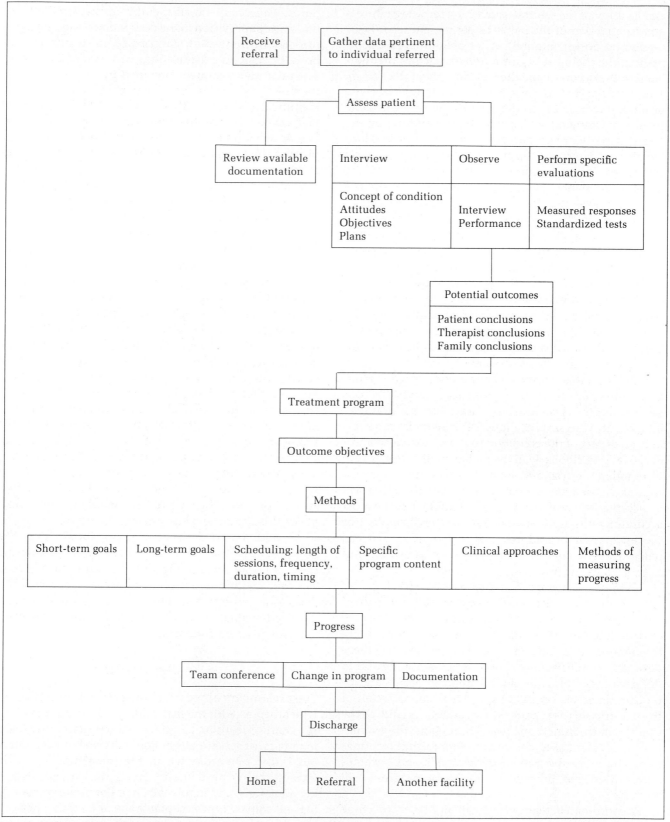

Figure 28-4. Occupational therapy flow sheet.

can be used effectively in the absence of other information.

By observing the patient's facial expression, the therapist can detect paralysis, drooling, spasticity, or confusion as well as alertness, fatigue, happiness, sadness, or pain. The position of the arms and legs can indicate spasticity, flaccidity, deformity, or pain. The sitting position can give indications of muscle imbalance, discomfort, or lack of voluntary control. Splints or slings also indicate some deficit in normal function. When walking into the room, the patient may display a gait produced by the use of braces, crutches, a prosthetic limb, a cane, or a walker or reveal a degree of paralysis not necessitating these aids. The skin may exhibit the effects of exertion or anxiety by appearing sweaty or red or becoming pale and clammy. Undue pressure from a splint or brace produces red or ulcerated marks or sores on the skin. If the therapist asks the patient to perform a task, the response can reveal hearing loss, muscle weakness, or incoordination.

Interview

The interview is a chance to get to know how the patient feels about what has happened, the effects on life and family, and the crucial priorities of the situation. Little may be known about the patient or the patient's condition. The interview (combined with observation) is the opportunity to find out information helpful to the therapist in planning the therapeutic program. Informal discussion leads to ease with the therapist and with the environment.

Most persons do not tolerate persistent questions about themselves at this point in their rehabilitation, but they may wish to share information regarding their problems in order to try to deal with them. The sincere therapist who observes the patient's reactions during the interview can often pick up valuable information about his or her interests and fears and can regulate the interview according to the reactions, attitudes, and tolerance exhibited.

The attitude of the therapist must be accepting if trust and confidence are to be inspired. The interview need not be rigidly formal, nor need it be completed in a single session. The initial contact marks the beginning of the relationship, which may last a long time, depending on rehabilitation needs. This beginning is crucial to the establishment of a good therapeutic environment, incorporating atmosphere, privacy, duration, acceptance, freedom of expression, and comfort.

Structured and Standardized Evaluation and Testing

Structured and standardized evaluation and testing procedures are objective methods with which to judge performance levels. Frequently, these methods are broken down into specific tests to be completed with specific equipment and in conformance with specific procedures. Examples include using a goniometer to measure passive and active range of motion, using a dynamometer to gauge grip strength, using a pinch gauge to register prehension pressure, or using an aesthesiometer to determine two-point discrimination.

Standardized tests for coordination include dexterity tests, such as the Crawford Small Parts Dexterity Test (Fig. 28-5), the Pennsylvania Bimanual Work Sample, the Minnesota Rate of Manipulation Tests (Fig. 28-6), and the Bennett Hand Tool Test. These tests and many others have norms or standardized measurements for comparing results. At times, however, the norms relate to normal performance and thus have selected use for the physically disabled person. Each test has a specific purpose and method of administration. If the norms are to be used in reference to the test score, administration of the test must be according to the instructions. For example, a quadriplegic, lacking a normal level of physical movements and sensory functions of the hands, may perform much lower on a coordination test if speed is an important factor, whereas if the speed factor is removed, he may perform with a high level of accuracy and tolerance. From the many tests available, it is essential to select those that will reveal the needed information so that explicit information can be given to team members as needed.

Tests of perceptual–motor function may include the

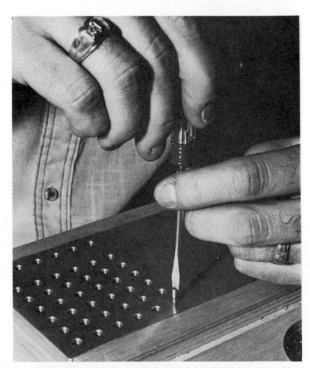

Figure 28-5. Crawford Small Parts Dexterity Test. A timed, standardized bimanual coordination test using small screws and a small screwdriver to complete transfer pattern to a metal plate.

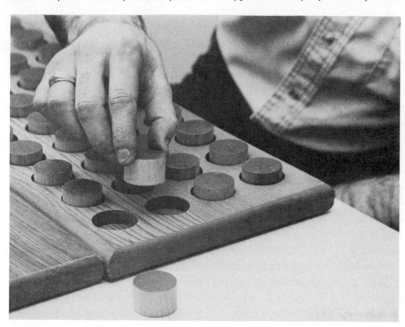

Figure 28-6. Minnesota Rate of Manipulation Test. A five-part timed, standardized test using unilateral and bilateral object manipulation patterns for transfer of wooden discs.

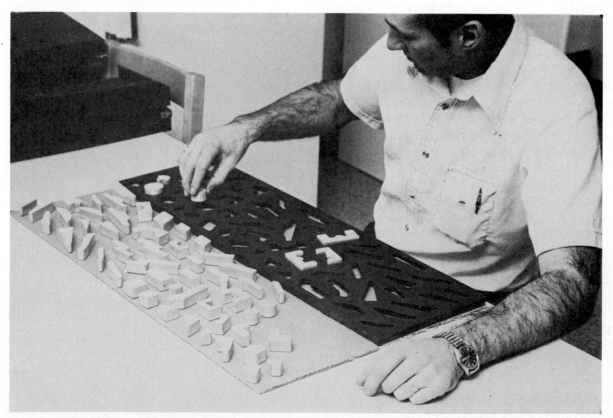

Figure 28-7. Minnesota Spatial Relations Test. A timed standardized unilateral test used to evaluate visual–motor perception and organization as the patient transfers objects one by one from one field to another.

Ayres Battery and the Frostig Battery, which are not standardized for an adult population, and the Minnesota Spatial Relations Test (Fig. 28-7). Treatment centers use a variety of specific tests to measure performance according to norms; the aforementioned are but a few of those commonly used. Further information on specific tests can be found in the chapter on evaluation.

Nonstandardized Assessment

In assessing general performance, the therapist evaluates how well the patient accomplishes a specific task. What are limitations of strength, coordination, or range of motion as indicated by ability in reaching for, grasping, or placing objects? (See Fig. 28-8). How well is the patient adjusting to limitations? This can be evaluated by observing the character of social interactions with other patients, mental tolerance of the social context and activity of the occupational therapy room, and ability to work with the spouse or therapist in reviewing self-care abilities in light of eventually going home, where the assistance of a family member may be needed.

Performance testing also involves the assessment of problem-solving ability in accomplishing a task comprising several steps. For example, a woodworking project may be used to test the perceptual–motor abilities of the patient with brain damage. The therapist observes the method of planning the project, signs regarding visual perception, eye–hand coordination, concept of verticality, and proper use of tools.

In performance testing, it is essential to set up the task so that, although difficult, it is within the patient's ability. The use of a familiar task in evaluation may be threatening because it causes the patient to become acutely aware of the loss of ability. Performance testing must include a balance of success along with evaluation of functional deficits. Otherwise, the client may become overly discouraged or negative toward the occupational therapist, and such an attitude can hinder progress.

Documentation

Accurate documentation is essential in the accumulation of specific testing results, impressions, and interpretations. Forms vary from setting to setting and are often under revision. A sample worksheet for general information gained from the interview or performance testing is shown in Figure 28-9. As stated, it is simply a structured format to assist the therapist in gathering and noting specific information for the overall assessment report. In many program settings, there are restrictions as to forms that are included in the formal chart documentation; therefore, the therapist devises forms to assist the informal gathering of information. This form is helpful in noting information for subsequent inclusion in the formal report, for communication to other occupational therapists or assistants working with the patient, and for general reference regarding the progress of the patient. Additional specific evaluation forms may be used, such as those for perceptual testing, range-of-motion testing, strength testing, and testing of self-care independence. The use of forms depends on the individual needs of the patient.

Treatment Planning and Process

As stated in the section on assessment, specific functional areas designated in occupational therapy treatment are described in the *Uniform Terminology for Re-*

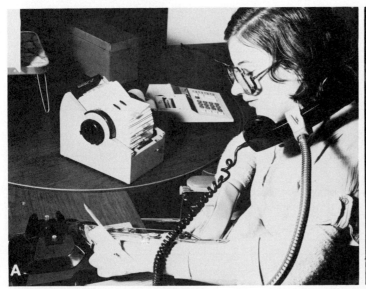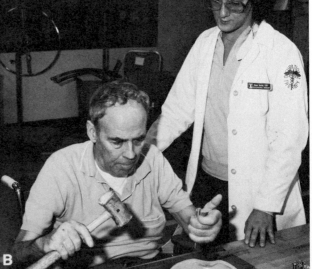

Figure 28-8. (*A*) and (*B*). Nonstandardized performance testing.

Admission Date: _____
Discharge Date: _____

Occupational Therapy Worksheet

Name: _____ Admission Date: _____ Room # _____
Address: _____ Diagnosis: _____ Duration: _____
Age: _____ Education: _____ Pertinent History: _____
Occupation: _____ O.T. Referral/Order: _____
_____ _____
Marital Status: _____ Dr.: _____ Date: _____
Children: _____
Other: _____ Precautions: _____
  House: Surroundings: _____ Entrance: _____
         # Floors: _____ Bedroom: _____
         Kitchen: _____ Bathroom: _____
         Architectural Barriers: _____
_____

Physical Evaluation:
    Upper Extremities: (ROM, strength, coordination, sensation, muscle tone, movement patterns, endurance)

      RUE: _____

      LUE: _____
      Bilateral: _____

      Functional Deficits: _____

    Trunk and Lower Extremities: (Mobility, sensation, muscle tone, sitting/standing tolerance, balance, gait)
_____

Mental Functioning Evaluation: (attention, awareness, judgment, behavior, retention, reception, abstract reasoning, cognition, problem solving)
_____

Perceptual Functioning Evaluation: (visual, auditory, motor planning, stereognosis, proprioception, perceptual motor correlation)
_____
_____

Functional Activity Evaluation:
  ADL: (position, balance, transfers, mobility, assistive devices used, motivation, perceptual deficits)
    Hygiene/Bathing/Grooming: _____

    Dressing: _____

    Self-feeding: _____

    Writing/Reading: (signature, tracing, copying, spontaneous writing and reading, dominance, field cut, neglect, eyesight)
_____

Homemaking: (food preparation, clean-up, safety, home modifications, assistive devices, positioning, responsibilities, financial management, work simplification, energy conservation)
_____
_____
_____

(continued)

Figure 28-9. Sample occupational therapy worksheet.

Occupational Therapy Worksheet (cont.)

Attitudes: (emotional status, self-concepts, behavior)

_____

Interests: (vocational, avocational, and social skills and abilities)

_____

Orthotic and Assistive Equipment: (type, date given, recommendations)

_____

Summary of Findings: (deficits, functional limitations, potentials, attitudes)

_____

_____

_____

_____

_____

Treatment Plan:
  Objectives: _____

               _____

               _____

  Methods: _____

               _____

               _____

  Duration/Frequency: _____

  Expected Outcome: _____

               _____

Date: _____   _____ OTR

                                       Signature

---

porting Occupational Therapy Services (see Appendix D). Major functional areas are:

1. Independent living/daily living skills, including physical and emotional skills and performance in work and play activity
2. Sensorimotor components, including neuromuscular behavior and sensory integration
3. Cognitive components, including orientation, conceptualization/comprehension, and cognitive integration
4. Psychosocial components, including self-management, dyadic interaction, and group interaction
5. Therapeutic adaptations, including orthotics, prosthetics, and assistive/adaptive equipment
6. Prevention, including energy conservation, joint protection/body mechanics, positioning, and coordination of daily living activities.

The *Standards of Practice,* also developed by the AOTA, provides a guideline for the implementation of the treatment programs based on the designated functional areas. Recommendations for documentation, standards of assessment and treatment, program de-sign, discharge planning, re-evaluation, and quality assurance are included in the *Standards.*

To hold onto the previous lifestyle and self-image and to struggle to regain them are inherent in the individual to some extent through all stages of rehabilitation. These energies and motivations are part of the vital force of life and the will to continue to control the context and freedom of one's existence and function. In their work on motivation, Heijn and Granger refer to "differential motivation" during specific rehabilitation programs to reflect this struggle "to preserve a prior adaptation without accepting the permanent changes imposed."[5] They further suggest that "motivation is like a vehicle that carries the patient through stressful times in order to achieve potential" and in order to achieve alternatives required by permanent disability.[5] They state that successful rehabilitation depends on "1) the patient's ability to adaptively master the emotional stress which is a frequent accompaniment of physical handicap, 2) his ability to renounce or modify highly valued activities, future plans, or relationships, and 3) his ability to implement feasible new plans and actions."[5]

The person referred to occupational therapy for

functional services may actually fear what he or she has become with regard to functional independence. In this case, there may be an underlying resistance to all positive approaches from others and to potential gains. The challenge for the occupational therapist and the occupational therapy assistant is to establish effective therapeutic intervention by developing an environment and relationships that will assist the patient to develop therapeutic performance.

When the occupational therapist develops the treatment plan, the patient is the prime component and must be included when choosing methods to achieve functional gains. This includes initial planning, changes based on progress, and feedback regarding performance. This consideration encourages the patient to take an increasing role in planning therapeutic activities and adaptations. If the therapist sees the patient first in the outpatient or home environment, prime consideration for the patient's views and maximum involvement with program planning is even more essential. In taking gradual steps toward responsibility in planning and self-evaluation, the patient develops self-awareness, confidence, creativity, problem-solving ability, and responsibility for his or her own health. The following are ways the patient can be included in the treatment planning and implementation:

1. Participating in the initial evaluation procedures and results; assisting with treatment plan design
2. Learning factual information from assessment results to use in planning the course of treatment
3. Involving the patient's interests, major current concerns, abilities and long-term goals in the plan
4. Planning short-term goals with the patient; obtaining commitment from the patient if feasible
5. Planning treatment modalities to include positive feedback to the patient to increase self-awareness and satisfaction from gains
6. Planning long-term goals with the patient with regard to implications of disability, financial boundaries, and medical and functional prognosis
7. Encouraging the patient to develop the ability to design treatment goals, to set priorities among treatment objectives, and to take responsibility for his/her own program.

Implementation of the treatment plan requires an environment conducive to the achievement of the objectives. When the patient can be involved in the planning, there is likely to be greater commitment to progress than when the therapist does all the planning. Where this involvement is not feasible due to the patient's lack of interest or inability to communicate, the efforts of the therapist should be directed toward increasing the involvement of the patient. The therapist orients the level of treatment to the patient's interest and level of ability to respond.

Beginning the treatment program with a short-term goal that is significant to the patient helps establish an effective relationship between the therapist or assistant and the patient. Use of passive range of motion or demonstrations aids in the teaching of active movements and encourages functional patterns. New or adaptive techniques and equipment should be demonstrated by the therapist in the same manner that the patient is expected to perform so that the patient can imitate the expected motion. Involvement in therapeutic exercise and activity provides increased productivity and a sense of purpose to the therapeutic regimen. The engagement of the patient in problem-solving, planning, and evaluation to meet treatment objectives aids in the accomplishment of the objectives. With appropriate and therapeutic feedback with regard to performance, the patient increases self-awareness and can relate the daily progress to the goals. The treatment plan itself should relate to the eventual goal of going home and being responsible for the continuity of care. Patient and family involvement in treatment facilitates continuity in the home following discharge from formal institutional programs. Long-term accomplishments are effected by day-to-day efforts in a succession of intermittent but progressive gains.

In order to escape the misery of accepting a disabling condition or a long-term progressive illness, the patient may deny its existence. Although physical or intellectual deficits may be obvious, the patient may still consciously or subconsciously deny the occurrence or implications of the condition. The occupational therapy program provides the patient with the opportunity to see herself or himself as a thinking, doing being. Through the performance of tasks directed toward achievable accomplishments, daily awareness of abilities and problems is encouraged. The task is directed toward self-accomplishment and self-awareness. In treatment, success and failure are both therapeutic. Failure can be tangible proof to the patient that he or she is denying inability. Although this failure may cause depression, hostility, or discouragement, it is only by knowing both strengths and weaknesses that the patient is able to see abilities currently possessed and abilities to be regained.

Independence of the patient in self-care activities is an area of concern and adaptation shared by the nurse and the occupational therapist. Self-care represents the most significant aspect of self-awareness and self-acceptance. During the initial stage of denial, the patient is effectively able to deny responsibilities, the body, and its functions. Concern is focused on physical sensations such as pain, positioning, and movement. The patient relinquishes responsibility for care of his or her body and may even be afraid of it, since the frightening effects of disease or trauma have made it an unknown.

During this period, it is important for those working with the patient to talk about the body, to reaquaint him or her with it, and to help him or her accept it. Gradually, the patient relearns how to relate to it through taking responsibility for bathing, grooming, eating, and dressing. Thus, the patient becomes aware of how the body feels and moves, as well as which parts may need more help or experience more pain.

During therapy sessions, movement is incorporated into self-care programs. The responsibility for assistance in independent self-care falls generally to the occupational therapist in collaboration with the nurse. The occupational therapist assesses the self-care problems. For example, inability to distinguish objects of different shapes or colors or to relate to vertical or horizontal positions may make the patient unable to determine the front, back, or sleeve of a shirt. A person with a flaccid arm cannot handle eating utensils in the usual manner and thus may have to learn how to cut meat one-handed, switch the fork to the nondominant hand, or use a plate guard. The occupational therapist analyzes these problems, determines the approach for handling them, and teaches techniques to be used in performing each activity. These techniques are then used in the patient's daily program.

With the physically disabled person, activities of daily living (ADL) generally comprise those necessary for basic self-care independence: bathing, hygiene, elimination, grooming, dressing, and eating. Consideration is given to such items as eyeglasses, hearing aids, dentures, prostheses, splints, slings, braces, and adapted clothing. The patient's abilities should be evaluated both with and without the adapted equipment to accurately assess levels of independence. For example, a patient who is unable to do buttoning without the use of a hand splint is "independent" with the hand splint; he or she is "dependent" without it. This is also true when special utensils or other equipment are required for eating without the assistance of another person.

The disabled person learns how to choose and retrieve clothing from drawers and cabinets, how to apply and secure assistive devices, how to use catheters, tampons, or suppositories as necessary, how to manage such items as soap, washclothes, nail clippers, combs, toothpaste, and make-up. In the process of eating, the patient learns the use of napkins, utensils, glasses, and cups, as well as how to take food from a serving dish and use salt and pepper.

Included in self-care is the use of the telephone, including how to dial the phone, answer it, take a message, and call for help. Those who need special equipment learn how to use it and how to obtain special operator assistance.

In some instances, the patient can accomplish self-care and eating tasks by performing them in a different manner rather than by learning how to use special de-vices or equipment. When devices are necessary (elastic shoe laces, Velcro closures, or elastic thread), or when a new skill must be mastered (one-handed shoe-tying or meat-cutting), all possibilities should be explored to ensure minimum reliance on, but maximum effectiveness of, the special equipment or the acquired skill. Effectiveness in self-care provides the patient with independence, which not only aids the patient, but also helps in family relationships. The accomplishment of self-care tasks leads to further successes, enhances motivation, and provides daily physical exercise.

The general mobility of the patient is a concern and adaptation shared by the nurse, the physical therapist, and the occupational therapist. As the patient must assume optimum position for function, an adapted transfer technique from bed to wheelchair or to walker or crutches may be necessary. Although the physical therapist may decide which technique the patient should use, a coordinated team effort is needed to assist the patient in the same technique for aid in learning; therefore, the occupational therapist needs to know transfer techniques.

Specific restoration of functional ability may precede or follow the development of self-care activity. Body exercise and sensory awareness developed during the accomplishment of daily tasks are correlated with specific activities also directed toward the restoration of functional ability. These activities include specific exercises to improve strength, range of motion, coordination, and function.

The terms *exercise* and *activity* are used here interchangeably, since it is felt that activity provides exercise and exercise can be provided through activity. An exercise modality may consist of a measured movement or a combination of movements.

Occupational therapy emphasizes active rather than passive exercises and utilizes the abilities of the patient to the maximum. Although assistive equipment (suspension slings, wheelchairs, lapboards, and splints) may help the patient passively, the *purpose* of their use is to achieve the maximum level of independent and active functioning. For example, the suspension sling may facilitate arm movement for a quadriplegic, enabling him or her to bring both hands together, to eat independently, to use a button board for practice, to write a letter, or to type schoolwork. A variety of assistive equipment may be needed to encourage arm and hand function and to prevent fatigue during exercise activities.

The treatment room provides an atmosphere of activity, with emphasis on productive achievement and encouragement to try. Activity is geared toward what is interesting, purposeful, and acceptable to the patient, so that he or she can see its relation to the overall rehabilitation goals. The patient may reject a treatment situation because of inability to do things done competently in the past. The patient may resent doing familiar tasks in an inferior way, performing the games of a child painfully and laboriously, or being unable to function to an expected or desired standard. For some of these reasons, the patient may become belligerent and refuse to participate in the therapy program. The occupational therapist must make every effort to involve the patient in planning appropriate treatment programs and activities.

The occupational therapist discusses vocational plans with the patient and focuses training objectives on areas related to vocational interests, aptitudes, and goals. For example, a patient who is attending school may wish to improve handwriting and note-taking skills. Job tasks may be simulated for the individual who can return to work. If new vocational goals are set, such as bookkeeping or mechanical drawing, proficiency in performing these tasks may be gained by using hand splints, special techniques, or adaptations.

Machinery that is available to the occupational therapist for clerical use or for the construction of assistive equipment can serve a dual purpose in providing both evaluation and training tools for the patient with physical or perceptual deficits. After a primary check to ensure safety in use, these tools can be used to provide information regarding physical ability, work habits, work skills, and problem-solving abilities.

In a hospital program, the occupational therapist may work with a vocational rehabilitation counselor in the formulation of vocationally oriented treatment. In a rehabilitation center, the vocational program may be separate from occupational therapy but may follow the prevocational exploration program provided by the occupational therapist. A vocational readiness program may be provided by the therapist or assistant on an outpatient basis, or the patient may be referred to a facility specially equipped to provide vocational testing and work-simulated tasks to determine realistic vocational areas for consideration by the patient. Many training programs in occupations are adapted to the needs of persons with physical limitations.

Avocational interests are explored in order to give the patient an interest in daily activity. Hobbies such as reading, writing, painting, and drawing can be pursued even though physical limitations may require use of adapted equipment. Avocational pursuits can also develop into economic benefits for the patient.

The occupational therapist can assist the patient in making satisfactory adjustment to a disability and in restoring self-confidence by concentrating on accomplishments and capabilities and also by providing opportunities for social interaction. The patient should be encouraged to participate in recreational programs and in the patient governing bodies active in many rehabilitation facilities.

To ease the fear of taking part in outside social activities because of "looking different," the patient should be encouraged to go on outings, such as bowling, baseball games, and movies, while still in the hospital. These activities make the patient begin to function as a member of a community in preparation for discharge. Upon discharge, each person should be encouraged to participate in social and community affairs and to attend functions that were part of his or her life before the injury or onset of disease.

The Team Approach

The ideal treatment approach to the patient with multiple problem areas, who is cared for by several persons or programs, is the *team approach*, in which formal and informal interaction is encouraged among all persons working toward developing and implementing a unified treatment program. This team includes the patient and family as well as specialists in the health field.

Team members are important sources of information and support for one another. For example, a patient may develop signs of extreme fatigue, such as sweating and difficulty in breathing, while in the occupational therapy area. The occupational therapist contacts the physician or the nurse for assistance in determining the cause and seriousness of the symptoms. The occupational therapist contacts the physical therapist to determine techniques for safe and successful transfer from one chair to another, for information about whether the patient will be safe standing to perform a woodworking project, or whether the patient can safely stand and walk in the kitchen for assessment of homemaking skills.

Occupational and physical therapists should coordinate muscle testing, range of motion, sensory testing, and assessment of physical tolerance and balance. The speech therapist and occupational therapist work together in designing treatment for the aphasic patient. Realistic vocational planning by the counselor is aided by the occupational therapist, who assesses the functional abilities of the upper extremities, the intellectual level of functioning in applied tasks, and the general physical tolerance. The physician aids in developing realistic planning in terms of the prognosis and the patient's mental approach to rehabilitation.

In the rehabilitation approach, there are generally overlaps in evaluation and treatment among such persons as physicians, nurses, occupational therapists, physical therapists, speech therapists, social workers, and vocational rehabilitation counselors. Overlaps can be useful in providing carryover of activities and exercises and continual monitoring of the patient's progress. Good communication among team members is necessary to encourage coordination rather than antagonism over "who does what." For example, the occupational therapist works with the physician, heeding the medical precautions on correct body positioning, optimal mental and physical tolerance of activity, and progression of pathological symptoms. A coordinated self-care program involves the cooperation of nurses and occupational therapists in planning daily hygiene, grooming, dressing, and eating programs. The occupational therapist coordinates the morning dressing program and general exercise activities with the physical therapy program so that physical gains are maintained throughout the day and fatigue is avoided. The speech therapist aids team members in effective communication skills for patients who have speech deficits. As the social worker deals with the patient and family, he or she needs to know the treatment programs and progress in order to interpret and convey this information to the family and to assist the patient in understanding the daily program. The vocational rehabilitation counselor relies on the occupational therapist's evaluation of functional ability to determine the need for further education, job return, training, placement, or relocation.

A functional delineation of roles among team members is essential for optimal communication and effective rehabilitation. The specific roles of each member of the team may vary in different treatment settings.

Discharge Planning

With the development of the team approach and the growth of rehabilitation, discharge planning has grown from the concept of placement or referral of a person following discharge to actual preparation for discharge by the patient and the rehabilitation team. The result of a well-coordinated team effort is effective referral or community re-entry, with all team members contributing to the plan. The most important member of the team is the patient.

Preparation includes medical considerations (continuation of medication, follow-up visits, plans for future treatment), provision of assistive equipment for home exercise functions and independence in daily living, counseling the family on the patient's self-care and general activity, and a home visit to determine the presence of architectural barriers and to evaluate the patient's potential for functioning there.

Discharge planning begins with the referral of the person to the treatment setting where the anticipated treatment program is to take place. Thus, the first information regarding discharge questions or expectations will appear in referral materials. The program following referral may diverge from the initial expectations and may result in further discharge planning. Thus, discharge planning becomes a continual process based on the condition of the patient at any given time, rather than simply a plan of where to go when a given program is completed.

After the referral information is gathered, evaluation occurs. This includes all team members and pertinent information needed for appropriate and optimum treatment of the patient, including information about the patient's home environment, lifestyle, educational level, and occupation. The patient and the team can create a treatment plan that will assist the patient in preparing to go home. Since the total treatment plan is geared toward meeting the needs of the patient on discharge, therapy can be seen as important for realistic discharge planning rather than as a program that bears no relationship to the most crucial problems of returning home.

Publications are available to aid the family and the recovering patient in postdischarge home programs that continue the rehabilitation process. As recovery may continue over a period of years, professional programs are transferred to the patient and family to incorporate into daily routines.

In planning long-range needs and placement, the therapist and the patient must consider such limitations as the following: no home to return to upon discharge; no financial coverage for outpatient services; no transportation available for outpatient services; and no family member to provide attendant care or homemaking services in the home following discharge.

Consumer groups provide many types of support and many opportunities for the disabled individual. National organizations established to benefit victims of a particular disease and to engage in specific relevant research projects publish information for professionals and consumers, hold educational meetings, and provide a forum for discussions. A list of organizations is included in Appendix J.

Consumer groups, which may include able-bodied friends and professionals, provide initial socialization opportunities at meetings. A person can meet others with the same disability or with similar problems. Discussions focus on common concerns, such as the legal rights of the disabled, architectural and accessibility laws, building codes, transportation needs, housing, employment, and educational opportunities. Attending such meetings can be encouraging and informative for both the patient and the therapist. Such meetings may be held in rehabilitation centers or hospitals, thus making preliminary information and experience available early in the adjustment process.

Summary

The process of functional restoration following a disabling condition embodies the totality of human potential. Assisting a person to build or restore his or her life to its fullest use and satisfaction is a philosophical mandate of occupational therapy practice. An essential member of the rehabilitation team, the occupational therapist works with the patient, family, and other professionals in a coordinated interdisciplinary team from admission of the patient to a therapeutic program to the optimum level of independent living at discharge. The patient may participate in programs in different settings before taking full responsibility for his or her continued health. Through this process, health professionals collaborate in a health-oriented approach to daily living.

Individual effects of disability are reflected in psychosocial and physical responses by a person, reaching into all areas of life and often requiring adjustment of familiar life patterns. Trauma and disease may result in dysfunctional manifestations through a sudden or gradual pathological process. Disability may be nonprogressive or progressive, temporary or permanent. The functional implications of the problem may be denied by the patient initially and require long-term intervention for acceptance of self and redirection of physical energies. Attitudes of individuals experiencing disability are affected by age, previous ability, achievements, lifestyle, family, status, self-concept, interests, and general responsibilities. The patient goes through a process from ability to disability to a regaining or refinding of abilities during rehabilitation. Attitudes have a significant effect on the rehabilitation process and its outcome. The disabled person draws on all personal resources.

The occupational therapist has a large variety of approaches, methods, and tools to use in assessing the deficits and potentials of a functionally limited person and designing appropriate treatment programs for functional restoration. Twelve principles are presented to assist the therapist in developing a comprehensive program. The occupational therapist utilizes the concept and components of a therapeutic environment, therapeutic relationships, and therapeutic performance to improve function. The activity factor is crucial to the constructive aspects of performance and the regaining of function through purposeful activity. Activity can aid in diagnostic, therapeutic, and restorative program objectives.

Personal and environmental adaptations are crucial to re-entry into the world of purpose and accomplishment. Architectural access to one's own home as well as to the buildings in the environment is essential. Functional recovery progresses through the final stages of community re-entry.

The initial contact between the patient and the occupational therapist is facilitated by a referral to services. Although this may come from virtually any professional on behalf of the patient, specific program and reimbursement restrictions may be incurred. Occupational therapy assessment and treatment areas include: (1) independent living/daily living skills and performance, (2) sensorimotor skill and performance components, (3) cognitive skill and performance components, (4) psychosocial skill and performance components, (5) therapeutic adaptations, and (6) prevention. The assessment process is related to the treatment process. Assessment requires the appropriate involvement of the occupational therapist and the occupational therapy assistant, as designated by the AOTA role delineation. Treatment content is identified by both the AOTA *Uniform Terminology* and the AOTA *Standards of Practice.* The assessment is performed using nonstructured, nonstandardized, and standardized methods, as well as by observation and interview. How the patient responds to the assessment and treatment procedures depends on the therapeutic relationship between the therapist and the patient and the degree of participation of the patient in the planning and implementation of the program. This aspect is essential to encourage the development of individual responsibility for continued rehabilitation on the part of the patient through the practice of problem-solving abilities.

There are many types of programs in which the occupational therapist provides services. Whatever the specific program, correlation of occupational therapy objectives and techniques with other programs in which the patient is involved is necessary for effective progress. Discharge planning is a team effort that involves the patient and assists the patient in developing healthy attitudes toward community involvement as a consumer and in maintaining healthy attitudes and activities in the independent environment.

References

1. Ayres AJ: Sensory Integration and the Child, pp 46, 64. Los Angeles, Western Psychological Services, 1979
2. Daniels S: In disability and sickness: A theory. Proj Health 1:1, 1981
3. Dunning H: Environmental occupation therapy. Am J Occup Ther 26:292, 1972
4. Entry-Level Role Delineation for OTRs and COTAs. Rockville, MD, American Occupational Therapy Association, 1981
5. Heijn C, Granger CV: Understanding motivational patterns: Early identification aids rehabilitation. J Rehab 40:26, 1974
6. Reilly M: Occupational therapy can be one of the great ideas of 20th century medicine. Am J Occup Ther 16:1, 1962
7. Vargo JW: Some psychological effects of physical disability. Am J Occup Ther 32:31, 1978
8. Williams WC, quoted in Richards MC: Centering, pp 79–80. Middletown, CT, Wesleyan University Press, 1964

Appreciation is extended to Martha Willis for critical review and to Patricia Curran for editorial assistance.

Functional Restoration: Neurologic, Orthopedic, and Arthritic Conditions

Elinor Anne Spencer

The focus of this chapter is major diagnostic and symptom complexes in neurologic, arthritic, and orthopedic conditions commonly seen by the occupational therapist in clinical and community settings. In the previous chapter, the impact of temporary and long-term manifestations of disabling injury and disease was presented to identify the functional implications, the factors affecting rehabilitation, the role of occupational therapy, and referral to occupational therapy services. The general context of assessment and treatment of the person suffering physical dysfunction was discussed. However, specific conditions call for modifications in the application of these concepts. In this chapter, assessment and treatment techniques may be associated with specific symptomatology in the text but may not be limited to those specified.

The occupational therapy program consists of three major areas: (1) *identification* of functional capacities and deficits through evaluation procedures in the assessment process, (2) *development* of functional capacity through the use of specific activities, and (3) *integration* of functional abilities into daily tasks. The occupational therapist and the occupational therapy assistant work together with the patient to plan and implement an appropriate program of functional restoration. The specific value of this program for the patient is enhanced by effective communication with all persons involved with the rehabilitation. Nonprofessional as well as professional persons, family, and friends are often included in the comprehensive approach to optimum functional restoration, regaining of a satisfying life-style, and setting and implementing of a positive future perspective. Components of the occupational therapy program include setting a therapeutic environment for function, facilitating therapeutic relationships, and establishing programs directed toward therapeutic performance.

Neurologic Conditions

Perhaps the most complex manifestation of functional deficits and the most difficult rehabilitation challenges arise from neurological conditions. Neurological dysfunction is caused by damage to the nervous system but may affect other body systems as well. Major sites of lesions in the nervous system are the brain, the spinal cord and nerve roots, the myoneural junction (between the spinal cord and the muscles), and the extremities. The specific clinical manifestations are determined by the location, type, and extent of the lesion. Symptom complexes are identified as the outcome of trauma or disease. Table 29-1 lists various neurological conditions

Table 29-1. *Correlation of Location of Lesion with Resultant Pathological Condition, Course, and Organic Manifestations*

Location	Pathological Condition	Course of Pathology	Manifestations
Brain	Cerebrovascular accident	Nonprogressive	⌈ Intellectual
	Head injury	Nonprogressive	Personality
	Multiple sclerosis	Progressive	Sensorimotor
	Parkinson's disease	Progressive	Emotional
			Communication
			Physiologic
			⌊ Functional
Spinal cord	Amyotrophic lateral sclerosis	Progressive	[Physical, physiologic, motor communication
	Poliomyelitis	Nonprogressive	⌈ Sensorimotor
	Guillain–Barré syndrome	Nonprogressive	Physiologic
	Spinal cord injury	Nonprogressive	Functional
Myoneural junction	Myasthenia gravis	Progressive	⌊ Motor comunication
Extremity	Peripheral nerve injury	Nonprogressive	[Physical, functional

(Note: bracketed manifestations apply to all pathological conditions listed in the group.)

according to the location of the lesion, the resulting pathological or diagnostic condition, the course of the lesion, and the gross areas of clinical manifestation.

The course of a neurologic condition may be *nonprogressive* or *progressive.* Sudden onset of a cerebrovascular accident (stroke) or head injury, spinal cord injury, Guillain–Barré Syndrome, polio, or peripheral nerve injury leaves immediate clinical signs. The symptoms of these trauma and disease effects are *stationary:* they do not increase. The maximum severity of the symptoms occurs at the time of onset. *Progressive* neurologic diseases include multiple sclerosis (MS) Parkinson's disease, myasthenia gravis (MG), and amyotrophic lateral sclerosis (ALS) among others. In the course of these diseases, which are discussed in this chapter, symptoms worsen over time, progressively diminishing functional capacity. Although there may be a similarity in the clinical assessment and treatment of specific deficits associated with these progressive diseases, the long-term pattern of treatment and personal psychological adjustment may differ.

Lesions in the Brain

Lesions in the brain are caused by *internal trauma,* such as cerebrovascular accident (CVA, stroke); *external trauma,* such as head injury; or disease, such as MS or Parkinson's disease. Lesions in the brain can result in: (1) personality changes and psychosocial challenges, (2) communication disorders, (3) cognitive distortions and intellectual deficits, (4) sensorimotor dysfunction, and (5) disruption of functional performance levels. The course is generally nonprogressive in the case of internal and external trauma but progressive in the case of disease. Secondary disability may occur as a result of inadequate primary assessment and treatment. Personality changes may interfere with the person's familiar behavior patterns, causing concern or disruption of family and personal relationships. Communication disorders may affect self-expression in oral or written form, understanding of auditory input, and interpersonal relations. Inability to communicate interferes with learning and interaction. Cognitive deficits may also interfere with communication, interpersonal relationships, and functional performance and development. The specific areas affected may be: understanding and using abstract concepts, perceiving environmental stimuli, and responding appropriately.

Sensorimotor symptoms of brain lesions are characterized by *upper motor neuron* (UMN) signs, which are caused by lesions in the corticospinal or pyramidal tract located in the brain or the spinal cord. The resultant conditions are spastic paralysis of the upper and lower limb on the same side (hemiplegia, hemiparesis), of both lower limbs (paraplegia, paraparesis), or of both upper and lower limbs (quadriplegia, quadriparesis, or bilateral hemiplegia or hemiparesis). The location of the lesion determines the location and the extent of the paralysis. Specific clinical signs in the extremities include loss of voluntary movement and control, increased muscle tone (spasticity), pathological reflexes, and loss of sensation. Lesions in the extrapyramidal system of the brain can produce disorders of muscle tone and involuntary movements, such as manifested in Parkinson's disease. Lesions in the cerebellum and its pathways can cause cerebellar ataxia, as seen with head injury, brain tumor, MS, and ALS.

Functional performance levels can be disrupted by personality changes, communication deficits, cognitive deficits, and sensorimotor dysfunction. Lack of understanding of movement patterns, functional planning, and the natural implementation of task activity may preclude independent performance, as can the presence of pathological sensorimotor functions.

The global objectives of the rehabilitation program for the person with a brain lesion are:

1. Integration of cognitive and sensorimotor functions
2. Restoration of the ability to interact independently and satisfactorily with the physical and human environments
3. Restoration of the ability to plan and implement personal objectives in an unstructured environment
4. Participation in personal and social productive living
5. Optimum reintegration into the home and community as an independently functioning member

To assist in the achievement of these objectives, the occupational therapist evaluates the functional assets and deficits with regard to the ability to perform self-initiated, purposeful, and productive activity and develops therapeutic programs to assist in developing these abilities. Sample objectives are to enable the patient to:

1. Develop cognitive–perceptual–motor function and sensory integration
2. Refine sensorimotor systems to increase volitional motor control
3. Increase attention span and activity tolerance
4. Decrease nonproductive behavior
5. Develop organizational and problem-solving abilities for functional activities
6. Improve ability to learn alternative methods to compensate for continuing deficits
7. Develop independence in self-care, activities of daily living, and homemaking skills
8. Improve skills for community re-entry

The therapist performs appropriate evaluation and treatment in all areas of functional disability according to the ability of the patient to respond.

Approach to Assessment and Treatment

One of the major functions of the occupational therapist is to help the patient adjust to both the symptoms and the general situation in the treatment setting. The patient needs to know why she or he has come to occupational therapy and what is expected. These explanations may need to be repeated for emphasis, clarification, and reminders as the patient improves to maintain a stabilizing continuity that compensates for fluctuation in moods and abilities. How the therapist uses words and voice tone must be focused on the level of receptivity but must at the same time show respect. When the patient is not capable of spontaneous speech, he or she may not respond vocally to questions, comments, or simple requests from the therapist. In such cases, a code system of communication may be worked out between the therapist and the patient. For example, the patient may be capable of indicating "yes" or "no" by closing the eyes, frowning, moving the head, or lifting an arm. Disorientation and confusion may also result from being unable to communicate.

The chronological order of specific tests of functional abilities, deficits, and potentials must be geared to the individual and relate to the capacity to respond. Initially, a person with brain trauma may exhibit intolerance for or incomprehension of the meaning of stimuli. The noise or movements of others may be distracting or produce fear. If the person suffers from blurred or double vision, he or she may have low visual tolerance magnified by visual perceptual distortions that give inaccurate information regarding objects and relationships in the environment. Symptoms related to physical pain, discomfort, and distorted body image and sensory feedback also hinder assessment procedures.

Therapeutic procedures begin with choosing and setting up the therapy environment to elicit maximum response from a person who may be highly distractable. The length and type of specific assessment and treatment techniques are determined by the person's mental and physical tolerance, cooperation, comprehension, and response. Thus, at the beginning, the therapist establishes a means of communication with the person who may lack speech or comprehension of instructions or who may be disoriented in time and space.

General Functional Considerations

Personality Changes and Psychosocial Challenges

The impact of physiological trauma influences the self-image, the perception of the meaning and reality of the resultant changes, and the ability to make appropriate adjustments. The regaining of the memory of the self-image and the integration of the past with the present and future is a continual process in rehabilitation that begins in the hospital and often continues throughout the life of the individual. Adjustment to changes in personality often requires specific programs of counseling to work through the emotional distortions experienced and expressed by the patient, family, and friends.

The patient's attitudes toward his or her medical condition and resultant functional abilities, the treatment setting, and the therapist may or may not be revealed on the first contact. Initial observations and evaluations by the therapist reveal information regarding the patient's general affect and behavior; attention span; distractibility; comprehension of oral, written, or demonstrated instructions; and memory of immediate, recent, sequential, or remote information and events. Because mental and physical tolerance may be limited, particularly early in the recovery, attention is focused on facilitating positive performance during evaluation. Techniques are changed or terminated during the session if the patient becomes overly stressed, discouraged, or fatigued. The therapist makes sure that every evaluation period has positive feedback for the patient regarding intact functions and progress.

Interpersonal contact with other patients facilitates the regaining of self-awareness and ego strength needed to meet the functional challenges of disability and to develop a positive self-image needed for meaningful social interaction with family and friends.

Communication Disorders

The ability of the patient to perceive himself or herself as a total functioning and worthwhile being relates to the ability to receive and use messages from the environment through sensory stimuli and through awareness and integrated interpretation of them. With deficits in auditory, language, or intellectual functions, the patient may demonstrate blockage in response to these stimuli. The therapist must determine what messages the patient does receive, to what extent, and how he or she can apply them to function. Accurate assessment of this depends on the creativity and skill of the therapist in using evaluation materials appropriately.

The patient may show deficits in the ability to express himself or herself both verbally and behaviorly in accordance with how he or she feels or with actual abilities. Verbal expression may be limited to uncontrolled, repetitious, or meaningless phrases, causing poor communication and confusion on the part of the patient and the therapist. Generally, the therapist must speak as if the patient has understood verbal communication, even if the patient appears not to understand. Depending on the amount of control the patient has over physical functions, he or she may use this avenue of expression, particularly if he or she has a language deficit.

Keeping in mind the environmental effects on the neurologically impaired patient, the therapist uses auditory stimulation therapeutically during evaluation and treatment. Verbal cues can be used supportively, as reinforcement, and for orientation. In the same manner, socialization can be used for functional auditory discrimination and localization as well as for verbal feedback. Music can be used for relaxation or stimulation during or after effort or as a rhythmic accompaniment to gross motor activity during the use of assistive equipment, such as a support spring suspension sling.

A variety of electronic devices and equipment is available to provide communication assistance for persons without expressive language ability (speech). With the severely physically disabled person in a wheelchair, the first consideration is evaluation of the sitting position and the physical abilities of the head, trunk, and extremities in order to determine the options for control of the devices. Scanning equipment can be mounted on wheelchair lapboards or standard tables, can be portable or console, and may be equipped with head pointers, strip printers, computers, training aids, and visual systems. Electronic aids can be useful in evaluation, training, and working. Catalog addresses are listed in the appendix for reference to these useful items, without which many severely physically disabled persons would have no means of communication or would be left with primitive measures below their intellectual abilities.

Cognitive Distortions and Intellectual Deficits

Cognition is knowledge and understanding of the environment gained through information-processing by the brain. It involves the mechanisms of perception, memory storage and retrieval of information, organization, and language expression. Cognitive behavior is related to the character and effect of interpersonal relationships. Difficulty in handling input of stimuli (reception, interpretation, organization, order of importance) can hinder ability to store necessary information in the brain for retrieval, resulting in poor concentration for intellectual processing or a deficit in long-term memory.

Basic orientation to objects and properties may be hindered by: (1) difficulty in recognition of an object when its position or relationship is changed, (2) lack of understanding of relationships between or among tasks, (3) lack of awareness of a picture, concept, or task, or (4) difficulty in sequencing of steps to complete a task. Deficits in orientation to place and time may accompany lack of insight into the present medical condition and resulting situation. Responding to time and space appropriately requires maintenance of a mental representation of material, leading to visual organization and memory.

When the patient comes for treatment, he or she should be oriented to the occupational therapy room, with furniture, people, and activities being pointed out and identified. The furniture can be used to relate form constancy and color and shape discrimination. Deficits in awareness of body image, movement patterns, and sensorimotor functions may show evidence in the neglect of intact functions. Awareness of the use of the body, neglect of intact functions, and actual use can be determined by the evaluation of sensory and motor functions. The use of the draw-a-person test, figure assembling tests, identification of body parts, and self-care assessment assists in determining the function of the total body awareness.

Activities involving movement that changes the plane of the head or body in space can be used to improve position and space concepts. Among these are games involving spatial concepts: shuffleboard (from the wheelchair or while standing), table shuffleboard, catching a ball or beanbag, hitting a ball suspended with the hand, dancing, or marching.

When denial or neglect of a visual field or extremity is shown, the patient should be encouraged to look at his or her body during exercises and activities. Cutaneous and verbal stimulation can draw attention to the extremity, and the patient should be encouraged to place an arm on the table even though he or she might not be using it actively in a task. Visual tasks such as object assembly, puzzles, reading the newspaper, writing, or copying encourage visual organization.

Before giving tests for visual perception, the therapist determines if the patient wears glasses or has a visual acuity deficiency. The patient is then asked to identify familiar objects or printed words. The therapist determines the patient's accuracy in color, size, and shape discrimination. Tests can be used to evaluate the function of figure ground, spatial relations, and form constancy. The patient is asked to read a sentence written in large letters on an advertisement from a magazine; he or she is asked to write his or her name. This identifies the ability to form letters and to interpret them; reading, writing, and block designs can be used to detect the presence of a field cut or neglect of the visual field.

Ability to write is tested by asking the patient to write his or her name. If the patient is unable to do this, the therapist gives assistance by forming the letters and asking the patient first to trace and then to copy them. Close observation reveals perceptual disorders in spatial relations, directionality, and concepts of form. If the patient is able to write spontaneously, the following activities should be checked: ability to copy letters and numbers, to do simple arithmetical problems, and to answer questions about a written paragraph. Problem-solving and construction abilities can be evaluated by assessing the ability to plan an activity or project and to follow step-by-step procedures to its completion.

Intellectual changes are manifested in decreased memory, inability to abstract quickly, and shortened attention span. A variety of signs of memory dysfunction may be exhibited, such as: (1) shallowness of thought, (2) disorganization or fragmentation of thought, (3) limitation to concrete (rather than abstract) thinking, (4) difficulty in retrieving information, (5) confabulation, (6) tendency to forget in the middle of a thought, (7) confusion of past and recent events, or (8) loss of past and future, with a tendency to live in the moment and general unfamiliarity as to identification

and purpose. Memory may show specific decrease in digit span, auditory and visual retention, awareness of routine and current events, retention of previously learned information, and recollection of personal past events and history. The difficulty in following written or oral instructions may be accompanied by distraction by visual and auditory stimuli, affecting accuracy and thoroughness in intellectual functions and resulting in low activity tolerance.

Sensorimotor Dysfunction

During evaluation and treatment, optimum body positioning is essential. The biomechanical and functional appropriateness of the patient's position for exercise and activity is vital, whether in bed, in a wheelchair or a regular chair, standing, or walking. The therapist should evaluate the patient's balance and awareness of position and then show the patient different positions that may be used comfortably and safely. If necessary, extremities are passively placed in the optimum position for active motion. Among the devices and concepts that aid the patient are: a mirror for visual feedback, use of gravity for ease of movement, repetition of movement for sensory awareness, sensory contact for reinforcement, bilateral use of the extremities for midline crossing and integration of two sides of the body, and supportive devices to minimize fatigue and maximize function.

The therapist touches the patient lightly to determine the patient's perception of the location of tactile stimulus. This is done from distal to proximal, because sensory and motor deficits are usually increasingly impaired from proximal to distal. The patient's vision is occluded. A blindfold should not be used, as this may frighten the patient. The therapist can perform the test either by covering the testing area or by placing the patient's arm under the table while testing, with the therapist sitting opposite the patient.

The patient's fingers are touched with rough and smooth objects to determine texture discrimination; familiar objects of various sizes, shapes, and weights are placed in the hand to determine stereognosis. In the case of hemiplegia, the uninvolved extremity should be checked first so that the patient understands what is being asked; then the affected hand and arm should be checked. This provides some positive input and feedback and encourages the patient regarding intact functions.

The therapist should also observe the position of the limbs at rest for signs of spasticity, edema, muscle weakness, or neglect. These can be noted in the posture of the patient while lying in bed or while sitting.

Safety precautions during motor evaluations are essential. Although the patient may say there are no deficits, the therapist evaluates thoroughly to make certain of the sensorimotor condition. In the assessment of the motor ability, activities can be provided to stimulate strength and coordination and to detect apraxia and more specific motor deficits. The patient's vision should be occluded when evaluating proprioceptive and kinesthetic functions.

The ability to perform the motor act may be more functional when the patient is asked to perform a particular task, such as reaching for an object in the therapist's hand or touching a part of his own body. The therapist evaluates both sides of the patient's body during motor evaluation. Except in cases of bilateral hemiplegia or factors such as previous fractures, arthritis, or neurological problems affecting the sound extremity, bilateral evaluation indicates the impairment on the affected side as compared with the sound side. For the confused patient, checking the passive range of motion of both extremities before requesting active movement may help to give a better understanding of the available range, as well as familiarize the patient with the active movement requested. Patients often do not understand technical terms, and demonstrations of instructions will relieve undesirable anxiety. This technique also helps the apraxic patient, who cannot initiate the voluntary motor act on request, although he or she may have the motor ability to perform the movement.

The therapist checks passive and active range of motion, strength, reflex activity, coordination, proprioceptive and kinesthetic functions, postural reactions, and bilateral coordination. These techniques are modified according to the position of the patient during evaluation.

Gradual controlled increase in stimuli in all activity should be provided. In all task-oriented activity, there is a variety of sensory input: visual, auditory, tactile, proprioceptive, and vestibular. Reinforcement of sensory cues assists memory development and orientation through repetition and familiarity; this increases awareness. Associations should be made between and among activities; for instance, the correlation between vertical–bilateral sanding and pulling up one's pants.

Application of stimuli to the skin of the involved extremity over flaccid muscles, using touch and moderate pressure, can result in improved sensory response and increased motor function. Passive cutaneous stimulation by the therapist, using stroking, pressure, brushing, and object pressure, stimulates sensation. Manipulation of shapes in both the affected and nonaffected hand encourages feedback from the normal extremity. Pressure over the muscle belly, joint, or tendon stimulates individual muscle response. Cutaneous stimulation from tools adapted with surface textures encourages security of grip and sensory stimulation. Rolling in bed during dressing and bathing stimulates body awareness. Self-stimulation and location of the affected extremity during self-care activities encourage range of motion, bilateral awareness and integration, and increased function.

Techniques of inhibition include warmth, slow stroking, gentle shaking or rocking, pressure on the insertion of a muscle, and joint compression. In addition, cool colors; soft, regular rhythms; and soft, even speaking tones can be used.

Biofeedback can be used by qualified therapists to provide motivation for potential movement, a means of facilitating specific weak muscles, relaxation of spastic muscles, and an awareness of muscle improvement or potential. In using biofeedback with activity, the therapist can combine two media effectively to enable the patient to have a more visual concept of muscle function for task completion. Biofeedback is particularly meaningful to the patient who has no sensation of muscle contraction and thus little active input to re-education. Information about which muscles are functioning and how much they are functioning is indicated by the biofeedback machine, as auditory or visual feedback is given in response to muscle contractions. With increased awareness, the patient is motivated to increase muscle activity, thus increasing the response and motivation. Active exercises used in conjunction with the biofeedback machine encourage understanding of muscular gains.

Feedback devices are available to provide the patient with knowledge of the results of muscle contractions not otherwise available to him or her, returning feedback on the performance of an activity. The electrogoniometer can accurately record joint range of motion while the subject is moving that joint. Another feedback device is a pressure-sensitive device which returns a light signal when a programmed amount of pressure is applied and gives a second light signal when a measured increment of pressure is applied. This feedback response may be activation of an electrical appliance rather than a light. Use of these devices provides an objective record of the performance to validate progress.[9]

Disruption of Functional Performance Levels

The loss of functions described in the preceding sections disrupts the performance of daily activities temporarily or permanently, depending on the severity of the trauma. Reattainment of the maximum performance level depends on the involvement of the patient in an activity-oriented rehabilitation program. In such a program, the patient focuses on the activity instead of the specific muscle or extremity function. The goals related to psychosocial, communicative, cognitive, or sensorimotor dysfunction are inherent in the appropriate therapeutic activity designed for the patient; thus, performing the activity should increase functional performance level.

Sensory stimulus is developed through adapted cutaneous contact with tools, the beater of a loom, or the handle of a sander. Sensory discrimination is stimulated through the adapted tools as well as by the use of materials such as clay, sand, or Theraplast. Gross motor reaching and throwing activities to stimulate proprioception and kinesthetic awareness (shuffleboard; beanbag, ball, and dart throwing) are useful. Use of the skateboard attached to the forearm for directed range-of-motion activities stimulates active upper arm movements. Adaptation can be made for holding a pencil and drawing patterns on paper or on a horizontal blackboard during directed skateboard movement.

Suspension slings and pulley systems incorporating weighted or counterbalanced resistance both support weak extremities and facilitate movement. They may be used in conjunction with activities to increase shoulder and elbow function. A functional hand splint may be added to encourage positioning and grasp. Activities such as weaving, woodworking, and, especially, sanding, planing, and filing can be adapted to incorporate movements, with gravity assisting for diagonal patterns and to encourage midline crossing.

Trunk stability and correct positioning are encouraged during all activities. Stability of the trunk and joints proximal to those being used is necessary for self-directed, goal-oriented, coordinated activity.

The self-care evaluation is done in the location and manner in which the patient is comfortable. Evaluation is done in privacy to prevent open discouragement if the patient is not independent in a task he or she previously could perform well. Evaluation of self-feeding skills can be done either in the occupational therapy room or in the patient's room, depending on the patient's desires and mental state. The use of the nondominant, sound extremity may be embarassingly uncoordinated, and practice may be needed to accomplish one-handed self-feeding. It is often desirable for the patient to gain skill in self-feeding before eating in a public place. Evaluation to determine the need for splints, assistive devices, and changes in methods in performing an activity accompanies the assessment of self-care skills. The therapist should observe the performance in self-care activities.

The careful evaluation of all self-care areas is essential to the patient's regaining self-esteem and respect through the retrieval of maximum independent functional ability. Attention to these areas assists the patient in regaining a sense of self-worth as well as in regaining his or her family role.

The provision of splints and slings for the brain-injured patient remains a controversial subject among physicians, occupational therapists, orthotists, and physical therapists. This controversy is caused by the variety of treatment approaches and settings available. Those using sensorimotor facilitation and inhibition techniques tend to discourage traditional splinting, because it may counteract the use of neurophysiological techniques. Use of *appropriate* splinting design is consistent with neurophysiological treatment techniques to reduce hypertonicity.

Splinting has four basic options of application: static or dynamic, volar or dorsal. The provision of assistive devices and splints should be carefully assessed and should correlate with other treatments, thereby providing the patient with the maximum advantage of all treatments and modalities available. When the functional deficits and potentials have been determined through comprehensive physical and sensory evaluation, consideration is given to the need for splinting to assist in restoration of function. Given appropriately, splinting can provide positioning against spasticity and resultant deformity, stimulation to muscle groups, increased sensory awareness, relief of pain or discomfort, and support of weak or malaligned extremities. Splints are generally prescribed to channel or enhance function or to protect nonfunctioning extremities for future functions.

Poorly designed and monitored splints can cause deformities. It is good practice to teach the patient when to wear the splint and when to take it off or to instruct someone else in this procedure. The patient should know the purpose of the splint, be aware of the need to check for pressure areas, and know whom to contact if it is not fitting properly.

In the restoration of upper extremity function, a static cock-up splint may be beneficial to support the weak wrist in a functional position both at rest and during activity. A C bar at the thumb web space to prevent atrophy and tightness provides effective functional positioning. Dynamic splinting using the long opponens with an outrigger system and finger cuffs encourages active use of the fingers during resistive functional exercises to strengthen palmar grasp, opposition, and prehension.

Orthokinetic splinting providing a combination of mobilization and support can be used for (1) relief of pain, (2) increase of muscle strength, (3) increase of range of motion, (4) muscle re-education, and (5) improvement of coordination. This type of splint uses a minimum of static coverage where inhibition is desired and acts as a facilitator of paralyzed extensor muscles through the use of a wide elastic straps over the forearm muscle bellies and tendons. The orthokinetic concept is a dynamic one; its purpose is function rather than immobilization.

An arm sling is commonly used both to support the flaccid arm and to prevent subluxation of the shoulder caused by excess gravitational pull on weak muscles during ambulation. When properly positioned, it also prevents edema of the hand. The patient who uses a wheelchair uses other devices attached to the chair to support and position his or her arm; an overhead suspension sling, a lapboard, an arm trough, or a padded wedge placed on a lapboard can prevent edema of the hand.

Positioning is very important; every effort must be made, both in bed and chair positioning, to prevent edema, contracture, and subluxation in the hand and shoulder. Although the arm sling is an easily recognizable means of support for the paralyzed arm, care must be taken *not* to use a sling that will cause shoulder pain, increase in adductor or flexor spasticity, or shoulder subluxation, which are results of poor design, application, use, or monitoring.

A balanced forearm orthosis or a suspension sling with an overhead bar can be attached to the wheelchair to support the arm and to facilitate movement. Both of these supports provide mobility to the extremity; therefore, it is important before using special equipment to distinguish whether the need is for static or dynamic support.

At times, a sling and a splint can be combined. However, it must always be remembered that patients can be harmed by the use of inappropriate equipment or by prolonged use, which can impede the return of function and maintain the individual at a dependent level.

The occupational therapist may or may not be directly involved in a specific evaluation of a person's fitness for driving following a debilitating disease or injury. Where there is a definite role, protocols are usually spelled out for each team member.

In the routine performance evaluation, the occupational therapist may obtain information relevant to the person's safety in driving with a disability. Such signs are excessive caution, slow reaction time, reduced visual acuity and perception, hearing deficits, tremors, retarded reflexes, and slower adjustment to stimuli. Behavioral changes such as agitation, impatience, impaired memory, spatial disfiguration, or mental confusion can be hazardous in driving. Use of drugs can make the patient susceptable to these impairments mentioned or cause drowsiness or dizziness.

The person who has had a stroke is often anxious to return to driving despite residual deficits, which he or she may or may not acknowledge. Inability to accept dependence on others may prompt the homebound person to resume driving, thus creating a hazard for himself or herself and for other drivers. Deficits in figure ground or color and form discrimination can result in faulty interpretation of signal lights and inability to distinguish these from other visual stimuli. Deficits in auditory discrimination or location can result in lack of pickup of warning horns or cautioning passengers.

Safe driving is the prime concern. Minor driving aids may be advantageous for the driver with cerebral palsy, a limb amputation, hemiplegia, paraplegia, or quadriplegia. Examples of these include steering devices attached to the steering wheel and change of side for the accelerator or gear shift column, turn signals, lights switches, and other controls. For the more severely handicapped person, a variety of hand control designs are available, as are other devices necessary for the person lacking lower or upper extremity mobility. Special adaptations for cars and vans are available, including ramps and lifts for vans, car-top carriers for wheelchairs, and clamp-downs, which permit a person to drive from a wheelchair. The upper extremity-involved driver may be assisted by hand splints to manipulate controls and to maintain grip strength.

Physically, a variety of adaptive devices are available to enable the disabled person to resume driving; however, careful assessment is necessary to determine any psychological or neurological factors that could preclude safety.

The occupational therapist may see the patient initially during the diagnostic period or further along during the course of rehabilitation or maintenance programs. After careful evaluation of abilities and deficits, the occupational therapist plans a program geared toward assisting the patient to achieve the highest functional level and to utilize assistive equipment as necessary to maintain independent and meaningful daily activity. The therapist assists the patient in adjusting to the disease or injury and in realistically accepting the changes. In learning how to adapt to these changes, the patient becomes better able to cope with daily living and planning in a postive way.

Specific Diagnoses and Conditions

Cerebrovascular Accident (CVA, Stroke, Shock)

The cerebrovascular accident (CVA) is a lesion in the brain commonly referred to as a stroke, an insult, or a shock because of its sudden onset. It results in paralysis of one side of the body (hemiplegia) or of both sides (bilateral hemiplegia). The lesion is characterized by an interruption of the blood supply to the brain tissues in a particular location caused by thrombus, embolus, anoxia, hemorrhage, or aneurysm. Precipitating factors may include hypertension, arteriosclerosis, or congenital artery wall weakness. Hypertension and arteriosclerosis contribute to the vessel breakdown or occlusion in the older adult, whereas congenital vascular weakness can result in an aneurysm, a common cause of hemiplegia in the young adult.

Vascular disease can cause a complete CVA with a full picture of hemiplegia or temporary symptoms from a transient ischemic attack (TIA) caused by vascular insufficiency. The TIA may result in brief and spotty impairment of neurological functions; it is frequently a warning of the likelihood of a more serious CVA in the future. The treatment of the patient with either a complete CVA or a TIA should be geared not only toward rehabilitation of the present problem but also toward prophylactic techniques to prevent further TIA or CVA.

Other causes of hemiplegia include external trauma (a blow on the head or striking the head during a fall), heart attack, and brain and spinal tumors. In these cases, the character of the condition may differ slightly from the cerebrovascular lesion, but, because many of the symptoms are similar, evaluation techniques and treatment procedures used in CVA can be applied.

The lesion in the brain that causes hemiplegia usually occurs in one hemisphere and affects the contralateral limbs and face. The result is designated right or left hemiplegia, according to the side of the body involved. It is essential to distinguish between the location of the CVA and the location of the hemiplegia: should the CVA occur in the left hemisphere, the hemiplegia will be on the right side of the body and vice versa.

Depending on which side of the brain is involved, there can be, in addition to motor and sensory deficits, impairment of perceptual and cognitive functions, of premorbid personality, of motor planning and problem-solving abilities, and of judgment (Table 29-2). Uri-

nary continence, motivation, and a sense of social awareness and responsibility may be lost.

A lesion can affect both hemispheres of the brain, causing bilateral clinical signs.

Impact
Whether the person is affected by the sudden onset of an internal CVA or by the shock of external head trauma causing hemiplegia, the results of the condition can have a devastating impact on his or her life. The adult patient may be going to school, completing vocational or academic training in preparation for employment, secure in employment, nearing the peak of vocational goals, nearing retirement, or retired. In all of these situations, the patient may suffer the threat of not returning to the previous lifestyle or occupation. The severity of the brain damage, the premorbid health conditions, the patient's attitude toward the condition and rehabilita-

Table 29-2. *Cerebrovascular Accidents and Their Effects*

Artery	Areas of Brain Affected	Manifestation
Internal carotid	Frontal lobe	Aphasia (dominant hemisphere)
	Parietal lobe	Contralateral hemiplegia
	Temporal lobe	Homonomous hemianopsia
	Internal capsule	
	Optic nerve	
Anterior cerebral	Anterior part of internal capsule	Contralateral monoplegia (leg)
	Tip of frontal lobe	Sensory loss
	Surface of cerebral hemisphere to parietal–occipital junction	Mental confusion
		Apraxia
		Aphasia (dominant hemisphere)
Middle cerebral	Convolutions of cerebral hemisphere	Contralateral hemiplegia (primarily arm)
	Lateral orbital–frontal region	Contralateral facial weakness
	Internal capsule	Aphasia (dominant hemisphere)
	Anterior thalamus	Homonomous hemianopsia
		Sensory loss
Posterior cerebral	Midbrain	Contralateral hemiplegia
	⅔ Temporal lobe	Hemianesthesia
	Middle occipital lobe	Homonomous hemianopsia
	Posterior internal capsule	Ataxia
		Tremor
Basilar	Pons	Symptoms from 3rd to 12th cranial nerves
	Medulla	Loss of proprioception
	Cerebellum	Cerebellar dysfunction
Cerebellar	Midbrain	Cerebellar ataxia
	Pons	Contralateral loss of pain and temperature
	Cerebellum	

tion, the support of the family, and the restoration of various functions are all factors in rehabilitation.

Functional Restoration

Psychosocial. Whereas the patient's developmental level prior to the CVA was that of an adult, the effect of the CVA may reduce the physical and mental levels to those of a child. The patient may be unable to accept the arduous recuperation of lost functions through specific "childlike" activities, such as strengthening of limbs and development of coordination; learning again to read, write, and speak; or developing independence in self-care and toilet functions. Frequently, the patient denies the full implications of self-involvement in the recovery of these functions; the patient may be unable to cope with the multitude of problems facing him or her and his or her family, or the patient may be suffering damage to those brain tissues that control motivation and adjustment. The adult hemiplegic tends to look back to normal functioning and impose premorbid standards on present abilities.

Sensorimotor losses are accompanied by changes in body image and personality, which affect both the patient and the family and can strain their relationship. Confusion resulting from brain trauma can leave the patient unable to establish self-direction and purposeful motivation or to understand simple conversations. The effects on the patient's personality may result in a change in values, affecting the level of performance. Because the older adult suffering a CVA has "all that has been gained to lose," one of the most difficult problems for both the patient and the therapist is overcoming the belief that the patient has "lived his life" and that there is nothing left.

The following factors contribute to disorientation, confusion, malfunction, and lack of progress:
1. Auditory deficit
2. Receptive or expressive aphasia
3. Impairment of spoken or written expression
4. Deficits in learning ability
5. Impairment of previously independent function
6. Denial and neglect of affected extremities and other functional deficits of the condition
7. Distortion of time and place affecting the individual's ability to perceive the future and to plan realistically
8. Loss of tactile sensation and motor function
9. Loss of proprioceptive and kinesthetic awareness, which hinders integration
10. Impaired bilateral extremity function
11. Apraxia (loss of voluntary motor activity), which hinders functional ability and motor improvement
12. Visual–perceptual deficits such as field cut (hemianopsia), visual neglect, or deficits in functional scanning, discrimination of color and form, figure ground

These deficits are not always present, at least not to the same extent.

Mention has been made of the devastating effect of hemiplegia on the person. Not all persons, of course, react in the same way to catastrophic illnesses or disabilities. Often, the reactions reflect premorbid taboos and fears. The patient's gains from rehabilitation are, to some degree, dependent on attitudes developed prior to the CVA.

The patient who is lacking in motivation and is depressed is difficult to rehabilitate and may become a burden to both himself and family. Often, the patient is the breadwinner or the homemaker, and the loss of ability to carry out these responsibilities affects both the patient and the family. The family may suffer financial hardships because of the hospitalization, and this may be a further worry for the patient. At times, the family finds it difficult to function without the hospitalized member and needs counseling to understand the course of rehabilitation and to solve the seemingly insurmountable problems of daily living.

The supportive benefits of group activity can be shared by the patient's learning about individual abilities and limitations in physical, communication, and social skills. In structured group activities, patients have the opportunity of working together in performing body movement exercises, projects, recreational activities, or perceptual games, thus stimulating motivation and encouragement. Group work diminishes fear of personal interaction with family and friends and aids in development of self-awareness and acceptance. Helping team members and receiving help restore self-confidence. In Figure 29-1, the therapist teaches the patient to use bilateral movements to stimulate sensorimotor sensitivity and function, right and left orientation, bilateral use of the arms, and trunk balance. During physical activity, patients talk with each other and the therapist, discuss what they are doing and how, and what they see in the outside environment. Visual perceptual tasks (Fig. 29-2) increase interest in the environment, and the change in atmosphere stimulates new interest and motivation. Group activity aids in integrating sensory, motor, and perceptual skills for improved performance in daily tasks. The peer support gained from group activity is distinct from one-to-one treatment and relates to social skills the patient will need to return home and to the community.

Communication. Both left and right hemiplegic patients show communication disorders in the early stages after CVA; however, the right hemiplegic tends to retain more severe deficits in speech, verbal reception, and language, because a lesion in the dominant hemisphere (usually the left) affects all language areas to some degree. Specific problems that occur are impairment in interpretation of the meaning of spoken and written

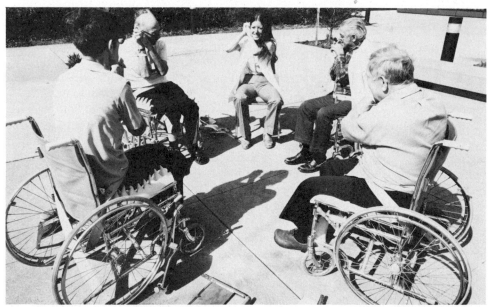

Figure 29-1. Group activity. The therapist demonstrates to patients how to grasp the hemiplegic hand with the sound hand and raise both hands up to touch the right ear. Activity is used for specified body movement and awareness.

words (receptive aphasia), impairment of the ability to use speech and to write communicatively (expressive aphasia), and impairment of motor function of speech (dysarthria). Distorted auditory reception, loss of hearing, and inability to locate auditory stimuli or to make meaning of them can affect the speech response. Apraxia is the impairment of the voluntary ability to use

the speech mechanisms; the patient may possess these functions but be unable to use them. Despite apraxia, the patient may be able to use his tongue, lips, or speech mechanisms for automatic and reflexive actions such as chewing or blowing.

The occupational therapist correlates the use of speech and written language in both instruction giving

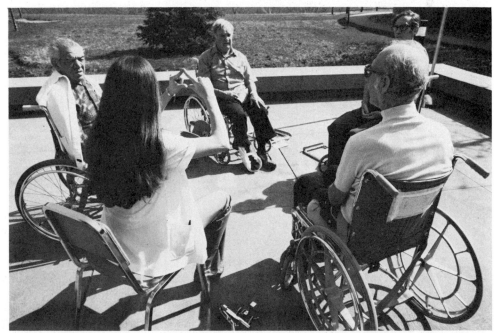

Figure 29-2. Visual perceptual task. The therapist makes the form of a triangle with her fingers and asks the patients to find a similar shape in the environment to stimulate body movement, awareness of the environment, and group interaction.

and writing exercises with the objectives and functional levels recommended by the speech pathologist. Consistency in language development is important for the patient's improvement and self-confidence, as well as for preventing confusion from overstimulation or overexpectation of functional ability.

Cognitive. With the disturbance in sensorimotor reception and expression, the hemiplegic patient frequently demonstrates impairment in abstract reasoning. The severity of this condition depends on the auditory, visual, and tactile abilities that remain intact. Sensory deficits may impede learning through auditory instructions, reading, imitation, and demonstration. The prognosis for restoration of independent function depends on the ability to receive and to organize information for learning and implementation. Careful evaluation of perceptual areas is essential to planning the patient's approaches to learning.

Visual. Double vision (diplopia), loss of half of the visual field (hemianopia), and neglect are three common manifestations of visual impairment. Loss of part of the visual field prevents the patient from seeing objects on

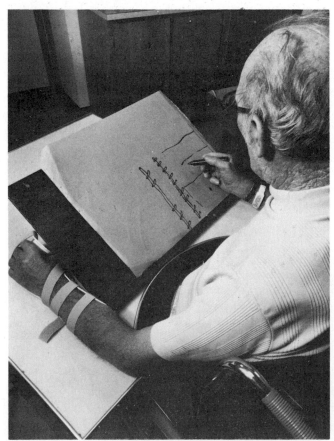

Figure 29-3. Patient with left-sided hemiplegia demonstrates left visual field neglect by drawing only on the right side of the paper.

the right or left side. Patients are unaware of this "cut" in the visual field until they realize that a paragraph makes little sense because they can read only half of it, until they drive their wheelchairs into the side of a doorway, or until they half dress, thinking the task has been completed.

Visual field neglect occurs when the patient ignores visual stimuli on the side of the hemiplegia when confronted with simultaneous stimuli from both visual fields (Fig. 29-3). This occurs when visual fields are intact.[10] Distortions in the perception of spatial relations (vertical, horizontal, oblique) result in difficulty in deriving meaning from visual stimuli and in using this information in intellectual functions.

Although diplopia can be controlled by an eye patch, it is often difficult for the patient to recognize and compensate for a field cut (hemianopia). Visual cues, practice, and memory of turning the head to the side of the limited field may be helpful.

Sensorimotor. A lesion in the brain, usually localized in one hemisphere, impairs motor function on the opposite side of the body. Complete (-plegia) or partial (-paresis) flaccid paralysis of the upper and lower musculature and facial muscles is manifested in the loss of active mobility of the involved extremities. Although passive range of motion is complete initially, gradual onset of spasticity presents the threat of increased muscle tone, impeding active range of motion and causing contractures and deformity. The severity of involvement depends on the location and extent of the lesion. Some patients begin to regain voluntary muscle power a few days following a CVA, whereas others experience no return for months or years and for some, the ability is never regained. Impairment of the dominant extremity necessitates a change of dominance and causes loss of bilateral coordination with a possibility of partial loss of strength and coordination in the sound extremity.

Sensory impairment is manifested in reduced peripheral reception of stimuli, tactile functions in the affected hand, and general sensory awareness. Manifestations of peripheral impairment include lack of sensation of cutaneous stimuli (temperature, touch, pain); inability to locate the area of stimulus; inability to identify the position of the extremity (proprioception); inability to identify a familiar object through tactile sensation (stereognosis); inability to effect the motor act (apraxia); inability to correlate purpose and accomplishment of tasks (ideational apraxia); and inability to carry out new purposeful activities while retaining the ability to perform routine activities (ideomotor apraxia). Lack of sensory functions and impairment of sensory receptors in the extremities affect motor functions by causing lack of feedback. Bilateral integrative functions are also affected by sensory deficits.

In all sensorimotor activities, it is important to evaluate the status of sensation and sensory function in the extremities before initiating exercises, activities, self-care, or splinting. Because one of the objectives of treatment is sensory integration and total body awareness and adaptation, the patient must be informed of the results of the sensorimotor evaluation.

A variety of treatment modalities and approaches is used to aid in the development of isolated and voluntary function of flaccid or spastic extremities. Because synergy patterns may develop following a stroke, the patient may have asymmetrical reflexes and sensorimotor behavior. Treatment techniques stemming from neurophysiological approaches to development of volitional extremity function are effective in occupational therapy programs or in combination with physical therapy. Facilitation and inhibition techniques used appropriately can stimulate independent function.

In the early stage of hemiplegia, the extremity tends to be flaccid, and a major concern is the positioning of the extremity to prevent deformity, contractures resulting from spasticity, and edema. If visual neglect and decreased sensation are present, the patient may be unaware of the arm's position or location. Splinting the extremity helps with visual and sensory awareness of the flaccid extremity and contributes to preventing the above problems. A simple cock-up splint can aid in wrist positioning for functional use of the extremity. A static forearm–hand splint can be used at night and during the day when the patient is not working with the extremity in therapy, functional activities, or self-regulated range-of-motion exercises. Snook suggests the use of a spasticity reduction splint, which incorporates the Bobath technique of using a reflex inhibiting posture (RIP) for positioning, using wrist and thumb extension, finger abduction, and extension of the interphalangeal joints.[13] This splint is designed to provide full pan volar support at fingers and thumb, with dorsal coverage on the forearm and carpal area of the hand. Finger separators are used to maintain finger abduction, with metacarpal flexion at 45° and wrist extension at 30°. A variation of the static forearm–hand pan splint is to set the wrist and fingers at maximum extension abduction stretch beyond the point of spasticity.

The splint is removed periodically for relaxation, inhibition, and facilitation techniques as appropriate to work toward isolated volitional movements. As the patient begins to regain function, the need for a splint is reassessed to determine wearing time and design alteration, allowing the hand freedom during the day for functional activities while maintaining or allowing for regained function.

A variety of splint patterns and recommendations are available for use with the patient with spasticity. In some cases, treatment techniques do not include splinting, and hence splinting should not be used. Attention to consistent and collaborative therapy techniques is essential for optimum success. The splint may or may not be desired in the therapeutic regimen.

Function. With sensory and motor loss in the arm and leg on the affected side of the body, the hemiplegic person functionally becomes one-sided. Activities such as rolling over in bed, eating, dressing, bathing, grooming, and two-handed activities are now limited by the paralysis of an arm and a leg. Not only are the specific peripheral functions impaired, but the sense of integration of the body is also affected. The patient may find it difficult to adjust to a necessary change in hand dominance. Activities requiring total sensorimotor awareness are affected. The patient may deny or neglect the functional implications of this condition and may grow to depend on others for assistance in daily functions and responsibilities. The rehabilitation program is geared both toward maximizing independence and toward family awareness and acceptance of the patient's level of function.

Functional activities for developing abilities are geared to the ability level of the patient in all areas previously mentioned: psychosocial, communication, cognition, visual, and sensorimotor. Treatment is directed toward the following goals:

1. Maximum active range of motion, strength, and coordination of the extremities
2. Maximum volitional unilateral and bilateral function of the upper extremities
3. Maximum independence in self-care activities
4. Use of assistive devices for increased function as needed
5. Awareness and acceptance of functional ability
6. Ability to achieve social interaction and basic communication (verbal or nonverbal)
7. Prevocational and avocational exploration and planning as appropriate

With the left hemiplegic patient, daily exercises and activities are directed toward increasing sensory awareness and carrying over this awareness into self-care functions. Exercises and activities should develop visual and proprioceptive awareness of the involved extremity, encourage turning of the head to the affected side to include the part missing from sight because of field cut or neglect, and increase the patient's proprioceptive awareness of the involved extremity through developing bilateral functions. Although distortion in body image concepts may hinder self-care independence, the practice of self-care techniques and activities can aid awareness and integration of bilateral functions.

The patient whose limitations in function are primarily in the motor areas (flaccid or moderately spastic extremities, for instance) can learn techniques of self-care fairly easily by using the sound extremities to assist the affected ones.

The occupational therapist assists both right and left hemiplegics in self-care feeding, dressing, bathing, and grooming tasks as soon as medically possible and incorporates these skills into the patient's daily program. The patient is also encouraged to use one-handed techniques and assistive devices, such as a rocker knife for cutting meat, Velcro attachments on clothes for ease of fastening, and elastic shoe laces. Bathing and grooming are assisted by long-handled sponges, bath mitts, and adapted nail clippers for one-handed use.

Use of neurophysiologically based movement and balance techniques are correlated with self-care activities to encourage developmental patterns of re-education of function, bilateral awareness, and adaptive behavior.

Family education in the patient's ability level and areas of need for assistance is essential. Sessions with the patient and his or her family help to show the latter what the patient has achieved, can do, and needs help in accomplishing. This helps to assure continuation of the patient's ability level upon return home.

The level of accomplishment in self-care skills and activities of daily living by the hemiplegic patient is largely dependent on *motivational, perceptual, judgmental,* and *sensory-integrative* factors. Although both right and left hemiplegic patients suffer motor paralysis or limitations, there are distinctions in the effects of the locations of the lesions. Functional areas largely affected by a lesion in the right hemisphere of the brain are those involving motivation, perception, judgment, and sensory integration. Therefore, the left hemiplegic patient may deny the affected extremities, have visual or sensory neglect or denial, have distortions in concepts of movement and spatial relations, have lost the concept of the motor act, or lack motivation for self-improvement. These deficits may be more of a hindrance to function than are motor paralysis and physical limitation. The left hemiplegic patient also is more likely to suffer difficulties in tasks such as seeing all the food on the plate or finding eating utensils, grooming the left side of the body, dressing the whole body, or walking than is the right hemiplegic patient. The right hemiplegic person, while also suffering motor paralysis or impairment, usually does not incur the problems with judgment encountered by the left hemiplegic person. However, the right hemiplegic person shows various degrees of communication disability.

The social implications for re-entry into the home and community include adjustment to permanent functional deficits, dependence on assistive equipment (braces, slings, wheelchair), and financial insecurity. The person may no longer be able to drive or to work because of visual and intellectual deficits. Developing a new lifestyle may be necessary.

For the young or middle-aged adult suffering hemiplegia, the effect on vocational potential can be serious, depending on skills previously attained and the impairment of intellectual functions. Return to a previous vocation depends in large measure on the type of job the patient was doing, the patient's status in the company, the understanding of the employer, and the patient's ability to regain salable skills. If return to employment is feasible, the occupational therapist includes prevocational assessment and planning in the treatment program and carefully and realistically assists the patient in reviewing alternatives.

Frequently, job competition is too great for re-entry of the worker with permanent hemiplegia. The worker who is no longer able to pursue a vocation suffers a loss in self-esteem, self-image, and status in the family and society. Prevocational evaluation for alternative job opportunities and training programs to learn new skills then become part of the rehabilitation program.

Head Injury

Head injuries are caused by direct trauma to the skull, with 70% occurring in traffic accidents and falls. Other common causes are industrial accidents, wounds, or direct blows. The resulting trauma includes concussion, contusion, laceration, or compression. Although both skull fractures and brain damage may occur, one can occur without the other. The resultant *state of the brain*, rather than the state of the skull, is the most significant effect of a head injury.

A variety of neurological symptoms and manifestations can result from head injury. Depending on the location and extent of the lesion, the symptoms may be of short duration, latent, or extended over a period of years. The outcome of rehabilitation is also related to the length of time the person was in a coma; the longer the coma, the poorer the prognosis.

Post-trauma manifestations include occasional loss of consciousness, dizziness, headache, or vertigo provoked by sudden changes in position; confusion and disorientation about time and place; convulsions; and emotional reactions such as combativeness. Behavior disturbances may be blatant, particularly during the initial recovery period. Personality disorders, amnesia, and delirium may also occur. These manifestations may be accompanied by intellectual deficits, blindness, diplopia, hemianopsia, olfactory dysfunction, and auditory deficits. Physical symptoms include quadriparesis, unilateral or bilateral hemiparesis, initial decerebrate rigidity, and speech deficits. Restoration of functional, intellectual, social, psychological, and physical manifestations may require years if the injury was severe.

The patient may demonstrate physical and mental deficits similar to those of a person who has suffered CVA: cognitive–perceptual–motor dysfunction, spasticity, disorientation, speech deficits, and disturbance of sensory motor integration. Mental manifestation and

Chapter 29 Functional Restoration: Neurologic, Orthopedic, and Arthritic Conditions **475**

personality changes are often more pronounced than those seen in CVA, even though these patients are generally much younger than the stroke victim. These deficits prevent the head-injured person from effectively interacting with the environment and may hinder rehabilitation. The patient may seem to have lost contact with his or her surroundings and to be able to focus only on the narrow, yet overwhelming, feelings, concerns, and behaviors imposed by the sudden disability.

The functional problems of the patient with brain injury fall into four general categories: (1) cognitive, (2) behavioral and emotional, (3) communicative, and (4) physical. The clinical picture represents a pattern of fluctuating symptoms in these areas, subject to frequent change influenced by internal and external stimuli. This fluctuation is evident throughout the recovery as the patient tries to adjust to the deficits imposed by the injury, to learn to decrease and eliminate handicapping effects, and to renew self-confidence through awareness and acceptance of the immediate and future level of function. In the early stages, therapeutic support during unknown or confusing occurrences is needed to allay anxiety until the patient gradually regains conscious control of feelings, behaviors, motivation, abilities, relationships, and daily activities.

Impact

The trauma of head injury causes significant personal impact. The patient must deal with the residual manifestations with whatever assets can be retrieved from the premorbid life experience. The following areas are common rehabilitation challenges of the brain-injured patient and are described briefly to give a general clinical picture of this patient; it must be remembered that not all patients show the symptoms, nor do they show them to the same extent. Premorbid characteristics of lifestyle, body health and type, achievement, attitudes, and goals may positively or negatively affect the functional outcome. Also, since many head injuries are caused by traffic accidents and falls, there may be accompanying physical disabilities, such as amputations, peripheral nerve injuries, paralysis, or fractures that add to the complexity of adequate treatment.

The long-term impact of brain injury may interfere with learning ability, cognitive integration, social interaction and status, self-esteem, and motivation for personal goal setting and achievement.

Functional Restoration

Recovery scales have been developed in an attempt to determine prognosis and to outline programs appropriate to the patient's abilities. Information from these scales aids in the coordination of goals and methods used by team members. There is some tendency to model scales on the developmental patterns of cognitive

or intellectual function, behavior, and social, motivational, and motor levels.

The DARSHI method (Developmental Assessment of Recovery from Serious Head Injury) uses four chronological segments of development to determine areas and levels of function:

1. 0–4 years, using functions from infant scales
2. 4–8 years, using items from the Stanford–Binet Intelligence Scale
3. 8–12 years, using tests for basic information processing, including sequencing, left and right differentation, and visual perception
4. Mature adaptive function, including concepts, skills, and information processing related to daily activity performance[5]

The Disability Rating Scale (DR) uses the following six categories from the Glasgow Coma Scale to rate the head injury according to specific functional area: (1) eye opening, (2) verbalization, (3) motor response, (4) feeding, (5) toileting, (6) grooming, (7) level of functioning, and (8) employability.[11] The Glasgow Coma Scale indicates eye, motor, and verbal response levels, whereas the Glasgow Outcome Scale consists of five stages related to the ability to work: (1) death, (2) persistent vegetative state, (3) severe physical and mental disability (cannot work), (4) moderate disability, (5) good recovery with continuing emotional problems but can work.[7,8]

Eson and colleagues state that the quality of neuropsychological recovery is highly variable in rate, pattern, and level of recovery of adaptive function. Levels of adaptive function are defined as follows: *early*—activities of daily living, self-care, and rudimentary social interaction; *middle*—conceptual and information-processing skills needed for social interaction and ability to initiate and carry out sustained, planned activities directed toward a goal; and *complete or near complete*—ability to seek and maintain employment and to participate in normal adult social and recreational activities without supervision.[5]

In the effort to plan and implement effective and appropriate rehabilitation for the brain-injured person, a variety of approaches have been developed by professional teams and researchers. Whatever the structure or organization of methods of treatment used by the occupational therapist, it is essential that they relate meaningfully to programs and techniques used by others in the daily care of the patient.

The program at Loewenstein Hospital Rehabilitation Center identifies three stages relative to the medical picture based on behavioral characteristics. The first phase is postcoma, characterized by dream-like disorientation in time and space, causing disturbances in establishing order and relationships within environmental stimuli. The second stage is behavioral, characterized by increasing consciousness of the outside world but continuing disturbance in interpreting and handling stimuli, resulting in anxiety and stress fatigue. In the third phase, the patient begins to enter a period of realism and experiences a series of conflicting but realistic changes in self-awareness, which result in a variety of emotional responses. During this stage, the struggle to identify with the external environment satisfactorily and functionally and to integrate external and internal experiences and meanings occurs.[14]

In its approach to rehabilitative management, the Rancho Los Amigos Hospital program describes eight progressive levels of cognitive functioning and behavioral responses based on developmental order: (1) no response (coma), (2) generalized response (inconsistent and nonpurposeful), (3) localized response (specific but inconsistent response to stimuli), (4) confused-agitated (heightened state of activity with decreased ability to process information), (5) confused, inappropriate, non-agitated, (6) confused-appropriate, (7) automatic-appropriate, (8) purposeful and appropriate. Beginning with the initial assessment, the treatment team determines at which level the patient is functioning and then administers treatment in accordance with this developmental pattern.[6]

The occupational therapy approach will depend on the rehabilitation program in the individual setting and the use of such scales as mentioned above.

In preparing for the functional assessment of the brain-injured patient, the therapist must think of the long-term effects of short-term care. This begins with the patient's first contact with the therapist. The initial interview should take place in an area physically comfortable, with few auditory and visual distractions. Input received during early periods may be stored for future use when the patient is more capable of volitional behavior; however, it is important to control the environmental input according to the patient's level of receptivity. Attention to therapeutic and functional positioning informs the patient of the therapist's concern for comfort, as well as conveying the expectation of active, functional use of his or her body. Repeated abnormal functioning can contribute to later weakness and deformities of both the trunk and the extremities.

Having evaluated the effect of the physical environment, the therapist observes the patient's social reactions to the therapist and to other people in the area. Through discussion with the patient and family, the therapist obtains a picture of what the patient was like premorbidly. This information helps in planning therapeutic programs related to the patient's interests. It is also important to know what accomplishments, failures, dreams, plans, and specific areas of activity played a significant role in the personal and social life prior to the head injury. Since the patient may suffer amnesia with regard to information about premorbid life or the injury,

or experience language deficits resulting in reception or expression inadequacies, questions regarding these areas may cause anxiety, irritability, or confusion. Gentle encouragement to discuss the accident assists the patient in clarifying and accepting the medical situation and in understanding why he or she is receiving treatment. This helps prevent the build-up of anxieties regarding the unknowns of the past, present, and future by providing an outlet for self-expression and discussion of changing feelings and concerns. In questioning the patient about the accident, the therapist provides the patient an opportunity to tell his or her side providing a check on the patient's accuracy of information.

The patient may experience the following symptoms during initial evaluation and treatment:

1. Postural dizziness: sensation of dizziness or disorientation caused by change of position or quick movements of the head; dizziness may also result from exertion or fatigue
2. Headache: intermittent or persistent headache, pain, feeling of pressure in the head
3. Fatigue: related to extent and length of time of physical or mental effort during activity
4. Eye strain: due to intensive light, contrasting colors, or movement of visual stimuli, weakness in focus or interpretation
5. Hypersensitivity to sudden, loud, or multiple noises or movements in the immediate physical area

The point at which the patient is seen by the therapist—in the acute stage of trauma, the early rehabilitation phase, the outpatient stage, or during home treatment—will determine the nature and extent of evaluation and the treatment progams appropriate. At all levels, continual communication between the therapist and the patient is essential with regard to changes in the treatment goals, progress, and his or her motivation and goals.

As noted above, treatment begins with assessment of a communication method, of sensorimotor deficits, orientation, and functional ability. The patient is then treated *symptomatically*, with the program directed toward self-awareness, awareness of objects, and initiation and accomplishment of purposeful activity. Development of motor strength and coordination is combined with activities to encourage social awareness and interaction with others. Graded intellectual and problem-solving tasks (reading, arithmetic, and writing) aid the patient in regaining function.

Treatment may begin with basic visual and tactile discrimination and sensorimotor activities such as self-care skills, exercise, activities, and games. Initially, the occupational therapist works with the patient in quiet surroundings, gradually increasing the auditory and visual stimuli. The patient is provided with activity simple enough to hold his or her interest. As physical and mental tolerance increase, the therapist can expand the complexity of the environment.

Psychosocial. The clinical response may be characterized by bewilderment, confusion, denial, anger, complacency, or hostility, with fluctuating changes in behavior related to the individual stage of self-awareness and the level of adaptation to self and environment. Short-term or chronic personality changes may occur, beginning with denial and vagueness in response or with hyperactivity, depending on the level of consciousness and the severity of injury to brain tissue. Disturbance in the ability to relate to the environment outside of himself and to time outside of the present may be apparent. Expressed desires and needs may relate to self-concerns and comforts.

The patient may represent a totally new person to his or her family. The therapist learns about the patient *as the person he or she has become* and is challenged to help the family understand and accept the person the patient now is. The family helps the therapist learn what type of person the patient was premorbidly so the therapist will understand the amount and type of change both the family and the patient are experiencing post-trauma.

The patient may demonstrate loss of inhibitions, distortions in judgment, personality changes, and denial of reality. He or she may lack awareness of the meaning of the present situation. Since the patient may be unable to differentiate appropriate and nonappropriate social behavior, he or she may benefit from techniques such as behavior modification, group process, reality orientation, and other psychodynamic methods of social adjustment and self-awareness.

In working with the patient suffering manifestations of brain injury, it is important to provide an atmosphere free from overwhelming and confusing input and challenges to the sensory systems. Reassurance regarding the program's content, duration, and expectations helps the patient relax enough to respond to specific treatment techniques. The therapist can limit anxiety by talking about the physical surroundings, what is going on, and feelings about where she or he is, what she or he is doing, and how she or he is doing. This helps with reality orientation, resocialization, and environmental adaptation.

Working through the stages of denial, anger, and depression to self-awareness and acceptance requires physical and emotional endurance and often results in fatigue or decreased motivation for continuing the struggle. When the patient is able and ready to begin to deal with the realities of the situation, discussions with the therapist about the injury help reassure the patient and may clarify what has happened, put present and future goals and concerns into perspective, promote self-understanding, and help the patient adjust to changes. As adjustment occurs, the patient is able to take on more responsibility in decision-making by planning and implementing daily schedules and evaluating progress.

The patient may have difficulty in adapting to people and things and may deny reality, forcing others to relate to him or her. Disturbance in self-awareness may allow fantasizing regarding both condition and behavior, and feelings of unfairness regarding the condition may be expressed. Striving for stability and control, the patient may react poorly to change and time, showing a tendency toward minimal social initiative, occasionally showing suspicion of other people who are attempting to help. Disorder in judgment may contribute to an emphasis on physical problems rather than on psychological difficulties relating to cognition and behavior.

Self-awareness develops through active involvement of the mind and body. Task-oriented individual and group projects can provide opportunities to develop and practice abilities and to reintegrate the positive and negative aspects of functioning. Group projects can extend participation in and responsibility for social activities by demonstrating productivity and skill. Group discussions provide social feedback as to acceptable and nonacceptable behaviors and provide opportunities to change behavior as necessary or desired.

The use of videotaping during activity gives the patient a visual picture of his or her physical and social behavior, which can be viewed privately, critically, and objectively. In viewing the group, the patient is able to distinguish between himself or herself and others and to engage in cognitive development. Working within the group helps the patient practice social skills useful in developing and maintaining successful contacts with family members, friends, and strangers.

Social awareness, visual tolerance, concentration, and cognitive functioning and adaptation are stimulated by participating in group discussions and activities, listening to the radio, watching television, playing electronic games, reading books, and reading the newspaper. Gradual increase in responsibility in social and productive activities helps to increase familiarity and function in the environment. In the rehabilitation process, it is important for the patient to be able to adapt to the distractions of the unfamiliar environments in the community in order to be socially adjusted and independent.

Communication. In using language to communicate with the patient and to stimulate functional response, it is essential that the occupational therapist follow the guidance of the speech pathologist in order to maintain consistency in the aspects and levels of the patient's language development.

Finding a means of response is the initial task of the occupational therapist. Use of physical demonstration followed by imitation by the patient may provide a means of communication for the patient with severe language deficits. Although unable to respond orally, the patient may be able to read and write words or symbols.

The patient who is unable to engage in normal verbal communication is often denied satisfying social interaction and opportunities for personal, educational, and social development. Selection of appropriate equipment for functional communication is preceded by an evaluation of other equipment being used, the cognitive level of function, and optimum body positioning.

Electronic and battery-operated communication aids can assist in the evaluation of deficits as well as in retraining programs to develop skills to apply to educational, vocational, and avocational pursuits. These aids are equipped with computer mechanisms providing feedback through a visual or auditory signal, indicating physical and cognitive functional abilities and levels. Devices can be activated by a variety of sources (head turning, mouthstick, light touch, breath control, muscle contractions, and pointing). Use of communication aids by the occupational therapist reinforces the efforts of the speech pathologist in developing physical and cognitive skills and in providing consistency of newly learned techniques. Head sets are useful in minimizing auditory distractions during retraining.

The occupational therapist provides input to the rehabilitation team regarding physical range of motion, strength, coordination, and endurance needed to activate the equipment, as well as with regard to the patient's ability to scan visual input effectively for use of the device. Strip printers or a typewriter may be included to provide additional feedback.

With the development of computer systems, electronic aids are increasingly available and adaptable to the disabled person in treatment, at home, or at work. The use of electronic games assists both the child and the adult in adaptation of these systems for practical purposes. A variety of communication aids can be mounted on a wheelchair or on a desk table and can be powered by rechargeable batteries for practical use. Specific information is available in equipment catalogues and from organizations, some of which are listed in Appendix J.

Cognitive. Memory deficits may prevent the patient from remembering or recognizing people or events from day to day; therefore, continual repetition of tasks and symbols might be necessary until memory is extended. Establishing routines of activity and expecting the patient to perform in consistent patterns may be useful, as may behavior modification techniques.

Memory is needed for visualization and learning. In working with a patient with a memory deficit, attention is given to determining the number of steps in a task the patient is able to store and retrieve. Exercises can be devised to test and practice memory for past events, types of things remembered, retention time, and carry-over to future planning. Planning and scheduling practice are increased by individual and group exercises in visualization of current events, future events, and carry-over from the day with application to planning. Organization of time is improved by the patient's taking responsibility for scheduling daily activities, accepting responsibilities with time limits, achieving carryover of activities, and reinforcing time and space concepts.

The level of mental tolerance is related to motivation, functional deficits, and amount of adaptation required to carry out instructions. The patient may display a short attention span, distractibility, and fear of insanity, particularly when blindness, disorientation, amnesia, or a combination of physical, psychological, and intellectual manifestations are present. Techniques to increase mental tolerance include relating a task to an interest area (sports, reading, cooking, or puzzles), using repetition to provide practice of specific skills to reinforce methods of performance, and providing feedback regarding ability. The program should be graded to gradually increase skill and challenge and should use time blocks to increase physical and mental tolerance. Through the therapeutic group experience, the patient gains a broader social reality focus, learns coping skills for working with others, and practices assertiveness training for self-confidence.

Performance may be hindered by general limitations in adjusting to environmental stimuli. Controlling such strong stimuli as the bright light of the sun, loud or sudden noises, or the distracting sounds of people talking is useful. For maximum selective response to the therapist, the patient may initially require an area void of visual and auditory stimuli. As tolerance for stimuli increases, the therapist gives meaning and relevance to gradually increased stimuli and assists the patient in focusing attention while in the presence of distracting sights and sounds.

Sensorimotor. The patient may be initially defensive tactually, hypersensitive, or apraxic or may demonstrate lack of coordination caused by tremor or ataxia. Spasticity may develop later in the recuperation period. Evaluation of reflex patterns revealing abnormal tone in the brain-injured patient shows three major patterns: (1) decerebrate rigidity or extensor pattern of all extremities, (2) decorticate rigidity flexor pattern in the arms, (3) a mixed pattern of upper extremity flexion and lower extremity extension. Increased muscle tone produces trunk rigidity, which may result in poor sitting balance.

Lack of control of the trunk muscles may also result in poor sitting patterns. The patient may be sensitive to touch and may lack volitional movement.

Before functional activity programs focusing on the upper extremities can be carried out effectively, the patient must be able to maintain a functional sitting position and balance without using the arms for support. Special equipment may be necessary to achieve this, including aids for position and control. Neurophysiological therapy techniques assist the patient in regaining head control, trunk rotation, equilibrium, trunk extension, trunk balance, and arm relaxation for independent isolated control and function.

Function. Since a patient commonly uses denial to avoid seeing the reality of an imposed traumatic situation, involvement in activity programs not only helps to increase strength, joint range of motion, coordination, and cognitive function but also provides feedback to the patient regarding his or her actual abilities. The focus is on the *increase in ability*. Activities are chosen to provide the patient the means to express anger and hostility, as well as to assist in the development of speed, accuracy, and competence in productive accomplishment of specific tasks.

Participation in individual and group physical activities assists the patient in adapting to and overcoming the effects of dizziness. Activities that necessitate changing body position in space (woodworking, gardening, shuffleboard, and ping pong) help in vestibular adaptation. Specific physical activities provide increased self-awareness and self-worth through increases in joint range of motion, strength, and coordination. The programs must be correlated with other functional areas such as perception, social interaction, behavior, and tolerance of environmental stimuli. In preparing for discharge, the patient needs to know what he or she can and cannot do safely and competently. The patient develops and practices physical functions in a compatible, supportive environment, encouraged to learn adaptation when necessary. Decreasing such symptoms as spasticity, contracture, apraxia, tremor, and pain is part of the physical restoration program used to increase functional abilities.

While in a treatment setting, the patient learns how to live in a controlled and structured environment. In preparation for discharge, the patient must learn how to adapt to other environments as well as how to exercise control over his or her goals and behaviors and plan daily activities and responsibilities. Independent attitudes and functions begin as self-care skills are developed, and the patient progresses to being responsible for scheduling time and organizing activities. The patient chooses clothes and retrieves them from drawers and closets and takes care of grooming and other needs preparatory for daily activities. Independence in the structured treatment setting prepares the person for discharge planning.

Other commonly needed skills, including using a pay phone and telephone book, reading a map, listening to and following directions, organizing appointments, applying for a job, and using a newspaper, can be practiced during individual and group outings.

The patient may maintain the delusion that going home will improve the condition or, conversely, that he or she is unwanted or unneeded at home. Family awareness of residual impairments and needs at discharge from the formal rehabilitation program is encouraged in predischarge orientation and guidance sessions. By attending predischarge therapy and group sessions with the patient and the therapists, the family members can see how they can assist with the program and how to welcome the patient back into family life. Sharing in group sessions with other families is helpful to both the family and the patient.

Family orientation to specific problems (memory deficits, reduced tolerance of external stimuli, physical or communications problems) is important before the patient begins resocialization with weekend visits at home. These visits often show the family and the patient both what has been accomplished and how much work remains to be done.

Outings from the treatment center or from home help the patient assume socially appropriate behavior regarding activities and interaction with others. Such activities may include those available through adult programs or church groups. Community activities include such familiar tasks as crossing streets, using money, finding restrooms, reading menus, ordering food, buying things in a store, and paying bills. Trials in doing these things help the patient to communicate and use patience with others.

The patient's educational and employment goals depend on overcoming intellectual and judgmental deficits as well as developing integrative abilities. Learning, retraining, work adjustment, and development of social skills and work habits may be necessary for vocational readiness.

The level of pretrauma intellectual functioning and the achieved educational level affect the regaining of vocational potential. In regaining the ability to return to work, the brain-injured person is more likely to be hindered by cognitive, behavior, and social difficulties in performance than by physical deficits. Regaining a positive self-image, independence in self-care, physical and mental tolerance, successful social contact and interaction, capability in cognitive and intellectual functioning, and acceptable work habits all contribute to vocational potential for the well-motivated person.

During functional retraining, the patient with vocational potential is provided with opportunities to work on familiar skills and those needed for his or her job. Levels of cognitive, social, behavioral, and physical function are determined through prevocational assessment techniques to evaluate the need for retraining or vocational redirection.

Return to work may begin on a part-time basis. Retraining and relocating may be necessary to ensure employment of the patient able to work in some capacity but unable to return to a previous occupation at the earlier level of performance. Although premature return to work requiring strenuous physical or mental effort is strongly discouraged, too long a rest from the routine of work may be detrimental to the person capable of employment.

Outpatient follow-up provides physical and psychological support during the transition from hospital or rehabilitation center to family and community reentry. Through this type of program, the patient can continue a therapy program outside the structured setting. This may help in adjusting to less structured surroundings and aid in developing confidence to plan daily activities and responsibilities.

Multiple Sclerosis

Multiple or disseminated sclerosis is a progressive disease of the nervous system. It begins with the destruction of the myelin sheath covering the nerve fibers, which interferes with the transmission of impulses and results in fatigue. The degenerated sheath is replaced eventually by sclerotic plaques or patches that affect the white matter of the brain and spinal cord. These plaques may also be found in the gray matter of the cerebral cortex and in the cranial and spinal cord roots.[4]

Impact

Characterized by intermittent exacerbations and remissions, MS may pursue its unpredictable course for many years. It usually affects young adults (ages 20 to 40) during their period of greatest potential and productivity. Although the cause of the disease is unknown, viral infections, pregnancy, surgery, and trauma may be precipitating factors. Change in climate, fatigue from overwork, and poor dietary habits have also been implicated. Nervous tension and irritability may precede the onset of physical symptoms, which may vary in intensity, character, duration, and location.

The clinical picture may be hemiplegia, paraplegia, or quadriplegia, and the patient's prognosis and life span are variable. Although the average life span of a person with MS may be 20 years, it can range from 3 months to 40 years; remissions can last as long as 25 years.[2] There may be long and almost complete remissions in the early stages of the disease. However, after middle age, the disease often progresses.

Symptoms appear in two general modes. The first is characterized by a single lesion or several isolated lesions that result in neuritis, double vision, weakness in a limb, or numbness in a part of the body. The second is insidious and is manifested as a slowly progressive weakness of one or all limbs. Accompanying spinal symptoms include spastic paraplegia, superficial sensory loss in the lower limbs and trunk, impairment of postural sensibility and sense of vibration, and spastic/ataxic gait.[2] Decreased sexuality, loss of self-esteem, and anxiety may be evident.

Common early signs of MS include nystagmus (lateral oscillation of an eye to one or both sides), slight intention tremor in one or both upper limbs, and exaggeration of tendon reflexes. These initial symptoms may disappear over a period of weeks or months, leaving only slight residual physical signs; however, the cumulative effects of multiple lesions later cause permanent changes in personality.[2]

The symptoms of advanced MS include scanning or staccato speech and slurring of syllables, nystagmus, dissociation of conjugate lateral movement of the eyes, weak and grossly ataxic upper limbs, paraplegia, contractures, sensory loss, incontinence, episodes of euphoria and depression, irritability, impairment of postural sensibility, and astereognosis.

Although muscular wasting or atrophy are rare, motor weakness may appear in the extremities, trunk, and face. The patient may experience a feeling of heaviness in the spastic extremities and may lose postural sensibility in limbs and trunk.

Incoordination is a frequent problem for the patient with MS. Intention tremor on involuntary movement is accompanied by muscle imbalance in hands and arms, and the tremor may develop in head movements during the later stages of the disease. When the patient must perform tasks requiring accurate movement, the tremor may increase, resulting in incoordination. Ataxia is evident in the gross movements of both the upper and the lower extremities.

The patient suffers sensory deficits manifested by numbness, impairment of positional and joint sense, fine tactile discrimination, hypersensitivity to contact, impaired postural sensibility and vibration sense, and astereognosis.

The ability to communicate orally may be hindered by dysarthria caused by spastic weakness or ataxia of the muscles of articulation. In some instances, the speech impairment may become so severe as to render the patient unintelligible.

In some cases, the patient with MS displays only ocular symptoms for many years. Although the patient's vision usually improves within a few weeks of the initial onset of symptoms, residual damage to the optic nerve is manifested in atrophy. Sporadic unilateral blindness or diplopia may occur.

Treatment includes graded resistive exercises to increase strength and coordination, gross motor activities to encourage general mobility and to increase chest excursion, fine patterns of movement for maintenance of productive abilities, maximum independence in self-care and ADL, and encouragement of motivation, self-esteem, and socialization.

Because the gradual development of rigidity and immobility are characteristic of Parkinson's disease, auditory stimulation such as music can be used to encourage body mobility through rhythmic marching, dancing, clapping, and singing, either individually or in groups. Participation in groups also provides needed support and encouragement to maintain mobility in spite of continuing symptoms.

Sports can be used for motivation, socialization, and movement; ball-throwing, ping pong, darts, and shuffleboard also increase strength and speed of movement in all extremities. In gross motor activities, balance, coordination, and breathing patterns are emphasized.

Manual activities can be used to maintain gross and fine coordination, strength, and concentration, since these are required for general self-care functions. Activities should be designed to encourage good posture, increase mobility, and stimulate successful accomplishment. Manual activities can also be related to assessing and developing vocational skills to enable the patients to keep their jobs. Although patients may experience a change in job activities or responsibilities, it is essential to maintain their daily work status as long as possible.

Broadening of social contact and activity interests helps encourage continuing mobility and productivity programs at home. Patient and family education aids in assuring the continuation of these activities. In order to assist the family and the patient in planning daily activity programs, the therapist can guide them to the resources of the National Parkinson Foundation, which is a valuable organization for the consumer, providing helpful information on the disease, on exercise, and on activities to maintain mobility.

Summary of Care for Patients with Brain Lesions

Lesions in the brain can result from trauma such as head injury or cerebrovascular accident and from disease such as multiple sclerosis and Parkinson's disease. Lesions can produce temporary or permanent functional deficits. The onset can be sudden or progressive. The particular clinical manifestations, in the form of dysfunction, depend on the part of the brain affected by the trauma or lesion. Symptoms that are commonly manifested, either temporarily or permanently, are personality and behavior changes resulting in psychosocial challenges, cognitive distortions, and intellectual deficits; sensorimotor dysfunction; and disruption of functional performance. Deficits in these areas can have a significant impact on the future functioning of the individual and may require lifestyle changes with regard to family and community life.

Treatment programs directed toward functional restoration and adaptive living begin with the hospitalization in the acute phase and progress through intensive rehabilitation to home assessment and carryover of therapeutic programs. Outpatient therapy and follow-up visits complete the medical monitoring of short-term care and become a pattern for the intermittent care of residual problems or exacerbations of progressive diseases. Effective functional restoration depends equally on psychosocial and physical rehabilitation. The occupational therapist makes an essential contribution in providing the patient with opportunities to develop the maximum level of functional ability, self-awareness, and acceptance through individual and social interaction and daily activity in the therapeutic environment. Programs are individually designed with the patient for maximum effectiveness.

Lesions in the Spinal Cord and Nerve Roots

Lesions in the spinal cord can be caused by both disease and trauma. One of the diseases is amyotrophic lateral sclerosis, in which the motor nuclei of the medulla, the corticospinal tracts, and the anterior horn cells of the spinal cord are involved. In poliomyelitis, the anterior horn cells are affected, and in Guillain–Barré syndrome, the lesion is in the nerve roots with possible lesions in the peripheral and cranial nerves. Of these lesions of the spinal cord, ALS is the only progressive disease. There is a high recuperative potential in Guillain–Barré syndrome, with minimal residual disability and the full benefits of high patient motivation and effort and an optimum formal rehabilitation program. In contrast, the recuperative expectation from polio is low, with permanent disability in the affected areas. Spinal ataxia or incoordination in the limbs may result from lesions in the spinal nerve roots. Clinical manifestations are stationary signs of sensorimotor and physiologic dysfunction which may involve the respiratory system, bowel, and bladder. These lower motor neuron diseases (LMN) are usually systemic and symmetric with the exception of polio, where widely scattered manifestations may be found in the limbs. LMN lesions result in loss of voluntary function, flaccid paralysis, sensory loss, and atrophy.

Injury to the spinal cord can result from transection, puncture, laceration, or compression caused by vertebral fracture or dislocation, which cuts or presses on the cord, or by a tumor. Upper motor neuron (UMN) clinical signs of spasticity are present. The manifestations are nonprogressive except in cases of secondary injury, and the extent of recuperation depends on the location and extent of damage. All of the diseases and trauma states mentioned above exhibit immediate sensorimotor and physiologic manifestations relative to the site and extent of the lesion(s).

Amyotrophic Lateral Sclerosis

ALS is a chronic systemic disease of unknown cause that affects the corticospinal system from the cortex to the periphery. It is characterized by degenerative changes that are most evident in the anterior horn cells of the spinal cord, motor nuclei of the medulla, and corticospinal tracts. The loss of nerve cells causes progressive wasting of the muscles, particularly those in the upper extremities and those innervated by the medulla.[4] The onset of ALS is gradual, and the disease is steadily progressive, with death generally within 1 to 6 years.[1] It is nonhereditary.

Impact

The symptoms may first occur either in muscles most used by the patient in his or her occupation or at the site of an injury.[4] Muscular atrophy usually begins in the intrinsic muscles of the hands and the arm musculature; the patient complains of weakness, stiffness, and clumsiness of the fingers. Although the onset usually is centered symmetrically in the upper extremities, it can vary in location and severity. Thenar and finger flexor atrophy generally precede atrophy of the extensors.

Weakness extends proximally from the hands to the shoulders. From the shoulders, the weakness moves to the tongue, where atrophy and paresis of the lips, tongue, and palate cause slurred speech, which eventually becomes unintelligible. The ability to swallow is also affected. As the extensors become involved, weakness in the trunk, loss of head control, and lower extremity paralysis occur; eventually, all reflexes are lost.

Functional Restoration

ALS is treated symptomatically to maintain nutrition, to prevent fatigue, to prevent respiratory infections, and to avoid exposure to cold. Drugs can be used to control problems in swallowing, spasticity, and respiratory and urinary infections.

The rehabilitation program includes moderate activity to maintain strength through muscle re-education and passive exercises to prevent contractures. The exercise program provides relaxation and alleviation of spasticity. Self-care techniques require the use of assis-

tive devices to substitute for the gradual loss of motor function, including respiratory failure. Gait training with braces is used when the patient can tolerate standing.

The occupational therapist provides both physical and psychological assistance in the development of coping skills. Therapeutic techniques and activities should be used with care to maximize functional benefit and minimize fatigue. Passive range of motion by the occupational therapist can provide relaxation in addition to maintaining maximum range of motion in the joints. The passive range-of-motion exercises should be followed by a short, active exercise period determined by the patient's muscle power.

Assistive equipment can help the patient retain as much function as possible and remain active as long as possible. A wheelchair, suspension slings, arm supports, and positioning aids can stimulate the patient to socialize, to care for himself or herself, and to engage in activities that provide a day-to-day enjoyment of life. Environmental control systems or attendant care may be necessary in the later stages of ALS, as the patient loses mobility in the extremities.

Poliomyelitis

Because of the extensive use of effective vaccines, poliomyelitis is no longer prevalent in children's hospitals or in adult rehabilitation centers. However, the occupational therapist occasionally encounters a patient who has had polio, which complicates the current admission for treatment. Also, in a prevocational or vocational program, the therapist may need to evaluate the functional ability of a client who has had polio.

Polio, an LMN lesion, is an acute infectious disease caused by a virus that can affect the anterior horn cells of the gray matter of the spinal cord and the motor nuclei of the brain stem.[2] The result is immediate widespread or localized muscular paralysis with subsequent atrophy. The paralysis may be asymmetrical and patchy, resulting in long-term paralysis in some muscles of one limb but not in others, causing an imbalance. Although the lower limbs are more often affected than the upper limbs, there may be complete or partial monoplegia, hemiplegia, paraplegia, or quadriplegia. Sensation is intact.

The symptoms include loss of cutaneous and tendon reflexes in the affected muscles, flaccid paralysis of the muscles affected, atrophy, subluxation of adjacent joints, general body weakness, respiratory and circulatory effects, and imbalance of muscle power. Contractures can occur in stronger muscles because of weakness of the antagonist muscles. Asymmetric paralysis of spinal muscles can result in scoliosis. Bone growth can be retarded in the affected limbs.

Impact

Polio results in immediate and long-term paralysis of muscles, necessitating the eventual use of substitutes for function. In extreme cases, the patient requires extensive functional devices and mechanisms for breathing; more commonly, the patient needs splints, arm supports, braces, or assistive devices for self-care and other upper extremity functions.

Functional Restoration

Medical treatment begins with immediate and complete bedrest; physical activity increases the risk of further paralysis. Hot packs are provided to relieve muscle pain, and the patient is positioned to protect the limbs from contracture and deformity. A tracheotomy may be necessary to provide an airway, and there may be a need for assistance in ventilation. Various types of respirators and ventilators are used and might be required throughout the patient's life.

During the phase in which the patient is receiving assistance in breathing, a *gentle* program of maintenance of passive and active functions is used. Massage, passive and active joint range of motion with graded resistance, splinting for prevention of contractures, and functional training follow as the patient regains physical tolerance. Surgical considerations include tendon transfers and arthrodesis to improve function and correct deformities.

The prime precaution in treating the patient with polio is to avoid muscle and body fatigue. Fatigue can result in further weakness, and, if the muscles are overworked, function can be lost. Aside from this serious problem, fatigue can cause the patient to miss hours of necessary treatment because of the debilitating effects. Respiratory and cardiac stress must also be avoided. Signs of labored breathing should be looked for, and, if necessary, the treatment should be terminated. The muscle function should be continually evaluated for signs of imbalance.

In order to maintain and increase the range of motion, endurance, and coordination, exercises and activities should be progressive and resistive and should be done symmetrically. Prevention of substitution patterns is important in the initial treatment program to encourage strengthening of weak muscles; however, when optimum muscle power has been reached, the patient may have to learn to use substitution patterns to assist in independent functions.

Arm supports and splints can be used both to minimize fatigue and to aid the patient in positioning weak extremities, particularly if there is shoulder girdle involvement. The balanced forearm orthosis (ball-bearing feeder) can be used for self-feeding, hygiene, upper ex-

tremity dexterity tasks, and other activities. Gravity can assist weak musculature. For the severely involved patient, provision of special equipment becomes essential for continuation of upper extremity functions. Devices such as an electric wheelchair, electric page turner, tape recorder, prism glasses, talking books, and special splinting can be helpful. With the proper equipment, the severely involved but well-motivated patient can adjust to adaptive functioning for daily activities and employment.

One of the most significant contributions the occupational therapist can make is in providing assistance through adaptive and supportive activities for maximum productivity and social involvement. Because the effect of the disease is permanent, the patient with severe upper extremity involvement must adjust to being assisted by complicated mechanical and electronic systems that substitute for or assist with arm positioning and hand activities.

Guillain–Barré Syndrome

Guillain–Barré syndrome is an acute distress of the nervous system that involves the spinal nerve roots, peripheral nerves, and, occasionally, the cranial nerves.[4] It is characterized by a hypersensitivity response of the peripheral nervous system, resulting in polyneuritis or inflammation of the nerves following a viral infection. The disease can affect either sex at any age. The acute phase of this LMN lesion involves the rapid onset of paralysis of the limbs with accompanying sensory loss and muscle atrophy.

The initial illness, followed by flaccid paralysis, may affect all four limbs at once or may begin in the legs and spread upward to the arms. It may involve muscles of respiration. The proximal and distal muscles of the limbs are usually affected symmetrically. Reflexes are diminished or lost, sensation is impaired in the extremities, and the muscles are tender, but not all sensory modalities are impaired.

Impact

The patient with Guillain–Barré syndrome, unlike the patient with polio, has a good prognosis for recovery. The factors affecting recovery are the premorbid physical condition, motivation, extent of return of muscle function, and the character of the rehabilitation program.

The prognosis is varied, and improvement may be sporadic. Almost complete recovery may be gained within 3 to 6 months or more, or the recovery may be incomplete with slight remissions, serious relapses, or a plateau. The patient may regain independent ambulation but retain some residual weakness and incoordination in all extremities, with some atrophy in the intrinsic muscles of the hands. The patient who makes slow progress may develop atrophy which, if unattended, can hinder the effective use of the hands in manipulative tasks. The patient with weakness and incoordination of the legs may require braces to substitute for the lack of strong muscles.

Functional Restoration

The patient generally benefits from an intensive rehabilitation program. With the initiation of rehabilitation techniques as soon as medical stability has been reached, activities are introduced to encourage active muscle use to prevent atrophy or wasting.

A common precaution in the rehabilitation program is the avoidance of fatigue in order to protect future function. Psychological support, practical use of returning musculature in productive activity, and social stimulation are essential if the patients are to become involved in the rehabilitation objectives. General rehabilitation goals include maintenance of nutrition, prevention of contractures, gradual diminution of the inital rest program, passive and active joint range-of-motion exercises for the affected extremities, activity for muscle strengthening and coordination, restoration of sensation, increase in activity according to the patient's tolerance, splinting to prevent deformity from atrophy and disuse, a self-care program to encourage independent functions, assistive devices to encourage functional use of extremities, and development of work tolerance for prevocational preparation.

The occupational therapist designs a program geared to the *gradual* improvement of active functions. Because the patient may be totally paralyzed when referred to occupational therapy, the first consideration may be to provide splints to maintain the functional position of fingers, thumbs, and wrists to prevent contractures from poor positioning. While on bedrest, the patient can benefit from the stimulation and encouragement of light social activities such as visits from family and friends, watching television, and supportive visits from the therapist, who engages the patient in positive conversation regarding his or her interests while performing passive range-of-motion exercises. It is important to maintain free joint motions of the wrist and fingers for grasping activities that use tenodesis function.

Early treatment is similar to that of the spinal cord-injured quadriplegic. The therapist must consider maintaining full passive joint range and encouraging active range against gravity. In addition, the therapist provides psychological support and social stimulation and encourages the patient to use special devices such as an electric page turner, which can provide the satisfaction of reading independently yet requires a minimum of movement to operate.

As the patient improves medically and begins to regain motor power, the occupational therapist provides activities that require increasing ranges of motion, coordination, and strength. The development of strength in specific muscles encourages the strengthening of other muscles.

However, as has been stressed, *care must be taken not to fatigue the patient.* Fatigue can be prevented by the therapist's providing suspension slings or arm supports for positioning and for facilitation of movement for hand functions. As the power begins to return and coordination improves, care should be taken to vary activities between gross and fine, resistive and nonresistive, so that maximum gain can be derived without undue fatigue.

Specific activities of the upper extremities should encourage coordinated movements while maintaining good body alignment to minimize the development of substitution patterns. The patient who is steadily improving needs assistive devices *only* to prevent fatigue and substitution; usually, these are not needed permanently. However, the patient whose progress is slower should be encouraged to use assistive equipment to gain strength and function.

From the beginning of treatment, self-care activities can encourage sensory and motor stimulation. Self-feeding and grooming can be started when necessary arm functions begin to return, even if a palmar cuff is needed to substitute for grasp. Dressing can be started when physical tolerance increases and the patient has sufficient active joint range of motion.

As the patient regains functions, the program should be upgraded to challenge strength and coordination. The patient should be encouraged to function independently whenever possible and to ask for assistance only when needed. Along with the physical therapist, the occupational therapist monitors the regaining of individual muscle control and checks for muscle atrophy.

Because the prognosis for the return of ambulation and functional upper extremity ability is generally good, the recovering patient is encouraged to participate in an activity program in which abilities for maximum independence can be developed. Recreational activities such as sports improve physical endurance and coordination. (For specific adaptation of activities, assistive devices, and self-care techniques, see the following section on spinal cord lesions.)

Spinal Cord Injury

Injury to the spinal cord results in temporary or permanent paralysis of the muscles of the limbs and the autonomic nervous system, usually manifested *below* the level of the lesion. Symptoms of a temporary nature are caused by compression of the cord without transection or puncture. Permanent paralysis is caused by fractures and dislocations that puncture or transect the spinal cord.

Spinal cord injury is caused by gunshot wounds, stab wounds, falls, automobile accidents, and sports accidents. The most common of these is the automobile accident, when forced flexion and hyperextension of the trunk results in fracture and dislocation of the vertebrae. The initial symptoms are: (1) spinal shock, (2) loss of sensation, (3) flaccid paralysis of the affected extremities, (4) incontinence of bowel and bladder, and (5) decreased reflex activity below the level of the lesion, followed by an increase in reflex activity. In many cases, secondary injury results from improper handling of the injured person at the scene of the accident and during transportation to the treatment facility.

Impact

The temporary or permanent implications to the injured person include the sudden interruption of the chosen lifestyle; severe loss of familiar bodily sensation, awareness, and volitional functions; and loss of bowel, bladder, and sexual controls, physical independence, psychological stability, social effectiveness, sexuality, financial security, educational goals, vocational skills and plans, avocational interests, personal expectations, and hopes for future content and planning.

Common problems that may occur periodically during rehabilitation are denial, anger, hostility, boredom, depression, lack of motivation, dependency, urinary tract infection, decubiti, weakness, atrophy, spasticity, and contractures.

Survival, disability, treatment, and function of the spinal cord-injured person depend on the level and extent of the lesion. *Quadriplegia* results from injury to the cervical and, possibly, the high thoracic areas of the cord and produces sensory deficits and muscular deficiencies of the upper extremities, trunk, and lower extremities. *Paraplegia* occurs from injury to the thoracic and lumbar cord areas and produces sensory deficits and muscular paralysis of the trunk and lower extremities. The terms *quadriplegia* and *paraplegia* refer to paralysis of the limbs, whereas *quadriparesis* and *paraparesis* refer to weakness of the limbs.

The level of segmental innervation determines the effect of the trauma. The extent of the injury determines the functional outcome. Muscles innervated by segments at and below the level of injury are affected. The sensory and autonomic systems may be involved; functional loss may be asymmetrical, depending on the location of the lesion. Although a functional estimate and expectation can be made on the basis of the level of the injury, other factors may retard or change the rehabilitation prognosis. Among these factors are respiratory complications, head trauma, other accompanying injuries, sensory loss, decubiti, damage to the vertebral column, urinary tract infections, spasm, and lack of motivation for recovery.

Functional Implications

The initial program for the person with a spinal cord injury is crucial to his or her total well-being and the beginning of the rehabilitation process, which may require adjustment to lifelong disability. It is a gradual, arduous, and sometimes painful progression from total dependence to the maximum level of independence; from the shock of functional loss to the acceptance of achievable abilities. Communication, planning, and coordination among team members are essential to ensure optimum rehabilitation outcomes medically and functionally.

Both the acute-care setting and the rehabilitation center provide medical care, carry out rehabilitation measures to prepare the injured person for future life involvement, provide therapy directed toward achievement of maximum levels of bodily movement and function, and implement psychological preparation for self-motivation for daily activity and goal setting. Rehabilitation is the preparation for setting and reaching achievable satisfactory goals. The initial rehabilitation period is a mere beginning to the new life the person will lead as a quadriplegic or paraplegic upon re-entry into community living.

In the early care, it is essential to prevent the patient from becoming either overly discouraged or overly hopeful. In discussing the medical condition with the patient, physicians may advocate informing the patient, immediately and clearly, of the chances of walking and of the degree of permanent paralysis to expect, in order to avoid false hope by the patient and family and to facilitate the rehabilitative process. In other cases, the physician may initially inform the patient that he or she will recover full functions or provide ambiguous answers to questions regarding functional loss in order to avoid psychological trauma. In the early stages of hospitalization, the patient tends to deny the extent of the injury. At this stage, denial serves as a valuable protective mechanism to avoid seeing the realities that must be faced eventually. In most cases, denial actually helps the patient through the devastating effects of the initial trauma and the long-term implications of disability.

Functional Restoration

Planning begins in the acute-care facility with protection of the flaccid extremities for future functioning, establishment of short-term and long-term goals, and gradual conditioning to enable the patient to tolerate an upright position. Establishment of maximum use of the upper extremities for self-care and productive activities aids the patient in acceptance of permanent paralysis and in preparation for functional wheelchair living. The therapist helps the patient develop physical and intellectual resources with which to combat the challenges of functional living and social interaction.

The goals of rehabilitation for the patient with spinal cord injury, regardless of the level of the lesion, include:
1. Recognizing and developing physical and intellectual capacities
2. Attaining the maximum level of self-care
3. Resuming satisfying relationships with family and friends and redeveloping social activities
4. Making realistic plans
5. Understanding the condition and accepting responsibility for continuing the rehabilitation process
6. Learning and following a therapeutic home program
7. Learning of and using available community resources
8. Resuming education and employment activities and plans

Involvement with his or her own plan helps the patient learn to take responsibility and enables the patient to develop an independent attitude toward his or her abilities. This involvement begins during acute-care hospitalization, continues during early rehabilitation, and progresses further if treatment continues at a specialized rehabilitation facility.

Positioning
Exercises and activities can be done in almost any position if both the patient and the equipment are properly situated. In preparation for productive activity, the patient should be positioned for optimum biomechanical advantage in function.

Bed. Upper extremity activities can be assisted by the use of an inclined lapboard in the supine and sitting positions with suspension slings attached to traction frames for early arm support.

To avoid the natural tendency of the flaccid extremities to yield to the pull of gravity, they are properly positioned in normal alignment using sandbags, pillows, or footboards to prevent the stretching of unused or weak muscles and the development of contractures of spastic muscles, which would limit future function of the limbs. Undue pressure on flaccid limbs from bed clothes is avoided, and the limbs should be visible to monitor positioning. Prism glasses enable the patient to see his or her extremities and to request repositioning if necessary.

Prone Position on a Circo-electric Bed. When the quadriplegic patient is prone (face down) on the Circo-electric bed, he or she can use gravity for shoulder flexion and elbow extension. A table is necessary to provide support in elbow flexion if the patient lacks lower arm functions. For the quadriplegic in a prone position, independent eating should be encouraged, using slings, a palmar cuff, and a nonskid mat and positioning the tray under the bed. Plateguards allow the patient to pick up the food independently.

Wheelchair Position. Good position is necessary. The patient is generally seated on a cutout seatboard with a gel, water, or air cushion for hip positioning and prevention of decubiti. The chair should initially have an extended back, adjustable arm, and foot support. A lapboard, suspension slings, or a balanced forearm orthosis can be attached to the wheelchair for the quadriplegic.

Standing Table. This device is used by the patient wearing braces to aid in trunk strengthening and balance, standing tolerance, and upright positioning. Activities done at the standing table may also be accomplished by some patients with sufficient balance by using a belt support to stand at a work table.

Skin Protection. Protection of the skin and prevention of contractures are essential for the patient with a spinal cord injury. Because sensation is lost below the level of lesion, the patient is unable to detect pressure from external objects and because of muscle paralysis is unable to change position easily. Thus, position changes must be made initially by nurses or attendants. The skin is susceptible to injury from the shearing force of sheets, pressure from footboards used for positioning, and the gravitational effect of the immobile limbs on the mattress. Decubitus ulcers (pressure sores) develop from local anemia caused by this pressure and appear over bony prominences. Even though air mattresses and water mattresses are used, and routine position changes are followed, decubitus ulcers can still occur. To avoid pressure sores, the therapist instructs the patient in the importance of turning in bed or shifting weight when seated in the wheelchair. As a patient becomes more mobile, instruction is given on how to check all vulnerable areas of the body, using a long-handled mirror to check the back, buttocks, arms, and lower extremities.

Self-Care
The daily accomplishment of self-care and other independent or assisted activities helps the patient maintain joint range of motion, strength, and physical and psychological endurance. The abilities and progress in these areas should be discussed with the family throughout the hospitalization and rehabilitation process so that they will encourage as much independence as possible.

The person with paraplegia is generally able to regain independent self-care activities and virtually all aspects of daily living. Depending on the level of the lesion and the manifestations, complications, and motivation for independent function, the person with quadriplegia is challenged with use of electronic assistive equipment, hand splints, and motorized or a specially equipped wheelchair to deal with disability in all four extremities.

Assistive Equipment

Adaptive equipment may be required for substitution of motion, compensation for decreased trunk balance, and assistance for reduced reach and grasp and for limitation in locomotion. Assistive devices may be needed to perform the self-care activities of personal hygiene, grooming, eating, and dressing. Although assistive equipment may increase functional independence, it may decrease desired sensory and motor function. Some patients refuse all assistive equipment; others want everything, even some that is not needed.

In most cases, the wheelchair becomes a way of life for the spinal cord-injured person. Therefore, it must be prescribed for individual comfort, safety, maneuverability, and independence. A poorly fitted wheelchair can contribute to deformity, muscle disuse, decubiti, and decreased motivation for function and socialization. The wheelchair needs of the paraplegic and quadriplegic patients are different.

The wheelchair should be ordered as soon as possible in the rehabilitation program to encourage the patient's early association with wheelchair living.

Avocational

Activities provided for restoration of specific upper extremity function can become outlets for avocational needs and interests. As the spinal cord-injured person works through adjustment to wheelchair living, avocational outlets are needed for venting feelings as well as for providing a sense of accomplishment. As new patterns of movement and skill develop, the patient can apply these to pursuing leisure activity at school or in the community. Many spinal cord-injured people have benefited greatly from participation in organized sports such as basketball, swimming, ping pong, and weightlifting. Competition contributes to resocialization, achievement, and increased sense of self-worth and confidence.

Educational

Vocational goals and discharge plans may include returning to school for the adolescent or young adult with a spinal cord injury. Therapists evaluate the campus for architectural accessibility by wheelchair to buildings, classrooms, bathrooms, cafeterias, and other areas. A system for carrying books, obtaining optimum work surfaces and heights, and notetaking may be needed by the quadriplegic student. Full involvement of the wheelchair-mobile person in all aspects of the educational environment is essential to acceptance by peers.

Driving

One of the most common social problems facing the wheelchair user is the lack of adequate public transportation. Therefore, it is essential that the paraplegic person become independent in using hand controls for driving, car transfers, and placing the wheelchair in the car.

Many quadriplegic individuals can drive with hand controls and a steering knob, although they may need assistance getting in and out of the car and most need help getting the wheelchair into the car. For these individuals, a van with a wheelchair lift is recommended. The person may need to transfer from the wheelchair to the driver's seat or passenger's seat once in the van, or the van may be equipped with clamps to secure the wheelchair in a position to allow the individual to drive. Predriving evaluation and training programs are available to guide the person in using safe techniques in purchasing an appropriate vehicle and in driving.

Prevocational

The employment potential of the spinal cord-injured person is not necessarily correlated with the injury and its residual manifestations. A person with a debilitating injury is able to return to work if he or she is motivated, possesses salable knowledge and skills, is offered reassurance from family and friends, and is able to find a job, although the patient may have to change former vocational goals. The occupational therapy program provides the opportunity to learn potential functional levels and to explore feasible vocational areas of interest. Prevocational evaluation determines the salable skills that the person has, can develop, or requires for vocational planning and preparation for appropriate vocational training.

Discharge Planning

The patient and family are included in the rehabilitation program as soon after hospital admission as possible and are fully informed of all of the stages of the rehabilitation process the patient will go through. The process begun in the hospital continues at home, in the rehabilitation facility, and in the community for as long as is necessary. The individual maintains a relationship with the rehabilitation team to achieve planned goals upon discharge through outpatient programs and follow-up.

During hospitalization, the rehabilitation team may encourage the patient to go home on weekends to begin to face the adjustments that will have to be made after discharge and to use skills acquired in the treatment facility in the home environment. These visits alert the family to the patient's capabilities, progress, and general program. It is from these visits that the patient, family, and therapist can work together on home planning and architectural renovations.

Specific Considerations: Quadriplegia

The initial treatment of the person with quadriplegia (paralysis in upper and lower extremities) is immobilization of the vertebral column by skeletal traction using head tongs or neck bracing. Traction is generally applied for 6 weeks, following which immobilization is continued with a neck support for 2 to 4 months.[12]

The patient's position while in traction is interchangeable (supine and prone) in a completely extended position for optimal protection of the spinal cord and musculature. The injured person may be placed on a Stryker frame bed, which rotates horizontally for position change to prone or supine, or on a Circo-electric bed, which can be turned from the horizontal to the vertical position on a 180° axis and be stabilized at any angle, allowing placement in the supine or prone position. These special beds are used to aid in the frequent change in body position essential to protect skin and limbs from decubiti. Change of position is made every 2 hours. The tilt-table is also used to assist in moving the patient passively from the horizontal to the vertical position. If the patient is not gradually acclimated to changes in space during the initial immobilization, he or she tends to become dizzy when assuming the sitting position following weeks spent in traction.

Early treatment of the quadriplegic patient in the acute stage of trauma consists of turning, massage for circulation and sensory stimulation, and passive range of motion exercises to maintain freedom of joint movement and to prevent muscular contractures and decubiti. Following the traction period, general conditioning exercises are provided, including proper breathing and training in rolling from side to side. Self-care is begun as soon as possible to relieve anxieties regarding nonsensitive and nonmoving body parts and to prevent dependency on others for any functions the patient is able to accomplish.

Evaluation

As previously mentioned, the level of segmental innervation determines the effect of trauma and the anticipated functional outcome (Fig. 29-4 and Table 29-3). In the acute-care setting, the quadriplegic patient is usually seen for initial evaluation while confined to bed. The following steps are recommended for the initial assessment of capabilities and functional deficits:

1. Review the chart for medical status, treatment prescribed, and bed position restrictions owing to the injury to the spinal cord and other areas.
2. Establish nonthreatening rapport with the patient on the initial visit, showing empathy and respect. Interview the patient about what happened, the medical situation, treatment plans, and schedule, asking for a description of concerns and priorities.
3. Evaluate active and passive joint range of motion, strength, sensation, coordination, general mobility, and function of the extremities and trunk.
4. Evaluate bed position for alignment of extremities and trunk for prevention of muscle stretching, shortening, and deformity and for the patient's awareness of position requirements.
5. Examine the extremities for reddened areas, which indicate pressure.
6. Determine the functional aspects of upper extremity sensation by requesting the patient to identify the location of and describe sensory stimuli and identify the location of the extremity during passive positioning.
7. Determine passive and active joint range of motion, identifying restrictions caused by trauma, pain, weakness, spasticity, contractures, or hypersensitivity.
8. Determine the need for hand splints to maintain body alignment for future function to prevent deformity and for sensory awareness and stimulation.
9. Assess the need for arm support to extend the functional positioning of the hands for use; assess the need for arm exercises in a supine position.
10. Talk with the patient about interests, abilities, past achievement, and primary concerns regarding the condition and its implications for his or her life.
11. Inform the patient of the results of the evaluation and discuss his or her personal goals; make treatment plans with the patient for short-term and long-term goals.

Treatment

Bed Phase. During all treatment in this phase, the patient should be encouraged to use *all* possible active movement to increase physical endurance, strength, and functional ability. By doing this, the patient becomes involved in his or her program and assumes some responsibility for rehabilitation. The therapist provides activities in which the patient is interested and psychological support throughout the treatment regime. The therapist coordinates occupational therapy with nursing and physical therapy personnel and other members of the rehabilitation team in order to aid the patient in gaining maximum function while suffering minimal fatigue and frustration.

Treatment considerations during the bed stage are as follows:

1. Monitor *bed positioning* daily for prevention of decubiti and contractures.
2. Gently *massage* and stimulate sensory receptors of the upper extremities for sensory awareness and tactual localization.

(list continues on page 494)

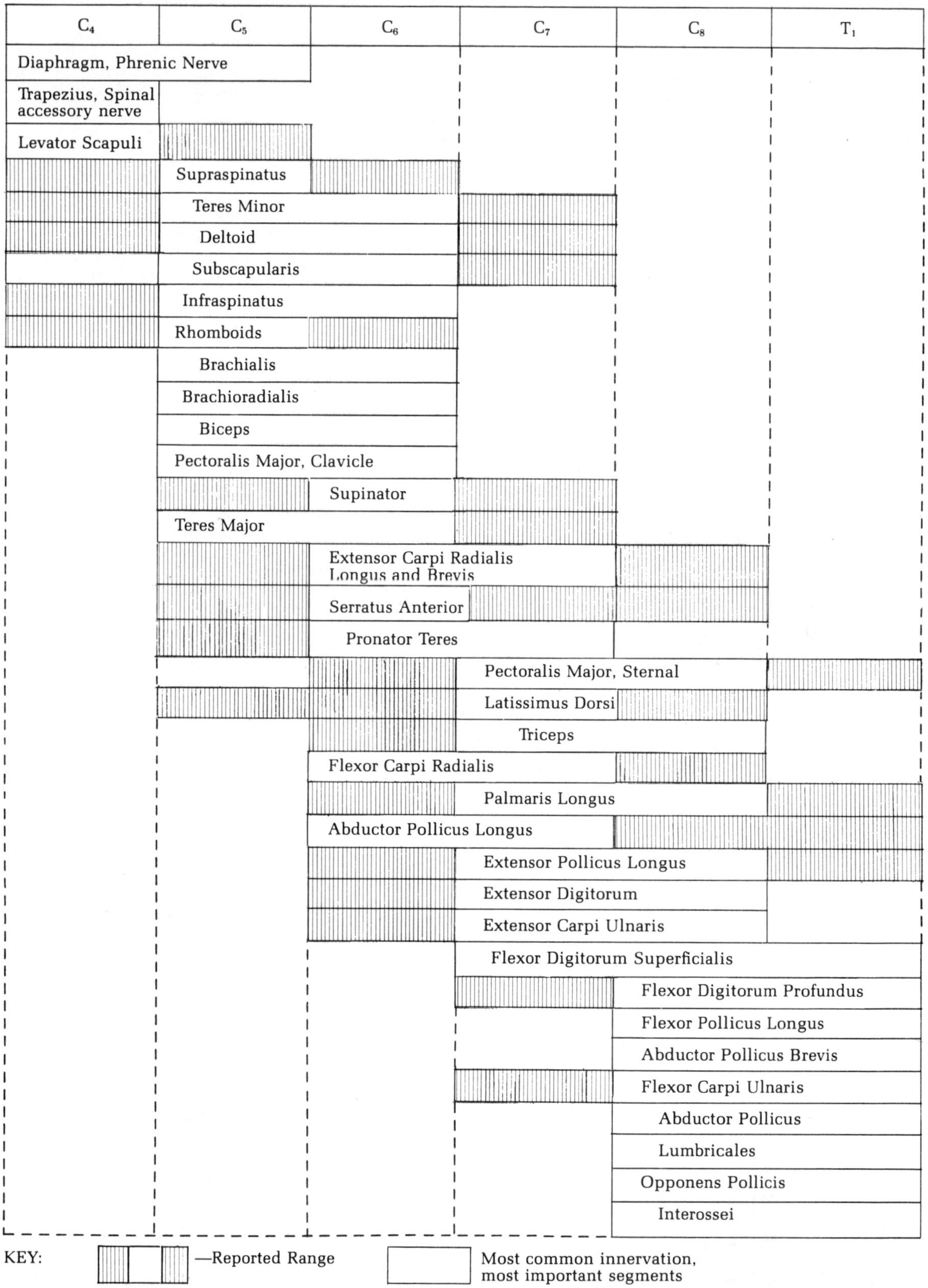

	C_4	C_5	C_6	C_7	C_8	T_1
Diaphragm, Phrenic Nerve						
Trapezius, Spinal accessory nerve						
Levator Scapuli						
Supraspinatus						
Teres Minor						
Deltoid						
Subscapularis						
Infraspinatus						
Rhomboids						
Brachialis						
Brachioradialis						
Biceps						
Pectoralis Major, Clavicle						
Supinator						
Teres Major						
Extensor Carpi Radialis Longus and Brevis						
Serratus Anterior						
Pronator Teres						
Pectoralis Major, Sternal						
Latissimus Dorsi						
Triceps						
Flexor Carpi Radialis						
Palmaris Longus						
Abductor Pollicus Longus						
Extensor Pollicus Longus						
Extensor Digitorum						
Extensor Carpi Ulnaris						
Flexor Digitorum Superficialis						
Flexor Digitorum Profundus						
Flexor Pollicus Longus						
Abductor Pollicus Brevis						
Flexor Carpi Ulnaris						
Abductor Pollicus						
Lumbricales						
Opponens Pollicis						
Interossei						

KEY: —Reported Range   —Most common innervation, most important segments

Figure 29-4. Segmental innervation of specified muscles in the cervical spinal cord from C4 through T1. There is commonly a range of innervation from two or three spinal segments, and there is a variation in people as to segmental innervation. In traumatic spinal cord injury, those muscles are affected that are innervated *below* the lesion. Bilateral symmetry of paralysis depends on the exact location of the lesion and its severity. For example, a transection caused by a fracture-dislocation of a vertebra may cause an oblique lesion or an incomplete lesion. Inflammation and swelling can contribute to a higher initial deficit.

Table 29-3. *Functional Implications of Cervical Cord Lesions.* *

Level of Lesion	Remaining Musculature	Active Mobility	Functional Loss	Functional Implications	Occupational Therapy Implications
C_4	Sternocleidomastoid Upper trapezius	Neck movements Shoulder elevation	Respiratory endurance Upper extremity functions Trunk sensation and control Lower extremity sensation and control General endurance General independent mobility	Total dependency in self-care Dependence on external devices for upper extremity movement and productive activity Confined to wheelchair Can propel electric wheelchair	Requires assistance in communication skills: tape recorder, electric typewriter (using hand typing sticks, headstick, mouthpiece, electronic communication board), electric page turner for reading, talking books (records) Uses externally powered (electric or CO_2) functional hand splints and arm supports for upper extremity activity in the wheelchair Can engage in light recreational and avocational activities for ROM, strength, interest, and motivation
C_5	Sternocleidomastoid Trapezius Rhomboids Partial rotator cuff Partial deltoids Partial biceps	Neck movements Shoulder elevation Scapular rotation, adduction Partial elbow flexion Weak or no sensory function	Ability to change from supine to prone position in bed Ability to achieve sitting position in bed Independent trunk control and sensation Lower extremity sensation and control Wrist and hand functions	Use of externally powered devices for arm and hand functions Assistive devices for self-feeding Dependency in self-care and transfers Can propel electric wheelchair	Devices described above may be necessary Dynamic tenodesis splints for writing, grasping, and other hand functions Mobile arm support, balanced forearm orthosis, or suspension slings for general upper extremity support and mobility Special equipment or devices for telephone, TV operation, eating, drinking Recreational and avocational activities for ROM, strength, interest, motivation

Level					
C$_6$	All muscles of C$_4$ and C$_5$ level Partial serratus anterior Partial pectoralis Partial latissimus dorsi Deltoid Biceps Partial extensor carpi radialis	All movements of C$_4$ and C$_5$ Scapular adduction, flexion, extension Weak trunk control Shoulder flexion Elbow flexion Wrist extension (tenodesis function for grasp) Weak sensory function in hand	Weakness in trunk control, affecting balance Lower extremity functions Weakness in grasp, release, and prehension	Can achieve sitting position in bed by using trapeze bar (above bed) or rope attached to foot of bed Can assist in wheelchair transfer Can propel regular wheelchair Can use assistive devices for self-care Fairly mobile arm control Weak tenodesis function	Dynamic tenodesis splints for hand functions Assistive devices for independence in self-care: razor holders, utensil holders, pencil holders, extended handles for reaching, dressing loops for pants, sliding board for transfers, devices for toilet needs (catheter and leg bag, suppository management) Friction adaptations to wheelrims or knobs for pushing wheelchair using thenar eminence of hand Typing sticks Push-ups in wheelchair for arm strengthening and prevension of decubiti Independent living skills Driving with hand controls and wheel knobs Vocational goals
C$_7$	All muscles of C$_4$, C$_5$, C$_6$ level Finger flexors Finger extensors	All movements of C$_4$, C$_5$, C$_6$ Moderate trunk control Functional grasp and release Sensory function of hand	Weakness in trunk control Weakness in intrinsic muscles of the hand and isolated finger functions Limited dexterity and general hand strength	Independent bed and wheelchair mobility Independent bed/wheelchair transfers Strong arm control Has grasp functions and coordination without splints Nonfunctional ambulation for standing and short distances	Assistive devices for toilet activities and lower extremity dressing Upper extremity activities for physical restoration without splinting Can drive with hand controls and do car transfer Independence in daily living and community involvement Vocational and avocational goals

* This information represents an average range of capability. Variations can be expected owing to individual spinal innervation and other factors.

3. Move the upper extremities in gentle, full *passive range of motion* daily to monitor changes in range, informing the patient when the extremity is moved, in which direction, and how many times. Encourage the patient to watch the extremity during massage and passive joint range of motion.

4. Precede active range of motion exercises by gentle *manual resistance* to joints and muscle groups in the hands and arms for sensory stimulation and motor facilitation.

5. Attach *suspension slings* to the traction bar above the bed to support the arms as well as to stimulate available active movements of the shoulders and elbows. Slings can be modified with springs to facilitate movement and to provide sensory feedback. The use of weights encourages increased muscle power.

   Use elbow and wrist straps to support the arms for maximum active movement and hand functions; use a palmar cuff with a pocket for insertion of a spoon or a pencil, enabling the patient to use the arms and hands in productive activity.

   Facilitate motion of all joints of the upper extremities by using gravitational assists such as suspension slings, the balanced forearm orthosis adaptations, weights, or a bed table.

6. Use *assistive devices* to facilitate and support movement; among these devices are a common bath mitt, a universal palmar cuff device to hold a fork for eating, a plate guard to aid in arm control while eating, and arm slings or positioners. These devices encourage exercise through active arm movement, increase body awareness, encourage self-esteem by providing independent function, and decrease dependency.

7. Provide *splinting* to prevent tightening of muscles and deformity. Restriction may be necessary to prevent flexion of the elbows, wrists, fingers, and ankles. It is essential to correlate the use of splints with manual therapeutic techniques. Provide initial static hand splinting progressing to dynamic splinting to stimulate tenodesis function as appropriate. Splinting stimulates sensory awareness and assists in channeling the muscles for function.

8. Set up an *electric page turner* on the bed table so that the patient can operate it with palm contact (Fig. 29-5) or with movement of the chin or shoulder if he or she lacks lower arm function.

9. Provide *prism glasses* to prevent the patient from developing eyestrain while viewing television; reading, seeing, and talking with visitors; or watching his or her limbs as the therapist moves them when the patient is supine (Fig. 29-6).

In the bed position, the following adaptations are possible:

1. Use the bed table to position objects for activities (books or visual puzzles) that can be performed by using prism glasses.

2. A table lapboard with a bottom edge can be placed over the patient's chest; this can be inclined and stabilized using projecting legs to hold reading materials and other items.

3. Commercial book holders are useful.

4. Suspension slings can be attached to the traction frames on the bed.

5. Slings, mirrors, and activities can be attached to the Circo-electric bed frame.

6. Objects for activities can be placed on a chair or low table for the patient who is prone on the Circo-electric bed. Food trays can also be placed on a chair.

During the bed stage, the patient is encouraged to adjust to the vertical position for sitting by using the tilt-table. This adjustment should be accomplished gradually. When cerebral spatial adjustment and physical tolerance increase to a sufficiently functional level, the patient progresses to the semi-reclining wheelchair and then to the fully upright position for continued adaptation to wheelchair mobility, sitting balance, and the use of the upper extremities.

The move to the wheelchair for daily treatment sessions is a significant one for the quadriplegic patient. This change in position requires vestibular adjustment as well as total body adaptation. The occupational therapy program changes to focus on evaluation of functional ability in this position and direction of therapeutic methods toward optimum sensorimotor performance achievements.

Wheelchair selection for the quadriplegic is crucial to daily health and function. A variety of chairs, controls, and accessories are available to meet the varied demands of individual capabilities, interests, and lifestyles. For the quadriplegic patient with a high cervical lesion and severely limited or nonfunctional reach and hand placement, electronic arm or head controls may be necessary. Electronic wheelchair and environmental control systems enable the severely disabled person to have independent wheelchair mobility and an element of independent function. With such systems, the disabled person can control appliances such as an electric bed, a call signal, a telephone or intercom, television, thermostat, or doors.

Quadriplegics with lower cervical lesions benefit from operating electric controls on wheelchairs or by using special accessories on standard nonelectric wheelchairs. For ease of maneuvering, the quadriplegic person may require knobs or plastic friction sheaths on the wheel rims for easier propulsion or a motorized chair with touch controls. The back should be higher than that of the paraplegic's chair, since the quadriplegic has

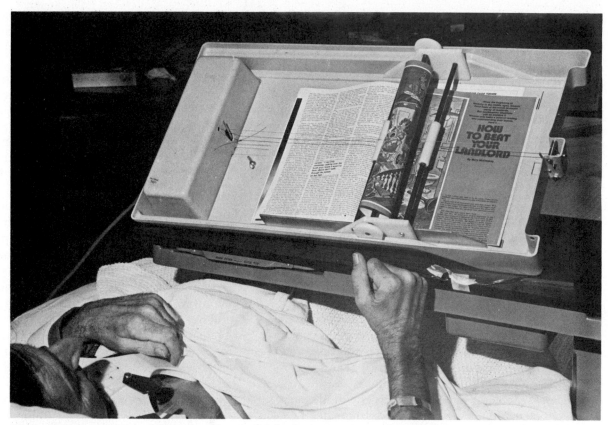

Figure 29-5. Patient with traumatic quadriplegia operates an electric page turner using palm contact with a microswitch attached to the bed table beneath the right corner of the machine. The page turner is inclined for increased ease in visibility from the patient's semisupine position in bed.

lost trunk control and needs extra support. A brake extension may be necessary for independence in locking brakes. Heel loops and leg rests are needed for foot and leg positioning, and a safety belt may be needed for balance. Although a wheelchair with a reclining back may be used at first to compensate for the quadriplegic's tendency to become dizzy, it is not recommended during later periods, as it can increase dependency on the reclined position, which limits upper extremity function.

Figure 29-6. Prism glasses prevent eyestrain during television viewing for the quadriplegic patient lying supine in bed. Foam cuff protectors are used to prevent skin breakdown from gravitational pressure of the mattress on the bony prominences of the elbows. Static handsplints provide passive thumb positioning to maintain adductor stretch for position of opposition. Arms are positioned in elbow and wrist extension to prevent flexion contractures.

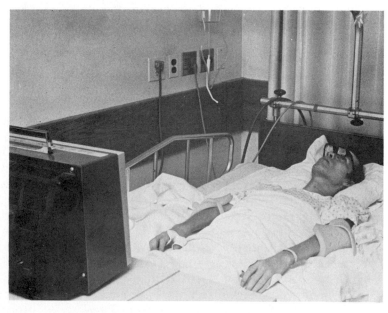

Wheelchair Phase. When the patient has progressed to sitting in a wheelchair, guidelines are determined for treatment planning. During all evaluation procedures, assist the patient in movements when necessary. Do not allow fatigue or discouragement. Emphasize what *can* be done and encourage the patient to accomplish it. Be explicit in instructions and demonstrate when necessary. Terminate the evaluation before the patient becomes fatigued and try to end with accomplishment. Talk with the patient regarding his or her interests so that the treatment program can include activities that are related to these interests and aid the patient in setting realistic long-term and short-term goals. The following evaluation areas are examined:

1. Joint range of motion: move the joints through complete passive range of motion, one at a time, being careful not to cause pain in sensitive joints, particularly in the shoulders and elbows. Give support to the flaccid or weak limbs by holding them carefully, always informing the patient of what is to be done. Measure the joint range with the goniometer. Check for spasticity and deformity in the upper extremities.

2. Muscle strength: provide gravitational assist if necessary to determine how much gravity the patient can resist. Give gentle resistance to joint movement to determine gross muscle strength and the presence of spasticity. Use a scale gauge to measure gross joint strength against resistance and a pinch gauge and dynamometer for grip.

3. Sensation: note the presence of pain during passive movement. Occlude the patient's vision; touch the skin lightly with your finger and determine if the patient responds to the stimulus. Progress from distal to proximal areas. To evaluate two-point discrimination, sharp touch, and localization of stimuli, touch the skin with a sharp object, such as a sharpened dowel stick or a two-point pressure gauge. Determine first whether the patient responds to the stimulus, can localize the stimulus, and can distinguish one from two stimuli. Place an object between the patient's thumb and fingers, move it around in the palmar area, and then ask for recognition of the object by its size, shape, and texture to determine stereognostic function.

4. Position sense (proprioception): move the body part to be tested gently in reciprocal movements and then ask the patient to identify the position of the limb when stopped. He or she may feel the movement but may be unable to identify the position without seeing it.

5. Patterns of movement: provide the patient with a reaching or grasping task to perform, for instance, picking up a 2 × 2–inch foam block, reaching to the shoulder, or reaching for an object held in the air. Observe the pattern of movement to determine functioning muscles and the presence of spasticity. Observe any substitution patterns the patient may use to the detriment of other muscles that should be strengthened.

6. Functional activities: determine the actual gross grasp, prehension, coordination, strength, and tenodesis function. Determine the ability to perform functional activities, such as picking up an object and placing it, reaching for an object, using two hands, writing, pushing and pulling objects, and turning the pages of a book. Use objects of various weights, sizes, and textures. Present tasks within the patient's functional ability as determined by joint range of motion, muscle power, sensation, position sense, and patterns of movement already observed and evaluated. Do not ask a patient to do impossible tasks.

7. Determine the trunk control for free movement of the upper extremities in isolated asymmetrical use and use in the ADL functions.

8. Evaluate the need for assistance devices or splints for restorative exercises and activities in addition to those needed for positioning and self-care activities.

9. Evaluate self-care and all ADL, including self-feeding, grooming, toileting, bathing, dressing, writing, clerical skills, and homemaking skills. The physical plan of the home must also be evaluated.

10. Prevocational evaluation: evaluate functions for job skills and employment potential when the patient has mastered upper extremity functional activities and ADL within his or her limits.

Self-Care. Although the quadriplegic patient may have little range of motion and muscle strength with which to accomplish self-care tasks, it is essential for him or her to use the available power to accomplish parts of tasks. Limitations in reach, grasp, strength, joint range of motion, respiration, and physical endurance are common. Assistive and substitutive techniques of adaptive body positioning, use of reflexes, and assistance from an attendant help in developing skills. Long handles to extend reach, palmar cuffs to substitute for hand grip, spring clips to provide sustained grip, loops on clothing, special devices for grooming, soap on a rope, bath mitts, and adapted equipment for grooming and make-up are readily available and often make the difference between ability and handicap. Often, the most limiting factor can be the patient's refusal to participate.

Functional Restoration. All activities should increase upper extremity joint range of motion, strength, physical tolerance, grasp, and psychological adaptation. These activities should include the use of assistive equipment to increase the patient's capacity to function independently and result in the realization of maximum capacities.

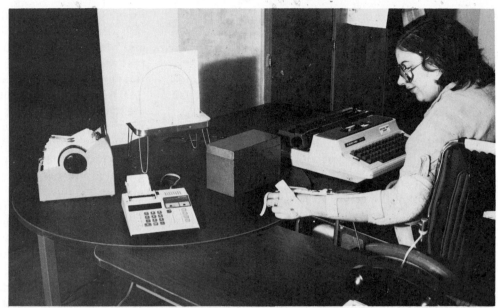

Figure 29-7. Quadriplegic patient used a tenodesis splint on her left hand to provide functional prehension and uses a revolving table surface that gives easy access to clerical equipment and supplies for effective organization of the work area.

Specially designed tables adjust to the height of the wheelchair, angled for easy access to work surfaces or on a rotating base (Fig. 29-7), assist the patient in optimum mechanical advantage for task accomplishment.

Manipulation of pegs and of other objects of various sizes, weights, and textures improves the grasp, reach, and ability to place objects. These can be presented in the form of peg games (HiQ, checkers, or chess) to elicit the patient's interest. The activity teaches isolated arm and hand functions and provides the patient with experience in using assistive equipment.

Constructive activities such as woodworking can be adapted to provide joint range of motion and strengthening of the upper arms and trunk muscles. If the patient has poor grasp, a palmar cuff, bilateral handles, or holding mitts can be used with tools for such tasks as sanding, sawing, planing, or drilling.

Diversional activities are provided for the pure fun of engaging in a game with another person while at the same time assisting the patient in gaining functional use of the upper extremities. These activities, such as checkers, chess, or Scrabble, can be done in bed or in a wheelchair. Arm support may be needed, as may hand splints, but the patient is able to engage in competitive activity and receive the rewards from it.

Suggestions for adapted activities for the spinal cord-injured person, with modifications according to lesion level, include:

1. Use of table-based power tools such as a small jigsaw, drill press, or printing press, which can have extended handles for easy reach and control
2. Use of handpower equipment, secured if necessary to substitute for the patient's lack of control
3. Vertical and adjustable angled chalkboards for gross arm and writing exercises
4. Use of ropes attached to loom harnesses to enable the patient to change the shed by using the arms, if the lower extremities are paralyzed
5. Special handles on the loom beater to provide supination or pronation exercises
6. Use of a pulley and weight system attached to the loom beater for strengthening upper extremities by providing resistance
7. Use of recreational activities for gross arm exercise: ball throwing, shuffleboard, shooting pool
8. Use of manual activities for sustained upper arm strengthening and light resistive hand use: painting, knitting, hooking
9. Use of activities for sensory stimulus and light resistive hand use: gardening using adapted planters at wheelchair level, forming and painting ceramics
10. Use of homemaking activities: cooking, cleaning, ironing

All activities offer possibilities for adaptation. Some of the activities mentioned are helpful to the paraplegic patient as well as to the quadriplegic patient, because they provide a means to increase strength, endurance, and balance for the trunk and upper extremities. The quadriplegic patient needs these functions for wheelchair manipulation and for performance of all activities. The paraplegic patient needs upper arm strengthening for wheelchair maneuvering over long distances, transferring, standing in braces, and walking with crutches. The build-up of maximum upper extremity strength is essential to the paraplegic. Engagement in an upper extremity activity program is crucial to the beginning of productivity from a wheelchair and leads to independence in daily living tasks, increased responsibility, and, eventually, employment. The paraplegic patient should experience all aspects of functioning from a wheelchair before leaving the rehabilitation setting.

Functional Splints. Early use of appropriate splints benefits the quadriplegic patient in providing muscle exercise, mechanical function for purposeful activity, and assurance that the patient is capable of accomplishing tasks.

The quadriplegic patient is provided with a tenodesis or flexor-hinge hand splint when he or she has achieved active hyperextension of the wrist. It is with active motion against resistance that the patient is able to channel movement through the splint into a strong and functional prehension grip (Fig. 29-8). The tenodesis splint uses the natural function of the finger flexor tendons to tighten in wrist hyperextension and to relax in wrist flexion. Although the patient may be able to effect this

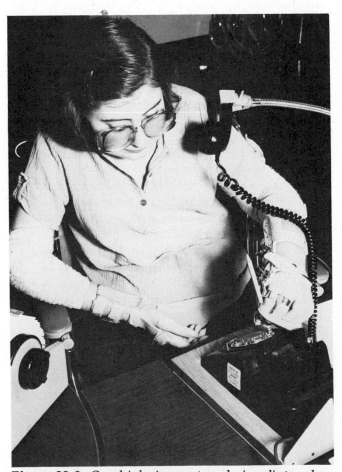

Figure 29-8. Quadriplegic uses tenodesis splint on her left hand to provide sufficient grasp strength to hold pencil used in dialing a telephone. Telephone is held by gooseneck holder attached to the table; it can be positioned easily.

function voluntarily with sufficient active wrist extension without the splint, grip sufficient for strong grasp and fine prehension may be lacking in thumb–finger prehension. The splint is applied to give power for the functional needs of prehension.

There are various forms of splints available; some are for trial and training, whereas others are for permanent use. Trial tenodesis splints may be made by the occupational therapist from thermoplastic materials. The patient is taught how to use the splint in active grasping and releasing and in coordination activities. The flexor-hinge hand splint is made by the occupational therapist or the orthotist for permanent use and is usually made of metal or high-temperature plastic. The patient may continue to use the splints if they aid in daily activities or may eventually discard them as muscle power and substitute functions are gained.

If the patient does not have active wrist extension against gravity and resistance, other types of hand–wrist tenodesis splints may be needed to provide the function of grasp. These may be electronically or carbon dioxide (CO_2) controlled. The use of these devices depends on the motivation of the patient, as they require tolerance to noise and the pressure of harnesses and special rigging as well as acceptance of complicated assistive equipment to substitute for natural functions.

Environmental Control Systems. The high-level quadriplegic who is unable to move his or her upper extremities for functional activity depends on teaching others how to perform needed physical tasks. In spite of this dependence, the severely disabled patient can find independence in environmental control and self-expression in written communication through the aid of environmental control systems (Fig. 29-9). Such systems enable training and practice in functional written communication skills for use in recreational activities, educational needs, or employment functions. Electronically controlled computer systems with typewriter mechanisms, auditory systems, visual feedback, and custom adaptations can be made for positioning and operation.

Specific Considerations: Paraplegia

Evaluation

Evaluation of the paraplegic patient in the initial post-trauma stage may be at the bedside if the patient is immobilized in traction and special equipment or has significant accompanying injuries. In evaluating the paraplegic, the therapist looks for variations in functional ability, which depend on the level of the lesion. Although the paraplegic may initially be immobilized, he or she demonstrates full functional use of the upper extremities in active range of motion, sensation, and hand use. While in bed and during the wheelchair phase, the patient will become accustomed to depend-

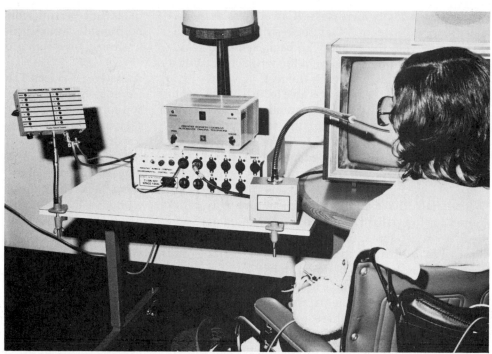

Figure 29-9. Quadriplegic using a mouth-operated environmental control system to activate lamp and television switches independently.

ing on the arms and trunk for mobility and function to provide leg positioning.

Specific areas of evaluation during the bed phase include:

1. Determine status, rehabilitation goals, and treatment being provided.
2. Determine medical restrictions on movement as noted in the chart with regard to the status of the spinal cord injury and other injuries.
3. Note the body position for proper alignment of the paralyzed trunk and lower extremities.
4. Evaluate the passive and active range of motion and strength of the upper extremities (which should be normal but may be weak).
5. If not medically restricted, evaluate trunk and lower extremity movement, noting areas of spasticity, weakness, paralysis, sensory loss, substitution, and compensation.
6. Assess need for an ability to use self-care devices to perform daily activities.
7. Interview the patient with regard to accident, medical condition and its impact, lifestyle, goals, and expectations.
8. Encourage the patient to discuss premorbid achievement, avocational and vocational interests, and plans.

Treatment

Bed Phase. While confined to bed, the paraplegic patient benefits from an upper extremity activity program to strengthen the arms and hands, to provide initial self-care assistance, to learn body image and self-awareness, to learn the extent of current functions, and to provide a sense of self-worth through accomplishment of achievable tasks on a daily basis. The longer the patient remains away from productive activity, the more difficult is his or her adjustment to the benefits of rehabilitation. The following activities and adaptations are suggested to encourage a positive attitude toward maintenance of restoration of productive abilities:

1. Inclined bed table, lapboard, and prism glasses for ease in performing upper extremity activity in bed
2. Devices with extended handles for reaching and self-care; a long-handled sponge for bathing; a reacher for picking up items
3. Increasing involvement in daily self-care program
4. Low-exertion upper extremity activities for active exercise of the arms while supine; reading, book games, manual activities
5. Activities that offer resistance in hand and arm functions to increase strength and to decrease mental frustration from inactivity; Theraplast, leatherwork, making models, copper tooling, macrame, loom weaving, and woodcarving

Barring the complications of decubiti and excessive spasticity, the paraplegic person is able to learn to be essentially independent in self-care. The high-level paraplegic may have some problems with lower extremity dressing because of trunk instability and loss of muscle strength for balance; however, various assistive devices can help in overcoming these problems.

Self-care activity increases self-awareness, responsibility, and self-esteem. When the restrictions on mobility are removed, the patient can begin self-care activities, such as bathing in bed or in the wheelchair using a long-handled sponge to reach the feet.

At this time, if the patient is able to turn in bed and to reach a sitting position, upper extremity dressing can be done in bed as tolerance for the sitting position increases. When the patient can sit for longer periods, lower extremity dressing in bed may be begun. For this, a long-handled reacher may be needed.

Wheelchair Phase. Some adjustment time may be required for the patient to regain a sense of balance and body use when first moving from the bed into a wheelchair. When this is accomplished, all bathing and grooming can be done before a mirror and upper extremity dressing can be done in a wheelchair. It is crucial to the rehabilitation of the paraplegic that he or she be encouraged to assume these responsibilities as functional ability is regained. Self-care activities not only provide independent functions but also provide important daily exercise in balance, strength, and coordination. Since fatigue may be experienced in the early accomplishment of these tasks, the treatment program must be coordinated with all other therapies. All rehabilitation team members are informed of the patient's level of accomplishment, so that efforts are coordinated toward the achievement of maximum independence.

Since functioning from a wheelchair will, in most cases, become a way of life for the paraplegic, it is essential that the chair be equipped to meet all physical, personal, and functional needs. The wheelchair should be heavy duty, but light weight for ease of lifting in and out of a car; should be as narrow as possible for easy passage through doorways and maneuvering in bathrooms; should have swing-away removable footrests for transfer and proximity to cabinets and work areas; and should have removable desk arms at a comfortable height for arm positioning, transfer, and proximity to tables and counters. A seatboard with a special cushion to prevent decubiti is sometimes used to maintain good positioning of trunk and hips. The foot pedals should clear 2 inches from the ground for safe travel over bumps and rough ground, the depth of the seat should extend to 2 inches proximal to the knee bend, and the back height should extend no farther than 3 inches below the axilla to allow free movement of the arms but provide needed trunk support. Pneumatic tires are often recommended for ease and safety over rough ground and for a comfortable ride. However, because these tires need to be checked for sufficient air pressure and do go flat occasionally, they are contraindicated when the patient is unable to attend to these functions or does not have access to someone who can help. Hard rubber tires may be more practical in this case. In most cases, the paraplegic person will be able to propel a wheelchair both inside and outside on smooth ground with ease, less easily on rough ground.

Assistive Devices. The paraplegic individual needs fewer assistive devices than does the quadriplegic person for independent living. He or she generally uses a seatboard and special cushion for the wheelchair, a transfer board, a long-handled reacher for dressing or retrieving objects from high places or the floor, and wheelchair accessories (drink holder, ashtray, and carrying bag). The patient who is able to transfer with or without a sliding board can practice this skill in occupational therapy by transferring to a regular chair. The chair should have both a firm back and a firm seat. Working from a regular chair increases trunk and upper extremity strength and mobility.

Activities and Skills. In the social and activity-oriented climate of occupational therapy, the paraplegic is able to use his or her arms fully in bilateral strengthening activities, increasing upper extremity coordination, balance, and physical tolerance for performing all productive activity from a wheelchair. The challenges of using cabinets, shelves, electrical outlets, standing electric machinery, and heavy hand tools help in developing skill and self-value in accomplishment. Group activities with peers and other patients (games, projects, discussions, planning) aid in self-awareness, social skills, and responsibility. Construction of assistive equipment such as seat boards, tub boards for transfer, and sliding boards aid in acceptance of their use by the patient and may provide opportunities to gain skills to benefit others as well (Fig. 29-10).

In many cases, the paraplegic patient will want to learn to use braces and crutches to walk; however, the braces are heavy, and walking requires much strength. Because of the cost in energy, the patient often resorts to the wheelchair for ease of travel; this occurs after a trial time that may last for months or years.

Life in a wheelchair, however, requires that all activities be done sitting. The patient will be dependent on the arms for mobility, vocation, and avocations. The resourceful paraplegic individual can do virtually anything from a wheelchair except climb steps, pass through narrow doorways, or reach appliances and counters that are too high.

The occupational therapy program consists of developing upper extremity productivity, which will lead to prevocational and vocational planning. Skills begun in occupational therapy during hospitalization can greatly assist the paraplegic person in accepting limitations and using abilities for developing salable skills and healthy attitudes.

With training, the paraplegic person can function independently in self-care from bed and wheelchair,

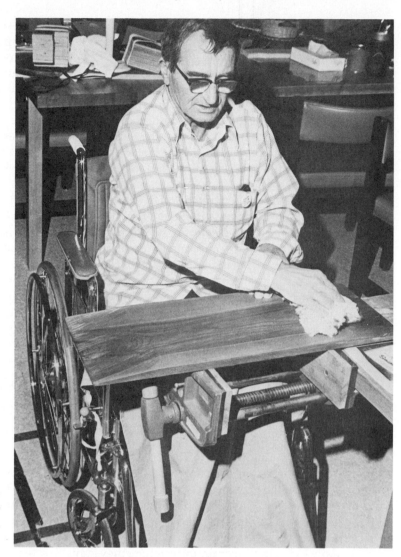

Figure 29-10. Assistive equipment. Paraplegic patient works on his transfer board for upper-extremity strengthening and adjustment to wheelchair living.

can perform household activities from a wheelchair, can transfer to and from the wheelchair, drive with hand controls, and perform vocational skills. The major problems will be those caused by architectural barriers outside of and within buildings, problems which impair mobility and make job-seeking extremely difficult.

Community Re-entry

In the occupational therapy program, opportunities for total independence in self-care, ADL, homemaking skills, manual skills, program planning, and evaluation of functional levels and progress assist the patient in developing abilities for successful community re-entry.

The spinal cord-injured person benefits from patient and family education sessions, weekend trials of self-care and social skills, group trips into the community during the formal treatment program, and education regarding the community resources available following discharge. The patient is able to participate in sports competition, social activities, conferences, workshops,

and other functions designed and sponsored by and for disabled people. Due to increased efforts to eliminate architectural barriers to disabled persons, wheelchair users are finding that, where individual motivations and efforts are demonstrated, they can re-enter communities in fully functioning capacities despite their physcial disabilities. In an accepting society, they are disabled, but they are not handicapped.

In suffering a spinal cord injury, the person immediately becomes involved in an interruption of lifestyle content and plans. The loss may be devastating or adjustment impossible. In accepting assistive equipment, the patient must accept loss of physical function and the use of mechanical substitutes. Energy level and motivation determine his or her priorities in the functional use of the remaining physical and mental abilities. Whether the patient can accept doing part of a task rather than the whole, can accept assistance, and can ask for help when needed are important elements in rehabilitation.

The person who must adjust to permanent spinal cord injury must accept continuing daily personal and social life in a wheelchair. From the onset, he or she begins to make choices, which often require compromise:

1. Whether to remain immobile and dependent or to become mobile and perhaps partially independent
2. Whether to use a shiny metal electronically operated hand splint to permit handling objects with strength and coordination or to be dependent on others to pick up objects because he or she lacks hand strength, coordination, and joint range of motion
3. Whether to use limited energy to push the wheelchair independently or to save the energy for other functions and use an electric wheelchair
4. Whether to stay home because many buildings are inaccessible to people using wheelchairs or to use community resources to determine those that are accessible and to fight to make more of the community barrier free
5. Whether to make the disability obvious to others by using helpful assistive devices for function or to remain dependent without independent functions to ensure self-worth through attention-seeking
6. Whether to do part of a task or to ask someone else to do all of it.

These are some of the choices faced by patients in planning for community re-entry. The therapist begins working with patients on adjustment, planning, and practicing new skills beginning with the evaluation. Early involvement aids patients in learning their capabilities and needs, enabling them to request help and monitor it effectively to strengthen them for the challenges of daily living in the community, where they may find rejection, lack of interest, and lack of help and where they must be able to use all of their remaining abilities and skills to deal with the challenges facing them.

Summary for Care of Patients with Spinal Cord and Nerve Root Lesions

In summary, disease and trauma affecting the spinal cord and its pathways can result in progressive or nonprogressive dysfunctional conditions. The progressive disease ALS presents a clinical pattern of diminishing sensorimotor stability and function in the extremities, which may include the motor functions of speech. In poliomyelitis, the immediate paralyzing effects are permanent. In Guillain–Barré syndrome, although there is an immediate paralysis, there is a good prognosis for substantial return of function during an intensive rehabilitation program. The functional manifestations and permanence of the initial paralysis due to injury to the spinal cord are dependent on the segmental level of the cord lesion and the type and extent of the injury. Significant differences in rehabilitation programs demonstrate the functional challenges met by the therapist in the evaluation and treatment of the patient with quadriplegia and paraplegia. The methods detailed in the information on these programs can be applied to similar dysfunctional manifestations in persons suffering from the diseases mentioned above.

The occupational therapy program provides the patient with the opportunity to focus on ability through specific muscle re-education, functional adaptation and performance, and planning based on awareness of his or her condition and capabilities. Mutual planning by therapist and patient, communication with rehabilitation team members and family, and adaptation of treatment modalities to the patient's lifestyle and preferences contribute to the potential effectiveness of the program. Effective community re-entry is enhanced by effective formal programs.

Lesions of the Myoneural Junction: Myasthenia Gravis

Myasthenia gravis (MG) is a progressive degenerative disease that affects the myoneural junction and is characterized by severe muscle weakness. Impairment of conduction of nerve impulses to muscles occurs because of a presynaptic or postsynaptic block at the receptors on the motor endplates caused by a lack of release of the neurotransmitter acetylcholine.[2] Abnormalities in the thymus gland and the body's immune system are suspected of being responsible.

Impact

Beginning with a gradual onset, this chronic disease is characterized by intermittent, abnormal fatigue of isolated muscle groups. In later stages, it results in permanent weakness of some muscles and atrophy of others. Although it can occur at any age, the disease usually affects young adults, with females being more commonly affected than males.

The most common symptom of myasthenia gravis is abnormal muscular fatigue, most frequently in the eye muscles, where it leads to ptosis (drooping of both upper lids) and diplopia (double vision). In addition, the patient may present weakness of the facial muscles; total eye closure; retraction of the angles of the mouth; weakness of the bulbar musculature necessary for chewing, swallowing, and articulation; dyspnea (shortness of breath); weakness in the trunk and limbs causing difficulty in balance and walking; and general fatigue. Initially, these symptoms are exacerbated when the patient is fatigued but may disappear following rest. The patient may also have a tendency toward respiratory failure and may demonstrate a high, nasal voice.

In the later stages of the disease, the patient experiences difficulty in swallowing and speaking. Eventually, he or she becomes bedridden and immobile with severe permanent paralysis.

Remissions (decrease in symptoms) and improvement in general muscle strength and function may be marked and can last for years. However, exacerbation or attacks of weakness caused by physical exertion, infection, or childbirth can occur. These fluctuations can be sudden and of unpredictable severity.

Functional Restoration

The therapist's prime concern in working with the patient with MG is to aid him or her in regaining muscle power and endurance; the therapist must take care not to cause debilitating fatigue. Because this disease is characterized by remissions, the recuperating patient may be able to regain functional abilities in the upper extremities, independence in self-care, and in some instances, be able to walk. If physical tolerance can be maintained during rehabilitation, the patient might be able to return to a nonexertive form of work. Overexertion must be avoided, and respiratory problems must be prevented. The patient should be encouraged to employ work simplification techniques, therapeutic breathing, and energy conservation during activities.

The therapist should provide gentle, nonresistive activites that are interesting to the patient. These activities should be creative and productive and should provide psychological and intellectual stimulation to maintain a concept of self-worth. During therapy, the patient may use a respirator to maintain breathing.

In the later stages of the disease, the bedridden patient may lack ability to use the arms. Should this occur, he or she can benefit from assistive equipment such as arm supports and splints to aid in positioning for function. Electronically controlled devices that substitute for nonfunctioning arms and hands can be activated by microswitches, minute body movements, chin controls, or breath controls. These devices can enable the patient to operate a tape recorder, record player, television set, radio, or telephone. They have been produced in the United States (Prenke Romich) and in England (POSUM). Although they are expensive to buy and to repair, they enable the severely disabled person with intact intellectual abilities to communicate with the outside world and to have control over his or her immediate environment. For example, systems can be devised for activation of heating systems, windows, doors, lights, and typewriters, in addition to those pieces of machinery mentioned above. A discussion of the social and intellectual stimulation that this equipment can provide

to the patient severely disabled with MG appears in Dorothy Clark Wilson's book, *Hilary.*[15]

Lesions of the Peripheral Nerves

Peripheral nerve injuries result from direct trauma to the extremity and affect all muscles innervated below the point of injury. Common causes include fractures, dislocations, crush injuries, compression, and lacerations. Primary impairments include sensory and motor dysfunction, contractures, deformity, and swelling. Continuing malfunction of the nerves can cause long-term or permanent muscle dysfunction, deformities of the hand, sensory loss, and trophic changes.

The occupational therapist encourages the patient to develop maximum functional use of the impaired extremity. Total body use is important in reintegrating the disabled extremity with the rest of the body; activities that are gradually upgraded in resistance encourage coordination, increase function, and augment general physical and mental tolerance of the condition. However, the occupational therapist must be careful not to overwork the patient; excessive exercise can cause edema in the affected extremity, creating stiffness in the joints, thus hindering range of motion. (For additional information, see Chapter 31).

Arthritic Conditions

Arthritis can affect a person of any age, has a variety of causes and effects, and can be of short duration or lifelong. It can result from local trauma or the aging process (osteoarthritis) or from systemic conditions (rheumatoid arthritis). Although it is commonly thought that arthritis is an affliction of the elderly, it may also be a disability of the young.

Degenerative joint disease (DJD) or osteoarthritis is the least-feared type of the disease. DJD most commonly affects the fingers at the interphalangeal joints, causing little or no pain. Other frequently traumatized joints are the ankles, knees, hips, and elbows. DJD often occurs in people who have been active in sports or those whose jobs have caused strain on their joints, or it accompanies the aging process, affecting the weight-bearing joints. The swelling associated with DJD is in the bony structure.

The treatment of DJD is generally local, consisting of rest of the affected joints to relieve pain and stress. Heat and therapeutic exercises may be prescribed in a gradually intensified program. The focus for the patient is on maintaining joint mobility and muscle power by carrying through a home exercise program, using assistive devices as needed to relieve joint stress, and developing individual work simplification methods to conserve joint functions in daily activities.

Other arthritic diseases involve the soft tissues surrounding the joints. Among these are lupus erythematosus, scleroderma, and rheumatoid arthritis. These diseases share the characteristics of joint inflammation, edema, decreased extremity function, and potential deformity. The occupational therapist may see all three in the clinical setting; however, the patient with rheumatoid arthritis is by far the most frequently referred. The therapist may see the individual with rheumatoid arthritis in both clinical and home care situations. Many of the methods of evaluation and treatment are applicable to persons with other conditions resulting in joint limitation and pain. The focus of this section therefore will be on assessment and treatment methods used for rheumatoid arthritis.

Impact

Rheumatoid arthritis is a progressive systemic disease resulting in inflammation, pain, and structural changes in the affected joints. Characterized by remissions and exacerbations, rheumatoid arthritis results in progressive limitation and deformity. Many persons are between the ages of 20 and 40 years. They exhibit swollen, reddened, and painful joints during and after excessive use. Because of the limitations imposed by the disease, the persons's functional ability, physical appearance, and mental and psychologic tolerance are affected. Treatment must be geared toward assisting the patient in combating the debilitating effects of the disease and in maintaining maximum independent functions. The occupational therapist aids the person in learning a self-directed program of joint protection and function to continue at home. Due to the intermittent nature of the disease, it may be necessary to change functional lifestyle patterns that may exacerbate the symptoms and result in joint destruction. Therefore, working with the patient to develop therapeutic daily functional patterns is an essential part of the program. Because the disease is progressive, the patient experiences a gradual decrease in functional ease and capacity due to decreasing strength, mobility, coordination, and painfree movement.

Functional Implications

The major clinical focus in rheumatoid arthritis is the joints, where there may be subluxation, dislocation, pain, swelling, stiffness, and deformity. Functional problems caused by arthritis arise from limitations in active and passive joint movement affecting reach, grasp, and coordination. Among the causes are internal joint damage, fear of pain, actual pain, and decreased strength and sensation, and deformity.

During the period of inflammation, the joint is vulnerable to deformity produced by repetitive stress causing malalignment. Muscles are strained and weakened during this time, giving less resistance to the development of deforming positions. If muscles become overstretched and shift position, they can actually maintain and strengthen the deformity. This is frequently seen in the ulnar deviation of the metacarpophalangeal (MP) joints due to lateral slippage of the long finger tendons. When this realignment occurs, continuous finger flexion encourages rather than counteracts the deformity.

The following precautions should be used while performing physical evaluations and during treatment of the patient with arthritis:

1. In the presence of dislocation and subluxation
   a. Avoid overactivity of the affected joints
   b. Avoid resistive exercises.
2. In the presence of pain and swelling
   a. Limit passive range of motion of the extremity during the acute stage of the disease
   b. Encourage active range of motion with resistance (as tolerated)
   c. Do not allow fear to develop
   d. Minimize strenuous activity and alternate activity with rest periods.
3. Avoid overexercise; work within the limits of joint pain, exertion, swelling, and general tolerance.
4. Prevent muscle atrophy
   a. Limit exercise to the maximum range of motion with regard to specific joint range
   b. Provide an activity in which the patient can work on strengthening muscles when he or she can work against resistance.

One of the preventative surgical procedures performed to combat the symptoms of rheumatoid arthritis is synovectomy. This procedure is performed early in the course of the disease to relieve pain and swelling of the joint, to release contractures, and to prevent arthrodesis of joints. Other surgical procedures include arthroplasty and joint replacement and are directed toward relieving pain, aligning joints, establishing function, and increasing range of motion. When a surgical procedure is considered, the occupational therapist should inform the surgeon of the patient's functional ability so that function is retained postoperatively. The patient's attitude and expectations regarding surgery are crucial to rehabilitation. Through careful evaluation of functional activities, the occupational therapist is able to determine an accurate picture of what the patient is incapable of doing because of deformity, pain, or muscle imbalance. It is important to communicate this information to the surgeon prior to surgery.

Functional Restoration

Assessment

The occupational therapist assesses the mental and physical tolerance by chart review, observation, and discussion of the patient's progress with members of the rehabilitation team. Evaluation sessions should not be prolonged beyond the effectiveness of both the patient and the therapist. During the session, the therapist provides encouragement and support; particular areas for consideration are the patient's stated concerns and apprehensions, medical condition, and resultant functional challenges. The occupation therapist varies the tests and activities so the patient can complete them without unnecessary pain, frustration, or joint stress. It is important that the therapist emphasize the patient's abilities realistically.

The following steps should be taken:

1. Examine the extremities for signs of redness, swelling, atrophy, discoloration, surgical scars, malalignment, joint deformities, hyperflexion, hyperextension, abduction, adduction, and ulnar deviation.
2. Examine the relaxed limbs for signs of atrophy, joint limitation, and discomfort.
3. Examine splints, braces, or other special equipment. Determine the patient's ability to use and care for the devices and evaluate their effectiveness.
4. Gently move the extremities through the passive joint range of motion, noting any subluxation, limitation, muscle tightness, or pain.
5. Ask the patient to move his or her extremities through all ranges of motion actively and to indicate if there is pain.
6. Check the muscle strength by providing resistance to active range of motion.
7. Provide activities that demonstrate the functional use of hands and arms:
   a. *Grasping* small objects such as coins, paper clips, a pencil, or a key
   b. *Lifting* heavy objects such as a hammer, using one hand, and a large can of sugar, using two hands
   c. *Reaching*, by placing a book on a shelf, turning on a faucet, or opening a drawer
8. Observe the use of the hands in task activities such as writing, removing a letter from an envelope, counting money (either change or bills), and finding a page in a book.
9. Evaluate self-care: bathing, grooming, eating, transferring from one position to another, walking, and carrying needed items.

The therapist should remain alert for signs of mental, psychological, or physical fatigue. The patient's confidence is gained by asking him or her to describe present needs, interests, and concerns and to discuss plans.

Treatment

General Principles

There are several basic principles of therapeutic intervention that can be used in working with the patient with rheumatoid arthritis, whether in an acute-care program, an outpatient program, or a home program. It is toward these objectives that the therapist instructs the patient so that the patient can maintain the long-term attention to self-care that the disease requires.

Control of the Rheumatoid Process
Anti-inflammatory and analgesic drugs are used to control the disease. Bedrest is essential during the acute phase and postoperatively in instances of severe destruction of the joints. Although procedures may succeed in retarding the rheumatoid process for a time, the patient may continue to have exacerbations of the disease. When the joints show a reduction of swelling and inflammation, the rehabilitation program can begin.

Joint Mobility Through Range of Motion
Passive and active joint range of motion of all extremities are essential for functional restoration. Passive and active joint range of motion techniques should be employed to determine the presence of pain and limitation. Active range of motion with resistance should be encouraged only after pain, swelling, and inflammation have been sufficiently reduced to avoid any risk of deformity.

Functional Training
The occupational therapist uses a functional training program to make the patient aware of both limitations and abilities. Analyzing the patient's daily activities can help the therapist provide specific self-care techniques and appropriate productive avocational activities in conjunction with joint protection.

Maintenance of Muscle Power
The patient with rheumatoid arthritis may exhibit weakness. Deformities may prevent functional use of muscles, and joint alignment may be continually challenged. Without adequate joint function, muscle power is reduced, but the use of a functional hand splint can properly align muscles, joints, and tendons. Activities requiring strength must be used carefully in the therapeutic program. Too much resistance can cause joint pain. The occupational therapist must avoid activity that will cause fatigue and must make the patient aware of limitations in strength.

Independence in Self-Care

Because of the existence of pain and joint limitations characteristic of arthritis, the patient may suffer deficiencies in self-care, may avoid dressing, or may request assistance in basic ADL. The therapist should encourage the use of self-care techniques as therapeutic exercises, employing assistive devices and special equipment to conserve energy and avoid further joint destruction.

Increase Physical and Mental Endurance

The person with rheumatoid arthritis is subjected to frequent hospitalizations. Exacerbations and remissions are common, and the patient displays the frustration caused by the inability to cope with family or job responsibilities. The therapist should encourage the patient to develop a regimen of alternate rest and work that will protect joints and conserve energy. The patient should also be instructed in the principles and use of joint protection techniques. Awareness of the nature of the disease can help both the patient and the family cope with the physical limitations that result from tension, overwork, or pain.

Assistive Devices

These devices should be used only to increase function or to protect impaired joints. They should be lightweight, simple to operate, and acceptable to the patient. They should encourage independent function. If the patient cannot use the device easily, he or she will discard it.

Home Program

The occupational therapist must stress the need for the patient to continue the therapeutic program at home. Among the elements of discharge planning are a home visit to determine architectural barriers, necessary rearrangement of furniture and toilet facilities, assistance with work space and appliances, and development of specific devices.

Specific Measures

The approaches to treatment must be individualized. The outpatient may be seen for the first time at the request of a physician for the construction of resting splints or splints to protect joints and to improve function, teach an energy-conservation orientation, and provide assistive devices. The outpatient often has a family to care for, a job to perform, or school to attend. With the implementation of various aids and programs the patient can perform tasks with greater ease and comfort and can gain the satisfaction of accomplishing chosen activities with less pain and stress. Following the remission of painful symptoms requiring medical treatment, the patient may need only a few treatment sessions. The homemaker can be assisted in organizing time and tasks to minimize tension. The employed arthritic person can be assisted in self-evaluation of job activities and can learn how to adapt equipment or arrange the work schedule. The student can learn ways to ease the strain of notetaking and of carrying books and equipment. The student should also be encouraged to participate in social activities and engage in recreation.

The inpatient is likely to be on bedrest during the acute stage of arthritis. Evaluation and initial treatment may be accomplished during this time. During the period of inflammation, there should be little stress on the joints, and daily activities of bathing and feeding should be assisted. Bathing can be simplified with the use of a bath mitt or a long-handled sponge. For meals, the patient can be provided with a fork with a built-up handle, a serrated knife, a large-handled plastic mug, easily managed food containers, and a rubber mat upon which to place plates.

Bed positioning is extremely important to prevent deformities and to encourage the most beneficial, comfortable, and successful means of functioning. The patient should use a firm mattress and should lie flat in the supine position with the arms and hands straight at the sides. A small pillow may be used if necessary. Lightweight covers should be used to minimize weight on sensitive limbs.

Prism glasses for television viewing or seeing visitors can minimize fatigue and eyestrain during this period. A book holder can be angled for bed use, and a lapboard placed in a comfortable position can be used for reading and writing. All items should be placed within easy reach.

During the period of bedrest, the patient often suffers pain from inflammation of the joints and requires encouragement and diversion more than active exercise. Exercise, when used, should *not* include resistance.

Poor positioning of the extremities may cause pain, poor alignment, stiff joints, deformity, and general discomfort. Thus, splints may be indicated during the acute inflammatory stage of rheumatoid arthritis. Note, however, that the provision of splinting for the patient with rheumatoid arthritis is both crucial and controversial. As Hollander wrote, "It is usually much easier to prevent a deformity in arthritis than to correct one." Some experts believe that no splint at all is preferable to a splint that causes decreased function or deformity. The purposes of splinting the arthritic are provision of support to diseased joints, alleviation of pain, prevention of deformity, maintenance and promotion of function, and establishment of functional alignment.

Splints are used at night to maintain the extremity in a static position, providing proper alignment of the joints without undue stress on them, and establishing a functional position for daily activities. Because the wrist is the key joint for hand function, stabilization and alignment of the wrist must be done prior to splinting of the fingers. The splint used at night can be a volar splint extending from the distal third of the forearm to the fingertips, with abduction and extension of the thumb. In some cases, the thumb may be left free, and the splint may terminate at the distal portion of the MP joints. This construction may be necessary to prevent stiffening of the phalangeal joints in extension, since they should be slightly flexed.

Daytime splints also maintain functional alignment of the wrist and fingers; however, the splints must be of different types from those used at night. If the pain is at the wrist, static positioning can stiffen the joints, and thus the splint must be removed and the joints allowed full range of motion several times during the day. Dynamic splinting must be controlled to prevent both pain from movement and deformity from poor positioning. The palmar aspect of the splint can terminate at the palm. Finger cuffs and rubber bands can be used to provide finger mobility with an outrigger for positioning and resistive activity. With this type of positioning, it is essential that the wrist be stabilized to minimize trauma to the finger joints.

After the occupational therapist has constructed the splint(s), they should be inspected to ensure that they provide proper support and comfort. Splints should be lightweight, cover a minimum of skin, and be easily applied or removed (Fig. 29-11). The patient must be advised to inform the therapist of areas of irritation and to use both passive and active range of motion exercises in conjunction with the use of the splint.

The importance of positioning continues when the patient is sitting in a chair, using a wheelchair, or walking. When the patient is able to sit in a chair for activity, attention should be given to proper alignment of the body. A high-backed chair should be used for trunk and head support. Feet should be placed firmly on the floor, and firm cushions should be used to raise the patient to a comfortable position. Good positioning minimizes strain, encourages mechanical advantages in function, and prevents deformities.

When the patient is in a wheelchair or is ambulatory, the occupational therapy program becomes more intensive. As soon as medically feasible, the patient can engage in light activities that employ maximum active range of motion. Needlework, Turkish knotting, light weaving, and painting can be used to strengthen the upper extremities and to increase joint range of motion and coordination. In occupational therapy, water can be used as a therapeutic medium to relax and soothe the painful extremity in preparation for passive and active joint range of motion exercise and activity. Careful massage of joint and tendon areas by the theapist helps to loosen up stiff areas for active movement. This limbering-up may be provided in the physical therapy session and is particularly beneficial if scheduled just before the occupational therapy session. In preparation for functional activity, the patient benefits from warmth and from the desensitizing flotation effect of this exercise. Doing grasping exercises of increasing resistance and coordination uses the warmth and flotation to advantage.

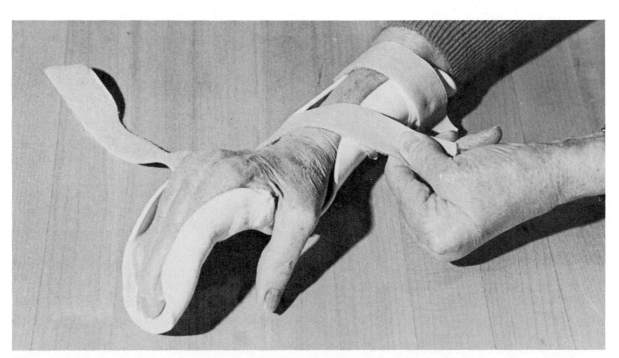

Figure 29-11. Patient with rheumatoid arthritis puts on her volar splint, which provides rest and functional positioning of the hand and wrist at night or during the day.

Joint Protection

Education in joint protection is an essential part of the occupational therapist's work. Because of pain and instability, some arthritic patients fear further damage to the joints and therefore avoid using them. On the other hand, an arthritic patient may deny the disability, avoid preventive precautions, and actually cause destruction and deformity.

Adopting the joint protection attitude and techniques can benefit the school-age child with arthritis; he or she can endure writing exercises by using custom-made hand, wrist, or finger splints and large square or rough-textured pencils for traction. Work surfaces and chair contour and height should fit the child comfortably and therapeutically to maintain stable, pain-free positioning for maximum performance.

The patient must become involved in the rehabilitation process, carrying over program principles learned during hospitalization. Among these principles of joint protection are:

1. Avoid positions that cause deformity. The therapist should encourage the patient to look carefully at the affected extremities to determine whether natural positions are resulting in redness, swelling, or pain. Tests for both passive and active joint range of motion should be discussed with the patient so that he or she recognizes how to avoid excessive strain during daily activities.

2. Avoid sustained positions. The occupational therapist should teach the patient that maintaining a fixed position places stress on specific joints. For example, the longer a person grasps an object, the greater the likelihood of pain and stiffness upon release of the object. The arthritic must be encouraged to change position or activities frequently, encouraging the reciprocal muscle movement to stretch tightened muscles and to relieve pressure on the joints.

3. Use the strongest joints for heavy work. Patients with arthritis must be taught to compensate for weakened joints and to try to develop bilateral capacity.

4. Do not start what you cannot stop. Arthritic patients are often characterized by ambition and a strong work ethic. These traits impair the ability to create a pace compatible with the disease. The occupational therapist must instruct the patient in energy conservation, organization of tasks, and awareness of fatigue.

5. Use joints to the greatest mechanical advantage. Certain activities can be done more easily in a standing position; among them are mopping a floor, mixing a cake, or washing one's hair. Among activities which are more easily done while seated are reading a book, working on a puzzle, doing needlework, or sewing. The crucial element here is not only putting the body in the most advantageous position but also preventing stress on other joints. If the mechanical aspects of different positioning for different activities are analyzed thoroughly by the therapist, the findings can be valuable in assisting the therapist in adapting positions and activities to increase function. Not using the body in a position that utilizes strong muscles and joints effectively may cause strain and even present a safety hazard.

6. The patient must be taught to respect pain. Although one can sometimes detect the signs of pain on someone's face or can learn of pain through the patient's complaint, pain itself is highly subjective. Tolerance for pain varies, and, when there is a sensory deficit, the perception of pain may be entirely lacking. In periods when the arthritis is active, the patient may complain of severe pain, and there may be visible inflammation of joints. In the stages following acute attacks, the pain must be considered when planning activity programs. It must be conveyed to the patient that joint protection is for the purpose of improving and maintaining function rather than restricting function. This is often misinterpreted, and the patient ignores the suggestions for optimal bodily functions in the presence of arthritis. Improper use of joints can increase pain. Lack of attention to position changes and activity changes can cause pain. Denial, frustration, or tension can cause improper use of joints and put undue strain on them. The patient must plan activities to maximize function and range of motion.

The occupational therapist teaches the patient the use of assistive devices and techniques that can aid in self-care and homemaking activities. For example, built-up handles, mitts, and rubber mats for cooking utensils aid the homemaker. Dressing can be assisted by the use of long-handled implements, and reachers can be used to grasp objects from the floor or from high places.

The arthritic patient's home can be made safe by the addition of railings at stairways, removal of heavy doors and scatter rugs, provision of easily managed latches on doors and cabinets, and arrangement of furniture and work areas for ease of movement and function. The occupational therapist can advise the patient in these labor-saving and safety factors.

In order to maintain muscle power and prevent deformity, the patient learns methods of using the muscles that maintain joint range of motion, strength, coordination, and body alignment. Therapeutic use of joints keeps the patient functioning with maximum use of muscles and prevention of deformity. The most effective way of performing protective exercises for preservation of joints and prevention of deformity is to incorporate these therapeutic positions and movements into daily living activities.

A daily plan of activities schedules them according to the degree of physical stress, enabling the patient to alternate work and rest activities, gross and fine motor functions, and sitting and standing to provide therapeutic change to maintain activity tolerance and realistic productivity according to the individual's needs, desires, and abilities.

Summary for Care of Patients with Arthritic Conditions

In summary, disease of the joints affect the overall mobility and function of the individual. Diseases may be local or systemic. Degenerative joint disease or osteoarthritis affects individual joints and is manifested as swelling in the bony structure. Treatment focuses on the relief of joint pain and stress. Rheumatoid arthritis, lupus erythematosus, and scleroderma are systemic diseases characterized by inflammation in the soft tissues of the joint, edema, pain, decreased function, and potential deformity. Because the patient with rheumatoid arthritis is frequently referred for occupational therapy services, assessment and treatment aspects of functional restoration with regard to this disease have been emphasized in this section. The principles of joint protection described aid not only the patient with rheumatoid arthritis but provide an optimum therapeutic approach to all patients with joint sensitivity resulting in decreased motivation and confidence in maximum daily functional activity.

The occupational therapist provides an essential service to the patient with arthritic manifestations by providing functional adaptation opportunities through assistive splinting, assistive devices, or adaptive methods that promote effective daily exercise and activity as well as the psychosocial benefit of continued optimum performance.

Orthopedic Conditions

In the acute-care setting, patients may be referred for occupational therapy with a variety of orthopedic problems such as fractures, muscle tears or lacerations, bone repair or replacement, and amputations. Referral depends on such factors as the length of hospital stay, the short-term or long-term functional implications, additional problems, the extent of functional disruption of independent lifestyle patterns and expectations, and recognition of the value of occupational therapy by the orthopedic surgeon. Treatment of patients with upper extremity conditions may be provided in an outpatient program.

Impact

The impact of a sudden fracture and the resultant temporary or permanent disability varies with the extent and complexity of the clinical manifestations. The range extends from the simple bone lesion requiring immobilization for a period of weeks to the more complex injuries involving bone, nerve, and muscle trauma. In such cases, therapeutic programs are directed toward regaining maximum functional ability through an adaptive program of daily exercise and activity. To accept the restrictions imposed on activity by casting, bracing, confinement to bed or wheelchair, and the new need for assistive devices to accomplish previously independent functions requires understanding of the condition, the course of recuperation, and the expected functional outcome on the part of the patient. Where there is immediate and sudden disruption of the continuity of lifestyle patterns, the patient's acceptance is enhanced by recognizing the functional value of his or her remaining abilities.

The patient with brain or spinal cord injury may also have sustained one or more fractures of the extremities. In this case, the more severe injury may complicate the healing and general care of the fractured limbs. If the patient exhibits communication deficits, behavior disturbances, or decreased sensation, it is important that he or she understand what the therapist is doing and why. Sensitivity may be increased or decreased. If splinting or assistive devices are used in the presence of a sensory deficit, the affected extremity or extremities should be closely monitored for fit, function, and pressure areas. Alternate therapeutic approaches may be necessary to facilitate passive and active joint range of motion in the presence of traction or additional therapeutic equipment.

Functional Restoration

Among patients referred to occupational therapy are those with hand injuries and persons with hip, back, and upper or lower extremity fractures that confine them to bed or cause them to be placed in traction. The evaluation differs depending on the type of injury and the extent of the immobilization. For example, a patient with a neck injury may be seen initially while he or she is in neck traction. If the spinal cord has not been injured, there may be weakness but not paralysis in the extremities. The patient with a lower back injury may have full upper extremity function but be confined to the supine position in bed and may have restrictions on back movements with or without lower extremity dysfunction. The patient with a lower extremity fracture may have full use of the arms but be confined to bed in leg traction, or there may be precautions against hip flexion. A person with an upper extremity injury may be in bed, in a wheelchair, or ambulatory.

In preparing to evaluate the patient, the occupational therapist should review the medical factors pertinent to the injury and the present medical condition. These factors include the type of fracture, length and type of immobilization; alignment and progress of bony union; presence and extent of nerve involvement; presence of infection; precautions for mobility, safe joint movement, and muscle stretching; and appropriateness of removal of supporting casts, braces, or splints during activity or exercise.

Evaluation includes passive and active range of motion of the joints proximal and distal to the immobilized joint(s); general mobility of all extremities; positioning alternatives; feasibility of the use of a wheelchair or of walking; and the existence of factors such as paralysis, trophic changes, edema, pain, fatigue, contractures, scar tissue, and psychological problems. The occupational therapist evaluates the level of functional ability and independence in ADL.

The general principles of treatment for the affected limb include:

1. Support of the injured part to relieve trauma, to prevent further destruction of tissue, to ensure proper alignment of the extremity, and to prevent pain from joint limitation
2. Prevention of disuse atrophy in the musculature surrounding the traumatized area by encouraging the patient to maintain strength, range of motion, and function
3. Provision of a therapeutic exercise program for re-education of muscles and joints
4. Encouraging normal functional return following immobilization through gradual use of the extremity in unilateral and bilateral activities
5. Assisting the patient's adjustment to any cosmetic and functional changes

A patient may have pain in the extremity caused by the trauma itself or by immobilization; such a patient may not be motivated to participate in a full program of exercise and activity. The therapist encourages the patient to become involved in rehabilitation in order to prevent deformities, pain, and substitution of motor patterns in the weakened limb.

The patient with upper extremity trauma may remain in the acute-care setting for a relatively short time but long enough for adequate setting of the fracture, healing of surgical sites, and stabilization of medical complications. Initial casting is usually done by the physician, but the occupational therapist may be requested to assist in preparing for future adjustment by splinting

in coordination with a functional exercise and activity program.

Specific Considerations— Upper Extremity

For persons with upper extremity injuries, the surgeon may request functional training for increasing joint range of motion, strength, and coordination; provision of assistive devices for self-care; static and dynamic splinting; and supportive activities for those in traction. The general rehabilitation goal is to return the patient to a maximum level of function and independence. The injury may have caused serious damage to the sensorimotor system, resulting in the loss of extremity function by blocking the conduction of nerve impulses. Depending on the location and severity of the injury, the patient may suffer a long-term disability. The rehabilitation program focuses on return of the capacity to use the extremity and development of sensory and motor function. Physical and cosmetic changes in the extremity may cause difficulties in the patient's psychological adjustment to disability.

Shoulder disabilities can occur postoperatively in cases involving tumor, traction, immobilization, fracture, or periarthritis. Clinical signs include pain, muscle atrophy, shoulder weakness, contracture of the adductors with inability to rotate externally, fear of movement, and stiffness. Following heat, massage, and whirlpool activity in physical therapy, the occupational therapy program includes graded activities to increase strength, joint range of motion, and function. Examples of such activities are the floor loom, printing press, woodworking, macrame, and basketry. The patient should be encouraged to participate in recreational activities such as shuffleboard, darts, bowling, and ball games to develop full use and integration of the injured extremity. The physical tolerance and fatigue level should be the gauges for gradation of the program. Prevocational evaluation becomes part of the treatment program for the patient who will be able to return to work. The occupational therapist works closely with the vocational rehabilitation counselor in identifying specific job-related abilities. The industrially oriented program is basically one of regaining work tolerance in a graded conditioning program.

For upper extremity injuries, activities such as using hand tools and power machinery, painting, and shoveling are used. The conditioning program should utilize productive work tasks, and activity time should be increased as endurance develops. However, the patient should be monitored for signs of pain, swelling, or fatigue. Home activity programs should be developed to encourage the patient to maintain a general conditioning program.

Patients who have a fractured *forearm or hand* may require a splint as a supportive device for strenuous activity. Unless there is peripheral nerve involvement from the injury, the orthopedic surgeon usually provides the initial splint. However, the occupational therapist may be asked later to provide a dynamic splint to encourage finger function. The most useful treatment is functional training in the use of the injured extremity. Productive activity is essential to the achievement of this goal. Graded manual activity and specific dexterity training in the affected hand are essential for the regaining of functional abilities. If the patient cannot regain adequate use of the hand through functional activity, counseling for alternative job training and placement may be required.

Patients who suffer residual effects from surgery (scarring or amputation) may need cosmetic adjustments. The occupational therapist counsels the patient, pointing out assets and helping him or her accept the additional trauma of cosmetic disfigurement.

Specific Considerations — Lower Extremity

When a patient has suffered a fracture of a lower extremity, the occupational therapy program begins with activities to provide support while the patient is confined to bed. When able to stand and put weight on the injured extremity, the patient can begin a program of standing tolerance and general reconditioning. Lower extremity active exercises include graded, resistive exercises of the extremity, coordination exercises, and use of the extremity together with the entire body.

Adaptations to the floor loom, printing press, bicycle saw, and woodworking equipment can aid in gradual increase in strength and coordination. Work-simulated tasks designed for the injured worker offer preparation for the demands of the job.

For the patient who has had a *back or leg injury*, work activities include weight bearing, lifting, carrying, climbing, and bending. Activities such as lifting, carrying weights, climbing ladders, shoveling, chopping wood, pushing a wheelbarrow, and pulling heavy objects are given and upgraded according to the patient's tolerance. Specific activities for strengthening a limb and increasing tolerance that are used for the patient having a lower extremity injury include balancing and exercising using adapted equipment such as a bicycle saw, treadle sander, lathe, or printing press.

The patient with a *fractured hip* or *hip replacement* is commonly referred to the occupational therapist by the orthopedic surgeon, rheumatologist, or physiatrist. The patient benefits from supportive activities, self-care training, assistive devices, home evaluation, and home adaptation.

During the bedrest stage following surgery, the patient may benefit from supportive activities that assist in psychological adjustment and divert attention from pain. When there is medical clearance for the patient to move around in bed, he or she should be encouraged to participate in morning hygiene and self-care. Because the patient may be restricted in the use of the hip joint in flexion and resistive movements, long-handled reachers and special hooks can provide assistance in dressing. When the physician concurs, joint range of motion of the hip should be encouraged during activity. However, the rehabilitation process must be gradual.

The patient may be discharged from the hospital before he or she has fully recovered from the injury or surgery; therefore, a home program should be established to protect the hip from further injury and to encourage participation in exercise and self-care activities. The occupational therapist instructs the patient in both protective precautions and the use of various devices that can assist in self-care. The patient should avoid bending the hip more than 90° and crossing the legs at the knees or ankles. A firm, knee-height, straight-backed chair with arm rests should be used. Reclining chairs are very difficult for the patient to get into or out of, can cause him or her to fall, and thus should be avoided. Toilet seat extensions and firm pillows in low chairs can ensure proper height for adequate transfer and comfort.

The patient should be advised to sleep in a supine position to promote good alignment of the hip joints. If the patient is accustomed to turning in bed, a pillow should be placed between the legs to inhibit movement.

Other aspects of the home program include instruction and advice in the use of assistive devices for bathing (long-handled sponges, soap on a rope, and nonskid safety strips in the shower), for dressing (long-handled shoehorn, stocking aids, elastic shoe laces, and reachers), and for other ADL. A walker bag attached to the crutch may be used to carry small objects. Cars with low reclining seats should be avoided, although a cushion may be used to raise the seat to a comfortable height.

In summary, patients referred to occupational therapy with orthopedic conditions involving the trunk, the upper extremities, or the lower extremities may be seen on a short-term basis while in the acute-care setting, or the treatment may continue into or begin in the outpatient setting. This will depend on the extent and severity of the lesion(s) and the resultant pathological and functional manifestations. Patients with orthopedic injuries may have accompanying neuromuscular deficits as well as damage to additional systems. The occupational therapist and the occupational therapy assistant contribute to the general functional program of the patient with particular regard to assistance in the regaining of sensorimotor, self-care, avocational, and vocational abilities. A significant aspect of the program is the assessment of the need for assistive devices and equipment for optimum function in the home as well as in the treatment setting, with specific recommendations for the provision of appropriate equipment.

Lesions in the Muscle: Muscular Dystrophy

Muscular dystrophy (MD) is a disease of the muscle cells that causes progressive degeneration of specific muscle groups. This disease is characterized by variation in the size of individual muscle fibers caused by initial swelling of muscle groups; the result is a pseudohypertrophic (enlarged) appearance. Although this false enlargement gives the appearance of a very strong extremity, it is caused by an excess of fat in the tissue and is eventually followed by atrophy.

Impact

The disease affects children, adolescents, or young adults. The most common type is pseudohypertrophic MD, which usually affects males and is inherited as a sex-linked recessive genetic defect. It may occur sporadically or may affect several siblings.[2]

Symptoms appear during the first decade of life; a previously normal child begins to walk clumsily, tends to fall, and has difficulty getting up after a fall. The characteristic pseudohypertrophy of the muscles manifests itself in the calves, glutei, quadriceps, and deltoids. These muscles are enlarged and firm to the touch, but they are usually weak. In some cases, this manifestation appears in the triceps and forearm muscles. The accompanying atrophy usually affects the proximal more than the distal muscles. Muscle impairment can cause weakness of the extensors of the spine, resulting in lordosis, weakness in the knees, and diminished tendon reflexes. While sensation and intelligence are unimpaired, the child with MD may be limited by the rapid onset of severe physical limitations and confinement to a wheelchair. Schooling may be interrupted, and the child's capacity to progress with his peers may be diminished.

Early signs of MD are manifested in the sloping appearance of the shoulders; this is caused by weakness in the shoulder girdle. Contractures are common in the later stages of the disease, caused by weakness in muscle groups whose antagonists remain comparatively powerful. An example of the developing contracture is seen in the patient who walks on his toes because of progressive weakness of the anterior tibial muscle and the tendency of the biceps femoris and hamstrings to shorten. When the patient becomes confined to a wheelchair, contractures occur in the trunk, causing postural changes.

Functional Restoration

Because MD results in a gradual loss of muscle power and control, the rehabilitation program is directed toward the maintenance of joint range of motion and strength through the continuation of self-care and functional skills. Contractures can be prevented through passive range of motion exercises, proper positioning in the wheelchair for arm function, active exercises and activities for the arms, and assistive devices.

As the weakness increases, assistive equipment such as arm supports is used to help the patient in reaching, self-feeding, and other arm and hand activities. Special devices may be needed for bathing and dressing and for diversional and productive activities. The therapist should also provide the patient with a home exercise program, which can maintain the existing muscle power and allow participation in various pursuits. Although the life span of the person with MD is shortened, he or she can continue a relatively normal life with the use of adaptive equipment and assistive techniques.

Conclusion

Human potential is realized through actual functional performance. A debilitating disease or injury can pose a devastating threat to the regaining of temporarily or permanently lost performance capabilities. The rebuilding of a lifestyle challenges the creative skills of both the therapist and the patient. From the reality base of dysfunction must come a mutually designed therapeutic program directed toward the achievement of health by elimination of barriers to well-being through the progressive understanding, implementation, and tolerance of adaptive processes necessary to reach maximum personal productivity and life satisfaction. Focus on ability, realistic integration of assets and deficits, and self-directed risking to take control of one's life are essential for a positive move toward mental and physical health. The patient or client must be in a continual process of gaining this control regardless of the medical prognosis or the progression of the disease or disability.

Appropriate timing in therapeutic interventions begins with respect for the patient's ability to relate to medical and therapeutic objectives and the challenge to integrate them into his or her short-term and long-term goals. It is therefore the therapist's responsibility to identify and work with the patient's goals as well as the therapist's goals and to elicit the patient's understanding of the direction and implications of all goals. There may be different priorities on the part of the provider and the consumer. Although the occupational therapist may be distanced from the patient in terms of studied knowledge and skill, it is the responsibility of the therapist to assure that the patient understands the clinical findings related to his or her dysfunction and the rationale for the treatment approaches appropriate to his or her situation. Although the consumer lacks the experience and skill of the provider, this should not thwart either the communication of information or attention to personal rights.

The engagement of an individual in activity is not sufficient as a therapeutic goal. The effect of a given activity on a person can be positive, negative, or neutral. The therapist is accountable for achieving a therapeutic result from the provision of activity or occupation. In order to derive healthful benefits from an activity or active involvement in treatment, an individual must participate in the choice, planning, and implementation of such activity. Activities must precipitate a transfer to the patient of control of his or her life decisions and patterns in an appropriately graduated program. This requires the development of positive moves from previous life experiences, a regaining of a sense of the familiar self, a recognition of the new situation, an integration of the old with the new, and an ability to engage in creative functional personal planning.

The health approach of occupational therapy requires a composite of areas such as psychosocial, physical, and functional performance to regain the capacity to control life planning for successful re-entry into independent community living as an individual. Toward these ends, the occupational therapist facilitates the ability of the patient or client to: (1) engage in problem-solving with regard to his or her situation; (2) analyze the situation to determine the information needed to make a dynamic plan to follow a path to implement in order to improve the life situation; (3) abstract and objectify information about oneself such as continuing medical challenges, and functional, social, and financial implications; (4) develop achievable plans with the therapist, the family, friends, and the medical team; and (5) achieve healthy perceptions of the self, trauma, functional status, and options. The occupational therapist assists in the patient's or client's ability to: (1) convert physical capacities into functional abilities; (2) determine adaptive aids and techniques needed for functions, and (3) plan optimal functional living with regard to energy levels, disease or condition limitations, and precautions imposed by disease, condition, or trauma. In the *psychosocial* area, the occupational therapist assists the consumer in: (1) understanding and accepting himself or herself and determining personal strengths and weaknesses affecting potential gains in self-development; (2) achieving psychologic independence for optimum self-awareness and planning; (3) relating to others with self-respect and respect for others; (4) interpreting needs for assistance from others, instructing others in appropriate and beneficial assistance, and accepting assistance from others; (5) accepting and planning beneficial social re-entry regardless of functional deficits or physical or social environmental barriers; and (6) benefiting from peer support and sharing experiential findings on an equal basis with others. The therapist assists with the ability of the patient or client to achieve self-esteem, risk-taking, self-motivation, a sense of humor, physical and mental endurance, and a positive healthy attitude. In the *functional* areas, the therapist assists the consumer with the ability to: (1) develop the scope of individual functional capacity; (2) develop maximum functional skills; (3) benefit from available human, physical, and informational resources; and (4) develop motivation to learn and pursue internal and external resources.

In *regaining control of one's daily life pattern,* it is essential for the patient to engage in: (1) determination of his or her objectives; (2) planning and implementation of an active trial-oriented approach to growth; (3) a new lifestyle context based on integration of the old and the new; and (4) a positive attitude toward the personal growth gained from experience. *Successful independent re-entry into community living* depends on: (1) the achievement of independent functions; (2) independent control of assisted functions, and (3) continual development of objectives and implementation for productive, satisfying, and healthy living.

The occupational therapist is in a unique position to provide essential services to patients in regaining a healthy perspective and involvement in life experiences following disease or trauma. Within the context of the philosophic base of occupational therapy and the availability of dynamic frames of reference, therapeutic theory, specific skills in clinical and community application of practice techniques, and adaptations are the mandates for responsible and essential therapeutic services.

References

1. Alpers BJ, Mancall EL: Clinical Neurology, 6th ed, p 598. Philadelphia, FA Davis, 1971
2. Bannister R: Brain's Clinical Neurology, 4th ed, pp 323, 329, 347, 392–394. London, Oxford University Press, 1973
3. Boyes JH: Bunnell's Surgery of the Hand, 5th ed, p 240. Philadelphia, JB Lippincott, 1970
4. Brain B, Walton JN: Brain's Diseases of the Nervous System, pp 494, 525, 595, 598, 814. London, Oxford University Press, 1969
5. Eson ME, Yen JK, Bourke RS: Assessment of recovery from serious head injury. J Neurol Neurosurg Psychiatr 41:1036, 1978
6. Hagan C, Malkmus D, Durham P: Communication Disorders Service (revised 11/15/74 by Malkmus D, Stenderup K). Downey, CA, Rancho Los Amigos Hospital, 1972

7. Jennett B, Bond M: Assessment of outcome after severe brain damage: A practical scale. Lancet 1:482, 1975
8. Jennett B, Teasdale G: Aspects of coma after severe head injury. Lancet 1:878, 1977
9. Morris AF, Brown M: Electronic training devices for hand rehabilitation. Am J Occup Ther 30:379, 1976
10. Mossman PL: A Problem-Oriented Approach to Stroke. Springfield, IL, Charles C Thomas, 1976
11. Rappaport M: Disability rating scale for severe head trauma patients. Presented at the Third Annual Conference on Head Trauma Rehabilitation: Coma to Community, 1980
12. Rusk H: Rehabilitative Medicine, p 321, ed 3. St. Louis, CV Mosby, 1971
13. Snook JH: Spasticity reduction splint. Am J Occup Ther 33:648, 1979
14. Stern JM: Cranio-cerebral injured patients: Psychiatric clinical description. Proc 7th Int Congr World Fed Occup Ther 1978, pp 81–84
15. Wilson DC: Hilary. New York, McGraw-Hill, 1973

Bibliography

A Guidebook to the Minimum Federal Guidelines and Requirements for Accessible Design. US Architectural and Transportation Barriers Compliance Board, 330 C St SW, Room 1010, Washington, DC, 20202, 1981

Abreu BC (ed): Physical Disabilities Manual. New York, Raven Press, 1981

American Occupational Therapy Association Publications Mart Catalog, Rockville, MD, 1980

Ayres AJ: Sensory Integration and the Child. Los Angeles, Western Psychological Services, 1979

Banerjee SN (ed): Rehabilitation Management of Amputees. Baltimore, Williams & Wilkins, 1982

Basmajian JV (ed): Therapeutic Exercise, 4th ed. Baltimore, Williams & Wilkins, 1984

Brooks NA: From rehabilitation to independent living. In Kottke FJ, Stillwell GK, Lehmann JF (eds): Krusen's Handbook of Physical Medicine and Rehabilitation, 3rd ed. Philadelphia, WB Saunders, 1982

Carle TV: The long term picture in spinal cord injury. In Kaplan PE (ed): The Practice of Physical Medicine. Springfield, IL, Charles C Thomas, 1984

Cromwell FS (ed): Occupational Therapy Strategies and Adaptations for Independent Daily Living. New York, Haworth Press, 1984

Cynkin S: Occupational Therapy toward Health Through Activities. Boston, Little, Brown, 1979

Demopoulos JT: Rehabilitation in fractures of the limbs. In Ruskin AP (ed): Current Therapy in Physiatry. Philadelphia, WB Saunders, 1984

Dorros S: Parkinson's: A Patient's View. Cabin John, MD, Seven Locks Press, 1981

Ehrlich GE (ed): Rehabilitation Management of Rheumatic Conditions. Baltimore, Williams & Wilkins, 1980

Erhlich GE (ed): Total Management of the Arthritis Patient, 2nd ed. Philadelphia, JB Lippincott, 1986

Electronic Aids for the Severely Handicapped: Wheelchair Control Systems. Prentke Romich Co., 1022 Heyl Road, Wooster, Ohio, 44691

Field EV (ed): Multiple Sclerosis. Baltimore, University Park Press, 1977

Flatt AE: Care of the Arthritic Hand, 4th ed. St Louis, CV Mosby, 1983

Flower A, Naxon E, Jones RE, Mooney V: An occupational therapy program for chronic back pain. Am J Occup Ther 35:243, 1981

Ford JR, Duckworth B: Physical Management for the Quadriplegic Patient. Philadelphia, FA Davis, 1974

Fraser C: Does an artificial limb become part of the user? Br J Occup Ther 47:43, 1984

Friedman LW: The Psychological Rehabilitation of the Amputee. Springfield, IL, Charles C Thomas, 1978

Gilfoyle EM, Grady AP, Moore JC: Children Adapt. Thorofare, NJ, Charles B Slack, 1981

Golden CJ: Diagnosis and Rehabilitation in Clinical Neuropsychology. Springfield, IL, Charles C Thomas, 1981

Gruen H, Medsger TA, White JF: Joint Protection Training for the Patient with Early Rheumatoid Arthritis. Basle, CIBA–GEIGY, 1980

Gurgold GD, Harden DM: Assessing the driving potential of the handicapped. Am J Occup Ther 32:41, 1978

Heilman KM, Valenstein E: Clinical Neuropsychology. New York, Oxford University Press, 1979

Heiniger MC, Randolph SL: Neurophysiological Concepts in Human Behavior: The Tree of Learning. St Louis, CV Mosby, 1981

Held JP: Rehabilitation of Head Injury Patients. In Ruskin AP (ed): Current Therapy in Physiatry. Philadelphia, WB Saunders, 1984

Jennett B, Teasdale G: Aspects of coma after severe head injury. Lancet 1:878, 1977

Jennett B, Teasdale G: Management of Head Injuries. Philadelphia, FA Davis, 1981

Kaplan PE (ed): The Practice of Physical Medicine. Springfield, IL, Charles C Thomas, 1984

Kottke FJ: Therapeutic exercise to develop neuromuscular coordination. In Kottke FJ, Stillwell GK, Lehmann JF (eds): Krusen's Handbook of Physical Medicine and Rehabilitation, 3rd ed. Philadelphia, WB Saunders, 1982

Krusen FH, Kottke F, Ellwood PM: Handbook of Physical Medicine and Rehabilitation, 3rd ed. Philadelphia, WB Saunders, 1982

Malick MH, Meyer CMH: Manual of Management of the Quadriplegic Upper Extremity. Pittsburgh, Harmarville Rehabilitation Center, 1978

Marquit S: Psychological Factors in the Management of Parkinson's Disease. Miami, National Parkinson Foundation, 1981

Mayer NH: Concepts in head injury rehabilitation. In Kaplan PE (ed): The Practice of Physical Medicine. Springfield, IL, Charles C Thomas, 1984

Najenson T, Groswasser Z, Mendelson L, Hackett R: Rehabilitation outcome of brain damaged patients after severe head injury. Int Rehab Med 2:17, 1980

Newcombe F, Brooks N, Baddley A: Rehabilitation after brain damage: An overview. Int Rehab Med 2:133, 1980

Nichols PJR: Rehabilitation Medicine: The Management of

Physical Disabilities, 2nd ed. Woburn, MA, Butterworths, 1980

O'Brien MT, Pallett PJ: Total Care of the Stroke Patient. Boston, Little, Brown, 1978

O'Sullivan SB, Cullen KE, Schmitz TJ: Physical Rehabilitation: Evaluation and Treatment Procedures. Philadelphia, FA Davis, 1981

Occupational Therapy in the Care of Spinal Pain Patients. Downey, CA, Professional Staff Association, Rancho Los Amigos Hospital, 1979

Olszowy DR: Horticulture for the Disabled and Disadvantaged. Springfield, IL, Charles C Thomas, 1978

Palmer ML: Manual for Functional Training. Philadelphia, FA Davis, 1980

Payton OD, Hirt S, Newton RA: Scientific Bases for Neurophysiological Approaches to Therapeutic Exercise. Philadelphia, FA Davis, 1977

Pedretti LW: Occupation Therapy: Practice Skills for Physical Dysfunction, 2nd ed. St Louis, CV Mosby, 1985

Product Inventory of Hardware, Equipment and Appliances for Barrier-Free Design, 2nd ed. Minneapolis, National Handicap Housing Institute, 1981

Redford JB (ed): Orthotics Etcetera, 2nd ed. Baltimore, Williams & Wilkins, 1980

Reed K, Sanderson SR: Concepts of Occupational Therapy. Baltimore, Williams & Wilkins, 1980

Reichel W (ed): Clinical Aspects of Aging, 2nd ed. Baltimore, Williams & Wilkins, 1983

Rowland LP (ed): Merrit's Textbook of Neurology, 7th ed. Philadelphia, Lea & Febiger, 1984

Roy R, Tunks E (eds): Chronic Pain. Baltimore, Williams & Wilkins, 1982

Ruskin AP (ed): Current Therapy in Physiatry. Philadelphia, WB Saunders, 1984

Sacks O: A Leg to Stand On. New York, Summit Books, 1984

Scheinberg LC: Multiple Sclerosis: A Guide for Patients and Their Families. New York, Raven Press, 1983

Sharpless JW: Mossman's A Problem Oriented Approach to Stroke Rehabilitation, 2nd ed. Springfield, IL, Charles C Thomas, 1982

Silverstone B, Hyman HK: You and Your Aging Parent. New York, Pantheon, 1982

Stern G, Lees A: Parkinson's Disease: The Facts. New York, Oxford University Press, 1982

Trombly CA (ed): Occupational Therapy for Physical Dysfunction, 2nd ed. Baltimore, Williams & Wilkins, 1983

Umphred DA: Neurological Rehabilitation, Vol 3. St Louis, CV Mosby, 1984

Vallbona C: Bodily responses to immobilization. In Kottke FJ, Stillman GK, Lehmann JF (eds): Krusen's Handbook of Physical Medicine and Rehabilitation, 3rd ed. Philadelphia, WB Saunders, 1982

Wilson DJ, McKenzie MW, Barber LM: Spinal Cord Injury: A Treatment Guide for Occupational Therapists. Thorofare, NJ, Charles B Slack, 1974

Wittmeyer M, Barrett JE: Housing Accessibility Checklist. Seattle, University of Washington Press, 1980

Wittmeyer MB, Stolov WC: Educating wheelchair patients on home architectural barriers. Am J Occup Ther 32:557, 1978

Wolf JK (ed): Mastering Multiple Sclerosis. Rutland, VT, Academy Books, 1984

Wright GN: Total Rehabilitation. Boston, Little, Brown, 1980

Appreciation is extended to the staff of the Harmarville Rehabilitation Center in Pittsburgh, Pennsylvania, and the Eastern Maine Medical Center in Bangor, Maine, for assistance with library resources and photographs in this chapter; to Martha Willis for her critical review; and to Patricia Curran for her editorial assistance and general encouragement.

CHAPTER 30

Functional Restoration: Amputation and Prosthetic Replacement *Elinor Anne Spencer*

It's not what you've lost that counts,
it's what you do with what's left.

McGonegal[7]

To be an amputee is to be without a limb or limbs as a result of congenital deformity, injury, or disease. Age, developmental level, sex, functional ability, vocational and avocational preferences, social status, psychological status, and financial factors affect surgical decisions, preprosthetic programs, and prosthetic replacement. A child born with a congenital anomaly generally develops bodily functions and body image while adapting to the anomaly during the growth process. Therefore, a prosthesis is an addition to the natural developmental process and must be incorporated into a meaningful relationship with the body to become a functional part of it. The older child, adolescent, or adult, having passed this developmental period, suffers an amputation as a loss that disrupts both the body image and the sensorimotor integration of previously developed bodily functions and skills. The traumatic amputee and the congenital amputee must adapt to the mechanical replacement of natural function and then incorporate its use into total body function for satisfactory prosthesis use. The circumstances of the loss, its meaning to the individual, and the functional consequences are thus different for the congenital and the traumatic amputee.

Regardless of the developmental level or cause of the amputation, effective prosthetic replacement depends on a coordinated team effort by the physician, nurse, physical therapist, occupational therapist, psychologist, social worker, prosthetist, educator or vocational counselor, patient, and family. To assure maximal team effort in the appropriate prosthetic replacement for the amputee, the following factors are essential:

1. The amputee must be able to accept the use and appearance of the prosthetic replacement in relation to personal lifestyle and daily needs.
2. The prescribed prosthetic components and design must be appropriate to the needs and expectations of the amputee.
3. The prosthesis must fit properly before functional training and use can begin.
4. The amputee must be able to tolerate the prosthesis physically for functional wear and use.
5. Fundamental elements of the prosthetic replacement program include: assessment, prescription, preprosthetic training, prosthetic checkout and care, prosthetic training, and follow-up.

The major focus of the first section of this chapter is on traumatic amputation and prosthetic replacement in the upper extremity (UE). Although the discussion relates to the adolescent or adult amputee, the materials and approaches can be applied to the child amputee as appropriate. Some discussion of pediatric considerations is given at the end of the section. Because the role of the occupational therapist includes preprosthetic and prosthetic assessment and training, major attention is given to these areas. The section includes surgical considerations, postoperative program, and prosthetic replacement.

The second section of the chapter discusses the lower extremity (LE) amputee. Generally, the specific preprosthetic and prosthetic assessment and training programs for the LE amputee are carried out by the physical therapist. During these periods, an LE amputee may be referred to the occupational therapist for functional standing tolerance and balance activities and for adaptation and training in self-care and homemaking, vocational, and avocational skills. In order to train the amputee in these skills adequately, it is necessary for the occupational therapist to have some awareness of the precautions and the objectives of the prosthetic training program. Ideally, the therapist participates in a credentialled training course. The role of occupational therapy in LE amputation and replacement as related to the preprosthetic program, the prosthetic program, and prevocational exploration will be discussed.

Upper Extremity Amputation and Replacement

The amputee rehabilitation program begins with the decision to amputate and ends with the successful functional and cosmetic integration of the prosthesis into the body schema. Whether the cause of the amputation is trauma or disease, the first step in the program is selection of the type and level of surgery and the psychological and physical preparation of the patient.

There are many causes of amputations. In the upper extremity, the most common is external trauma caused by industrial machinery, burns, or firearms. Other causes are prolonged infection such as osteomyelitis, severe neuromuscular impairment such as injury to the brachial plexus, or tumors.

Prior to the operation, the necessity of the amputation, the expected result, the postoperative conditioning program, the possibility of difficulties in adjustment, and the prosthetic training program are explained to the patient. When feasible, presurgery exercise and activity to strengthen specific muscles that will be needed postoperatively for prosthesis operation assist both physical and psychological adjustment to the total process. Such programs include all humeral and scapular ranges of motion (ROM) and forearm rotation.

Surgical Considerations

During surgical amputations, all possible bone length, soft tissue, and skin are saved.[3] This practice stems from the belief that the lower the amputation, the better the function will be both with and without the prosthesis. The importance of structural length and support of the bone(s), the length and strength of cut or damaged muscles, and the sensory properties of adequate skin coverage bear out the practicality and necessity of preserving tissue. Regardless of the level of the amputation, the muscles involved directly or indirectly in the function of the amputated part are affected by the loss. In addition to providing adequate tissue to withstand the pressure of the socket during prosthesis use, maximum sensation is preserved to provide sensory feedback during prosthesis function. The loss or distortion of sensation is the greatest limiting factor to prosthesis use and will be discussed further in this chapter.

Both during and after surgery, an effort is made to form the stump in such a way as to maintain maximum function of the remaining tissue and to provide maximum use of the prosthesis. Blood vessels and nerves are pulled down, cut, and allowed to retract so that they do not interfere with the amputee's use of the prosthesis by causing pain in the stump when the device is used.

Either a *closed* or an *open* amputation may be done by the surgeon. The open amputation allows free drainage of material, minimizing the possibility of infection before closure. The immediate closed amputation may reduce the period of hospitalization, but it also reduces free drainage and increases the danger of bacterial growth. When a closed amputation is performed, either immediately or following sufficient drainage, the maximum amount of tissue is saved. However, regardless of the surgical method used, the stump must be strong and resilient and must have a snug, comfortable contact with the socket of the prosthesis, for the amputee will exert much pressure on the stump while using the device.

Levels of Upper Extremity Amputations

Amputations are generally defined in relation to the fingers, wrist, elbow, and shoulder. The levels indicate both the surgical level and the type of prosthetic replacement expected.

Amputations at the joints are referred to as *disarticulations* (*i.e.,* finger, wrist, elbow, or shoulder disarticulation). Amputations below the wrist across the metacarpal bones are referred to as *transmetacarpal*. At this level and below, amputations are referred to as *partial hand*. Should the amputation occur between the wrist and the elbow, the level is referred to as *below elbow* (BE), and

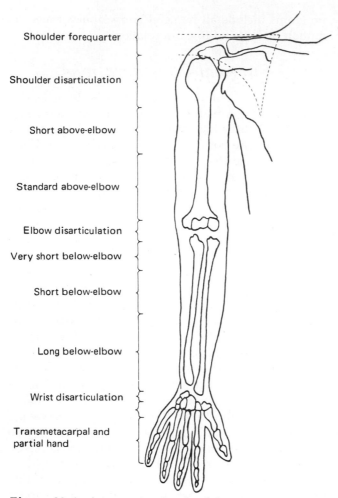

Shoulder forequarter

Shoulder disarticulation

Short above-elbow

Standard above-elbow

Elbow disarticulation

Very short below-elbow

Short below-elbow

Long below-elbow

Wrist disarticulation

Transmetacarpal and
partial hand

Figure 30-1. Amputation levels of the upper extremity.

amputation between the elbow and the shoulder is referred to as *above elbow* (AE). Amputations at the surgical neck of the humerus (distal to the humeral head) to
the shoulder articulation are referred to as *shoulder disarticulations.* Amputations above the shoulder joint involving the clavicle and scapula are referred to as *forequarter* (Fig. 30-1).

Although there are general types of prostheses for
each level of amputation, each prosthesis is medically
prescribed for the person's individual needs, and the
artificial limb is custom-made and individually fitted.

The higher the amputation, the more the amputee
must depend on the prosthesis for replacement of bodily
function. The shorter the stump, the greater the coverage of the stump socket, thus adding weight, limiting
proximal joint functions, and limiting sensory contact of
the extremity. With the progressive prosthetic replacement of joint functions, the prosthesis gains weight and
challenges the amputee to increasingly complex motions of the amputated and sound extremity to accomplish functional replacement.

Sensation and Pain

Following traumatic injury and surgery to an extremity,
the amputee may experience a variety of sensory
changes. Initially, the individual experiences the pain of
sudden trauma and then of surgery. Because the sensory
representation of the amputated limb remains in the
brain after the limb has been removed, a sensation of the
missing part, or "phantom sensation," can be triggered
or reinforced by sensory input from elsewhere in the
body.[3] The sensation may be described by the amputee
as a tingling sensation, an actual sensation of the hand
or foot, or a sense of gripping or clenching. Although in
most cases phantom awareness is painless, it can become intolerable if sensed as actual pain. Traumatic
crush injuries are prevalent causes of painful phanton
sensations such as burning or cramping. Phantom pain
can lead to postsurgical problems for the amputee; if
serious, it may warrant surgical revision of the stump.
Continuation of phantom pain can lead to difficulties in
accepting, tolerating, and using a prosthesis. In addition
to supportive counseling, the most effective compensations for phantom sensations are: (1) early preprosthetic
use of the amputated extremity in daily activity, (2)
stump desensitization to build tolerance to sensory contact and assure prosthetic readiness, and (3) early prosthesis fitting.

Pain can also result from edema, infection, or neuroma in or around the amputation. The nerve tissue
neuroma or tumor forms a painful mass in the stump.
The pain increases on contact of the stump with the
prosthetic socket and is unrelieved by the prosthetist's
revisions of the socket. Surgical revision may be recommended.

The sensation in the stump is important in the amputee's rehabilitation. For optimum prosthesis use, adequate skin coverage is essential. The presence of scar
tissue, fragile skin areas, and bony prominences can
hinder the development of sensory tolerance of the
pressure needed to operate the control system.

If a hand has been amputated and the patient has
been fitted with a prosthetic prehension device, he or
she no longer experiences functional sensation in the
area that has been amputated. Although he or she has
sensation in the stump, it is functionally lost when the
prosthesis is put on. Therefore, he or she will have to
depend on visual cues to use the terminal device (TD) to
handle objects. Sensation can also be a problem if the
socket is ill fitting or if the stump is not well-formed at
the distal end. Therefore, the amputee must adjust to the
pressure of the socket on the stump. He or she also must
become used to the pressure of the harness on the
shoulders and to the weight of the prosthesis.

The amputee may also have to accept a new body
image; this is difficult for some amputees because major
changes in their body images will occur with the loss.

Some amputees may be disturbed by this change in body concept and may have subsequent difficulties in prosthetic training. To be functionally useful, the prosthesis must be integrated into the body schema and must become a part of the individual.

Partial Hand Options

A major consideration in the traumatic partial hand amputation is whether to leave remaining healthy hand tissue or to amputate. Decisions involve careful evaluation of the integrity of the remaining tissue, as well as of sensory, motor, functional, and cosmetic aspects. Further amputation may be postponed. This area of consideration demands individual and creative design in the skillful provision of functional and cosmetic components relative to the amputee's needs.

The partial hand amputee may or may not need or want a prosthesis.

In the effort to save as much tissue as possible, the surgeon can often save parts of the hand for motor function and sensation. As shown in Figures 30-2 and 30-3, full function can be maintained for the grasping of tools and general coordination and sensation with partial amputation of the fingers. In this case, there is complete function of the metacarpophalangeal joints for adequate positioning of the fingers, and strength is preserved in the muscle tendons as in fingertip sensation.

Levels of amputation are generally classified as transphalangeal, thenar, transthenar, or transmetacarpal, with or without the thumb. Surgical reconstruction of the hand or part of it may be feasible to maintain functional structure and sensation and to avoid prosthetic or orthotic replacement.

Complete amputation of the fingers necessitates prosthetic replacement to provide grasp and prehension. Figures 30-4 and 30-5 show the use of a functional replacement to enable the amputee to use tools. The amputee shown here has normal function and sensation in the thumb. Cosmetic replacement can also be provided by a glove with soft or firm fingers that can be manually positioned for function and appearance. A custom glove may fit over a passive partial hand replacement molded from the sound hand and fabricated as desired. It may be supplied with or without a zipper for ease in wearing. It can also be designed with freckles, veins, and hair to provide a natural appearance.

Limb Replantation

Limb replantation, or the immediate surgical rejoining of the traumatically amputated part, has been done with varying success. Replantation has not yet proved effective in providing a functional body part. The best results have been found with simple digit replantations.[3]

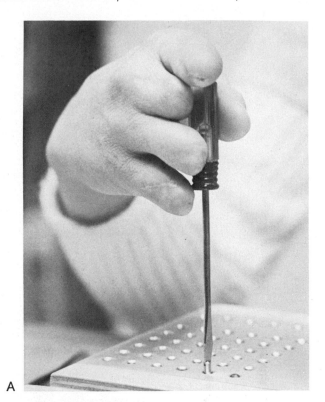

A

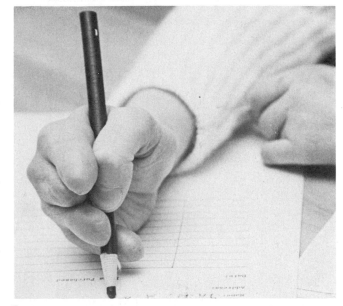

B

Figure 30-2. *(A)* Amputee grasps a small screwdriver between the partially amputated fingers and the remaining thumb. *(B)* The amputee with full use of the thumb is able to write normally with adaptive grasp by the partially amputated fingers.

It is generally accepted that prosthetic replacement is limited as an acceptable substitute for natural appearance and function of the lost part and that the replacement will always remain a substitute. The conventional prosthesis has the disadvantage of being mechanical

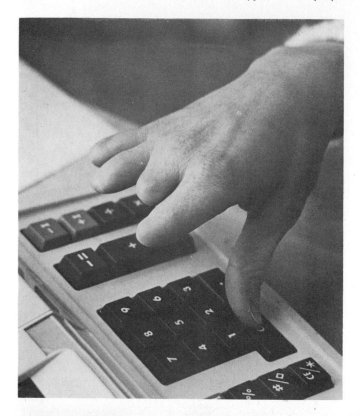

Figure 30-3. The individual had partial finger amputation by an industrial machine. Full mobility at the metacarpophalangeal joints and complete sensation enable the amputee to use a calculator effectively.

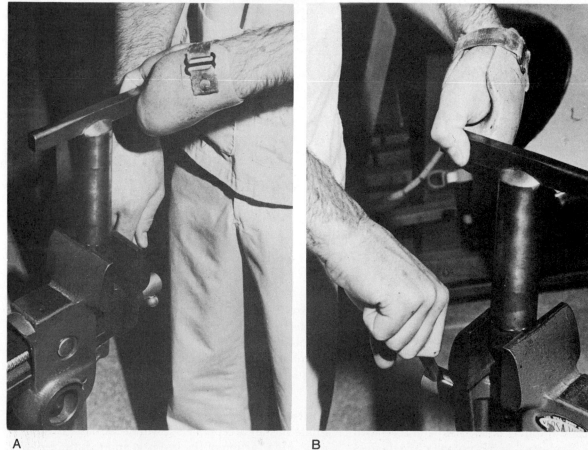

A   B

Figure 30-4. (*A* and *B*) This partial hand amputee uses a prosthesis to replace the fingers and to provide opposition to the remaining thumb for grasping.

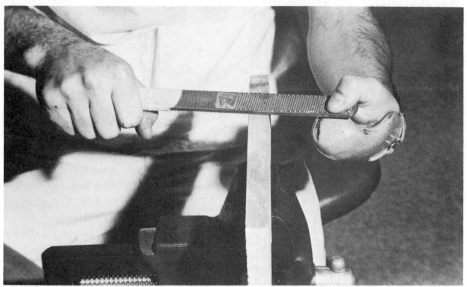

Figure 30-5. This patient wears a partial hand prosthesis to hold tool for bimanual wood filing.

and lacking sensory feedback and general function. Periodic breakdown of devices and the cosmetic challenge to self-image are further disadvantages.

Replantation has been done when immediate medical attention is available and when the amputated part of the limb can be salvaged and replaced safely. Success depends on vascular continuity and nerve and tendon repair. Fibrosis and atrophy can occur, however, and the replanted part may be limited in function and sensation.

Figure 30-6 shows an amputee who has functional amputated digits of her right hand and a hand replantation of her left arm at the wrist. In this case, a 1-inch

prehension range was achieved; however, digital sensation is minimal. The amputee uses her hand as a functional assist, and she enjoys the relatively normal cosmetic look. Since amputees are likely to have different opinions regarding cosmetic value and function, it is important to find out how the amputee feels in regard to the replacement alternatives.

Cineplasty Procedure

A second surgical procedure may be performed following the healing of the first to provide the amputee with

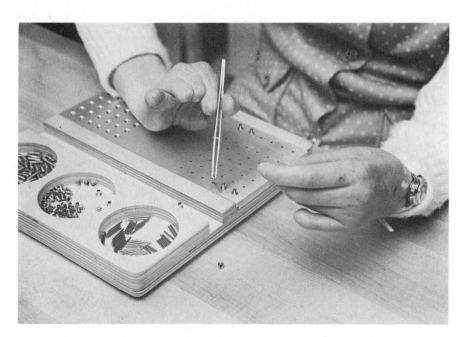

Figure 30-6. Bilateral amputee uses right partially amputated fingers to grasp tweezers. The left hand is a replantation and has limited pinch function and acceptable cosmetic value but lacks functional sensation.

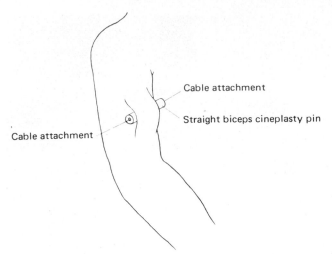

Figure 30-7. Biceps cineplasty tunnel with straight cineplasty pin.

cable control by the biceps or pectoral muscle and to provide increased sensory feedback during prosthesis use. This procedure, called a cineplasty, is done to eliminate the cumbersome figure-eight shoulder harnessing, which can interfere with heavy work, as well as to increase sensory feedback from the TD. The more common of the two sites for cineplasty is the biceps muscle. A surgical tunnel is made through the muscle into which a plastic pin is inserted, and the control cable is attached to both ends of this pin. The prosthesis is then controlled by contraction and relaxation of the biceps muscle (Fig. 30-7).

Because the tunnel must be kept clean, there is a considerable chance of infection if the amputee does not take sufficient care of his or her hygiene. Additionally, the amputee who has had a cineplasty procedure must be able to accept the cosmetic effect of the tunnel through the biceps muscle.

Cineplasty is no longer a common surgical procedure in UE amputation. Modern myoelectric systems are providing the patient with increased functional and cosmetic prosthetic integration. Improvement in harness and socket design have increased the efficiency of prosthetic suspension. Elimination of the conventional harness for general use of the BE prosthesis is feasible with the myoelectric components as with the cineplasty prosthesis. For heavy work, a conventional harness is still used, even with the cineplasty prosthesis.

Postoperative Program

Psychological Adjustment

In assisting the amputee in adjusting to his or her condition and in becoming motivated to learn the function and care of the prosthesis, the occupational therapist must recognize the amputee's psychological reactions to his or her situation. If the patient feels guilt or shame regarding the amputation, his or her relationships with family and friends may be affected, presenting difficulties. He or she may be depressed and may refuse to cooperate with the training program. On the other hand, the amputee may be interested in compensating for the loss by learning as much as he or she can about the prosthesis, by accepting change, and by demonstrating eagerness to learn.

During the postoperative and preprosthetic periods, the patient will usually automatically use the sound extremity. If the dominant extremity has been amputated and the patient is forced to use the nondominant extremity for grasp and placement of objects, he or she may have some incoordination. In this case, he or she can benefit from activities to improve the fine coordination of the previously nondominant arm. The amputee who has suffered loss of the nondominant extremity may be less motivated to use the prosthesis, for he or she will depend on the dominant extremity.

It is important to stress bilateral activities to help the patient adjust to limitations in reaching and in holding large objects as well as to aid the development of bimanual coordination. Involvement in activities aids in the healing of the stump and in learning to use the prosthesis.

Physical problems may affect or hinder the prosthetic training program with either UE or the LE amputee. Such problems are the length of the stump, its skin coverage, its sensitivity (*i.e.*, presence of hypersensitivity or edema), its healing, the condition of the skin, and the presence of infection. For example, an amputee with either a very long stump or a very short one may find the design of the various components of the prosthesis unsatisfactory cosmetically or functionally.

Becoming familiar with the prime concerns of the amputee with regard to vocational and social needs as well as self-esteem begins with the initial contact between the patient and the therapist. Careful attention is given to combining the components needed and desired by the individual. Careful initial evaluation, preprosthetic preparation, and prosthetic training in all areas of function are necessary for acceptance and use of the prosthesis by the amputee. The therapist's positive attitude toward the amputee, his or her stump, his or her fears, achievement of lost function, and cosmesis through prosthetic replacement reinforce the patient's attitude. Most important is the provision of opportunities for the patient to use the prosthesis in all appropriate activities and to socialize with others in the process. Involvement of family members in the training program is essential.

Immediate and Early Prosthetic Fitting

It is generally recognized that early fitting of the prosthetic socket and components aids in effective prosthetic adjustment, wear, and use. When the amputee is provided with a working prosthesis before the sutures are removed, it is referred to as "immediate fitting." This postsurgical fitting is a temporary prosthesis made with a rigid cast socket to which controls and components are attached for early use training. Immediate fitting, in addition to shortening the time between the amputation and the wearing of the prosthesis, hastens the control of edema, lessens postsurgical pain, encourages conditioning of the stump, and provides more rapid use of the controls and the prosthesis. The plaster dressing and conventional harness and controls are applied at the time of surgery or during the immediate postoperative period. The plaster casts are changed as the stump shrinks. Provision of this type of immediate prosthesis encourages a positive approach from the patient and early learning of appropriate muscle use and control movement.

The "early fitting" prosthesis is similar to that applied in the immediate fitting, consisting of a plaster cuff with components and a control system similar to those of the permanent prosthesis. Early fitting is done after healing and removal of sutures and relief of swelling. Bender states that application of the prosthesis soon after the amputation reduces pain and edema in the stump, facilitates healing, and ensures a minimum waiting time until a permanent prosthesis can be fitted.[1] Some physicians and therapists think it is more desirable to fit several temporary prostheses rather than to wait for several months for the arrival of the permanent one.

Postoperative care of the amputee with or without a temporary prosthesis includes ROM, compression wraps of the stump with Ace bandages, vigorous muscle contractions for circulation to reduce edema, and progressive resistive exercises. For the AE amputee, mobilization of the shoulder; elevation, abduction and adduction of the scapula; and flexion and extension of the humerus are emphasized. For the BE amputee, flexion and extension of the elbow and supination and pronation of the forearm are stressed. Stump care, shrinkage, and temperature and tactile contact are combined in the general desensitization program. The therapist encourages use of the stump in daily activities, with washing, massage, rubbing, and tapping to help desensitize it as well as to help decrease the patient's fears of handling the amputated extremity. The use of a temporary prosthesis helps to toughen the stump through sensory contact and pressure during exercise of control movements.

If the BE amputee has a long forearm stump, utensils can be fitted into the Ace bandage compression wrap to encourage bimanual use of the extremities or secured to the stump with Velcro cuff adaptations to enable the amputee to use the extremity in functional activity. A temporary cuff can be devised from plaster or leather to which utensils or a prosthetic hook can be attached. A figure-nine harness and a temporary cable can be devised to stimulate a control system.

The AE amputee is encouraged to carry such items as towels or newspapers or other objects between his stump and body to regain sensory awareness of the stump, to use the shoulder musculature, and to initiate use training.

Prosthetic Replacement

The occupational therapist is a principal team member in the prosthetic training program; with sufficient expertise, the occupational therapist can recommend the type of prosthesis appropriate for the amputee. The occupational therapist monitors the amputee's adaptation through the preprosthetic and prosthetic period, checking the prosthesis for fit, comfort, and optimal function.

The most important factor in prosthetic replacement is the choice of components and control system to suit the functional and emotional needs of the amputee. Patient and family education are as essential as a therapeutic prosthetic training program directed toward return to school or employment, family, home, and community.

The prescription of the prosthetic replacement and the acute and rehabilitation program routines vary according to the treatment team, patient needs, and facility. The material included in this section gives a general view of approaches to the needs of the amputee with regard to the type of prosthetic replacement provided.

Partial Hand Replacement

As mentioned in the discussion of surgical considerations, the partial hand replacement often requires individual adaptive considerations according to the type and extent of the injury and the extent of the remaining functional parts. The occupational therapist provides ROM, sensory stimulation and desensitization, and functional adaptation and use. The amputee may have a prosthesis to provide the function of the thumb or the fingers to achieve a functional grip. The occupational therapist may be requested to devise a temporary adaptive device and to recommend a permanent design for an orthotist or a prosthetist to fabricate. Because the partial hand amputee may prefer to utilize the remaining sensation in the digits, the training program may be one of muscle re-education, sensory discrimination, coordination, and adaptive hand use. Unilateral and bilateral activities are provided for skills training. Prevocational and avocational areas are explored with the patient through occupational therapy. Figure 30-8 shows the use of a temporary orthotic device by an amputee to replace both the thumb and the fingers.

Conventional Prosthesis

The conventional prosthesis is the traditional means of prosthetic replacement. Using a basic figure-eight or -nine harness across the shoulders for suspension of the

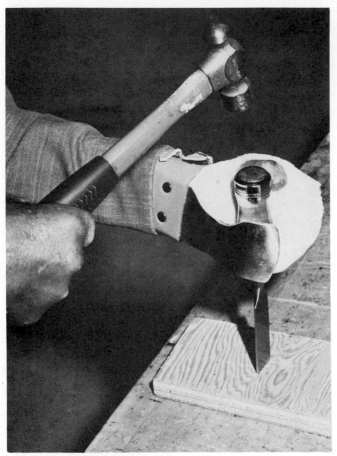

Figure 30-8. Partial hand amputee used an orthotic post to assist firm grasp of the chisel.

plastic laminate socket, hook, or hand, the prosthesis is operated by a cable control system attached at the TD (artificial hook, hand), the socket, and the harness. The sources for the operation of the prosthesis are within the gross movements of the affected extremity and the shoulder of the sound extremity. Control from the sound extremity can be assistive in cases of high amputations and decreased efficiency for prosthetic controls in the amputated extremity. The BE amputee uses unilateral or bilateral scapular excursion or abduction and adduction and shoulder flexion for operation of the TD; the AE amputee uses biscapular abduction and shoulder flexion for TD operation and shoulder extension for operation of the elbow lock; the shoulder-disarticulation (SD) amputee uses chest excursion for all functions.

The preprosthetic period is the time between the amputation and the fitting of the prosthesis. This is the period of getting ready for the prosthesis. In the following discussion, the program described is that in which an immediate or early fitting has not been prescribed and there is a delay between the surgery and the provision of the permanent prothesis, during which time the stump heals and the amputee learns and applies stump wrapping for shrinkage and densitization and engages in exercises and activities to prepare for prosthetic use.

Preprosthetic Training Program

A successful preprosthetic program hastens physical and psychological adjustment to the prosthesis and minimizes problems in wearing and using the permanent prosthesis. In this period, it is important to counsel and guide the amputee regarding both the acceptance of his or her condition and the acceptance of the mechanical device that must substitute for natural motor power, sensation, and physical appearance. Counseling sessions with the amputee should also include his or her family and friends in order to involve them in the training program.

Generally speaking, the longer the stump, the more the amputee can do both in the preprosthetic program and in the prosthetic training program. With a well-healed, healthy stump, the amputee has a good purchase power on the socket and security in its fit. In the case of a BE amputation, the longer the stump, the more active supination and pronation the patient is likely to have. This situation will assist him or her in positioning the hook for grasp and placement of objects. Also, if the stump is long, either AE or BE, it is more useful to the amputee; he or she has a tendency to use it more frequently, thus maintaining normal ROM and strength.

When medically approved, passive and active strengthening activities are started by the physical therapist and the occupational therapist to encourage maximum use of the stump, maximum ROM, and maximum use of muscles, especially those of the arm and shoulder. A well-planned preprosthetic exercise program contributes to successful adaptation and provides strong muscles for the training in isolated motions needed for control and use of the prosthesis.

Following the amputation, the loss of the weight of the missing part causes a shift in the amputee's center of gravity. Atrophy of the musculature on the side of the amputation, scoliosis, and compensatory curves may occur if the patient does not have proper exercise. Therefore, the beginning exercise program is geared toward correcting faulty body mechanics and providing the amputee with sufficient ROM and strength to operate the prosthesis.

The first step is to establish good rapport with the patient so that it will be possible to help him or her work through the necessary adjustments and learn independence in daily living with the aid of an artificial limb. The relationship between the therapist and the patient is a very important one, for the therapist must understand the patient's attitudes toward the prosthesis in order to help him or her accept and use it. The amputee may have fears of being different, may question the attitudes of others, and may even question himself or herself about possible inadequacies.

Before the amputee receives the prosthesis, he or she must develop strength and tolerance in the stump. Therefore, as soon as possible following the amputation, exercises are begun to maintain and, if necessary, to regain normal passive and active ROM in the joints proximal to the amputation (Fig. 30-9). Since the hospital stay may be short, these exercises are designed so that they can be done in outpatient situations in the clinic. Although exercise may be painful to the patient, it is important to maintain and encourage maximum movement and use of the extremity during healing in order to prepare the amputee for the prosthesis, to prevent weakening of muscles through disuse, and to encourage shrinkage of the stump.

After complete healing, the stump is massaged to encourage circulation, to prevent adhesions from scar tissue, to reduce swelling, to encourage desensitization, and to prevent the patient from fear of handling the stump (Fig. 30-10). Bandaging with an elastic Ace bandage or "shrinker" is done several times per day to encourage shrinkage and shaping. Wrapping should be done carefully with attention to tightness, avoidance of unnecessary folds, and complete, even coverage of the stump to ensure comfort. Bandaging should be done

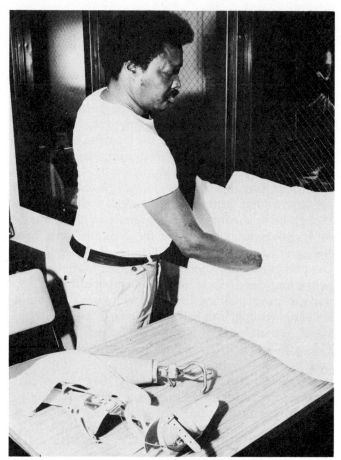

Figure 30-10. To desensitize and improve pressure tolerance of the distal stump in preparation for socket contact, the amputee punches a soft pillow with increasing arm force.

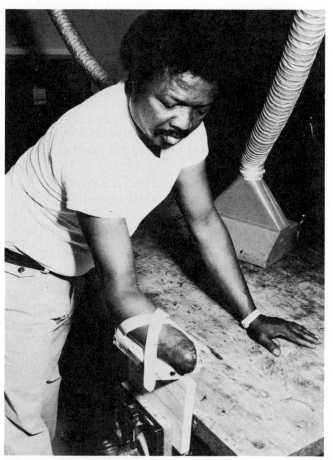

Figure 30-9. Below-elbow amputee benefits by early active use of the amputated extremity in sanding with an adapted sanding block. The patient gains early awareness of the use of his arm, and pressure on the sanding block helps desensitize his stump.

from the distal to the proximal end. Care must be taken not to bandage so tightly as to produce muscle atrophy.

To encourage the use of the stump, the occupational therapist may strap utensils to it which are used in activities of daily living (ADL). Such utensils may include a knife, fork, or toothbrush. The amputee should be encouraged to use the individual implements in ADL.

The shrinking and shaping of the stump are also hastened by provision of a temporary prosthesis in the form of a leather or plaster cuff to which utensils can be attached for functional use of the extremity.

In this period, maximum use of the arms should be encouraged in both unilateral and bilateral exercises and functional activities. Additionally, since posture can be affected by the loss of a part, balance and posture exercises are necessary to prevent substitution patterns; these exercises help make the amputee aware of his or her new body image.

Although the preprosthetic program can be enhanced by the use of a temporary prosthesis, the amputee's tolerance determines when it may be applied. The temporary prosthesis aids the amputee in overcoming the initial psychological shock of amputation in the following ways—it provides a temporary replacement for the length of the missing arm; it provides him or her with a degree of independence, because a fork or a tool or other utensils may be attached to it to provide functional use of the amputated extremity; it aids in cosmetic lengthening of the stump; and, most significantly, it is a device with which the amputee can perform bimanual and bilateral activities. One of the most important parts of the training program lies in the amputee's early involvement in activities that show results.

At this time, the amputee should be encouraged to use the sound arm in one-handed activities, even though he or she may not be naturally motivated to do so. If the amputated arm was the dominant one, he or she may have temporary difficulties in accepting the loss and in using the nondominant arm. In this case, he or she may need exercises to develop coordination patterns in the remaining limb. Activities such as eating, dressing, writing, and bathing may be difficult with the nondominant hand. It is important at this time to provide a program to encourage successful one-handedness in daily activities.

For the amputee with a cineplasty, the biceps muscle becomes the motor for the prosthesis, thus providing the link between the muscle and the prosthetic mechanism. Because the cineplasty provides increased arm ROM and the amputee is free of a harness, it allows the amputee to hold the prosthesis in any position without affecting the operation of the TD. For maximum use of the cineplasty prosthesis, it is necessary to have a 1½ to 2-inch excursion of the surgical tunnel. Routine exercises to maintain this excursion include isolated muscle exercise of the biceps, isometric contractions and holds, and sufficient relaxation for the excursion and the opening of the TD. The cineplasty prosthesis is reported to improve the dexterity and sensitivity of the amputated limb by the physiological use of the stump muscles.

In preparing the patient for prosthesis wear and in providing the prosthesis appropriate to the patient's needs and expectations, the occupational therapist must consider several important questions. First, does the patient need it? This will depend on the patient's limitations as a result of the amputation, his or her vocational and avocational needs and interests, and his or her attitude toward the value of the prosthesis. Second, what does the amputee need it for, and will he or she wear it? This depends largely on the patient's attitude toward the loss of the limb and of function and the relationships of the amputee with other people. Third, does he or she need and want function or cosmetic acceptance or both? Finally, what is most important to him or her in home life, at work, in hobbies, and in social life? Following the preprosthetic program, or near its end, these questions are seriously considered in order to prescribe the appropriate prosthetic components for the maximum benefit to the amputee. At this point, the rehabilitation team comes together for consultation.

Prior to the prescription, the physiatrist measures the stump and examines the patient. The parts and controls of the prosthesis are determined by many factors: ROM, strength, length, skin coverage and appearance, incision site, shoulder strength, and job requirements. Ideally, the physiatrist prescribes the prosthesis at the amputee clinic in the presence of the rehabilitation team and the patient and with the consultation of those who will be training the patient to adjust to and to use the prosthesis. At this time, if not before, the occupational therapist can acquaint the new amputee with the various components and harnessing that he or she is likely to have and perhaps can introduce him or her to another amputee who has completed the training program and is using a similar prosthesis successfully.

The accompanying preprosthetic evaluation form can be used by the occupational therapist as a guide to the appropriate components (hook and hand) for the amputee (Fig. 30-11). If the patient has not remained in the hospital during the postoperative, preprosthetic period, the evaluation form is helpful in determining his or her limitations and needs in terms of strengthening the extremity and trunk for prosthesis wear and use. Should an amputee return to the hospital's amputee clinic for prescription of a new prosthesis, this form is helpful in evaluating whether he or she should be given the same type of prosthesis or whether different components would be more helpful. The occupational therapist can also assess the amputee's needs for further training, especially if he or she has not used the prosthesis extensively in daily activities.

It is important to stress bilateral activities to help the patient adjust to limitations in reaching and in holding large objects as well as to aid the development of bimanual coordination. Involvement in activities aids in the healing of the stump and in learning to use the prosthesis.

The bilateral amputee usually chooses the side with the longer stump to become the dominant side. Sometimes, he or she is trained in the use of one prosthesis at a time. However, because the two prostheses have a common harness and the body must adjust to the weight and balance of both mechanical devices, the bilateral amputee may start the training program with both limbs, concentrating on one at a time.

Prosthetic Components

The basic components of the conventional prosthesis are a plastic laminate socket, the TD, a wrist unit, the harness, and a control system. All UE prostheses have these components, with variations for individual amputation and functional levels and needs.

Occupational Therapy Pre-prosthetic Evaluation

Name: _____ Date: _____

Address: _____ Telephone No. _____

Age: _____ Dominance: _____

Date, cause, and type of amputation: _____

_____

Level of amputation: _____ Length of stump: _____

Prosthesis: #1 _____ #2 _____ #3 _____ #4 _____

Type of present prosthesis: _____

Occupation: _____

_____

Date last worked: _____

R.O.M. in shoulder: _____ elbow: _____ wrist: _____

　　supination-pronation: _____

Strength in shoulder: _____ elbow: _____

Pain in stump: _____

Phantom sensations: _____

Current use of limb without prosthesis: _____

Use of previous prosthesis: _____

Attitude toward new prosthesis: _____

　　a) function: _____

　　b) cosmesis: _____

Additional remarks: _____

_____

_____

Prescription at clinic: _____

_____

Prosthetist: _____ #Training sessions: ____

　　　　　　　　　　　　　　　　　　　Signed: _____

Figure 30-11. Sample preprosthetic evaluation form.

Plastic Laminate Socket

The intimate fit between the socket and the stump must be snug and comfortable to ensure tolerance and optimum prosthesis use by the amputee. The socket may be either single-or double-walled. A BE amputee has a double-walled socket consisting of an inner wall that conforms to the stump and an outer wall that provides length and contour to the forearm replacement. The wrist unit is laminated onto the distal end of the forearm socket. Since the forearm socket can be used by both the AE and the BE amputee to carry objects (*i.e.,* a coat, a handbag, or packages) as well as to push or to pull large or heavy objects, it is made of strong plastic resins that are light and durable.

Because overall weight and bulk must be minimized for the AE or SD amputee, a single-walled forearm socket , or shell, is used for these prostheses. The socket provides length and contour to the forearm replacement. A double-walled socket is provided for the upper arm stump.

The Munster-type socket was devised mainly for the short stump of the BE amputee to eliminate problems of fit, security, and poor leverage that were prevalent with

the conventional split sockets, which are difficult to fit on this type of amputee. It consists of a single double-walled forearm socket that extends just proximal to the olecranon process posteriorly and fits around the biceps tendon anteriorly. The socket is preflexed at approximately 35°, thus limiting complete flexion and extension of the elbow. However, even with this disadvantage in ROM, the fit is adequate for lifting and holding.

The more distal the socket coverage on the forearm, the more active supination and pronation the amputee will have with the prosthesis on. Extending the socket length proximally increases stability of the prosthesis for functional use.

The upper arm unit of the AE prosthesis is a double-walled socket with the locking elbow unit laminated onto the socket. Since the AE amputee lacks independent elbow flexion and extension, these are provided mechanically by an elbow unit, which is activated, locked, and unlocked by the cable control system. A turntable at the joining of the locking elbow unit and the upper arm socket can be manually moved for internal and external rotation of the forearm, enabling the amputee to work with the hook directly in front of the body or out toward the side. The forearm shell is attached

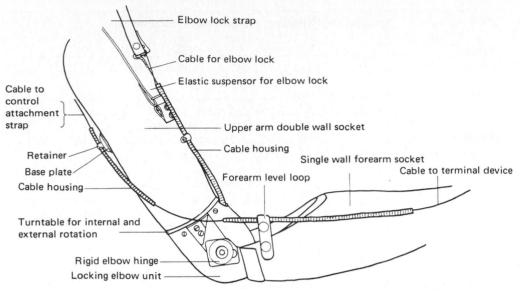

Figure 30-12. Conventional right above-elbow prosthesis with locking elbow unit.

to the locking elbow unit and the upper arm socket (Fig. 30-12).

The SD prosthesis has a supporting socket portion that sometimes extends to the anterior and posterior aspects of the shoulder, depending on the level of the amputation. Frequently, a passive abduction hinge joint is added at the shoulder for ease in manually positioning the arm and donning clothing.

Hinges provide functional alignment and positioning between the forearm and the upper arm socket or the harness. In addition, the flexible Dacron or leather hinges used in the BE prosthesis allow active rotation of the forearm with a minimum of restriction. In the AE prosthesis, the steel hinges provide rigidity for the mechanical elbow joint to ensure strength, durability, and dependability.

A *stump sock* is worn by the amputee to absorb perspiration, to provide warmth, and as padding for comfort and fit of the socket. An AE amputee frequently uses the short sleeve of a T shirt in place of the stump sock. Use of an underblouse or T shirt can alleviate discomfort from the harness straps in beginning training sessions.

Terminal Device

The most significant component of the prosthesis is the TD, which provides function, cosmesis, or both.

A cosmetic TD, used principally for appearance, may be as simple as a flesh-colored glove used to cover a partial hand. Aside from being used to hold light objects or to position objects by pushing or pulling, this device may have little functional value. However, its psychological value is unquestionable.

A second type of cosmetic TD is the functional hand that can be attached to the wrist unit of most UE prosthesis (Fig. 30-13) and is operated by cable control. The functional hand consists of a plastic spring-controlled device with fingers that are controlled in flexion and extension at the metacarpophalangeal joints by the control cable of the prosthesis. The thumb can be placed manually in either of two positions: to grasp small objects or to grasp large ones. A plastic glove fits over the hand, presenting a natural appearance. The gloves are available in a variety of skin tones. Functional hands have either voluntary opening or voluntary closing mechanisms activated by cable control, and they may either lock in position or be free-wheeling or nonlocking.

The hook is the most functional of the TDs. It is made of either steel or aluminum, and it is canted or lyre-shaped. It is either locking or nonlocking, with either voluntary opening or voluntary closing capacity (Fig. 30-14). The hook may be lined with Neoprene, to protect objects while the amputee is grasping them, or serrated, to improve grasp. The needs of the amputee determine the weight, length, design, and function of the hook chosen by the rehabilitation team.

Many kinds of hooks are available to provide for diverse needs. Among them are aluminum hooks required for AE and SD amputees who need minimum weight of the prosthesis, steel hooks for BE amputees requiring durability, farmers' or carpenters' hooks for ease and safety in tool handling, and narrow opening hooks for use in laboratory or office work. Special hooks also are available for bowling and for holding a baseball mitt. Special adaptations are available for ease in grasping tools or in driving.

A series of children's hooks are available that have rubber or plastic parts to increase cosmesis and to pre-

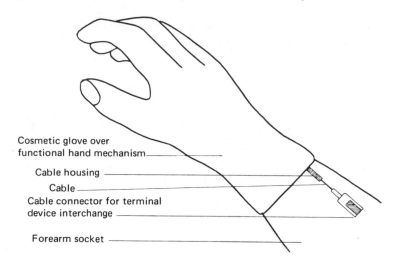

Figure 30-13. Functional hand with cosmetic glove and cable attachment.

vent harm to objects while the child is using the prosthesis to play.

Hooks and functional or cosmetic hands are generally interchangeable through the common wrist unit attachment laminated onto the forearm socket.

Wrist Unit

The TD (hand or hook) is connected to the forearm socket (or shell, as in the AE or SD prosthesis) by the wrist unit. This unit allows interchange of cosmetic and functional TDs and rotation for TD position change for functional variations. There are three basic wrist units: locking, friction, and oval.

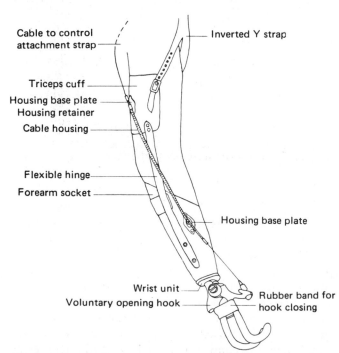

Figure 30-14. Conventional right below-elbow prosthesis.

The advantage of the *locking* unit is that it prevents the hook from rotating during heavy industrial work. By pushing a button on it, the amputee manually operates the unit, which allows the position of the hook to be changed by rotation. The hook can easily be ejected for interchange of hook and hand.

The *friction* unit has threads, and the hook must be screwed into the unit. Although this procedure is more time consuming than that of the locking unit, the hook can be positioned more easily for specific tasks. Either the locking or the friction unit can be used with both BE and AE prostheses.

The *oval* unit is a special thin unit for a wrist disarticulation prosthesis. It is used where the length of the components must be minimal in order to make the length of the amputated arm conform to that of the sound extremity.

A *flexion* unit is available for placement of the hook in three wrist flexion positions for increased function. It is a manually operated device, and it is usually prescribed for the bilateral amputee for added versatility in TD positioning. One activity that is aided by this device is shaving; it helps as well in other activities close to the body.

Terminal devices and wrist units have standard connections. When the desired type of TD has been chosen, one needs simply to determine the type and size of the wrist unit to accompany it. Usually, the wrist unit is chosen according to the way in which the amputee will use the prosthesis in ADL and at work.

Harness

The harness attaches directly to the socket. Its function is to provide stable support of the prosthesis to facilitate the amputee's wearing and using of it, to provide attachment for the control cables, and to assist the cables in the operation of the prosthesis. Basically, the Dacron straps are formed in a figure-eight pattern with extra straps added as needed for better support or additional control function. For ease in use, the figure-nine harness is used with the BE Munster prosthesis. For the wrist disarticulation amputee, a simple cuff socket and a figure-nine harness may suffice.

The shoulder saddle harness (Fig. 30-15) is used for the BE amputee to minimize stress from the axillary loop used in the figure-eight harness; this stress occurs on the sound arm during heavy work. The shoulder saddle is fabricated of leather, Dacron, or polyethylene. Shaped like a saddle, it rests over the shoulder of the amputated side, and it is attached to the prosthesis anteriorly and posteriorly, bearing the weight of the axial load rather than transmitting the pull to the sound axilla.[1] A chest strap is used to secure the saddle in position and to attach control cables.

Use of the saddle harness enables the amputee to lift heavier loads with the prosthesis and to gain complete ROM. There is less discomfort for the amputee because the saddle covers larger and stronger weight-bearing

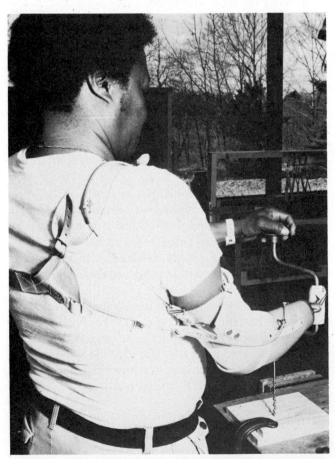

Figure 30-15. Right below-elbow amputee uses conventional below-elbow prosthesis with shoulder saddle harness over the right shoulder to assist in freedom of movement for bilateral wood-working procedure.

areas over the shoulder. The chest strap also distributes pressure over a larger body surface, thus preventing problems from tight pull of the axillary loop in the sensitive axillary area of the sound arm.

Control System

The control system determines the functional value of the prosthesis for the amputee. The control cable of the TD is attached to the device and to the harness. This cable is guided along the socket and cuff or the upper arm socket by retainers that hold it in the most advantageous position for ease of function. Terminal device operation is generally accomplished by forward flexion of the shoulder. During the training period, the amputee practices this isolated motion, and eventually he or she is able to operate the hook or hand with minimal physical strain.

For the AE amputee, this basic TD control cable also serves in flexion and extension of the mechanical elbow when the elbow unit is unlocked. It is activated by forward shoulder flexion. At times, additional joint motions are used in this cable operation because of limitation of shoulder control or strength, to provide smooth operation of the prosthesis, and to enable the wearer to achieve maximum function of the mechanical arm and hand in reach, grasp, release, and hold. These motions may be shoulder abduction and adduction, scapular abduction and adduction, or shoulder flexion of the unamputated arm.

The second basic cable operates the elbow lock. It is attached internally or externally to the elbow unit, and it extends to the anterior deltoid–pectoral strap of the harness. A combination of shoulder elevation, depression, external rotation, and extension is used both to lock and unlock the elbow unit.

Control cables for the SD and forequarter protheses are attached to the humeral or scapular part of the upper arm socket, and their exact design and function are determined by the needs of the individual amputee.

During the training period, the amputee is carefully instructed to isolate the patterns of joint and muscle movement that control the operation of the prosthesis. (The instruction process will be discussed in the section on prosthetic training.) The extent to which the prosthesis provides the amputee with increased function depends on the quality of the fabrication of the prosthesis, its fit, the comfort and limitations of the wearer, and the range of mechanical function. The amputee's limitations may be physical, psychological, or social. The range of mechanical function of the prosthesis includes grasp, release, hold, push, pull, and reach, which, depending on the control by the wearer and the types of prescription components, can be extensive.

Prosthetic Checkout and Care

Before the amputee begins his or her training program, members of the rehabilitation team examine the prosthesis to make sure that it conforms to the prescription and that it is mechanically sound. In performing the checkout of the prosthesis, the occupational therapist evaluates its fit and comfort for the wearer and checks the motion and function of the components. Should adjustments be needed in any part of the prosthesis, the rehabilitation team makes recommendations to the prosthetist. The amputee should not begin the training program with an uncomfortable or mechanically mediocre device. The physician gives the final approval of the prosthesis.

At the time of the checkout, which occurs during the first training session, the occupational therapist begins to acquaint the amputee with prosthetic terminology. The amputee learns the names of the parts and their functions and learns the proper attachment of the harness and the components so that he or she can keep the prosthesis clean and can interchange the TDs efficiently.

In instructing the patient in the care of the prosthesis, the occupational therapist teaches the proper use of the hook, wrist unit, and cable system. The amputee is instructed to use just enough motion to open or close the hook, to watch for worn rubber bands, to avoid putting unnecessary strain on the cable, and to watch for spreading of the housing and excessive friction between the cable and the housing. The socket should be kept clean with soap and water; the stump socks should be washed daily; and the harness should be washed at least once a week. Leather parts can be cleaned with saddle soap. If the tips of the Dacron harness straps begin to fray, they can be sealed at the edge by singeing with a match.

The amputee should be instructed to use only cable control to operate the functional hooks and hands. Manual operation may damage the mechanism. The amputee should also be warned never to use the TD for such activities as hammering nails or removing screws, because this can tear threads and damage hook neoprene.

The cosmetic gloves on the functional hand are perishable. It is important to guard the glove against tearing, because it protects the hand mechanism from dirt and wetness. Also, these gloves soil easily, can be stained or marked if laid on dirty surfaces, and darken with age. Substances such as certain foods, ink, newsprint, and chemicals can damage the glove and lessen its cosmetic effect. The occupational therapist should recommend that the amputee keep the hand in a plastic bag when it is not in use. The amputee should be warned against oiling parts of the prosthesis or removing the glove from the hand, and he or she should be counseled to return to the prosthetist for any assistance needed.

Prosthetic Training Program

A successful training program for an amputee requires the coordinated efforts of a rehabilitation team that includes the surgeon, nurse, physiatrist, physical therapist, occupational therapist, social worker, prosthetist, rehabilitation counselor, and psychiatrist or psychologist. A coordinated effort of these persons is necessary for appropriate prosthetic replacement and training in the use of the prosthesis.

At the beginning of the training program, the prosthesis should be put on over a lightweight shirt so that the occupational therapist and the amputee can see the prosthesis function and so that it is not hindered by tight clothing. The amputee should become accustomed to using the mirror as a guide to learning the correct positioning of the harness straps in back and in learning control motions.

Loose clothing is recommended for the amputee to facilitate putting on, wearing, and using the prosthesis. Clothing with front fastenings, Velcro closures, and wide shirt cuffs are helpful. The use of a button hook (Fig. 30-16) designed especially for the amputee can assist him or her in fastening the sleeve button on the sound side. Sewing the buttons on with elastic thread enables the amputee to leave the button fastened when removing the shirt, even if the cuffs are narrow, for the cuff will then stretch enough to allow the hand and arm to be removed from the sleeve. When putting on the shirt, the amputee should put it on the amputated side

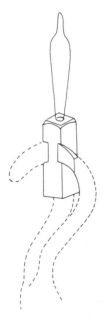

Figure 30-16. Amputee buttonhook.

first. One-handed shoe tying and special closures can simplify dressing.

There are two approaches commonly used in training amputees. In one, the training program is directed toward developing the maximum potential level of performance. With this approach, a unilateral amputee learns fine coordination with the prosthesis, so that he or she can have maximum use of it even in case of an injury to the remaining extremity. The other approach differs in that the amputee is trained to use the prosthesis only as an aid in bimanual activities. Regardless of the approach, activities should be suitable to the amputee's needs. The occupational therapist should encourage the amputee to indicate any additional and special training that he or she desires.

The training period serves as a try out of the efficiency of the prosthesis and the practicality of the components for the amputee's individual needs and permits adjustment to correct any malfunctions of the device. The length of the sessions should be increased as the amputee's tolerance and adaptation increase. He or she must master prosthesis use before combining it with the remaining extremity in bimanual activities and before wearing it outside the clinic. Wearing it outside the clinic overnight is advised for the first out-of-clinic experience. This is preferable to having the amputee wear it at home for an entire weekend. Training with the hand should be delayed until use of the hook has been mastered unless only a hand has been provided.

The general goals of training include: (1) independence in self-care and ADL, (2) return to former work or to a better job, (3) improved appearance, (4) return to hobbies and recreations, and (5) mastery of new skills.

Certain factors affecting the amputee's capacity to learn may, unfortunately, be detrimental. They include poor habits uncorrected in preprosthetic training, lack of motivation, lack of sensory feedback from the nonsensory prosthesis, time needed for training, age, inability to learn, and lack of a sense of accomplishment. The occupational therapist must attempt to minimize these factors.

The positive attitude of the amputee is important; he or she must want to learn. The occupational therapist must encourage the amputee to have positive attitudes toward the prosthesis, such as considering it as a tool, a device to conceal his or her disability, an improvement of his or her body image, and a substitute for loss. Since it is important for the amputee to eventually integrate the prosthesis into his or her bodily function, he or she must become acquainted with it as a potential part of the self, both functionally and cosmetically. The amputee should have a feeling of success after each training session.

Early successful training in the use of control motions can enable the amputee to feel that he or she will be successful in future training activities. He or she

should be cautioned against using the opposite shoulder to control the device and should be taught to operate the prosthesis with the amputated extremity as much as possible. Control motions should be minimal to save strength and, thus, to extend the time during which the amputee can wear and use the prosthesis.

Sensation is a natural guide to motor control; we recognize objects by shape, texture, size, and movement. However, the amputee must often substitute vision for sensation (*e.g.*, using visual cues to determine the amount of hook opening). He or she combines this with the sensation of cable tension to provide visual-sensory training, using the perception of both position and force. The proprioceptive sensation in the stump and the arm can aid here. He or she also uses auditory cues, such as the clicks in the elbow lock, hand, and hook, for efficient operation of the prosthesis.

During the first session, it is important to acquaint the amputee with the actual function of the hook by teaching exercises for opening and closing it. Since many voluntary opening hooks are prescribed for amputees, let us use them as an example.

Following the cable pull by shoulder flexion, the cable tension is released by shoulder extension, and the hook is pulled closed by its rubber bands, which yield 1 pound of pressure each. The standard number of rubber bands is usually three or four, although eight or more may be used for the BE amputee for added grip strength. (Figure 30-17 shows a device for applying rubber bands.) The amputee begins his or her training by learning to isolate the control motions needed to activate the hook. Then, using visual cues and sensing in his or her shoulder the resistance of the rubber bands, the amputee learns how to control the opening of the hook. In order to minimize the energy expenditure needed to use the hook, the amputee should be encouraged to open the hook only slightly beyond the size of the object he or she wishes to pick up—just enough to grasp it. The amputee should practice with objects of different sizes and weights. Additionally, drills requiring the grasp of objects of different forms, textures, and materials are necessary for the amputee to learn the basic motions used in operating the hook (Fig. 30-18). Since some materials are light, breakable, or easily crushed (*i.e.*, a paper or plastic cup), it is important to teach the amputee to employ a minimum of pressure by maintaining tension on the cable during grasp. The amputee should also learn to operate the hook in different planes of arm movement, so that he or she will achieve maximum functional use.

These drills for grip control should be extended to other components of the prosthesis. The amputee must learn how to position the TD at the wrist unit, how to operate the elbow unit, how to use the turntable, how to coordinate the elbow lock and elbow flexion and extension, and how to position the shoulder. In these drills,

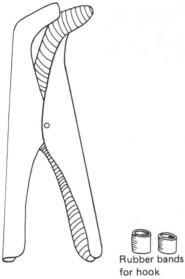

Figure 30-17. Band applier for voluntary opening hook.

the use of the TD is combined with a number of gross arm functions. The amputee learns the grasp, placement, and release of objects on shelves, tables, and the floor and learns to depend on the grip of the hook or functional hand (Fig. 30-19).

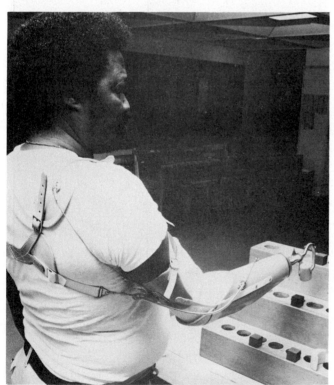

Figure 30-18. Amputee practices control of hook opening and closing in grasp, release, and placement of blocks of various shapes.

During this early drill period, use of the sound extremity should be encouraged. During the rest periods, the amputee should be encouraged to practice unilateral activities as well as bilateral ones. It is through these more complicated coordination activities that the prosthesis begins to be functionally integrated into the bilateral UE activities of the amputee. Although the unilateral amputee may already have become independent in ADL during the preprosthetic period, there are many things that we are accustomed to doing with two hands. For example, the amputee may find it difficult to cut meat, button a sleeve, tie shoes, or wrap a package with one hand. The prosthesis may help him or her accomplish these things, or the occupational therapist may discover that additional adaptive devices are needed.

Whatever the problem, the occupational therapist should encourage the amputee to become skillful in the use of the hook and to devise ways to increase independence in function. Participation in woodworking, sewing, weaving, or other avocational activities can be motivating for the amputee, can provide coordination and strength, can show how his or her prosthesis can help in doing things, and can aid in integrating the prosthesis into bodily function (Fig. 30-20).

Using a worksheet checklist of activities accomplished can be helpful in recording the amputee's progress in training both in the clinic and at home. Since there are many activities the patient will do at home that cannot be simulated in the clinic, the therapist should continue to encourage the amputee to do new things at home following each training session and to report successes or difficulties with the new tasks. In this way, the therapist is able to assist the patient not only in controls, training drills, and activities but also in tasks and responsibilities in the routine of daily living. Thus, the program becomes relevant to each amputee's needs. The categories on the worksheet should include basic prehension activities, dressing and grooming (including putting on and taking off the prosthesis), eating and social skills (using keys and opening an umbrella), homemaking, clerical activities, and activities related to vocational and avocational interests.

Another aid is a prosthetic training board with common objects (locks, light switches, pencil sharpener) attached to it.

Recreational activities during the preprosthtic and prosthetic training periods provide general body conditioning and assist the development of a new image for the amputee.

Because industrial accidents are a frequent cause of UE amputations, a prevocational assessment should be included in the training program to assist the amputee in recognizing capabilities in prosthetic function and in deciding whether he or she can safely return to the former occupation or whether he or she needs to consider a change of occupation and additional vocational

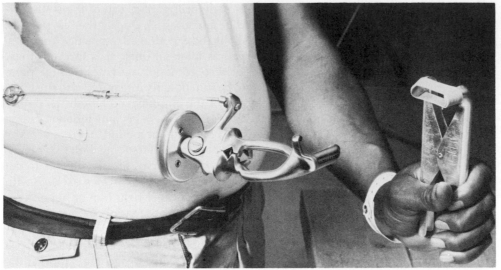

Figure 30-19. During initial prosthetic training, the amputee learns to apply bands to the voluntary opening hook to increase grip pressure of the hook.

training. Specific tasks related to the individual's type of work should be included in the prosthetic training program; for example, assessment of safe and efficient handling of tools, power equipment, and heavy and light materials. Work tolerance can be assessed with timed job-simulation tasks (Figs. 30-21 and 30-22).

Prevocational considerations include training in general household activities. Training in the accom-

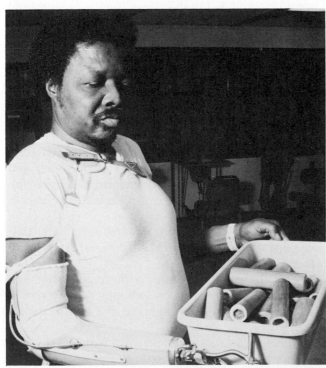

Figure 30-20. The unilateral amputee practices bimanual activities to learn how to use the prosthesis as a functional assist. Here, it is not necessary to open the hook, but it must be positioned properly on the object to assist in carrying a heavy load.

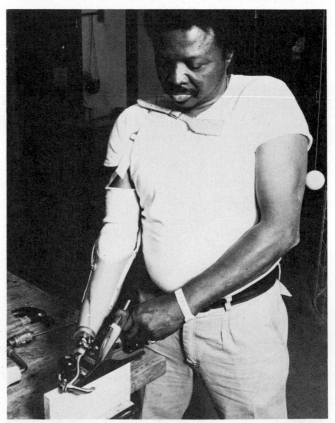

Figure 30-21. Practice with bilateral grasping and use of common construction tools improves coordination and bilateral integration. Here, the amputee uses a steel carpenter's hook with serrated edges for firm grasp.

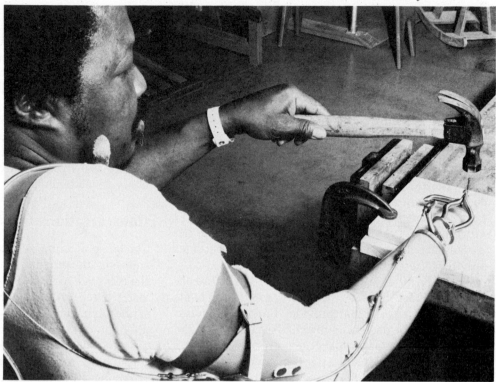

Figure 30-22. The below-elbow amputee is able to position the carpenter's hook to hold a nail for hammering.

plishment of homemaking tasks such as meal preparation, cleaning, and household repairs is included. Child care is also included as appropriate.

In assisting the amputee to return to the former job or to redirect his or her vocational goals, the occupational therapist works closely with the vocational counselor and the employer. Use of standardized tests and work-stimulated activities are an important part of the program for assessment of attitudes, aptitudes, work habits, and skills.

Pediatric Considerations

"Movement puts the child in relationship with his surroundings so that through this relationship the child can have an effect upon his environment as well as be affected by his environment."[4]

Depending on the nature of the condition, a child with a congenital skeletal deficiency may develop adaptively without prosthetic replacement of the missing parts and often without the need of symmetry. Although the lack of a prosthesis during this period may not be a concern for the child or the parents, a prosthesis may become necessary or desirable later so the person can participate as fully as possible in individual and group activities with peers. If the provision of a prosthesis is postponed beyond early development, there may

be tremendous psychological, physical, and social problems in adjusting to wear and use.

For the congenital amputee, the prosthesis is ideally prescribed at 6 months to 1 year of age. It is prescribed as soon as possible after a traumatic amputation. This is essential for the young child to prevent the natural development of habits that might be detrimental to early adaptation and integration of a prosthetic replacement for optimum present and future function.

The training program of the child amputee must involve activities natural to his or her level of development. Early fitting during the prewalking period aids the child in developing gross bilateral coordination and balance in integrated trunk and extremity activity.

During the first year of development from the horizontal to the vertical position in bodily reflexes, the child learns body parts, their extent, and their use through imitation, trial, adaptation, and accomplishment.

Education and training are vital for the family to encourage psychological adjustment to the prosthesis and to teach the importance of putting on and removing the prosthesis, checking the skin for irritation, and encouraging positive play activities using the prosthesis. Children are often hindered by parental distractions during training sessions, so times should be scheduled for the child alone as well as for the child and parent together. This results in effective training for prosthetic function and for family education. The most successful method of teaching a child prosthetic function is through play; consideration of the age and attitude of the child is essential.

The child with a congenital limb deficiency may first be fitted with a semirigid passive Robin-Aids mitt with a Munster-type socket with preflexed elbow and figure-eight harness control. This prosthesis can be used for gross bilateral use and initial balance activities. This cosmetic device is preparatory to the functional one. At 6 months, a mechanical element is added to the prosthesis. Natural development of movement in time and space, supplemented by guidance in the use of appropriate components, can be incorporated into the child's body image and can assist functional use in further development. Between 12 to 18 months, the child becomes ready for a functional TD with cable control.

A Child Amputee Prosthetics Project (CAPP) device may be provided. This is a voluntary opening TD made of nylon and Kraton that provides function and cosmesis and can be used until the child is eight years old. An alternative is the voluntary opening, covered child's split hook with a protective plastisol covering. The AE amputee may use a preflexed socket until 2 years of age for ease in using the TD and for bilateral proximity in holding objects and body balance while using the prosthesis.

As the child plays wearing the cable-operated prosthesis and notices the hook opening and closing, he learns to control this action. With early fitting, the child generally has a hook by 2 years of age. The smallest hand is for a 5-year-old. "Children become aware of the purpose for changing the position of the forearm during the third year of life. They learn to operate the prosthetic controls and apply them to functional activities during the fourth year of life."[9]

In her discussion of AE prosthetic training of the young child, Shaperman notes five developmental factors related to learning control use:
1. Ability to see some purpose for positioning the forearm and willingness to explore new uses for this positioning
2. Ability to follow oral instructions and perform drills
3. Ability to meet the physical requirements for consistent operation of the dual-control system
4. Possession of a well-fitting, well-functioning prosthesis and availability for therapy
5. Experience of some previous success in using the prosthesis.[9]

The principles of training the child amputee include:
1. Begin with early minimal and simple prosthetic coverage.
2. Engage the child in gross sensorimotor activities to develop body awareness and use of the prosthesis.
3. Correlate training activity with prosthetic skill and developmental level.

4. Provide and train in control use as appropriate to the child's development, receptivity, comprehension, and physical functional ability.
5. Involve the family in the training program.

Whether the child benefits from prosthetic replacement depends on functional capacity, ingenuity, integration, and family support. It is important that the child with a congenital deficiency be provided with a prosthesis before starting school. Generally, a new prosthesis is provided every 4 years to accommodate growth and functional development.[1]

Considerations in Bilateral Amputees

The bilateral amputee faces not only the functional and cosmetic adjustments of the unilateral amputee but also the complete loss of sensory contact with objects while using the prostheses. Prosthetic replacement is prescribed according to the level of amputation. Particular attention is given to minimizing weight and to providing ease of bilateral operation of the elbows and TDs through the control system. For ease in putting on and removing the prosthesis by the amputee, as well as for its security and adjustment, the two prostheses are secured to a common harness system. A wrist flexion unit is helpful on one side for added mechanical positioning.

Because sensation is essential to the *blind* bilateral amputee, the Krukenberg surgical procedure may be done if the individual has a long BE amputation of either or both arms. This procedure involves separating the radius, ulna, and accompanying musculature to enable the amputee to achieve grasp and release through supination and pronation of the forearm. Sensation is maintained as grasp is achieved without an external prosthesis. Some amputees can achieve independence with this procedure.

Cineplasty Prosthesis

Because the clinical use of the cineplasty procedure is diminishing, discussion of this procedure, training program, and prosthetic replacement will be brief.

Preprosthetic Training Program

The preprosthetic training program for the amputee with a cineplasty begins with the initial amputation and training. The amputee participates in the stump wrapping and desensitization procedures to prepare for socket contact and functional use of a conventional prosthesis. During this period, the amputee learns the gross arm control motions to develop general strength, coordination, and prosthetic tolerance.

The cineplasty prothesis differs from the conventional prosthesis in that rather than using joint motion or muscle expansion to control the prosthesis, the patient operates the prosthesis by the biceps or pectoral muscle through which a surgical tunnel has been made. A pin through the tunnel is the anchor for the cable system, and the muscle contraction and relaxation provide the motor for the prosthesis by directly affecting the opening and closing of the TD. For maximum use of this type of prosthesis, it is necessary to have a 1½- to 2-inch excursion of the muscle within the surgical tunnel. Preprosthetic exercises focus on developing this excursion range and muscle strength. This is done by isolated muscle exercise, isometric contraction and relaxation patterns, and adapted activity using these exercises. Adaptations can be effectively designed by the use of pulleys and weights to facilitate muscle contraction and relaxation to develop the muscle excursion needed to operate the cable system (Fig. 30-23). Exercise adaptations are attached to the medial and lateral ends of the cineplasty pin. When the amputee contracts the muscle, the contraction can be measured by a ruler placed along the cineplasty area. Thus, the amount of progress toward the needed muscle excursion can be monitored by both the therapist and the patient.

An essential part of the preprosthetic program is the care of the surgical area. The occupational therapist teaches the amputee to develop a routine of daily cleaning of the tunnel with alcohol, cleaning the cineplasty pin upon removal from the tunnel, and observing the surgical area for redness or skin breakdown due to pressure during prosthetic wear and use. It is essential to maintain optimum opening of the tunnel to ensure function of the cable system, as well as to maintain the

muscle excursion for efficient prosthetic operation and function.

Prosthetic Components

The components of the cineplasty prosthesis are essentially the same as those of the conventional prosthesis with the exception of the cable system and the harness. The harness provides additional support and comfort for the wearer but is not necessary for the function of the prosthesis. Thus, the harness may be eliminated except for the amputee who needs to perform heavy work with the prosthesis. This person wants added security from the harness, particularly to support the added weight of heavy-duty hooks for the functional/cosmetic hand. For the biceps cineplasty amputee, a triceps cuff may be strapped around the upper arm (Fig. 30-24). This cuff is attached to the forearm socket with flexible hinges.

The same choice of TDs is available for the cineplasty as for the conventional prosthesis. The combination of the isolated muscle function for TD operation and the use of the voluntary closing Army Prosthetic Research Laboratory (APRL) hook and hand increase the sensory feedback from TD function for the amputee with a cineplasty. With biceps control, there is some simulation of sensation in TD use that has been reported to improve dexterity and sensitivity of the amputated limb and replacement. The control system for this prosthesis consists of two cables attached to the medial and lateral ends of the plastic pin inserted into the surgical tunnel. These cables eventually join in a common adjustment plate, and another cable extends from this point to the TD device, which is operated by muscle contraction pulling on the plastic pin (Fig. 30-24).

Prosthetic Training Program

Prosthetic training begins with exercises and adaptive activities to develop the necessary muscle excursion for TD operation. When the amputee receives the prosthesis, the occupational therapist checks it for conformity to the prescription, fit, and function. The amputee then follows a functional training program such as that described for the conventional prosthesis to learn TD operation. The cineplasty allows increased arm range of motion due to the elimination of the harness. Because the arm position does not determine TD operation, there is a more rapid adjustment to positioning of the extremity for TD function.

Myoelectric Prosthesis

Developments in the use of myoelectric controls for prosthetic and orthotic replacements of lost limb functions have been steadily increasing in clinical application. A major significance of myoelectric prosthetic con-

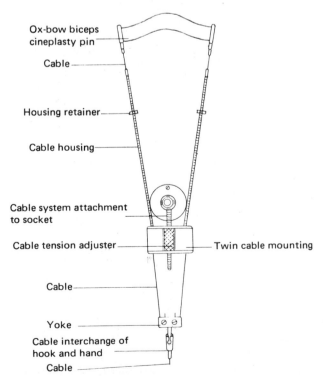

Figure 30-23. Biceps cineplasty cable control system.

Ox-bow biceps cineplasty pin

Cable

Housing retainer

Cable housing

Cable system attachment to socket

Cable tension adjuster

Twin cable mounting

Cable

Yoke

Cable interchange of hook and hand

Cable

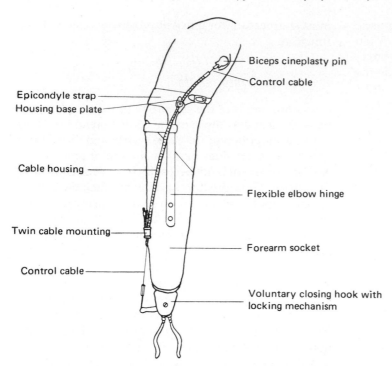

Biceps cineplasty pin
Control cable
Epicondyle strap
Housing base plate
Cable housing
Flexible elbow hinge
Twin cable mounting
Forearm socket
Control cable
Voluntary closing hook with locking mechanism

Figure 30-24. Right below-elbow cineplasty with voluntary closing hook.

trol is the use of signals from the neuromuscular system to activate specific component functions.

By approaching the amputee and prosthetic replacements as a complete unit or system, research and clinical teams are integrating natural and artificial elements.[11] In the effort to assist the amputee in achieving both efficient and natural function and appearance, combinations of conventional and myoelectric components may be considered within the same prosthesis, particularly for amputation or skeletal deficiencies above the elbow. Myoelectric components and controls are available for operation of cosmetic/functional hand, wrist rotation, and elbow flexion and extension. These are available for unilateral, bilateral, BE, and AE amputees.

Preprosthetic Program

Ability to isolate and control the muscle sites and to develop strength and speed of muscle contraction determines effective prosthetic use. Assessment of surface EMG muscle sites for control of a prosthesis is made using the myotester. Further training with the myotester helps the amputee develop signal levels and reliable isolation of potential myoelectric control sites. This may be done using bench-mounted units such as the terminal device and the wrist unit.[11] A temporary plaster prosthesis may be used to determine the preliminary ability of the amputee to use myoelectric controls implanted in the socket. Efficiency of muscle control is established through use of the temporary prosthesis until the permanent one is ready for fitting and training. Preprosthetic activities also include practice in unilateral functional activities with the sound or remaining ex-

tremity, particularly if it is nondominant. Assistive devices for independent living skills may be beneficial during this period.

Identification of muscle sites and the number required for prosthetic operation depend on the level of the amputation and the ability of the amputee to isolate and use the muscle contractions. For example, a BE amputee may use either a single site or two sites for TD operation. In the dual control, extensor muscle contraction may be used to open the TD, and flexor muscle contraction may be used to close it, thus simulating normal body associations. The AE amputee may use biceps contraction for prosthetic elbow flexion and triceps contraction for prosthetic elbow extension, with cocontraction of these muscles to open and close the hand.

Passive, manually operated shoulder, elbow, and wrist components may be used. Cosmetic and functional electric hooks, hands, and elbows are commercially available. Electronic controls and batteries are stored within the sockets or the hand of the prosthesis or externally (Fig. 30-25).

Prosthetic Components

A myoelectrically controlled prosthesis or component operates by using the electric potential produced by a contracting muscle to activate a battery-driven motor that operates a prosthetic component. Proportional control of the motor by regulation of the extent or speed of muscle contraction can affect the force or speed of the movement of the component.[6]

Myoelectric prostheses are provided to children and adults both experimentally and clinically. In both cases,

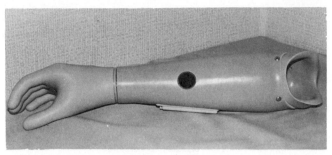

Figure 30-25. Complete below-elbow myoelectric prosthesis with cosmetic/functional terminal device, external battery pack, and double-walled forearm socket.

the candidates are chosen for optimum success in myoelectric wear and use. Since the myoelectric prosthesis is expensive, both in initial provision and in maintenance, proximity of the amputee to the prosthetist, adequate funding, vocational appropriateness, and available prosthetic checkout and training are essential considerations. During the initial prosthetic prescription, factors such as the level of the amputation, the condition of the limb, the number of limbs involved, the extent of power, and the control in the remaining limb and body are assessed.

The positive aspects of the myoelectric approach are:
1. Utilization of natural muscle stimuli for component operation
2. More accurate control with less energy output from the amputee
3. Elimination of the shoulder harness
4. Ease in full-range of isolated extremity movements
5. Improved natural control and cosmesis
6. Decreased body movement to control prosthesis

The negative aspects of the myoelectric approach are:
1. High expense of controls, components, and repairs
2. Requirement for skilled repair in the event of breakdown
3. Limited number of suitable candidates
4. Noise of component operation
5. Daily battery charge required
6. Lack of proprioceptive feedback from harness
7. Added weight
8. Efficient control sites necessary
9. Muscle fatigue

Good candidates for myoelectric replacement have the following attributes:
1. A healthy attitude toward the disability
2. A desire for myoelectric control
3. Commitment to following the procedures and fulfilling the responsibilities for myoelectric wear and care
4. Healthy skin and stump for effective socket and electrode contact

5. Fair muscle function in the arm to produce electrode signals for component operation

During the evaluation and prescription, the amputee is introduced to the advantages and disadvantages of conventional and myoelectric control relative to his or her capabilities, interests, objectives, and readiness for prosthetic replacement.

Sockets are single or double walled, depending on the level of amputation. Generally, the harness is eliminated and the prosthesis is self-suspended on the extremity. In the BE prosthesis, a supracondylar suspension, using bony prominences, or a Munster-type socket high on the forearm, is used for secure fit and comfort. In the Munster-type socket, there is no supination and pronation available in active movement, and elbow flexion and extension are limited. The AE socket or APS uses atmospheric pressure suspension.

Preliminary temporary fittings assist the amputee in adjusting to prosthetic replacement and use. Early and permanent fitting of the myoelectric controls involves locating suitable sites for the electrodes, casting for electrode placement locations, provision of the permanent socket with electrode emplacements, provision of the component system, controls, battery pack, on/off switch, and pigmenting. Since provision and maintenance of myoelectric controls and components are expensive, the amputee may first be provided with a conventional prosthesis with harness control to determine individual feasibility for myoelectric wear and function. In order to best meet the individual needs of the amputee, combinations of cable driven and myoelectric components can be used as feasible and appropriate for optimum function and cosmesis.

It may be advisable for the amputee to have two prostheses so that one is available should one be in need of repair. This is to prevent the efficient prosthesis user from the inconvenience of not having the functional and cosmetic benefits of the prosthesis available to him or her at all times. As with the standard prosthesis, there is a big difference between learning the control system of the myoelectric prosthesis and actually using the control system to perform functional activities. Prosthetic wear requires a gradual adjustment, acceptance, tolerance, and use.

Prosthetic Training Program

Prosthetic training is done on either an inpatient or an outpatient basis and begins with a preprosthetic program of isolating muscle contractions to produce signals for training in specific component operation. The prosthetic training program includes the following:
1. Checkout of the fabrication, fit, and efficiency of the prosthesis
2. Evaluation of the amputee's ability to control the prosthesis

3. Specific training in general component use and coordination
4. Instruction in the care and operation of the prosthesis
5. Training in self-care activities
6. Use of prosthetic and natural upper extremity motions in bimanual and bilateral functional activities

During all stages of training, the therapist monitors and discusses progress and problems with the patient to ensure optimum success in prosthetic wear and use. Social interaction with other amputees assists him or her in adjusting and problem-solving.

The extent of daily use of myoelectric controls is dependent on conservation of the battery's energy during nonuse. This is accomplished by a manual switch that is turned on to use the controls and turned off when the amputee removes the prosthesis or during long periods when control use is not necessary. To avoid blockage between the electrode contact and the muscles, a stump sock is not worn. The amputee is taught to examine skin areas on removal of the prosthesis to monitor irritation from the socket and to keep the socket and parts clean.

Wear and successful use of the prosthesis depend on an appropriate prescription and effective training with adequate periodic follow-up and monitoring of the function of the prosthesis.

During the training program, patients share experiences and meet individual needs through group discussions. As prosthetic replacement of function is a personal and individual adjustment, patients are encouraged to take part in planning the program by talking about individual expectations, goals, problems, and ideas regarding their prosthetic replacement.

Pediatric Considerations

In providing prosthetic components to the child with a congenital or a traumatic amputation, it is essential to consider his or her developmental level. The sooner the prosthesis can be fitted, the better. Sorbye reports that children between the ages of 2½ and 4 years are the most suitable for the BE myoelectric prosthesis and that all children should be able to learn to use one.[10] He advises that a change from the standard or split hook prosthesis be made before the child is 4 years old to avoid problems of adjusting to a change in the prosthesis and the control system.

Candidacy for myoelectric replacement in children depends on personality, maturity, and the interest of the child and his family, since all will be involved in learning the system and in monitoring prosthetic wear and use with regard to training. Sorbye states, "The children teach themselves how to open and close the prosthetic hand within a few minutes from the initial application, over 2½ years of age."[10] Training programs emphasize two-handed activities and involvement in developmental activities appropriate to the age and maturation of the child. Whether the child amputee benefits from the prosthesis depends on his or her functional capacity and ingenuity.

Endoskeletal Modular System

The endoskeletal modular prosthetic system is designed primarily for cosmesis provided by a central inner tubular (pylon) support covered with a soft, pigmented polyurethane foam to give natural contour and soft appearance. A nylon stocking covering is stretched over the foam. A variety of interchangeable components are available to meet the needs of the amputee. The modular arm includes a nonfunctional cosmetic hand, passively activated elbow, and shoulder units. Harness and control cables can be eliminated, because the components are operated manually with the sound hand.

Future Considerations

Research is continuing into more effective control systems and sites and the development of components that better simulate natural movements and functions. Efforts are being made to lessen weight, to improve locking and grasping mechanisms in the hand and the hook, to improve the glove material, and to increase the overall cosmesis of the prosthesis. Specific considerations are development of a more efficient elbow unit, rerouting of the cables to the inside of the arm, improved appearance, higher operating efficiencies, and decreased wear on clothing. There is also interest in providing active wrist rotation.

The experimentation in electric control is directed toward providing the amputee with a total coordination pattern and better integration of the total body system. The aim is to provide a link between the person and the prosthetic device by using a stimulus from the person's energy to activate the prosthesis. Another idea is the use of phantom sensations to aid in the control of the BE prosthesis, using the signals from the forearm muscles for prehension and forearm rotation (pronation and supination). This method does not apply to the AE amputee, since the forearm muscles are gone and the power source muscles are removed from the terminal device.

Unlike the advances in the development of mechanical and electronic prosthetic components and control systems, development of prosthetic replacement of lost sensory functions has been slow, forcing the amputee to depend on visual and auditory monitoring for effective operation of standard cable-operated and myoelectric prosthesis. There is much effort toward the provision of sensory feedback regarding prosthetic hand functions such as perception of grip strength and stability, kinesthetic information regarding hand and arm position, or movement and perception of the actual force in the joints of the prosthesis. Gross sense of the extremity in space exists, but there is poor sense of hook pressure for grip. Harness and cable stress and movement give a gross indication at times for hook opening and closing.

The harness system used in controlling the components of the conventional body movement or joint-operated prosthesis provides the amputee with proprioceptive awareness or feedback regarding the function of the prosthesis; this is lacking in the myoelectric prosthesis, which is not suspended or operated through a body harness. Although visual cues are necessary to guide the accurate manipulation of objects with the TD, the amputee learns to perceive hook operation to some degree by harness and socket tension, the weight of the prosthesis, material coverage of fabrication, and the sound of the control and components in operation. When an external power source is provided, this information from the control cable is unavailable, because a much smaller and more delicate movement is required to open a valve or trigger a microswitch, providing less feedback from the controlling mechanism.[6] Findings such as these have led to development of artificial feedback systems.[5]

Research continues in the incorporation of such artificial feedback mechanisms within myoelectric prostheses to provide increased sensory integration of the prosthesis and the remaining arm, proprioceptive awareness of position and movement, and perception of the degree of force in the joints of the prosthesis and detection of change in the grip of the TD. In addition to myoelectric electrodes, strain gauges or stimulating signals have been used to cause a tingling sensation in the stump indicative of the force in the prosthetic grip, changing as the pressure changes to provide control information through sensory feedback.[2]

Shannon and Agnew state that the presence of the sensory feedback is appreciated by subjects and enables them to hold objects confidently even when the object is obscured from vision.[8] Other considerations in providing sensory feedback include vibrations within electric systems, electric currents indicating the magnitude of the force applied, information regarding the speed of prosthetic hand closure, and tactile and joint position information.

In addition to the prohibitive cost of these experimental devices, another problem with an external power source is replenishment of the power. Efforts to produce designs that will simulate characteristics of normal muscle functions continue in hopes of achieving integration of the device and the person.

With the continuing research into the use and application of external power, the concept of "man-machine," or the integration of the person and the assistive device, is often cited. Since the physician and prosthetist recognize the need for an engineer who can provide devices operated with external power, the engineer or specialist in bioengineering has become a member of the rehabilitation team.

Lower Extremity Amputation and Replacement

Amputations of the lower extremities are generally more common than those of the upper extremities because of the high incidence of peripheral vascular disease and traumatic injuries to the lower limbs. The psychological reactions of the UE amputee, mentioned earlier, pertain also to the LE amputee. Since age, body build, physical and medical condition, vascular supply, and motivation are factors in the rehabilitation of the LE amputee, there are some patients for whom a prosthesis is contraindicated. These persons are encouraged to maintain maximum independence and mobility with the aid of a wheelchair, crutches, and other necessary assistive devices. The amputee for whom a prosthesis is appropriate can usually look forward to partial restoration of basic functions, independence in self-care, and the opportunity to return to work of some kind.

Role of Occupational Therapy

Basically, the detailed study of LE function, preprosthetic preparation, prosthetic prescription, checkout and training, and the management of problems encountered by the amputee are handled by the physician and the physical therapist. However, there are many ways in which the occupational therapist can contribute to the functional rehabilitation of the LE amputee. In a general hospital or a rehabilitation center, the occupational therapist may actually work with as many or more LE than UE amputees. The occupational therapist assists with both the preprosthetic and prosthetic programs for general physical conditioning, psychological and functional adaptation to the loss of a body part, and the regaining of maximal functional independence in self-care and general mobility. To provide effective therapeutic programs for the LE amputee, the occupational therapist needs to participate with the physical therapist, the physician, the prosthetist, and other professionals in a coordinated team approach.

Preprosthetic Program

Passive and active exercises of the lower extremities are performed or supervised by the physical therapist during the early postoperative period. The nurse or physical therapist teaches the amputee to bandage the stump to encourage shrinkage and forming for prosthetic fitting.

Proper positioning of the body in the wheelchair is important to prevent contractures in the joints proximal to the amputation, scoliosis, and edema, all of which could hinder successful prosthetic function. In the case of a below-knee (BK) amputation, the use of a seatboard adapted for the individual amputee can be used in a regular chair or a wheelchair to maintain the knee in passive extension with knee flexors stretched while the amputee is performing activities in a sitting position.

The LE amputee may be referred to occupational therapy in the preprosthetic or the prosthetic phase of training. In either case, the occupational therapist should become familiar with the medical aspects of the patient's care and the goals of the rehabilitation program. Pertinent information obtained from the chart or staff members should include:
1. The location, type, level, and cause of amputation
2. The condition of the stump and amputated extremity
3. General body condition
4. Any precautions and complicating conditions
5. Previous prosthetic replacement, if any
6. Recommendations for passive and active positioning of the joints of the amputated extremity
7. The appropriate amount of standing and walking and the degree of safe support needed by the amputee

Throughout the preprosthetic and prosthetic training, the amputee may go through changes in attitude and behavior as he or she gradually realizes the extent of the loss and its effect on his or her life. Continual counseling is often necessary to help the amputee adjust to the amputation, the change in body image, and the wear and use of the mechanical device to substitute for natural function. He or she must also adjust to working with his or her arms, gearing himself or herself to abilities rather than disability, finding new interests, and socializing in the new situation.

The seatboard mentioned previously can be made by the amputee as part of an UE exercise program. It can be made of ½- or ¾-inch plywood that conforms to the measurement of the inside of the chair seat; one side extends to the end of the amputee's stump. The extended side should be narrow enough to prevent interference with the comfort of the sound leg in a sitting position and at the same time should provide passive extension of the knee of the amputated leg. The seatboard should be padded sufficiently for comfort, and particular attention should be paid to such sensitive areas as the end of the stump.

In this preprosthetic phase, the amputee may come to occupational therapy either in a wheelchair or walking with crutches. A variety of treatment techniques can be used. Since balance and UE and trunk strength will be important in prosthetic use, maximum function of these areas is encouraged. Insofar as the amputee can tolerate the exercise, his or her sitting tolerance and balance is challenged by the use of UE activities. Although at first a patient with a high above-knee (AK) amputation or bilateral leg amputations may need to hold onto the chair with one hand to support himself or herself in a sitting position while using the other hand, he or she should be encouraged to depend on the trunk for balance to leave both arms free for UE activities. As UE strength and confidence in balance increase, ROM and resistance required for manual activities should be increased to further challenge trunk balance. Activities such as wordworking, weaving, and printing may be adapted to the amputee's individual needs. An activity in which the patient has a vocational or avocational interest may provide motivation so that he or she can increase tolerance of the given position and redirect energies from anxieties regarding his or her condition toward purposeful activity. Activities at this stage are directed toward the amputee's achieving independent function of the arms and trunk while seated in a wheelchair.

Another aspect of independence is self-care tasks, including bathing and care of the stump, transfers, and dressing. A unilateral amputee should have little or no difficulty in this area. However, aids such as grab bars for bath and toilet, a transfer board or tub seat for bathing, and a raised toilet seat can be helpful as the amputee adjusts to a new body image and copes with the problems of balance. Phantom limb sensations can be a complicating factor if the amputee suddenly moves to get up and forgets that he or she cannot stand on the amputated limb, even though feeling is there. Continued physical and psychological support is necessary in these instances to minimize fear and to encourage confidence. Dressing is usually easier from a sitting position on the bed. Front fastenings and loose clothing help minimize frustrations.

Maximum independent function should be encouraged both with and without the prosthesis. For example, the amputee should be encouraged to stand on the sound leg in front of a table for short periods of time. This will encourage hip extension of the amputated side, and it will develop balance. However, attention must be paid to the amount of standing time so as not to encourage scoliosis.

Therapists have found that immediate postoperative fitting of a prosthesis or the use of a temporary pylon and the working prosthesis after the amputee's scar tissue has healed is beneficial to the training program. The temporary pylon provides early replacement of the amputated limb to encourage functional activity while the stump is being conditioned and the permanent prosthesis is being made.* The pylon consists of a plaster stump socket to which a pylon is attached to provide length

---

* For specific designs of the pylon, see Jones MS: *An Approach to Occupational Therapy,* Chapter 6. London, Butterworths, 1964.

and base support to the amputated leg. With the pylon, the patient can stand and ambulate soon after the amputation.

A working prosthesis is permanently attached to the machine that the amputee will use for exercise (*i.e.*, to the foot-powered lathe or the bicycle jigsaw). It also consists of a stump cuff that is laced up the sides for ease in putting on and that provides a comfortable fit for different persons. It is open at the distal end to eliminate pressure on the end of the stump.

When the patient has put the cuff on the stump, he or she fits the pylon shafts into the cuff. As the base is attached to the bicycle jigsaw or the lathe, the amputee is able to operate these machines and thus engage in active exercise of the amputated limb. The working prosthesis can be used with a foot-powered floor press, treadle sewing machine, or loom if properly adapted to the needs of the amputee. ROM and resistance can be graded, and the amputee can engage in an activity requiring coordination, balance, and strength of all four extremities and the trunk.

It must be remembered that at first the amputee fatigues more rapidly, even in maintaining sitting and standing positions, and that until tolerance increases, energy is directed toward these basic functions.

Prosthetic Training Program

The LE amputee depends on the prosthesis for support in standing and walking. It is important that the prosthesis be appropriately prescribed, that it fit comfortably, and that it provide adequate functional assistance. The prescription and mechanical function of the prosthesis are checked thoroughly by the physical therapist. Function of the parts, how the amputee should put on the prosthesis, and how he or she should use it are taught by the physical therapist.

Independent locomotion depends on the fit and comfort of the prosthesis as well as on the general condition and tolerance of the amputee. Some may be able to discard their wheelchairs fairly soon. However, the amputee with poor tolerance of the prosthesis or a poorly fitting one may need the security of the wheelchair for a long time. In either case, the occupational therapy program can benefit the amputee by encouraging work in the treatment room doing activities in a standing position when he or she can tolerate it. Even if the amputee is still dependent on the wheelchair early in prosthetic training, he or she must eventually adjust to the mechanical, insensitive prosthesis by learning to judge where it is relative to the rest of the body, and he or she must learn how to function with it.

When the amputee receives the prosthesis, most of his or her attention will be on the fit and use of it. Since he or she needs rest from ambulation training, he or she continues in an occupational therapy program for UE strengthening and prosthetic tolerance. The activities outlined in the preprosthetic period are continued. At this point, they are done with the prosthesis on unless the amputee is resting the stump or it has been irritated by the prosthesis. His or her program is geared toward encouraging acceptance of the prosthesis (to function in activities challenging UE and LE coordination and function), prosthetic tolerance, development of ADL independence, UE and LE exercise, realization of his or her capacities, and vocational and avocational guidance.

The prosthesis wearing time is gradually increased according to the comfort and tolerance of the socket in sitting and standing positions. The amputee must adjust to the sensation of bilateral weightbearing and the sensitivity of the stump to the hard edges and base of the socket. According to his or her tolerance and balance, the amputee can decrease the support he or she uses while standing. Engagement in UE activities in a standing position, which provides a wide range of motion and resistance, helps to challenge and to increase standing balance. Walking to cabinets to get and replace materials or tools and walking around tables and machines should be encouraged to increase functional independence. Carrying articles from place to place also challenges balance and independent function. Aids such as a cart with wheels or a tray can minimize the stress of carrying items.

In ADL, the patient now learns to incorporate the prosthesis into bodily activities. He or she learns at what point in dressing to put on the prosthesis so that it will aid, rather than interfere with, ease and speed in dressing.

An important part of the prosthetic training program is helping the amputee realize his or her capabilities. In the occupational therapy environment, tasks may be set up both to improve the amputee's tolerance and function with the prosthesis and to relate to the requirements of his or her job.

Prevocational Exploration

Amputation may prevent a person from returning to a former line of work, and this may be a great source of anxiety. In such cases, the occupational therapist can provide valuable information to the vocational rehabilitation counselor regarding the functional capabilities of the amputee. Information regarding interests, intelligence, physical abilities and skills, work tolerance, work habits, and general motivation for achieving new skills assists the counselor in investigating possibilities for the employable amputee in vocational planning.

Through formal prevocational performance evaluation using standardized dexterity tests, interest tests, and work-simulated tasks, the occupational therapist is able to provide an indication of motivation and readiness for vocational exploration. Through simulated work activities, the therapist is able to assess general work habits, comprehension, problem-solving ability, social compatibility, quality of work, and work tolerance.

Summary

Amputations of the upper and lower extremities may be due to congenital deformity, injury, or disease. A variety of options are available for prosthetic replacement in the attempt to meet the developmental, psychological, physical, social, and functional needs of the amputee.

In UE amputations, surgical procedures are directed toward saving as much bone and soft tissue as possible so that the amputee can gain optimum benefit from the prosthetic device. Prosthetic components are custom prescribed by the rehabilitation team to form the most functional type of prosthesis according to the level and type of amputation. Residual sensation and pain affect adjustment to the prosthesis and eventual wear and use.

The postoperative program begins with psychological adjustment to amputation and orientation to the preprosthetic and prosthetic training program. Immediate or early fitting of a temporary prosthesis enhances general conditioning of the stump as well as psychological and functional adjustment.

Whereas the provision of cineplasty prosthetic systems is being phased out, the myoelectric systems are becoming more widely used. Nonetheless, the conventional prosthesis remains the traditional, most reliable, and most economical prosthetic replacement. Both conventional and myoelectric systems are prescribed for children. Research and development are attempting to provide a system that enables the amputee to relate to the insensitive prosthetic replacement in a manner that yields optimum integration of natural and replacement functions, with maximum sensory feedback.

The occupational therapist contributes to the preprosthetic and prosthetic training program and general adaptation of the LE amputee.

References

1. Bender LF: Prostheses and Rehabilitation after Arm Amputation, pp 34, 57, 157. Springfield, IL, Charles C Thomas, 1974
2. Brittain RH, Santes WF, Gibson DA: Sensory feedback in a myoelectric upper limb prosthesis: A preliminary report. Can J Surg 22:481, 1979
3. Cummings V, Alexander J, Gans SO: Management of the amputee. In Ruskin AP (ed): Current Therapy in Physiatry, pp 212, 213, 219. Philadelphia, WB Saunders, 1984
4. Gilfoyle EM, Grady AP, Moore JC: Children Adapt, p 1. Thorofare, NJ, Charles B Slack, 1981
5. Herberts P, Korner L: Ideas on sensory feedback in hand prostheses. Prosthet Orthot Int 3:157, 1979
6. Robertson E: Rehabilitation of Arm Amputees and Limb-Deficient Children, pp 42, 44. London, Bailliere Tindall, 1979
7. Russell H: The Best Years of My Life, p 17. Middlebury, VT, Paul S Erikson, 1981
8. Shannon GF, Agnew PJ: Fitting below-elbow prostheses which convey a sense of touch. Med J Aust 1:243, 1979
9. Shaperman J: Learning patterns of young children with above-elbow prostheses. Am J Occup Ther 33:304, 1979
10. Sorbye R: Myoelectric prosthetic fitting in young children. J Clin Orthoped Rel Res 148:36, 1980
11. Stein RB, Charles PD, Hoffer JA, et al: New approaches for the control of powered prostheses particularly by high-level amputees. Bull Prosthet Res 17(10):52, 1980

Bibliography

Agnew PJ, Shannon GF: Training program for a myoelectrically controlled prosthesis with sensory feedback system. Am J Occup Ther 35:722, 1981

Banerjee SN (ed): Rehabilitation Management of Amputees. Baltimore, Williams & Wilkins, 1982

Cummings V, Alexander J, Gans SO: Management of the amputee. In Ruskin AP (ed): Current Therapy in Physiatry. Philadelphia, WB Saunders, 1984

D'astous J (ed): Orthotics and Prosthetics Digest Reference Manual. Ottawa, Edahl Productions, 1981

Dickey RE, Stieritz L: Amputation and impaired independence. In Abreu BC (ed): Physical Disabilities Manual. New York, Raven Press, 1981

Ey MC: Experiences with myoelectric prostheses: A preliminary report. Inter-Clinic Inform Bull 17:15, 1978

Ey MC, Helfgott S: A temporary thumb prosthesis. Inter-Clinic Inform Bull 17:9, 1978

Fraser C: Does an artificial limb become part of the user? Br J Occup Ther 47:43, 1984

Friedman LW: The Psychological Rehabilitation of the Amputee. Springfield, IL, Charles C Thomas, 1978

Herberts P, Korner L, Caine K, Wensby L: Rehabilitation of unilateral below-elbow amputees with myoelectric prostheses. Scand J Rehabil Med 12:123, 1980

Madruga L: One Step at a Time: A Young Woman's Inspiring Struggle to Walk Again. New York, McGraw–Hill, 1979

Mastro BA, Mastro RT (eds): A Review of Orthotics and Prosthetics. Washington, DC, American Orthotic and Prosthetic Association, 1980

Murphy EF, Horn LW: Myoelectric control systems—a selected bibliography. Orthot Prosthet 35:34, 1981

Orthotics/Prosthetics (information packet). Rockville, MD, American Occupational Therapy Association Division of Professional Development, 1979

Pedretti LW: Occupational Therapy Practice Skills for Physical Dysfunction. St. Louis, CV Mosby, 1981

Prosthetics Yes . . . Bionics Maybe ??? (review of Third World Congr Int Soc Prosthet Orthot), Whitestone, NY, National Amputation Foundation, 1977

Review of Visual Aids for Prosthetics and Orthotics. Committee on Prosthetic–Orthotic Education, Division of Medical Sciences, National Academy of Sciences, National Research Council, Washington, DC

Rosenfelder R: Infant amputee: Early growth and care. J Clin Orthop Rel Res 148:41, 1980

Shaperman J, Sumida CT: Recent advances in research in prosthetics for children. J Clin Orthop Rel Res 148:26, 1980

Talbot D: The Child with a Limb Deficiency: A Guide for Parents. Los Angeles, UCLA Child Amputee Prosthetics Project, 1979

Taylor CL: The biomechanics of control in upper-extremity prostheses. Orthot Prosthet 35:7, 1981

Thompson RG: Evaluation of the amputee. In Kaplan PE (ed): The Practice of Physical Medicine. Springfield, IL, Charles C Thomas, 1984

Whipple L: Whole Again. Ottawa, Caroline House Publishing, 1980

Appreciation is extended to the Eastern Maine Medical Center and the Harmarville Rehabilitation Center for resources used in work on this chapter; to Ed Collins, Ron Gregory, and Patricia Marvin for photographs; to Barry Kaufman for line drawings; to Martha Willis for critical review; and to Patricia Curran for editorial assistance.

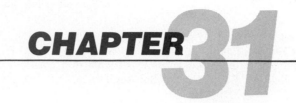

Hand Rehabilitation

Maureen Moylan Syler

Hands are the eyes for those who cannot see,
the words for those who cannot hear,
and the tools by which we sustain our lives.

Maureen Moylan Syler

History of Hand Rehabilitation

The history of hand rehabilitation can be traced to the 16th century, when incising and draining of wounds was first reported. By the 17th century, an Irish surgeon, Abraham Colles, was doing work on nonarticular fractures of the distal radius. DeQuervain, in 1895, defined stenosing tenosynovitis at the first dorsal compartment of the wrist; Sudeck, in the early 1900s, described the symptomatology now recognized as reflex sympathetic dystrophy; and Kanavel, a young surgeon during the industrial revolution, treated patients who had work-related injuries.

During World War II, Sterling Bunnell, who later became known as the father of hand surgery in the United States, addressed the growing need for hand services when he established nine hand centers within the General Army Hospital. This helped to advance the specialization of hand surgeons. While advances in hand rehabilitation were occurring in the United States, Charles Wynn-Parry in England and Eric Moberg in Sweden were also working to increase knowledge in this field.

In the early 1950s, Bunnell was instrumental in founding the American Society for Surgery of the Hand.[5] As the specialty of hand surgery grew within the ranks of orthopedists, plastic surgeons, and general surgeons, so too did the need for specialized therapists to deal with the complex problems of hand injuries. The ranks of occupational therapists and physical therapists soon grew with support and direction from the American Society for Surgery of the Hand, culminating in the founding of the American Society for Hand Therapists in 1978.

Today, the modern hand treatment team consists not only of the surgeon, therapist, and patient, but also of the rehabilitation counselor, social worker, vocational nurse, and employer. Patients requiring the services of a hand specialist include those with an acute inflammatory process, degenerative joint disease, sports-related injuries, congenital anomalies, fractures, tendon injuries, nerve lesions, soft-tissue injuries, and devascularizations.

Evaluation

When the patient is first seen by the physician, a thorough history of the problem is ascertained. The physician will order various tests such as arthrograms, radiographs, topography, and others when necessary to ensure an accurate diagnosis. Unless surgery is indicated, a noninvasive conservative approach will be elected.

When introduced to the rehabilitation phase, the patient often feels concerned about the outcomes. Thus, the therapist must be well versed in the anatomy and physiology of the hand and also in medical terminology, pathology, and the social implications of the disease process.

Evaluation begins during the initial visit. The therapist can learn a great deal by observation:

How does the patient carry and present the injured extremity?

What does the patient say about the injury?

Does the patient talk about the injured part as a separate entity?

Has the patient developed a psychological disassociation?

How does the patient qualify and quantify the discomfort he or she is experiencing?

At this time, the therapist begins to establish a therapeutic relationship with the patient. This includes alleviating the patient's anxiety, reassuring the patient, and answering his or her questions.

Patient History and General Information

Initially, the therapist must ask the patient several questions regarding the injury: how did it occur? when? and does it involve the dominant hand? The therapist also must ask about the patient's occupation. Additional questions include:

What is the patient doing at home to care for the involved extremity?

Has the patient been injured before?

Will the patient have difficulty attending therapy?

Does the patient have someone at home who can assist him or her?

Prior to the initial testing, the therapist explains to the patient which test(s) will be performed and the information that will be gathered. This helps the patient know what to expect during testing and to plan his or her responses to questions. At this point, it will be valuable to ask the patient how much he or she understands about the diagnosis and what information the physician has relayed. The therapist must use his or her knowledge of pathology in order to explain clearly and simply the nature and prognosis of the injury to the patient. Various illustrated educational materials and three-dimensional models can be used to instruct the patient in the anatomy of the arm and hand.

Range of Motion Tests

The patient is placed in a comfortable position, supporting the extremity proximal to the specific joint that will be tested. The therapist gently examines the hand prior to taking specific measurements and notes any deformities or dermal abrasions. When recording range of motion (ROM), the therapist must always define it as active or passive and include the date of the test.

Active Range of Motion

Active ROM is joint motion that results from an active muscle contraction. Using a goniometer, the therapist records the degrees of active mobility for each involved joint. It is important to note any attempts by the patient to use trick motions or substitution such as moving a finger with an adjacent digit instead of moving it independently.

Passive Range of Motion

Passive ROM is joint motion that results from an external force moving the joint through its arc of motion. Passive mobility is measured and recorded in degrees at both ends of the range. Where limitation occurs, it is important to ascertain whether this is due to a tight joint structure or to tendinous tightness. Joint tightness will cause a fixed position no matter what plane the joint is in, whereas it is generally accepted that tendon tightness will vary in degree depending on the placement of the digit in space.

Total Active Motion and Total Passive Motion

Total active motion is derived by subtracting the total degrees of extension for a digit from the total degrees of flexion of that digit. It is becoming more common to record total active motion (TAM) and total passive motion (TPM) for each digit and use these to gauge improvement. An example of a record of total active motion of the involved index finger is given in the box on page 548. Where limitations inhibit full flexion, many therapists measure composite flexion of the digit by having the patient flex the finger to the maximum and then measure the distance from the pad of the involved digit to the distal palmar crease. This number is recorded on the hand therapy evaluation form as centimeters from the distal palmar crease (Fig. 31-1).

Example of a Record of Total Active Motion

Metacarpophalangeal joint (MP)	=	0°–75°
Proximal interphalangeal joint (PIP)	=	20°–100°
Distal interphalangeal joint (DIP)	=	0°–65°
Total flexion		= 240°
Total extension		= 20°
Arc of mobility		220°

Subtracting the extension from the flexion, the arc of mobility for the involved digit is found to be 220° This is the TAM for that specific digit.

Edema

A volumeter may be used to compare fluid displacement bilaterally. A carefully calibrated volumeter is filled with 500 ml of water. With the involved extremity supinated, the patient submerges it in the volumeter until the cleft between the middle and ring fingers rests on a stationary dowel. The displaced fluid flows into a container, where it is measured and the amount recorded. The fluid is replenished to 500 ml, and the same procedure is then followed with the uninvolved extremity. This assessment may be required before, during, and after treatment to monitor edema elicited by activity or to evaluate edema as it is affected by the time of day.

Sensation

When nerve function is impaired, numerous sensory evaluation tests can be conducted. The most common tests are listed below, with the corresponding testing instruments shown in Figure 31-2.

Protective Sensation

Protective sensation is tested with the forearm in supination and with vision occluded. The patient is touched with the point or the closing clasp of a safety pin, and the patient describes each stimulus as either sharp or dull. It is important to remember that the most intensified area of sensory nerve endings is in the distal pads of the digits. The therapist must employ several random stimuli to the involved, as well as the uninvolved extremity to ascertain whether protective sensation is intact, impaired, or absent. If the patient correctly identifies the stimuli, it is assumed that protective sensation is intact. If the patient's responses to the stimuli are inconsistent, sensation is recorded as impaired. If the patient is unable to identify any of the stimuli, sensation is considered absent.

Vibration Sense

The patient is seated comfortably with the forearms and hands supported and at rest in a supinated position. The therapist tests the hands bilaterally for perception of the vibration of the 30 HV tuning fork and the 256 CPS tuning fork. The 30 HV fork is used first, because it will be perceived before the 256 CPS fork can be. Returning ability to perceive the 256 CPS fork indicates progression in regeneration of the nerve.

Testing with the tuning fork is initiated by tapping the fork on the table and then applying it proximal to the anticipated site of the lesion. The uninvolved extremity is tested first to enable the patient to compare sensation in the intact area with the area that has been injured. Once the uninvolved extremity has been stimulated, the tuning fork is tapped on the table, and the same stimulus is given to the involved extremity. After the stimulus has been applied proximally, the tuning fork is moved distally, and the patient is asked to respond when the sensation of the vibration changes as well as when the sensation of vibration is absent.

Another method for assessing vibration is to tap the tuning fork and apply it first to the uninvolved extremity and then to the same spot on the involved extremity, using constant touch as opposed to moving touch. The patient is asked to respond to the stimulus by indicating if it is the same as the uninvolved extremity or different, and, if different, how it is different.

Light Touch

The patient is seated comfortably with the forearms supinated and vision occluded. Monofilaments are selected from largest to smallest, and the stimulus is applied to the volar surface of the hand. The patient is asked to indicate the specific point at which he or she felt the touch of the filament. As long as correct responses are recorded, progressively smaller filaments are used. When the patient becomes unable to make correct responses, the size of the preceding monofilament is recorded. The patient's sensitivity to monofilaments has been correlated with the return of protective sensation as well as with the return of two-point discrimination.

Two-Point Discrimination

Two-point discrimination is widely recognized as being positively correlated with sensory return.[3] The patient is seated with the supinated forearm supported and vision occluded. With calipers or a molded paper clip calibrated in millimeters, the patient first receives a stimulus of one or two points on the uninvolved extremity (which is used as a sensitivity reference). When evaluating the involved extremity, the therapist begins with the caliper tips 10 mm apart and applies the instrument longitudi-

Hand Therapy Evaluation

Name: _____   Dominance: _____   Occupation: _____

HX Diagnosis: _____

_____

Surgeries: _____

Range of Motion			Right or Left (circle)							
Date										
Shoulder 0-160		Ext/Flex.								
160		Abd.								
90		Int. Rot.								
90		Ext. Rot.								
Elbow 140		Flex.								
0		Ext.								
Forearm 90		Pro.								
90		Sup.								
Wrist 65		Ext.								
60		Flex.								
25		Rad. Dev.								
25		Uln. Dev.								
Index 0-90		MP	to	to	to	to	to	to	to	
0-120		PIP	to	to	to	to	to	to	to	
0-80		DIP	to	to	to	to	to	to	to	
Middle		MP	to	to	to	to	to	to	to	
		PIP	to	to	to	to	to	to	to	
		DIP	to	to	to	to	to	to	to	
Ring		MP	to	to	to	to	to	to	to	
		PIP	to	to	to	to	to	to	to	
		DIP	to	to	to	to	to	to	to	
Little		MP	to	to	to	to	to	to	to	
		PIP	to	to	to	to	to	to	to	
		DIP	to	to	to	to	to	to	to	
Thumb 0-60		MP	to	to	to	to	to	to	to	
0-90		IP	to	to	to	to	to	to	to	
		web space								
Tam										

Strength		R	L	R	L	R	L	R	L	R	L	R	L	R	L
Date															
Grip	Power														
	Tip														
Pinches	Lateral														
	Palmar														

Composite Flexion To Palm In CM.

Date		I	M	R	L	I	M	R	L	I	M	R	L	I	M	R	L

Circumferential Measurement In MM.

		I	M	R	L	I	M	R	L	I	M	R	L	I	M	R	L
Date	PIP																
	PP																

Figure 31-1. Hand therapy evaluation form of the Austin Hand and Upper Extremity Rehabilitation Center, Austin, Texas.

nally from distal to proximal for the length of the injured area. It is important not to make the skin blanch with the stimulus. The patient is asked to distinguish between being touched by one or two points. After each correct response, the caliper measurement is reduced until the patient is unable to distinguish two points of contact. This measurement is recorded, and the testing proceeds to the next digit.

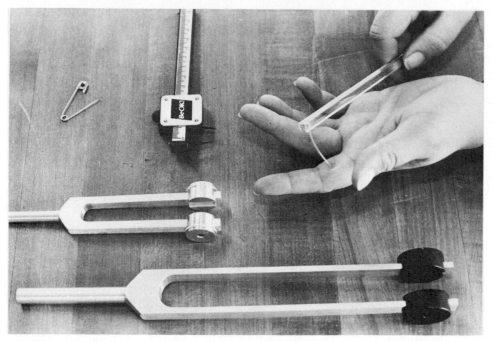

Figure 31-2. Sensory evaluation instruments; from top left: safety pin, 2-point calipers, Von Frey monofilaments, turning forks.

Moving Touch

The eraser of a pencil is used for this evaluation. The patient is positioned with the supinated forearm supported, and the eraser is placed proximal to the lesion and moved distally. The patient is instructed to report when the sensation changes and when the stimulus is no longer felt. As the data are compiled, sensory mapping is done on the patient's sensibility evaluation chart (Fig. 31-3). As a rule, sensory evaluations are repeated every 4 to 6 weeks.

Strength

The Jamar dynamometer and the pinch meter (Fig. 31-4) permit reliable and reproducible measurements. In using the dynamometer to measure hand grasp, the gripping handle is placed on the third notch, and the patient is seated with the arm adducted at the side, the elbow flexed to 90°, and the forearm in midposition. The patient is asked to squeeze the handle with maximum effort after being told that the handle will not move but will exert a force on the dial that registers in inch-pounds of force. Both the involved and the uninvolved hands are tested with three attempts, and an average of the three scores for each hand is recorded. If there is a question about the validity of the patient's effort, the clinician can take measurements on each notch, which, when plotted, should form a bell-shaped curve with the first and last positions being the weakest. When administering the test, the therapist must be sure

that the patient's arm is not supported, because this will cause inaccurate readings. The therapist must always use the same dynamometer when reassessing the patient's strength.

When using the pinch gauge, there are three prehension patterns the clinician assesses:

Pad-to-pad, which is between the thumb and index finger

Palmar or three-jaw chuck, which is thumb opposed to the index and long fingers

Lateral or key pinch, which uses the pad of the thumb against the lateral surface of the index finger at the level of the PIP joint

Activities of Daily Living

An informal interview will usually reveal if the patient is having difficulty with activities of daily living (ADL), the most common being with personal hygiene and communication skills. However, actual performance of activities should be done to determine the extent and type of deficits. The more involved the medical problem, the more extensive the therapist's assessment should be.

Coordination a..d Dexterity

Many standardized tests are available to evaluate fine motor coordination. Some of these are the Lafayette Grooved Pegboard, Crawford Small Parts, Purdue Peg-

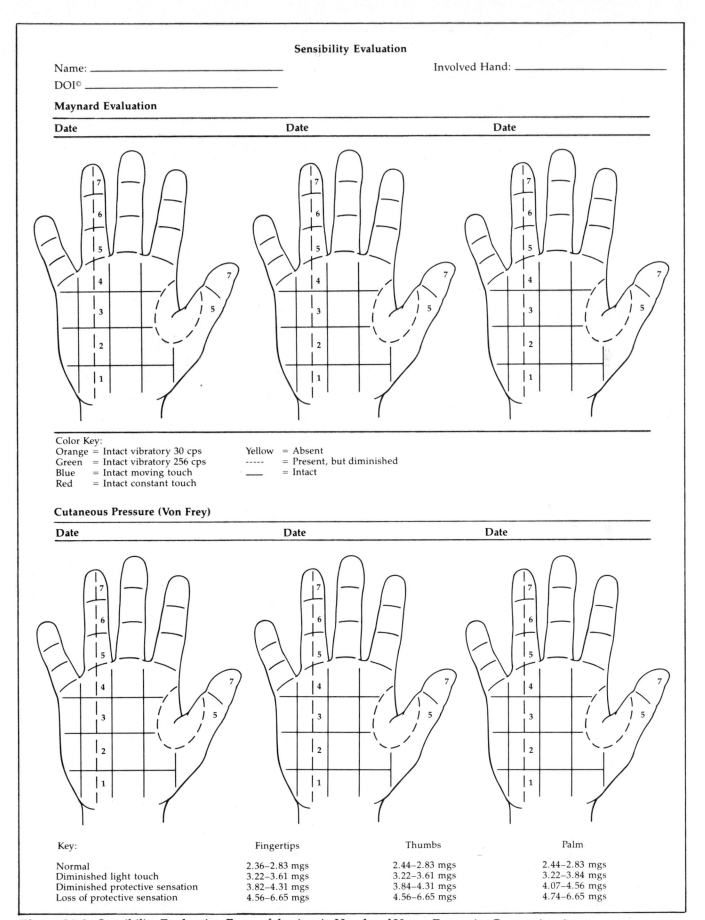

Sensibility Evaluation

Name: _____   Involved Hand: _____

DOI© _____

Maynard Evaluation

Date _____   Date _____   Date _____

Color Key:
Orange = Intact vibratory 30 cps   Yellow = Absent
Green = Intact vibratory 256 cps   ----- = Present, but diminished
Blue   = Intact moving touch   ____ = Intact
Red   = Intact constant touch

Cutaneous Pressure (Von Frey)

Date _____   Date _____   Date _____

Key:	Fingertips	Thumbs	Palm
Normal	2.36–2.83 mgs	2.44–2.83 mgs	2.44–2.83 mgs
Diminished light touch	3.22–3.61 mgs	3.22–3.61 mgs	3.22–3.84 mgs
Diminished protective sensation	3.82–4.31 mgs	3.84–4.31 mgs	4.07–4.56 mgs
Loss of protective sensation	4.56–6.65 mgs	4.56–6.65 mgs	4.74–6.65 mgs

Figure 31-3. Sensibility Evaluation Form of the Austin Hand and Upper Extremity Center, Austin, Texas. *(Figure continues on page 552.)*

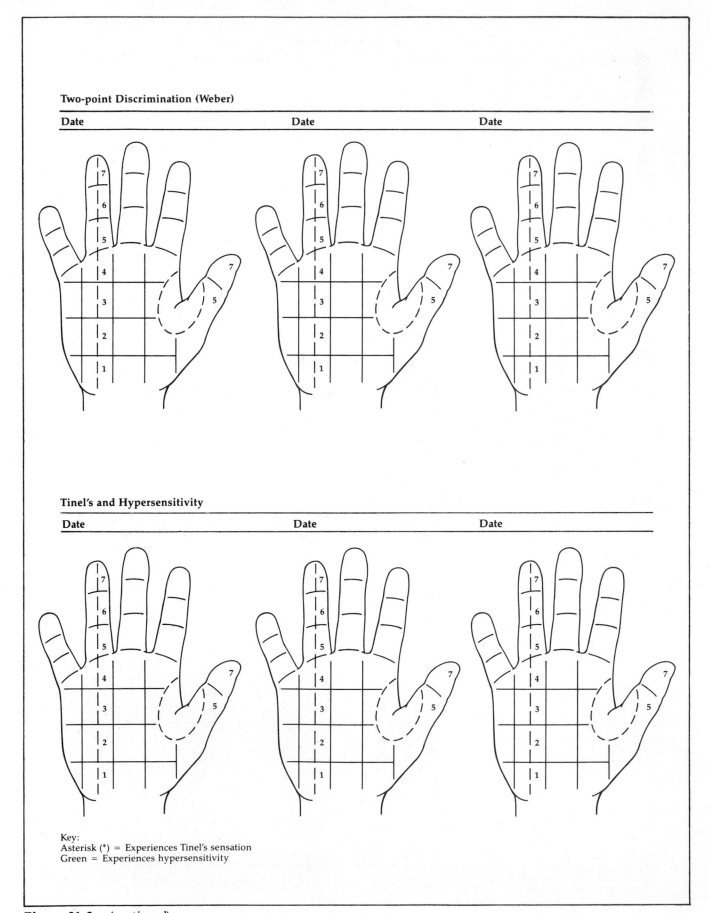

Two-point Discrimination (Weber)

Date   Date   Date

Tinel's and Hypersensitivity

Date   Date   Date

Key:
Asterisk (*) = Experiences Tinel's sensation
Green = Experiences hypersensitivity

Figure 31-3. *(continued)*

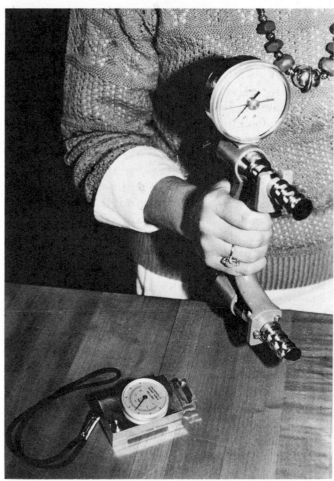

Figure 31-4. Jamar dynamometer (top) and pinch gauge.

board, Minnesota Rate of Manipulation, and the Pennsylvania Bimanual Dexterity Test (see Fig. 31-15). Within the realm of the occupational therapist's training, there are also such tests as the Jebsen Hand Function Test and the Moberg Pick-Up Test, to name only a few.

When administering a test, not only must the therapist be concerned with the time and the number of correct responses the patient is able to make but also with observations of the patient. Much can be learned about coordination by observing:

Substitution patterns that the patient uses to achieve a certain result
Ability of the patient to follow directions
The patient's oral responses during the test
The patient's general attitude

The testing procedures and reasons for their use should be thoroughly explained to the patient. This will help to allay any fears or concerns the patient has regarding performance and test results.

Psychosocial Aspects

Initially, one of the most difficult areas in rehabilitation is loss of a body part or the presence of a visible deformity. Early in the evaluation process, the patient may go through all the stages of grieving for the lost part just as he or she would mourn the loss of a loved one. It is important to listen to what the patient says during the evaluation, especially those comments concerning the nature of the injury. There may be anger directed at the patient's employer or fellow employees if the patient feels that someone else is directly or indirectly responsible for the injury. If there is poor communication between spouses, the patient can harbor a great deal of anger, feeling that his or her spouse is unable to understand or appreciate what has happened. When dealing with a patient who has noticeable deformities, loss, or mutilation, it is important to clarify, before treatment begins, whether the patient is comfortable and has grown accustomed to the appearance of the extremity.

It is reassuring to observe the amount of support that can be elicited from fellow patients. Camaraderie develops between patients that helps to ease anxieties. Many patients have gone through the same experience, have made the necessary changes, and can share with those who are just starting the rehabilitation process.

Nerve Injury and Repair

Neuroanatomy

Any discussion of the mechanism of nerve repair must begin with definitions of terminology and an understanding of basic neuroanatomy.

The basic component of any major nerve is the nerve fiber, which may be visualized as a single tube made up of either sensorimotor or sympathetic fibers. Nerve fibers may be bunched together into what is called a *funiculus.* The funiculus is a well-defined bundle of nerves in which the individual nerve fibers or axons are separated by a substance called *endoneurium.* The funiculus is also surrounded by a type of connective tissue called the *perineurium,* which acts as a sheath to isolate the funiculus into a well-defined bundle of nerves. Several funiculi may come together to form a *fascicle.* The fascicles are separated by another connective tissue sheath called the *epineurium,* the outermost sheath of a nerve.

Classifications

The classifications of nerve injuries now in use are those of Seddon and Sunderland. Seddon categorizes nerve injuries as neurapraxia, axonotmesis, and neurotmesis.[12] Sunderland uses a numerical grading system (1 to 5) to categorize nerve injuries, and these grades correspond with Seddon's classifications.[13]

Neurapraxia, as described by Seddon, is a conduction block of the nerve and is the same as a Sunderland type 1 injury.[12,13] Axonotmesis, according to Seddon, is loss of continuity of the axons but not of the surrounding endoneurium. Axonotmesis corresponds to a Sunderland type 2 injury. Seddon describes neurotmesis as a cut nerve; Sunderland divides this category into types 3, 4, and 5 injuries. Type 3 injury refers to the loss of continuity of axons and endoneurium, with the epineurium intact. Type 4 refers to the additional loss of axons, endoneurium, and perineurium, leaving only the epineurium intact. Type 5 refers to the transection of the entire nerve bundle.

Processes of Nerve Injury and Repair

When considering what happens when nerves are injured and repaired, it is important to look at the nerve as simply a tubular structure that has been divided into two parts. Changes occur in each part, and these are crucial to the actual repair process.

When the nerve is transected or injured somewhere along its tubular path, the central nerve body progressively enlarges over the first 3 weeks. The enlargement on the proximal portion of the nerve is thought to be caused by increased production of protein by the central nerve cell body. This protein migrates along the axon or tube of the nerve to the site of the injury.[4] It is thought that, in some way, this protein substance is used in the repair of the axon. Approximately 7 days after the axon has been divided, sprouting begins that appears to be an attempt by the axon to bridge the gap at the site of injury. If these axon sprouts are able to join with the distal ends of the cut axon, then nerve repair can occur.

On the distal portion of the cut nerve, a different process is occurring, and time appears to be critical. Once the distal end is separated from the central nerve body, the axon begins to undergo neuronal destruction, called *Wallerian degeneration*. During this process, which occurs over a period of 6 weeks,[13] the basic molecules of the nerve break down and are digested by surrounding cells. Eventually, the destruction becomes complete and is accompanied by atrophy, which minimizes the possibility of subsequent regeneration.

Another important factor in nerve repair is the state of the tissue the nerves are supposed to stimulate. There appears to be a considerable difference in the response to an interruption of the nerve supplies to muscle cells or to sensory end organs. The muscle cells begin to atrophy about 3 to 4 months after the nerve supply has been interrupted. After approximately 2 years, the destruction may be so extensive that the muscle fibers are actually disintegrating. There is no conclusive evidence that external electrical stimulation can alter this course within the muscle cells; the only demonstrated way to halt the cell destruction is to re-establish nerve stimulation. If this is not achieved within 24 months after the injury, degeneration is probably irreversible.[1]

The situation with the sensory end organs appears to be quite different. Even after a period of 1 year, repair of a sensory nerve should provide at least protective sensation to the involved area.[10] The age of the patient appears to be particularly important; younger individuals have a greater response to repair of a sensory nerve than do older ones. In addition to the factor of time, which appears to be most important in the repair of motor fibers, other factors play a role in the eventual outcome of nerve repair. These factors include the general condition of the tissue, the nutritional status of the patient; absence of crushing around the injured nerve site; and the vascular supply.

The Nerves of the Hand

Each of the major nerves of the hand will be described in this section, including the muscles innervated, the primary function of the nerve, the results of nerve damage, and the treatment of nerve injuries.

Median Nerve

Anatomy and Actions

The muscles innervated by the median nerve are the pronator teres, palmaris longus, flexor carpi radialis, flexor digitorum superficialis, flexor digitorum profundus to the index and long fingers, flexor pollicis longus, pronator quadratus, lumbricals 1 and 2, and all of the thenar muscles in the hand except the adductor pollicis, the deep head of the flexor pollicis brevis.[8] The primary functions of the median-innervated muscles are coordination, dexterity, manipulation, and prehension.

A patient with a low median lesion develops an "ape hand," with loss of opposition of the thumb and palmar abduction of the thumb. A high median lesion, in addition to this damage, also causes loss of interphalangeal joint flexion of the thumb and the first and second digits and a weakness in grasp due to loss of the flexor digitorum superficialis moving the proximal interphalangeal joint in the third and fourth digits. The sensory loss involves the volar aspect of the thumb and index and middle fingers, with variations to the ring finger volarly.

Treatment of Injuries

When treating a patient with median nerve involvement, the therapist must deal with the serious loss of

Motor Evaluation Form

Normal	Poor + −	
Good + −	Trace	
Fair + −	Zero	

Name: _____

DOI: _____

Median Nerve

Pronator
FCR
FDS
½FDP
FPL
Pronator
Lumbricals

Pronator Teres							
FCR							
FDS							
½FDP							
FPL							
Pronator Quadratus							
Thenars 　FPB (sup. head)							
APB							
Opponens							
½Lumbricals							

Ulnar Nerve

FCU
½FDP

Hypothenars
Lumbricals
Interossi

FCU							
½FDP							
Hypothenars 　ABD. Dig. Min.							
Opponens Dig. Min.							
Flexor Dig. Min.							
½Lumbricals							
Interossei 　1st							
Adductor							

Radial Nerve

Triceps
Brachio-
radialis
ECRL
ECRB
Supinator
EDC
ECU
APL
EPL
EPB
EIP
EDM

Triceps							
Brachioradialis							
ECRL							
ECRB							
Supinator							
EDC							
EDM							
ECU							
APL							
EPL							
EPB							
EIP							

Figure 31-5. Motor Evaluation form of the Austin Hand and Upper Extremity Center, Austin, Texas.

sensibility as well as of the motor components. It is important to go through sensory mapping of the hand and instruct the patient in vital sensory precautions to compensate for the loss of protective sensation. The patient must realize that caution must be taken in dealing with hot and cold, especially when the individual smokes. With the loss of the sense of light touch, the patient cannot discern the pressure needed to hold items and may frequently drop things. The patient will need to *see* what needs to be picked up due to the loss of stereognosis. Skin lesions can appear on the areas of sensory loss, and these will take longer to heal because of the diminished vascular supply.

Following the sensory evaluation, the patient's ROM should be assessed as well as grip and pinch strength. A manual muscle test may be necessary to establish baseline motor function, which is recorded on a motor evaluation form (Fig. 31-5).

If the neuropathy involves the dominant hand, splinting and ADL adaptation may be required. The usual splint for a median nerve disruption is a C bar, also known as a web spacer (Fig. 31-6), which places the thumb in direct alignment with the second metacarpal to aid in prehension and to prevent contracture in the web space. In ADL, a writing assessment may be required, or the patient may need to be trained in alternate ways to hold the writing utensil. In addition, various dressing activities may be practiced, such as fastening buttons and zippers.

The most common problem involving the median nerve is *carpal tunnel syndrome.* The median nerve runs through the carpal tunnel along with nine tendons. The relatively small size of the canal and the rigidity of the surrounding cavernous structure and the flexor retinaculum can put pressure on the nerve, compressing it until it is pinched off like a garden hose. This may occur if the patient has diabetes, rheumatoid arthritis, congestive heart failure, or kidney dysfunction; is in the third trimester of pregnancy; or is obese. Impedance of the nerve will prevent it from firing and will cause night pain and paresthesias. The patient's primary complaint is pain at night, with a tingling sensation in the involved area that wakes him or her. If the skin over the carpal tunnel is tapped, the patient will report a tingling or shocking feeling running to the digits known as a positive Tinel's sign.

To further assess the problem, the physician will perform Phalen's test. This test is done with the elbows comfortably flexed and the forearm supinated. The examiner places the hand at the maximum amount of flexion at the wrist for 60 seconds. The physician then asks the patient if there is any difference in the feeling in one hand or the other. The patient will have a positive Phalen's test when he or she feels a numbness or tingling in the involved hand. To further confirm the diagnosis, the physician may order a nerve conduction study or an electromyograph (EMG).

A conservative approach may be recommended to the patient, in which case the therapist will evaluate the hand and may be requested to apply a forearm-based volar wrist cock-up splint to maintain the wrist in approximately 20°–25° of extension leaving the thumb and fingers free (Fig. 31-7). This splint, by extending the wrist, opens the carpal canal and alleviates the pressure. The splint is worn primarily at night and intermittently during the day.

The physician may administer a steroid injection or request physical therapy using phonopheresis with micronized hydrocortisone. A home program is then outlined, using Theraplast exercises to strengthen the in-

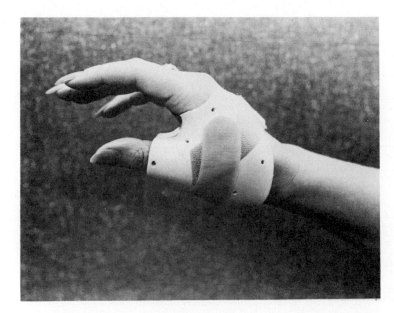

Figure 31-6. Median nerve splint supports the thumb in opposition and maintains the web space.

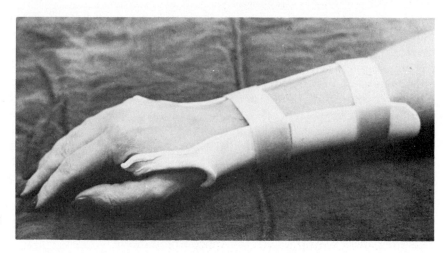

Figure 31-7. Forearm-based volar wrist cock-up.

trinsic and thenar muscles and to increase the general strength of the hand. After a carpal release, the patient may require therapeutic intervention, including modalities to decrease scar sensitivity, massage to soften the scar tissue, exercises to increase composite motion, functional activities to improve coordination and dexterity, exercises for general hand strength, ADL adaptations, and a home program.

Ulnar Nerve

Anatomy and Actions

The ulnar nerve begins in the forearm with innervation of the flexor carpi ulnaris and the ulnar half of the flexor digitorum profundus. Within the hand, it innervates the abductor digiti quinti and the flexor digiti quinti, lumbricals 3 and 4, the three volar interossei, the four dorsal interossei, the deep head of the flexor pollicis brevis, and the adductor pollicis in the thumb.[8] The primary functions of the muscles innervated by the ulnar nerve are to provide grip strength, leverage, and metacarpal mobility.

An ulnar nerve lesion produces a pseudo-claw hand.

(A true claw hand is produced by both median and ulnar nerve lesions.) The sensory involvement produces loss on the volar and dorsal surface of the small fingers, with a variation of the ring finger and possibly the middle finger.

Treatment of Injuries

As with the median nerve, the therapist must first address the sensory loss. Although this loss does not have the same impact on function as does median nerve injury, it must still be mapped, and the patient must be instructed in sensory precautions. Following assessment of ROM, grip, and pinch, the therapist may conduct a manual muscle test to more clearly define the extent of involvement.

The splint most frequently required is a hand-based splint with a lumbrical bar (Fig. 31-8). The function of the lumbrical bar is to prevent hyperextension of the metacarpal phalangeal joints of the ring and small fingers in order to allow the extrinsic extensors to fully extend the fingers and, thus, prevent contractures of the metacarpophalangeal joint in extension.

For ulnar nerve injury, ADL activities usually in-

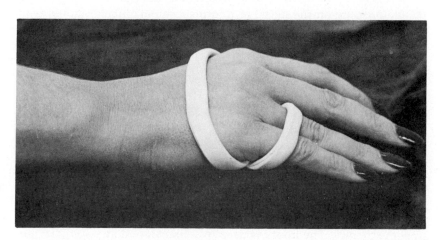

Figure 31-8. Ulnar nerve splint supports the dorsum of the digits to decrease clawing and allow the extrinsic extensors to extend the remainder of the digit.

clude more gross motor activities than are needed in patients receiving rehabilitation for injuries of the median nerve. The most common site of involvement for the ulnar nerve is at the elbow, which results in an ulnar palsy. The cause may be a fracture or dislocation in the elbow or compression of the ulnar nerve in the olecranon fossa.

Because of the tight fit of the ulnar nerve at the elbow and the structure of the cubital tunnel, a positive Tinel's response will be elicited with palpation or percussion at the cubital tunnel; however, it is important to check both extremities to determine the intensity. A positive Froment's sign can be elicited when the therapist places a piece of paper on the lateral edge of the index finger and asks the patient to grip it with the entire length of the thumb. Due to the loss of the first dorsal interosseus and the adductor pollicis function, the patient holds the paper with the flexor pollicis longus muscle and the interphalangeal joint of the thumb pulled into flexion, as opposed to tight adduction of the proximal phalanx. Nerve conduction studies will indicate a slowed conduction rate and will help to determine the level of involvement. When the elbow is placed in flexion, the patient will report pain and paresthesias, similar to the Phalen's test for the median nerve.

A second site, involved less frequently, is Guyon's canal. The condition is called *ulnar tunnel syndrome*. This canal is located adjacent to the carpal tunnel, and damage is more frequently associated with trauma such as repetitive blows to the base of the palm. The therapy intervention is prophylactic splinting for the elbow during sleep. By keeping the patient's elbows fully extended, the splint prevents compression of the nerve while the patient is in sleeping positions.

Neuritis in this area may also benefit from steroid injections or phonopheresis. Due to the loss of sensation, the patient needs to be instructed in sensory precautions and instructed in work-simplification techniques to decrease repetitive trauma. Hand and wrist strengthening will also be involved using Theraplast and weights for general reconditioning.

If surgery at the elbow is indicated, it most often is to relieve pressure on the nerve or to transpose the ulnar nerve out of the cubital tunnel. Sometimes, the operation also involves removal of the medial epicondyle. The surgeon may choose to place the nerve anteriorly into the antecubital fossa, where it will be amply padded. Following surgery, the patient rarely requires therapy except for a home program for motion, general reconditioning, and work simplification.

Median and Ulnar Involvement

Effects

This injury significantly affects the function of the entire upper extremity. The injury is usually a direct lesion at the level of the wrist or is secondary to brachial plexus injury. Nerve involvement is further complicated by direct laceration of adjacent tendons, resulting in a true claw hand. A low lesion produces total anesthesia of the palmar surface, leaving it susceptible to injury from hot and cold. With the imbalance of the intrinsic and extrinsic musculature, the metacarpophalangeal joints hyperextend and the interphalangeal joints flex. The median-innervated thumb then folds into extension, and the patient develops a flattening of the palmar arch that further hinders the use of the extrinsic muscles. If the site of involvement is higher, forearm pronations will be affected or lost and the entire hand will be useless, with no ability to grasp.

Treatment of Injuries

Treatment of an injury with median and ulnar involvement calls upon the therapist to use all of the tools at his or her disposal. First, one splint must be constructed to replace lost function and another to prevent contractures. A hand-based dorsal positioning splint is required, with a lumbrical bar to facilitiate extension of the interphalangeal joints and a C bar to promote opposition. A night-time forearm-based volar positioning splint is constructed with the wrist at 30° of extension, the metacarpophalangeals flexed to 60°, the interphalangeals extended, and the thumb opposed (Fig. 31-9). Because of the lack of sensation in the hand, great care should be taken in constructing any splint: if the palmar arch is not maintained and pressure is placed on the heads of the metacarpals, pressure sores will form.

Sensory evaluation must be done very carefully, and instruction in sensory precautions is a primary concern. The patient will need to inspect the hand for injuries and to care for the nails on a daily basis. With direct nerve lesions, prominent trophic changes will occur that affect the quality of the skin. The most obvious atrophy is the loss of sweat gland function, followed by loss of flexor creases, papillary depth, and pencil-pointing of the pads of the fingers. The wrinkle test is done to determine the degree of nerve injury: the hand is placed in water for 5 minutes and then dried; where nerve function is absent, there will be no wrinkling of the skin.

It is important to get a baseline sensory evaluation, as well as to perform a manual muscle test and ROM evaluations. A sensory test is not indicated until 6 weeks postinjury when the tendon and nerve are both repaired. The healing of the tendon must be handled very carefully. The average rate of regeneration of a nerve is 1 mm per day, or approximately 1 inch per month. Re-evaluations are best done on a monthly basis and should include both sensory and motor status, as well as ROM and grip strength. The Jebsen hand function test is used to assess returning gross hand function. In order to prevent tendon shortening as well as joint contractures, it will be important for the therapist to encourage the pa-

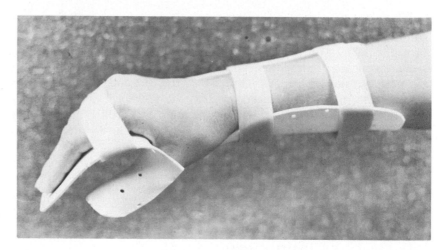

Figure 31-9. Forearm-based volar positioning splint.

tient to follow through with a home program involving active and passive ROM and functional activities.

Radial Nerve

Anatomy and Actions

Three motor branches of the radial nerve arise in the lower third of the upper arm. The first branch innervates the brachioradialis, the second the extensor carpi radialis longus, and the third the extensor carpi radialis brevis. In the forearm, the radial nerve innervates the supinator and the extensor digitorum communis, the extensor carpi ulnaris, the abductor pollicis longus, the extensor pollicis longus, and the terminal branch of the extensor indicis proprius.[8]

The characteristic hand position after a radial nerve injury is that of a drop wrist, along with loss of the ability to extend the wrist, the metacarpophalangeal joints, and the thumb. A high lesion causes weakness in forearm supination.

Treatment of Injuries

Radial nerve damage is perhaps the easiest nerve injury to address. The sensory loss is all dorsal and does not have the same ramifications as in injuries of the median and ulnar nerves. However, the sensory branch of the radial nerve does become superficial distally at the level of the radial styloid, and injury in that area can produce a painful problem that is easily aggravated.

Of primary concern is the restoration of function by means of a dynamic splint. The splint of choice is a dorsal forearm-based wrist cock-up that immobilizes the wrist in 20° to 30° of extension. Next, an outrigger is applied, and finger cuffs are attached to the proximal phalanx of the involved digits, holding the metacarpophalangeal joints in a neutral position (Fig. 31-10). An extension outrigger also may be indicated for the thumb.

The most common site of disruption of the radial nerve is at the humerus, where the nerve spirals around the bone. It may be a secondary injury from a fractured humerus or a primary lesion from compression of the

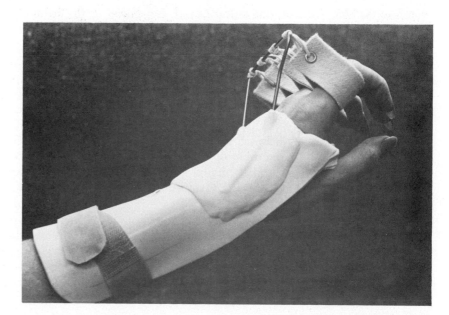

Figure 31-10. Radial nerve splint. Wrist is supported at 30° extension and MPs at neutral so that intrinsics can complete digital extension.

radial nerve (Saturday night palsy). Compression and contusion will usually be followed by spontaneous return of function; however, until this occurs, the hand requires splinting. If the patient is in a cast for a fractured humerus, an outrigger may be applied to the cast and affixed with additional plaster. At first, the therapist may think that the fingers are beginning to extend and that recovery has begun, when in fact the patient can fully extend the fingers using substitution patterns such as the tenodesis effect of wrist flexion or by letting the tightness in the extensor tendons give the illusion of full extension. By watching the patient, the therapist can quickly become aware of substitution patterns.

Summary

When dealing with nerve injuries, the therapist must be especially prudent about educating the patient to sensory precautions in order to prevent further injury. Accurate measurements must be kept that detail sensory and motor return, as well as changes in active and passive ROM over time. As regeneration occurs, the patient will benefit greatly from an activity program to enhance coordination, dexterity, strength, and mobility. At this point, craft activities become more pertinent to treatment. Some of the more appropriate ones involve leatherwork, macrame, copper tooling, woodworking, and beadwork. Not only can a patient see and feel improvement with these activities, but bilateral involvement will increase, and ADL tasks will be enhanced. Where there is loss of sensation, it is easy to neglect the affected part because of the absence of sensory feedback. Activities that enhance bilateral involvement challenge the sensory system and keep the patient cognitively aware of the injured part.

Tendon Injury and Repair

A tendon is composed of long strands of an extremely fibrous protein called *collagen*. Throughout this fibrous mass, there is a sparse number of cells called *fibrocytes*. It is believed that these fibrocytes are somewhat inactive under normal conditions.

Injury and Repair

One of the first changes after a tendon is injured is the noticeable increase in the number of cells at the site of injury. These cells appear to be inflammatory and are probably brought to the site by the surrounding blood supply.

Considerable controversy exists in the literature regarding the mechanism of tendon repair. It was formerly thought that the entire process was dependent on cells that come to the site from the blood.[11] It is now believed that the collagen for the repair process is produced by both the fibrocytes and the cells from the blood.[9]

As with nerve repair, several factors have a considerable effect on the outcome. The quality of the tendon injury is important, in that cleanly cut tendons will have a greater chance of healing if appropriately repaired than will those that are crushed or avulsed. Similarly, any process that delays healing, such as contamination by foreign material or an infection, will impede healing. Ultimately, the single most important factor appears to be the blood supply from the surrounding tissue: if the tendon and the tissue receive less than the normal blood supply, then tendon healing will be seriously hindered.

Treatment of Injuries

Tendon lacerations, of both flexors and extensors, account for the largest percentage of patients in hand clinics. Much has been learned regarding restoration of function following tendon injuries through the work of such surgeons as Kleinert, Duran, and Houser. Rehabilitation following tendon repairs has greatly changed: dynamic splinting is initiated within the first week, in contrast to the treatment protocol used in the 1960s and early 1970s, which required 4 weeks of immobilization.

Flexor Tendons

On the volar surface of the hand, there are five zones. Injuries to zone 1, including tendon advancements of the flexor digitorum profundus, usually cause little difficulty. The tendon repair can be done by end-to-end anastomosis if the distal tendon segment can be retrieved for the suture.[5,7] If not, the proximal end of the profundus is reinserted into the phalanx through a drill hole in the phalanx, and pull-out wires are attached proximally, dorsally, and distally through the fingernail.

Zone 2, often called "no man's land," includes both the flexor digitorum profundus and the flexor digitorum superficialis in each digit and extends to the level of the distal palmar crease. In this area, synovial sheaths surround the gliding tendons and keep them lubricated as well as nourished. Following primary suture of the zone 2 tendons by the surgeon, the hand is splinted with a forearm-based dorsal blocking splint, with the wrist placed in 30° to 45° flexion, the metacarpophalangeal joints in 45° to 60° flexion, and the interphalangeal joints left free (Fig. 31-11). The dorsal component of the splint maintains a flat surface to allow the digits to move into full interphalangeal extension. The hand is placed in bulky compressive dressings at the time of surgery, and then a dorsal plaster is applied for 1 to 3 days.

When the patient arrives at the hand center, the bulky dressings are removed, and a sterile dressing change is performed. The therapist devises a forearm-based dorsal blocking splint from a thermoplastic mate-

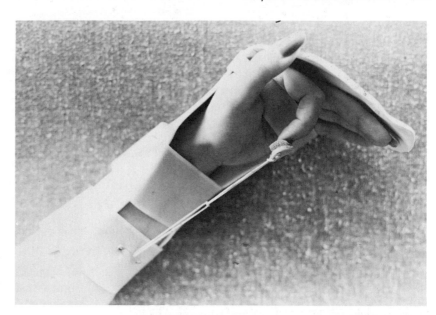

Figure 31-11. A forearm-based, dorsal blocking splint used with Kleinert traction for early mobilization of primarily repaired flexor tendons.

rial that keeps the wrist flexed. Dynamic traction is established with elastic bands from the tip of the digit to approximately 3 to 4 inches proximal to the wrist flexion crease. During surgery, the surgeon may put a large suture through the nail to which a rubber band is applied for the dynamic traction; if the surgeon has not done so, Velcro or a millinery hook can be affixed to the nail with Superglue in order to attach the elastic traction to the nail.

The patient is instructed to extend the digit ten times per hour, making sure that it reaches the length of the dorsal platform that is in extension (the Kleinert technique).[10] This exercise allows the tendon to move passively while preventing joint stiffness. The contraction of the extensor muscle allows the flexor to relax by means of reciprocal inhibition and thus alleviates the internal tension at the repair site. It is also important to keep the finger in flexion when at rest to prevent any sudden impact or jerking that could disrupt the repair. The therapist must always instruct the patient not to use the uninvolved digits. Because the profundus and superficialis move all four digits, the internal contraction needed to use one digit will elicit tension in the muscle and thus place pressure on the repair site. To prevent stiffness in the distal interphalangeal joint, the traction device may be set up with a pulley system, or the digit may be moved passively into full extension.

Duran and Houser advocate a program of controlled passive motion (CPM) after a repair in zone 2. The hand is placed in a splint with the wrist in 20° of flexion, the metacarpophalangeal joints flexed 60°, and the interphalangeal joints extended. The proximal interphalangeal joints are moved passively through flexion and extension. This protocol, as well as the Kleinert mobilization technique, are followed for 4 weeks, at which time the dorsal splint is removed and a wrist cufflet with continued rubber band traction is applied. At this time, the patient may go through full digital extension with the wrist at neutral. By the sixth week, all devices are discarded, and the patient is working on active ROM exercises. The active ROM program involves blocked mobility at the metacarpophalangeal and proximal and distal interphalangeal joints. Composite flexion is achieved through various functional activities that enhance finger flexion. Such activities may include moving graduated marbles in the palm of the hand, Theraplast exercises, or a Knavel table for mass strengthening. If proximal interphalangeal flexion contractures are present, the therapist may begin extension splinting between the eighth and twelfth weeks. At this time, the therapist begins a strengthening and weight program using Theraplast.

Zone 3 is the area from the midpalm to, but not including, the carpal tunnel, zone 4 is the wrist area (including the carpal tunnel), and zone 5 is the forearm area. Lesions in zones 3, 4, and 5 usually involve several tendons and possibly nerves. The extent of the repair dictates the postoperative immobilization. As a general rule, the repair is left immobile for 3 weeks. The patient is fitted with a forearm-based dorsal blocking splint with the wrist at 30° flexion, the metacarpophalangeals at 60° of flexion, and the interphalangeals extended. The therapist starts the patient on active and passive motion exercises at 4 weeks and progresses with therapy as stated for other flexor tendon injuries. In zones 3 and 4, finger traction may still be necessary, as per physician preference.

As with tendon repairs in zone 2, flexor tendon repairs are impeded by the formation of scar tissue. Fibrin unites the tendon and holds it taut. The scar that develops internally is not discrete enough to attach only to the involved tendon but firmly affixes itself to all surrounding structures, whether skin, tendon, or fascia. The combination of healing and scarring is a challenge for the therapist and patient, because scar tissue formation is essential for the healing of the tendon. Ideally, the Kleinert mobilization technique and the controlled passive technique of Duran aid in the remodeling of the scar in order to elongate the fibers and permit motion. Even though these techniques are used, adhesions usually impede function, especially at the bifurcation of the superficialis in zone 2.

It is often beneficial to use topical heat, as this relaxes the hand and makes massage of the scar more comfortable. The massage is usually done in circular fashion to make the scar more supple and malleable. The therapist follows this with blocked or isolated joint motion activity to work each tendon individually. When these exercises are followed by functional activities, the therapist can capitalize on scar management and mobility. Some therapists also use biofeedback and functional electrical stimulation to enhance the rehabilitation program. As always, the therapist needs to be sure of the surgeon, the patient, and herself or himself. The greatest potential for improvement will be realized if the patient is thoroughly educated regarding the healing process, if the activity program is carefully tailored to individual needs, and if the patient is involved in his or her own therapy.

Flexor Tendon Grafts

When there is a significant injury requiring major reconstruction, it may be necessary to do free tendon grafting to the flexors instead of a primary repair. The procedure requires implantation of a flexible silicone rod. Often called "Hunter's rod,"[5] it is inserted into the flexor canal of the involved digit and attached to the dorsal stump. Placing the rod in the tendon bed allows a smooth canal to evolve. This operation is stage I. While awaiting stage II of the procedure, it is important to monitor the individual in a comprehensive program of active and passive ROM to maintain joint mobility. If a contracture exists, it may be necessary to do dynamic or serial splinting in order to correct this deformity prior to the insertion of the tendon. Since there is no active motion in the stage I digit, often "buddy taping" will keep the fingers moving by passive association with the neighboring digit[5] (Fig. 31-12). However, if the patient is too vigorous, synovitis may develop, requiring immobilization. The therapist must observe the patient for early detection of this complication.

Stage II of the flexor tendon graft involves the actual replacement of the missing tendon. A length of tendon is removed from an associated tendon, usually the palmaris longus. The length required is removed from the donor muscle, attached proximally to the silicone rod, and then drawn distally through the canal by removal of

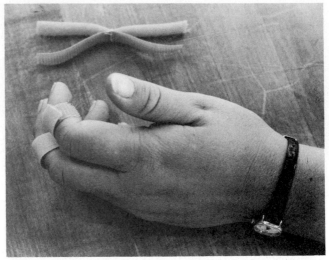

Figure 31-12. Velcro buddy splint is used to protect a weakened finger or to move adjacent finger passively.

the rod at the distal tip. Once this is done, the proximal and distal sites are sutured. The patient then follows the treatment protocol developed for zone 2 repairs of flexor tendon injuries.

If it is necessary to use buttons on the fingernails to hold the tendon reattachment in place, the Kleinert dynamic exercises may be contraindicated and the use of controlled passive motion may be more appropriate. An important fact to remember is that, as a free graft, the tendon initially has no circulation. It may therefore be slower to heal and should be dealt with in a conservative manner.

Flexor Tenolysis

Despite increasingly sophisticated surgical techniques and aggressive rehabilitation programs, some patients will have limited mobility because their tendons and the surrounding tissues have become entrapped in scar tissue. Passive ROM far exceeds active ROM. It is important during this time to maintain passive ROM to facilitate the early motion exercises necessary following a flexor tenolysis.

After approximately 6 months, when it is evident that no progress has been made, the surgeon may choose to dissect the scar tissue impeding the motion (tenolysis). Once this is done, the tendon glides freely, and therapy will begin immediately. Following this operation, the body will once again lay down scar tissue to heal the area. Therapy begins immediately using elevation and ice packs to control edema followed by active and passive ROM exercises. Theoretically, as new scar tissue appears, active ROM stretches that scar in a linear fashion and elongates the fibers to allow increased mobility. Although the tendon has been freed, it is important to remember that this operation leaves the tendon weakened by loss of the supporting scar tissue and, thus, vulnerable to rupture if motion exercises are too vigorous or resistive. As the patient progresses, more modalities are added weekly to the ROM program.

Three to four weeks after surgery, motion becomes more difficult to achieve because new scar is forming. This is an important time to emphasize patient re-education so that he or she does not become frustrated because the motion does not come as easily as it did immediately after surgery. Six to eight weeks after tenolysis, resistive exercises may be started along with a strengthening regimen.

Extensor Tendons

Extensor tendon injuries are complicated by many factors. An extensor tendon is thinner and has a weaker structure than a flexor tendon.[5] Also, due to the fact that the lymphatic system runs dorsally and the skin is intimately related to bone, any scarring or injury to the dorsum of the hand can have serious ramifications with regard to edema.

Crushing injuries with no structural damage often produce swelling of the fingers and the dorsum of the hand. Elevation, effluent massage, gradient-pressure garments, and active ROM are indicated for treatment. A volar positioning splint may also be required to maintain the metacarpophalangeal joints in flexion and the interphalangeal joints in extension, since edema usually holds the hand in the reverse position. Splinting can be done in combination with compressive strapping, such as with Velfoam, but never with an Ace bandage because it affords uneven tension, can restrict circulation, and can cause distal swelling. Active ROM makes the intrinsic musculature contract, forcing residual fluid from the tissue. The pumping action of the extrinsics in a contract–release fashion helps the fluid move distally to proximally. The therapist must always keep in mind that the body fluid carries fibrin, which will be deposited and increase the scarring.

A *mallet finger deformity,* the most common injury to the distal tip of the digit, is caused by forced hyperflexion of the distal interphalangeal joint. There is a disruption of the terminal tendon of the extensor digitorum communis, which may be associated with loss of the bone fragment from the distal phalanx. This injury is seen in sports-related accidents. Depending on the degree of damage, the digit may be splinted in 15° of hyperextension for 6 to 8 weeks, or surgical pinning in this position may be required.

Jamming injuries to the proximal interphalangeal joint, as well as those produced by forced flexion, can precipitate development of a traumatic *boutonnière deformity.* The forced flexion at the joint can disrupt the central slip of the extensor tendon and subsequently allow the tendon's lateral bands to migrate volarly along the lateral and medial borders of the joint. Although initially the flexion at the joint is not significant, prolonged flexion can cause further migration of the lateral band, which then allows the distal interphalangeal joints to go into a hyperextended position in order to balance the internal tension on the associated tendon group. With early intervention consisting of proximal interphalangeal extension splinting for 6 to 8 weeks, surgical reconstruction may be averted. Although the length of the proximal and middle phalanges is difficult to splint, great care must be directed to allow free metacarpophalangeal and distal interphalangeal mobility during proximal joint immobilization.

Injuries to the metacarpophalangeal joint often impede the gliding of the dorsal expansion (also known as the dorsal hood). A most difficult complication to deal with is that of an extensor tendon lag. When the scar tissue is adherent to the structures surrounding the joint, the muscle force on the tendon is exerted at the adhesion site and not transmitted distally. This constricture allows the development of an extensor lag. A lag greater than 30° is said to be a functional deficit. The associated functional motion of the digit is then hindered by allowing the interphalangeal joints or the metacarpophalangeal joints to flex, but composite digital flexion is unattainable. When contractures such as this exist, it is important to be able to discern the difference between a contracture involving the joint and one secondary to scar tissue or a deficit in the excursion of the tendon itself. If the finger is placed in extension at the metacarpophalangeal joint and the proximal interphalangeal joint presents with a 30° loss of extension, the digit should be brought into metacarpophalangeal flexion with reassessment of proximal interphalangeal extension. If the finger, now brought into metacarpophalangeal flexion, allows the proximal joint to go into additional extension, this indicates limitation of tendon excursion according to the tenodesis theory. If the contracture of 30° persists in the proximal interphalangeal joint once the metacarpophalangeal joint is flexed, this is considered joint tightness.

The traditional approach to monitoring repairs of extensor tendons has been to immobilize them in composite extension for 4 weeks (Fig. 31-13). At this point, active ROM exercises are begun, and the patient makes progress over the next 4 weeks, leading to increase of muscle strength by 8 weeks postrepair. If at this time extensor contractures exist, dynamic splinting to correct these deformities may be initiated. With the ever-advancing knowledge of tendon healing and scar proliferation, however, many physicians are using early dynamic traction for mobilization of the extensors.

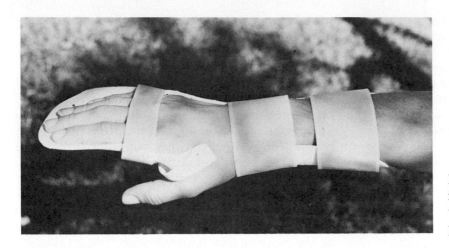

Figure 31-13. Modified volar positioning splint for composite extension of the wrist and fingers to allow healing of repaired extensor tendons.

Fractures

Fractures run the gamut from simple and nondisplaced to compound and comminuted. A simple nondisplaced fracture will produce low-grade swelling with pain and tenderness upon palpation and pain with motion. A fracture that is displaced will likewise produce pain, swelling, and tenderness, but there will also be a deformity along the course of the bone, as well as false motion and crepitus. Fractures can be more complex if they include surrounding soft-tissue injury, involving the nerves, tendons, or the vasculature.

The Process of Bone Healing

The torn ends of the fracture, periosteum, and the bone fragments at the fracture site supply granulation tissues. These tissues proliferate and differentiate into fibrous connective tissue, fibrocartilage, and hyaline cartilage, all of which bridge the fracture site. The fractured bone begins to form a complex structure known as a callus (osteogenesis). Callus develops from the periosteum and is of major importance because of the small arteries, veins, and capillary complex in the periostium. The bridging of the fracture begins at the external borders and progresses interiorly until the gap is united. Healing time differs with the extent of the damage and associated soft-tissue injury and the age, nutritional status, and general health of the patient.

Complications of healing include nonunion, which may be due to inadequate contact of bone ends or to avascularity. Nonunion is diagnosed when, after 3 months, no signs of healing are evident on radiographs. Another complication, malunion, arises from a problem with alignment or shortening sustained at the time of the original injury.

Forearm Fractures

Perhaps the most common fracture of the forearm is *Colles' fracture*, which results from falling on an outstretched hand. The force of impact affects the distal radius, producing a disruption in continuity as well as dorsal displacement. The traditional position to attain adequate reduction is placement of the wrist in flexion immobilized in a short arm cast. As reviewed earlier, the wrist in flexion may impinge on the median nerve, so these patients should be watched for symptoms of acute carpal tunnel syndrome. There also may be trophic changes that alert the therapist to another complication known as reflex sympathetic dystrophy[6] or shoulder–hand syndrome. The primary signs are:

Low-grade edema in the fingers and hand
Erythema dorsally at the proximal interphalangeal and metacarpophalangeal levels
Shiny skin with loss of flexor creases and distension of skin folds
Heightened pain with motion of the digits

Therapy is indicated early in the healing process to decrease edema and pain and to increase motion. The use of a transcutaneous electrical nerve stimulation (TENS) unit for pain management has proven beneficial. Once the patient is out of plaster, mobilization of the remaining joints of the wrist and forearm begins. Establishing a therapeutic relationship with the patient prior to cast removal may lessen his or her anxiety.

When dealing with postmenopausal women, the therapist must always be alert to the osteoporotic changes that can reduce bone density. Initially, a deformity of the forearm involving decreased supination, thought to be secondary to the patient's protective splinting of the upper extremity, can cause problems with hand-to-face actions.

A less common fracture of the forearm is known as the Smith's fracture and is a reverse Colles' fracture. It occurs in younger patients and is usually secondary to falling on a flexed wrist.[5] The Smith's fracture is different from a *Barton's fracture*, which includes a subluxation of the wrist and an articular disruption of the radius.[5]

Carpal Fractures

The carpus is made up of eight carpal bones that articulate proximally with the radius and distally with the metacarpals. The proximal row consists of the scaphoid, the lunate, the triquetrum, and the pisiform and the distal row consists of the scaphoid, the trapezium, the capitate, the hamate, and the trapezoid. Thus, the scaphoid is the only bone spanning both the proximal and distal rows.[5] Any force transmitted through the carpal bones leads to fractures more commonly in the proximal row. Fractures of the scaphoid or the lunate occur most frequently and have significant complications. The scaphoid has limited healing potential owing to its circulatory distribution: the blood supply is dorsal and lateral with dimished capillary infusion to the proximal portion. The scaphoid may take up to 6 months to heal.

During healing, the involved area should be protected with a thumb spica, which originates in the forearm and supports the wrist in extension with the thumb in opposition. Avascular necrosis or a nonunion of the bone may require surgical intervention with intercarpal fusion.

The lunate, which is adjacent to the scaphoid, is well protected by the surrounding carpals and so is fractured less frequently. The lunate, too, may undergo avascular necrosis, in which a slow degeneration of the bone occurs. This is known as *Kienbock's disease.*

Although not a fracture, osteoarthritis of the carpometacarpal joint of the thumb is of significant concern. This is a common site of osteoarthritis, causing pain and decreased ability to use the thumb.

The trapeziometacarpal joint is important because it is impossible for a person not to use the thumb. The sustaining ligaments become lax as the joint surfaces change. In normal flexion and extension of the thumb, the joints and ligament are under no significant stress; however, in opposition, there is a rotary force, and this component is stabilized only by the ligaments.[5] Stresses are unequally distributed throughout the joint surface. Bony disruption at this joint usually necessitates a forearm-based splint for support and relief of discomfort. It is imperative to do an ADL evaluation and then teach the patient joint conservation and work-simplification techniques. Because the interphalangeal joint is not involved in the disease process, it can be left free for controlled pinch activities.

Metacarpal Fractures

The most common metacarpal fracture is the *boxer's fracture* involving the fourth and/or fifth metacarpal and usually sustained when a clenched fist impacts an opposing mass. The force of impact causes a fracture in the area associated with the neck of the metacarpal bone. As the bone fractures, it angulates dorsally, causing the knuckle to become depressed and a large mass to form.

After having the fracture reduced and placed in an ulnar gutter splint for 4 to 6 weeks, the patient usually requires rehabilitation for mobilization of the metacarpophalangeal joint. Due to calcification, the extensor digitorum communis and the extensor digiti quinti may become entrapped in the callus, inhibiting free motion. Depending on the proximity of the fracture to the joint, metacarpophalangeal motion may be blocked in the cast, leaving residual stiffness.

For the metacarpal of the thumb, the most common fracture is a *Bennett fracture,* an interarticular fracture of the base of the first metacarpal. As with all articular fractures, accurate reduction is essential, and this minimizes the incidence of osteoarthritic changes. Because the abductor pollicis longus attaches to the large metacarpal shaft and the ulnar collateral ligament fastens to the smaller fragments, these fractures can be unstable and may require open reduction and internal fixation.

Ligament Injury

As discussed earlier, eight bones make up the carpal complex, but there are 21 articular surfaces interconnected by a vast maze of ligaments. Of these injuries, the *scapholunate ligamentous dissociation* can prove to be most debilitating. The injury may not show up on initial radiographs. Upon resumption of normal activity, the patient complains of chronic wrist pain that is localized on the radial half of the wrist. Repeat radiographs may show a widening space between the scaphoid and the lunate, 2 mm being within normal limits. As these two bones migrate horizontally, the scaphoid also begins to rotate.[5] If more definitive testing is required, an arthrogram may be done. Contrast medium is injected into the carpus, and radiographs are taken. If any of the contrast material escapes from the carpal complex, it will be revealed on the films, confirming the diagnosis.

Another common ligamentous problem is a tear in the triangulofibrocartilage ligament uniting the ulna with the carpus of the triquetrum. This injury causes pain with rotation of the forearm, allowing the ulna to subluxate around the radius. This also may not be clearly defined on plain radiographs, necessitating an arthrogram. The splint of choice for this injury when managing the patient in a conservative program is a near-circumferential ulnar gutter splint to decrease the ability to rotate and to reduce pain.

Gamekeeper's thumb, a tear in the ulnar collateral ligament, may result in an avulsion of a bone fragment of the metacarpal. The diagnosis can be made at this metacarpophalangeal joint by application of lateral stress bilaterally to establish the degree of instability. A hand-based thumb spica can be worn for conservative management. If the fragment is unstable, surgery will be necessary.

Overview of Treatment

Great strides are being made in the repair of hand injuries with advances of the microsurgical techniques. This specialization has allowed intricate reconstructive operations, such as replantation of amputated appendages and revascularization of free muscle flaps, to name but a few. The therapist must stay current on surgical techniques and update treatment modalities.

Evaluation

It is necessary to be aware of the anatomy, physiology, kinesiology, neurology, and ergonomics of the body. By listening to the patient, one can pick up valuable insights:

How the patient perceives himself or herself
How the patient perceives the injury
How the patient relates to the environment
If the patient has a support system

Modalities

In rehabilitation of the hand, many treatment procedures are applicable. Some type of topical heat or cold applied prior to treatment facilitates the formal exercise program, which is guided by the therapist. However, in some instances, such as Duran's exercises of controlled passive motion, topical applications may be contraindicated. Where a nerve lesion exists, great care must be taken with the insensate parts of the hand. The steam heat from hot packs can cause blisters in nerve-deprived areas. The therapist needs to explain that extra padding will be used to decrease the intensity of the heat. The patient can be taught to monitor the heat with the uninvolved hand. This also helps to involve the patient in his or her treatment.

Effluent massage may be used to decrease edema, act as a relaxant, and precipitate stretching exercises. As a rule, massage is done with the body part slightly elevated and proceeds from distal to proximal as if applying a leather glove. Rotary massage may be the treatment of choice in a dressing-scar management situation. When adhesions involve scarring of structures, such as skin or underlying tendons, the skin must be mobilized in all directions. Using pressure with massage softens the underlying scar bed. Lotion is beneficial to the general quality of the skin. When doing massage, the therapist can elicit scar tension and, through massage, aid in relaxing the scar to allow for elongation of the fibers.

Use of the modalities of heat and massage and other physical therapy techniques which are generally not taught in occupational therapy curricula must be learned through special coursework following basic professional education in order to meet licensure restrictions in many states.

Range of Motion

When doing active and passive ROM, it is important always to do blocked flexion and extension exercises. By supporting the phalanx proximal to the flexor crease, the distal interphalangeal joint can be moved individually from the proximal interphalangeal joint. The reason for blocked motion is to allow excursion of each specific tendon. This process is carried out for all joints of the fingers and thumb. Composite flexion exercises that follow blocked motion are then enhanced.

Functional Activities

Once the initial treatment is completed, it is important to follow with graded functional activities incorporating the motion that the therapist is striving to improve. When the patient is set up with supervised activity, he or

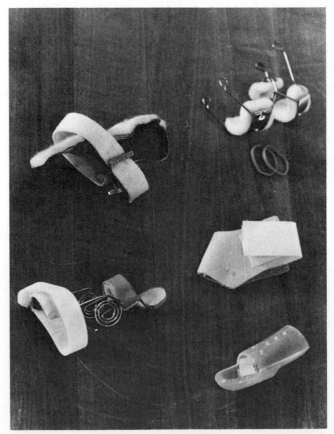

Figure 31-14. Prefabricated splints commercially available for digital motion; from top left: joint jack, reverse finger knuckle bender, LMB flexion strap, Stack splint, Capener. Many others are also available.

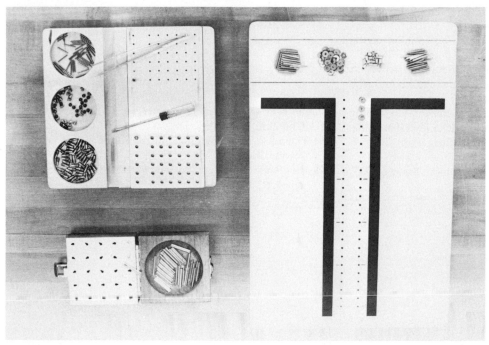

Figure 31-15. Coordination tests used in prevocational evaluation; from top left: Crawford's Small Parts, Purdue Pegboard, Lafayette Grooved Pegboard.

she can see functionally what improvement has been made. This can be an excellent way for the patient to ventilate, in a nonthreatening way, his or her frustration, anxiety, and, in some cases, anger. Activity analyses done in the core curriculum by students start the problem-solving approach to adapting activities best suited to achieving the intended goal. In many cases, this is the patient's first experience with successful utilization of the involved extremity and provides an incentive to continue.

Splinting

When splinting is indicated, the goals may be protection, support, or correction. Various splints are commercially available (Fig. 31-14); however, attention must be given to the fit so that the splint will not impede motion in the associated joints. A custom splint fabricated from thermoplastic materials should afford correct fit when tailored to the patient's specific problem. Splints can be static or dynamic and, if static, can be used in a serial fashion by modifying them to accommodate the progress made in therapy.

The cosmetic status, which was discussed earlier in the therapeutic program, culminates in the use of pressure garments or silicone molds to control edema. Jobst garments are commercially available, as are Isotoner gloves. Customizing of Lycra–Spandex material to accommodate smaller areas has also been beneficial.

As the time for discharge draws near, preparation for return to work should be initiated (Fig. 31-15). Many patients have a smooth transition to the previous routine, but there will be those who need assistance with an occupational change. To facilitate this, inclusion of the rehabilitation counselor in the therapeutic team is essential. On-site job evaluations may be indicated to adapt the environment to facilitate resumption of job responsibilities. Treatment may then continue through work hardening, prevocational evaluation, vocational assessment, and vocational retraining.

References

1. Bowden REM, Gutmann E: Denervation and reinnervation of human voluntary muscle. Brain 67:273, 1944
2. Dawson DM, Hallett M, Millender LH: Entrapment Neuropathies. Boston, Little, Brown, 1983
3. Dellon AL: Evaluation of Sensibility and Reeducation of Sensation in the Hand. Baltimore, Williams & Wilkins, 1981
4. Ducker TB, Kempe LC, Hayes GJ: The metabolic background for peripheral nerve surgery. J Neurosurg 30:270, 1969
5. Hunter JM, Schneider LH, Mackin EJ, Callahan AD: Rehabilitation of the Hand, 2nd ed. St Louis, CV Mosby, 1984
6. Lankford L: Operative Hand Surgery, Vol 1. London, Churchill Livingston, 1982
7. Lister G: The Hand: Diagnosis and Indications, 2nd ed. London, Churchill Livingston, 1984
8. Markee JE: Nerve Blocks and Nerve Lesions: Brochure for

Students. Durham, North Carolina, Duke University School of Medicine, 1955.

9. Matthews P, Richards H: The repair potential of digital flexor tendons. J Bone Joint Surg [Br] 56:618, 1974

10. Onne L: Recovery of sensibility and sudomotor activity in the hand after nerve suture. Acta Chir Scand Suppl 300, 1962

11. Potenza AD: Critical evaluation of flexor tendon healing and adhesion formation within artificial digital sheaths: An experimental study. J Bone Joint Surg [Am] 45:1217, 1963

12. Seddon HJ: Three types of nerve injury. Brain 66:237, 1943

13. Sunderland S: Nerves and Nerve Injuries, 2nd ed. New York, Churchill Livingston, 1978

Bibliography

Ariyan S: The Hand Book. Baltimore, Williams & Wilkins, 1980

Green DP: Operative Hand Surgery, Vol 1 & 2. London, Churchill Livingston, 1982

Strickland JW (ed): Symposium on Flexor Tendon Surgery. Hand Clin 1 (1) 1985

Wynn–Parry CB: Rehabilitation of the Hand. London, Butterworths, 1973

CHAPTER 32

Burns *Maude H. Malick*

The United States continues to have one of the highest fire death rates among the major industrialized nations of the world. More than 7,000 persons die each year in fires or as a result of thermal injuries, although this figure has dropped to approximately half the number of 10 years ago. Safety legislation is thought to have played a major role in this decrease.

Approximately 80% of all fire deaths occur from residential fires. The majority are caused by smoke inhalation. Fire in the home remains the largest cause of accidental death among children up to 14 years of age. It is estimated that a fire occurs every 10 seconds in the US, with someone being burned every 17 seconds.

Approximately 2 million adults and children seek medical attention for thermal injuries annually, 70,000 of which are severe enough to necessitate hospitalization. Approximately 20,000 persons have a total body surface involvement of 25% or more. Of these, 17,000 adults and children are referred or admitted to specialized burn facilities. Of the 32,000 children admitted to a hospital, approximately 21,000 require intensive care.

Types of Burns and Initial Treatment

The major cause of residential mortality is careless smoking, which accounts for more than 25% of deaths in houses and 30% in apartment buildings. Almost 4,000 injuries are reported annually from upholstery and bedding fires. However, heating and cooking continue to predominate as types of home fires, followed by smoking and arson. Among children, hot-liquid scalds are the most frequent type of burn, generally caused by pulling over appliances or pans. The elderly remain the largest group at risk, possibly due to their slow reaction time to a burn. Flame burns involving fabric ignition account for the majority of their injuries.

Statistics from the National Burn Information Exchange* indicate that the mortality rate is four times higher in patients in whom burns are associated with clothing. Twenty-four percent of the patients sustaining clothing-related burns die in the hospital as compared with only 6% of patients whose clothing did not burn. The National Consumers Bureau has now made it mandatory for children's clothing to made of nonflammable fibers.

The electrical burn is seen more in males than in females, and the extent of injury is dependent on the number of volts to which the body has been subjected. In more than 75% of electrical burns, the upper extrem-

---

* The National Burn Information Exchange is a service of the American Burn Association. The current address is given in Appendix J.

ity has been injured or involved. The number of amputations from electrical burns is extremely high, with accompanying increased morbidity. The mortality rate is highest in those suffering severe electrical injury, and it is caused primarily by respiratory and cardiac arrest than by the burn.

The primary objective in dealing with all thermal burns is to extinguish all flames, remove smoldering clothing, and position the patient horizontally, because standing often results in smoke inhalation. In chemical burns, the area should be immersed or washed with large amounts of water to dilute the agent.

The initial application of cold to minor burns is extremely helpful in reducing pain and edema, provided it is applied soon after the injury. Care should be taken not to use large cold compresses when transporting patients for long periods of time, because severe hypothermia may result, interfering with capillary perfusion and viability of the injured areas.

The burned areas should be covered with a clean material. Ointment or other remedies should not be applied, so that an accurate assessment of the injury can be made at the initial medical facility. The extensively burned patient should not be given water, because aspiration or water intoxication may jeopardize the patient's life.

Anatomy and Physiology of the Skin

The skin is the largest organ of the body. It is made up of three layers. The outer layer, which is called the *epidermis,* is approximately 60μm to 120μm thick, except on the palms and soles of the feet, which are from 0.5 mm to 0.8 mm. There are no blood vessels, capillaries, nerve endings, or lymphatics in the epidermis. Directly beneath the epidermis is the *dermis,* which is five to ten times thicker than the epidermis. This layer contains lymphatics, capillaries, nerve endings, hair follicles, sweat glands, and sebaceous glands. These are embedded in a *ground substance* that also contains collagen fibers, fibroblasts, reticulin, and elastin fibers lying in smooth parallel formations. The *subcutaneous tissue* lies directly beneath the dermis and epidermis.

In addition to providing a covering for the bony framework of the body and the life-sustaining organs, the skin serves the following purposes:

1. It protects against infection by maintaining a physical barrier that keeps out bacteria and other organisms. It has a bacteriostatic and bactericidal capability that can destroy small numbers of bacteria that penetrate the skin.
2. It prevents loss of body fluids. The structure of the skin is such that it can assist in maintaining the delicate fluid balance that is required by the body, avoiding dehydration.
3. It controls body temperature. The increase and decrease of evaporation of water from the sweat glands act as a temperature control. The sweat glands excrete excess water with small amounts of sodium chloride and cholesterin and traces of albumin and urea.
4. It is an organ of sensation. The nerve endings within the dermis distinguish light or excessive pressure, pain, and low or high temperatures, thus allowing the individual to avoid damage. The sebaceous glands protect the skin by the secretion of oils that soften and lubricate it. Vitamin D is made when the sunlight reacts with the cholesterol compounds within the skin.
5. It is cosmetic. The skin varies in pigment and texture, from one race to another and from one individual to another. These variations serve as a means of identification.

All of these purposes should be taken into consideration in determining the extent of the burn and its trauma to the patient in both its physical and its psychological components.

Classification of Burns

The extent of the total body burn should serve as the basis for the selection of the treatment facility. Burns of up to 15% of the total body surface can be adequately handled in community hospitals and those up to 25% in general hospitals. If more than 30% of the body area is burned, the patient should be taken to a burn center. Minor burns include partial-thickness burns of less than 20% of the total body surface and full-thickness burns of less than 10%. If the patient is to be transferred to a facility with more advanced services, the evacuation should be carried out as early as possible. All patients with burns of the hands, perineum, and face should be admitted to the hospital.

The severity of the burn is determined by its size and depth, the age of the patient, his or her medical history, and the part of the body burned. Only after these factors are determined can the proper decisions be made about disposition, treatment, and prognosis.

The extent of the area burned can be determined in several ways. In adults (16 years or older), the "rule of nines" applies, and is adequate for most clinical purposes (Fig. 32-1). For infants and children, the burn estimate diagram and table have been modified. A detailed diagram should be completed only after the blisters and dirt have been removed, because dirt and debris of normal skin often have the appearance of burned skin.

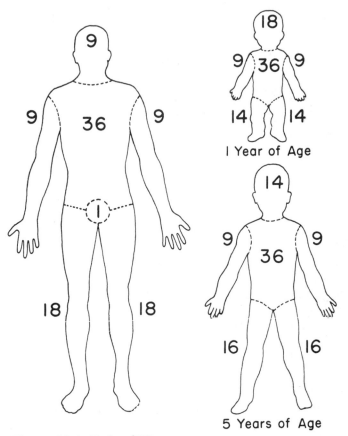

18

9 36 9

14 14

I Year of Age

9

9 36 9

18 18

I

14

9 36 9

16 16

5 Years of Age

Figure 32-1. Rule of Nines.

The rule of nines aids in estimating the percentage of burn, for it divides the body surface into areas of approximately 9% or multiples of 9%. The head and neck represent 9%, as does the upper extremity; the lower extremity and the front and the back of the torso each represent 18%; and the perineum represents 1%. The rule is modified for children from birth to 1 year of age, allowing from 18% to 19% for the head and neck and 13% for the lower extremities. One percent is subtracted from the head and neck and added to the lower extremity for each year in ages 1 to 10. At the time of definitive

care, a more accurate estimate of the extent of the burn is made by using a table that more precisely relates to the changes of body proportion with maturation.

Burn injuries are arbitrarily classified as minor, moderate, and severe (Table 32-1). Minor burns rarely require hospitalization. Patients with full-thickness burns of less than 2% not involving critical areas may be treated as outpatients until they require hospitalization for skin grafting. Noting that a patient's hand is about 1% of the total body surface can be useful in estimating the area of the burn on admission. The following criteria can be used to determine the degree of the burn:

Superficial (first-degree) burns (Fig. 32-2) are confined to the epidermis and are characterized by erythema that blanches under pressure. There can be slight pain and edema but no blistering. The superficial burn can heal in a week because enough epithelial cells remain in the skin to provide new dermis.

Partial-thickness (second-degree) burns involve the dermis and are characteristically more painful and sensitive to pinprick, with blisters and considerable subcutaneous edema. The treatment of partial-thickness burns is directed entirely toward the prevention of infection. Bacterial infection can seriously interfere with healing and can change a partial-thickness burn into a full-thickness injury.

Deep partial-thickness burns are burns in which the epidermis and part of the dermis are dead. The deep dermis is injured but alive, and it will provide tissue for spontaneous healing. The hair follicles and sebaceous glands are destroyed. Only the deepest parts of the sweat glands in the epithelium will survive. Small bits of epithelium will suffice for re-epithelianization on the surface, although it occurs more slowly than in the superficial partial-thickness burn. This type of burn is sometimes referred to as deep thermal burn.

Full thickness (third-degree) burns involve the destruction of the full thickness of the skin with possible muscle, tendon, and bone damage. Spontaneous

Table 32-1. *Means of Classifying Severity of Burns*

	Minor	*Moderate*	*Severe*
Percent partial thickness	Less than 15%	15% to 30%	More than 30%
Percent full thickness	Less than 2%	2% to 10%	More than 10%
Hand, face, feet, and perineum	Not involved	Not involved	Involved
Age	Of little significance	Of little significance	Less than 18 months; more than 65 years
Etiology	Of little significance	Minor chemical and electrical burns	Major chemical and electrical burns
Complicating illnesses	Of little significance	Of little significance	Cardiac, renal, and metabolic involvement

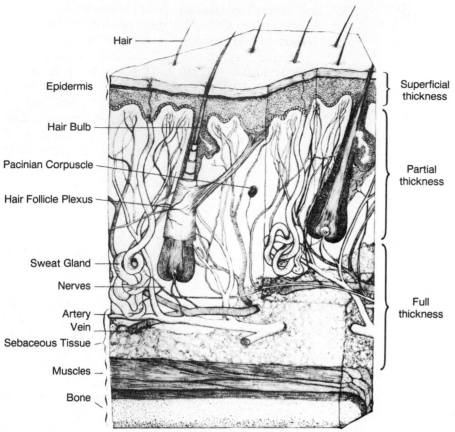

Figure 32-2. Cross-section of the skin showing the depth of burn in relation to skin damage.

healing is not possible. Grafting is usually necessary after the necrotic eschar has been removed. The area of full-thickness burn is usually dry and unblistered; it is depressed below the surface of the surrounding burns; and it is transparent, with thrombosed vessels in its depth. The burn is pain free and insensitive to pinprick. Deep flame burns and some electrical burns may appear charred or black. Doubtful depth areas are leathery, waxy-white or red, and nonblanching, with subcutaneous edema. Occasionally, blisters occur. Pinprick sensation can be absent. These burns usually destroy the full thickness of skin in children and areas of thin skin such as ears, eyelids, and inner forearm in adults. The swelling and pain associated with burns of the preorbital area, perineum, and both hands and feet frequently make outpatient nursing difficult.

Other Major Burn Damage

Respiratory Tract

Respiratory-tract injuries are one of the major causes of death in burn patients. In considering causes of respira-

tory distress in the acute burn, keep in mind that only a few patients with facial burns require an artificial airway or ventilatory assistance and then only rarely during the first 24 hours. The oral airway is necessary if the patient is comatose, and close observation for signs of airway obstruction is necessary. If the patient has evidence of facial burns with singed nasal hairs and soot about the nose and mouth, careful monitoring is required. A tracheostomy should be performed only if absolutely necessary.

Body Fluid

When a burn occurs, there are changes in the distribution of the body fluid. Depending on the temperature and the duration of heat causing the burn wound, a certain depth of injury or tissue death occurs. In minor burns where a thin layer of epidermis and dermis are exposed to heat for a short time, the changes will be minimal, and they may include redness with a separation of the outer layer of epidermis caused by blistering or slight edema. With prolonged exposure to heat, the capillary bed and the deeper tissues are destroyed. This trauma causes increased capillary permeability or a thrombosis in severe wounds. As capillary permeability increases, fluid leaks into the interstitial spaces, and interspatial fluid is increased. This is called *edema*. The lymphatic system would normally carry away the increased fluid, but when the burn is large, there is a great deal of plasma leak, and the lymph system is rapidly overloaded. The lymphatic system may also have been damaged by the heat.

In minor burns, reabsorption occurs at the same rate as accumulation of fluid, so edema does not occur. When massive edema does occur, immediate surgical measures may be needed to avoid vascular constriction.

Limb Ischemia

Escharotomies may be needed both to relieve pressure and to prevent limb ischemia. Edema developing under circumferential full-thickness burns in an extremity may produce a rise in interstitial pressure sufficient to cause cyanosis of the distal unburned skin, impairing capillary filling and producing progressive neurologic deficits. Medial and lateral incisions of the eschar only to relieve pressure are painless when made through third-degree burns, and they should be performed promptly if the signs of ischemia develop. In electrical burns, fasciotomy occasionally is necessary to relieve pressure. With increasing edema, a circumferential full-thickness chest burn may significantly restrict the motion of the thoracic cage, requiring an escharotomy for relief. This is especially likely in children, who may become exhausted by the increased ventilatory effort.

Role of the Occupational Therapist

During the first 72 hours after a severe burn injury, the patient is in burn shock. During this period, the burn team's duty is to stabilize the many internal and external changes caused by the thermal insult. As a result of the burn and loss of skin, the body has lost its ability to protect itself against infection, to maintain fluid balance, and to prevent heat loss. Although most burn units maintain approximately 80°F room temperature, heat shields are also often used to maintain body heat.

The occupational therapist plays an important role in the initial phase of burn management by preventing soft-tissue contractures, which are the major cause of loss in joint function and distorted skeletal positioning. Because of burn trauma and heat loss, the patient quickly assumes the flexed, adducted fetal position for comfort and warmth. This position directly causes contracture deformities resulting from the shortening of healing tissues across and around the joints of the burned parts of the body. These contractures restrict full range of motion, and their strong flexor pull can cause

grotesque distortions of the extremities, most notably around the face and neck, especially when anterior neck and face burns exist. The impending contractures can be prevented by careful positioning at the time of admission, daily monitoring of positioning and splinting, and active exercises.

Positioning and Splinting

Proper bed positioning must be initiated immediately on admission in order to prevent deformity (Fig. 32-3). In general, the position of extension must be maintained, accompanied by frequent short periods of active exercise as practical during dressing changes and tubbing. Placing the joints in extension maintains the overlying burn scar at its maximum length so contractures can be prevented. This extended position must often be accomplished by the use of extension splints across the major joints. These apply traction to the healing tissue in the form of an opposing force (Table 32-2). When evaluating the need for splinting, consideration should be given to areas where the burns involve a joint or where they are lateral to the flexor surface of a joint. Uninvolved joints should be free to prevent tendon shortening and stiffness.

Exercise

All of the joints should be exercised daily, preferably using active motion rather than passive motion to prevent stiffness. Active motion contributes to the maintenance of muscle mass and strength, while passive mo-

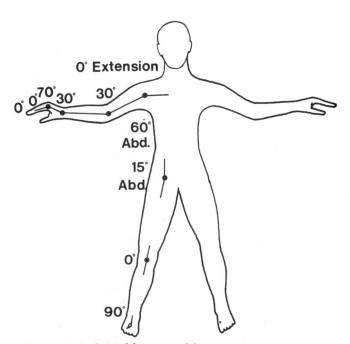

Figure 32-3. Initial burn position.

Table 32-2. *Directions for Positioning and Splinting*

Body Part	Positioning	Splinting
Neck	Slight extension No pillows should be used Mouth of patient should be able to be closed	Soft cervical collar Rigid (low-temperature thermoplastic neck conformer) (Fig. 32-4)
Shoulders	Arms abducted 60° to 90° with slight internal rotation	Traction or axillary splints may be used Small pillow between scapulae will encourage external rotation
Elbow	Full extension when anterior surface of arm is involved Elbow should be ranged with exercise and/or activity during the day and positioned at night in full extension	Three-point extension splint can be worn over dressings (Fig. 32-5)
Hips	Whether prone or supine—neutral extended position Legs should be abducted 15° from the midline	Abduction position can be accomplished by positioning drop foot splints approximately 12 inches apart A bar placed between the knees attached to the three-point extension splints will maintain abduction
Knee	Full extension to 5° flexion	Three-point extension splints for night use (Fig. 32-5)
Ankle	90° (normal standing position) prevents shortening of the Achilles tendon	Foot board—drop foot splints When using a posterior splint, the heel must be suspended to prevent pressures sores. When prone, position patient so that foot hangs over edge of the mattress. Extension splints can be attached to tennis shoes to aid in positioning
Spine	A straight-line position to prevent scoliosis, especially with lateral body burns	
Hands	Wrist 30° extension or dorsiflexion Metacarpophalangeal joint 70° flexion Proximal and distal interphalangeal joints full extension Thumb abducted and extended to maintain web space (Fig. 32-6)	Functional pan splint placing interphalangeal joints in full extension maintaining ''burn'' position

tion prevents tendon adherence as well as tightening and shortening of the joint capsules. Passive motion should be gently executed and never pressed beyond tissue resistance. This is especially pertinent in electrical burns, where the extent of internal trauma cannot be assessed initially.

All wounds should be carefully cleaned, debrided, and dressed at least twice daily. Splints must be thoroughly washed and dried before reapplying. Low-temperature splints such as those made of Orthoplast, Kay-Splint, and Polyform can be gas autoclaved or wiped with alcohol. Exercise, self-care activities, and a night splint regimen must be followed until the burned areas heal and pressure garments can be worn. However, areas that have undergone skin grafting must remain immobilized until the grafts have taken, usually 3 to 4 days postsurgery. Gentle active mobilization may begin 5 to 6 days postsurgery while maintaining night splinting for the first 3 to 4 days following graft adherence.

Pressure Stretch Techniques

A study conducted at the Shriners' Burns Institute in Galveston, Texas showed that more than 80% of patients who have partial- and full-thickness burns will develop hypertrophic scarring throughout the burned areas after new skin and grafts have healed (Fig. 32-7). If the development of scar hypertrophy is not controlled, crippling disfigurement is likely as a result of severe contractures and the unchecked formation of thickened, knobby, red scar tissue. In normal burn wound healing, there is a great increase in vascularity to form the granulation tissue the body uses to restore the damaged skin. Studies conducted by Dr. Hugo Linares at the Shriners' Burns Institute indicate that the granulation tissue has an increased number of *fibroblasts*, which are the cells that synthesize mucopolysaccharides and collagen fibers for the new connective tissue.

In the development of normal skin dermis, fibro-

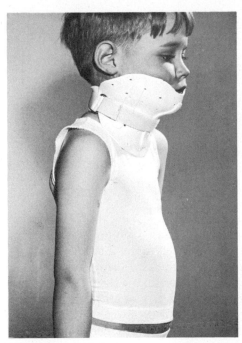

Figure 32-4. A rigid low-temperature thermoplastic cervical collar.

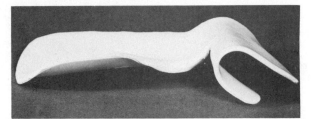

Figure 32-6. Functional position splint for the thumb.

blasts appear irregular in shape and flat with a lumpy surface. In contrast, the fibroblasts that appear within the reticular layer of a hypertrophic scar are spider-shaped with rounded nodular bodies. These fibroblasts produce an excessive amount of collagen fibers that adhere to one another in an irregular pattern. The nodules of compact collagen permit little or no interstitial spacing because they fill the middle and lower reticular layers of the dermis. The collagen filaments entwine in ropelike fashion (Fig. 32-8). In addition to forming nodules of irregular shape, a hypertrophic scar will synthesize collagen at more than four times the rate of normal skin. It is this pile-up of collagen-filled nodules that gives rise to the rigid, thickened hypertropic scar that later can cause disfigurement and contractures.

It has been known for some years that the application of controlled, consistent pressure to the surface of an immature hypertrophic scar will, in time, reduce the scar and leave a smooth, pliable skin surface. But the problem of how pressure could be applied and maintained throughout the maturation of the scar persisted. Pressure dressings and elastic Ace wraps were tried, but all of these materials slipped, bunched up, constricted, or fell off.

The Jobst Institute in Toledo, Ohio, developed a special Dacron Spandex elastic fabric to be used in the con-

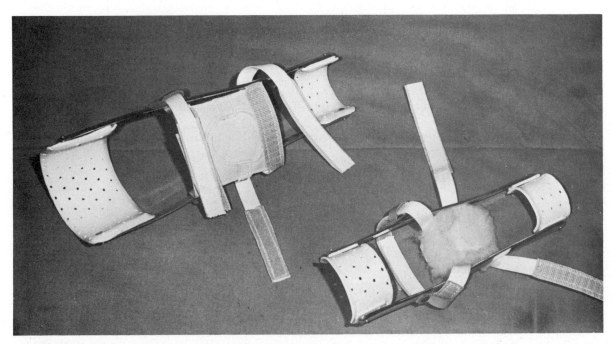

Figure 32-5. Three-point extension splints can be used for elbow and knee extension.

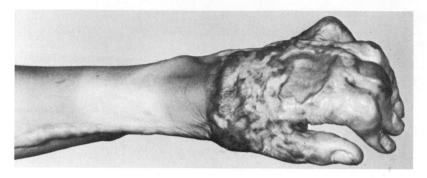

Figure 32-7. Scar hypertrophy on a healed burned hand.

struction of carefully fitted pressure-gradient garments. Garments constructed of this fabric, when accurately measured and fitted and consistently worn, maintained adequate pressure to prevent hypertrophic scar formation in burn patients. In addition, the multidirectional stretch of the fabric allowed any natural movement of the body. There are now several manufacturers of pressure garments specifically designed for burn patients. They are custom engineered and constructed for each patient to provide a consistent gradient pressure over the scar areas. The garment can be engineered to apply specific pressure directly over the burned areas, including the entire body (Fig. 32-9). Often, one body area will be grafted or will heal several weeks before the rest of the body is ready for measuring. These areas should be measured, and garments should be ordered as early as possible (Fig. 32-10), leaving the large unhealed areas for measurement later. Compression dressing such as Tubigrip can be used in the interim.

Healed burns that are ready for measurement can vary greatly in color from a deep purple to a pink. The measurement and fitting of pressure-gradient garments may begin as soon as these open areas of newly healed scar tissue are reduced to the size of a dime. In other words, any graft site, whether it is a patch or mesh, should be almost completely healed before measurement. A minimum of 7 days postgraft should be allowed before measurement is considered. Donor sites should also be dry and well healed before garments are fitted. (These areas must also be maintained under a pressure garment, since they have the potential of becoming hypertrophic as well.)

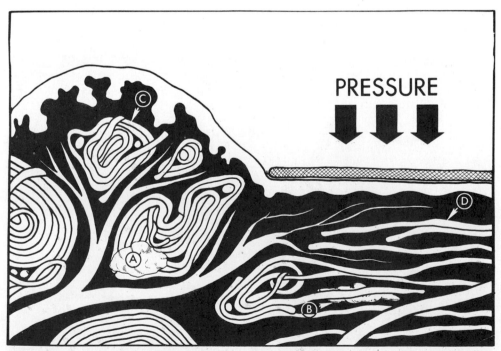

Figure 32-8. Effect of pressure on healing scar tissue. *A,* Fibroblast in hypertrophic scar; *B,* Fibroblast in nonhypertrophic scar; *C,* Ropelike collagen filment in hypertrophic scar; *D,* Linear parallel arrangement of collagen filament in nonhypertrophic scar.

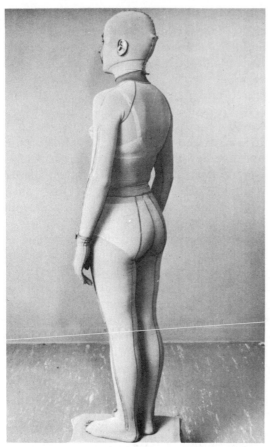

Figure 32-9. Jobst pressure-gradient burn garment.

The pressure garments must be carefully measured and designed in order to provide adequate pressure over the burned areas and still allow normal body mobility. When ordering garments, full-length zippers should be designated whenever a burned extremity is involved. In this way, all shearing effects can be eliminated when the garments are donned. Zippers may be omitted or shortened on later orders.

In order to be wholly effective, the pressure garments must be worn consistently 24 hours a day for 12 to 18 months or until full scar maturation. The patient and his or her garments and splinting should be evaluated on a regular outpatient basis (every 2 weeks and later monthly) in order to monitor the pressure and position management.

Even with the success of pressure techniques, certain body areas have additional needs. The areas around the nose and mouth and the concave body areas require interface molds to maintain consistent pressure. Rivers has written about the use of Uvex face molds to apply definitive pressure to remodel the facial scars (see Bibliography). Silastic elastomer can be worn in a flexible mold under the pressure garments to apply adequate pressure to specific areas such as the face, anterior chest, feet, and axilla. This Dow Corning product fills the concavity that occurs with normal movements when wearing pressure garments. Both have proven highly successful.

The pressure stretch techniques are essential to soften, smooth, and maintain elastic skin during the maturation process and to prevent hypertrophic scarring and subsequent contractures. Pressure on hyper-

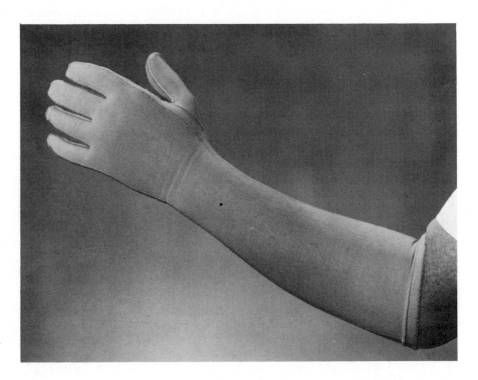

Figure 32-10. Jobst pressure-gradient gloves.

trophic skin will continue to be effective until the scar reaches maturity; that is, the number of capillaries is diminished and the skin no longer blanches with light pressure. Adequate pressure can reduce the scarring, soften the hypertrophies, and encourage elasticity. In this way, joint mobility is gained, and severe contractures can be avoided.

The Burned Hand

The burned hand is of major concern to the occupational therapist. The burn occurs most frequently because the hand is used to extinguish a fire. Dorsal hand burns are the most frequent and the most disabling. Dorsal burns tend to produce a deformity that consists of hyperextension of the metacarpophalangeal joints, flexion of the interphalangeal joints, adduction and extension of the thumb, radial deviation to the wrist, and wrist flexion. The resulting flattening of the transverse and longitudinal palmar arches renders the hand nonfunctional. All of these deforming positions will develop into contractures unless the hand is appropriately exercised, splinted, and treated.

The basic burn splint should be designed individually to prevent the development of hand deformities. In addition to preventing wrist flexion, the splint prevents metacarpophalangeal joint extension deformity and proximal interphalangeal joint flexion contracture commonly called the claw deformity (Fig. 32-11). The extensor tendons that lie on the dorsum of the hand are so poorly protected that they are extremely vulnerable to injury as they cross the proximal interphalangeal joint. The classic boutonnière deformity is seen all too frequently. When the wrist is held properly in extension, the metacarpophalangeal joints tend to flex because of the effects of gravity and the tension on the intrinsic muscles. This position allows the intrinsic muscles to act on the interphalangeal extension. However, the most vulnerable joint in the hand is the proximal interphalangeal joint.

If direct burn damage to the extensor mechanism or through proximal interphalangeal joint flexion causes the middle extensor slip to be caught between the unyielding eschar and the underlying heads of the proximal and middle phalanges, partial destruction of the extensor mechanism will result. The lateral bands of the joint can be shredded or can slip volarly, causing the hand to assume the typical burned-hand deformity. For this reason, careful positioning of these two sets of joints is mandatory, and no fist clenching is permitted until the stability of the extensor mechanism is assured. Internal splints with Kirschner wires can be used to prevent the development of metacarpophalangeal, interphalangeal, and thumb deformities in extreme cases.

The main indication for internal splinting is destruction of a tendon by the burn or bacterial invasion. This injury most frequently involves the extensor mechanism over or just proximal to the proximal interphalangeal joint. Careful external splinting judiciously monitored can prevent flexion deformity. If the flexion deformity is not corrected, the pull of the flexors, mainly the strong sublimis, will cause the proximal interphalangeal joint to flex, often more than 90°. Thumb adduction will also occur unless the thenar web space is maintained and the thumb placed in the position of abduction and opposition.

Palmar burns produce contractures and deformity pulling toward the location of the injury. Dorsal splinting or contoured palmar pan splints (Fig. 32-12) that hold the hand in full extension should be considered.

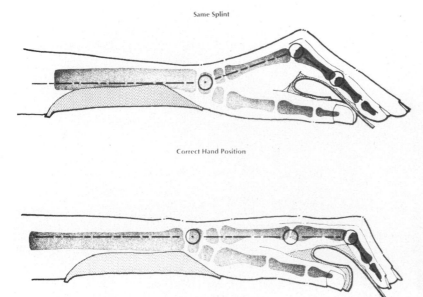

Figure 32-11. Burn functional hand splint. If the splint is allowed to slip forward, a claw deformity can result.

Wrist flexion contractures and deformities can easily arise with accompanying adduction and flexion contractures of the thumb.

Dynamic splinting may be required to do corrective positioning, to counterbalance flexion contractures, and to apply a slow traction pull. Splints are indicated for a metacarpophalangeal flexion deformity. Early adduction contracture of the thumb may be an indication for dynamic splinting. If the thumb contracture persists, resulting in the adduction deformity, early surgical intervention is often employed.

Often, direct-pressure contour pan splinting is required to soften, stretch out, and oppose existing contractures (Fig. 32-13). Progressive contour pan splinting can stretch out an immature (pink) scar in order to reach maximum extension and motion in a joint. Further definitive pressure may be obtained by including an elastomer insert within the splint.

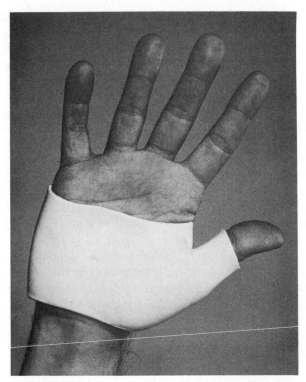

Figure 32-12. A palmar extension pan splint can be used to soften scar tissue and correct web-space contractures.

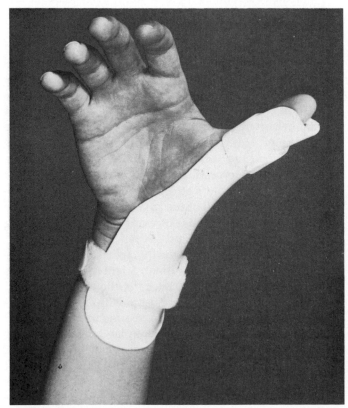

Figure 32-13. A pressure contour splint can correct deformity.

Treatment Plan

When the course of occupational therapy is planned, the following factors must be considered: the depth and location of the burn(s), any associated injuries, extent of total body injury, the extent of injury to the hands, the age of the patient, and patient cooperation. Age is of particular importance. Most children are unable to understand or cooperate in a program of active motion, but they can understand carefully planned play and self-care activities. The hands of children can be splinted for prolonged periods without producing undue stiffness. Even after numerous days of static splinting, the full active range of motion can be regained within a few days. Elderly patients often lack the strength or comprehension to carry out exercises for active motion, so careful splinting and monitoring must be instituted. Early self-care activities can provide the motivation for movement. The members of the burn team or hospital staff should encourage cooperation and should repeatedly emphasize correct positioning and active motion. Staff and patient education must be ongoing to aid in the prevention of deformity and to encourage early functional return.

Early self-care activities such as eating and personal hygiene should be started as soon as the patient is medically stable. Sometimes, adaptive devices may be needed, but they should not be used unless absolutely necessary. Many problems related to functional loss of joint motion and anatomic deformities can be alleviated through normal use of the extremities and activity. Strength will return in weakened and atrophic muscles, especially with early ambulation and normal daily movements of the body. Adhesions of tendons and surrounding structures will also be released through continuing activities of daily living. Time is an important factor. Capsular structures, shortened by poor positioning or inactivity, can be stretched when appropriate activities are planned.

The occupational therapist should work toward full self-care independence and increase in extremity function, physical endurance, and muscle strength. A homemaker checkout should be required to see if any additional training is required such as work-simplification and energy-conservation techniques. Bilateral activities should be stressed, and easy-flow work patterns should be established. Self-care activities can be used as therapeutic exercise.

Early ambulation with good posture should be encouraged. If extensive leg burns exist, wrapping with Ace bandages using the figure-eight technique may be indicated to alleviate pain caused by blood rushing to the lower extremities. If the patient has had skin grafts to the legs, bedrest must be maintained for 10 days. Even though venous circulation has returned to the graft site and the graft appears stable, adequate arterial blood flow will take longer to become established. The patient may be allowed to stand and move about with Ace wraps after 10 days to encourage ambulation and proper foot positioning to eliminate heel cord contractures. Leg pressure garments should be considered. Active motion in the form of exercise, self-care activities, planned activities, and ambulation will improve muscle strength, free adhesions, and stretch skin and joint contractures.

A variety of graded work and recreational activities that include leatherwork, weaving, and woodwork projects can be programmed to increase range of motion, to develop work tolerance, and to increase personal independence.

Psychological Considerations

The emotional aspects of burn care deserve careful consideration because the patient suffers not only devastating physical trauma but also overwhelming psychological stress. The occupational therapist, as a member of the burn team, will need to aid in the identification and management of psychological problems. Age, personality, family support, and social and economic factors influence the manner in which the patient handles his or her problems.

The fear of death is real for the burn patient in the face of immobility, prolonged and intense pain, separation and isolation, loss of control over one's fate, and association with dying patients. The fear of mutilation and disfigurement can be traumatic, especially as body changes occur throughout the treatment process. Especially threatening are fears of disfigurement experienced by patients with facial burns. Genuine grief must be recognized as the patient faces discharge with the loss of an acceptable body image and fear of nonacceptance by the outside world.

The patient's self-perception has an impact on the individual's personality, and feelings of hostility and grief can develop. The patient must also be able to cope with emotional stress, not only in relation to feelings toward the self, but also in relation to feelings toward the individuals and circumstances concerned with the accident.

Disruption of one's life and separation from the family can cause complex problems, especially if hospitalization is for a considerable length of time. The patient may develop, as a substitute for familial emotional support, new methods for gaining gratification and reward. The severely burned patient frequently is in conflict over dependence *versus* independence. Some patients find it difficult to accept forced dependency and to develop necessary trust in others.

Long-term hospitalization and convalescence put a strain not only on the patient but also on the attending medical team. Each surgical procedure must be interpreted carefully. Strong anxiety in the patient must be recognized, especially in relation to the patient's perception and interpretation of the injuries in light of plans and goals.

When massive burns exist, the patient often has a hospital stay of more than 90 days, and he or she faces a longer term of continuing medical procedures. Many times, these procedures are carried out in a rehabilitation unit or center, which is an appropriate site for agressive rehabilitation. Transfer to a rehabilitation area also gives the patient a feeling of progress. A physical medicine evaluation should be made early in the acute-care stage; management by a physiatrist in a rehabilitation center then can be recommended and planned.

Initially, the therapist is involved as part of the burn team in the identification of physical and psychological problems and in planning the management of those problems. Development of rapport and an interpersonal relationship betwen the therapist and the patient is of vital importance. A kind but realistic approach will be most helpful to the patient in coping with the numerous problems as they become apparent. The therapist can be effective by interpreting the problem realistically and reducing the patient's stress by providing sound emotional support. Much of the anxiety can be alleviated by giving the patient a sense of worth and by maintaining interpersonal relationships.

At the first encounter, the therapist should introduce himself or herself to the patient, orient the patient to his or her environment, and interpret the therapist's role. During treatment, the therapist aids the patient by explaining what procedures and treatments are necessary and by defining medical terms in lay language. In this way, a sound rapport and respect can be developed between the patient and the therapist. Thus, the patient can more easily express feelings, and he or she will be more amenable to re-establishing personal independence and cooperation throughout the longer phase of rehabilitation and scar maturation.

Counseling should be directed toward a return to normal activity as quickly as possible, with the importance of follow-up visits stressed. Often, the family and friends must be counseled to aid in interpreting and understanding the patient's reactions and feelings. This is especially important when there are feelings of grief or hostility. Group therapy sessions are important for the psychological rehabilitation of the patient. In these sessions, the patient should be allowed to express fears and anxieties openly. Here, he or she can discuss possible solutions with others in the same situation. The social worker and psychologist should be members of group therapy sessions. The family should be included in discussions with the patient in order to discern ways of handling situations that they will encounter after the patient returns to the home, job, or school.

Nutrition

Nutrition must be carefully monitored and modified so that the catabolic phase of metabolism is corrected. The patient should be in positive nitrogen balance or anabolism, which promotes healing. This positive nitrogen balance is necessary, and it must be maintained through a high-calorie, high-protein diet. The patient must recognize that good nutrition with a well-balanced diet is necessary for tissue repair and maintenance of strength during the rehabilitation period.

Follow-Up Program

A schedule for close outpatient follow-up is necessary to check and to maintain a good outpatient protocol. In this way scar maturation, joint problems, pressure garments, and need for reconstructive procedures can be monitored (Fig. 32-14). The social worker should be active in the outpatient program to monitor the home situation, to provide home-care services as needed, to give emotional support, and to provide for equipment and transportation needs. Should reconstructive surgery be indicated, whether it be functional or cosmetic, the patient must understand the need for the procedures and the need for time to pass before many of these procedures can be accomplished. The surgeon and the physiatrist should work together to correct deformities in order that the patient may gain maximum function.

The most frequent areas of reconstruction are the webbing of the hands, thumb adduction, wrist flexion, axillary contractures, facial contracture, and posterior knee contractures. Children require the most reconstruction because their scar tissue may not grow as rapidly as developing bone.

The American Society for Burns Recovered, Inc., is a national organization formed to aid burned individuals and their families to cope with ongoing problems. The national office is in Orange, New Jersey. Local chapters

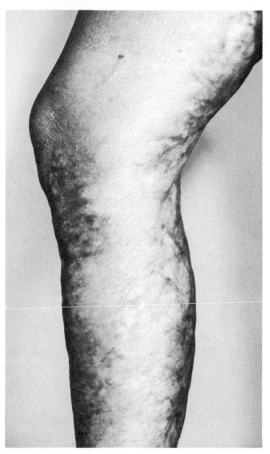

Figure 32-14. A blanched mature burn scar can be attained with proper pressure on the scar areas. Close outpatient follow-up is necessary to maintain the schedule.

have been formed in most major cities in which burn units are located.

Bibliography

Artz CP, Moncrief JA, Pruitt BA: Burns — A Team Approach, pp 466–478. Philadelphia, WB Saunders, 1979

Bruster JM, Pullium G: Gradient pressure. Am J Occup Ther 37:485, 1983

Giuliani CA, Perry GA: Factors to consider in the rehabilitation aspect of burn care. J Phys Ther 65:619, 1985

Malick MH, Carr J: Manual on the Management of the Burn Patient. Pittsburgh, Harmarville Rehabilitation Center, 1982

Malick M, Carr J: Flexible elastomer molds in burn scar control. Am J Occup Ther 34:9, 1980

McGourty LK, Givens A, Fader PB: Roles and functions of occupational therapy in burn care delivery. Am J Occup Ther 39:791, 1985

Rivers EA, Strate RG, Solem LD: The transparent face mask. Am J Occup Ther 33:108, 1979

Appreciation is extended to Clare McDonald, Dip. C.O.T., of Harmarville Rehabilitation Center for her contribution.

CHAPTER 33

Sensory Loss—
Blindness and Deafness *Ann Starnes Wade*

Vignettes*

Alice is a totally blind child who attends public day school with seven other blind, multiply handicapped children ages 3 to 7. Like the others, she is developmentally delayed in adaptive and social–emotional skills, but Alice can hear, she has clear if sometimes echolalic speech, and she walks and enjoys swimming and using many items on the playground. She is moderately tactually defensive, frequently refuses to trail the wall with her hand, and has difficulty making transitions from one situation to another. Jack, a classmate, is deaf, partially sighted, nonvocal, and delayed in all areas of development as a result of rubella syndrome. He is classified as deaf–blind and multiply handicapped, and he displays some autistic-like behaviors. Jack walks with a broad-based gait, using his residual vision to find food as well as to avoid obstacles. He knows and uses signs for drink and eat. Both children appear to crave vestibular stimulation. Occupational therapy services are included in these children's programs because their teacher has requested them within the guidelines of federal and state special education standards. Teacher, therapist, classroom aides, and those families who can

work collaboratively with Alice, Jack, and some of their classmates. Direct occupational therapy services are provided individually on an average of two half-hour periods per week, usually in the occupational therapy department but also in halls, classrooms, and, occasionally, at a swimming pool. Developmental and sensorimotor integration approaches are used to attain psychosocial and cognitive–perceptual–motor goals. □

Mary is 6 years old, recently enrolled in a residential school for the deaf. Having no other physical disability, she is unlikely to be referred for occupational therapy. A volunteer recently reprimanded Mary, in sign language, when Mary kicked the volunteer, apparently for not providing undivided attention. The volunteer, a skilled worker with adult deaf in another setting, later discussed with the occupational therapist the tendency of some deaf adults to interrupt, to be dependent, and to expect instant gratification; both see the need to stop this trend during childhood by: (1) teaching developmentally appropriate self-management, play, work–study, and social skills; (2) communicating effectively with the children as persons of worth; (3) setting reasonable limits with consistency among houseparents, teachers, volunteers, support staff, and parents; and (4) adding responsibilities and privileges as students become

---

* Modified to protect confidentiality.

ready. These are areas where the occupational therapist may serve as consultant, member of a task force,
as one of the providers of continuing education and
sometimes as direct service provider.   ☐

Mr. James recently lost his vision in a laboratory
accident. He is wondering how he will function,
declaring that he cannot do anything now that he is
blind, that he must find some work other than his
profession of medical technology, but what . . . and
how . . . His wife and parents are upset, not sure
how to help, and nearly as shocked as Mr. James.
Now past the medical crisis, he is due to be discharged
from the hospital within a week to 10 days. Occupational therapy, social work, and nursing are involved
in treatment and discharge planning, under the
leadership of the ophthalmologist.   ☐

Mrs. Turner is a blind, diabetic woman proud of
her Mexican-American culture, her numerous young
grandchildren, and her independence. She is receiving
physical and occupational therapy in a southern
rehabilitation center. Her left leg was amputated due
to diabetic gangrene 6 months ago, and she wants to
walk with a "wooden leg" rather than be confined to
a wheelchair. She also wants to return to her two-
room cottage rather than live with one of her children.
Coming from a rural area to this metropolitan one
and a rehabilitation center whose mostly Anglo-
American staff all seem to be under 30, she is attempting to manipulate the situation in order to cope
with so much strangeness.   ☐

Mrs. Reed is a deaf widow with marked arthritic
deformities that confined her to a geriatric chair in an
intermediate-care facility (nursing home) that serves
many deaf residents. Because of her arthritic hands,
Mrs. Reed's sign language and approximate rather
than accurate finger-spelling are difficult to receive.
Her "gerichair" tray was adapted with an alphabet
and a few symbols to clarify communication and to
make possible some communication with nonsigning
people. Until she had eye surgery to improve her
vision, she needed the 1¼-inch-high letters to enable
her to receive others' messages too. Since surgery and
with new corrective lenses, she can see to receive
American Sign Language, to write, and to read what
others write or print at an elementary level. She also
communicates by tracing words or letters with her
finger when pencil, paper, and laptray are not available or when her fingers are too painful to hold a
pencil. Mrs. Reed often uses her left hand to help position her right hand more correctly for certain letters
of the manual alphabet. Having recently discovered
that she can slowly maneuver a regular wheelchair
within the building, Mrs. Reed and the staff are
preparing a new, narrow laptray that will permit both

communication and mobility. Her improved vision
enables use of smaller letters and the addition of
some frequently used words including her name, address, and phone number. Nursing personnel, the
activities director, and the occupational therapist have
shared ideas and services with this spunky woman.   ☐

Mr. Williams is an elderly bachelor who has
Usher's syndrome, which rendered him deaf at birth
and gradually, during middle adulthood, blind. Other
family members are unable to maintain close contact,
so he has been in a residential facility for the deaf and
deaf–blind. Because of a strong desire to regain his
independence, Mr. Williams received and completed
orientation and mobility training and training in safe
independent living through state rehabilitation
services for the blind. This involved the client, an
orientation and mobility specialist, a rehabilitation
teacher of the blind, and a certified interpreter for the
deaf. Mr. Williams receives sign language and finger-
spelling by placing his hands over the signer's hands,
with occasional clarification by tracing numbers in the
palm of his hand. He signs and finger-spells, sometimes accompanied by an approximation of speech
that can give some clues or, when he is excited, be
confusing. In meetings, he sometimes needs to be reminded by contact signing not to use his voice while
signing, since he cannot see or hear when the meeting
formally begins nor when people try to "shush" him.
He uses a timer-activated vibrating pad under his
pillow as an alarm. This gentleman's personal organization skills are good, but he does want and need
sighted, signing help for checking the cleanliness and
colors of certain clothing, for shopping, for learning
current news, for keeping up with sporting events,
and for reducing his sense of isolation. Having been
blind for about 15 years and institutionalized for 10 of
these, he is relatively unfamiliar with inflated prices
and with changes in technology, marketing, and so
forth. Occupational therapy and social work services
have been needed for psychological and physical
reasons between the completion of independent living
training and his actually moving into an apartment.
(Independent living training had been arranged
before the facility employed an OTR). Purposeful
activity, which appealed to him, mainly in the nature
of making salable items such as rake-knitted hats and
scarves, woven rugs, and hand-rubbed wooden
pieces, has helped him wait more patiently, sleep and
feel better, use less chewing tobacco, and earn a little
pocket money. (When sighted, he had supplemented
his factory wages by hand-crafting items.) Shopping,
cooking, eating, and cleaning up are important for
reality of prices, for personal satisfaction, and for
refinement of skills. A joint effort of personnel is
helping him establish the habit of writing messages
and lists, following established channels for personal

assistance rather than seeking help or conversation from staff each time he thinks of something. These behaviors will enhance relationships both in his current environment and in the independent living apartment complex for elderly, deaf, and physically disabled persons. Covered by state funds, the rehabilitation teacher will review training and reorient him as soon as he has moved to the apartment. Social work and occupational therapy services will discharge him when he moves, but volunteers will assist him biweekly to shop, bank, place items for sale through a senior citizens craft outlet, attend deaf–blind club functions, and handle other activities. □

Significance of Visual and Auditory Senses

Both vision and hearing are *distance* or *distant* senses. These are primary channels by which most individuals gather information and receive pleasure from the environment without making physical contact with it. *Near* senses, of touch, movement, taste, and smell, are also important; information transmitted by touch–tactile, kinesthetic–proprioceptive, gustatory, and olfactory channels requires either direct contact or, in the case of olfaction, closer range. Particularly during infancy and early childhood, the individual seeks to touch, manipulate, taste, and smell himself or herself and the surroundings, as well as to look and listen. Vision and hearing become increasingly sophisticated and reliable in the course of normal development. The match between near and distant sensory data gathered and integrated during early exploration and manipulation of the world gradually enables the child to identify human and nonhuman sounds, objects, scenes, and events through visual and auditory information. The contributions of visual and acoustic senses are understandably great both in the development and continuation of communication skills; perceptual–motor ability, including purposeful manipulation and mobility within one's environments; psychosocial function; and cognitive capability. This should not imply that a blind or deaf person cannot develop and use all residual and intact senses to their full extent, only that acquisition of such skills presents challenges to the individuals, their families, and the professional persons who work with them.

Nature of Visual and Auditory Problems
Deficits in Vision

Types and Causes

The legal definition of blindness in the United States is visual acuity that cannot be corrected to better than 20/200 feet or 6/60 meters. That is, the legally blind person, even with maximum correction, cannot see the Snellen or similar chart with the stronger eye from a distance of 20 feet or 6 meters any better than a person with normal visual acuity can see it from 200 feet or 60 meters. An individual may also be considered legally blind if he or she has no peripheral vision; that is, if the visual field is restricted to less than a 20° angle so that he or she sees no more than what a fully sighted person might see through a tube or tunnel.[10,21]

Legal definitions of blindness allow people with a wide range of visual problems and abilities to be classified as blind. Total blindness, the complete inability to see, accounts for about 20% of these.[13] A person may be legally blind yet have some *near visual acuity*, corrected or uncorrected, sufficient to read ordinary newsprint, large print, or something in between the two. Normal near visual acuity can be described as 14/14, achieved by accurately reading the 14th, or smallest print line on a Jaeger test type reading card at a distance of 14 inches.[10] Unless there is an eye disease that contraindicates this, there is apparently no damage to the visual system even if the individual must hold a book or object only a few inches from the eyes. Each individual will vary in the manner and effectiveness with which he/she uses his or her visual acuity.

A blind person may have *no awareness* of environmental light, may have *light perception,* which is awareness of light versus dark, or may have *light projection,* which is the ability to indicate the light source.[21] The capacity of a legally blind person to perceive enough visual information to permit safe independent movement in the environment is called *travel vision.*[8]

About a half million people in the United States have been classified as legally blind, but another million visually impaired persons do not meet the criteria for legal blindness. It is appropriate, more accurate, and positive to say that these visually impaired persons are "partially sighted" or have "low" vision, reserving the term "blind" for persons who have no sight.

A person legally blind in one eye may not be classified as such if acuity in the other eye is greater than 20/200. These individuals, as well as those with scotomas, amblyopia, color blindness, and central nervous system disorders of visual perception, also warrant attention for their problems. Since a person may not qualify for additional tax deductions and other benefits unless *legally blind,* the classification can be significant for financial reasons.[42]

The primary causes of blindness are diabetic retinopathy (the leading cause of adult blindness), glaucoma, cataract, retinitis pigmentosa, detached retina, macular degeneration (the leading cause of visual loss in the elderly), rubella (especially maternal), retrolental fibroplasia, and, in Third World countries, trachoma, a preventable contagious disease of the eye exacerbated by malnutrition and poor hygiene. These conditions are described and discussed in terms of prognosis and implications in a useful 1979 publication of the American Foundation for the Blind.[42] Other visual problems may be due to injuries, malignancies (especially retinoblastoma), and conditions and diseases affecting the central nervous system *in utero,* in childhood, or in later life.

Some visual-field deficits are of psychogenic origin. Ordinarily, as a person steps back from an item he or she is viewing, the visual array expands accordingly. Similarly, the person with organic tunnel vision can see more as he or she moves farther from the subject or scene. In contrast, persons with psychogenic field deficits characteristically do not perceive an expanded visual array at a greater distance but continue to identify only the original subject matter.[10]

Previously sighted persons who lose their vision are generally referred to as the *adventitiously* or *newly blind.* Those born without sight or with severely impaired vision are known as *congenitally* blind. Whenever a sensory loss occurs, it tends to be isolating and to effect a type of sensory deprivation. The impact on development must receive particular attention to avoid severe secondary handicaps.

The Blind Child's Development

As long as a blind infant can hear, smell, or feel his or her mother often enough in some meaningful way, the infant will come to recognize her. If stimuli typical of mother are absent, even though the little one is within her vision, to the infant, she is absent. In fact, until the infant develops object permanence, mother ceases to exist. Ordinarily vision plays a significant role in the development of object concept, but if the blind infant has sufficient opportunity and encouragement to use and refine the other senses while manipulating and responding to human and nonhuman objects, the milestone will be reached. The blind child's abilities to hear and to begin to associate words with objects and events and to move, explore, and manipulate objects become particularly important to the development of object recognition and permanence, relationship-building, and concept formation.

Fraiberg and associate psychiatrists[15] have studied the development of blind and sighted children. They found that otherwise normal, totally blind infants: (1) tend to lie passively in their beds with their arms abducted to each side, elbows flexed 90°, and the hands at head level; (2) can distinguish parents from a stranger by the age of 6 to 8 months even when all are silent and the stranger attempts to hold the infant just as the parents did (this is within the normal range, or nearly so, of discrimination of strangers, which begins at approximately 24 weeks[16]); (3) *does not spontaneously reach* for objects unless shown by auditory input, from tapping of

the toy on table or floor, that the object they have just been holding or touching is within reach; (4) can localize sound at about 10 months of age; and (5) begin to creep *only after they can both localize sound and reach.* Finally, blind children develop the apparently innate smiling response as do sighted infants, but they do not further develop or maintain true smiling in infancy, except occasionally for the mother, probably because imitation and reinforcement of the smile are not possible. Interpersonal relationships between parents and the blind infant can be affected by this apparent lack of facial responsiveness on the part of the infant, as well as by the parents' shock at discovering their child cannot see.

More recently, Fraiberg[14] has reported that sensorimotor and emotional development are dependent on a good mother–child relationship in the early months and years. Given that not-easily-established good relationship, some blind children are in fact able to smile spontaneously and appropriately. Fraiberg and her associates emphasize the need to work with and through the mother to assist the development of a positive relationship with her child and to stimulate crucial development throughout the sensorimotor period. Without that stimulation, Fraiberg has found that blind infants and young children may achieve static postures but may lack purposeful mobility and hand skills and may lag in language, intellectual development, and social development.

Deficits in Hearing

Types and Causes

Deafness has been defined as the inability to hear and understand speech through the ear alone. This definition and the following classifications have been used for the 1971 National Census of the Deaf Population and in the Model State Plan for Rehabilitation of Deaf Clients.[36] There are now approximately 16 million hearing-impaired persons, of whom about two million are deaf.[11]

The person who cannot hear and understand speech may be described according to the phase of life at which deafness occurred. An individual is said to be *prelingually* deaf, if he or she did not have or lost hearing prior to the development of speech, or *prevocationally* deaf if he or she became deaf before reaching 19 years of age. *Adult* deafness refers to loss of hearing ability at or after age 19. The earlier deafness occurs, the more severely handicapping it is likely to be; however, regardless of age of onset, loss of hearing is usually accompanied by emotional problems. Schein, editor of the Model State Rehabilitation Plan, cautions that the size of the deaf population has grown and that it shifts in regard to growth rate. He calls attention to the unusually large number of young deaf adults due to the rubella epidemics of 1964–1965, producing the "rubella bulge," and to the fact that many deaf workers currently have "jobs in declining industries or occupational categories."[36]

Hard of hearing is the term for hearing impairments less severe than deafness. In childhood, these may affect language development, with effects of later onset depending upon one's occupations and on what is done about the problem.

Intensity or loudness, the amplitude of sound waves, is measured in decibels (dB). Ordinary conversation registers approximately 60 dB. The frequency of sound waves, known as pitch, is usually measured in cycles per second or hertz. The lower-pitched sounds are those such as *o* in *go, d* and *g* in *dog;* higher tones include *f* in *puff, s* in *say, school,* and *this.* Adequate auditory perception of speech requires hearing between 500 and 2000 hertz (low to high, respectively), but frequencies from 16 to 16,000 hertz are audible to persons with normal hearing. Early hearing impairment may first be detected when testing for sounds at 4000 hertz. Loss is usually gradual and may go unnoticed or undiagnosed for some time. If audiometric tests reveal an average auditory loss of 16 dB for frequencies of 500, 1000, and 2000, the individual is considered to have a *beginning hearing impairment.* A person is classified as *deaf* when the average auditory loss is 82 dB or more for those frequencies.[10]

There are two major categories of deafness. In *middle ear* or *conduction* deafness, when sounds are conducted by air rather than bone, there tends to be greater difficulty in hearing lower frequencies. This type of impairment may respond well to treatment. The greater problem in *perception* or *nerve* deafness, which is usually permanent and less frequent, is for the higher frequencies, whether sound is conducted by air or bone. If the hearing impairment involves the cochlea, slight increases in sound intensity may, through recruitment, be perceived as much louder, even to the point of pain.[10]

Deafness may be attributed to hereditary nerve lesions, brain defects, birth trauma, congenital (maternal) rubella, maternal ingestion of certain medications during pregnancy, and early infections such as cerebrospinal meningitis and encephalitis.[23,39] Premature infants, the athetoid cerebral palsied, and those whose blood type is incompatible with their mother's Rh-negative type have a higher incidence of deafness than other infants.[23] Otosclerosis, which may first be identified during adolescence, is the primary cause of deafness among active adults.[10] Continuous loud noises can damage the inner ear, but there are no conclusions regarding intermittent intense noise. The incidence of deafness increases with the age of the population. Although more women than men have otosclerosis, more men than women have hearing loss due to all causes.[2,10]

The Deaf Child's Development

If all other senses are intact and appropriately stimulated, the nonhearing child will develop object recognition, object permanence, and interpersonal relationships based on visual, manual, and physical exploration and the internal and external results of these experiences. Communication through smiling, other facial expressions, body language, gestures, and possibly sign language will be the basis for the young child's "labeling" of objects, events, and feelings. Later, more formal manual signs, finger-spelling, lip or speech reading, printed words, and symbols may supplement the infant's language. If the nonhearing child's back is turned or the child is not visually attending in the parent's direction, the child's inability to respond to his or her parent's words or footsteps as one or the other approaches may affect their relationship. However, when the child does see them, their appearance may be acknowledged with a genuine smile and animation. Particularly before a definite diagnosis of deafness, the young child may be perceived and treated as stubborn, withdrawn, peculiar, or retarded as a result of apparently fluctuating attention.

There is some evidence[25,37] that if the deaf infant is reared by deaf, signing parents, he or she will likely achieve greater emotional stability and maturity than the deaf child who develops in an environment where communication and understanding are usually inadequate, as is often the case with hearing parents.

Most prelingually deaf persons without other physical disabilities ultimately develop keen visual and manual abilities, but receptive and expressive oral and written language has usually fallen far behind. A small percentage may learn, laboriously, to speak and/or to speech read, but the deaf who learn these at a more adequate level usually had at least some hearing through the language development years. Some deaf never develop sign or oral language but communicate by means of gestures, signs that have meaning only among immediate family or group members, pictures, and demonstration. This is not necessarily an index of intelligence or lack of it but does greatly complicate communication with both deaf and hearing persons.

Inability to hear conversation and other environmental sounds tends to result in some fear of the unknown even among the sophisticated deaf, and often in the suspicion—sometimes well-founded—that others are talking about them or preventing their knowing all that is being said.[28] Failure to communicate in a language that *all* group members can understand *all the time* may severely retard ego development in the prelingually and prevocationally deaf and may offend and isolate the adult deaf. Such are the observations of *deaf leaders* in the field of deaf rehabilitation.[28]

Besides the lack of self-confidence found in many deaf persons, it has been said that some deaf have a "gimme" attitude that takes the form of overdependency on or exploitation of hearing and successful deaf individuals. It may be that this expectation of instant gratification is due in part to the inability to hear all the planning, problems, and preparation associated with events, services, and purchases that simply seem to appear. Overprotection and paternalism at home and in the service arms of society may also erode motivation and incentive. These, then, are problems that compound the common problem of most deaf—that of a communication gap, or chasm, with hearing society, including many in medical and rehabilitation services.

Deaf–Blindness or Blind–Deafness

Types and Causes

Both combinations of deaf–blindness and blind–deafness are included in the heading because some libraries catalog according to the second term, even though most use the first. Some professional workers in this field use the word order to designate which condition occurred first.* Since most persons with combined hearing and visual losses are congenitally deaf persons who become blind,[42] the term *deaf–blind* is usually employed. Often, there is residual vision, as well as visual memory, on which to capitalize in rehabilitation. As suggested in the preceding sections on visual and hearing deficits, the combined loss of both distant senses may be due to hereditary or congenital causes, to infections, or to central nervous system trauma, and it may ultimately accompany or be complicated by the aging process.

Usher's syndrome is a combination of congenital deafness and *retinitis pigmentosa* that, although hereditary, results in gradual rather than congenital loss of vision. There is no known cure other than prevention through genetic counseling. It is found in about 50% of the deaf–blind population.[42] Many of these persons will have sign language and writing skills, and many have some functional speech, although they cannot hear. However, the loss of vision will necessitate slower signing, received tactually in the hands or within whatever possible field (tunnel vision) of vision the person may have. Corrective and magnifying lenses may help; however, blindness may become total.

If the person was blind before becoming deaf or hard-of-hearing, he or she may continue to use Braille, good English, and voice; he or she may function with auditory memory but will be cut off from some or all external auditory stimulation. Amplification should be explored.

The major cause of deaf–blindness in children is maternal rubella during the first trimester of pregnancy.[42] Because of the other organs affected by the rubella virus, some of the deaf–blind children suffer cardiac problems, motor and/or mental retardation, hyperactivity, and in some cases, autistic-like behaviors.[9]

The Deaf–Blind Child's Development

The world of the infant who is both deaf and blind consists only of those human and nonhuman objects that can be felt, smelled, tasted, and manipulated. Fortunately, many deaf–blind individuals have some vestige of one or the other distant sense, so that residual vision or hearing, however small, can be used to aid in motivation, orientation, exploration, and satisfaction. Recalling the tendencies toward passivity of blind infants and the attentional problems of deaf infants, one has some notion of the probable need to *bring* the world to the deaf–blind infant and vice versa in a manner appropriate, acceptable, and meaningful to the child. Until touched, this infant may receive no stimuli that say someone or something is near. Medical staff and parents may not initially have been aware of the profound sensory loss, and thus they may have found no reason to handle the newborn differently from any other full-term or premature infant.

Mouchka,[24] the knowing parent of a deaf–blind child, who has also had experience with other similarly handicapped youngsters, noted that these infants behave differently in three ways: (1) they do not respond to any apparent stimuli but remain passive; (2) they consistently respond vigorously, protectively, and hypersensitively to any attempt to handle them; or (3) they cry most of the time whether they are being handled or left alone. These findings correlate with reports from parents and caretakers of other deaf–blind children and with those of Chess and associates,[9] psychiatrists who have studied children handicapped as a result of the rubella syndrome. Additional cardiac and neurological problems can compound the sensory deficits and can make homeostasis even more precarious, which may explain the extreme sympathetic nervous system responses of some multihandicapped children as well as the apparent vegetative state of others. Before object recognition can be attained, there must be homeostasis and sufficient meaningful sensory information to permit the infant to sense and respond to the mother or another object. A trusting relationship is based at least in part on sufficient appropriate stimuli that the infant can somehow perceive as safe, satisfying, predictable, and dependable. The demanding and frustrating roles of parents of such handicapped children require ongoing

---

* Personal communication with Marguerite Moore, Registered Interpreter for the Deaf and Instructor, Columbus, OH, July 1981.

acknowledgment, support, and guidance by empathetic, creative, and competent health care professionals.

Object recognition and permanence, relationships, and communication can be developed slowly through vestibular, tactile, and proprioceptive experiences appropriate for the infant, and as the little one becomes neurologically and motorically able to tactually and kinesthetically experience and explore self, mother, father, crib, food, toys, and larger environment, augmented by relevant sensory information through all possible channels. Consistent tactual symbols and signs, tactile–kinesthetic rhythms, motions, and vibrations will gradually become representative of objects and events experienced, contributing to language development and the establishment of trusting relationships with others who can use the language.

Educational programs for deaf–blind children have accepted any child whose disabilities prevent his/her benefiting from programs offered the blind or the deaf child. Generally speaking, the most progress has been made by children who become adventitiously disabled, rather than the congenitally deaf–blind. Legislation enacted after the 1964–1965 epidemics has helped prepare more special education teachers, habilitation programs, sheltered workshops, and centers that offer "therapeutic work" and independent living services to those functioning at too low a level to cope with even sheltered employment.[36,42]

Occupational Therapy Services to Persons with Impaired or Absent Distant Senses

Nature of Clients Served by Occupational Therapists

Data from the American Occupational Therapy Association's 1982 member survey (about 50% response) indicates that fewer than 1% of OTRs and COTAs serving clients checked visual or hearing disabilities as being among their clients' three most frequently occurring health problems. (Visual disabilities—OTRs 0.3%, COTAs 0.3%; hearing disabilities—OTRs 0.1%, COTAs 0.2%.[1]) This is likely to include therapists who practice in schools, rehabilitation centers for the blind, special hospital units, and possibly some nursing homes. However, it is also probable that the majority of occupational therapists encounter among their clients with various health problems at least a few persons who are *also* blind, partially sighted, deaf, hard of hearing, or a combination.

Nine occupational therapists from various places in the United States responded to my inquiry in "Member Hotline" of the April 1981 *Occupational Therapy Newspaper*[26] regarding where and how occupational therapists and occupational therapy assistants were serving blind, deaf, and visually and hearing impaired persons. Five OTRs worked in state or local residential or day schools or school systems serving deaf or deaf–blind or deaf–multiply handicapped children ages 0–22, with one of these schools employing a COTA to work with visually impaired students. Two of the five OTRs' roles specifically included some consultation and direct service in the areas of prevocational assessment and life adjustment. Two OTRs, from separate residential schools for the mentally retarded, indicated that many residents have some type of visual handicap. An OTR employed by a society for the blind, serving adults from 17 to over 90 years of age, reported a caseload of mostly newly blind who were referred for development of self-confidence and refinement or development of remaining senses. Other services there included a deaf–blind program and treatment emphasizing sensory integration for many congenitally blind and some newly blind. A public health OTR indicated that of 12 clients at the initiation of the visiting occupational therapy program, four were legally blind and a fifth was visually impaired. Their primary diagnoses were multiple sclerosis, cerebrovascular accident, quadriplegia, and cerebellar degeneration. All were homebound and confined to wheelchairs. The therapist reported close coordination with a society for the blind.

Although as therapists we may be more familiar with frail elderly persons, we encounter among colleagues, clients, and their families and ours persons who, as they approach age 65, frequently experience noticeable decreases in vision, hearing, or both. The greatest percentage of visual and auditory impairments affect the elderly whether or not they have other problems. (See the chapter on gerontology for more information on this population.)

One occupational therapist's thesis delves into the need for occupational therapy involvement in the rehabilitation of the visually impaired (not totally blind) adult patient, who she believes is already part of the general occupational therapy caseload.[5] She found that, of the 61% of 180 Missouri occupational therapists who responded to a resource questionnaire, 89% had encountered one or more visually impaired patients in the course of practice. She further stated that only 19% reported that they felt they were able to offer comprehensive services to those clients. To that end, she prepared a guide for occupational therapy with the low-vision patient, including problems, aids, roles of occupational therapy, and the inexpensive equipping of an occupational therapy clinic to meet needs of these clients with or without additional health problems.[6]

A review of American Occupational Therapy Association materials indicates that some other OTRs and a COTA working with the blind and partially sighted also find sensory integrative treatment approaches relevant[4,30] or have been moved to share insights into sensory problems of the elderly[22] and treatment methods for blind and visually impaired persons.[35,38] Public Laws 94-142 (Education of All Handicapped Children Act) and 95-602 (Rehabilitation Act Amendments of 1978) have broadened the scope of services available to handicapped children and adults, including the visually and hearing impaired, blind, deaf, and multiply involved. This has implications for occupational therapy within educational, sheltered workshops, independent living, and other rehabilitation settings. To date, the adult deaf population is the most underserved due to a communication gap.

Special Considerations for Occupational Therapists Serving Visually and Hearing Impaired Persons

Attitude and Personal Preparation

The occupational therapist and other team members must have healthy, realistic, and flexible attitudes toward blindness and deafness and must see the potential for developing or redeveloping and maintaining satisfactory functioning by persons with these problems. Positive and realistic attitudes can be facilitated through reading biographies, professional literature, and journals or newsletters published by groups of visually or hearing impaired persons and especially by interacting with blind and deaf persons. Besides the selected bibliography, agencies and organizations are listed in Appendix J so the reader may write for general or specific information, publications, or perhaps a film.

For a more personal, subjective experience, one can wear a blindfold, opaque sunglasses, or earplugs designed to reduce industrial or other noxious sound. This simulated disability can provide insights if it is maintained in a variety of situations for at least several hours, but the wearer must remember that this is only a very temporary disability and it is not conducted to win praise or instant rapport with a client. The experience can approximate some experiences of adventitiously lost sight or hearing, but it cannot provide as much understanding of the circumstances of congenitally blind or deaf persons, because the learner will not erase his visual memory or language development. Occupational therapy students who simulate disabilities including the sensory ones must be careful to do so responsibly, either explaining the purpose to laypersons or being consistent and behaving appropriately from the time they leave class or home in the role of a disabled person until they return.

Communication and Interaction

If the deaf or deaf–blind client is known to use sign language and finger-spelling, and if he or she does not read and write understandably, the therapist should arrange in advance for a certified interpreter. Exceptions to this are if: (1) the resident has understandable speech and the therapist can sign and finger-spell well enough to introduce self, state the purpose of the visit, and ask or answer the necessary questions; or (2) the therapist has good receptive as well as expressive skills for American Sign Language (AMESLAN, ASL) or manual English, whichever the client uses. Basic vocabulary is the same in ASL and signed English. In ASL, however, word order in short sentences may vary; articles are omitted; actual time sequence determines order of phrases or clauses; verb tense is indicated by context or by use of words like "finish, yesterday, tomorrow"; one sign concept is used to represent several English words; much facial and body language is used to show meaning; and few words are finger-spelled.[32]

A certified interpreter may be located through the Registry of Interpreters for the Deaf. Usually, the interpreter will sign with the deaf person for a few minutes to determine receptive and expressive skills so the interpreter can use the most appropriate method and vocabulary when interpreting for the therapist. I prefer to introduce myself, explain that I am learning to sign but am slow, introduce the interpreter, and then proceed with my business. The therapist asks questions and gives information to the deaf persons through the interpreter who will sign to the client in the style needed, moving the lips without voice while doing so, although one may request vocalization also to understand concepts. When the client signs a response, the interpreter will "reverse interpret," speaking to the therapist, also converting ASL to English if necessary. Interaction between the client and therapist is confidential unless otherwise agreed with client. Interpreters as well as therapists have codes of ethics.

For any ongoing program with the signing deaf and deaf–blind, it is my opinion and experience, shared with many others in the field, that the personnel must learn to sign. Most deaf and deaf–blind persons are patient with slow reception of their signs and finger-spelling (Fig. 33-1). Some enjoy teaching new signs, and nearly all receive hearing persons more readily when we are obviously trying to communicate in their language.

Although many deaf adults use combined sign language, facial and body expression, and lip reading with or without speech (referred to as total communication or simultaneous method), some deaf persons do not express or receive signs or speech well. Formal assess-

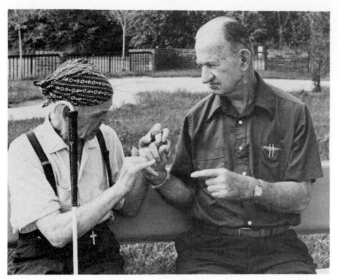

Figure 33-1. The deaf–blind person is receiving his companion's fingerspelling tactually with his left hand while fingerspelling with his own right hand. (Photo by Ann Wade, with permission)

ments of language skills are likely to be conducted by other professionals, but the occupational therapist should discern what communication methods the client can use effectively for daily and emergency needs, such as transportation, job, exchanging information, and locating resources. One listens to and watches the client, communicating with him or her by voice, pencil and paper or magic slate, illustrations (pictures or on-the-spot drawings), touch, sign language, demonstration, or gesture.

Deaf and hard-of-hearing persons may read lips as well as facial expressions (speech read), but much of English is not discernible to lip readers. One must be careful to articulate carefully yet not to exaggerate lip and tongue movements when speaking to a lip-reading person and to be certain to face the person with the light on the speaker's face while keeping hands away from the mouth. Body and facial language need to be consistent with signs and/or speech.

Mindel and Vernon,[23] a psychiatrist and a psychologist accepted by the deaf community, have suggested that many deaf persons tend to use a mannerism reminiscent of the age at which it is natural and acceptable to communicate without words. The mannerism is the smile, which for the sighted but deaf infant can be reinforced and is one of the foundations for a warm relationship with parents and others. Rather than conveying a true feeling of pleasure, however, a deaf person of any age may smile (or nod) at the speaking, hearing person both to conceal the fact that he or she did not understand all of the spoken message and to avoid embarrassing the speaker. Hearing persons also may nod or smile for the same reasons, or to denote interest or acceptance, whether or not they understand or agree.

Such mixed messages, however well-intended, may be the basis for grave misunderstandings and mistrust, especially when two parties use different language and cannot readily clarify points.

If the person wears a hearing aid or is hard of hearing, one should modulate the voice, speak slowly and distinctly, near the better ear if this seems helpful, and project the voice without shouting. In groups, a microphone or public address system assists the hard-of-hearing. Persons dependent on sign language or speech-reading must have an unobstructed view of upper body or head of speaker.

Two-way manual communication requires free hands and mental and visual (or tactile for the deaf–blind) attention. It is advisable to wear a garment that provides both pockets and a noncompeting but contrasting background for the hands. This is particularly important for partially sighted deaf signers, as is one's location. Persons with tunnel vision may need to be about 3 feet from the signer in order that the visual field can include the entire area where signs are made. Finger-spelling must often be slower. If the individual must use peripheral vision, as is true for macular degeneration and pupils dilated to see around a small cataract, standing or sitting slightly to the preferred side may help prevent a stiff neck. Presbyopic individuals will prefer greater distance than myopic persons, and some will require more light on the signer than others. The principles of visual field, light, and placement of therapist and hands apply to anything the hearing or deaf low-vision client needs to see.

Unless the partially sighted or blind person is known to have a hearing loss, he or she will appreciate being spoken to in a distinct, well-modulated voice no louder than required for ordinary conversation. The speaker should identify himself or herself to the blind client when entering the room unless definitely known by voice when speaking to the person by name. In conversation with more than one other person present, remarks and questions should be prefaced by the name of the person being addressed. Procedures or actions should be explained to the blind person before they actually begin. One must be precise but concise so the person can readily understand and remember or visualize what is described or asked. It is important to check one's facts and carefully report exact information, since the blind client cannot check for himself.[33] Reliable data and follow-through foster trust. Blind persons, as well as the deaf, are too frequently given reason to distrust, regardless of the motives of others.

Braille books, Twin Vision (type and Braille) children's books and talking books in record, reel, and cassette form are available through the Library of Congress's free lending program.[41] Recorded books can be played on machines provided free by the local agency. Many persons who become blind as adults prefer not to learn Braille, so the talking book program is particularly helpful. It includes fiction and nonfiction, both general and professional. Many retail stores and libraries now offer a wide range of topics on audio cassettes; these are usually read or spoken with greater vocal expression than talking books, which allow the listener to supply personal interpretation such as the reader does with printed page. Deaf–blind persons must generally rely on Braille to read books independently, but there are some labeling and personal information systems that use raised letters or larger tactile symbols (Fishburne) so the deaf–blind persons can mark containers, note and/or read short instructions, addresses, etc.[13,19]

For low-vision persons, magnifying glasses and monocular lenses, adequate indoor and outdoor lighting, and large-print books and magazines can be of great help. Light, bright colors on oven controls, door sills, and step edges may be useful. Studies of the reduced visual perception of the elderly have shown that signs that consist of white or bright yellow letters and symbols against a dark background are more easily read than the reverse.[27] Because of the yellowing of the lens, colors in the blue, green, or violet range become more difficult to distinguish, making it advisable to use bright colors of red, orange, and yellow.

Code book and separate medical and school emergency communication cards to facilitate essential messages between deaf and nonsigning persons are available through the National Association of the Deaf. Communication boards and cards can be helpful for nonsigning, possibly illiterate, or aphasic deaf. These are listed in some educational, speech and language, and general rehabilitation materials catalogs, but they can also be made by the OTR or COTA, preferably with the client. Picture/word selection should be undertaken in collaboration with the client, family, and nursing personnel. To my knowledge, the deaf do not use Blissymbols unless there is some other disabling condition that prevents signing and reading words. Blissymbols are printed symbols in various combinations designed to be an international conceptual communication system now used with some severely handicapped, nonvocal persons although originally designed as an effort toward world peace.[7,17]

Telecommunication devices (TDD) are more common and somewhat less expensive than previously. These devices enable persons to type messages on special typewriters that convert each letter or symbol to an audible signal, transmit it by telephone (as do some other computers), and then reconvert the signals to a typed message. Typing skill and use of some keys especially for TDD need to be learned by persons who use this equipment. Many transportation and other agencies now list a TDD number as well as the regular phone number so that the deaf may communicate directly. For the deaf–blind who use Braille, there are some TDDs with additional devices that convert Braille to signals and back.[19]

Mobility

For blind and deaf–blind individuals, development or restoration of mobility is of great importance. Independent travel skills should be taught by specially trained teachers called orientation and mobility specialists. A full course in orientation and mobility requires approximately 180 hours for the adventitiously blind person.[20] Prior to or along with the course, family, friends, workers, and the blind person should be taught the correct way for the blind to use a sighted guide. The guide walks about a half step ahead of the blind partner, who grasps the guide's arm just above the elbow (Fig. 33-2).

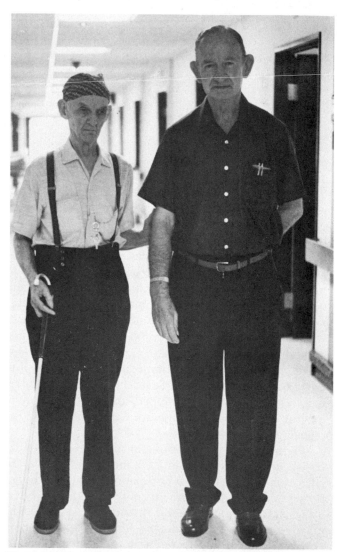

Figure 33-2. When they begin to move, the blind gentleman will drop back a half step, maintaining grasp at or just above his companion's elbow. White cane technique was adequate for navigating hall independently in spite of obstacles, but a crowded lobby and walk outdoors are more comfortably managed when his friend serves as sighted guide. (Photo by Ann Wade, with permission)

Both hold their upper arms close to their bodies for more effective detection of movement. It becomes less necessary for the guide to alert the partner to curbs, stairways, turns, and stops since the blind person can detect these through the guide's movements. Obstacles such as doorsills, uneven pavement, or ice should still be identified and located for the blind person; sights and landmarks along the way can be described for enjoyment and enlightenment. The client should also practice detecting changes in surfaces underfoot, and localizing and identifying sounds and scents. Some blind persons may eventually use guide dogs. Special training courses are available for this.[18] Dogs can also serve to alert some deaf persons to significant sounds, and they can be trained by their owners or others to obey manual as well as spoken commands.

Meaningful and Purposeful Activity

Selection of Activity

Certain considerations have already been described in discussions of object concept and general development, deficits in vision and hearing, and communication. Activity selection is important in assessment as well as in relation to client's goals and needs. For assessment purposes, interviews must be validated and supplemented by performance that will indicate what type of functional or potentially functional residual vision and hearing are present, under what circumstances (if any), and how the other sensations are received, perceived, and used for function. Age- and stage-appropriate pursuits and natural performance should be combined with whatever specific sensory testing is needed to glean just enough information on visual, auditory, tactual, kinesthetic, proprioceptive, vestibulogravity, olfactory, and gustatory senses. The more severely visually or auditorially and multiply handicapped the person, the more careful and creative the therapist must be to find the resources the person has.

For treatment purposes (or consultant recommendations), those activities that have most relevance to the client's major life tasks or occupations are the most appropriate. Those that have the most immediate survival value or that spark interest or motivation should be given priority. From that perspective, re-establishing contacts with employer, creditors, and significant others by telephone, tapes or typing, and direct contact could be most relevant for a newly blind worker with adequate verbal, tactile, and social skills. Depressed, apathetic, or dependent clients are a special challenge. Learning to problem solve while trying familiar and adapted methods of self-care is an appropriate multifaceted activity. Pursuing a work-related activity rather

than a craft could enhance worker image and, if performed with one or more others in an appropriately structured situation, could also enable development or resumption of interpersonal skills. If individuals lack abilities to enjoy themselves, play, recognize and abide by reasonable limits, or feel comfortable with others, then play or leisure activites including games, crafts, and hobbies in an atmosphere of fun and acceptance have much merit.

Within those major activities or pursuits, the occupational therapist must assist the client to use residual skills to the maximum and to compensate with other senses, with items on hand, and with modified or adapted methods or materials. Therefore, activities should be selected that incorporate one or more of these requirements at the appropriate degree of difficulty for challenge or comfort and success. It is wise to begin with something the client has indicated is a priority, or at least an interest, and to use it to increase rapport as well as to reinforce positively the use of intact senses while working on a familiar or desired task. The tasks should lead, especially initially, to the strengths of the person, such as capitalizing on the oral/verbal and auditory abilities of the blind person. Activities such as discussing news and playing word games or crossword puzzles with the therapist can then augment tactual abilities to learn to dial or press the numbers for telephone calls, to use a tape recorder, and to identify coins. Likewise, the deaf person could demonstrate visual and manual skills by visual inspection and sorting of products, materials, or job samples relevant to him or her or by performing some mechanical or sewing task, either of which should be introduced by demonstrated, written, or illustrated directions and the communication method he or she

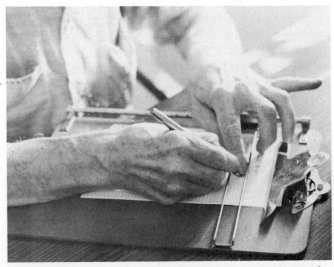

Figure 33-3. With the aid of the Marks writing guide plus his own kinesthetic, tactile, and visual memory abilities, the blind man prepares a grocery list. (Photo by Ann Wade, with permission)

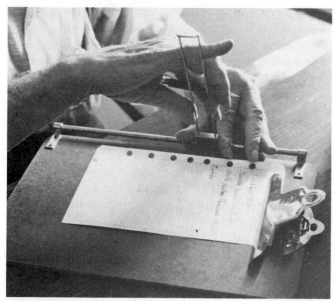

Figure 33-4. The guide bars are moved down the page at regular intervals as determined by notches in the rod on left side. A movable piece on the guide bars can be set where script stops, helpful when patient is interrupted before completing a line or paragraph. (Photo by Ann Wade, with permission)

uses. Hair care, shaving with an electric razor, stuffing envelopes, or pinching the dried leaves from a sturdy plant could enable the deaf–blind person to succeed with tactual-kinesthetic skills, as could tactual inspection of wood products or roller bearings for slight rough spots. Learning to use compensatory methods and aids and to evaluate their worth should occur in the context of activities important to the partially sighted, blind, hard-of-hearing, deaf, or deaf–blind person (Figs. 33-3 and 33-4).

Presenting and Teaching a New Activity

Careful preparation is needed before instructing any client or client group in an activity, but some aspects should be stressed. Therapists must be clear on the number and sequence of steps in the process, the most concise but precise words or sign concepts to use, the actual performance of the task according to directions with the materials and tools available, and the constraints and consequent compensatory methods required by the client. It facilitates understanding through visualization and handling to have samples not only of the finished product but also of each major step in the process if this is at all feasible and applicable.

In presenting the task or end-product activity, therapists should relate the process, materials, or product to something the individual has done previously, and they should state the goal or purpose that may or may not be the same as the final result or product. Time must then be given for the visually or hearing-impaired client to examine the examples and materials. Then, each step with an example, if applicable, is introduced and taught one at a time. *Deaf* persons need time to watch the instructor and then to examine the example while communication ceases until the person is ready for the next step. Demonstrating that step may be the best method for the client to show that he or she understood and can follow the directions, and it may also be the best reinforcement of learning. As with other learning situations, check to see if there are questions about that step in the process before proceeding. *Blind* persons need explicit directions in a minimum of words before and/or while handling the example, with careful attention to left, right, over, under, and texture, because they will rely on visualization and memorization as they learn. Again, successful or corrected completion of each step as presented enables learning by experience. The *deaf–blind* client requires signed and/or finger-spelled, Braille, or other tactual instructions, with time to examine and manipulate examples and materials, with or without actual physical guidance of the hands but definitely with ongoing supervision to be certain of understanding and successful action. The process is most time consuming for the deaf–blind; one instructor–volunteer for each of these persons in the group is initially almost essential. Patience is needed during the entire process with any sensory-impaired client and with oneself; careful advance preparation will maximize patience and effectiveness, but the therapist will still need to be flexible for various unforeseen difficulties or on-the-spot adaptations.

When the therapist becomes familiar with the client's demonstrated learning style and abilities, it may be advantageous to assist the client to continue the activity independently without the therapist being present. Key examples and cards for steps, written or Brailled in a style understood by the client, can facilitate this. Later, the client may learn independently through video or audio tape-recorded, Brailled, or printed and illustrated magazines or instructions.

Organizing Materials

To compensate for little or no vision, it is essential that the partially sighted, blind, or deaf–blind person have good organizational abilities or at least the habit of maintaining consistent arrangement of belongings and appointments. Although not imperative for the deaf or hard-of-hearing, prompt and orderly management of things and affairs at home and on the job are attributes of effective persons.

If materials feel the same but are different colors,

each color must be kept in a separate container, or be labeled in some manner if large, like clothing. The containers may be distinguished by Braille, Fishburne, or other tactually perceived label; by an assigned number of rubber bands around the container; or by the shape or other property of the container itself. During a supervised activity, it may be sufficient to designate the contents of separate and identical containers by their locations on the table. Rather than searching through numerous containers for dissimilar items, it also is sensible to sort and label groups of like items. Labels may be affixed to rubberbands that may be placed on new cans when old are empty. Clothing may be identified by patterns of French knots sewn in a consistent location in like garments or by small abbreviated aluminum Braille labels similarly tacked, or even by safety pins or order of hanging or placing in drawers. File folders, papers, and addresses may be marked and organized using tactile and common-sense systems. Color-coded files, labels, and large print may be sufficient for partially sighted persons. It is important for safety as well as convenience that foods, cleaning products, grooming items, and medicines be unmistakenly identified, labeled, and separately organized. Work simplification principles are useful to all persons, but they may be applied according to personal need and preference.

Locating, Ordering, Purchasing and Obtaining Materials

Many deaf, blind, or low-vision clients need help initially in locating a source of a particular item or service, whether it be groceries, food, information, craft, recreation, personal, or work needs. The client should then record the location, independently or with assistance, in a method that they may independently retrieve and pursue. He or she might travel to stores or services by bus, feet, car, or cab or write, type, or telephone an order and pay for it in the most advantageous way. There are some individuals who will need considerable help in these areas, but it is possible for many to become independent given the right location, funds, mobility, communication, and money management skills. Teachers, occupational therapists, social workers, and others have important functions, along with family members, to teach and expect the maximum amount of responsible independence.

Activity Applications

The preceding paragraphs on organization and procurement of materials and services apply particularly to Mr. Williams, Mr. James, Mrs. Reed, and Mrs. Turner, described in the vignettes. The women will need either to write for materials or to telephone, with the deaf woman using a TDD; otherwise, they will need public or private transportation by bus or van equipped with a wheelchair ramp or lift operated by someone else and with appropriate help at their destinations. The blind amputee could transfer from her wheelchair, and therefore, she could use a car with driver–helper; but arthritic deaf Mrs. Reed is unable to bear weight for standing or sliding-board transfer, so she needs to remain in a chair to avoid difficult two-person transfer into a car.

Before he was ready to function at home again, newly blind Mr. James had to regain confidence in himself, orient himself to his surroundings and belongings, and gain mobility within his immediate environment and with a sighted guide. In situations like this, personal care is particularly important, because it is comprised of familiar and repeatable skills, it influences and reflects the self-concept of the person, and it influences others' attitudes toward the individual and toward blindness. Personal care, including bathing, hygiene, dressing, and care of teeth and hair, are more likely to be routine, automatic, and quickly resumed. With encouragement, Mr. James began to manage these at bedside, and then in the bathroom with stand-by assistance a few times from a therapist or orderly. Mr. James was encouraged to use good posture, to look or turn directly toward the one to whom he is speaking, and to interact with sighted, blind, and partially sighted individuals. He decided to extend his right hand when meeting others to invite their handshake. Problem solving with the client about difficulties helped his success and also set the tone for rehabilitation. Skills requiring stereognosis and kinesthesis, like eating and all related activities (*i.e.*, buttering bread, cutting meat, and managing salt, pepper, and sugar) were taught and practiced in his room or in occupational therapy (walking there using therapist as sighted guide), because Mr. James was sensitive about being clumsy and messy. He progressed rapidly, and he soon taught his family that visualizing the plate as a clock face assists communication about the location of food and other items, such as meat at six o'clock and water glass in line with one o'clock.

Analysis of his skills and the requirements of his job began in the hospital with the therapist. He and the social worker contacted his employer and services for the blind before discharge, so that he knew what to expect in terms of cooperation, workers' compensation, and assistance. He expressed some interest in computer programming and medical writing, either in the context of his medical technology profession or related areas. Although Mr. James' supervisor seemed hesitant, he indicated willingness to cooperate if professionals and James would tell him what to do.

Applying the section on meaningful and purposeful activity to Alice and Jack, those blind and deaf–blind developmentally delayed children (see first vignette), are in need of appropriate self-care and play skills and other adaptive behaviors. They require much tactile cuing. Alice requires oral preparation and instructions, whereas Jack needs to have his visual attention directed to items, actions, and simple signs; both then receive tactile and kinesthetic demonstration through the teacher's or therapist's assistance throughout the activity. Therapist and child should be in the correct position for independent dressing and other performance once the procedure is learned through corrective and positive feedback, and occasional appropriate reward (hug, treat, favorite activity). The children should also learn where clothing, soap, towels, toys, and so forth are consistently and conveniently stored so they can become able to obtain and replace materials. Sensory clues to the activities should also be emphasized, such as hearing, seeing, feeling water running, scents of soap or food, time of day (before or after certain meal, daylight or dark, chime of clock), sounds or sights of toys, and dishes. It is important to assist these children to be independent in small components of tasks, if not in the entire task, so that they can perform increasingly adequately and they can be meaningfully self-directed. Routines are helpful, if not imperative to begin with, but should be varied slightly once learned so that the child can accept some flexibility and can transfer learning to other situations. Some sensory integrative treatment strategies are also employed to influence appropriate tactile and vestibular functions and to facilitate achievement of developmental tasks and self-management.

Other Media and Methods

Occupational therapists also use games and crafts to assist a person to develop confidence and tactile, kinesthetic, and auditory skills. Braille or Fishburne labeled cards, Braille dice, Scrabble letters, Bingo cards, and games such as adapted checkers, chess, and Chinese checkers are useful. Many large dice and dominos have deep-enough depressions for dots that the person can determine numbers by feeling the pattern and counting the depressions. However, Sevel and Hart noted that their eye patients found a raised spot easier to distinguish than a depression.[40] The American game "Cootie" (British "Beetle") are assembly-type games that can be played tactually.

Patterns may be cut in fabric, paper, Styrofoam, leather, or wood by attaching a firm cardboard or plastic pattern with paper clips, pins, or rubber cement, with the blind or partially sighted person then following the edge with one or more fingers and guiding regular or electric scissors, coping saw, or safety handle knife. If the person is diabetic or incoordinated or has peripheral neuropathy, the therapist will observe precautions and avoid sharp tools. Templates can be used successfully for tracing or for applying glue and sand, beans and

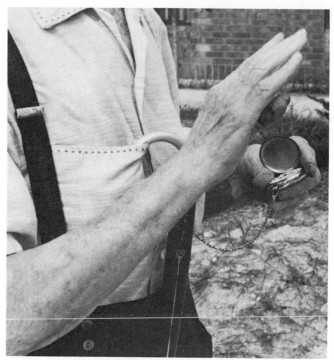

Figure 33-5. A Braille pocketwatch enables its deaf–blind owner to perceive tactually that the time is five after four. (In this photo, the owner is conveying the "four" to another person.) Note that the cane has been hooked in chest pocket to free hands yet make retrieval certain. (Photo by Ann Wade, with permission)

gravel. Ceramics and papier-maché offer opportunities to create, and they can be glazed or painted by pouring, dipping, spraying, or brushing as the person and therapist decide, depending on ability. When working with materials that may be easily dropped, such as beads, it is helpful to work over a tray or box lid so that objects may be retrieved by the worker.

Special tools, clocks, games, and other Brailled or tactually usable items for the blind are listed in the Braille and typed catalogs of the American Foundation for the Blind. A variety of items will be carried by local vision centers or rehabilitation centers for the blind (Fig. 33-5).

The telephone company will install a special receiver on the conventional telephone so that the user may amplify the incoming message by turning a dial. Lights, fans, and vibrators sensitive to sounds are used by some people who need an alternate means of perceiving doorbell, telephone, TDD or alarms, and infant or invalid calling. These are available through security-system retailers and some hearing-aid dealers.

Vocational Considerations

Deaf and blind persons, like many disabled persons, are good and reliable workers when they have been successfully oriented, and they often have lower absenteeism than nonhandicapped persons because they value their jobs. The deaf tend to be *underemployed;* that is, employed for tasks or positions that do not use all their education and capabilities and that therefore do not pay well.[37] It is often difficult for deaf who are multiply disabled, ethnic minority group members, or low achievers to find employment; they especially need intensive and creative habilitation. Although deaf persons are usually excluded from medical professional education and subsequent qualification and employment as registered nurses, therapists, physicians, and technologists, they are pursuing education for work in some health careers.[31] Communication continues to be the greatest problem, with earlier overprotection and immature attitudes complicating the situation. Deaf persons in service work need to find an appropriate way to let clients know that they do not hear and in what manner the employer and other persons can catch their attention and communicate. Technology is improving; for example, blood pressure can be read by a computerized stethoscope, which reports the results like a digital watch or clock, thereby eliminating the need to listen except to check discrepant results.

Rusalem cautions against restrictive lists of occupations suitable for the blind.[34] If lists are open-ended and allow for individual interests, abilities, and modifications of certain job methods, they may be a reasonable starting point. Technological advances are opening doors for blind workers, with computerized "voices" for output of some machines. Blind and partially sighted persons can be found in a full range of occupations, from the professions to unskilled labor, although some positions within a field are not feasible (*e.g.,* medicine). Persons already working in one field may find it possible to return to that work following loss of vision, if the employer can be convinced that it is acceptable and cost-effective. If the specific functions are not amenable to adaptation to blindness, there is often some other position in the same company that the blind person can assume. Since returning to the established workplace may be faster than changing jobs, it may be psychologically as well as financially beneficial.

When developmentally blind and deaf or visually or hearing-impaired persons obtain work, their job-related personal–social skills may need more attention and improvement than do the actual tasks. Self-care, management of personal affairs, social behavior, general work habits, transportation, and communication should be assessed and improved as needed. Groups or individual adolescents and adults might benefit from using some or all of the chapters in *Career Planning for the Blind,* copyrighted by Hadley School for the Blind,[12] and the therapist should find *Coping with the Unseen Environment*[34] useful for vocational rehabilitation. Occupational therapists and related personnel serving deaf and severely handicapped deaf will find pertinent and practical information in the *Proceedings of the National Forum VII* on *Careers for Deaf People* (1974)[3] and in the final report of a grant to Crossroads Rehabilitation Center on *A Program for the Severly Handicapped Deaf.*[29] Both stress the need for personal and career development and work adjustment training, with the former also emphasizing the need for deaf school children to be helped to develop the ability to think for themselves, learning to recognize and set goals, to problem solve, and to give as well as take. The Crossroads program includes objectives, methods, forms, research data, and descriptions of all aspects of the program, including a variety of living arrangements and representative case studies. The *Model State Plan for Rehabilitation of the Deaf* indicates needs and the current state of the art. Although not specifically mentioning occupational therapy, except as it can be understood under medical rehabilitation, the plan described can use occupational therapists with deaf experience to help implement.[36] For generic occupational therapy information, the reader is encouraged to refer to Chapter 18, Section 1.

Role of Occupational Therapy with Family and Agencies

Blindness and deafness are accompanied by profound isolation. Partial loss can also disrupt meaningful interaction with the human and nonhuman environments. Communication channels must be kept open, reopened, or discovered to enable the individual to give and receive understandable messages about feelings, needs, support, and information. Adventitious loss or diminution of sight or hearing will of course be mourned, with the individual passing through any or all of the stages of reaction to loss. Without family support and professional help, however, the person may plateau at early stages or may regress. The premorbid personalities of the individual and family members and their attitudes toward blindness and deafness will affect adjustment to the sensory loss as well as the family's treatment of the individual (*i.e.,* rejection, overprotection, ambivalence, embarrassment, and encouragement). Congenital loss will not be mourned initially by the individual, but it will certainly affect parent(s) or other primary care-givers, who may initially experience shock, denial, anger, embarrassment, mourning, or rejection of the infant. The congenitally handicapped child may begin to experience these reactions to disability when he or she begins school or when coping with many other problems during adolescence, at which time it is so important to be like one's peers. Even if peers are similarly disabled, by this age, the young person is aware of things that nondisabled teenagers can do such as driving a car, conversing easily in a group or on the telephone, and being more independent generally.

Whether the occupational therapist is serving the

client directly or as a consultant, it is important to ascertain that the client and significant others' needs for emotional support and guidance are being recognized and met in the most appropriate way. This may require that a specific professional be designated; that *could* but does not have to be the occupational therapist. Interagency cooperation may be needed to assure that this is taken care of. If client or family is not ready to acknowledge a problem or need for help, the avenue to help should nevertheless be kept open, with the client group knowing how to contact the agency or a trusted person within the agency and with nonforcing contacts from professionals at reasonable intervals. This seems particularly important when there is a blind or deaf–blind infant involved, because initially, the best stimulation can be provided through the mother who is very likely to need support, guidance, and some physical relief from other tasks. Without visual experience, early sensorimotor development can be easily retarded unless the mother or caring mother substitute consistently provides the handling and nurturing that the baby needs.[14] Professional personnel who may visit in the homes of blind or deaf clients include public health nurses and therapists, caseworkers, family interventionists, visiting teachers, and rehabilitation teachers for the blind. Some parent organizations or groups of low-vision, blind, hearing-impaired, or deaf individuals might send representatives to offer support and socialization opportunities (Fig. 33-6). Professional personnel must be careful to protect confidentiality by asking the client and support representatives independently for permission to introduce, without giving specific information until both parties agree, and then not providing more than

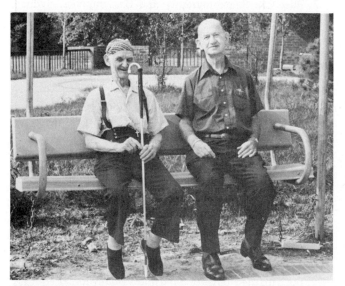

Figure 33-6. Movement in a sturdy swing, fresh air, sunshine, and companionship are enjoyed by these deaf friends, one of whom is also blind. (Photo by Ann Wade, with permission)

essential and approved information. Depending on the individual center and state, services for persons with impaired or lost vision, hearing, or both may be comprehensive and nonstereotyped or less than that. For example, some states and facilities may be much more progressive in the types of prevocational and vocational exploration and rehabilitation available and in the type of job placement and follow-up. Regardless, the occupational therapist can cooperate with state and local agencies as needed for the client, with the ultimate goal being the realistic coping and satisfactory quality of life for the blind, deaf, partially sighted, hard-of-hearing, or deaf–blind person in his or her environment.

Additional Opportunities and Responsibilities Related to Visual and Hearing Losses

Prevention of Unnecessary Sensory Losses

Along with others in the field, occupational therapists need to practice as well as to teach such preventive measures as inoculation against rubella for all females of child-bearing age; avoidance of harmful medications during pregnancy; careful handwashing before and after contact with individuals who may carry herpes or cytomegalovirus, which in some instances can infect the fetus or neonate and cause multiple handicaps; precautions against the handling of cats and litter boxes by pregnant women (because cats may transmit toxoplasmosis that may produce deaf–blindness and mental retardation in the developing infant); annual ophthalmologic examinations for diabetic individuals; and at least biannual examinations for all persons 40 years old and above for glaucoma and cataract, as well as for refractive errors and other possible eye diseases or conditions; wearing of safety goggles; careful use of cyanoacrylics; protection of the ears against prolonged industrial, traffic, and other loud sounds; and adequate vision and hearing screening and prompt eye and ear examination by medical specialists, especially for individuals with injuries, communication, and learning problems and other disabilities.

Public and Professional Education and Awareness

Through reading, viewing films, TV and radio productions, and by becoming acquainted with many capable blind, deaf, and deaf–blind persons, occupational therapists, professional colleagues, and the general public can learn that blindness and deafness do not have to be such isolating disabilities. They will likely recognize and reduce their own possibly stereotypic thinking and begin to appreciate the range of characteristics and methods—some special, some ordinary—that are found among successful persons who have visual, auditory, or combined handicaps or losses. We can share positive attitudes and knowledge of compensatory methods and materials with families and other professionals and paraprofessionals. By complimenting TV stations that use interpreters or captions to inform the deaf, and by acknowledging those networks and producers who participate in *closed-caption* programming (available only on sets that have a user-purchased closed-caption converter) and the newspapers and guides that indicate such programs, the deaf and those interested in them can reinforce current efforts. Similarly, public acknowledgment or information about talking-book programs, radio reading services for the blind, and services available through the library and telephone company are educational and encouraging to the providers.

More Effective Use of Resources

The Practice Division of the American Occupational Therapy Association has a packet of information on Hearing Impaired/Visual Impaired that therapists can request and share. Other major resources are listed in Appendix J and in many of the books cited in the references and bibliography. To make these and the many other resources available to visually and auditorially limited persons, their families, and therapists, each of us can maintain a file of potentially useful information and also can be willing and able to direct questions to others who may be better sources than we. Mutual sharing, rather than a defensive stance regarding what occupational therapy can do, seems to be healthier and more beneficial to clients and ultimately even to our profession. Prompt, clear requests or referrals for further assistance to the client, with a follow-up check, may make the critical difference in whether a client achieves independence and whether the family receives timely and appropriate counseling.

Summary

The principles and treatment approaches in occupational therapy as a whole definitely apply to our work with clients who are additionally or solely blind, deaf, or deaf–blind. Some methods must be modified, and certain materials are available to facilitate some processes. Attitudes of the client, family, and professional personnel serving the client are one significant determining factor in prognosis for rehabilitation. Preparation for working in these areas includes specific learning about visual and hearing impairments and treatment methods, examining, and if necessary, improving one's attitude toward the disability and developing sufficient skill to communicate understandably with the client. All occupational therapists need great patience, empathy, ability to know when and how to take a psychological approach different from the supportive one with some clients, and sufficient creativity and ingenuity to modify procedures to suit the needs and personality of the individual client. When the reader meets a client who has a sensory problem, with or without other problems, it is hoped that it will be a challenging and beneficial experience for both parties.

References*

1. American Occupational Therapy Association, Operations Research Division, Rockville, MD, August 1982
2. Atchley RC: The Social Forces in Later Life: An Introduction to Social Gerontology, p. 54. Belmont, CA, Wadsworth Publishing, 1972
*3. Austin GF (ed): Careers for Deaf People. Washington, DC, US Department of Health, Education and Welfare. Office of Human Development, Rehabilitation Services Administration, 1974. (Also available from National Association of the Deaf.)
*4. Baker–Nobles L, Bink MP: Sensory integration in the rehabilitation of blind adults. Am J Occup Ther 33:559, 1979
5. Baron L: The adult low vision population: An area of concern for occupational therapy. Master's thesis, Washington University, St Louis, August, 1981
*6. Baron LS: The Adult Low Vision Population: A treatment guide for allied health professionals, 1985. Available from Leslie Baron, 5602 Green Springs Drive, Houston TX 77066 (includes updated page inserts)
7. Bliss CK: Semantography and Blissymbolics. Sydney, Australia, 1965
8. Bourgeault SE: Blindness–a label. Visually Handicapped 6:1, 1974
9. Chess S, Korn S, Fernandez P: Psychiatric Disorders of Children with Congenital Rubella. pp 82–87, 120–130. New York, Brunner–Mazel, 1971
10. Chusid JG: Correlative Neuroanatomy and Functional Neurology, 19th ed, pp 304, 312–316. Los Altos, CA, Lange Medical Publishers, 1985
*11. Combs A: Hearing Loss Help: How You Can Help Someone with a Hearing Loss . . . and How They Can Help Themselves, p 19. Santa Maria, CA, Alpenglow Press, 1986
12. Crawford FL: Career Planning for the Blind: A Manual for Students and Teachers. New York, Farrar, Straus and Giroux, 1966. (Available in regular and large print, Braille, and talking-book form.)
*13. Dickman IR: Making Life More Livable: Simple Adaptations for the Homes of Blind and Visually Impaired Older

* Asterisked items are recommended as resources.

People, p 5. New York, American Foundation for the Blind, 1983

*14. Fraiberg S: Insights from the Blind: Comparative Studies of Blind and Sighted Infants, chapters 5 and 6, and p 273. New York, Basic Books, 1977

15. Fraiberg S: Parallel and divergent patterns in blind and sighted infants. Psychoanal Study Child 23:264, 1968

16. Gesell A, Armatruda C: Developmental Diagnosis: Normal and Abnormal Child Development, 2nd ed., p 435. New York, Harper & Row, 1969

17. Helfman ES: Blissymbolics: Speaking without Speech. New York, Elsevier/Nelson Books, 1981

18. If Blindness Occurs: Practical Suggestions for Those Who Live or Work with Newly Blinded Persons (booklet). Morristown, NJ, The Seeing Eye, Inc. (This agency also lends a film on the subject.)

*19. Kates L, Schein JD: A Complete Guide to Communication with Deaf–Blind Persons. Silver Spring, MD, National Association of the Deaf, 1980

20. Koestler FA (ed): The Comstac Report: Standards for Strengthened Services, p 231. New York, National Accreditation Council for Agencies Serving the Blind and Visually Handicapped, 1966. Cited in Lydon and McGraw: Concept Development for Visually Handicapped Children, rev. ed, p 5. New York, American Foundation for the Blind, 1973

21. Lowenfeld B: Our Blind Children: Growing and Learning with Them, 3rd ed, pp 9–10. Springfield, IL, Charles C Thomas, 1971

22. Maloney C: Sensory losses common to elders. General Session #121, Official Program for 1981 Annual AOTA Conference, Denver

23. Mindel ED, Vernon M: They Grow in Silence: The Deaf Child and His Family. pp 25–30. Silver Spring, MD, National Association of the Deaf, 1971

24. Mouchka S: The deaf–blind infant: A rationale for and an approach to early intervention. In Proceedings from the Fourth International Conference on Deaf-Blind Children, August 1971, at Perkins School for the Blind, Watertown MA, pp 212–225

25. Norris C (ed): Letters from Deaf Students. Eureka, CA, Alinda Press, 1975. (Booklet available from National Association of the Deaf.)

26. Occupational Therapy Newspaper, The American Occupational Therapy Association. Member Hotline, Rockville, MD, April, 1981

27. Pastalan LA: Lecture–demonstration at Ohio State University, Industrial Design Program, Columbus, 1976. (See also Dr. Pastalan's "Empathic Model" described in Dickman: Making Life More Livable,[13] pp 84–89.)

28. Pettingill DG: Adjustments of the deaf. Printed address before a workshop, Understanding the Deaf Client, 1964. In Deaf Adults, collection of papers on problems of deaf people. Silver Spring, MD, National Association of the Deaf

*29. A Program for the Severely Handicapped Deaf: Final Report of RSA Service Grant 30-p-65000/5; a section 301(b)(1) project. Indianapolis, IN, Crossroads Rehabilitation Center, 1978. (Available from National Association of the Deaf.)

30. Ramm P, Charles S, Clark J, McCammon M: Sensory integration programming for the visually impaired, 0–22 years. Institute described in Official Program for 1981 Annual AOTA Conference, Denver, p 23–24

31. Rawlings B, Karchmer MA, DeCaro JJ, Egelston-Dodd J (eds): College and Career Programs for Deaf Students. Washington DC, Gallaudet College, National Technical Institute for the Deaf, Rochester Institute of Technology, NY, 1986

32. Riekehof LL: The Joy of Signing: The New Illustrated Guide for Mastering Sign Language and the Manual Alphabet, pp 11–12. Springfield, MO, Gospel Publishing House, 1978

33. Rouse DD, Gruber KF, Bledsoe CW: Occupational therapy for blind patients. Am J Occup Ther 10:252, 1956

*34. Rusalem H: Coping with the Unseen Environment: An Introduction to the Vocational Rehabilitation of Blind Persons, p 97. New York, Teachers College Press, 1972

35. Schaefer, KJ, Specht TR: A light probe adapted for use in training the blind. Am J Occup Ther 33:640, 1979

*36. Schein D (ed): Model State Plan for Rehabilitation of Deaf Clients: Second Revision. pp 2, 25–27, 31–36. Silver Spring, MD, National Association of the Deaf, 1980 (See also p 31 regarding Title VII of PL 95–602).

37. Schein JD: The deaf community. In Davis H, Silverman SR (eds): Hearing and Deafness, 4th ed., pp 513, 522. New York, Holt, Rinehart and Winston, 1978

38. Seltser CG: A COTA initiated program for visually handicapped patients: Therapeutic interaction with blind and visually impaired patients. COTA Forum topic and General Session #5, Official Program for 1981 Annual AOTA Conference, Denver, p 36

39. Sereni F, Principi N: Clinically harmful consequences of drug administration to the pregnant woman and the infant. In Ziai M (ed): Pediatrics, 2nd ed., pp 55–58. Boston: Little, Brown, 1975

40. Sevel D, Hart JA: Occupational therapy for the hospitalized eye patient. Am J Occup Ther 22:339, 1969

41. United States Library of Congress, Division for the Blind and Physically Handicapped, Washington, DC

*42. Yeadon A, Grayson D, Mulholland ME: Living with Impaired Vision: An Introduction, pp 10, 21–29, 55–62. New York, American Foundation for the Blind, 1979

Bibliography

American Foundation for the Blind: An Introduction to Working with the Aging Person Who Is Visually Handicapped. New York, 1977

Bolton B (ed): Psychology of Deafness for Rehabilitation Counselors. Baltimore, University Park Press, 1976

Caird FI, Williamson J: The Eye and its Disorders in the Elderly. Bristol, John Wright & Sons, 1986

Gloor B, Bruckner R (eds): Rehabilitation of the Visually Disabled and the Blind at Different Ages. Baltimore, University Park Press, 1980

Gregory S: The Deaf Child and His Family. New York, John Wiley & Sons, 1976

Harley RK, Henderson FM, Truan MB: The Teaching of Braille Reading. Springfield, IL, Charles C Thomas, 1979. (For material on prereading—tactual, auditory, physical, emotional and intellectual readiness, as well as for Braille itself.)

Harrity R, Martin RG: The Three Lives of Helen Keller. Garden City, NY, Doubleday, 1962

Haug O, Haug S: Help for the Hard-of-Hearing: A Speech Reading and Auditory Training Manual for Home and Professionally Guided Training. Springfield, IL, Charles C Thomas, 1977. (Some pointers for hearing persons and information about care of hearing aids.)

Hill AE, McKendrick O, Poole JJ, Pugh RE, Rosenbloom L, Turnock R: The Liverpool Visual Assessment Team: Ten Years' Experience. Child Care Health Dev 12:37, 1986

Hurvitz J, Carmen R: Special Devices for Hard of Hearing, Deaf, and Deaf–Blind Persons. Boston, Little, Brown, 1981

Moersch MS: Training the deaf–blind child. Am J Occup Ther 31:425, 1977

Neisser A: The Other Side of Silence: Sign Language and the Deaf Community in America. New York, Alfred Knopf, 1983

Ogden PW, Lipsett S: The Silent Garden: Understanding the Hearing Impaired Child. New York, St Martin's Press, 1982

Rouse D, Gruber K, Bledsoe C: Occupational therapy for blind patients. Am J Occup Ther 10:252, 1956. (As timely now as then.)

Scott E, Jan J, Freeman R: Can't Your Child See? Baltimore, University Park Press, 1977

Sonksen PM, Levitt S, Kitsinger M: Identification of constraints acting on motor development in young visually disabled children and principles of remediation. Child Care Health Dev 10:273, 1984

Sperber A: Out of Sight: Ten Stories of Victory over Blindness. Boston, Little, Brown, 1976

Spradley TS, Spradley JP: Deaf Like Me. Washington, DC, Random House, 1978. (Epilogue 1985 by LL Spradley; paperback by Gallaudet College Press, 1985.)

Woodring J, Gregg J: Occupational therapy in the rehabilitation of the blind. Am J Occup Ther 9:136, 1955. (Still relevant.)

Wright D: Deafness. New York, Stein and Day, 1969 (Personal account followed by sections on history and treatment of deafness.)

Yoken C: Living with Deaf–Blindness: Nine Profiles. Washington, DC, National Academy of Gallaudet College, 1979. (Available from National Association of the Deaf.)

Appreciation is extended to Columbus Colony for Elderly Care, Inc., and Columbus Colony Housing, Westerville, Ohio—caring, communicating facilities for deaf and deaf–blind and older persons, sponsored by Ohio School for the Deaf Alumni Association and funded in part by the US Dept of Health and Human Services; to multiply handicapped students, families, and staff in the Columbus Public Schools and beyond; to Elaine Ainsworth, OTR; Leslie Baron, OTR; Barbara Boyer, AOTA, Operations Research; Arlene C. Finocchiaro, OTR; Mike Hillis, OTR; Arlene Innman, OTR; Marguerite Moore, Interpreter and Sign Class Instructor; Cay Reilly, OTR; Suzanne Onderdonk, OTR; Crystal Overholt, OTR; Joyce Vargo, teacher; and others, for responding to my questions for the 6th edition; and To Teddy Kern, OTR, for her interest and ability. Special appreciation to Leslie Baron, OTR, and special thanks to the gentlemen who graciously allowed me to take their pictures in order to teach occupational therapy students some of the things that visually and hearing impaired persons can do.

CHAPTER 34

Pediatric Occupational Therapy *Patricia Ann Ramm*

Therapists share with parents a fascination blended with a curiosity about the nature of children's behavior and development. As ever-increasing numbers of occupational therapists enter the field of pediatric occupational therapy, there is a need for comprehensive material on this subject. But to provide such requires that a wide range of considerations be addressed.

Basic to the topic of pediatric occupational therapy is the need to understand human functional systems and their interrelationships. The blending of this understanding with knowledge about the variety and types of pathologic or disabling conditions that make an impact on young children forms a foundation for understanding the effect of these conditions on children's functional abilities and behavior.

Functional disorders or differences stemming from disease or other causes have an intimate relationship with the child's dynamic developmental process, and they further expand the complexity of this topic.

Gilfoyle and Grady's theoretical framework of spatiotemporal adaptation has provided a major contribution to pediatric occupational therapy. The continuum of acquiring integrated sequences of movement as a means of gaining skilled performance is fundamental to the subject of this section.

This broad yet intricate subject would nevertheless suffer unless thought is given to the influence and interrelationship that parenting and caregiving have on the child's state of health and function. Bonding, parenting skills, cultural values, health practices, and health knowledge are but a few of the crucial factors that need equal consideration.

Basic professional preparation of occupational therapists is an important factor as well. There is professional agreement that the basic premise of occupational therapy necessitates that the therapist's first level of preparation should be as a generalist. Further, at the present time, the field of occupational therapy has no professionally identified specialization. Despite this, the practice of pediatric occupational therapy presents an immediate challenge to the entering or inexperienced therapist to respond swiftly and effectively to children's needs for services requiring highly specialized skills. Admittedly, this is not unique to occupational therapy pediatric practice alone, but it is a growing and expanding factor in this area of practice.

For example, in the area of pediatric occupational therapy assessment alone, the number, type, and complexity of examinations that therapists are providing is greater than in any other specific area of occupational therapy practice. A number of valuable occupational therapy pediatric screening and assessment mechanisms are now being readied by testing and standardization. Use of advanced occupational therapy assessment and diagnostic procedures has and will continue to result in exciting advances and expansion of occupational therapy pediatric services. Yet the status of pediatric occupational therapy practice is such that many unusually demanding and specialized skills are required of the entering therapist if quality care is to be assured.

In most areas of occupational therapy, changes are occurring in settings where services are being provided. This is especially so in pediatrics. The reasons for such changes are the major advances in medical science and litigated human rights guarantees.

Though pediatric occupational therapy services primarily address the human condition, such services often face impositions based on the condition of the service setting. It would be true to say that the parameters of the professional services are closely tied to the delivery system or type of health service system available to the therapist. Though the traditional role of pediatric practice continues to exist in acute- and convalescent-care hospitals, large numbers of therapists are extending pediatric occupational therapy services to advance functional performance of children in community and educational programs. Viewing pediatric occupational therapy on a developmental continuum relating to the model depicted by Johnson expands the subject's perspective to include prevention, early detection, remediation, treatment, restoration, referral, and health maintenance as components of that practice.[5] This perspective underscores the variety of facilities and service

settings that therapists are encountering in this field of practice. Home settings, neonatal intensive care units, well-child clinics, infant–parent centers, private or public school programs, regional educational service centers, specialized pediatric intermediate-care units, and state-sponsored schools for the deaf and blind are appropriately utilizing occupational therapy services. Experienced pediatric occupational therapists are developing their own private clinics specializing in services for children with learning disabilities, and they are finding their services well utilized.

Each of these examples, including hospital-based programs, offer uniquely important, though differing, opportunities for practice. Settings vary in structure from informal to highly technical and complex systems. It is the ethical responsibility of each therapist to offer occupational therapy knowledge and skill appropriate to the client's needs, despite the constraints of settings and service systems. It is an equally important responsibility of each therapist to use the occupational therapy knowledge base to work collaboratively in attaining the overall constructive mission of each particular health delivery system. Expanded examples of indirect but valuable pediatric occupational therapy services include the following:

1. Screening of populations to identify the children who need services
2. Consulting with other related professionals or agencies who need services
3. Educating parents, teachers, and caregivers to influence children's development.

In this chapter, children are viewed in a variety of

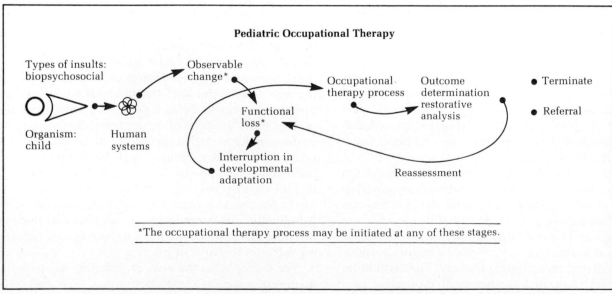

Figure 34-1. A model depicting the interrelationship of the occupational therapy process to biopsychosocial insult to human (child) funtion.

dimensions — as unique human beings living with different kinds of parents and families and living in different kinds of conditions — the whole of which is affected by physical, emotional, or social insult. To avoid any tendency to oversimplify or fragment the topic, a schematically based model (Fig. 34-1) is presented to depict the relationship of occupational therapy to children, their family, or a caregiver, when the children are experiencing a human system dysfunction. The model indicates broad types of insults and emphasizes the key functional systems therapists most frequently address. Included in this diagram are initiating points for occupational therapy services and linking of restorative analysis or outcome determination for termination, referral, or continued services with or without change.

The Developmental Process

Movement and subsequent adaptation to one's environment are at the heart of human development. Gilfoyle, Grady, and Moore discuss adaptation as an organized process of modification in which a child assimilates everything that is happening, accommodates to these experiences, and associates, differentiates, and integrates the new experiences with those previously acquired.[4] Most of the many theories of development tend to agree that development is a continuing process that results from biological advancement and the effect of environmental factors.

Ayres has described development and behavior on the basis of neurophysiological processing and organization.[1] This developmental theory, sensory integration, is "the process of organizing the sensations in the nervous system." Her theory stresses that "the greatest sensory motor organization occurs during an adaptive response to sensation and that a well-organized adaptive response leaves the brain in a more organized state."[2] Ayres' extensive writings and research on her theory have strongly influenced occupational therapists' practice in pediatrics, as have Gilfoyle, Grady, Bobath, Rood, Reilly, and Llorens. Ayres' emphasis on the natural patterns of development is depicted as a reflection of sensory organization, or an organization of sensations both from the body itself and from the surrounding environment.[1]

There is a common order or pattern of sensory integration usually seen in children's development. All children, regardless of race or culture, follow this developmental pattern of performance. The acquisition of gross and fine motor milestones is depicted later in this chapter in the Infant Parent Training Program (IPTP) assessment. Developmental maturation is also presented in Figure 34-3 by means of reflex patterns and the adaptation facilitated by this nervous system maturation process.

The basic principles of the developmental process are as follows:

Development is cephalocaudal and proximal – distal.
Reflexive movement promotes voluntary functions.
The brain and nervous system function holistically as maturation occurs.
Smooth motoric patterns are due to sensorimotor feedback mechanisms.
These feedback mechanisms are ongoing and contribute to progressively more complicated developmental patterns.
Each individual has a maturation pattern that is uniquely its own based on genetic, biological, and environmental factors.
Development is dependent on the integration of sensory reception including sight, sound, smell and taste, movement and gravity, touch, and muscle and joint reception.
Without the automatic integration of these senses, interference in development will occur.
Disorder in the motor milestone pattern suggests developmental deviation.

In some cases, deviations in development are obvious, but in many cases, the deviations are far more subtle. For example, it is obvious when a young child has poor balance and low muscle tone; therefore, the child is not attaining walking skills by the outer limit of 6 months. It is much less obvious, however, when a child does attain walking skills at the age-appropriate level but has significantly poor background postural control, sits with a rounded back and the head propped at a work table, and displays a mild delay in acquisition of prehensile skills.

Therapists should be keen observers of young children, noting the quality of movement in achieving sitting, rolling, creeping, kneeling, squatting, and walking skills. Frequently children with discrete developmental disabilities will attain skills but will exhibit marked though discrete differences. Close observation will reveal postural deviations and the inappropriate presence of primitive reflexes (nonobligatory). Stress and sometimes hand tremor will be noted as the developmentally deficient child attempts prehensile skills with some success, though obviously in an immature manner of usage of the upper extremeties. To the observing therapist, it appears as if the child does not have a clear body percept and has difficulty organizing objects in space. Frequently, parents and teachers of such children are confused by the child's irregularity in performance skills and assume those skills could be attained if the child tried harder.

In dealing with such children, it is essential that occupational therapists possess not only the skills and knowledge of the developmental process but also the ability to communicate the underlying reasons for such deviations in development clearly to the parents and teachers in a constructive way and to lead parents, in particular, to learn how to help their child attain a well-integrated system of development. Protecting the child from undue external pressure, reducing frustration and feelings of failure, reducing confusion about self-identity, and increasing the child's willingness toward tasks by staging more successful experiences is the collaborative task of parents and therapists.

Insult

In this model, the human organism under consideration is the young child. Insult factors have been categorized into three major components that are biological, psychological, or social in nature. Children and adults alike rarely experience an insult that is isolated and that does not have related overall consequences to the human being. Biological insults often relate to physical dysfunction stemming from disease, injury, or genetic, structural, or chemical factors. Psychological and sociological factors are entwined and are frequently indigenous to the pediatric occupational therapy process. Psychologically, harm may occur to any child regardless of economic condition and opportunity. Social disadvantages have a complex effect on children both negatively and in some cases paradoxically, because of the human support mechanisms that may be available. These support mechanisms may provide an impetus for advantageous change—whether psychological, social, or both—through health-providing services.

Human Functional Systems

A simplification of key human systems used in the conceptual models are listed together with the function of each system in Table 34-1. Included are observable change outcomes when such systems are insulted. This list of changes is representative but should not be considered all-inclusive.

The Pediatric Occupational Therapy Process

The occupational therapy process is complex and must be ordered in terms of achieving improved functional and behavioral goals if the therapist is to achieve beneficial outcomes for pediatric clients and their families. Figure 34-2 depicts the various stages of the process.

The subsequent discussion of these stages is in general terms. Chapter 35, entitled "The Occupational Therapy Process in Specific Pediatric Conditions" provides the following:

Case discussion
Schematic drawing of the individualized child-oriented problems and treatment or intervention program
Narrative or graphic information illustrating and describing an appropriate occupational therapy evaluation, plans, and goal-setting/objectives
Procedures for accomplishing these identified goals
Readjustments that are further discussed and diagrammed in some cases

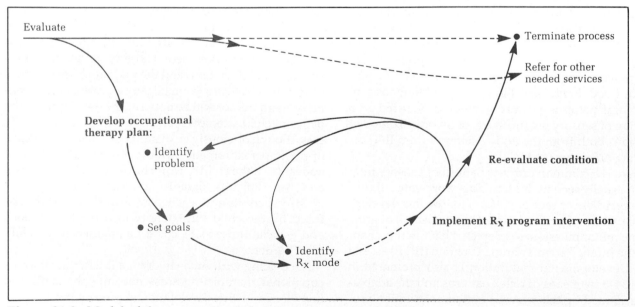

Figure 34-2. Model of the occupational therapy process with children.

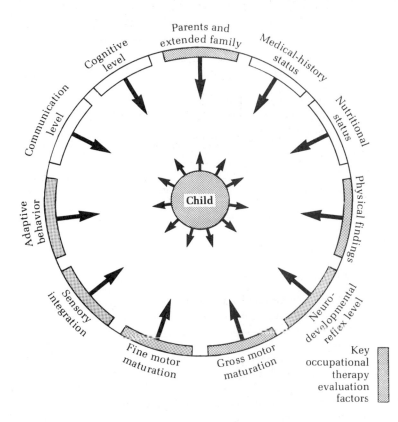

Figure 34-3. A diagram of key interrelated factors that affect children's development and behavior.

Evaluation

The key to the occupational therapy process is evaluation. A diagram that identifies key factors that influence children's health and developmental potential is presented in Figure 34-3. In the broadest sense, this diagram is a reminder that while on one hand the occupational therapy evaluation addresses a great number of these factors (see Fig. 34-3); on the other hand, the information this process yields closely relates to information being processed by other involved professionals or persons. The effectiveness of the evaluation process will be augmented if a true climate of collaboration and coordination is present.

Fundamentally, the evaluation process in any endeavor is the foundation for any change in effectivness. In pediatric occupational therapy, the emergence of great numbers of useful evaluation instruments or tools that have differing types of focus demands therapists' careful attention. It has been suggested by Lewke[6] that therapists and other health providers often err in the appropriate selection of evaluation measures. An error of this nature will diminish the effectiveness of the occupational therapy process. Therefore, it is essential that therapists correctly administer the test measures that are standardized with proven validity and reliability, that they clearly understand the population studied and the intended use for such tests, and that proven measurements of error be considered. Table 34-2 presents useful tests and measures and the categories that each test measures or addresses. A description of features and sources of many of these tests is included in Chapter 16.

Often, a therapist finds that decisions about the treatment plan for the child will need to take into account less tangible influences identified through observation and judgment of the child, the family, and the child's environment. Sample questions that guide the therapist's investigative thinking into these less tangible but fruitful avenues of consideration are:

What is the child's state (excitation) level primarily? Is there a lack of or marked increase in the alteration of the child's state level?
Are there significant alterations in the child's level of comfort?
Are the child's coping patterns maladaptive?
Is the family coping pattern effective?
Is the family structure supportive?
Is there a grieving process present in the family or possibly the child? Is it acute, anticipatory, or delayed?
Is there a potential for injury, trauma, or further complication?
Is there a need for or a lack of knowledge about the child's condition?
Is there noncompliance with the helping process? If so, why?
What is the level of parenting skills?
Are there nutritional alterations?

(list continues on page 608)

Table 34-1.   *Key Human Systems and Their Functions*

Human System	Function	Observable Changes
Circulatory/Cardiovascular	Oxygenation	1. Dyspnea (difficulty with breathing, especially during feeding) 2. Edema (fluid retention) 3. Cyanosis (bluing of nailbeds, lips, or fat) 4. Fatigue 5. Underweight and/or poor weight gain 6. Pallor 7. Unexplained vomiting 8. Shallow, grunting, or rapid breathing 9. Cough 10. Clubbing of fingers 11. Wheezing 12. Periodic apnea 13. Gagging 14. Flaring of nostrils
Gastrointestinal/Urinary	Digestion/absorption/filtration/elimination process	1. Obesity or poor weight gain 2. Milk intolerance 3. Edema 4. Nausea/vomiting 5. Anorexia (poor appetite) 6. Diarrhea/constipation 7. Fever 8. Abdominal/flank/suprapubic tenderness 9. Lethargy/weakness 10. Abnormal skin texture
Endocrine/Metabolic	Maintenance of homeostatis	1. Poor weight gain 2. Abnormal growth patterns 3. Excessive thirst/urination 4. Abnormal skin texture 5. Sweating 6. Abnormal activity (state) levels (*i.e.,* hypo-,hyper-) 7. Alterations in attention/attention behavior
Musculoskeletal	Structural framework	1. Joint abnormality 2. Asymmetrical posture 3. Stiff/difficult movement 4. Pain in joints on movement or handling 5. Swelling of joints 6. Inability to feed effectively (poor sucking ability) 7. Lack of smooth, coordinated movement 8. Congenital abnormalities
Neurological	Regulation of behavior/physiological function	1. Seizures 2. Tremor 3. Alterations in sensation 4. Hypotonia (ragdoll) 5. Hypertonia (stiff) 6. Sudden "startle-like" movements 7. Jerky random movement 8. Attention/alerting disturbances 9. Sleep pattern disturbances 10. Lack of smooth coordinated movement 11. Congenital abnormalities 12. Visual impairment, hearing deficiency, muteness 13. Poor feeding

Table 34-2. *Frequently Used Tests and Measures by Categories*

	Developmental	Motor Function or Reflex	Sensory Integration	Neuro-Physiological	Other (specify)
Barraga Diagnostic Assessment Procedure (of Efficiency of Visual Function)	X				X(Use of vision in visually impaired children)
Bayley Scale of Infant Development	X				
Callier-Azusa Scale	X				X(Assessment of multihandicapped children)
Central Institute for the Deaf Preschool Performance Scale	X	X	X		
Denver Developmental Screening Test–Revised	X				
Developmental Assessment for the Newborn or High-Risk Infant	X	X	X	X	
Beery's Developmental Test of Visual Motor Integration			X		
Gesell Developmental Tests	X				
Gestational Age Assessment	X				X(Cutaneous musculoskeletal)
Goodenough–Harris Drawing Test			X		X(Cognitive maturation)
Illinois Test of Psycholinguistic Abilities			X		X(Cognitive)
Joint Mobility		X			X(Musculoskeletal)
Miller Assessment for Preschoolers	X	X	X	X	X(Learning potential
Minneapolis Preschool Screening Instrument	X	X			
Neonatal Behavioral Assessment Scale (Brazelton)	X	X	X		
Neurological Assessment during the First Year of Life (Amile–Tison)	X	X	X	X	
Ordinal Scales of Infant Psychological Development (Uzgaris–Hunt)	X	X	X		
Parent Denver Questionnaire	X				X(Parent stimulation)
Pre-Term Behavioral Assessment Scale (Als–Brazelton)	X		X	X	
Reflexes in Motor Development (Crutchfield, Barnes, Heriza)		X			
Southern California Sensory Integration Tests	X	X	X	X	
Southern California Postrotary Nystagmus Test			X		

Is there dysrhythm in the sleep–rest cycle of the child, mother, or caregiver?

Is there sensory or social isolation?

Are thought processes impaired?

Is there a communication impairment?

Again, these questions are presented as samples to encourage and direct therapists to address fully less tangible but important factors that often clarify the occupational therapy plan and the ordering of therapeutic goals.

To complete the evaluative stages of the occupational therapy process, the therapist must address and synthesize a multiplicity of data collected relating to the child's status:

1. Physical
2. Neurodevelopmental
3. Motor performance
4. Sensory integration
5. Adaptive behavior

Figure 34-4 is an example of a comprehensive evaluation tool useful in the identification of a young child's developmental abilities.[3] This type of assessment enables therapists to pinpoint levels of reflex maturation, sensory integration, and gross and fine motor skill attainments in daily living skills as a basis for planning the occupational therapy program. This data must be viewed and interrelated with information about the child's social, cultural, and familial condition. From this synthesis, a tentative plan of treatment should be followed by problem identification objectives and treatment procedures. This synthesizing process is frequently the most complicated stage of work for therapists. If this stage of work is well executed, the ordering of occupational therapy processes, goals, objectives, and procedures will advance the child's functional ability to the highest level of expectation.

The Reflex Process

Knowledge of reflexes and proficiency in reflex examination are key to the pediatric occupational therapist's understanding of infants' and children's normal and abnormal movement patterns as well as the status of nervous system integrity. The therapist's knowledge of the reflex process aids in predicting the future function of a child when abnormality is noted. This knowledge will aid the therapist in determining the approximate developmental age of the child and in directing the treatment plan.

According to Easton, "normal motor coordination is based to a huge extent on reflexes. They may probably underlie all or most volitional movement in man."[6] It is important to conceptualize reflex behavior as a process in which sensory input (stimuli) initiates limited reac-

tions (movement), which then create more sensory input, resulting in further actions and ultimately coordination of these chains of reaction as the basis for all volitional movement.[4]

Reflexes and reactions are classified as:

1. *Primitive reflexes,* which begin developing *in utero* and are present at birth. These reflexes are strongly evident and have an effect on the distribution of postural tone throughout the body.
2. *Prehensile reactions* occur at birth and differentiate man from other primates. Reaching is incorporated in the prehensile reaction.
3. *Righting reactions* allow the child to move from a horizontal position to upright and provide control in the midline position.
4. *Equilibrium reactions* are tonic and phasic reactions that develop after righting reactions and provide control of posture despite changes in the center of gravity. These reactions, when efficient, are the center of mature movement and human adaptable function.

Table 34-3 describes neurophysiological reflex processes and the influence on movement and adaptation consisting of primitive reflexes, prehensile reactions, righting reactions, and equilibrium reactions based on data previously developed by Crutchfield, Barnes and Heriza. As noted, each reflex or reaction is described by name, position of the child, type of stimulus, location of stimulus, response of child, adaptation factors, neurological origin, and reflex age range.

The Occupational Therapy Plan

The occupational therapy plan evolves from the evaluation process that identifies strengths and weaknesses that the child is experiencing and that may influence the child's world. Problems should be clarified as stated goals. Many times, broad goal statements will be needed as a guide in the overall occupational therapy plan. To achieve these major goals, therapists must delineate more specific short-range goals or objectives that can be clearly stated as measurable objectives. From such objectives, treatment procedures and modes can be planned to implement the objectives and to adjust procedures in an orderly way.

Adjustment of therapeutic goals, objectives, and methods for attaining such are based on the success or lack of success in reaching these treatment objectives. Objectives achieved or not achieved require careful examination by occupational therapists providing direct services, as well as by supervisors and administrator–managers of occupational therapy service programs. Therapeutic goal achievement may be directly related to the quality of the service provided or may be complicated by other factors inherent in the service system.

(text continues on page 626)

Infant–Parent Training Program
Sensory Motor Integration Assessment[3,7]

Code: 1 + 5 = Present in increasing strength

A = Absent

(#) = Abnormally present

(A) = Abnormally absent

Child's name _____
Birthdate _____
Diagnosis _____
Referral source _____
Examiners _____

	Date	C.A.	M.A.	M.Q.
Test 1				
Test 2				
Test 3				
Test 4				

I. Neuromuscular Reflex and Gross Motor Development

Position	Reflex	Grading 1 2 3 4	Gestational age/wks 28 32 34 35 36 37	Age in months 0 1 2 3 4 5 6 7 8 9 10 11 12 13 15 18 21 24 30 36 48 60	Comments
	I. Primitive				
1. sup	Rooting				1.
2. sup	Sucking				2.
3. sup	Traction				3.
4. sup	Moro				4.
5. sup	Crossed extension				5.
6. sup	Flexor withdrawal				6.
7. sup	Plantar grasp				7.
8. pr	Galant				8.
9. sup	Neonatal neck righting				9.
10. vert	Plantar placing legs				10.
11. vert	Neonatal positive support				11.
12. vert	Spontaneous stepping				12.
13.	Tonic labyrinthine prone				13.
14.	Supine				14.
15. vert	Plantar placing arms				15.
16.	ATNR				16.
17. sup	STNR				17.

Figure 34-4. Infant–parent training program assessment (*continues on following pages*).

609

Infant-Parent Training Program
Sensory Motor Integration Assessment[3,7]

Code: 1 + 5 = Present in increasing strength

A = Absent

(#) = Abnormally present

(A) = Abnormally absent

Date	C.A.	M.A.	M.Q.
Test 1			
Test 2			
Test 3			
Test 4			

Child's name _____

Birthdate _____

Diagnosis _____

Referral source _____

Examiners _____

I. Neuromuscular Reflex and Gross Motor Development

Position	Reflex	Grading 1 2 3 4	Gestational age/wks 28 32 34 35 36 37	Age in months 0 1 2 3 4 5 6 7 8 9 10 11 12 13 15 18 21 24 30 36 48 60	Comments
	II. Prehension Reactions				
18. sup	Palmar grasp				18.
19. sup	Avoidance reaction				19.
20.	Instinctual grasp				20.
	III. Righting Reactions				
21.	Labyrinthine righting prone				21.
22.	Supine				22.
23.	Tilting				23.
24.	Optical righting prone				24.
25.	Supine				25.
26.	Tilting				26.
27. sup	Neck righting				27.
28. sup	Body righting				28.
29. pr	Landau				29.
	IV. Equilibrium Reactions				
30. vert	Visual placing arms				30.
31. vert	Visual placing legs				31.
32. sit	Protective extension forward				32.
33. sit	Protective extension sideways				33.
34. sit	Protective extension backwards				34.
35. vert	Positive support				35.
36.	Equilibrium prone				36.
37.	Equilibrium supine				37.
38. sit	Equilibrium sitting				38.
39.	Equilibrium quadriped				39.
40.	Equilibrium standing				40.
41. std.	Staggering reaction (protective)				41.

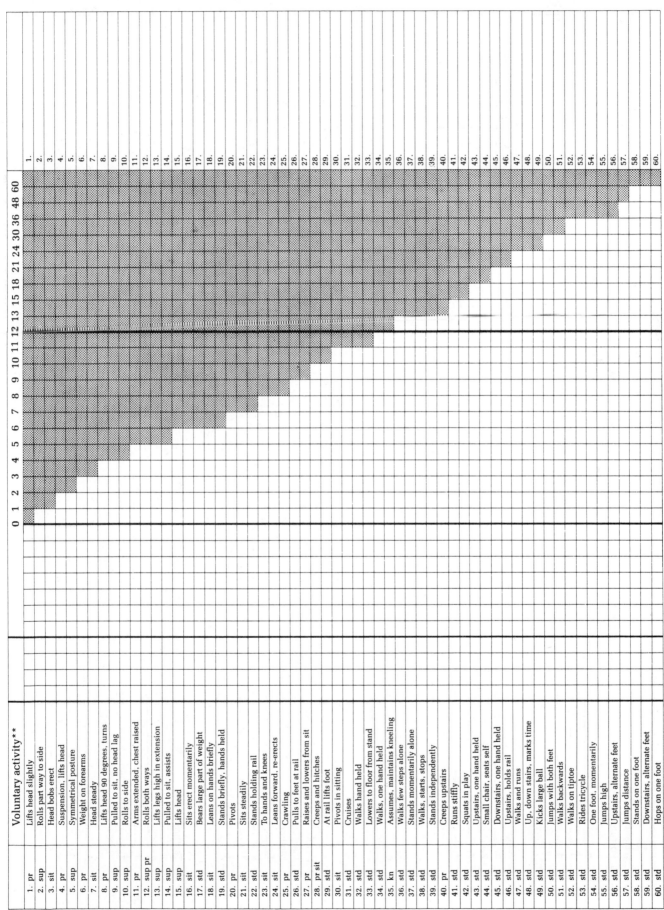

	Voluntary activity**	0 1 2 3 4 5 6 7 8 9 10 11 12 13 15 18 21 24 30 36 48 60	
1. pr	Lifts head slightly		1.
2. sup	Rolls part way to side		2.
3. sit	Head bobs erect		3.
4. pr	Suspension, lifts head		4.
5. sup	Symmetrical posture		5.
6. pr	Weight on forearms		6.
7. sit	Head steady		7.
8. pr	Lifts head 90 degrees, turns		8.
9. sup	Pulled to sit, no head lag		9.
10. sup	Rolls to side		10.
11. pr	Arms extended, chest raised		11.
12. sup pr	Rolls both ways		12.
13. sup	Lifts legs high in extension		13.
14. sup	Pulled to sit, assists		14.
15. sup	Lifts head		15.
16. sit	Sits erect momentarily		16.
17. sit	Bears large part of weight		17.
18. sit	Leans on hands briefly		18.
19. std	Stands briefly, hands held		19.
20. pr	Pivots		20.
21. sit	Sits steadily		21.
22. std	Stands holding rail		22.
23. sit	To hands and knees		23.
24. sit	Leans forward, re-erects		24.
25. pr	Crawling		25.
26. std	Pulls to feet at rail		26.
27. pr	Raises and lowers from sit		27.
28. pr sit	Creeps and hitches		28.
29. std	At rail lifts foot		29.
30. sit	Pivots in sitting		30.
31. std	Cruises		31.
32. std	Walks hand held		32.
33. std	Lowers to floor from stand		33.
34. std	Walks, one hand held		34.
35. kn	Assumes, maintains kneeling		35.
36. std	Walks few steps alone		36.
37. std	Stands momentarily alone		37.
38. std	Walks, starts, stops		38.
39. std	Stands independently		39.
40. pr	Creeps upstairs		40.
41. std	Runs stiffly		41.
42. std	Squats in play		42.
43. std	Upstairs, one hand held		43.
44. std	Small chair, seats self		44.
45. std	Downstairs, one hand held		45.
46. std	Upstairs, holds rail		46.
47. std	Walks and runs		47.
48. std	Up, down stairs, marks time		48.
49. std	Kicks large ball		49.
50. std	Jumps with both feet		50.
51. std	Walks backwards		51.
52. std	Walks on tiptoe		52.
53. std	Rides tricycle		53.
54. std	One foot, momentarily		54.
55. std	Jumps high		55.
56. std	Upstairs, alternate feet		56.
57. std	Jumps distance		57.
58. std	Stands on one foot		58.
59. std	Downstairs, alternate feet		59.
60. std	Hops on one foot		60.

**Criteria based on Hoskins, T.A., Squires, J.E., Dev. assessment, Phys. Ther., 53:117-126, 1973.

Figure 34-4. (*continues*)

II. Physical Findings

A. Posture

1. _____
2. _____
3. _____
4. _____

B. Muscle tone

1. _____
2. _____
3. _____
4. _____

C. Range of motion

1. _____
2. _____
3. _____
4. _____

	Date	C.A.	F.M.A.	F.M.Q.
Test 1				
Test 2				
Test 3				
Test 4				

D. Adaptive appliances

1. _____
2. _____
3. _____
4. _____

E. Other findings or comments

1. _____
2. _____
3. _____
4. _____

III. Activities of Daily Living

A. Feeding

Method

1. _____
2. _____
3. _____
4. _____

Quantity

1. _____
2. _____
3. _____
4. _____

Texture

1. _____
2. _____
3. _____
4. _____

Sensitivity

1. _____
2. _____
3. _____
4. _____

Assistance devices indicated _____

Reflexive feeding

	Grading			
	1	2	3	4

0–life   1. Gag reflex
            2. Rooting
            3. Suckling

1–5 mos.   1. Tongue protrusion
            2. Bite reflex
            3. Suck—swallow

Voluntary feeding

	1	2	3	4

4 mos.
1. Lip closure
2. Sucking
3. Anticipates food on sight

6–9 mos.
1. Vertical chewing
2. Holds own bottle

9 mos.
1. Rotary chewing
2. Lateral tongue movement
3. Tongue protraction
4. Tongue retraction
5. Tongue to palate
6. Finger feeding

12 mos.
1. Grasps spoon (picks up)
2. Drooling controlled except at meals
3. Drinks from cup (if held)

15 mos.
1. Holds cup; quickly tips
2. Inserts spoon in dish; poor filling
3. Spoon to mouth; may turn over

18 mos.
1. Fills spoon with food
2. Drinks from cup, 2-handed
3. Diff. inserting spoon
4. Considerable spilling

2 yr.
1. Drinks cup, 1-hd. repl. cup
2. Feeds self from spoon
3. Automatic swallowing

3 yr.
1. Feeds self c̄ spoon; may spill some

4 yr.
1. Feeds self with fork

B. Dressing

	1	2	3	4

1 yr.
1. Cooperates in dressing
2. Removes socks (from toe)

2 yr.
1. Removes shoe (untied)
2. Pushes down pants and removes

C. Grooming

2 yr.
1. Washes, dries hands (partl.)
2. Wipes face

D. Written communication

	1	2	3	4

1 yr.
1. Discr. use of crayon

18 mos.
1. Spontaneous scribbling

2 yr.
1. Vert.-horiz. patterns

3 yr.
1. Copies circles
2. Copies vertical
3. Copies horizontal
4. Imitates X

Comments

1. _____
2. _____
3. _____
4. _____

Figure 34-4. (*continues*)

613

IV. Upper Extremity Functional Activities

A. Prehension and bilateral hand usage

			Grading			
			1	2	3	4
1–4 mos.	1. Both hands fisted	R				
		L				
	2. Mass motor activity reac.	R				
		L				
	3. Hands open	R				
		L				
	4. Plays regarding hands	R				
		L				
	5. Brings hands to mouth	R				
		L				
4–8 mos.	Voluntary grasp pronation					
	1. Palmar	R				
		L				
	2. Ulnar	R				
		L				
6 mos.	Eye-hand coordination					
	1. Arms used, shoulder cont.	R				
		L				
	2. Raking grasp	R				
		L				
	3. Transfers object	R				
		L				
7 mos.	1. Radial palmar grasp	R				
		L				
8 mos.	1. Lateral pinch	R				
		L				
9 mos.	1. Crude pincer grasp	R				
		L				
10 mos.	1. Pikes finger in hole	R				
		L				
12 mos.	1. Precise pincer	R				
		L				
	2. Bangs 2 obj. together	R				
		L				
	3. Supinated grasp develop.	R				
		L				
	4. Reaches for large object, both arms	R				
		L				
12 mos. con't.	5. Brings 1″ cube over another					

		Grading			
		1	2	3	4
15 mos.	1. Places objects in and out of container				
18 mos.	1. Builds 3-blk. tower				
	2. Tosses ball undir.				
	3. Puts peg in 1″ hole				
	4. Turns pg. 2-3 at time				
2 yr.	1. Turns pg. 1 at time				
	2. Strings beads (1″)				
	3. Builds 6-blk. tower				
	4. Throws				
	5. Hand pref. R L				
3 yr.	1. Builds 9-blk. tower				
	2. Assists with 1 hand				
	3. Screws lid on jar				
	4. 10 pellets in bottle (30 sec.)				
	5. Grasps w/extended wrist and good thumb opposition				
	6. Turns door knob with forearm rotation				
	7. Imitates cube bridge				

Comments:

1. _____

2. _____

3. _____

4. _____

V. Sensory Integration

A. Tactile processing

Comments ___ 1. ___ 2. ___ 3. ___ 4.
Seeking ___ 1. ___ 2. ___ 3. ___ 4.
Avoids/withdraws ___ 1. ___ 2. ___ 3. ___ 4.

B. Postural adaptation

Comments ___ 1. ___ 2. ___ 3. ___ 4.
Seeking reinforcements ___ 1. ___ 2. ___ 3. ___ 4.
Withdraws/insecure ___ 1. ___ 2. ___ 3. ___ 4.
Phasic/lacks midline
  stability ___ 1. ___ 2. ___ 3. ___ 4.

C. Bilateral motor integration

Comments ___ 1. ___ 2. ___ 3. ___ 4.
Midline ___ R-L ___ L-R 1. ___ R-L ___ L-R 2. ___ R-L ___ L-R 3. ___ R-L ___ L-R 4.
Head rotation ___ 1. ___ 2. ___ 3. ___ 4.
Trunk rotation ___ 1. ___ 2. ___ 3. ___ 4.

D. Motor planning

Comments ___ 1. ___ 2. ___ 3. ___ 4.
Moves to pursue object
  efficiently ___ 1. ___ 2. ___ 3. ___ 4.
Mounts efficiently ___ 1. ___ 2. ___ 3. ___ 4.
Reproduces imitative ___ 1. ___ 2. ___ 3. ___ 4.

E. Visual processing

Comments ___ 1. ___ 2. ___ 3. ___ 4.
Eye preference ___ R ___ L ___ R ___ L ___ R ___ L ___ R ___ L
Fixates on light ___ 1. ___ 2. ___ 3. ___ 4.
Uses neck rot. to pur. ___ 1. ___ 2. ___ 3. ___ 4.
Isol. eye move. to pur. ___ 1. ___ 2. ___ 3. ___ 4.
Eyes follow past 90° ___ 1. ___ 2. ___ 3. ___ 4.
Converges ___ 1. ___ 2. ___ 3. ___ 4.
Midline disturbance ___ 1. ___ 2. ___ 3. ___ 4.
Quality of ex. ocular
  pursuit ___ 1. ___ 2. ___ 3. ___ 4.
Postrotary nystagmus ___ 1. ___ 2. ___ 3. ___ 4.
  ___ L 1. ___ L 2. ___ L 3. ___ L 4.
  ___ R 1. ___ R 2. ___ R 3. ___ R 4.

Figure 34-4. (*continues*)

F. Auditory-language processing

Comments _____
         _____

	Grading			
	1	2	3	4
1 mo.				
3 mos.				
4 mos.				
6 mos.				
9 mos.				
10 mos.				
24 mos.				
30 mos.				
36 mos.				

1 mo.   Responds to sound

3 mos.   Vocal noise, resembles speech

4 mos.   Turns to noise and voice

6 mos.   Distinguishes angry/friendly voice

9 mos.   Comprehends a few gestures

10 mos. Comprehends and waves "bye-bye"

24 mos. Attains 50 word vocabulary or 2-word sentences;
         Im. absent models; pretends; reconstructs memories

30 mos. 3-word sentences

36 mos. Adult grammatical structure

G. Comments:

1. _____

2. _____

3. _____

4. _____

Figure 34-4. (end of figure)

Table 34-3. Neurophysiological Reflex Processes and the Influence on Movement and Adaptation

	Reflex (See) (references below)	Position	Stimulus	Location	Responses	Adaptation	Origin	Reflex Age Range Initiation	Reflex Age Range Inhibition
Primitive Reflexes									
1.	Rooting (15, 33)	Supine	Light Tactile	Mouth	Opens mouth; rotation extension, and flexion of head follow	Search for breast or bottle in the direction of the stimulus	Pons	28 weeks' gestation	3 months
2.	Sucking (12, 33, 37, 39)	Supine	Light Tactile	Oral cavity	Close mouth, suck, and swallow	Obtain nourishment, develop tongue movement, and, later, produce sound	Trigeminal nerve	28 weeks' gestation	2–5 months
3.	Traction (46)	Supine	Proprioception	Forearms	Total flexion of upper extremeties	Momentary grasp with total flexion of UE leading to voluntary reach and grasp	Pons	28 weeks' gestation	2–5 months
4.	Moro (1, 2, 5, 9, 19, 20, 34, 35, 36, 37, 39, 41, 46)	Supine	Sudden change of head position > 30° extension (proprioception)	Head and trunk	1st: UEs extend and abduct; hands open and LEs may extend. 2nd: Flexion and adduction of UEs; hands close; may cry	If persists, will interfere with head control, sitting equilibrium, and protective reactions affecting adaptability of child for movement in space	Brainstem; medulla 1	28 weeks' gestation	5–6 months
5.	Crossed extension (1, 4, 11, 24, 28)	Supine	Noxious tactile	Ball of foot	1st flexion, then extension and adduction of opposite LE	Preparation for reciprocal LE use; persistence indicates pathology and interference in reciprocation and in walking	Spinal	28 weeks' gestation	1–2 months
6.	Flexor withdrawal (1, 2, 4, 16, 27, 34, 37, 39, 45)	Supine	Noxious tactile	Sole of foot	Withdrawal with flexion of hip and knee; dorsiflexion of foot with toe extension	Protection or defense. If persists, will interfere with weight-bearing in standing	Spinal	28 weeks' gestation	1–2 months
7.	Plantar grasp (31, 47)	Supine	Firm pressure	Ball of foot	Grasps with toes (flexion)	If persists, interferes with standing and walking; may evoke toe walking	Spinal	28 weeks' gestation	4–9 months
8.	Galant (8, 38)	Prone	Noxious tactile	Along paravertebral column from 12th rib to iliac crest	Incurvature of spine to same side	Organizes for trunk adaptation. If persists, interferes with symmetric stability of the trunk, independent sitting, standing. May lead to scoliosis	Spinal	32 weeks' gestation	2 months

(continued)

Table 34-3. Neurophysiological Reflex Processes and the Influence on Movement and Adaptation   (continued)

Reflex (See) (references below)	Position	Stimulus	Location	Responses	Adaptation	Origin	Reflex Age Range	
							Initiation	*Inhibition*
9. Neonatal neck righting (6, 27, 30, 31, 33, 37, 38, 41)	Supine	Proprioception to neck rotators	Neck rotators	Log rolling—supine to side	Rolling on body axis from back to right and left sides. Persistence delays segmented rolling and other developmental milestones, especially bilateral integration	Mudulla	34 weeks' gestation	4–5 months
10. Plantar placing of legs (21)	Vertical	Proprioceptive	LEs; dorsum of feet (stretch)	Placing of feet; flexion of hips/knees; dorsiflexion at ankle followed by LE extension & support on surface	Correlates to spontaneous stepping—primitive form of ambulation and stepping over objects	Spinal	35 weeks' gestation	2 months
11. Neonatal positive support (1)	Vertical	Proprioceptive	LEs; soles of feet	Partial weight bearing with hips & knees flexed & ankle plantar flexion in contact with floor surface	Prerequisite for stepping. Preparation for motion; not static. Weight-bearing	Spinal	35 weeks' gestation	1–2 months
12. Spontaneous stepping (1, 40)	Vertical	Proprioceptive and tactile	LEs with body inclined forward	Positive support then walking (coordinated & rhythmic with heel touching first)	Prerequisite for walking	Spinal and brainstem	37 weeks' gestation	2 months
13. Tonic labyrinthine (3, 17)	Prone	Head/face down in relation to gravity	Prone; head midline	Increases flexor tone of neck, UEs, & LEs	Contributes, when integrated, into a supportive framework of nonstressful movement	Inner ear—otlitic utrilical maculae	Birth	6 months
14.	Supine	Head/face up in relation to gravity	Supine; head midline	Increases extensor tone of neck, UEs, & LEs	If persistent, interferes with head control, coming to sit, rolling, creeping, and standing	Intermedulla		
15. Plantar arms placing (21, 34, 43)	Vertical	Proprioceptive (stretch)	UEs; dorsum of hands	Placing of hands: Flexion of shoulder and elbow, then fingers and wrist abduct and extend. Followed by extension of elbows & shoulders for UE support (infants may remain fisted)	Requisite for supporting body weight on forearms and extended arms	Spinal or brainstem	Birth	2 months

618

16.	Asymmetrical tonic neck (3, 6, 8, 17, 22, 23, 25, 28, 42, 44–49)	Supine	Proprioceptive (stretch) visual for infants	a) Neck muscles (rotation) b) Gaze to induce neck rotation	a) Extension of UEs and LEs on face side; flexion on skull side b) As above, but not obligatory	Contributes to the supportive framework of nonstressful movement Persistent obligatory presence indicates pathological state, inducing lack of symmetrical posture, reach and grasp, normal rolling, unsupported sitting, and a deficiency in walking. Globally, a lack of ability to develop motorically. Structural deformity (*i.e.*, scoliosis); hip subluxation (skull side). Nonobligatory presence interferes in motor planning, bilateral integration, and reading comprehension.	Atlanto-occipital and axial joints to upper cervical roots, integrating at medulla	Birth	4–6 months
17.	Symmetrical tonic neck (10, 28, 30, 31, 41)	Prone	Proprioceptive	Neck muscles, flexion and extension of neck	With neck flexion, UEs flex and LEs extend; with neck extension, UEs extend and LEs flex	Works strongly with asymmetrical tonic and tonic labyrinthine reflexes to influence tonic postural stability. Prolonged influence interferes with reciprocal creeping, sitting, standing, and walking	Same as for asymmetrical tonic neck reflex	4–6 months	8–12 months

Prehension Reactions

18.	Palmar grasp (42, 47)	Supine	Proprioception (palmar pressure)	Pressure on ulnar surface of palm	*"Catching phase,"* quick flexion and adduction of fingers. *"Holding phase,"* sustained finger flexion	Primitive precursor to coordinated voluntary grasp. If persists, will interfere with releasing and the development of prehension and hand skills	Subcortical	Birth	4–6 months
19.	Avoidance (43)	Supine, sitting or standing	Light tactile stroke	Dorsum or ulnar surface of hands	Fingers open; move away from stimulus	May cause overpronation of forearms, flexion of wrist, abduction extension of fingers. If persists, will strongly reduce tactile exploration and hand usage	Subcortical	Birth	6–7 years

(continued)

619

Table 34-3. Neurophysiological Reflex Processes and the Influence on Movement and Adaptation *(continued)*

	Reflex *(See references below)*	Position	Stimulus	Location	Responses	Adaptation	Origin	Reflex Age Range	
								Initiation	Inhibition
20.	Instinctive grasp (19, 28, 30, 31, 41)	Supine, sitting or standing	Light tactile proprioception	Ulnar or radial border of hands	Orientation of hand and fractionation of total grasping reflex for voluntary grasping patterns	Facilitates radial palmar grasp, thumb–2–3 finger grasp, and voluntary pincer grasp	Subcortical	4–11 months	Persists

Righting Reactions

	Reflex *(See references below)*	Position	Stimulus	Location	Responses	Adaptation	Origin	Reflex Age Range	
								Initiation	Inhibition
21.	Labyrinthine head righting *prone* (8, 28, 29, 37, 41)	Prone	Otoliths of the labyrinthine	Neck, without vision	Orients head (in space and to ground) in an upward position by neck extension	In general, automatic reactions that allow for normal standing position and preserve balance in the process of changing from prone or supine to fully upright position. Prerequisite for head control in the normal upright position. Initially, infant uses this reaction to clear the head in the prone position. In general, suppresses primitive abnormal reflexes and facilitates normal movement for sitting, creeping, standing, and walking	Red nucleus midbrain	Birth–2 months	Persists
22.	Labyrinthine head righting *supine* (8, 28, 29, 37, 41)	Supine	Otoliths of the labyrinthine	Neck, without vision	Orients head (in space and to ground) in an upward position by neck flexion				
23.	Labyrinthine head righting *tilting* (8, 28, 29, 37, 41)	Vertical	Otiliths of the labyrinthine	Neck, without vision	Orients head (in space and to ground) in an upward position by tilting of head				
24.	Optical righting *prone* (8, 26, 37, 39, 43)	Prone	Vision versus labyrinthine	Neck, with visual receptors	Orient head in space in an upright position in extension	As in labyrinthine head righting, need the subsequent motor development requiring head control in the normal upright position	Cerebral cortex, especially occipital	2 months	Persists
25.	Optical righting *supine* (8, 26, 37, 39, 43)	Supine	Vision	Neck, with visual receptors	Orients head in space in an upright position in flexion				

No.		Vertical	Vision						
26.	Optical righting *tilting* (8, 26, 37, 39, 43)			Neck, with visual receptors	Orients head in space in an upright position in lateral tilting				
27.	Neck righting (11, 30, 31, 34, 41)	Supine	Proprioceptive (stretch)	Neck–lumbar rotation	Body alignment in rotation on axis with segmentation. Shoulder–thorax rotation followed by trunk–pelvic rolling	Facilitates rolling for pursuits and for proceeding with head control to sitting, creeping, standing, and walking. Deficiency may indicate poor bilateral integration	Midbrain	4–6 months	5 years
28.	Body righting (11, 30, 31, 37, 40)	Supine	Proprioceptive (stretch) and tactile	Pelvis rotation with hip flexion	Trunk (thoracic rotation) on body axis with segmentation; pelvic–trunk rotation followed by shoulder–thoracic rotation on body axis	Facilitates rolling for pursuits and for proceeding to sitting, creeping, standing and walking. Deficiency indicates diminished bilateral integration	Red nucleus of the midbrain	4–6 months	5 years
29.	Landau (3, 8, 13, 18, 30, 31, 34, 37)	Prone	Proprioceptive (stretch)	Neck extensors	Increases prone extension tone	Dissociates flexor posture and assists neck extension in prone (especially pivot prone) coming to sit, and standing. Absence is associated with motor weakness and mental retardation. Early or exaggerated Landau is associated with spasticity or increased muscle tone. Delay in Landau will retard the development of prone extension, sitting and standing, and related developmental adaptations	Diffuse	3–4 months	12–24 months

(continued)

621

Table 34-3. *Neurophysiological Reflex Processes and the Influence on Movement and Adaptation* (continued)

Equilibrium Reactions

Reflex (See references below)	Position	Stimulus	Location	Responses	Adaptation	Origin	Reflex Age Range	
							Initiation	Inhibition
30. Visual placing arms (34, 43)	Vertical	Visual (advance UEs/hands toward supporting surface)	Hands	Flexion of shoulder/elbow followed by extension of elbow/wrist/fingers for support	Needed for weight-bearing on forearms and extended arms; also for accurate placing of hands, creeping, and visual reaching and grasping	Cortical	3–4 months	Persists
31. Visual placing legs (8, 34, 43)	Vertical	Visual (advance LEs/feet toward supporting surface)	Feet	Hip and knee flexion followed by dorsiflexion of the ankle and LE extension for support on surface	Needed for LE weight-bearing on knees and feet and for accurate placing of LEs in creeping, knee activity, and standing/walking	Cortical	3–5 months	Persists
32. Protective extension *forward*	Sitting	Vestibular and proprioceptive	Displace body forward	Flexion of shoulder with elbow, wrist, and finger extension	In general, protects body from harm when center of gravity of the body is displaced. Facilitates support with extended arms in sitting and is used to attain weight-bearing activities with UEs	Midbrain, basal ganglia, brainstem with cortical input	6–9 months	Persists
33. Protective extension *sideways* (1, 8, 14, 29, 30, 31, 34)	Sitting	Vestibular and proprioceptive	Displace body sideways	Abduction of shoulder with elbow extension and abduction of the fingers	Sitting with arm support and protection against falling sideways. Needed for rotation in sitting		7 months	Persists
34. Protective extension UEs *backward*	Sitting	Vestibular, proprioceptive, and visual	Displace body backward	Total extension of shoulder, elbow, wrist, and fingers with finger abduction	Sitting with arm support, rotating body on its axis, and protection from falling backward. Prolonged Moro may interfere with this development		9–10 months	Persists
35. Positive support (6, 7, 28, 34, 43)	Vertical	Proprioceptive, vestibular	Ball of feet	Hip abduction with external rotation, knee extension with dorsiflexion of ankles (cocontraction)	Facilitates weight-bearing/standing and provides generalized support (not rigid) for activity and movement. Increased obligatory extensor tone with hip abduction and plantar flexion of ankle indicates pathologic influence and prevents normal gait, sitting, and stair walking. Structured deformity may occur secondarily to increased extensor tone	Midbrain or thalamus	6–9 months	Persists

622

36.	Equilibrium *prone* (6, 29, 30, 31, 32)	Prone	Vestibular, proprioceptive, and visual	Displace the body, in prone laterally	Curvature of the spine, concave to the side being stressed or upward side, with abduction & extension of the extremities. Head turns toward upward side	In general, equilibrium reactions are automatic reactions which preserve body's center of balance when the supporting base is unstable. Also, equilibrium facilitates movement and postural adaptation to different gravitational changes	Cortical	5 months	Persists
37.	Equilibrium *supine* (31)	Supine	Vestibular, proprioceptive, and visual	Displace the body, laterally in supine	Curvature of the spine, concave to the side being stressed or upward side, with abduction and extension of the UEs			7–8 months	Persists
38.	Equilibrium *sitting* (31)	Sitting	Vestibular, proprioceptive, and visual	Displace the body in sitting, to the right and left, forward and backward	Curvature of the spine, concave to the side being stressed or upward side, with abduction and extension of the UEs	Stable, prone, and supine with beginning sitting equilibrium are necessary for sitting without support		7–8 months	Persists
39.	Equilibrium *quadruped* (31)	Quadruped	Vestibular, proprioceptive, and visual	Displace the body on all fours	Curvature of the spine, concave to the side being stressed with increased UE and LE extension on stressed side	Stable prone, supine, and sitting equilibrium with beginning equilibrium in quadruped are needed for creeping	Cortical	9–12 months	Persists
40.	Equilibrium *standing* (31)	Biped	Vestibular, proprioceptive, and visual	Displace the body in standing	Curvature of the spine, concave to side being stressed with abduction and extension of UEs and LEs	Stable equilibrium in quadruped and beginning biped standing reactions are needed for standing and walking. Delayed or deficient equilibrium reactions will interfere with all forms of volitional movement and restrict mobility and adaptability.	Cortical	12–21 months	Persists

(continued)

Table 34-3. *Neurophysiological Reflex Processes and the Influence on Movement and Adaptation* *(continued)*

Reflex (See references below)	Position	Stimulus	Location	Responses	Adaptation	Origin	Reflex Age Range — Initiation	Reflex Age Range — Inhibition
41. Staggering reaction (protective) (14, 16, 29, 42)	Biped	Vestibular, proprioceptive, and visual	Displace the body in biped position forward, backward, and sideways	One or more steps in direction of displacement to maintain balance	Perfected staggering ensures safe independent walking and recovery from loss of balance in concert with protective reactions of UEs.	Brainstem, midbrain, basal ganglia with cortical input	15–18 months	Persists

Development of Prehension

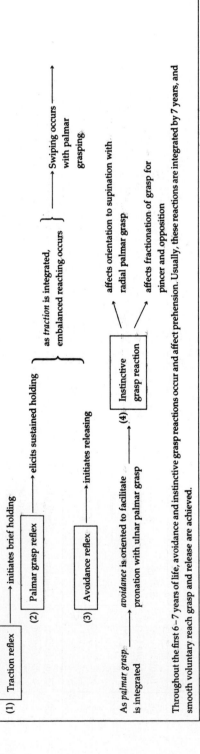

Throughout the first 6–7 years of life, avoidance and instinctive grasp reactions occur and affect prehension. Usually, these reactions are integrated by 7 years, and smooth voluntary reach grasp and release are achieved.

Reflex* References

1. Andre–Thomas, Chesni Y, Saint–Anne Dargassies S: The Neurological Examination of the Infant. Clin Dev Med, No. 1, 1960
2. Andre–Thomas, Autgaerden S: Locomotion from Pre to Post Natal Life. Clin Dev Med, No. 24, 1963
3. Ayres AJ: Sensory Integration and Learning Disorders. California, Western Psychological Services, 1972
4. Beintema DJ: A Neurological Study of Newborn Infants. Clin Dev Med, No. 28, 1968
5. Bench J, Collyer Y, Langford C, et al: A comparison between the neonatal sound-evoked startle response and the head-drop (Moro) reflex. Dev Med Child Neurol 14:308, 1972
6. Bobath B: A study of abnormal postural reflex activities in patients with lesions of the central nervous system. Physiotherapy 40:259, 1954
7. Bobath B: Abnormal Postural Reflex Activity Caused by Brain Lesions. London, William Heinemann Medical Books, 1971
8. Bobath B: The very early treatment of cerebral palsy. Dev Med Child Neurol 9:373, 1967
9. Bobath B: Motor development, its effect on general development, and application to the treatment of cerebral palsy. Physiotherapy 57:526, 1971
10. Bobath K: The Motor Deficit in Patients with Cerebral Palsy. Clin Dev Med, No. 23, 1969
11. Bobath K, Bobath B: Cerebral Palsy. In Pearson P, Williams C (eds): Physical Therapy Services in the Developmental Disabilities, pp 31–185. Springfield, IL Charles C Thomas 1972
12. Connor FP, Williams GG, Siepp J: A Program Guide for Infants and Toddlers with Neuromotor and Other Developmental Disabilities, Experimental Edition. New York, United Cerebral Palsy Association, 1976.
13. Cupps C, Plescia MG, Houser C: The Landau reaction: A clinical and electromyographic analysis. Dev Med Child Neurol 18:41, 1976
14. Easton TA: On the normal use of reflexes. Am Sci 60:591, 1972
15. Farber S: Sensorimotor Evaluation and Treatment Procedures for Allied Health Personnel. Indianapolis, Occupational Therapy Curriculum, Indiana University Medical Center, 1974
16. Fiorentino MR: Reflex Testing Methods for Evaluating CNS Development. Springfield, IL, Charles C Thomas, 1963

17. Fukuda T: Studies on human dynamic postures from the viewpoint of postural reflexes. Acta Otolaryngol (Suppl 161) 1960

18. Gilfoyle E, Grady A: A developmental theory of somatosensory perception. In Henderson A, Coryell J (eds): The Body Senses and Perceptual Deficit. Boston, Boston University, 1973

19. Goldstein K, Landis C, Hunt W, et al: Moro reflex and startle pattern. Arch Neurol Psychiatr 40:322, 1938

20. Gordon MG: The Moro embrace reflex in infancy: Its incidence and significance. Am J Dis Child 38:26, 1929

21. Halsay HJ, Allen N, Chamberlin HR: Chronic decerebrate state in infancy. Arch Neurol 19:339, 1968

22. Hellebrandt FA, Waterland JC: Expansion of motor patterning under exercise stress. Am J Phys Med 4:56, 1962

23. Hirt S: The tonic neck reflex mechanism in the normal human adult. Am J Phys Med 46:362, 1967

24. Humphrey T: Some correlations between the appearance of human fetal reflexes and the development of the nervous system. Prog Brain Res 4:93, 1964

25. Ikai M: Tonic neck reflex in normal persons. Jpn J Physiol 1:118, 1950

26. Illingworth RS: The Development of the Infant and Yound Child: Normal and Abnormal, 6h ed. Edinburg, E & S Livingstone, 1975

27. McGraw MB: The Neuromuscular Maturation of the Human Infant. New York, Hafner Publishing, 1974

28. Magnus R: Physiology of posture. Lancet 2:531; 585, 1926

29. Martin JP: The Basal Ganglia and Posture. Philadelphia, JB Lippincott, 1967

30. Milani–Comparetti A, Gidoni EA: Pattern analysis of motor development and its disorders. Dev Med Chil Neurol 9:625, 1967

31. Melani–Comparetti A, Gidoni EA: Routine developmental examination in normal and retarded children. Dev Med Child Neurol 9:631, 1967

32. Molnar G: Motor deficit of retarded infants and young children. Arch Phys Med Rehab 55:393, 1974

33. Mueller HA: Facilitating Feeding and Prespeech. In Pearson P, Williams C (eds): Physical Therapy Services in the Developmental Disabilities, pp 283–310. Springfield, IL, Charles C Thomas, 1972

34. Paine RS: Evolution of postural reflexes in normal infants and in the presence of chronic brain syndromes. Neurology 14:1036, 1964

35. Paine RS: Neurological examination of infants and children. Pediatr Clin North Am 7:471, 1960

36. Parmelee AH: A critical evaluation of the Moro reflex. Pediatrics 33:773, 1964

37. Peiper A: Cerebral Function in Infancy and Childhood. New York, Consultants Bureau, 1963

38. Robinson RJ: Assessment of gestational age by neurological examination. Arch Dis Child 41:437, 1966

39. Saint–Anne Dargassies S: Neurological maturation of the premature infant of 28–41 weeks' gestational age. In Falkner F (ed): Human Development, pp 306–325. Philadelphia, WB Saunders, 1966

40. Saint–Anne Dargassies S: Neurological symptoms during the first year of life. Dev Med Child Neurol 14:235, 1972

41. Schaltenbrand G: The development of human motility and motor disturbances. Arch Neurol Psychiatr 20:720, 1972

42. Tokizane T, et al: Electromyographic studies on tonic neck, lumbar and labyrinthine reflexes in normal persons. Jpn J Physiol 2:130, 1954

43. Twitchell TE: Attitudinal reflexes. Phys Ther 45:411, 1965

44. Twitchell TE: Minimal cerebral dysfunction in children and motor deficits. Trans Am Neurol Assoc 91:353, 1966

45. Twitchell TE: Normal motor development. Phys Ther 45:419, 1965

46. Twitchell TE: Reflexes and normal development. Presented at the Pediatric Symposium, University of North Carolina at Chapel Hill, Chapel Hill, 1970

47. Twitchell TE: The automatic grasping responses of infants. Neuropsychologia 3:247, 1965

48. Twitchell TE: Variations and abnormalities of motor development. Phys Ther 45:424, 1965

49. Waterland JC, Hellebrandt FA: Involuntary patterning associated with willed movement performed against progressively increasing resistance. Am J Phys Med 43:13, 1967

Alterations in the therapeutic plan made because of the lack or partial attainment of objectives should address the following questions:

Within the goal or objective-setting process, were the benefits (or objectives) realistically attainable?

Within the skill level of the service provider, were the goals–objectives achievable?

Within the structure and scope of the service delivery system, was the attainment of the goals–objectives possible?

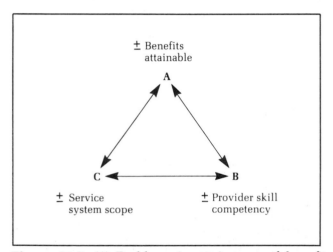

Figure 34-5. *(A)* Problems in attainment of benefits often relate to realistic goal setting. Competent evaluation and ability to synthesize information and to prioritize client needs are a primary consideration. *(B)* Deficits in the actual skills of providers, once identified, often can be addressed through staff education, whether group or individual, and when possible through hands-on experience. Above and beyond actual therapeutic competency, therapists need to consider less tangible factors of performance. Competent skills and sensitivity in touching, handling, communicating, and initiating voluntary movement with young children supersede all other treatment procedures in importance. Some therapists possess these abilities innately. Others are conscious of the importance of such skills and may find the greatest help in acquiring them through experience with therapists who demonstrate or provide models of such skills. *(C)* The reality of present pediatric occupational therapy practice in enlarging areas of the service delivery system was discussed in the introduction to this section. The lack of attainment of therapeutic goals because of service delivery limitations should be analyzed on the following basic factors: (1) Can the system be modified so that treatment objectives and procedures can be implemented? (2) If the system cannot be modified, and direct treatment measures based on sound objectives and goals are unrealistic, further consideration should be given to the value of consultative or educational process. Refer to the chapter on health systems in this text for further information.

Figure 34-5 is presented to assist and encourage this type of feasibility analysis as a means of refining and improving therapeutic planning for more effective treatment results.

Occupational Therapy Models of Treatment

The roles of the registered occupational therapist (OTR) and the certified occupational therapy assistant (COTA) in pediatric occupational therapy are clearly interrelated at all levels of professional performance—referral or assessment, screening or evaluation, and treatment planning and execution.

"The Delineation of Entry-Level Roles of OTRs and COTAs" document was developed and adopted by the American Occupational Therapy Association (AOTA) Representative Assembly in 1981. This document describes the roles in terms of tasks for both professional levels and reflects the present general practice of occupational therapy, which can easily be related to pediatric occupational therapy. This document, which includes definitions of terms used in our practice (previously adopted officially by AOTA) and a glossary of role-delineation terms, is a very suitable guide for developing standards of practice for individual pediatric occupational therapy programs or departments. Further, it could be very useful in developing job descriptions for occupational therapy personnel that clearly specify the roles of both the OTR and the COTA and their interrelationship in a particular pediatric setting. This document states that the OTR is responsible for knowing and understanding the COTA role and functions. It also points out the requirements of supervision of the COTA by the OTR. (See Appendix H.)

The following is a description of the process of an evaluation of a 4-year-old boy by an OTR and COTA team. The OTR has worked 3 years and the COTA 1 year since graduation at an outpatient treatment center for children. The child was referred to the center by the child's pediatrician following a parent conference about the child's behavior during a routine medical checkup. The physician's preliminary diagnosis is attention deficit disorder with possible gross and fine motor delay. A written referral was received by the OTR, who contacted the parents the same day to gather their key concerns and set up a convenient appointment to evaluate the child and conduct an initial parental conference.

The OTR informs the COTA of the new client's appointment for evaluation at their daily patient/client conference meeting. The COTA records the appointment in the master schedule, because the routine includes keeping the schedule current, tabulating changes, and daily attendance records. Also at this meeting, the OTR indicates the evaluation processes to be used, consisting of sensorimotor components, cognitive components, and activities of daily living.

Following the meeting, the COTA informs the department secretary of the new client's schedule and level of evaluation. The secretary prepares a folder for the child's records containing the specific testing instruments and places the folder in a daily file in preparation for the evaluation date.

On the date of the evaluation, the COTA pulls the folder and meets briefly with the OTR for any update. In this case, a social worker's report has been received of a home visit interview with the mother and father about the child's condition. Both therapists review this one-page report and are then notified of the arrival of the child with his parents. Parents and child are greeted by the therapists. The OTR receives the parent's completed history and questionnaire and escorts the parents to a conference room adjacent to the testing area. The COTA escorts the child, who willingly separates from his parents at the sight of the testing room, which has been arranged by the COTA in readiness for testing with special interesting toys and games to put the child at ease. The COTA has been trained specifically to observe the child while he engages in these activities and to collect data on gross and fine coordination, orientation to task, concentration, attention, and memory.

In the meantime, the OTR explains the evaluation process to the parents in detail and gets feedback from them about their concerns. The OTR escorts the parents to an observation area, where they will be able to watch the evaluation. The parents are put at ease and are given some idea of the length of the examination and a note pad to record their reactions, if any, or any points of information they feel are relevant to the examination.

The OTR enters the testing area and becomes acquainted with the child as formal testing is initiated. The OTR administers both nonstandardized and standardized evaluations while the COTA records the data on the protocol sheets or evaluation forms that the COTA has been trained to use. The COTA also assists by making all testing equipment available and removing it as needed unobtrusively to avoid distracting the child's attention from a task.

When the OTR has completed this phase of examination, the COTA gives the data collected back to the OTR and then engages the child in structured tests of several daily living skills and performance as indicated by the OTR. The OTR scores the standardized tests and meets once again with the parents for a closing conference about the evaluation. Together, they schedule a later in-depth conference about the findings, interpretations, and recommendations regarding appropriate occupational therapy services.

The COTA provides the OTR with the data on those daily living skills performances with a brief report on the data. The OTR documents all the data and interpretations and completes a report for the referring physician and the parents. Using all available data, the OTR, with the assistance of the COTA, develops a preliminary plan of long- and short-term goals to improve the quality of the child's functional status.

This, along with the evaluation report and functional status, will be reviewed with the child's parents at the time of the conference. The COTA will attend the conference and play an integral part in the occupational therapy treatment under the direction and, in some cases, supervision of the OTR.

This description stresses the interrelationship of OTRs and COTAs in the the pediatric evaluation process for efficiency and efficacy. It also stresses that the responsibility of the OTR is to plan the evaluation, to administer standardized and nonstandardized tests, and to analyze and synthesize the evaluation data. It also stresses the importance of developing a structured format of related data collection to be conducted by the COTA who has received specific training in these methods and has demonstrable skills in collecting, summarizing, recording, and reporting the data to the OTR supervisor.

References

1. Ayres AJ: Sensory Integration and the Child. Los Angeles, Western Psychological Services, 1979
2. Ayres AJ: The Development of Sensory Integrative Theory and Practice. Dubuque, Kendall/Hunt, 1974
3. Barnes MR, Crutchfield CA, Heriza CB: The Neurophysiological Basis of Patient Treatment, Vol. 2. Morgantown, WV, Stockesville Publishing, 1978
4. Gilfoyle E, Grady AP, Moore JC: Children Adapt. Thorofare, NJ, Charles B Slack, 1981
5. Johnson JA: Delegate assembly address—April 19, 1976. In Hopkins HL, Smith HD (eds): Willard and Spackman's Occupational Therapy, 5th ed, p 111. Philadelphia, JB Lippincott, 1978
6. Lewke JH: Current practices in evaluating motor behavior of disabled children. Am J Occup Ther 30:403, 1976
7. Hoskins TA, Squires JE: Developmental Assessment. Phys Ther 53:117–126, 1973

Bibliography

Brazelton TB: Neonatal behavioral assessment scale. Clin Dev Med No. 50, 1973
Buros OK: The Ninth Mental Measurements Yearbook, Vol. 1 and 2. Highland Park, NJ, The Gryphon Press, 1985
Clark PN, Allen AS: Occupational Therapy for Children. St Louis, CV Mosby, 1985
deQuiros JB, Schrager OL: Neuropsychological Fundamentals in Learning Disabilities. San Rafael, Academic Therapy Publications, 1978
Entry-Level Role Delineation for OTRs and COTAs. Rockville, MD, American Occupational Therapy Association, 1981

The Occupational Therapy Process In Specific Pediatric Conditions *Patricia Ann Ramm*

This chapter discusses specific pediatric conditions that occupational therapists often address. These specific diagnostic topics are presented by means of the conceptual model, in most cases, so that equal emphasis is placed on the cause of the condition, the characteristics of the condition and the manner in which an individual child within his or her living condition is affected. Preliminary history, background, and evaluation information are blended in the evaluation stage to advance the actual implementation of the therapeutic intervention or treatment process. In most conditions, an illustration of the appropriate treatment processes is presented in relation to the therapeutic goals and objectives. Frequently, further evaluation and adjustments to the plan, goals, and methods are also presented to clarify the therapeutic process as an ongoing system.

Neonates or High-Risk Infants

Rapid advances in the field of neonatology and the institution of neonatal intensive-care units (ICUs) have significantly improved the survival rate of critically ill neonates.[24] Following a decade of research in the 1970s on the outcome of these infants who required specialized medical intervention in the neonatal period, it became apparent that these infants were at risk for later problems in motor, cognitive, language, or social–emotional areas. Occupational therapists, as well as professionals from other related health fields, began to intervene while the infant was in the neonatal ICU with the intent of minimizing developmental delays in the later years.

An infant is considered high risk for developmental problems if he or she suffers from prenatal or postnatal medical complications. These infants generally fall into two categories: the *premature infant*, who has a low birthweight (less than 2500 grams [5 pounds]) and a shortened gestational period (less than 37 weeks); or the *full-term* or *post-term infant* (greater than 38 weeks of gestation) with specific medical problems. The shorter the gestational period and the lower the birthweight, the greater the chances for medical difficulties requiring intensive-care treatment.

The Neonatal Intensive-Care Unit

A first visit to a neonatal ICU can be a shocking experience. The observer is struck by the high activity level of the staff, the abundance of equipment, and the size and appearance of many of the infants.[15] Infants are continuously monitored for their respiratory and cardiac status and therefore have many leads for machinery. It is common to see infants with a variety of intravenous lines.

Because of the type of medical treatment these infants receive, with the emphasis on life-saving techniques, the atmosphere can appear overstimulating for the infants. In some units, there is bright lighting, a variety of sounds from machinery, alarms from monitors, telephones, voices of staff members and visitors, and cries of infants. In addition, infants are often subjected to many noxious testing procedures such as frequent needle punctures for blood work.

Professionals concerned with the developmental growth of the infant should be aware of the possible side-effects that the environment of the ICU may have on the overall development of the infant. Efforts are now being made to further understand how this early experience affects the child's development and how to alter the environment to create a more natural and developmentally conducive setting.

Medical Problems of Premature and Other High-Risk Infants

Premature infants can suffer from a variety of medical problems in many body systems: respiratory, cardiovascular, metobolic, nutritional, immunological, and ophthalmological.[26]

One of the major problems for premature infants is that of respiratory deficiency. The respiratory muscles are small and poorly developed; the thoracic cage is soft and compliant. Some of the common respiratory deficits that often require the infant to breathe by means of artificial ventilation (respirator) are atelectasis, failure of the lungs to expand fully; hyaline membrane disease (HMD), inadequate fetal lung development; respiratory distress syndrome (RDS), a disorder characterized by grunting, chest retractions, nasal flaring, tachypnea, and cyanosis; bronchopulmonary dysplasia (BPD), chronic lung disease resulting from a direct toxic effect of oxygen on the lung; and apnea, a transient lack of breathing.

In the cardiovascular system, infants can have patent ductus arteriosus (PDA) which is a common cause of congestive heart failure. These infants can have subsequent nutritional and breathing difficulties. Because premature infants have weak capillary walls, they are vulnerable to hemorrhage, especially in the brain. Many infants suffer from intraventricular hemorrhage of various magnitudes. These infants are more at risk for neurological sequelae.

Metabolic problems such as hyperbilirubinemia, metabolic acidosis, hypocalcemia, and hypoglycemia may have some neurological manifestations: hyperirritability, jitteriness, or convulsions. Nutritional problems may interfere with the infant's normal feeding patterns

and weight gain. Some premature infants suffer from necrotizing enterocolitis (NEC), which affects the small intestine and colon.

Infections often delay the infant's growth and recovery in the newborn period. Some premature infants suffer from pneumonia, septicemia, meningitis, or urinary tract infections.

The most common ophthalmological problem among premature infants is retrolental fibroplasia (RFL). The incidence of this problem has declined substantially with the control of oxygen doses; however, occurrence is still noted. These infants have opaque tissue behind the lens which may lead to poor visual acuity, retinal detachment, or blindness in various degrees.

Additional medical problems can be manifested in any infant, whether premature or full-term. Neurological difficulties, such as asphyxia and seizures, can occur and have a direct impact on the developmental outcome. Congenital anomalies, such as genetic disorders (*e.g.,* trisomies) or congenital limb defects may necessitate neonatal intensive care. Some infants have difficulties during the birth, which may result in head injuries, nerve paralysis, or orthopedic problems.

The Role of the Occupational Therapist

Clinical practice in a neonatal ICU is a specialized area of pediatric intervention. Experience in infant evaluation and treatment, knowledge of normal and abnormal development, and an understanding of the medical problems of high-risk infants are prerequisites for providing services in this highly complex area.

The occupational therapist can serve in at least two capacities, depending on the organization of a particular neonatal ICU: direct service to the infant and family, or consultation and teaching to the staff of the unit.

Direct Service to the Infant and Family

In providing direct service to the infant and family, the occupational therapist is a member of an interdisciplinary team and coordinates the evaluation and intervention plan. Following assessment, the therapist may institute a treatment plan that involves the nursing staff and the infant's family as much as possible. A significant contribution to the child's plan occurs at discharge and in follow-up. At this point, a plan is set in motion to enable the family to meet the continued needs of their infant.

Consultation and Teaching

In some settings, the occupational therapist may function primarily in a teaching capacity, making specific recommendations to the staff working with the infant in order to facilitate normal development. The therapist may take an overall approach by instructing staff in aspects that can be generalized to most infants, or a more specific approach by relating the discussion to the needs of an individual infant. Regardless of the approach, the difference between the direct service role and one of consultation is that in the latter the therapist does not necessarily work with each infant on a continual basis. Rather, the therapist serves as a resource to the team working with the infant.

Assessment and the Occupational Therapy Plan

The Referral Process

The criteria for referral of an infant for an occupational therapy assessment may vary according to the organizational structure of different neonatal units. In some units, the program may be one of developmental support, where most infants receive an enrichment program that is not solely dependent on whether the infant is displaying developmental deficiencies. In other programs, referrals are based on the identification of specific problems in the infants. Some of the general categories where problems may be detected are:

1. *Feeding.* Many premature infants have particular difficulty learning how to feed from a nipple. This may be manifested in the inability to suck, leaking of liquids during sucking, gagging, or generally poor control in the oral-motor area. These characteristics may also be present in the full-term infant who has suffered a neurological insult or who has another medical problem causing disturbances of the feeding mechanism.
2. *Abnormal muscle tone and posturing.* These problems may be present in infants with neurological deficits. The infant may show poor head or trunk control, inability to move because of increased or decreased tone, asymmetrical movement patterns, exaggerated primitive reflexes, and abnormal postures (*e.g.,* opistotonus) that may interfere with normal motor development.
3. *Difficulties adapting to the environment.* Infants may have disorganized behavior manifested by their inability to orient to visual, auditory, tactile, or vestibular input. They may be irritable, hyperexcitable, or lethargic and difficult to arouse to an alert state.

Preassessment Considerations

Medical Precautions

In many neonatal units, only infants who are considered medically stable will be referred for an occupational therapy assessment. However, it is of utmost importance that the therapist realize that these infants are still critically ill and that the therapy assessment should be conducted only after the therapist has consulted with the medical team and is fully aware of the medical contraindications. Involvement should be a team approach, and the therapist's assessment should be placed in order of priority within the infant's health care plan.

There are two main precautions that therapists should consider when working with a critically ill neonate: the importance of temperature regulation and the infant's tolerance level. Infants are often kept in a temperature-controlled environment in an Isolette. The medical staff should be consulted to determine whether the infant can be treated outside the Isolette, or whether the therapist should handle the infant inside the Isolette to maintain the proper body temperature. Second, many infants can tolerate only minimal handling. The therapist should be aware of the signs of fatigue or overstimulation (*e.g.,* color changes, changes in breathing rates, irritability) and accommodate the infant.

Correcting for Prematurity

In assessing the development of premature infants, the chronological age is adjusted by subtracting the number of weeks of prematurity to account for the immaturity of development. For example, if an infant is 2 months old and was 8 weeks premature, the corrected age is newborn.[23]

The Structure of the Neonatal Assessment

The purpose of the occupational therapist's evaluation is to identify areas of neuromotor, sensory, oral-motor, and adaptive development that are delayed or abnormal so as to plan an intervention strategy. The assessment should be based on how normally developing premature and full-term infants behave according to developmental expectations. Therefore, an in-depth understanding of infant developmental and adaptive behaviors is a prerequisite for neonatal assessment.

The following format has been derived from the neonatal assessments of Brazelton,[12] Als,[1] and Stern.[30]

Neuromotor

The neuromotor assessment includes an observation of *muscle tone* while the infant is in the supine, prone, sitting, and standing positions and while the infant is rolled in both directions and brought to the sitting position. The therapist notes resistance or lack of resistance to movement.

The therapist observes the *types of movements* the infant exhibits and describes the patterns used. The therapist notes whether the infant moves with flexor or extensor patterns, whether the infant's movement is symmetrical or asymmetrical, and whether the infant has excessive movement or limited movement.

Developmental motor abilities are observed. The infant is evaluated according to the expectations for his or her age. In the neonatal period, emphasis is on the acquisition of head and upper extremity control.

The neuromotor assessment includes examination of neurological *reflexes and reactions* such as the asymmetrical tonic neck reflex, the Moro, automatic walk, hand and toe grasp, placing reactions, righting reactions, and clonus (see Chapter 34).

Sensory

The therapist observes the infant's visual, auditory, tactile, and vestibular responses. In the visual area, the therapist notes the infant's ability to focus on and follow visual stimuli such as a face or graphic design (*e.g.,* black-and-white bull's-eye configuration). Auditory awareness and localization are noted as the infant attends to the sound of a bell. Tactile and vestibular reactions are observed throughout the examination. Notation is made of the infant's changes in behavior as he or she is touched or moved. Specifically, the therapist determines whether the infant is sensitive to types of touch (*e.g.,* light or firm), and whether the infant is fearful or easily startled by movement.

Oral-Motor

The oral-motor assessment includes observation of the infant in nutritive (during feeding) and nonnutritive (sucking when not feeding) situations. During nutritive sucking, the infant must coordinate sucking and swallowing with breathing. The therapist notes the quality of the infant's sucking, the amount of liquid consumed, and the length of time it takes for the feeding. Oral reflexes, such as bite, gag, and rooting, are examined. Particular attention is given to the overall movement patterns of the infant during feeding, because abnormal posturing and muscle tone influence feeding quality and function. In the nonnutritive situation, further information is gathered about the quality of sucking and whether a difference is noted in swallowing when milk is eliminated.

Adaptive Development

The term *adaptive development* refers to the infant's ability to organize sensory stimuli and respond to changes in the environment. Sometimes, this is referred to as "organizational behavior." Observations are made as to the infant's ability to collect oneself when coming in and out of sleep, in moving out of an irritable state, and in response to stress. The therapist observes what triggers the infant's distress and the mechanisms used by the infant to regain a quiet state. This is observed throughout the assessment.

Additional Considerations in the Assessment Process

In addition to the observations made while handling the infant, the therapist should determine what the environment offers the infant. How is the infant positioned because of the medical interventions? Who handles the infant and how? If applicable, how is the infant picked up, carried, fed, and played with? The information about the environment assists the therapist in interpreting whether the infant's behaviors truly reflect the child's neurological make-up or are partially associated with influences from the environment.

The Occupational Therapy Plan

On the basis of the assessment, infants who demonstrate deviations in their behaviors require an intervention program. The goals and methods of the program are coordinated with the medical care of the infant and are communicated to the staff working with the infant and, if possible, to the parents. The frequency of treatment is dependent on the infant's capacity to be handled, as well as on the organizational structure of the specific neonatal unit.

Developmental Treatment on a Neonatal Intensive-Care Unit

The primary goal of occupational therapy intervention is to maximize the infant's developmental growth.[2] Normal development can be enhanced by providing the infant with carefully selected sensorimotor experiences appropriate for the infant's developmental age. The therapist makes changes in the ICU environment by promoting handling, sensory experiences, and social interactions that may be beneficial to the infant's development. Throughout the hospitalization, an extremely important goal is the facilitation of parent–infant attachment. Gradually, the parents need to become more comfortable with their infant for development to progress.

The treatment areas of neuromotor, oral-motor, sensory, and adaptive behaviors are closely interrelated and usually coordinated in the treatment plan. For the purpose of discussion, they are outlined separately.

Intervention for Neuromotor Problems

Treatment of infants with a variety of movement problems focuses on enabling the infant to sense normal movement reaction and respond automatically.[27] For some infants with abnormal muscle tone, the abnormal tone is changed to a more normal state with facilitation of appropriate movement responses. For infants who can be handled outside the Isolette, the therapist may work with the infant on the lap to improve mobility of the trunk, head control, weight shift, symmetry, and righting reactions. More often, however, these goals are accomplished by the manner in which the infant is handled and positioned on a daily basis.

Handling is the manner in which the infant is picked up, carried, held, changed from one position to another, diapered, dressed, and positioned or moved during feeding, sleeping, social interactions, and playing. This is the main avenue through which the infant can receive and respond to tactile, proprioceptive, and vestibular stimuli that may influence the motor system. Because it encompasses the infant's daily care, appropriate handling should be determined early in the infant's program and carried out by the primary caregivers (*e.g.,* nurses, physicians, therapists, and parents).

The following are examples of ways to handle an infant to promote neuromotor development.

Picking Up the Baby

For the infant who tends to arch into extension patterns, the goal is to interrupt the extension and facilitate flexion and rotation responses. The infant would be gently but firmly guided into flexion while coming from the supine position to a semisitting position in the arms of the person picking up the infant (Fig. 35-1).

Social Interaction and Play

For the infant who displays jitteriness or asymmetry, the parent or caregiver should lay the infant in the lap lengthwise so that the parent's legs form a soft, hammock-like surface in which the infant can be positioned in semiflexion. This position gives the infant guided support that may reduce the startling responses and enable the head to remain in the midline. In this way, the infant may even bring the hands to the mouth for the first time.

Positioning is often an adjunct to the neuromotor program because it serves to reinforce the goals of handling. For some infants, medical objectives dictate the

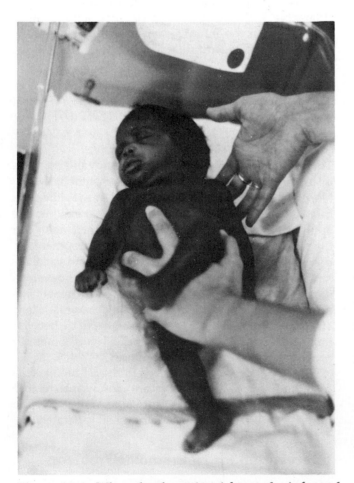
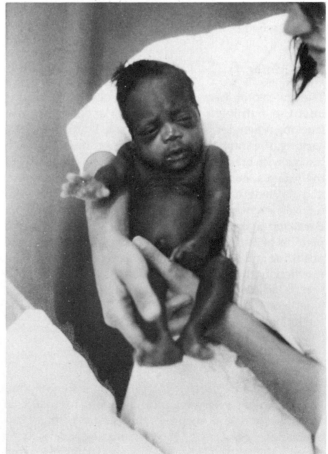

Figure 35-1. When the therapist picks up the infant, she guides the infant into a flexed position.

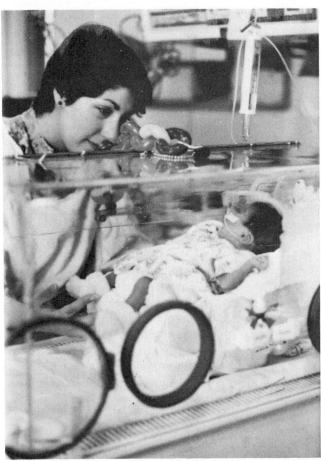

Figure 35-2. The critically ill neonate on a respirator is positioned for short periods in a custom-made infant seat to allow more upright and slightly flexed posture.

manner in which they are positioned. For example, the infant on a respirator may be placed in a supine position, with the neck in hyperextension to allow for optimal airway opening. This position may reinforce extension responses and make it more difficult for the infant to bring the arms forward or bring the hands to the mouth. To promote more flexion responses, the therapist may recommend the sidelying or prone position with the use of rolls or pillows to maintain the position. The sidelying position may facilitate symmetry and flexion.

Positioning can be accomplished with custom-made infant seats for the infant who should be more upright. This is particularly advantageous if the infant requires constant temperature control and cannot be handled outside the Isolette for long periods of time. The infant could be cradled by a seat if he or she cannot be held in the caregiver's arms (Fig. 35-2).

Intervention for Oral-Motor Problems

The oral-motor program for an infant who is having feeding difficulties influenced by abnormal muscle tone or disorganized behavior is highly complex. Much of the success of a feeding program is dependent on the knowledge and skill of the person feeding the infant. As in other areas of treatment of the neonate, the therapist prescribing the feeding program requires specialized training and experience.

There are at least four aspects to the oral-motor or feeding program: optimum positioning to facilitate head, neck, and trunk alignment, which influences oral-motor control; normalization of oral muscle tone and facial sensitivity; appropriate choice of nipples or feeding utensils; and manual assistance, such as gentle jaw control, to facilitate oral control. The feeding program requires constant coordination with the nursing staff and should be incorporated into the parent program when appropriate.

Intervention for Sensory and Adaptive Problems

Providing enrichment for visual, auditory, tactile, and vestibular development can be incorporated into the neuromotor, oral-motor, and adaptive development treatment areas. During handling of the infant there are numerous opportunities to engage the infant in visual play and language stimulation. Toys can be placed in the Isolette to stimulate visual focus. It is unknown what amount of stimulation is appropriate for these young infants; therefore, the therapist should be sensitive to the infant's behavioral signs to know whether to increase or decrease the amount of input.

Tactile experiences can be provided during handling by the therapist assisting the infant in exploring body parts. For example, the therapist can facilitate hands-to-mouth or hands-to-feet movements. Gentle but firm touch may provide the infant with a sense of security.

Proprioceptive input through swaddling, weight-bearing positions, and holding can facilitate calming for infants who may be overreactive or irritable. For these infants, this type of intervention often influences the level of alertness and promotes attention to other stimuli, such as auditory and visual.

Vestibular input should be carefully given through handling and moving in space (rocking). The infant is usually swaddled to ensure behavioral organization and then given slow, rhythmical, predictable rocking up and down. This is particularly helpful for the fussy, disorganized infant but should be done only with extreme caution by a therapist who has a deep understanding of the effect of the sensory systems on behavior. The therapist should be well acquainted with the medical contraindications for vestibular input.

Parent Involvement

Most parents of critically ill neonates are in an extremely fragile emotional state. They are going through a difficult period of trying to understand what has happened and worrying about the fate of their infant. The therapist can offer support to the parents by guiding them in interactions with and handling of the infant. The goal is to help the parents feel comfortable when handling their infant in order to enable them to be spontaneous and to provide proper nurturing. Instruction to parents should be gradual and conclude with a discharge plan and home program. Sensitivity to the parents' emotional needs and learning styles is crucial in helping them learn about their infants.

Discharge Plan and Follow-up

The discharge plan, coordinated with the other disciplines working with the infant and family, summarizes the continued needs of the infant and sets a follow-up plan in motion. It should include a description of the infant's current functioning, treatment recommendations when appropriate, a description of the parent program, and an appointment for a follow-up re-evaluation if possible. Treatment goals change considerably within the first year of life; therefore, regular re-evaluation is advisable to assure appropriate home management and parent education and support.

Case Study

Janet was a premature baby (32 weeks) born to a 34-year-old single mother. This was the mother's first pregnancy and she had received prenatal care in the last month of pregnancy only. Janet's weight at birth was 1304 grams (2 lbs, 10.2 oz) and was considered nearly appropriate for her gestational age. She exhibited neonatal distress, body temperature irregularities, apnea episodes, and complications of minor seizures during the first month. She was placed on a respirator to support her breathing, and progressed during the first month to initial feeding by nipple and largely weaned from the respirator by 37 weeks. At this point, she was referred by the medical staff for occupational therapy assessment. The staff had noted stiffness of the extremities, hyperirritability, and continuing difficulty taking liquids from the nipple. The staff also noted that Janet's mother was grieving over her child's condition and seemed very uncomfortable in the nursery and handling her daughter.

During evaluation of Janet at 37 weeks (3 weeks before the child's due date), the therapist noted that Janet had increased muscle tone, a tendency to arch into extension, and hyperactive reflexes. Sensory findings included inconsistent orienting to visual and auditory input. Tactile and vestibular input appeared to increase her extensor responses, and she startled easily. Her oral-motor functioning showed normal re-

flexes; however, she was slow to feed and tended to lose liquid when she sucked. In the adaptive area, she was irritable; however, when bundled, she calmed easily. Her mother was insecure and fearful when holding her (Fig. 35-3).

The occupational therapy program included the following:

1. Handling activities to normalize muscle tone, facilitate head control, decrease extension responses, and facilitate flexion responses such as hands to mouth
2. Instruction to the medical staff and mother on how to pick up, hold, feed, and play with Janet so as to interrupt extension responses, decrease startling, and encourage visual and auditory orientation
3. Suggestions of alternatives to supine lying for sleep to encourage flexion; for example, sidelying with a soft towel roll resting against her back
4. Initiation of a feeding program that encouraged proper positioning and manual techniques to increase her oral-motor control
5. Initiation of parent involvement with regular meetings with Janet's mother to demonstrate how to hold her so that she became less irritable, less extended, and more socially responsive; provision of emotional support, as well as practical suggestions on how to relate to her small infant; suggestions for visual and language enrichment and social interaction activities; guidance in following through on her feeding program

Once the combined efforts of the occupational therapist and nursing staff were under way in therapeutic handling, positioning, and the adapted feeding program, significant changes began to be noted in Janet's state and nutrition. The child's mother responded well to the instructions for handling and feeding from the occupational therapist and was soon successful in these strategies with her child, which led to improved social interaction between the mother and child. □

Summary

As occupational therapists approach the rapidly advancing field of neonatology, their unique contribution to this service is to assist the infant at risk who has a frail, fragile beginning in a complex medical center environment where survival is in many ways in opposition to normal human development and adaptation. The therapist is charged to act as an agent in promoting the tenuous development of the neonate despite complications and moment-to-moment fluctuations in the infant's medical stability. But certainly, the larger challenge for the occupational therapist and medical staff is helping

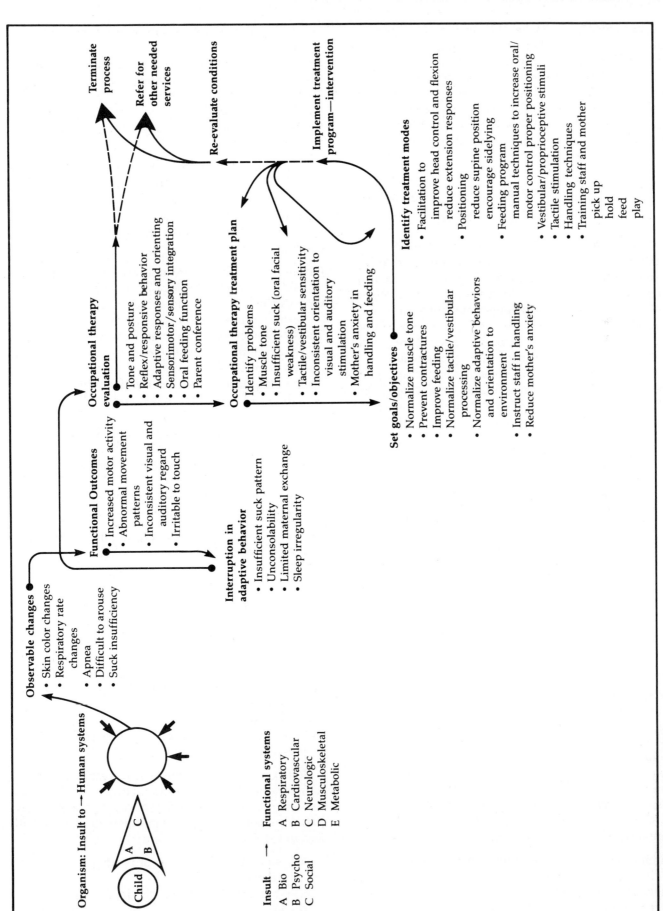

Figure 35-3. Case study: Janet.

the surviving infant make the transition from the ICU toward an integrated family unit. Acting as a supportive agent to the infant and family, the occupational therapist should provide direct treatement service (or by other related means as appropriate—consultation, teaching demonstrations, home visits) with the action occurring in the hospital as well as through discharge planning or follow-up care in the clinic or at home.

Congenitally Blind or Visually Impaired Child

Occupational therapists involved in the evaluation and treatment of young children with suspected developmental disabilities will in all probability encounter within their referral population a significant number of children who exhibit visual impairment or who are congenitally blind. In some cases, children who were born prematurely and who are younger than 12 months of age have a visual deficiency and a prognosis that is clouded or incomplete. In some cases, therapists encounter a baby who seems visually handicapped, but who has not been so identified. Because of the advances in survival of high-risk neonates (in which birth may occur as early as 24 weeks' gestation, with a birth weight of 16 oz or less), and because of the increased incidence of visual impairment in these cases, the previous discussion of neonates is directly applicable to the early experiences of the child and family. Survival of the baby is the overwhelming goal and desire for parents. Preoccupation with the child's circulation, respiration, and nourishment status preclude consideration of the consequences of impaired vision on the child's development.

As the child reaches physical and medical stability, parents can address their concerns about the child's development and to what degree visual impairment will hamper the child's potential. The occupational therapist serving a blind or visually impaired child and family has an important opportunity. Careful developmental assessment and critical interpretation are needed. Many congenitally blind or visually impaired children exhibit multisensory integrative problems, and their neurophysiological development differs from that of the sighted child in certain predictable patterns. Helping the child to achieve developmental gains directly, and also helping parents to recognize and enhance their vital contributions to the young child's development, is the thrust of occupational therapy in this field of endeavor.

General physical sensory variations of young congenitally blind children include:

Diminished muscle tone accompanied by poor joint stability in some cases
Irregularity in neurodevelopmental reflex presence and maturation

Delayed or partial acquisition of gross and fine motor skill
Irregularity in somatosensory and vestibular processing
Sensitivity to or misunderstanding of sensory stimuli
Means–ends (motor output)
Gestoral–imitation
Cause–effect (inductive reasoning)
Spatial relationships

Sensitivity to or misinterpretation of sensory stimuli by the child can be determined by the therapist during the assessment process and by information provided by the parents and by observation. Those senses under suspicion are listed with observable behaviors as an outcome:

Olfactory—Poor appetite or adversive behavior to certain foods on the basis of odor
Oral Tactile—Difficulty in accepting variations of food texture or feeding instruments
Tactile–Discomfort with touch contact, especially to certain clothing, dressing process, bathing, cuddling, and comforting
Tactile Proprioceptive—Voluntarily withdraws from support of self with upper and lower extremities from a surface
Tactile Proprioceptive–Vestibular—Responds negatively to unfamiliar handler, especially to imposed movement in space, or generally is earthbound by strong preference
Auditory—Frightened frequently by unfamiliar voices and environmental sounds

A lack of early mutual visual attention of the infant and parents may disrupt early bonding communication links between the child and parent.

Through neurodevelopmental reflex testing, a therapist gains much needed information. Therapists frequently need to review the basis of reflex testing. Through this understanding, the therapist is assisted in determining the child's response to:

Light and firm tactile stimuli
Proprioceptive stimuli
Spatial organization
Reaction to surface
Optical organization of space (when some vision is present)

Reflex testing, combined with vestibular testing, allows the therapist to understand the child's processing and organization in a definitive way. Some of the discrete variations in reflex maturation most frequently seen in the first years of life are:

Prolonged Moro reflex to loss of position
Prolonged avoidance reflex
Deficient labyrinthine head righting reflex, especially prone

Delayed or absent Landau reflex

Poor or disordered proprioceptive placing reflexes, both legs and arms

Delayed support mechanisms

As a consequence, equilibrium reactions in all planes and protective extension reactions are delayed. The attainment of gross motor milestones frequently varies in a particular order. The following may be observed:

Diminished oral/facial weakness

Diminished head/neck performance against gravity, especially in prone extension with neck rotation to left or right

Diminished prone extension performance on forearms and hands

Delay in prone progression; creeping and hitching

Deficiency in active transitions of coming and lowering to both sit and, later, stand

Delays in squatting in play

Delays in walking freely and running

Delays in all gross motor tasks requiring discrete midline stability

Figure 35-4 illustrates contrasts in motor performance of congenitally blind children and sighted children.

The attaining of fine motor skill is strongly dependent on somatosensory processing efficiency. If efficiency is present, many fine skills occur in an orderly fashion; however, even in these cases, the use of instruments for eating is characteristically delayed, though cup use is not.

When sensorimotor integration deficiency is present, and especially in the case of somatosensory deficiency, the early developmental understanding basic to skill attainment may or may not occur in a disorder. Problem domains include:

Object permanence

A lack of visual feedback regarding socially appropriate behavior needs consideration. Efforts to provide al-

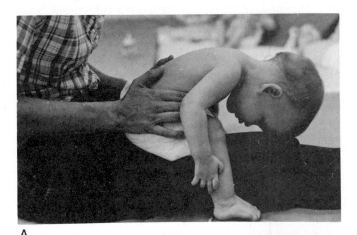

A

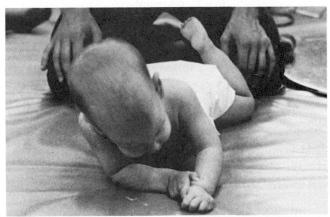

B

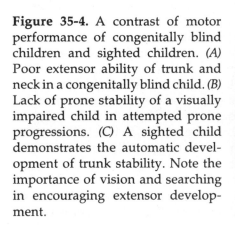

Figure 35-4. A contrast of motor performance of congenitally blind children and sighted children. *(A)* Poor extensor ability of trunk and neck in a congenitally blind child. *(B)* Lack of prone stability of a visually impaired child in attempted prone progressions. *(C)* A sighted child demonstrates the automatic development of trunk stability. Note the importance of vision and searching in encouraging extensor development.

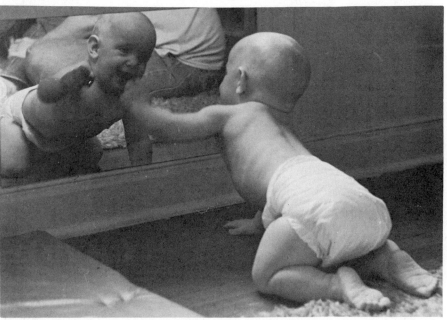

C

ternate methods of gaining such understanding are needed on an ongoing basis.

A lack of visual feedback of nonverbal communication influences overall appropriate behavior and assumes pragmatic ideation. As verbal communication develops, literal approaches and interventions may promote more appropriate developmental behavior. Auditory motor transactions can be stress producing and may have a negative influence on behavior and adaptation.

The better the therapist's ability to understand and communicate to the parent the unique nature of the development of their congenitally blind or visually impaired child, the greater the possibility of correctly developing a plan of treatment that incorporates the parent in the process. This joint effort improves the prognosis for success in the development of skills

Case Study

History

Beth was born prematurely at a gestational age of 22 weeks, weighing 1 lb, 11 oz. After birth, her weight dropped to 1 lb, 6 oz. Along with prematurity, she was found to have respiratory distress syndrome complicated by marked cardiac dysfunction, and there was little hope for her survival. However, treatment and nurturing offered through the services of a hospital neonatal intensive-care and nursery program advanced her physical–medical status over a 5-month period so that she was stabilized for discharge to her parents.

Parental Information

Beth's parents were reared and lived in a rural setting 60 miles from Beth's medical support system. Her parents were in their late 30s. The family also included two boys aged 14 years and 7 years. The oldest had a mild hearing impairment. Both parents had long wished for a baby girl, and Beth's mother had experienced several miscarriages in this attempt prior to her pregnancy with Beth. In general, Beth's parents were experienced and comfortable in their parenting role and responsibility. They were obviously solicitous in their attitude toward their children. In general, their management expectation of their children was to encourage useful orderly behavior. The family attended church regularly, and church values were a part of their daily life. It is important to know that Beth's mother was an efficient manager of the household and that she carried the chief responsibility for that and the children's care.

Beth's mother was quick to note and question Beth's visual attention when Beth was discharged home. Within 2 weeks of discharge, Beth had a complete visual examination that revealed her to be cortically blind due to retrolental fibroplasia. The mother's grief over her daughter's blindness was and continued to be a major factor of concern in infant–parent treatment programming.

Figure 35-5 depicts the initial occupational therapy program.

Occupational Therapy Program

An initial occupational therapy evaluation was conducted when Beth was physically stable and her neonatologist felt her resistance to infection was satisfactory. Her chronological age was 13 months (gestational age 9½ months). Beth required considerable restriction from contact with others outside the home in order to prevent her exposure to respiratory diseases for 8 months after discharge from the hospital. As a consequence, her mother experienced limited social contact during this period. Her examination was conducted at a community infant–parent program and was the first real opportunity for the parents to express their needs and concerns about their child's development.

Examination of Beth revealed the following information. She appeared pale and small and her skull was elongated due to positioning during her hospitalization. She was quiet when unattended. She alerted to sound but did not orient. The mother felt Beth could distinguish between low and high sounds. She was fearful of low voices and was afraid of being picked up by male family members, including her father. During testing, she displayed fussiness when handled, and she withdrew from light touch stimuli. She strongly objected to being placed in the prone position.

Physically, she was weak and floppy. All reflex responses were underactive; no pathologic tone condition was noted. Primitive tonic neck reflexes prevailed, though her tonic labyrinthine prone reflex was absent. Labyrinthine righting was demonstrated in supine but was absent in prone and tilting responses. There was no Landau reflex. Proprioceptive reflexes such as plantar and palmar placing were weakly present. Neck and body righting were stronger. Tactile-related reflex testing produced an avoidance of limbs, but some slight evidence of instinctive searching with her hands was noted. The most dynamic response in testing was her Moro response of complete embrace to loud sound and loss of position (backwards 45°). Some slight incurvature of the spine was seen in prone equilibrium testing, which was her only advanced reaction. Her reflex profile was that of a 5-month-old child, with certain exceptions often seen in congenitally blind children, as described earlier.

Gross motor skills were displayed to a 5-month level, except for raising the chest on extended arms and head lag in pull to sit. She rolled both ways and

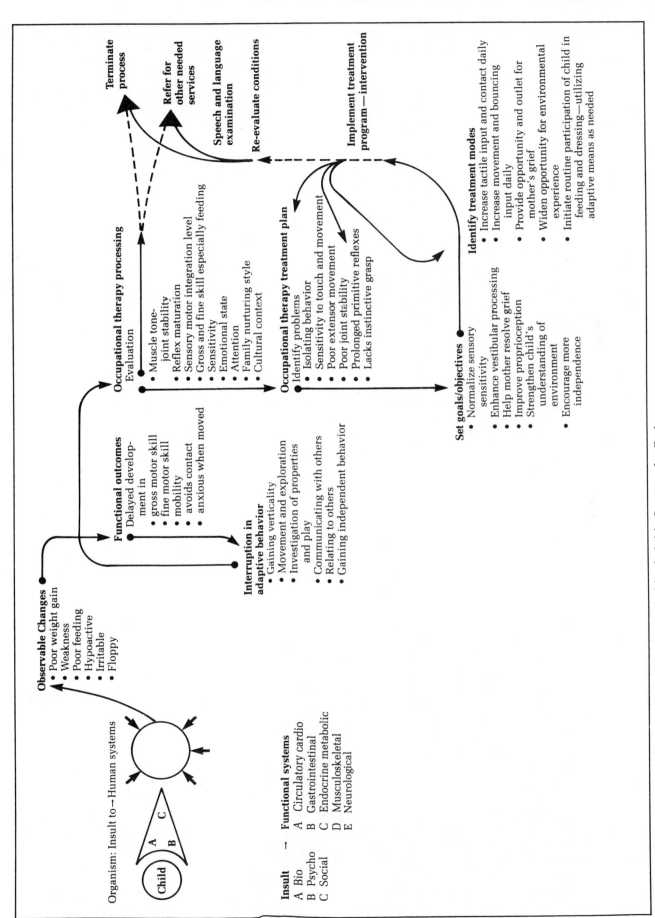

Figure 35-5. Occupational therapy with a congenitally blind child. Case study: Beth.

lifted her legs in extension, but could not sit independently even momentarily. Her gross motor quotient compared to her gestational age was 55%.

Her fine motor skills were quite depressed. She had no palmar grasping reflex, tending not to grasp generally, though she could bring her hands to her mouth and was scheming to use the thenar eminences of both her hands plus her two feet to prop her bottle while her mother fed her. No swiping behavior was present, and instinctive hand use was limited to feeding time, where she reached briefly for bits of food and occasionally for her spoon. The mother was encouraging Beth to search for parts of her body, particularly her feet. She was teaching Beth to assist in pulling off her socks.

Optokinetic testing produced no response, but blinking occurred to testing. No resting nystagmus was present, and there was no response to postrotary nystagmus testing. The mother felt that Beth might have some light perception. Beth's alerting to odors was minimal. She registered little interest in toys other than musical or chiming ones. She disliked fuzzy and furry toys.

The mother was quite open in expressing her concerns about her daughter, including:

1. A frustrating hope that Beth might see some day. She cried as she said, "Oh, if she could only see her pretty dresses."
2. Worry over Beth's poor appetite and slow weight gain. She also found feeding time frustrating because of Beth's picky appetite.
3. A fear of Beth's delicate health
4. Fear that when Beth cried or fussed, she was experiencing pain due to eye pressure, despite the lack of medical support to this belief.

Following the evaluation, the parents and staff held a planning conference to determine goals and objectives that would assist Beth's development. Because the family lived a distance of 60 miles from the infant–parent center, and considering Beth's somewhat fragile condition, the decision was made to arrange a home treatment program. A home therapist would provide treatment to Beth and train the family in appropriate therapeutic interventions. Weekly visits were provided, and an occupational therapy program was implemented (see Beth's Occupational Therapy Program–13 months).

Re-evaluation

At the next regularly scheduled 3-month evaluation, Beth, now 16 months old (gestational age 13 months), demonstrated some substantial gains in development. She showed marked improvement in behavior, including less fussiness and crying. The mother felt the remaining crying episodes were occurring when

Beth was hungry. The family was now enjoying Beth because she was happier and responsive to them when handled or touched. Beth now had a good appetite and was accepting a variety of foods. Reflex maturation was seen in inhibition of the Moro reflex and avoidance. Tonic neck reflex presence was diminishing, while improved labyrinthine righting and emergence of equilibrium response in prone, supine, and sitting were emerging. Good positive support of the lower extremities and instinctive grasp were noted. She was placing and protecting with the upper extremities forward and to the side. Reflexively, Beth was now programmed for gains in gross motor patterns and improved mobility.

Her neck strength and organization were improved. She no longer demonstrated head lag; she could sit steadily and lean forward, and re-erect. Her performance on the floor was markedly improved. She not only raised her chest in prone on extended arms, but she could also pivot 90° to right and left. As Beth became more comfortable in her world, she used rolling to explore her world. Gross motor skills were at a 7-month level.

All goals in feeding and dressing were accomplished. She was finger feeding, holding her bottle, accepting cup use, and assisting a little with spoon feeding. She quite automatically removed her shoes and socks and was far easier to dress. Her upper extremity skills included swiping, reaching, and transfer, and she had crude pincer skill and voluntary release. She did not bang two objects together, but she did bang on a surface and demonstrated crossing midline ability.

Her response on the postrotary nystagmus test was hyporeactive. There was no change in her visual status. The mother and father discussed their continued hope for eye surgery to help Beth see.

Changes and upgrading of Beth's home program were discussed with the family. A treatment plan was implemented during the next 4-month period of treatment (see Beth's Occupational Therapy Program–16 months, page 643).

At the next regularly scheduled 4-month evaluation, Beth at age 20 months old (gestational age 17 months) demonstrated continued developmental gains in most parameters; her gross motor age was 12 months and her fine motor skills were in a range of 12–18 months' level. Other advances were as follows:

1. Improved overall communication and minimal crying behavior overall. More use of gestures to make her needs known. No expressive speech
2. Reflexive maturation with good equilibrium in prone, supine, sitting, and quadruped positions
3. Improved mobility by means of prone progression, with emerging creeping and hitching, able to mount and lower from couch

(list continues on page 646)

Beth's Occupational Therapy Program: Chronologic Age—13 Months; Gestational Age—9 Months, 15 Days		
Therapeutic Goals	Objectives	Examples • Methods • Modes • Procedures
I. Normalize tactile sensitivity as a means to reduce isolating behavior.	IA. Increase child's contact with family members, objects of significance in the home.	IA. 1. Swaddle the child before child is handled by family other than mother. Play soothing music while handling. 2. Give firm rubdowns daily, especially before handling or tactile contact play. Emphasize palms of hands. 3. Encourage child to explore family members' facial features and hands. Encourage self touch. Use bells on ankles and wrists. Name body parts as child explores. 4. Encourage child to touch and hold objects common to child's daily experience. Name first then offer touch experience. Ex.: food, clothing, toys, mother's things, father's things, and brother's items. 5. Encourage Beth's exploration of hands/arms, feet/legs, face and skull with a manual vibrator. 6. Explore Beth's response to vibrating surface, especially when child demonstrates prolonged crying with cause.
II. Enhance vestibular processing as a means to improve adaptive behavior.	IIA. Child will increase tolerance to movement.	IIA. 1. Jigglers will be added to child's crib legs. 2. Mother will manually turn child slowly 10 x's to right and left; mother will tilt child in all directions 5 x's; mother will lower child 10 x's while holding the child erect. (Use swaddling if poorly tolerated). 3. Mother will gently swing child in a hammock on a basinette mattress. Child should be in prone or supine position. In prone chest wedge should be used.
III. Help mother resolve grief.	IIIA. Channel mother's grief.	IIIA. 1. Provide time to listen to mother's feelings about Beth. 2. Give mother emotional support as needed.
	B. Reduce the mother's anxiety about her child.	B. 1. Encourage mother to share home therapy program with other family members.

(continues)

Therapeutic Goals	Objectives	Examples • Methods • Modes • Procedures
		2. Encourage mother to share feeding responsibilities with father and older brother.
		3. Encourage family to resume previous socialization and leisure activities.
		4. Encourage mother to have ½ day/week away from care duty.
	C. Increase mother's knowledge about development in children with visual impairments.	C. 1. Encourage mother to communicate with other parents of visually impaired children.
		2. Provide information and sources of information on visually impaired children's development.
IV. Improve proprioception as a means to increase mobility.	IVA. Child will achieve raising chest on extended arms during playtime on own initiative.	IVA. 1. Bounce child in crib in prone, supine supported sitting and puppy with elbow support in extension. Add quadruped over bolster as stabilizer is achieved in puppy.
		2. Move bouncing activity to suspended hammock with spring as child's tolerance increases.
	B. Encourage rolling as a means to an end.	B. 1. Encourage rolling on a padded surface 3-5 x's to right and left. Use bottle as a lure, or a musical toy.
V. Strengthen child's understanding of her environment.	VA. Identify rooms of household by means of distinctive sounds.	VA. 1. Have mother examine each room in household and add noise factor to each room. Ex.: wind chimes at backdoor, radio in bedroom, TV in den, in backyard, etc.
	B. Plan a daily routine in which Beth is exposed to all areas of household.	B. 1. Child will spend time in kitchen, laundry room and bathroom, bedroom, garage-backyard and front porch.
VI. Encourage more independence.	VIA. Child will eat with more independence.	VIA. 1. Child will hold bottle during feeding.
		2. Child will have opportunity to finger feed a portion of every meal.
		3. Child will drink from a cup with lid and will place hands on cup to steady.
		4. Child will hold spoon and take tastes from spoon with help.
	B. Child will cooperate in dressing and assist.	B. 1. Child will remove socks.
		2. Child will reach and co-contract during dressing process.

	Beth's Occupational Therapy Program: Chronological Age — 16 Months; Gestational Age — 12 Months, 15 Days	
Therapeutic Goals	Objectives	Examples • Methods • Modes • Procedures
I. Continued normalization of tactile sensitivity as a means of encouraging improved adaptive behavior and socialization.	IA. Child will initiate touching and tolerate being touched.	IA. 1. Continue firm rubdowns daily. 2. Continue vibratory play. 3. Continue use of vibrator board as a calming means.
	B. Encourage improved tactile discrimination and localization.	B. 1. Play sticky tape game; place sticky tape on varying body locations, have child pull off tape. 2. Continue to have child contact self and others. Name first then have child touch these body parts. 3. Continue and expand contact with objects common to household and child's experience. 4. Encourage tactile searching for objects using sound clues.
II. Enhance vestibular processing as a means of improving mobility, function and adaptive behavior.	IIA. Child will tolerate swinging.	IIA. 1. Child will swing in a suspended hammock in all directions for 5-10 minutes (3 sec. arcs). Positioned in prone, supine and sitting.
	B. Child will tolerate tilting and respond.	B. 1. Child will tilt on a moderately firm surface in prone, supine, puppy and supported quadruped. (Use well inflated rectangular air cushion on 2 inch mat.) Use slow rate, wait for response.
	C. Child will tolerate sliding and initiate movement in sliding.	C. 1. Child will slide down an incline plane on stomach, on back and seated. C. 2. Child will use prone progression down incline plane. To be done 2 x's each or more if desired.
	D. Child will demonstrate improved response to angular vestibular stimulation.	D. 1. Child will turn slowly in hammock seated, side-lying and supine 12 x's in one direction followed by ½ turns in the reverse direction.

(continues)

Therapeutic Goals	Objectives	Examples • Methods • Modes • Procedures
III. Improve proprioception as a means to increase child's mobility.	IIIA. Child will move in prone progression automatically during play time and as a means to end. B. Child will maintain supported quadruped independently. C. Child will initiate creeping and hitching for 2 feet before lowering into prone progression for means to end. D. Child will stand supported by rail, 2 hands, child will raise one foot at rail and take initial side steps.	IIIA. 1. Child will wear weighted vest and cuff weights during proprioception activities. Weighted pockets Weighted cuff A,B,C. 1. Child will bounce in a suspended hammock with spring on a firm surface in sitting puppy position, and quadruped with limited support. D. 1. Add supported kneeling and standing, bouncing as skill emerges.
IV. Strengthen child's understanding and orientation to home setting as a means of gaining increased function, mobility and independence.	IVA. A child will move and search for centers of interest in each of the principal rooms in the home setting.	IVA-B-C. Orientation Process This orientation process is appropriate for child who has reflex organization for movement, either by prone progress or creeping and hitching. (Skull sensitive children may prefer to move backwards creeping. Because this is detrimental to orientation, it should be inhibited.) Reciprocal prone progression Creeping and hitching Backward (discouraged) A. 1. As tactile sensitivity subsides and child is exploring objects and toys, particularly objects with sound should be kept in a box. The box should initially be stationed under or near the child's bed. Noise from jigglers on bed will help the child locate the box and facilitate search. The box should be kept without variation is the same location until child is automatic in locating the box. *(continues)*

Therapeutic Goals	Objectives	Examples • Methods • Modes • Procedures
	B. Child will move and search the parameters of each room she frequents.	B. 1. Then the box should be used to orient the child to the entrance(s) to the room and the parameter (walls) of the room. Once the child can trace the room in one direction, the pattern can then be reversed. As the child accomplishes this in one area, a similar process is used in other principal areas.
	C. Child will move and search out pathways leading from one room to another.	C. 1. Box of interest should be placed to encourage child to search and move through spaces requiring change of direction to right and left, and reversed patterns. Varying floor surfaces aid the child to distinguish areas. Scooter board movement may be used to facilitate this progress.
V. Encourage development of more independent funcion in daily living skills.	VA. Child will eat independently with supervision.	VA. 1. Child will hold cup with lid and drink without assistance. 2. Child will spoon feed as a principal means of feeding with some spilling with adapted spoon and bowl. 3. Child may use fingers to discriminate foods and eat with fingers foods that are appropriate.
	B. Child will initiate undressing skills and assist in dressing.	B. 1. Child will remove shirt overhead, and push off pants from hips, at bath or bed time.
VI. Continue to encourage resolution of mother's grief over time.	VIA. Continue to channel mother's grief into useful pursuits.	VIA. 1. Continue the processes described in initial program Goal III A, B and C.

4. Improved searching ability within her own bedroom, living area, and kitchen. Family and staff were elated with her increased evidence of orientation as her mobility advanced.
5. Though all self-help skills were continuing to advance, she tended to cling to manual searching of foods in self-feeding with a slow acceptance of the use of utensils for feeding.
6. Improved prehension and instinctive grasping, good opposition. More abilities to place objects, stack objects. Recognizing familiar objects by touch

Both staff and family felt Beth's gains in sensory integration were fundamental to her major increases in function and improved adaptive behavior. The family expressed more confidence in Beth's future, but at the same time they were pursuing eye surgery for Beth in the next several months. The surgery was to attempt to reattach the retina of the right eye. If the operation was successful, the ultimate that could be achieved would be an increase in Beth's light perception. (Note: The surgical process was subsequently carried out as planned, but it failed to improve Beth's vision.) Beth's family continued to work conscientiously with the therapist in advancing Beth's development.

Over the following year and a half, Beth made great strides in gaining gross motor and fine motor skills. Though she was a happy child who learned to sing songs and imitate what she heard, language development, especially expressive speech, was slow. Her enrollment in a nearby special class for visually handicapped children at age 36 months was a turning point for Beth. Subsequently, Beth's ability to communicate markedly improved, which greatly enhanced Beth's potential for learning and functioning. □

Brachial Plexus Injury

A brachial plexus injury to a child at birth will result in damage to the peripheral nerves from injury to their roots at the site. The most common type of brachial plexus injury is of the upper arm, known as *Erb's palsy*, which involves the upper trunks of C5–C6. A less common type of brachial plexus injury is of the lower arm and hand, or *Klumpke's type*, which involves the trunks of the C8–T1 level. The child with these injuries has deficits in the musculoskeletal and neurologic systems of a lower motor-neuron lesion type, involving both the motor and the sensory nerves of the involved arm.

The child with an Erb's type of palsy characteristically keeps the arm in an adducted and internally rotated position, with little to no elbow flexion and little shoulder motion. Hand muscles are usually active, but the child has little opportunity to experience the normal adaptations to developing use of the hand due to the limited arm motion. There are various degrees of injury, with different amounts of residual muscle strength and a potential for return in the first year or two of life. Often, the child has little opportunity in those early years to experience inherently normal patterns of arm and hand movement and, as a result, learns to make little use of both hands in play. It is often easier for the child to develop the use of one hand to the neglect of the other than to try to use a hand that neither moves nor feels normal. This works to the detriment of strengthening returning muscle power and developing use of residual muscles in bilateral play, self-care, and other functions.

Occupational therapy intervention at an early age can contribute to the potential for improved muscle function by careful positioning of the arm for optimum muscle protection and strengthening. Equally important is the contribution of the program to helping the child develop functional use of the arm in play by positioning the arm to permit the child to see and use the arm and hand in early infant play. It is also important to help the parents work with the child for optimum gains, to learn to handle the child correctly to foster good arm use, and to learn to accept the residual deficits. Accepting the fact that the child will generally have some permanent deficits is not easy for the parents, but the occupational therapist may enhance parents' acceptance as they become involved with the child in the treatment program.

Case Study

Pat was found to have a brachial plexus injury at birth. She was referred to the occupational therapy service at 6 weeks of age. She maintained her right arm at an adducted and internally rotated position with elbow extension. Wrist and finger motion was limited. Her primary hand position was fisted, a normal position for a baby of her age. There was no marked passive limitation of motion in her arm, and she tolerated her mother handling and ranging her arm. Her lack of response to handling the right arm indicated a possible deficit in sensation. Normal infant patterns of motion at this age generally include some elbow flexion, arm abducted slightly away from the side, and some external rotation, particularly in startle and crying reactions. In her case, these patterns were lacking. Tone and motion patterns in the left arm and hand were normal, as were her head, neck, and leg reactions. Figure 35-6 depicts the occupational therapy process as planned for this child and her family.

This was the first child of a young mother. The father did not take an active role in the child's program, and the mother at first seemed unable to comprehend the need for a treatment program for her child. Fortunately for this child, a grandmother was

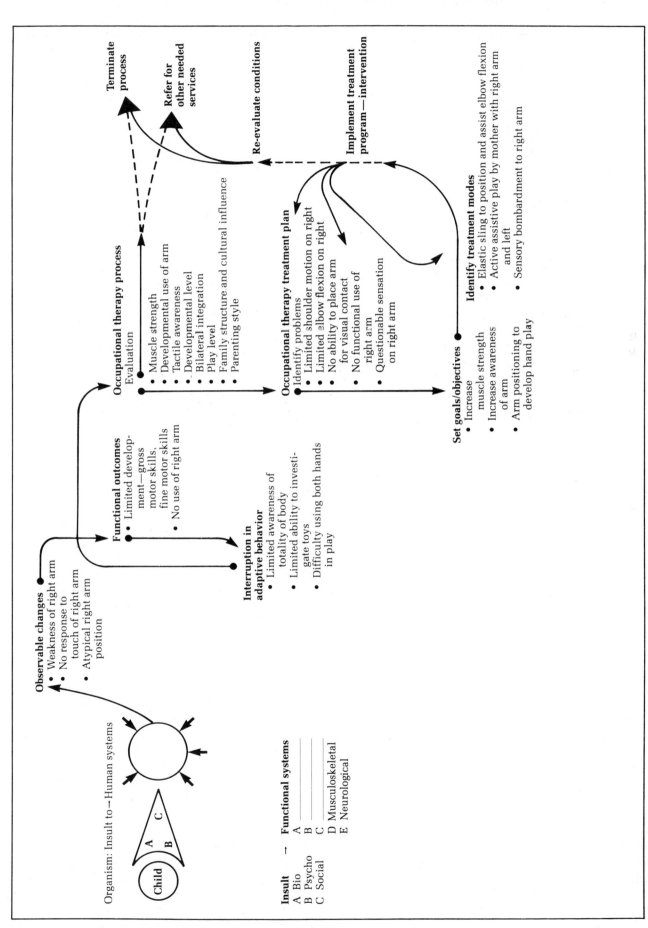

Figure 35-6. Occupational therapy program with an infant with a brachial plexus injury. Case study: Pat.

part of the extended family and took over the major responsibility for guiding the child's program at home. By the third and fourth visits, the mother had grown in her ability to comprehend and work with the therapy program and with the child.

Problems noted in this child were:

1. Limited active shoulder and elbow flexion musculature in right arm
2. Possible lack of sensation and no ability to place her arm where she visually compensated for lack of sensation
3. No ability to use her right arm in normal random waving motions.

The goals and objectives for the occupational therapy program were as follows:

Goal 1: Increased Muscle Strength in Right Arm
 Objective: Develop sufficient muscle strength in shoulder and elbow to enable Pat to place her arm in a position for hand use by the time she is 8 months old.
Goal 2: Increase Sensory Awareness in Right Arm
 Objective: Pat will be aware enough of her right arm to turn when someone touches her right hand by the time she is 8 months old.
Goal 3: Increase Functional Use and Awareness of Right Arm in Total Body Scheme
 Objective: Achieve a position for her right arm that would place her hand so Pat will be able to engage in some hand play between her hands.

The mother was instructed in a home program of (1) passive ranging of the right arm, (2) positioning of the right elbow in flexion by pinning an Ace bandage loop sling to the child's clothing and placing her right arm in the sling with elbow flexed for one half of the day, (3) positioning of the arm in abduction and slight external rotation by use of pillows when the child was lying on her back in bed, (4) sensory stimulation to the right arm by means of rubbing and stroking many times a day, and (5) maintenance of equal play by the mother with the child's right and left arms. The mother was also encouraged to prop Pat's right arm under the child's chest when she was on her stomach and to encourage Pat to lift up her head and push up with her left arm.

The child was re-evaluated 6 weeks later, when she was 3 months old. She had developed better use of her shoulder in that she was swinging her arm through about one-fourth of the range of motion of the left arm. Her elbow was kept in a slightly more flexed position, but no elbow flexion was seen actively. More finger flexion and extension was seen, but she had increased in her tendency to keep a tightly clenched fist rather than losing this reflexive posture as she had done in the left hand. She also

maintained her wrist in a sharply extended posture that is not normal for this age. She had continued to move through other developmental milestones, such as lifting her head well when prone, slight tension of her neck when pulled to sitting, relaxed hand on left, and momentary grasp on a rattle.

Additional problems noted since the initial evaluation included an increased wrist hyperextension tendency and a clenched fist hand. Because of these additional problems the following objective was added:

Goal 1:
 Objective 2: Develop a hand that is relaxed and slightly open at rest and one that Pat is able to open and close around toys.

Treatment instituted was the wearing of a special cock-up orthosis that prevented wrist hyperextension. The orthosis positioned her fingers in extension at the metacarpal phalangeal joints to encourage active finger extension. The mother was advised to have Pat wear this orthosis for 1½ hours three times a day. She was also advised to continue with the previous home program, with special emphasis on helping Pat move her right arm along with her left arm in play activities.

Pat was re-evaluated at 6 months of age. At that time, she was making excellent use of her right arm in reaching activities. Arm and shoulder motion was not normal, but her efficiency in reaching for toys was almost equalized between right and left. Her right hand was relaxed most of the time, with tension noted primarily in the thumb and index finger. She demonstrated palmar grasp with the right and used the right hand together with the left for holding larger objects. Elbow flexion still lagged behind, and all bilateral arm motions were accomplished with the extended right elbow. Supine with her right elbow propped in a slightly flexed position, she was able to flex her elbow slightly using the biceps occasionally. In all other positions, she was unable to activate the right biceps. When prone, she supported herself with the right and left arm equally. She had not started to creep or crawl, so use of her right arm in this pattern was not evaluated. Problems still noted were:

1. Lack of right elbow flexion unless maximally assisted
2. Lack of full arm raising on the right
3. Slight difficulty in opening thumb and index finger on the right

Additional objectives were developed as follows:

Goal 1:
 Objective 3: Develop elbow flexion sufficiently for her to bring objects toward her.
 Objective 4: Continue to develop free opening and closing of her right hand, especially thumb and index finger, sufficiently to allow her to handle toys.

Goal 3:
> *Objective 2:* Monitor use of right arm in developmental activities so that, as growth and development cause the need for more complex hand activities that require two hands, Pat is able to make sufficient use of the right hand to accomplish the developmental task.

The mother was again instructed in a home program, with the focus now being on propping the right elbow in a bent position and helping Pat make use of the slight biceps action that is present. The child was not ready for a walker at that time; however, an overhead sling with spring assist was to be added to encourage elbow flexion. Developmental activities of propping on both elbows; reaching out with both hands; and handling, dropping, and picking up toys were to be encouraged. Re-evaluations at regular 2- to 4-month intervals were scheduled until maximum benefits are achieved. □

Spina Bifida

The child born with spina bifida starts life with a limited number of opportunities to experience the full spectrum of sensorimotor experiences that contribute to normal growth and development. The child has no bowel or bladder control and various degrees of sensory and motor loss to the lower extremities and trunk. The child may also have some degree of hydrocephalus and may have a shunt to drain the cerebrospinal fluid to another part of the body.

The implications of this disability include a variety of losses of normal developmental experiences and the opportunity to experience normal developmental adaptation. The spina bifida child has limited mobility and therefore misses out on many of the normal experiences of movement, such as rolling over, rocking on his or her stomach, creeping, crawling, running, and jumping. The child may frequently be sick, and parents are necessarily more cautious and careful in handling the child. This will further limit the child's opportunities for movement, such as being bounced and swung around, and for normal social interactions with parents and peers. Sensation is also deficient in a portion of the body, so the child is receiving less than normal sensation from which to learn about his or her body and the world around.

These basic deficiencies in normal experiences, if not treated, will delay development, especially in those areas that are strongly dependent on normal tactile and vestibular input, such as eye control, integration of the two sides of the body, and good motor planning. When these problems are coupled with an untreated hydrocephalus that results in neurological deficits, the child's delays can result in marked learning deficits. Occupational therapy intervention at a young age can provide the child with an opportunity to experience some normal tactile and vestibular responses that will enhance the child's normal growth and development and will prevent developmental delays that would result in learning problems in later years.

Case Study

Mary, diagnosed as having spina bifida at birth, was first seen by the occupational therapist when she was 4 years old. Figure 35-7 depicts the occupational therapy program plan. The systems involved were circulatory, intestinal–urinary, musculoskeletal, and neurological. Mary presented no hydrocephalus. The observable changes in Mary were:
1. No active foot and ankle muscles, poor knee muscle strength, good hip muscle strength. She walked with bilateral long-leg orthoses and a walker.
2. No sensation from the knees down
3. No bowel and bladder control
4. Frequent infections of the urinary tract and respiratory system

Evaluation
The initial occupational therapy evaluation revealed the following functional losses and interruption in developmental adaptation:
1. No response to postrotary nystagmus test after 10 seconds of spinning, nor any response after a repeat test of 20 seconds' duration
2. No ability to achieve a correct prone extension holding pattern to overcome the dominance of the tonic labyrinthine reflex when prone. This deficit would be expected in her legs due to lower extremity weakness, but she also could not lift her head and shoulders and was very frightened of the position.
3. No protective extension or parachuting reaction
4. Poor attention to tasks. She frequently talked rather than attending to assigned play activities.
5. Limited experience on normal playground equipment. She was still frightened of most new play activities that involved total body motion.
6. Eye tracking was nonexistent. She did not even attempt to pursue the object by moving her head, as many 4-year-olds will do.

Fine motor skills were at age level, as were self-care skills. She even attempted the difficult task of putting on her long-leg orthoses. The family was very supportive and had attempted to seek medical advice at an early age. As a result, urinary tract infections had been kept at a minimum. She had been referred to a physical therapist by 10 months of age, but this was

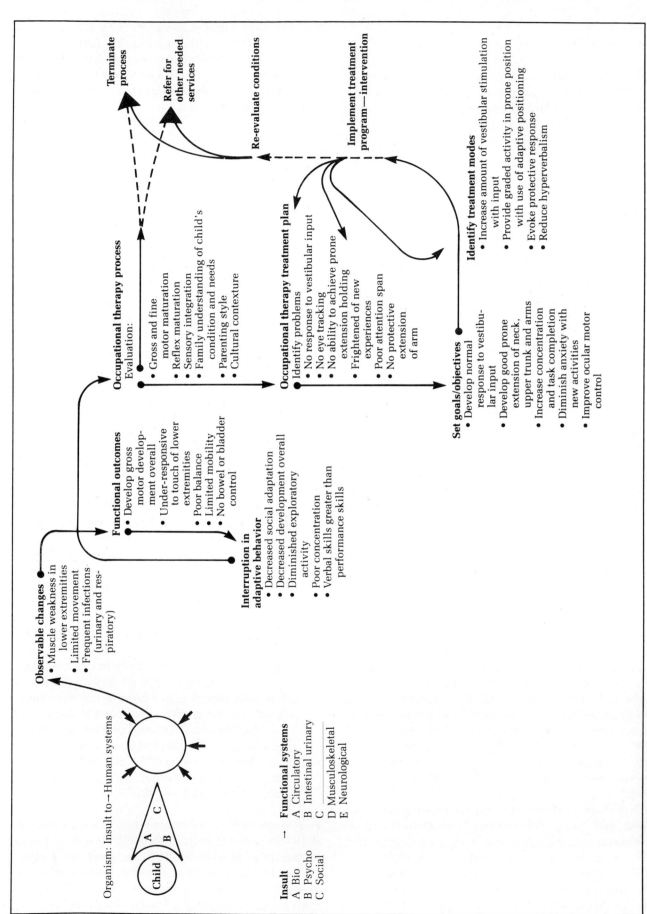

Figure 35-7. Occupational therapy program with a spina bifida child. Case study: Mary.

her first referral to an occupational therapist. There was a younger brother in the family, and play between Mary and her younger brother was normal for the ages of the two children in spite of the fact that Mary was more confined and limited in her activities.

Occupational Therapy Program

Occupational therapy intervention was necessary to achieve the following goals and objectives:

Goal 1: Child Will Develop Improved Vestibular Responses to Movement.

Objective: Mary will show slight nystagmus after 6 months of treatment.

Goal 2: Child Will Integrate Primitive Reflexes As a Means to Achieving Normal Adult Reflex and Movement Patterns.

Objective: She will be able to lift her shoulders, arms, and head when prone for 10 minutes and will be able to play in this position with moving activities for 10 minutes without fatigue.

Objective: She will be able to throw her arms out protectively four out of five times when turned upside down.

Goal 3: Child Will Develop Improved Eye-Tracking Ability.

Objective: She will be able to eye track smoothly horizontally three times and vertically three times after 3 months of treatment.

Objective: She will be able to eye track diagonally smoothly two out of three times after 6 months of treatment.

Goal 4: Child Will Develop Attention to Performance Tasks at Her Age Level.

Objective: She will be able to follow therapist's oral directions in the treatment sessions three out of four times without extraneous conversation.

Objective: She will be able to play appropriately with a toy of her own choice for 15 minutes.

Mary was treated weekly in an outpatient treatment center, and a home program was designed for the parents to use between treatment sessions. Her therapy program consisted of a variety of vestibular activities including spinning in a hammock, riding a scooterboard, swinging in an infant swing that supported her unstable legs, rocking in a ''Play All'' toy, and being bounced on a spring horse. Due to the weakness in her legs, she could not bounce herself on the horse.

She was also started in a program that would encourage the development of a good prone extension holding pattern by positioning her on a scooterboard, which was adapted to accommodate for some of her

structural deformities. Her hips were tight in flexion, and her lower back was lordodic. This caused her to be angled in an uncomfortable position downward when prone, contributing to her dislike of this position. By wedging her hips and upper trunk, she was placed in an optimum position to foster good upper trunk and head extension. By propelling herself on the scooterboard very rapidly, she was able to stimulate more automatic head lift. This treatment procedure was also designed to encourage better eye tracking.

Her parents were shown how to design a similar scooterboard for home use. They were supportive of the need to build this equipment and used it at home as a supplement to the weekly occupational therapy session. After the parents watched and helped with the child's treatment program for several treatment sessions, the family was provided with a home program to be carried out daily with Mary. The child's younger brother enjoyed the same activities, so peer play time was used to provide the optimum activities to enhance this child's development. By using the peer play time for the exercise program, less attention was drawn to the special treatment. This avoided the conflicts frequently arising in family situations when one child receives special treatment.

After 3 months in the program Mary was able to:

1. Lift shoulders, arms, and head when prone for 10 minutes and play in this position for 20 minutes without fatigue
2. Consistently throw both arms out to protect herself when turned upside down
3. Attend to assigned performance tasks for 20 minutes
4. Eye track horizontally five times smoothly

She had not made any gains in correct nystagmus following spinning nor had she gained any vertical or diagonal eye tracking. Her treatment program was revised to increase emphasis on the activities for these two areas, and she continued in the outpatient program for 6 more months. She was referred to the school-based therapist when she entered school at age 5. After a year in school, the school-based therapist reported that Mary had continued to make gains in eye tracking and attention span and was having no trouble in the regular classroom. At 6 years of age, she still did not show any nystagmus response to spinning for 10 seconds. She continued on a home program of stimulation to her vestibular system. The school-based therapist re-evaluated her progress frequently and made suggestions to the family, but Mary was not provided with direct occupational services because her classroom performance was excellent.

Although at 6 years of age this child still shows a neurological deficit in motor and sensory control of her lower extremities and a significant lag in her vestibular processing, the occupational therapy intervention enabled her to reach a more balanced level of growth and development allowing her to function in the regular classroom. Attention span and eye tracking deficits seen at age 4 could have hampered classroom performance without the intervention and remediation provided through the occupational therapy program.   ☐

Down Syndrome

Basic and general understanding of children with Down syndrome is clouded by long-standing misinformation. Despite more advanced methods, both lay persons and professionals often lack sufficient current information about this condition, characteristics of development, and specific developmental potential. Advances in cytogenetic studies do enable physicians to provide a more timely and accurate diagnosis. Accurate Down syndrome identification does clarify whether the genetic insult is hereditary or an accidental mutation. These advances are of great importance to Down syndrome children and the parents. Nevertheless, for parents of newborn or young Down syndrome children, the paucity of help in learning to parent their child and in understanding the development of their child is a major problem. Occupational therapists have an important early and long-range role in assisting both the parents and the Down syndrome children to attain their individual developmental potential. Certain physical characteristics of children with Down syndrome are classic and familiar:

Shortened limbs and fingers
Slanted eyes with skin fold over eyelid
Small mouth with enlarged protruding tongue
Simian line
Speckled iris
High incidence of congenital heart defects
Increased incidence of leukemia
Mental retardation

Other physical characteristics of importance to the child's development, though less well known, are:

Floppiness at birth and generalized low muscle tone prevalence in early years. Note: special weakness of trunk flexors and, in general, poor muscle cocontractibility
Hyperextensible joints, especially the hips, limbs, and digits
Poor muscle tone of oral-facial mechanism
Increased and prolonged tactile sensitivity with diffuse tactile discrimination deficiency
Increased sensitivity to gravitational adjustment
Hyporeactive postrotary nystagmus
Poor bilateral motor coordination

Because of the altered sensory integration, the following variations often occur in neurodevelopmental reflex maturation:

Diminished suck reflex
Accentuated gag reflex
Diminished palmar reflex
Prolonged exaggerated Moro reflex
Prolonged flexor withdrawal and avoidance reactions of hands and feet
Delayed proprioceptive placing of limbs and "air sitting" response to positive support testing
Poor optical righting, especially supine reactions
Poor body righting
Delayed equilibrium responses, especially quadripedal and standing

Some of the motor problems that are outcomes of these conditions are:

A general delay in gross motor milestone attainment based on body instability, weakness, and, often, fear of imposed handling or imposed touch sensation
Skull sensitivity, also feet and hands sensitivity
Prolonged head lag in coming to sit
Child avoids weight bearing on feet — air sits or retracts lower extremities
Child often incorporates creeping with knee extension pattern
Child may have hyperextended knees, pronated feet in walking pattern

Some characteristics are shown in Figure 35-8.
Other predictable outcomes based on these Down syndrome variations in development are:

Difficulty in early feeding ability with later selectivity in foods basically tied to gag reflex influences and poor chewing ability
Delays in prehension overall
Delays in finger feeding due to sensitivity of hands to messiness
Splintered hand skill development, with some compensation because of delayed or organized mobility.

In general, children with Down syndrome are classically dyspraxic based on vestibular somotasensory dysfunction.

Case Study

Jane, a 20-month-old child with Down syndrome, had a history of delayed development, recurrent respiratory infection, and allergies, despite general good health. Jane had received comprehensive developmental services prior to initial evaluation.

Jane's parents were newly located following the completion of their graduate studies in applied

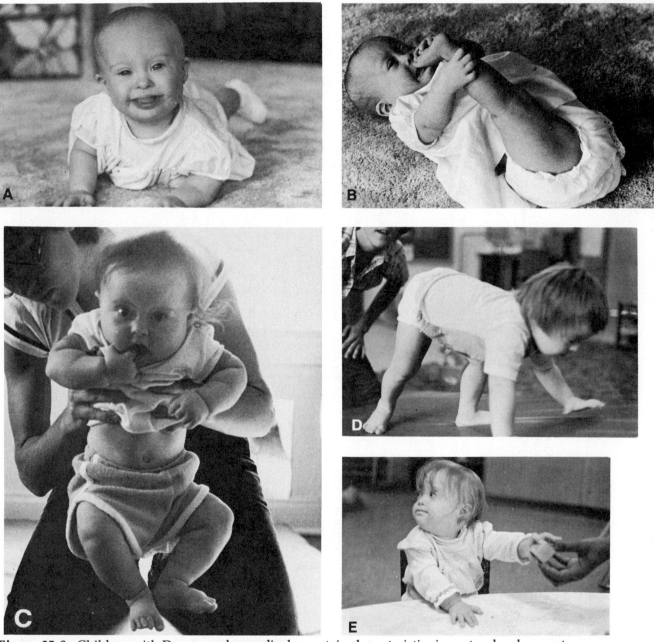

Figure 35-8. Children with Down syndrome display certain characteristics in motor development or performance. *(A)* Oral–facial weakness. *(B)* Hyperextensible joints, especially hips. *(C)* Diminished proprioception and tactile sensitivity seen in delayed positive support of lower extremities. *(D)* Extended knee creeping compensating for diminished proprioception and joint stability. *(E)* Poor attention and concentration in fine skill performance.

sciences. Both parents were in their late 20s. Each had secured promising positions in the field of their study. They had little experience in handling or caring for young children, Jane being their first and only child. Both were equally committed to their careers and their child. Communication between the parents seemed good. Household responsibilities were shared equally by the parents. The father demonstrated innate nurturing skills, while the mother, an assertive person, seemed less at ease. The father assumed equal

or more responsibility for Jane's care. Both held high expectations for their child's individual development and high expectations for those providing services directed toward such goals. They demonstrated good coping skills related to Jane's high-strung behavior and frequent temper outbursts. They initiated a request for developmental services, including occupational therapy services from a community infant–parent training program. Figure 35-9 depicts that process.

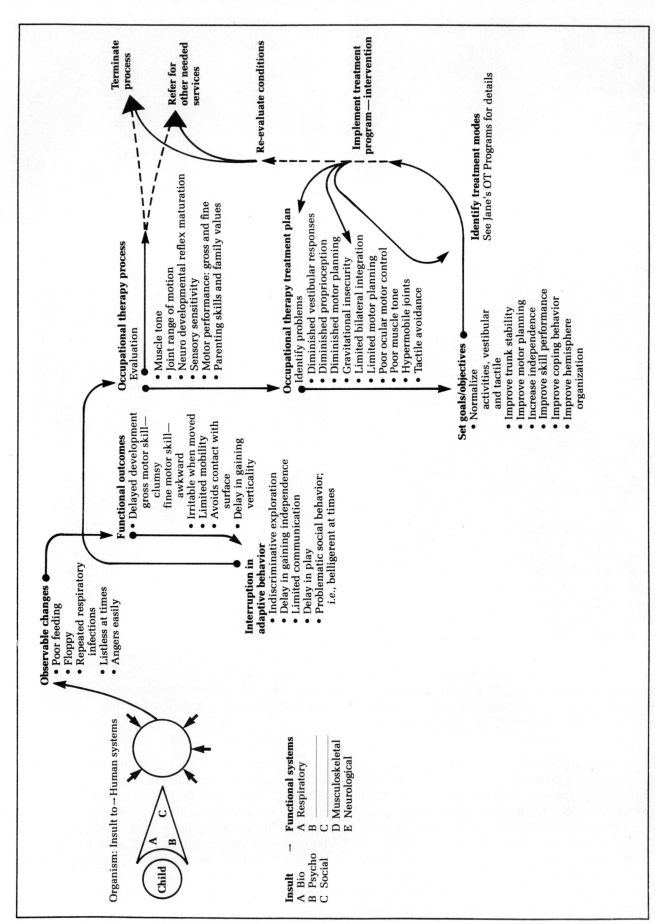

Figure 35-9. Occupational therapy with a Down syndrome child. Case study: Jane.

Occupational Therapy Program—
Initial Evaluation

During the initial evaluation of Jane at 20 months, she was noted to have moderately low muscle tone with hyperextensible joints in the limbs and digits. A key problem area was identified in the markedly limited mobility of the child. The child could sit with a fairly straight back when placed and could roll to right and left, but was delayed in independent coming to and lowering from sit. When pulled to sit, she assisted but still demonstrated head lag during the first 45° of movement. Delay was also noted in lower extremity weight-bearing and support. The child avoided surface contact by air sitting more than 50% of the time. She had recently gained pivoting in prone and had emerging skills in reciprocal progression in the prone position. Reflexively, she continued to show some hand and foot avoidance, though instinctive grasping was moderately present. She had poor placing of hands and absent visual placing of legs. The overall gross motor level was 6 to 7 months, with a motor quotient of 35%, indicating significant deficiency.

In contrast, fine motor performance was in advance of gross motor. In feeding, she had a good appetite and was eating a wide variety of foods, chewing fairly well, was independent in cup use and finger feeding, and was able to help with spoon feeding. In dressing, she was generally cooperative and was able to take off socks and untied shoes. In general manipulation, she banged blocks together, reached for large objects, approximated a 1-inch cube over another, and threw a ball undirected. She was beginning to discriminate a crayon and used it appropriately. She was using the right and left hands equally well and was just beginning to automatically cross the midline with the right. In general, her fine motor skills clustered at 12–15 months or roughly 60%–75% of chronological age expectancy. Sensory factors of significance were:

Tactile avoidance, with diffused and poor discrimination; oral sucking behavior; irritability to light touch on the back of the neck, abdomen, hands, and feet
Proprioception—under registered—seeking such on her own limits
Vestibular processing—poor postural organization with diminished response to postrotary nystagmus testing; alarmed and irritated by linear vestibular input when imposed
Visual processing—visually attentive but lacked smooth ocular motor performance, depending on neck rotation primarily; convergence limited, with midline interruptions
Visual search relating to object permanence judged to be at 8 months, and in obtaining objects, she could push away an obstruction to obtain a wanted object

Motor planning—limited gross motor planning in evidence, though fine motor planning included imitation of repetitive simple gestures and in some cases she was examining, letting go, and initiating some "give me" transactions

A treatment and educational planning meeting was held with the parents following completion of the child's evaluation. Evaluation results were explained, along with the identified problems, goals, and objectives.

The proposed treatment and educational modes or procedures to assist in achieving short-range goals were explained, including suggested home program activities. Though the parents agreed to the plan that focused on improving Jane's sensorimotor integration and adaptive behavior, they questioned whether more emphasis should be placed on cognitive activities. Staff provided further explanation of the need for sensorimotor organization for their child as a basis for cognitive development, explaining that in Jane's case, improved sensory integration would reduce her sensitivity and would lead to improved mobility, understanding, and function. There was agreement that Jane would attend daily classes at the center that would provide sensorimotor integration intervention, along with speech–language, educational, and social developmental activities. Home programming with parent training was agreed to as well. Formal re-evaluation was tentatively scheduled for 3 months after initiation of programming activities.

The outline of the treatment plan (see Jane's Occupational Therapy Program–20 months) includes major therapeutic goals, with specific objectives and suggested modes or procedures. Ongoing adaptation or adjustment of these procedures is required as objectives are achieved or when methods appear to be inappropriate or ineffective. Jane's attendance at the center was regular. Home programming visitation by the center's therapist was highly irregular due to parent cancellation. The reason given for the numerous cancellations of home visit appointments was work-related conflicts.

Re-evaluation

Jane was 24 months old at the time of re-evaluation. She continued to have hyperextensible joints and moderately low muscle tone, but she had made major gains in mobility. Improved motor planning for movement transitions were seen in new skills in raising and lowering from sit and from sit to hands and knees. The ability to creep and hitch were demonstrated with some instability. Because of this instability, she continued to use reciprocal prone progression as her chief mode, which was at that time a very efficient skill. Though she continued to air sit 25% of the time, when handled she showed emerging lower extremity positive support and was standing at a rail

(text continues on page 658)

Jane's Occupational Therapy Program: Chronological Age—20 Months

Therapeutic Goals	Objectives	Examples • Methods • Modes • Procedures
I. Normalize tactile sensitivity as a means to increase gross and fine motor function/mobility.	IA. Child will air sit infrequently (1 of 10 x's) when lowered in handling.	IA. 1. Apply firm tactile stimulation generally to child 2 x D. 2. Provide manual otolithic stimulation in all positions including supported standing to tolerance. 2 x D.
	B. Child will weight bear in standing hold to rail.	B. 1. Using external motivator, child will be assisted in transitional movement to achieve standing during purposeful play. 5x during a 30 minute period.
	C. Child will explore familiar objects using both instinctive and voluntary grasp with avoidance interference.	C. 1. Child will search for objects partially hidden in a box containing styrofoam stuffing, crumbled foam or pan of water for 10 minutes.
II. Improve proprioception especially trunk stability, as a means to increase gross motor function/ mobility.	IIA. Child will maintain static quadruped position during activity.	IIA,B,C. 1. Using a weighted vest and cuff weight, child will bounce on a flexible surface such as an air mattress with assist, 5–10 minutes. Other means of bouncing is a firm padded board in hammock on springs. When in quadruped be sure palms are flattened. Weighted/ vest Cuff weights Firm surface suspended/ by hammock & spring
III. Normalize gravitational insecurity and improve vestibular processing to enhance adaptive behavior.	IIIA. Child will tolerate swinging.	IIIA. 1. Child will swing on suspended pendulum swing with spring seated for 5 minutes (3 second arcs)
	B. Child will tolerate tilting.	B. 1. Child will tilt on firm surface in prone, supine, sitting and puppy position.

Therapeutic Goals	Objectives	Examples • Methods • Modes • Procedures
	C. Child will initiate and tolerate sliding.	C. 1. Child will slide down an incline plane on stomach and in seated position 2 times minimal or more frequently to desire.
IV. Improve motor planning as a means to increase gross and fine motor function.	IVA. Child will attempt to imitate complex gestures. B. Child will raise and lower from sitting. C. Child will move to hands and knees.	A. 1. Child will attend to task demonstration and initiate movement grossly. B&C. 1. Using external motivator, child will perform these transitional movements during play activities 5 times during a 30 minute period.
V. Improve bilateral integration.	VA. Child will cross midline right and left in seated activities. B. Child will cross midline in prone activities.	VA. 1. Child will place objects in a receptical to right of midline with left hand and vice versa 10 times. B. 1. Child will turn, while prone, using alternating hands, to right and left in hammock.
VI. Improve ocular motor control.	VIA. Child will track object using eye muscles with minimal rotation.	VIA. 1. While lying supine, child will follow a slowly swinging 3″ ball of contrasting colors.
VII. Improve the level of independence in activities of daily living.	VIIA. Child will eat with minimal assistance. B. Child will partially remove shirt and pants.	VIIA. 1. Child will be fitted with secured scoop dish and spoon with handle of ⅝″ diameter. Spoon should be bent slightly to compensate for poor supination stability. 2. Child should use feeding equipment at school and home daily. Assistance may be needed in practice of filling spoon. B. 1. Child will practice removing button shirt or loose T-shirt over head in 1 minute D, at school and home with encouragement. 2. Child will practice removing pants from knees when seated, in 2 minutes with encouragement D, at school and home.

and beginning to lower to sit. She could pivot in sitting and no longer showed head lag in coming to sit. The key changes in reflex status were seen in lessening plantar grasping; less avoidance of hands and feet; improved visual-labyrinthine righting in supine; improved placing of limbs, especially her hands and arms; improved equilibrium in prone supine and sitting; and emergence of protective reactions sideways. Gross motor skill level had reached 11 months, with a gross motor quotient of 42%.

Improved fine motor skill was also apparent. Jane now demonstrated independent spoon and two-handed cup use, though she was quite messy and needed a watchful eye at mealtimes to prevent chaos. She was beginning to wipe her mouth. In dressing, she was able to partially remove upper and lower garments. She was beginning to scribble with a stubby crayon. Her pincer grasp was precise as was opposition, and she could now release a block carefully, place a peg in a hole, and on occasion leaf pages one at a time. She was continuing to use some oral exploration, but she tended to rotate and examine objects more often.

Sensory integration factors of significance were:

Tactile avoidance — now less pervasive but continued to be noted, especially with lower extremities and feet; continued oral seeking behavior, at times; poor tactile discrimination now noted in two-point discrimination

Proprioception continued to be under-registered — continued to be sought by herself; changes were noted in her improved willingness to allow others to control her excessive drive. Poor concentration seemed to be linked to poor proprioception and cocontractability

Vestibular processing — improving postural organization with continued hyporesponsiveness to postrotary nystagmus testing; no longer alarmed by linear vestibular input when imposed — but now sometimes angered; now seeking angular vestibular stimulation

Motor planning — improved gross motor planning as reflected in gross motor milestone attainments; able to get off chair; fine motor planning and imitation level include clapping, waving bye-bye, imitating two gestures in twinkle-twinkle, making faces spontaneously and on occasion in imitation.

Resetting Goals, Objectives, and Methods

A joint parent–staff meeting was held following Jane's reassessment at 24 months. The parents were encouraged by Jane's advances in mobility and skill gains. They were concerned about Jane's behavior because of her continued temper outbursts that sometimes occurred in handling, often when the child was unable to get her needs met, and in some cases when expectations required Jane to "be still" for any

length of time. Jane's parents were worried about her limited concentration. The staff explained the related nature of sensory integration dysfunction to irritable behavior and anger, to poor organization, and hence, to poor concentration. The staff urged that they be given more opportunity to assist the parents in home management techniques and sensory integration opportunities. The parents agreed to make a more concerted effort to organize a supportive home program and to meet regularly with a home program therapist. The adjustments in goals, objectives, and methods are presented in Jane's Occupational Therapy Program – 24 months.

Subsequent re-evaluations of Jane at age 29 months and 34 months and conferences with parents confirmed the achievement of motor skills to 85% of age expectancy in fine and gross function. She was moving freely in space at home and outdoors, was running stiffly, squatting in play, mounting stairs, and descending while using a rail. On occasion, her parents did carry Jane, but principally for their own convenience or when Jane was tired. Jane could self-feed fairly well and undress with ease, and she was learning to unfasten. She was partially toilet trained. She was concentrating for longer periods; working simple puzzles; stacking blocks to seven high; and imitating vertical, horizontal, and circular patterns with chalk and crayon on a vertical and horizontal surface. Jane's skill performance was not splintered but generalized. She was playing with dolls symbolically and demonstrated many skills in her use of objects in symbolic play. Her construction of objects in space such as arranging chairs at a table, ordering large plastic boxes, and using objects for intended purposes was expanding daily. Parents and staff noted with satisfaction that as tactile, proprioception, and vestibular processing normalized, Jane had not only gained skills, but her stormy behavior had subsided, and she was far easier to manage. An extra bonus was Jane's markedly improved ability to follow oral instructions for motor output. Overall communication was advancing as well.

Staff and parents agreed to continue Jane's program with an upgrading of sensorimotor integration objectives until age 36 months. They also agreed that Jane could profit from a combination of early childhood programming (to continue needed therapeutic measures) with normal 2+-year-old nursery experiences. The transition to this was a fairly smooth one for Jane and her family. At age 48 months, a follow-up indicated continued sensorimotor integration, good mastery of skills overall, and, in particular, good visual–motor integration. This marked gain in ability to copy symbols was only one of a number of evidences that gave support to a hopeful future for Jane's academic potential and overall development. □

(text continues on page 661)

Jane's Occupational Therapy Program: Chronological Age—24 Months

Therapeutic Goals	Objectives	Examples • Methods • Modes • Procedures
I. Improve the continuity of the treatment program.	IA. Train parents in skills necessary to provide sensory motor integration programming as a part of their daily life pattern.	IA. 1. Hold planning meeting at child's home, review the new therapeutic objectives and procedures and how they will promote development. 2. Determine those procedures the parents will be able to incorporate over time. 3. Help parents obtain, construct or install equipment or supplies needed for program. 4. Teach by demonstration and example those techniques judged to be of greatest value to parent and child. 5. Have parents assist in procedures, then demonstrate the procedure independently. 6. Give genuine praise for effort, be alert to caution about procedures. 7. Give particular consultation, and demonstration method for controlling behavior during therapeutic procedures and in general daily living encounters.
II. Continue to normalize tactile sensitivity to improve gross/fine motor function/mobility.	IIA. Child will not exhibit air sitting when lowered in handling. B. Child will cruise independently and walk with hands held. C. Child will explore unfamiliar objects instinctively or voluntarily without avoidance.	IIA. 1. Continue to apply firm tactile stimulation generally. 2. Continue otolith stimulation, especially in kneeling and supported standing (5 min). B. 1. Using external motivator child will move independently in biped using furniture for support or hands of therapist during purposeful play. C. 1. Child will search for objects varied in texture and use. Place objects on shelves at different heights that require child to maintain kneeling or standing for 10 min.

Therapeutic Goals	Objectives	Examples • Methods • Modes • Procedures
III. Normalize gravitational insecurity and improve vestibular processing to enhance adaptive behavior.	IIIA. Child will increase tolerance to swinging.	IIIA. 1. Child will swing on platform in prone, supine, seated and puppy position for 5 minutes (4 sec. arcs).
	B. Child will increase tolerance to tilting.	B. 1. Child will tilt on a firm surface in the quadruped, kneeling and in supported standing 5 minutes D.
	C. Child will increase tolerance to sliding.	C. 1. Child will slide down inclined plane on a metal disc facing forward, backward and sideways; also in puppy position forward and backward to tolerance D.
IV. Improve proprioception, especially trunk, shoulder girdle and hands.	IVA. Child will propel herself with use of upper extremities.	IVA. 1. Positioned in seat or prone position in hammock, child will pull herself through space by means of suspended theraband strip 10x's 2x D.
	B. Child will place hands more effectively and initiate backwards protective extension.	B.*1. Child will use protective extension when moved while seated on carpeted barrel. 10x's D. *Continue use of cuff weights and weighted vest.
V. Improve motor planning as a means to increase gross and fine motor function	VA. Child will attempt to copy therapist's demonstrated gestures in goal directed task.	VA. 1. Child will pull bead on string, stack blocks 3–6 high, turn crank on toy, spin large top.

Therapeutic Goals	Objectives	Examples • Methods • Modes • Procedures
VI. Improve bilateral integration.	VIA. Child will demonstrate use of assisting hand. B. Child will cross midline in 2 step activities.	VIA. 1. Child will remove cap from pen, hold jar while unscrewing lid, hold bead while stringing same with dominant hand. B. 1. Child will move forward on scooterboard in prone position through a simple maze requiring turns of 180° to right and left using alternating hands. 10 feet trip 2x's.
VII. Improve ocular motor control.	VIIA. Child will track and converge as a part of a purposeful task.	VIIA. 1. Child will push and catch a 6″ ball while seated 10 x's D.
VIII. Improve the level of independence in activities of daily life.	VIIIA. Child will eat independently without supervision. B. Child will completely remove shirt and partially remove pants.	VIIIA. 1. Using adaptive feeding equipment, child will feed all meals routinely with less spilling. B. 1. Child will remove button shirt or loose T-shirt at nap time and bath time. B. 2. Child will take off pants when below hips.

Autism

Children with autism demonstrate a marked deviation in development, exhibiting classic characteristics of which pediatric occupational therapists need to be aware. Autism was first identified as a distinct syndrome by Kanner.[14] Through Kanner's work, other researchers intensified efforts to identify etiological factors and characteristics of the condition and to determine which treatment or methods of treatment were effective. To date, research has yet to identify the exact physical cause of autism.

Children with autism display unusual social developmental characteristics. Often, they are unable to relate appropriately to their parents, siblings, peers, and others they encounter in their environment. They often display an indifferent or detached behavior. Their language may be delayed or absent. Often, a deficiency is noted in reception or registration. In many cases, symbolic representation in expression is lacking, and the child's expressions are limited to echolalic production. In other cases, expressive language organization is disordered, and characteristically, pronoun references are poor. Because of the lateness, absence, or peculiarity of the child's ability to communicate, initially parents often seek professional help from physicians, psychologists, social workers, and speech pathologists. In other cases, parents seek help for their child because they recognize that their child is not relating to them (the parents) and that he or she has unusual behaviors — in some cases very obsessive — that prevent the child from advancing in acquiring generalized function.

More recent investigators of autism (Ornitz and Ritvo) have identified neurophysiological disorders as a major factor in autism, focusing on sensorimotor and perceptual motor processing as contributing factors.[22] Ornitz raises pertinent questions about the relationship of vestibular processing efficiency to autism.[20,21] Recent researchers in the field have recognized the inadequate ability of children with autism to process, organize, interpret, and respond to sensory information. Pediatric occupational therapy skills/services are specifically related to the improvement of such processing deficiencies as a means of promoting improved functional and behavioral/adaptive outcomes. As such, autism evaluation and treatment should include occupational therapy services. The treatment of this disorder should include the services of occupational therapists because of their therapeutic skills in developing such sensorimotor organization for functional behavioral advancement.

Specific characteristics identified in autism[22,25] include:

Onset prior to 30 months of age

Perceptual and sensory processing disturbances as a possible result of distorted sensation, faulty modulation of sensory input, and impaired discriminative ability

Deviations in the rate of development marked by periods of rapid growth, followed by plateaus

Inability to relate to others noted in such behaviors as aversion to physical contact, delay or absence of social smile, and lack of anticipation of being picked up

Unusual relating to objects with a need to "maintain sameness" (Kanner) in the environment, leading to rigid, inflexible, and controlling personality traits; frequently, manipulation of toys is inappropriate and maladaptive where spinning, twirling, rubbing, and feeling of them is common

Speech and language disorders marked not only by delayed development but also by abnormal features, including echolalia, pronoun reversal, and monotonous and atonal quality expressing little emotion; language-related functions in general are seriously impaired, including symbolic play, abstraction, understanding of gestures and written language, sequential tasks (primarily temporal in nature) and meaning in memory processes

Unusual motility or spontaneous motion patterns, either intermittent or continuous, repeated in serial fashion; included hand-flapping, finger-flicking, and toe-walking

Mental retardation is diagnosed in a high percentage of autistic children, as most cannot perform adequately on IQ tests and generally perform throughout life as mentally impaired individuals

Seizure disorders are likely to become manifested with increasing age, even in those with normal EEGs and neurological examinations early in life

"Soft" neurological signs often found, including low muscle tone, poor coordination, drooling, short attention span, hyperactivity, hypoactivity, and hyperreflexia

Efforts to identify possible explanations for this complex, behaviorally and clinically defined syndrome have led to inconclusive findings. Some authors have investigated parental traits and socioeconomic conditions,[10,16] noting a preponderance of highly intellectual, obsessive professional parents lacking in emotional warmth. However, most investigators now agree that central nervous system dysfunction is the basis for autism. Consideration given to prenatal and perinatal causes, association with viral diseases, genetic factors, and biochemical and metabolic elements has not produced a significant explanation of etiology. These factors continue to be studied in hopes of finding not only the reasons for the occurrence of autism but additional modes of intervention to increase the functional capacity of individuals involved.

The prognosis for children with autism in developing functions necessary for independent living is more hopeful for the mildly involved and those with fewer complicating and associated disorders, such as mental impairment and other developmental delays. Higher IQ, earlier language development, and earlier demonstration of appropriate play seem to be indicators of a more hopeful outcome.[17,18] However, the number who can live and work unaided is small, with most requiring assistance and supervision throughout life.

Intervention strategies are as varied as the possible causes and include behavioral approaches, milieu therapy, play therapy, neurodevelopmental treatment approaches, and pharmacotherapy provided in medical and educational settings.

Of particular interest to the occupational therapist who applies neurological and developmental principles in treatment is the disordered sensorimotor integration often displayed by children with autism. Responses to stimulation can be elevated or reduced in various instances in the same child. Children with autism may lack response to painful stimuli; to lack or have a delayed startle response; to lack visual attention to new events within the environment; or to be unaware of auditory input. In contrast, the therapist may note exaggerated responses to sensory stimuli that create observable stress in the child, who attempts to avoid or block out the sensation. The child who seeks to whirl and rock himself in one instance may display fear of vestibular activity in another. Oral-tactile sensitivites are noted in the child's aversion to foods of thick consistency and/or rough texture. Avoidance of certain odors may occur, yet the child may smell objects in his hand prior to mouthing them in exploration.

Seeking of stimulation is a commonly observed trait, especially of apparent input to the tactile, proprioceptive, and vestibular systems. Rubbing and twirling of objects in the fingers, probably to produce tactile stimulation, is noted in some children with autism. One adult reports a great need for heavy pressure, finding comfort and relief from stress when receiving significant amounts of such pressure input.[13] Rocking, head-rolling and head-banging, twirling, and hand-flapping may be methods of stimulation through proprioceptive and vestibular channels. Becker[8] reports Ayres' observations that children with autism seek joint traction to a degree that most individuals would find painful.

Auditory and visual input may also be sought in unusual, yet persistent and obsessive ways. Generally, it appears that there is preference for input through the proximal senses (somatosensory, vestibular, gustatory, and olfactory) over the distal senses (auditory and visual) for environmental exploration. If sensory modulation is inadequate, even information through the early-evolving tactile, proprioceptive, and vestibular systems may be of little value if the child cannot make sense of those inputs in forming the basis for advancing social, movement, and learning strategies. These sensory channels are the primary focus in applying the theoretical principles of sensory integration as occupational therapists attempt to enhance the foundation for increasingly sophisticated adaptive functions.

In investigating responses to sensory input as predictors of outcome in sensory integrative therapy, Ayres and Tickle found that those children with autism who were hyperresponsive or oriented to certain types of stimuli showed greater gains in treatment than those who were hyporesponsive.[7] It is suggested that children whose nervous systems are receiving some sensory input, but who fail to organize that information, have an advantage over those who do not register the information because of an inability or failure to orient to stimuli. It seems easier in therapy, through controlled sensory input, to help modify information that is entering the child's brain than to activate new or nonfunctioning neural circuits.

Children typically learn through movement and play, gaining information about themselves, about objects in the environment, and about themselves in relation to objects and others. Movement is basic to learning, laying the foundation for precepts, concepts, and abstract reasoning in addition to establishing the child's self-identity. Black and associates found that within a confined area equipped for gross motor activities, children with autism engage in more imitative play and display more appropriate play behaviors than in spaces where no objects or other smaller toys are presented.[11]

In the latter situations, more repetitive and solitary behaviors are noted.

Planned and controlled sensory input used in active play helps to facilitate more appropriate and adaptive behaviors in children and offers the occupational therapist a vital mechanism by which to impact on a child's total growth and development.

Case Study

Raymond, age 5 and autistic to a moderate degree, was born prematurely at 6 months' gestation. He remained on a respirator for 2 months before he was physically stable enough to be held by his parents. His mother reported that toxemia occurred during her pregnancy. Both parents are teachers and concerned about their child's needs, although they lack understanding about the implications of his handicap, as they expect him to eventually be like other children his age. They have become more aware of the severity of his disorder since the birth of their second son, now 10 months old. The younger child is developing at a typical rate and appears to be free of any dysfunction. There is no reported history of familial disorders such as autism.

Raymond attends a special-education program for severely emotionally impaired students five afternoons a week. He has used repetitive echolalic speech for approximately 2 years, and he lacks ability to make his needs known appropriately through verbal means. Raymond seldom makes eye contact and prefers to work in isolation at any task in which he becomes engrossed. He does not spin objects, nor does he exhibit hand-flapping or body-rocking, but he is an occasional toe walker.

Raymond's behavior, noted as hyperactive, distractible, compulsive, and sometimes aggressive, prevents him from being a candidate for standardized sensory integration and intelligence tests. Although Raymond's sensitivity hampers such testing, clinical behavior indicates an obvious presence of ability to perform simple tasks.

Obsessiveness in play is a noted characteristic as Raymond places objects adjacent to one another in a continuous line and becomes markedly disturbed if their order is disrupted. He usually puts toys and objects in his mouth upon picking them up before manipulating them to any extent with his hands. Other than these behaviors, play is disorganized and inappropriate for most tasks.

Observation and interpretation of his activities reveal a decided craving for tactile stimulation, as he is often noted to rub objects on his arms, legs, stomach, face, and hair as he handles them; however, he is extremely aversive to touching by other people. When overly aroused, he chooses to wrap himself in a blanket and hide in a confined space while sucking his thumb. Low muscle tone and poor cocontraction are noted, with hyperextensibility of fingers and elbows, scapular winging, and lordotic trunk. Raymond lacks adequate tonus of the flexor muscles, preventing him from ever holding on to a person who is carrying him. This problem has also been noted when he has been carried in piggyback fashion. Slight head lag is observed when he is pulled to sit. He refuses to play in a prone-lying position for any period of time, probably as a result of inadequate extensor tone that would allow him to perform against gravity. He is unable to maintain the quadruped (all-fours) position for creeping; instead, he rests on his heels and scoots along the floor to maneuver. He prefers to move while upright and generally runs rather than walks. He occasionally performs activities such as swinging, rocking, or jumping, which may enhance input through the vestibular system, but this does not seem to appeal to him as much as tactile input through self-stimulation.

Raymond eats most foods and can adequately handle a spoon, fork, or cup but often stuffs large quantities in his mouth at one time. He likes to smear food on his face and head while eating. Except for feeding, toileting, and some undressing, he is dependent in self-care.

Treatment Goals and Objectives

Children with dysfunction who are motivated usually have an inner drive that can be tapped for increasing self-direction. Occupational therapists should provide the opportunity for the child to achieve success while being appropriately challenged. This process leads to increased adaptive capacity and enhances the child's confidence and self-concept. Ayres emphasizes that therapists follow the child's cues, offering in treatment the type and amount of sensory input that he or she seeks and needs in tasks geared to his or her developmental level.[5]

Children like Raymond, who are not well directed by internal sources and who demonstrate poor orientation and sensory modulation, require particular sensitivity to their behavior as indicators of their sensorimotor needs. The ability of the therapist to interpret their activity as an outward expression of a disorganized and dysfunctioning central nervous system is the key to the therapeutic process. Therapists may be required to impose cautiously more external control and direction on the child with autism who lacks the innate ability to direct himself. Therapists should observe developmental principles, working in early developmental positions (prone, supine,

and quadruped) and initiating activities with the child in a gradual sequential order. Changes from one task to another should be at a pace that respects the child's needs and ability to learn and benefit from an activity.

An occupational therapy summary interpreting Raymond's behaviors indicated the following key problems:

1. Decreased attention span includes limited eye contact, distractibility, and hyperactivity
2. Inadequate modulation of tactile input, as evidenced by his craving for stimulation yet aversion to touch and stimulation by others
3. Signs of poor neuromuscular status, including:
   a. Low muscle tone in flexors and extensors
   b. Poor cocontraction
   c. Instability in early developmental positions
4. Inappropriate play due to lack of adequate sensorimotor foundation and as seen in immature manipulation and use of objects and obsessive behaviors
5. Inadequate social skills resulting from all problems as noted

Major Occupational Therapy Goals (in Order of Priority/Progression)

1. Decrease arousal, including hyperactivity, distractibility, and aversion to touch
2. Increase attention span
3. Increase physical stability through facilitation of muscle tone and cocontraction, especially of midline trunk and proximal joints
4. Improve visual attending and eye contact
5. Enhance tactile discrimination
6. Facilitate play behavior through appropriate use and manipulation of objects

Treatment Methods with Suggested Procedures for Achieving Goals

1. Decrease arousal through inhibitory methods that calm the central nervous system including:
   a. Decreased environmental auditory and visual stimuli
   b. Slow rhythmical movements provided by manual rocking
   c. Proprioceptive input through resisted activities, joint compression, and traction working against firm object or gravity
   d. Pressure–touch on body as tolerated, given manually, such as swaddling child, rolling child in a blanket, or sandwiching child between mats
2. Facilitate total body flexion. The flexed position is one of the first total body patterns to occur in infancy. It is seen as an important element in de-

velopment for organizing the child through symmetrical bilateral movement. Hands or feet may be engaged at the midline and provide the experience of self-exploration through touch and movement. Awareness of self and understanding of body movements are further enhanced and guided through vision, leading eventually to coordinated action of eyes and hands together.[28] The flexor pattern then is critical to the development of midline behavior and organization, beginning with the eyes and including symmetrical extremity movements, especially with the integration of the ATNR at 12–16 weeks. Example: move child on bolster using prone position; encourage improved holding while riding piggyback.

3. Enhance physical stability by increasing muscle tone and cocontraction, especially of midline trunk, and proximal muscles, through:

   a. Linear vestibular input (provides input to the spinal tract supplying extensors). Example: prone forward motion in hammock or on inflated ball

   b. Proprioceptive input as applied through resistance, compression, and traction. Example: quadruped position on firm surface pushing forward against moderately firm surface

   c. Reinforcement with above, through prone play where resistance of the extensors to gravity is maximally enhanced

   d. Resisted sucking activity (the first cocontraction pattern in infancy). Example: vary the resistance of child's suck effort by lengthening straw or thickening the liquid used

4. Provide appropriate tactile stimulation to enhance discrimination. Avoid light tactile input that is arousing and that could lead to aversive reactions. Emphasize firm touch–pressure and proprioceptive input as tolerated. Ayres has also found that vestibular stimulation can help to organize and modulate tactile functions, depending on the responses of the child, through common connections within the central nervous system.[3] Example: linear vestibular input—up-and-down, back-and-forth, and side-to-side movements seem to be more organizing.

Summary

Progress over a 3–6 month period of therapy was seen in Raymond's decreasing destructive behavior toward himself and others. He improved in tolerance to the prone position and to activity while in that position. Some reduced tactile self-stimulation was noted on a gradual basis. Further, an increase in overall stability was noted, leading to improvement in his organization base and his potential for function. ☐

Sensory Integrative Dysfunction: Developmental Dyspraxia

Certain categories of sensory integrative dysfunction have been identified[4-6,29] in which disorders of the tactile, proprioceptive, and/or vestibular systems are suspected to contribute to disruption in typical developmental processes. Such system disorders are manifest in deviations in movement, behavior, and learning.

Developmental dyspraxia seems to be the most frequently observed sensory–integration disorder. This dysfunction is seen in an inability to plan and to execute movement patterns of a skilled or nonhabitual nature. Praxis, or motor planning, is a uniquely human function that relies on an understanding of one's own body and how it operates within and relates to the external world. This type of understanding is based on appropriate and adequate input and processing through the channels of the tactile, proprioceptive, and vestibular systems. These systems are the first to mature and function in infancy and continue as movement feedback mechanisms. The focus of this discussion of dyspraxia relates to problems beginning early in life, stemming from a disorder in the developmental processes rather than that of an individual whose dyspraxia is the result of a traumatic injury later in life.

Several aspects of human movements are basic to understanding the concept of motor planning,[6] including:

Those that are automatic and reflexive
Those that are an inherent part of the human repertoire of movement strategies
Those that require motor planning

The latter leads to the acquisition of specific skills and the ability to learn new, unfamiliar, and complex tasks. Postural reactions fall within the first category, where processing of sensory input produces automatic responses without conscious effort to changes in position. These reactions, directed primarily by the brainstem, may be ineffecient in the child with sensory integrative dysfunction, because they are based on assimilation of sensory information.

Certain movement patterns, such as creeping and walking, are an inherent part of human development. The human nervous system is programmed in such a way that these actions occur during the normal course of development as maturation allows. The child may need stimulus to execute motor planning strategies when first demonstrating these acts, but generally children acquire these abilities without having to be shown how to do them. The child with minor nervous system disorders, such as sensory–integrative dysfunction, may show few problems in achieving these motor milestones.

As a child masters certain skilled tasks, there is a need to concentrate and direct energy toward the specific movement sequences necessary to complete these tasks. This involves the complex assimilation and integration of sensory input at several levels of the CNS in order to organize an appropriate motor response for the task. With repeated effort, the child eventually develops skills that become familiar and that can then be repeated rapidly as needed without great concentration. These skills comprise a certain motor skill "library." For example, most dressing tasks require children to initially direct great attention to the task. Eventually, the ability to initiate and complete these acts rapidly and without much thought is gained. The dyspraxic child often experiences a paucity of skills, although once the child has learned a skill, he can usually perform it well under familiar conditions.

Motor planning demands attention that enables the brain to direct movements in a specific manner. This is a highly complex function in childhood because it depends on processing and organization throughout the central nervous system, from the brainstem to the cerebral hemisphere. When a new or unfamiliar aspect of a learned skill is presented, motor planning is generally required in order to deal effectively with that aspect and to complete the task. For example, the child may learn to skip a rope with practice and become quite efficient at it. Introducing some change, such as skipping rope backward, requires the programming of some different actions and demands attention and concentration in order to learn the task. Eventually, with practice, most children become efficient at this altered activity. The dyspraxic child may need more practice or may fail to learn the task because he or she cannot put all of the components together.

Performance of skilled tasks, even those that have been learned and are slightly altered, present the greatest problem to the dyspraxic child. When motor planning problems are a result of sensory integrative dysfunction, the child often lacks the input needed to develop an understanding of his body, his movements, and his ability to impact effectively on the environment through movement; this presents the occupational therapist with a complicated therapeutic picture.

Because the child with developmental dyspraxia experiences a decreased capacity to impact on the environment, he may feel overwhelmed and powerless, failing to recognize himself as an animated being. Emotional lability is common. The child often cannot figure out how to get into or out of unfamiliar motor situations. He may avoid competitive activities where inadequacy would be obvious. The child may lack imagination and may fail to initiate active play. One may note a stubborn or uncooperative attitude resulting from a need to avoid change.

In summary, the following are identifying characteristics of developmental dyspraxia:
1. Difficulty in performing skills not previously mastered, where motor planning is required.
2. Sensory processing deficits, often in the tactile system, and occasionally in the vestibular and proprioceptive systems.
3. Low muscle tone, generally poorer in flexors than extensors. Flexor muscles are used primarily for phasic and skilled movements, while extensors serve tonic and postural functions.
4. Generally poor coordination, accident proneness, and disorganized movement. The child exhibits excessive concentration when approaching a new skill. Inefficiency and awkwardness of movements are noted.
5. Emotional instability, easily frustrated; appears to have an unwillingness to change.
6. Generally normal onset of developmental motor milestones but delay in acquisition of skills such as dressing and appropriate manipulation of toys (blocks, puzzles, etc.). Deficient skills are noted overall, with the child relying on a few learned skills that have been acquired through considerable effort and practice.

Case Study

Michael is 6 years old, the third child in a family of four children, and the only boy. The mother indicated that there were no problems during pregnancy and delivery, but she felt there was something different about Michael compared with her other children. She reported that he seemed to maintain a distance from other people and preferred remaining in his crib to being held and rocked. He was a very quiet baby, and though only moderately active, he achieved most motor milestones within the age-expected ranges. He was breast-fed for 8 months, and solid foods were introduced at 6 months. He indicated particular food preferences and tended to avoid eating meats and vegetables. He disliked bathing, hair-washing, combing, and brushing his teeth. The father noted that Michael was found crying several times as a baby when caught in corners or on furniture and when Michael could not independently get himself moved out of these situations. He was resistant to any boisterous play compared to his siblings, and he was severely distressed if jostled or swung in the air. As a toddler and preschooler, he was happier looking at books or being read to, and he is now beginning to read. His parents are interested in helping Michael but find him a confusing and frustrating child. They have sought family counseling because they feel responsible for his unhappy disposition.

Michael was referred to occupational therapy by his kindergarten teacher. She reported that Michael seemed to be a bright child, but he hesitated to become involved in activities with his peers. He had difficulty holding and using tools, such as crayons, pencil, or scissors, and often destroyed his papers or threw them away. On the playground, he made use of most of the available equipment, but he refused to participate in group games. Crying and pouting were commonly observed, with occasional temper tantrums when a situation became too frustrating. Michael has been referred to the school social worker for evaluation and has received speech therapy services for severe articulation problems.

An attempt was made in occupational therapy to evaluate Michael's sensory integrative abilities through the Southern California Sensory Integration Tests, but he could not maintain his attention long enough nor adequately follow directions to obtain reliable results on this assessment. The therapist found that clinical observation of performance in exploratory play and assessment of neuromuscular status and reflex integration was necessary to determine his strengths and weaknesses, while additionally trying to establish rapport with him. A developmental history was also obtained from his parents.

Clinical observation revealed several problems. Michael refused to remove his clothing, would not lie prone on any surface, and balked at new experiences of a variety of types. Slight hypotonicity was noted upon palpation in combination with hyperextensible fingers and elbow joints. His ability to track moving objects visually was poor. Movement on uneven surfaces evoked fearful reactions, and he would not allow himself to be picked up. In nonstructured exploratory play Michael was cautious but curious about the toys and equipment, and he manipulated many of them. When concentrating intently on a task that he was trying to learn, he appeared to be thinking through each step and often drooled or squinted in the effort. His awkward movements suggested poor body awareness that was further evidenced by his inability to change position quickly or efficiently move around objects. He often collided with equipment and tripped over toys. When he attempted to retrieve a ball that rolled under a table, Michael, in unplanned and slow sequence, turned himself around, climbed on the table, then got down and crept sideways on the floor before he could accomplish his goal. It was obvious that he had no idea what maneuvers his body should follow toward successful completion of the intended act.

Treatment Goals and Objectives

Michael's performance and behaviors were evidence of disordered sensory and motor abilities. The following problem areas were addressed through occupational therapy programming:

1. Impaired sensory processing functions
   a. Tactile system problems, as evidenced by aversion to handling and grooming, possible avoidance of textured foods, and sensitivity to uncovering his body
   b. Poor proprioceptive mechanisms, as shown in low muscle tone and inability to make use of and learn from his movements. Speech articulation problems may reflect both tactile and proprioceptive problems, leading to poor awareness of oral movements
   c. Inadequate vestibular activity, as seen in his fear of displacement from the earth, poor visual tracking, low muscle tone, and inefficient righting and equilibrium reactions
2. Impaired neuromuscular status and reflex integration noted, with low muscle tone and deficient postural reactions
3. Severe motor planning problems, as evidenced by his inability to move efficiently and skillfully through even simple motor tasks and the need to direct intense concentration on performance. Tool manipulation difficulties were a reflection of this condition
4. Behavior problems and inadequate social skills

Major Goals in Occupational Therapy

1. Decrease in aversion to touch, handling, and movement
2. Enhance functions of the tactile, proprioceptive, and vestibular systems
3. Improve postural reactions
4. Enhance motor planning ability
5. Decrease inappropriate behaviors (Although this was the reason for the referral, this goal is related to the first four major goals.)
6. Improve self-concept

Treatment Methods and Suggested Procedures and Achieving Goals

1. Decrease aversive reactions through
   a. Proprioceptive input in resisted activities. Example: In quadruped position, child pushes or pulls weighted objects.
   b. Pressure–touch as tolerated; avoid light tactile stimuli that are interpreted as uncomfortable. Example: A large inflated ball is rolled over child in prone or supine position.
   c. Movement in slow, gradual ranges using calm,

rhythmical input. Example: Child is rocked over ball, or rides pendulum swing while his feet touch the floor.

2. Enhance sensory system function as aversion decreases, emphasizing the following:
   a. Proprioceptive input. Example: Give manual joint approximation or traction to child or encourage push-off wall activity in different positions on scooter board.
   b. Discriminative tactile activities. Example: Taking clue from child noted to exhibit improved tolerance to varying floor surfaces while walking barefoot, increase other opportunity for tactile exploration (environmental) by feet and hands.
   c. Careful graded (gradual) movement. Example: Encourage movement on a variety of objects to the point that the child initiates climbing activity.

3. Build midline stability as the basis for postural reactions. Trunk stability must be achieved first and is facilitated through increased muscle tone via vestibular input, especially linear stimulation, and tactile and proprioceptive stimulation. Example: Tapping and vibration (myotendinous junction). Resistance to and movement against gravity is advance through proprioceptive and vestibular mechanisms. Example: Linear stimulation in the following directions (*i.e.*, up and down, back and forth, and side to side movement). All activity should encourage an automatic unconscious control of body. These procedures lead to enhanced movement around and away from the body axis.

4. Enhance motor planning built on somatosensory and vestibular processing and adequate postural reactions. Use simple movement activities and increase complexity that child can complete with success while being appropriately challenged. Add skills to the child's repertoire. Follow the child's cues, and present tasks appropriate for his abilities. Do not force him to perform.[5] Example: Encourage child to go under a table, or go under table and chair, crawling. Have child build a simple bridge-like structure with large blocks and then maneuver through the structure by crawling or by means of a scooterboard.

5. In reducing demands made on the child and allowing him success in his play, self-concept is enhanced, and frustration is reduced. As ability to successfully impact on and interact with the environment increases through sensorimotor and cognitive channels, the child's behavior can be more appropriately and productively directed so he has less need to act out.

Summary

Although certain substantial changes in Michael's sensory–integration process and behavior were achieved in a 3- to 6-month period, the identification of his problems had an even greater impact on his parents and family. Their ability finally to understand the reasons for their child's performance difficulties and behavioral reactions markedly improved their ability to help Michael. As the result of improved parenting, Michael demonstrated improved coping skills (less crying and sulking) and better ability to verbalize his feelings of frustration. Teachers, therapist, and family could observe the outcome of improved motor planning seen in his ability to engage in more creative and imaginary plan in general and use of tools and materials. He still avoided most children's games because of a lack of ability to organize game procedures and to predict outcomes at such a level. ☐

Child Abuse and Neglect

For centuries, child abuse or neglect has been known to exist in various degrees with a certain tolerance by society. Herod's destruction of males, the degradation and forced use of children as laborers during the industrial revolution, and, more notably, the descriptive work of Dickens are reminders of the exploitation of children. During the last two decades, child abuse has become a major concern in the United States, with most states adopting laws that require the reporting of medical incidents of child abuse while providing immunity for those reporting abuse in good faith. Once the reporting of child abuse was required by law, the extent of the problem began to reach both public and professional attention. By record, child abuse is the second most common cause of death of young children in the United States. Two-thirds of the child abuse or neglect incidents occur with children 3 years or younger. Permanent brain damage or other handicaps result in approximately 25% of the cases reported.[31]

Child abuse occurs by physical abuse or neglect, sexual abuse, and emotional abuse or neglect, and though they may occur in combination, physical abuse has the clearest diagnostic base and is the most frequently reported. The incidence of physical neglect, whether deliberate or unwillful, is more difficult to determine because of the influence of poverty or lack of means to provide adequate child sustenance. The incidence of sexual abuse is the least reported, whether assaultive or nonassaultive. Defining and managing abuse that is emotionally based is by far the most difficult because of the limited reportable physical evidence. The variation in cultural and social expectations of children further complicates the issue of what is truly emotional abuse or neglect. Failure to thrive and various learning disabilities have definitely been linked to emotional abuse and neglect—an important consideration for occupational therapists.

Physical abuse occurs most frequently to children 0 to 3 years of age. Sexual abuse, whether male or female, may occur at any age, but is more frequently seen in the school-age or adolescent girl. Emotional neglect or abuse is nonrestrictive to age.[31]

In general, occupational therapists considering this particular problem may find more than one area of potential useful service. Because the characteristics of adults involved in child abuse have been identified, therapists' services may need to be directed toward identifying individuals with high risk for abusing, or assisting in determining whether abuse has occurred, or, even more importantly, developing interventions to benefit families involved in abuse. The occupational therapist's evaluation of young children with a known or suspected history of abuse or neglect is strongly recommended because of the child's potential for short- or long-range problems in learning and adapting.

Characteristics of Abusive or Neglectful Parents

Parents are the most frequent abusers of children, though relatives, stepparents, or guardians may also be involved.[19] Basically, abuse is an outcome of past or present problems or stresses that the abusive parent has little control or ability to deal with, such as:

1. Lack of maturity—young parents with unmet needs often lack understanding of their children's behavior or needs.
2. Unrealistic parental expectations of the child, or the child may have *special needs* that prevent the child from meeting parents' expectations.
3. Unmet emotional needs of parents—parents may have problems relating to adults and may expect the child to satisfy their need for love, protection, or self-esteem.
4. Frequent family crises—incidental or ongoing financial, emotional, or physcial problems can explain abusive behavior in parents.
5. Lack of parenting knowledge or skill—many abusive parents know little about the various stages of child development, and often they have no model of successful family patterns from which to draw.
6. Poor parental childhood experiences—often, abusive parents were reared in a physically or emotionally traumatic pattern.
7. Family social isolation—abusive families often lack any support network of friends or family to help with simple or complex problems encountered in rearing small children.

8. Alcohol- or drug abuse-related activity limits parents' ability to rear children effectively.

Signs of Physical Abuse or Neglect

Therapists may have an opportunity to assist in the acute identification process of abused children. Key factors are listed:

Evidence of repeated, multiple, or significant injuries
Parental delay in seeking medical care for the child
Child has a vacant stare and lies very still when approached.

It is important to note that physicians have the key role in determining physical abuse. Medical diagnosis of physical abuse of children has been greatly refined. Radiologic laboratory studies of blood coagulation help establish a profile of present or past abuse patterns. But it is the responsibility of therapists to be alert to evidence of abuse and neglect and to have an understanding of the relevant laws governing their particular state.

In general, therapists need to become familiar with the types of skin and subcutaneous tissue changes, whether bruises, burns, scalds, or wasting, that are typical of abused or neglected children. Injuries to ears, nose, mouth, and head follow unusual and identifiable patterns that differ from usual accidental patterns. An excellent reference for such information is *Clinical Symposia: The Abused Child.*

Other visible signs of abuse or neglect should include children who are undernourished, inadequately clothed, or left unattended. Sometimes, these children will exhibit aggressive negative behavior on a constant and repetitive basis. Other children exhibit excessive withdrawal behavior and may be unable to relate to others, especially other children.

Occupational Therapy with Abused or Neglected Children and Their Families

Occupational therapists have an important role with parents who are abusive/neglectful or who have the potential for being so. Therapists' goals with such parents should be to:

Establish and maintain regular, not threatening, contact with the family
Promote a sense of parental adequacy
Support strengths of the parent–child relationship
Strengthen parents' understanding of their child and capability in child handling and nurturing; children's motor developmental process; nursing, feeding, and nutritional skills

Encourage improved child-rearing skills

Be alert to signs indicating continued abuse and, in such a situation, take appropriate action

Often, a therapist can appropriately use her or his skills in handling, feeding, and promoting gross and fine motor development, and demonstrating alternate approaches to behavior control as a model for parents.

Occupational therapy skills are even more directly related to services for children who have experienced abuse or neglect. Children, especially those 3 years or younger, who fail to thrive or grow in size, who have a developmental disability, or whose behavior is withdrawn or maladaptive, are at high risk for abuse or neglect or may be the result of neglect. Often, mental retardation is a factor—cause or result—in abused and neglected children.

The occupational therapists' evaluation of abused/neglected children should be complete. Frequently, therapists are asked to determine the motor developmental status of the child as baseline information when the question of abuse is being investigated. Sometimes, the therapists may be asked to develop an intervention program that would augment the child's motor development or improve behavior regardless of the domicile determination. In many cases, the therapist may have the opportunity to provide services to the child and parent or caseworker. When the abusing parents are judged to be temporarily or in fact incapable of controlling their abusive behavior, the occupational therapist's role may be more as an evaluator and guide to agency personnel who will sponsor the care and service to the abused or neglected child.

In any event, the occupational therapy assessment of abused and neglected children under 4 years of age should address:

1. Neurodevelopmental reflex maturation levels
2. Gross motor developmental skill levels
3. Fine motor developmental skill levels
4. Developmental level in activities of daily living
5. Sensory integration, including tactile, proprioceptive, kinesthetic, vestibular, and ocular organization

The referral of a child with a history of abuse or neglect to an occupational therapist suggests that the child is exhibiting significant behaviors of concern. In young children, these observable behaviors may include:

Overly compliant behavior

Social withdrawal; may not make eye contact

Lack of autonomy, with little exploring behavior or asserting behavior

Acting-out aggressive episodes, leading to alienation—isolated state

Apathy–helplessness

Retarded growth

Other concerns leading to referral are:

Hyperactivity—tendency to become overstimulated easily

Poor concentration and attention

Suspected mental retardation

Delay in developing daily living skills, especially irregularity in feeding habits

Delay in developing gross and fine motor skills

The occupational therapist examiner should review the referral of an abused or neglected child carefully in light of the person, professional, institutional/agency referral service, or case manager. The purpose of the referral must be addressed during the child's evaluation. But it is the ethical responsibility of the therapist to determine primarily the child's developmental, functional, and adaptive behavior levels and status as a means of identifying the child's individual needs. A summary or report of the evaluative process should include recommendations for improving the child's status as appropriate, while addressing directly the purpose of the referral. In some cases, the therapist may be asked to address the question of parent ability or effectiveness in caring for the child.

It is important to note that the opportunity and feasibility for direct occupational therapy services may, in some cases, be limited or unnecessary. Often, recommendations and advice to the referring service about the child's strengths and weakness, how to encourage improved functional ability in motor performance, adaptive behavioir, concentration, or other areas of concern may be the major contribution of the occupational therapist. When treatment is strongly recommended, the therapist needs to state that opinion clearly and to work assertively to eliminate barriers to the provision of needed services.

Case Study

History and Background

Gabriel, a child of Hispanic extraction, experienced severe infantile abuse from both his natural mother and his stepfather. The identification of four separate incidents of untreated bone fractures inflicted during his first year of life led to the removal of Gabriel from his parents by the state human resource department. Subsequently, he became a ward of the state. Gabriel had six different foster home placements during the following 18 months. These placements were, in some cases, in homes where Spanish was spoken and, in other cases, where English was spoken.

By the time Gabriel was 2½ years old, his behavior and limited communication skills were recognized as a problem. Specifically, he was hyperactive and hard to control and had a speaking vocabulary of three to five words. At that age, he underwent psychiatric, otologic/audiologic, and speech/language examinations. He was labeled mentally retarded due to environmental deprivation, functioning at an overall 18-month level.

By the time he was 35 months old, the state human resources department referred Gabriel for occupational therapy evaluation. His current foster parents were considering adopting him. Both the state agency and the foster parents were seeking definitive information about the child's development. The couple was in their early 30s; the foster mother was a certified kindergarten teacher who was not employed at that time. The father was a state agency employee. The foster parents reported specific concerns about Gabriel's communication, poor concentration, and behavior at meal time. Whenever food was presented, Gabriel responded by gorging himself; this was a special concern of the foster parents. The occupational therapy process is depicted in Figure 35-10.

Occupational Therapy Program

Gabriel's occupational therapy assessment consisted of an evaluation of:

General physical findings, including muscle tone
Reflex maturation
Gross and fine motor skill attainment
Daily living skill performance
Sensory integration and sensitivity
Visual motor integration
Adaptive behavior

The findings of the assessments were as follows:
1. Historically, the child was adequately nourished and small in stature. His normal muscle tone was low, but joint stability was adequate. No deformity was observable.
2. The child demonstrated delays in higher level reflex maturation and exhibited certain primitive reflex patterns of a nonobligatory nature. Midline stability was diminished, and balancing was poor.
3. Gross and fine motor skills had advanced to 24 months, a gain of approximately 6 months' motor maturation since his examination at chronological age 30 months.
4. Despite poor concentration, the child performed certain daily living skills fairly adequately to a 30-month-old level, such as removal of garments. He was clumsy in performance and awkward in those skills requiring dexterity. The foster parents reported the child had difficulty remaining seated during mealtime, and they were dismayed over the child's continued gorging of foods despite their efforts to discourage these behaviors.
5. Sensory–integration testing indicated tactile processing was deficient in discrimination and

localization. Diminished vestibular responses were noted in postrotary nystagmus testing. Proprioception and motor planning ability were deficient. On the K. E. Beery Developmental Test of Visual Motor Integration,[9] he scored an age equivalence of 30 months. He was noted to be significantly tactilely defensive and underreceptive to movement and spatial organization.

Additional factors relating to hemispheric specialization included:

Lack of specialization for preferred hand or eye usage
Poor contralateral use of right or left hand

Six adaptive behaviors during testing were significant:

The child was overstimulated and became disruptive if confined for fine skill performance activity.
He overresponded to gravitational testing and demonstrated increased falling behavior, apparently on a sensoral need basis.
Auditory motor organization was poor (*i.e.*, poor response to verbal directions for action).
Once overstimulated or angered, the child seemed to sustain this intensified state level for a fairly long time, lacking the ability to calm himself or to respond to efforts to help him be calmed.

The foster parents reported difficulty in scheduling the child's rest patterns. It was difficult for the child to take afternoon naps, and bedtime was a nightly battle, with erratic early morning waking also a part of the problem. The foster parents did feel that Gabriel was showing some improvement in understanding them on a verbal basis and by other more subtle factors. They also felt that Gabriel was showing signs of settling into a less frantic pattern of behavior, but they expressed concerns about the prognosis for improved behavior.

Following completion of the child's evaluation, an interagency family conference was held. The results of communication and occupational therapy evaluations were shared with the foster parents. Information about overall developmental level and potentials were discussed, along with the speech pathologist's findings. The occupational therapist encouraged both agency and foster parents to consider the child's developmental delay as one that could be altered by structuring the child, continuing improved nutrition, and giving sensory–integration treatment enhanced with language and educational therapy. The conference recommendations were favorable, indicating a general expectation for the child's increased ability to function in a nearly normal capacity if the child had the opportunity for bonding with caring parents who could provide a structured nurturing environment. The opportunity and need for occupational therapy to

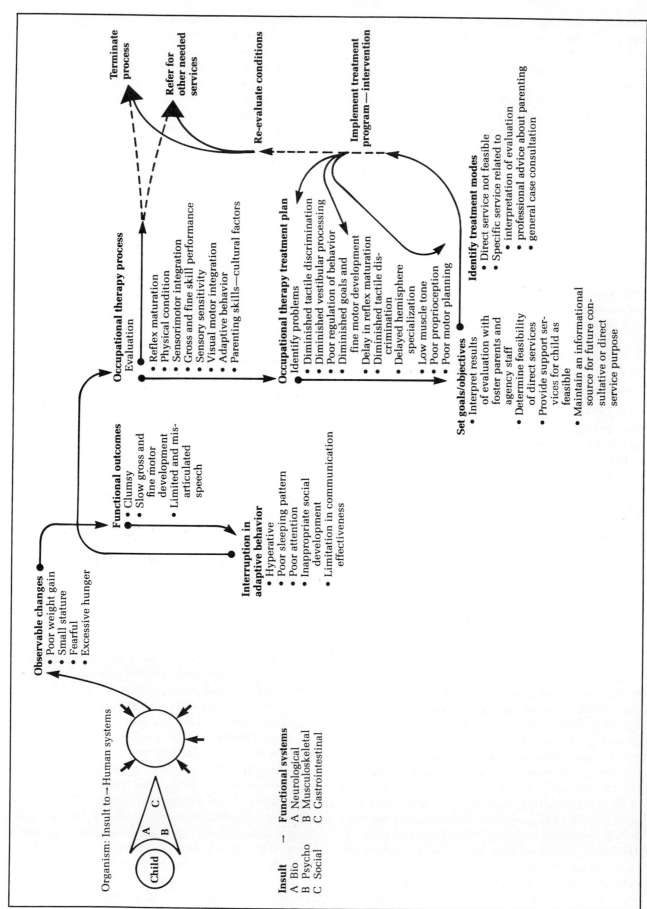

Figure 35-10. Occupational therapy program with an abused child. Case study: Gabriel.

CHAPTER 36

Cerebral Palsy *Margaret V. Howison*

The occupational therapist who works with cerebral palsied children must focus attention on the integration of the many aspects of a child's development. These include the physical, sensory, perceptual, emotional, cognitive, cultural, and social aspects discussed in Chapter 4. It is necessary to understand normal developmental sequences before evaluating and treating the individual with cerebral palsy. This chapter presents a problem-solving rationale for occupational therapy intervention for individuals with cerebral palsy. It is based on a neurodevelopmental approach to human development and treatment. The emphasis is on infants and children. However, many basic concepts apply to working with adult cerebral palsy patients.

Historical Perspective

Although cases of cerebral palsy have been mentioned throughout recorded history, it was not until 1843 that William John Little of England (1810–1894) first discussed what he called "infantile spastic paralysis," which became known as "Little's disease." In 1862, Little presented an accurate paper on the etiological factors of cerebral palsy. This described the problem as one resulting from prenatal, natal, and immediate postnatal influences.[22]

For many years, cerebral palsy was treated from a surgical perspective that was based on surgeons' experiences in treating poliomyelitis.[22] The enthusiasm for surgical intervention to correct deformities, to provide stability, and to improve motor control waned as assessment showed that deformities recurred or new ones developed.

In 1932, Winthrop M. Phelps (1894–1971) began developing a new approach. Phelps had been influenced by Bronson Crothers' work in the field of pediatric neurology. Phelps's theory included the necessity of exercise, muscle training, and bracing in the treatment of cerebral palsy.[22] He gradually moved away from the use of surgical intervention, except in cases of bone deformities in older children. Phelps eventually coined the term cerebral palsy to distinguish the condition from mental retardation.

Since Phelps' era, various nonsurgical approaches have evolved emphasizing neuromuscular training. They include neuromuscular reflex therapy, developed by Fay and Doman–Delacato; neurodevelopmental treatment, developed by Bobath; the neurophysiological approach, developed by Rood; and proprioceptive neuromuscular facilitation, developed by Kabat, Knott, and Voss (Chapter 8, Section 2).

Persons involved in the fields of neurology and psychology have studied early disorders more carefully. This has led to a closer study of the early stages of development. At the same time, people working in the areas of neonatalogy and pediatrics have enhanced knowledge regarding the newborn and the newborn's neurological status. These changes and increased interest have led to both earlier diagnosis and more successful treatment of cerebral palsy.[7]

Modern sophisticated obstetrical and neonatal care, together with the practice of referring at-risk infants for treatment before they are 1 year old, may lessen the number of severely involved individuals. These children may be able to lead relatively normal and productive lives. This same sophisticated neonatal care is also saving infants who at one time would not have survived. These children may be very severely involved and present a new challenge to the occupational therapist.

Definition, Incidence, and Etiology

Cerebral palsy is defined as a nonprogressive lesion of the brain occurring before, at, or soon after birth that interferes with the normal development of the immature brain. The resulting impairment of the coordination of muscle action with an inability to maintain postures and balance and to perform normal movements and skills is common to all cases.[8] Because the parts of the brain are interrelated, there may be many associated neurological abnormalities, such as sensory deficits, speech problems, sensory integration deficits, intellectual impairment, seizure disorders, and emotional problems.

Cerebral palsy occurs in approximately two per one thousand live births.[15] Thirty percent of incidences of cerebral palsy seem to be caused by prenatal complications, 60% by perinatal complications, and 10% by postnatal complications.[8]

Cerebral palsy may be inherited. Other *prenatal* causes are infection such as toxoplasmosis, rubella, and cytomegalic inclusion disease; prenatal anoxia (lack of oxygen) caused, for example, by an umbilical cord around the neck; prenatal cerebral hemorrhage (abnormal bleeding) caused by maternal toxemia or direct trauma; problems such as kernicterus resulting from Rh incompatibility; metabolic disturbances such as diabetes; harmful exposure to x-rays; bleeding in the first trimester; drug toxicity such as from vitamins A and D; or multiple conceptions.[3]

Perinatal causes include anoxia from respiratory obstruction, placental abnormalities, maternal anoxia, hypotension, or breech delivery; trauma or hemorrhage from disproportions and malpositions, forceps application, induced labor, sudden pressure changes in a precipitate delivery, prolonged labor, or cesarean delivery; and prematurity.[3]

Postnatal causes include trauma from skull fractures, wounds, and contusions of the brain or from subdural hematomas; infections such as meningitis, encephalitis, and brain abscesses; toxicity from lead, arsenic, and coal tar derivatives; vascular accidents such as from congenital aneurysms or hypertensive disorders; anoxia from CO_2 poisoning, strangulation, or hypoglycemia; and neoplasms or the developmental effects of tumors, cysts, or hydrocephalus.[3,15]

Development
Basic Components of Normal Development

Before the occupational therapist can successfully treat an individual with cerebral palsy, knowledge of normal development is essential. The therapist should be able to differentiate between what is (1) *normal* at a given age, (2) *primitive* or normal at one age but abnormal at another age, and (3) *abnormal* or not seen in the normal child at any period of development.

Normal movement is built on the development of righting, equilibrium, and protective extension responses or reactions. A righting reaction brings one up in space, an equilibrium or balance reaction keeps one in space, and a protective extension response occurs when one goes beyond the point of balance. The occupational therapist must be familiar with the normal components of movement that make up these three reactions in order to evaluate and treat patients in a functional, creative way.

An infant's first movements are primitive and gross. They are not purposeful, nor are they cortically controlled.[17] These motions help to establish a range of motion in joints so that the muscles around the joint can develop control. In time, random movements develop into symmetrical, bilateral movements of the arms and legs; both arms or both legs move together. This symmetrical activity then breaks down to dissociate one extremity from the other; one extremity is able to move independently of the other. All development progresses from head to foot as the extensor and flexor components of movement develop. The proximal muscles develop first to give midline and trunk control, with the distal muscles developing later. A combination of head to foot and proximal to distal development brings in the diagonal components of movement essential for righting and equilibrium responses.

Bly, a physical therapist, has studied the development of normal components of movement. She describes four general characteristics of movement: there must be (1) *a point of stability,* (2) *a point of mobility,* (3) *weight shift,* (4) *a reaction to weight shift.*[5]

A point of stability refers to the base of support or what is maintaining a child in a given position. The hips are the point of stability in sitting; the feet support the standing child; the hands and knees maintain the creeping child. Stability may be either external or internal. External, or positional, stability is found when the child uses his or her anatomical structures to broaden the base of support. Two examples of this are when the child "circle sits" with hips abducted and externally rotated with knees flexed and feet touching each other, and when the child sits with hips in wide abduction with knees extended. Internal stability is present when the child develops both muscle and joint control.[5] This is the mature stability necessary for functional movement.

The second characteristic of movement is *a point of mobility.* This identifies the place where movement is required; for example, the joints involved in a motion. When one lifts an arm, the point of mobility is in the shoulder and the point of stability is in the hips.[5]

The third characteristic of movement is *weight shift.* Every movement causes a weight shift that may be anterior, posterior, lateral, or diagonal. A sitting child reaches forward; this necessitates an anterior weight shift. An infant shifts his weight backwards to lift his head and chest off the surface; this is a posterior weight shift. He moves his weight from one elbow to the other; this is a lateral weight shift. He transfers his weight to one side in order to reach out with the opposite arm; this is a diagonal weight shift. It is necessary to know the direction of weight shift in order to elicit a righting reaction. Weight shift may be initiated by muscle action, visual stimulation, and head turning. If a child has steadied himself with a positional point of external stability, he will not be able to shift his weight effectively.[5] Internal stability is important for this component of movement.

The fourth characteristic of movement is *reaction to weight shift.* One child may react by falling, demonstrating lack of control. Another may use a righting reaction in which her head and trunk come into alignment. She may use protective extension by stretching out her arms. Another may use a balance or equilibrium response to keep himself in space.[5]

While the infant's development progresses from head to foot and from proximal to distal control, he or she acquires the extensor, flexor, lateral flexor, and rotational components of movement necessary for righting, equilibrium, and protective extensor responses. Before an infant can gain control of a joint, full range of motion and muscle elongation must occur. Developing full range of motion and elongation of muscles are two key points in treatment planning. When an infant is born, he

or she comes from the compact environment of the womb where the neck and back extensor muscles have been elongated. For this reason, the infant's first controlled movements are of extensor muscles.[5] An infant's extensor development will normally stay several months ahead of its flexor development.

When prone, the neonate uses neck retraction to lift and turn the head. The side to which the head is turned is the side that is weight bearing. The infant's arms are flexed, adducted, and internally rotated; the elbows are behind the shoulders. He or she has posterior pelvic tilt; the legs are adducted, flexed, and externally rotated with the feet in dorsiflexion. The newborn has a traction and grasp reflex response.[17]

When supine, the neonate does not have the flexion needed for controlled movements. The hips, ankles, knees, and elbows spring back when passively extended;[6] this is called *physiological flexion.* The neonate's head is not in the midline, but it is also not fully rotated to the side. When eating or crying, the infant's head tends to be in the midline, turned toward the side bearing more weight. When pulled to sit, a newborn has total head lag. When he or she is held in a sitting position, the head flops forward. The neonate's shoulders are forward with the arms flexed, adducted, and internally rotated with the hands clenched into fists. He or she is able to bring the back of the hand to the mouth but not in the midline. He or she still has posterior pelvic tilt, and legs are flexed and adducted with slight outward rotation. Because of the neonate's posterior pelvic tilt, he or she kicks in the air.[17]

Within 3 months, the infant has developed sufficient prone extension to lift his or her head up to 90° and is able to rotate it freely. The infant now has early proximal control of both horizontal abduction and adduction that allows forearm weight bearing with proprioception into the shoulders. The elbows have come forward and are in line with the shoulders. This allows the infant to have upper extremity external rotation. The 3-month-old infant has lumbar extension with the pelvis down. Hip extension has decreased, but the infant's hips continue to be flexed, abducted, and externally rotated.[6]

When supine, the 3-month-old assumes more symmetrical positions. Neck flexors have developed, so the head is held near the midline. The infant's eyes converge. He or she brings the arms together on the chest, but does not reach out in space. The infant pulls at his or her clothing. There is controlled internal rotation of the arms and forward flexion. The infant's legs tend to assume the "frog-legged" position, in which there is increased hip external rotation and abduction and the feet are together. When kicking, more of the foot hits the surface.[6]

When sitting, the 3-month-old infant holds his or her head up. Increased back extension has developed that is reinforced by scapular adduction and humeral extension. The infant tends to lean forward because of low muscle tone in the lower back and hips.[6]

At 6 months of age, the infant has well-developed neck extension when prone. He or she pushes up on extended arms. The narrower base of support and neutral shoulder rotation allow the infant's hands to point straight ahead. The 6-month-old maintains an extended arm position to shift weight to one side while reaching out with the opposite arm. The infant may be able to push backwards on the abdomen. A child of this age extends both legs vigorously to play in or use this newly developed extension pattern.[17]

When supine, the 6-month-old infant demonstrates increased flexor control by touching the feet with the hands. The baby reaches out in space with extended arms. He or she transfers objects from one hand to the other. He or she can roll from supine to prone.[6] When pulled to a sitting position, a 6-month-old lifts his or her head independently and pulls with the arms. Increased flexor control lets the child flex the legs at the hips and counter-balance with knee extension.[6]

This overview of gross motor development in newborn, 3-month-old, and 6-month-old infants illustrates some components of movement and their relationship to the next level of development. In summary, extension is normally well developed in the neck at 0 to 4 months, the midback by 3 to 4 months, the hips by 5 to 6 months, the knees by 6 months, and the feet by 6 to 8 months. As stated earlier, flexors usually lag behind extensors. Flexion is normally present in the neck by 5 months, abdominals by 6 to 7 months, and hips by 7 to 8 months. Lateral flexion is controlled in the neck by 4 months and in the trunk by 5 to 6 months. Rotational components are usually developed in the upper trunk by 4 to 5 months, lower trunk by 6 to 7 months, and the sitting position by 10 months.[17] The components of movement guide the therapist in preparing treatment plans for assisting the cerebral palsied child to attain the appropriate developmental milestones.

Normal and Abnormal Blocks

There are four major areas where the normal infant may have a temporary block in development: the neck, shoulders, pelvis, and hips. If the infant has not developed sufficient control of an area, the development may be blocked distal and/or proximal to that point.[4] As mentioned previously, persons with cerebral palsy may maintain some primitive movement patterns. A block in development which was normal at 3 months of age may be seen in the older child and adult and be a part of primitive or abnormal motor development pattern. Awareness of these blocks can guide the therapist in evaluating and planning treatment.

Neck Blocks

There are two types of neck blocks: neck *hyperextension* and neck *asymmetry.* Neck hyperextension is extension of the occiput on the atlas and is normally seen in the 1- to 3-month-old infant. Hyperextension is normally counterbalanced by the development of the neck flexors and leads to elongation of the neck. Head extension is balanced by head and cervical flexion. The child with cerebral palsy may show primitive and abnormal development when flexor control is insufficient to counterbalance extension. This may result in the neck's never becoming elongated. Also, head extension is never balanced by head flexion (chin tuck), although cervical flexion develops.

Neck asymmetry causes the head to be turned to one side. It may occur in combination with neck hyperextension. There is a lack of symmetrical development of the flexors necessary to bring the head to the midline and to suppress the stimulation of the asymmetrical tonic neck reflex. Neck asymmetry is normally seen in the infant until the age of 3 to 4 months, when flexors develop and bring the head to the midline, allowing symmetry to develop, the eyes to converge, and the hands to come together. Children with cerebral palsy may show primitive and abnormal development when they do not have symmetrical development of their flexors. They may have poor midline control of their heads. Their eyes may have difficulty converging, and their hands often do not come together. Also, cerebral palised children may have difficulty bringing their hands to their mouths and faces, which decreases the tactile stimulation they experience.

Shoulder Blocks

Because shoulder development is directly related to neck development, the presence of a neck block may cause a shoulder block to occur. There are two types of shoulder blocks: *scapulohumeral tightness* and *scapular adduction.*

Scapulohumeral tightness is normal in infants from 1 to 3 months of age, when the elbow is normally held behind the shoulder in prone. As the upper trunk flexors and scapular stabilizers develop, the infant's arms move forward so that the elbow is in front of the shoulder. This causes elongation of the muscles between the scapula and humerus. This is only possible after the scapula has become proximally stabilized on the chest wall. This allows scapulohumeral dissociation that permits upper extremity external rotation and forearm supination and pronation and that allows fine motor development of the wrists and fingers. When this does not take place in the child with cerebral palsy, the arms cannot move forward because of poor development of flexor control that causes tightness of the muscles between the scapula and humerus. The upper extremities are kept internally rotated. No dissociation occurs between the scapula and humerus, causing them to move as a unit. This inhibits the development of fine motor control in the upper extremity.

In the normal developmental sequence, scapular adduction reinforces back extension and stability. It is normal in infants aged 4 to 5 months when they are placed in prone suspension. This is seen in the Landau response. It is later seen in the initial stages of sitting, standing, and walking independently. It is always counterbalanced by equal trunk flexor control. If this normal balance does not occur, primitive and abnormal development may result. Because of poor scapulohumeral dissociation, scapular adduction causes the arms to retract. The scapular muscles do not become stabilized on the trunk, preventing dissociated upper extremity function. Lack of dissociation prevents the arms from coming forward for forearm support and prevents upper extremity function in unsupported sitting and upper extremity function in standing and walking.

A child with neck and shoulder blocks often compensates in ways that lead to abnormal development. These compensations are usually seen in sitting. A child with poor head control elevates the shoulders to provide head stability that further limits the possibility of lateral head righting and head rotation. The shoulders will become tighter and their mobility more limited when they are elevated. This increases neck hyperextension, humeral adduction, and humeral hyperextension. Neck hyperextension limits downward gaze, which leads to a forward jaw thrust, and makes lip closure more difficult.

Pelvic Blocks

There are two types of pelvic blocks: *anterior pelvic tilt* and *posterior pelvic tilt.* Anterior pelvic tilt, or lordosis, can be seen in a prone 4-month-old infant. When the infant reaches 4 to 5 months of age, anterior pelvic tilt is balanced by the abdominal muscles. Later, the abdominals and hip extensors work together. This elongates the iliopsoas muscles. When supine, anterior pelvic tilt can be balanced when the infant puts his or her hands on knees, feet in the mouth, and hands on feet in the air. It is muscular control of the hips that provides stability for prone forearm weight shifting. In a cerebral palsied child, anterior pelvic tilt stays strong because it is not opposed, and this may cause primitive and abnormal development. Abdominal muscles may not develop; the iliopsoas muscles are never elongated. The lower extremities stay abducted, flexed, and externally rotated in a frog-like position with no hip stability. Supine balancing activities may never occur. Low extensor tone in the hip muscles may cause the child to flop forward when

placed in a sitting position. A cerebral palsied child may circle sit, using legs for positional stability. This causes the child to use neck and trunk hyperextension to lift the head and trunk. The child may also compensate by "W" sitting, with the hips internally rotated and the knees flexed, allowing the child to sit between his or her legs. This provides a broad base of support but may lead to dislocated hips. He or she uses anterior pelvic tilt to lock the lower extremities into a position that stabilizes the pelvis. This may cause the child to hyperextend the trunk. The child's legs may remain abducted when standing. Because there is insufficient hip control to shift weight, the child compensates by abnormally adducting the hips and keeping the feet wide apart. Adducted thighs rather than trunk control give the child external stability. He or she shifts weight by using lateral trunk flexion to the weight-bearing side instead of elongating the weight-bearing side of the normal balance reaction.

Posterior pelvic tilt results from normal cocontraction of the abdominals and hip extensors. If this cocontraction does not develop, the child with cerebral palsy will lack hip joint mobility. Spastic hip extensors may become shortened and may lack mobility. This, in turn, limits the hip flexion; when a child tries to flex the hips, the pelvis is pulled back during sitting, which increases extensor tone in the trunk. This may throw the child backward. The child compensates by pulling the trunk forward into abnormal flexion. This leads to abnormal hip adduction and eventually to strong internal rotation of the hips. Long sitting (sitting with the legs extended forward) is difficult and nonfunctional for the child with a posterior pelvic tilt. He or she may resort to "W" sitting, which gives a more functional stable position. He or she keeps the pelvis back, thighs together, and feet apart for a wide base of positional support.

Hip Blocks

There are two types of hip blocks: *pelvic femoral tightness* and *hip extension adduction.* Pelvic femoral tightness is normal for infants from 3 to 4 months of age. Their legs are abducted, flexed, and externally rotated in a frog-legged position. This position changes when the iliopsoas becomes elongated and the development of normal hip extension, adduction, and internal rotation on a stable trunk allows the legs to come together. Lower extremity dissociation develops through a weight shift and elongation of muscles on the weight-bearing side. If the child with cerebral palsy continues to experience a pelvic femoral tightness hip block, his or her legs will not come together and will remain in a frog-like position. There is no lower extremity dissociation or weight shifting capability.

Normal hip extension and adduction occur as a result of the development of hip extensors with good abdominals, and hip adductors with good extensors. These are balanced by hip flexors and abductors. All of these are working together on a stable, integrated trunk. The child who has cerebral palsy may have an unstable trunk because he or she does not have good abdominals. Without a stable trunk, normal hip extension and adduction cannot occur. The legs may extend and adduct instead as a result of abnormal trunk flexion.

The Child with Cerebral Palsy

Classification by Muscle Tone

There are four types of cerebral palsy: spasticity, athetosis, ataxia, and flaccidity. All are characterized by abnormal muscle tone. Most cases are mixed and do not fit into a clear-cut diagnostic classification. Often, it is more meaningful to the therapist to refer to the type of muscle tone rather than a concrete classification. The superficial muscle tone is often not the same as the underlying tone. When the superficial muscle tone is inhibited, the underlying tone is often low.

Spasticity

Spasticity refers to extreme and above normal muscle tone. Spastic individuals usually have quadriplegic, diplegic, hemiplegic, or sometimes paraplegic involvement.

The severely spastic person has high muscle tone with little change in degree. There is constant cocontraction of muscles that inhibits relaxation while awake or asleep. Because they tend to assume a few abnormal postures, these individuals are more vulnerable to deformities including scoliosis; kyphosis; flexion deformities of the hips, knees, and fingers; forearm pronation contracture; subluxation of the hip; and shortening of the heel cords with inward or outward turning of the foot (equinovarus and equinovalgus, respectively). Movement occurs only when strongly stimulated. This movement is labored and remains within a limited range of motion. Primitive spinal patterns are often completely inhibited by tonic reactions. Startle reactions are common in many cases. Tonic patterns are seen in the tonic neck and tonic labyrinthine reflexes and also in a positive supporting reaction. Associated reactions can be felt, but little movement is observed. Righting, equilibrium and protective extension reactions are often absent, but neck righting may be present.

The individual with moderate spasticity may have normal to high muscle tone, is usually able to move around, and may be able to walk. The degree of high tone is negatively influenced by the amount of stimula-

tion received from effort, emotion, speech, and sudden stretch. More spasticity is seen in the agonist than in the antagonist muscles and more occurs distally than proximally. Deformities may develop from the maintenance of abnormal postures, the use of stereotyped abnormal patterns, and the associated reactions in lesser involved parts. These deformities may include kyphosis, lordosis, hip subluxations or dislocations, flexion contractures of hips and knees tight hip inward rotators, tight hip adductors, and heel cord shortening with foot rotation.

Although the moderate spastic possesses a greater range of motion, it is usually not complete throughout every range. Learned skills are performed in primitive and abnormal patterns without selectivity of movement. Total movements may be in synergies or patterns. There may be voluntary use of spinal and tonic reflex patterns for purposive movements. Primitive spinal patterns of total flexion or extension are common. A strong startle response is usually present. The tonic neck and tonic labyrinthine reflexes and positive supporting reactions are often present. Reactions in the form of associated movements are strong. Some righting reactions may be present. Equilibrium reactions are often developed in sitting and kneeling positions, but not in standing and walking positions. An individual's size and weight may eventually necessitate the use of a wheelchair. As a child grows bigger, he or she may become more spastic because of the increasing effort needed to move around.

The mildly involved spastic individual often is able to stand up despite incomplete righting and equilibrium responses. Because of his or her level of movement, deforming factors are minimal. This child seems motor driven and is often difficult to treat. As the child's speed builds up, muscle tone and tension increase. Mildly spastic children may have more diplegic and hemiplegic involvement. They learn to compensate for their problems effectively while still young.

Athetosis

Athetosis refers to muscle tone that fluctuates from low to normal and, in some cases, to high. Usually, there is quadriplegic involvement, but sometimes there is only hemiplegic involvement. It is rare for an individual to have pure athetosis. It is often combined with spasticity, tonic spasms, or chorea movements.

Individuals with athetosis like to move. They often maintain abnormal and persistent primitive patterns of movement. One compensation they may make involves the use of an asymmetrical tonic neck reflex to attain stability. The reflex pattern often involves the right side with the right arm extended and the left arm flexed. They will use the left hand for functional activities. Individuals with athetosis cannot hold their heads in the midline because of this primitive reflex. The head is used to control gross motor movements. If the head is turned, the rest of the body will assume the appropriate asymmetrical tonic neck reflex position. Because athetoid individuals have no gross motor midline, they have difficulty developing a visual midline involving head, hands, and eyes. This negatively influences perceptual skills.

Because an athetoid child has better control of the feet than of proximal muscles, he or she will start to develop extensor tone from the feet up rather than from the head down. The neck and shoulders may be locked into neck and shoulder blocks to assist in stabilization.

Low fluctuating muscle tone allows a broad range of motion in all joints. Joint dislocation may result from this hyperextension. The shoulders, especially, may dislocate easily and painlessly. When this occurs, it is difficult to attain joint stabilization.

Athetosis with Spasticity

The athetoid with spasticity seems to have moderate spasticity in proximal areas and athetosis in distal areas. Muscle tone fluctuates between normal and high. Deformities are less frequent than in the spastic type but may occur as flexor deformities in the hips, elbows, and knees. There may be some cocontraction in the proximal joints. Such individuals often lack selective movement and grading of muscle action. There is some control throughout the midranges. Postural patterns are similar to those of individuals with moderate spasticity. Primitive spinal patterns are present but modified by involuntary movements. There are strong influences of the tonic neck reflexes (symmetrical and asymmetrical) and the tonic labyrinthine reflexes. Although usually present, righting reactions are unreliable because of the intermittent influence of tonic reflexes.

Athetosis with Tonic Spasms

In the athetoid individual with tonic spasms, muscle tone changes from low to high. Lack of cocontraction causes excessive extension or flexion. Strong postural asymmetry influenced by tonic neck reflexes that are more exaggerated on one side may cause deformities to develop. These may include scoliosis, kyphoscoliosis, dislocation of the hip on the skull side, and flexor contractures of the hips and knees if the individual has been sitting for long periods. Occasionally, the hips, fingers, or lower jaw sublux. There is almost no voluntary control of movements because of strong intermittent tonic spasms. Extreme postures of flexion or extension are assumed. There seems to be more involuntary movement in distal areas than in proximal parts. Because the individual either is in tonic spasm or has low muscle tone and is unable to move, primitive spinal patterns are usually not present. Strong tonic patterns are seen in the asymmetrical and symmetrical tonic neck reflexes and the tonic labyrinthine reflexes. Righting, equilibrium, and protective extension reactions are absent.

Choreoathetosis

The individual with choreoathetosis has muscle tone that fluctuates from low to normal and from low to high. There is no cocontraction. Deformities are rare, but there is a tendency to subluxation of the shoulder and finger joints. There are extreme ranges of motion with no grading of midranges. The large jerky involuntary movements seem to be more proximal than distal. The hands and fingers are weak, but often coordination is good in free movement. There is a lack of selective movement and fixation of movement. Primitive spinal patterns are present but modified by the athetosis. There are intermittent tonic reflex patterns. Righting and equilibrium reactions are present to some extent, but coordination is abnormal. Protective extension of the arms is abnormal and often absent.

Pure Athetosis

The individual with pure athetosis has muscle tone that fluctuates from low to normal. There are rarely any deformities. There may be some transient subluxations of the shoulder and finger joints, and there is lack of cocontraction. Twitches and jerks of individual muscles or even of muscle fibers are seen. Slow, writhing involuntary movements that are more distal than proximal and lack of fixation are characteristic. Primitive spinal patterns are present but modified by athetosis. These patterns are less primitive and more selective than in choreoathetosis. There is rarely any tonic reflex influence. Righting, equilibrium, and protective extension reactions are present, but involuntary movements interfere with them.

Ataxia

Ataxia refers to muscle tone that fluctuates from below normal to normal. Usually, there is quadriplegic involvement. It is rare to see a case of pure ataxia. Children with ataxia may look normal at rest, but, in severe cases, they experience tremors when awake. Intention tremors and nystagmus are common.

Because ataxic individuals lack a point of stability, muscular coactivation is difficult for them. They do not like to move. They use primitive rather than abnormal patterns with little reflex influence. This causes gross, total patterns of movement. They have difficulty grading movements within a small range, and they will often overshoot targets. They use ''fixing'' or will stabilize themselves against any point of contact to gain stability.

They use their eyes to keep their heads in the midline. If they look to the side, they may lose their balance.

These children may have developed righting responses, but these are uncoordinated, exaggerated, and poorly utilized. Equilibrium responses may be developed, but they are not coordinated. Ataxic children may be slow to move to regain their balance, and their movements are poorly timed and not smooth. They use protective responses to fix or lock themselves into stable positions. They walk on the medial borders of their feet with their legs abducted to provide a wide base of support. They may reach out with their toes to feel their way and then bring their legs over their feet. Ataxic children use a flexor component to help stabilize themselves. If thrown off balance, they pull into flexion to protect themselves.

They may fix or stabilize with their mouths, which causes slow, thick speech. They may fix or stabilize their tongues between or against their teeth to know where it is. The tongue, like the head, is held in the midline with little lateralization or interplay. During feeding, ataxic children may hold their lips against their gums to keep track of where they are. They may have difficulty coordinating suck–swallowing and breathing.

Flaccidity

Flaccidity is characterized by fluctuating low muscle tone. This may be seen in either an infant or a toddler. Initially, the child is flaccid but later, with maturation, he or she may be classified as spastic, athetoid, or ataxic. Involvement is usually quadriplegic.

These children have little to no sensory or stretch feedback to stimulate movement and therefore stay passive. Because they may not be able to move, they may respond only with their eyes. Because they have no head control, their eye movements may not be smooth unless they are supine. It is important to check for eye brightness. These babies do not cry much, and when they do, the sound is shallow and low. They are considered "good" babies and therefore often get less attention and experience less interaction with adults during their crucial first 6 months of life.

The physiological flexion seen in the normal neonate does not occur. Infants of this type may look like premature infants. However, they do not build up muscle tone as "preemies" do; they may stay flaccid until 2 years of age. The longer the child is flaccid, the greater the probability of mental retardation. As this infant matures, it is important to watch for signs of spasticity or athetosis. The infant who fixes or stabilizes his or her shoulders and lower back may become spastic; the infant who fixes or stabilizes in trunk extension may become athetoid.

The child may first attempt to move when in extension. If the flaccid child does not become spastic or athe-toid, he or she will learn to fix using extension to come up against gravity. This occurs most frequently when the child is propped in a semireclining position and pushes back into the surface using extension. When supine, the child will play in extension. The child's hips go into outward rotation, attaining a frog-like position. Because this child spends much time supine, tonic labyrinthine reflexes become strong and pull him or her further into the surface. When prone, the flaccid child may not lift the head. As extensor tone develops, the child seems stronger; however, flexion does not develop at the appropriate rate. The flaccid child has a flat, narrow chest and a poor, shallow breathing pattern. Any respiratory infection may be life threatening.

Some infants stay flaccid until 6 months of age. Then the process is reversed, and by 18 months, they may have passed the appropriate developmental milestones. These infants are usually more responsive to their environment and seem more visually alert.

Associated Neurological Abnormalities and Problems

Occupational therapists must be aware not only of the motor implications of cerebral palsy but also of other problems and neurological abnormalities that may be associated with it. Most children with cerebral palsy have anywhere from two to seven additional disorders.[22]

It is estimated that 50% of children with cerebral palsy have *disturbances of vision.* This may result from a lack of eye coordination that occurs especially when there is quadriplegic involvement. There may be internal or external squints or strabismus. This may be alternating or fixed and may cause lack of accommodation. Lack of conjugate movement may cause an impairment of stereoscopic vision. The child may not be able to move his or her eyes and thus must move the head. Strong neck retraction may limit the athetoid child's ability to look down. A strong asymmetrical tonic neck reflex may fix the eyes or may prevent the eyes from moving over the midline. Total blindness may be caused by the increasingly rare retrolental fibroplasia and by optic atrophy. It is likely that the cerebral palsied child who is also hemiplegic will have visual field deficits from optic radiation.[8]

An estimated 25% of children with cerebral palsy have some type of *auditory disturbance.* The most common auditory problem is high frequency deafness. This is most likely to occur as a result of neonatal jaundice suffered by the athetoid child, but it is also common in the spastic child. There may be auditory imperception or agnosia.[8]

Speech disturbances are seen in approximately 25% of cerebral palsy cases.[22] The most common problem is dysarthria, which is pseudobulbar palsy seen in the spastic, athetoid, and mixed types. Aphasia is rare. Apraxia of the mouth, throat, and larynx may cause an inability to speak.[8]

Impairment of stereognosis is common in the individual with hemiplegic involvement. There may be a more subtle global problem with the spastic quadriplegic child.

Sensory integrative disorders are seen in approximately 14% of individuals with cerebral palsy.[22] Apparently, the incidence is higher among spastic children. This may be the result of a brain lesion, of the child's inability to explore the environment, or of learning disorders.

An estimated 50% to 75% of children with cerebral palsy have *below-average intelligence.*[15,22]

Seizure disorders are seen in approximately 25% of cerebral palsy cases.[15] Any type of seizure may occur, but seizures are usually generalized. Seizures are more common with hemiplegia of postnatal origin. They are rare among athetoid children.[15]

Emotional problems are common among children with cerebral palsy. They are often compounded by emotional immaturity, since these children tend to be dependent on their families because of physical dependency or isolation from normal children. The degree of acceptance of and adjustment to disability is primarily the result of both the problem itself and the reactions of the child with the immediate environment of parents and family.[8]

Some individuals with cerebral palsy exhibit a *weak self-image;* their ability to feel a sense of self-worth or responsibility may be minimal. They may experience difficulties in group situations and in interpersonal relationships. They may withdraw from social interactions.

A few studies have been done on the personality traits that may accompany cerebral palsy. It seems that athetoid children tend to have less emotional stability and to be "explosive." Spastic children seem to have obsessive–compulsive personality traits and may find it difficult to adapt to new situations.

In some cases, the associated problems are more limiting than the motor abnormalities.

Assessment

Accurate assessment of the individual with cerebral palsy is essential for functional treatment planning. Thorough evaluation should be done to determine the child's developmental levels. The physical, sensory, perceptual, emotional, cognitive, cultural, and social components of development should all be considered.

The occupational therapist should be aware that there is no single evaluative tool that defines the many abnormalities seen in the cerebral palsied child. Instead, there are many tools that can be used in combination. A

correctly selected combination results in a more accurate evaluation. The following are evaluative tools that the occupational therapist should be able to utilize. Many of the tools that may be used with the cerebral palsied child are discussed in the chapter on assessment. A few especially useful tests have been singled out and are listed below.

1. *Developmental Programming for Infants and Young Children—Early Intervention Developmental Profile*[21] and *Pre-School Developmental Profile* by Rogers and D'Eugenio[21] is one of the more comprehensive evaluation tools. It assesses children from birth to 6 years of age in the areas of gross motor development, self-care, perceptual and fine motor development, and language and cognition.
2. *Denver Developmental Screening Test* by Frankenburg and Dodds[13] screens children for developmental delays. It assesses children from birth to 6 years of age in the areas of gross motor development, language, fine motor development, adaptive behaviors, and personal–social behaviors.
3. *Bayley Scale of Infant Development* evaluates the young child in motor development, language, and cognitive skills.[2]
4. *Pre-Speech Assessment Scale: A Rating Scale for the Measurement of Pre-Speech Behaviors from Birth through Two Years* by Morris[18] evaluates the normal and abnormal characteristics of feeding and prespeech behaviors.
5. *American Academy of Mental Deficiency Adaptive Behavior Scale* by Nihira, Foster, Shellhaas, and Leland[20] serves as a guideline for development of a life tasks program for the young adult and adult.

Intervention

The treatment of the individual with cerebral palsy is a 24-hour-a-day process. The treatment team may consist of the occupational, physical, and speech therapists; the physician; the psychologist; and the nurse. The family is an integral, active part of the treatment team. In addition, the child often sees a pediatrician, neurologist, developmental pediatrician, orthopedist, physiatrist, and psychiatrist. To this team, the occupational therapist brings his or her skills in developmental assessment and individual problem solving. The child is viewed as a total being.

Before any evaluation or treatment can be effective, a mutual respect and acceptance needs to grow between the individual and the therapist. Children need to know that they are cared about; that they are important, and that they are unique.

The occupational therapist identifies the physical needs, emotional or maturational level, intellectual level, and specific interests of each person. The therapist, in conjunction with the family and, if possible, the child, then plans an individualized program and presents a choice of several appropriate activities. In choosing activities, the therapist considers the cultural background, age level, physical ability, interests, and the functional level of the child.

Home programs are an essential part of the treatment process. The goals and activities that make up these programs must meet the needs not only of the children but also of their families. One family may be able to follow an elaborate treatment program, whereas another family may be able to do only one small activity. If the activities are too complicated or too time consuming for their capacity, family members may feel overwhelmed and do nothing.

Many remediation techniques may be combined with age-appropriate activities. Besides toys, games, books, and crafts, everyday practical activities may be suggested. These activities may include helping to mix cookies, knead bread, fold laundry, hang up clothes, dry unbreakable dishes, or dust. The activity may simply be playing in a cabinet of pots and pans. All of these are normal developmental experiences that an individual with cerebral palsy may miss. The occupational therapist, in his or her unique professional role, plans a therapeutic environment that includes these activities in conjunction with treatment.

The family of a child with cerebral palsy may experience many emotional strains and practical problems. Occupational therapists must be sensitive to this and should help families cope with these difficulties. Parent support groups are an important part of the entire treatment process. These groups bring together families who have gone through or are going through similar problems and feelings. Group members may be able to help each other through difficult times and to new adjustment levels.

Occupational Therapy Treatment

General Occupational Therapy Treatment Principles and Remediation Techniques

The treatment principles and processes that will be presented here are based on the neurodevelopmental treatment (NDT) method based on the works of Dr. and Mrs. Karl Bobath.[17] Many others have pursued the NDT approach and have continued to build upon the Bobaths' work. The basis of the NDT approach is to establish the balance necessary to be upright in space. This balance is built on the development of normal righting, equilibrium, and protective reactions.[17] It is necessary to look at the components of the righting, equilibrium, and protective responses needed for functional movement. By

definition, the cerebral palsied child has high, low, or fluctuating muscle tone. When abnormal muscle tone is inhibited, the righting responses inherent in most children may be able to develop. The child is a motor–sensory–motor being: in moving, the child gains the proprioceptive feedback that prompts him or her to move again. Initially, the therapist should provide the components of movement the child needs. Later, as the child begins to develop inner control, the therapist decreases external control. The extent to which the individual with cerebral palsy responds to treatment is directly related to the amount of brain damage sustained. For this reason, some show more progress than others. Most will respond to some degree based on their innate ability.

The NDT program does not emphasize primitive and abnormal reflexes. Rather, it seeks to facilitate the normal components of movement that provide a solid basis for motor development and integration. When such components are missing, primitive patterns persist, and abnormal reflexes are dominant.

The occupational therapist's goal is to inhibit abnormal and primitive movement patterns and to facilitate normal righting and balance responses. The concepts of normal development on which a treatment program is based have been presented throughout this chapter. They include:

1. A muscle must be elongated before it can work.
2. A joint must have full range of motion before internal control can be developed.
3. Weight bearing throughout a joint for proprioceptive feedback is necessary to develop weight shift.
4. Weight shift and a reaction to weight shift are essential for development.
5. The capability of movement normally develops from head to foot and from proximal areas to distal areas.
6. Normal components of movement are the foundation of a treatment program.
7. Treatment must be symmetrical; that is, both sides of the body are treated regardless of the degree of involvement.

If the occupational therapist applies these basic concepts, he or she should be able to problem solve and to provide a functional treatment program for a child with cerebral palsy regardless of the type of muscle tone.

The therapist may want to use various pieces of therapeutic equipment to assist in moving and manipulating the child. These may include therapy balls that range from 1 to 4 feet in diameter. Rolls or bolsters may range from 3 inches to 24 inches in diameter and may be several feet long. Wedges, large stuffed animals, and many other devices may be used. The best equipment the therapist has available is his or her own body. For example, the therapist's legs may be used as bolsters or inclined planes. A child will sometimes accept the warmth of the therapist's body when he or she will not accept a ball or bolster.

Although treatment concepts in this chapter refer to the "child," the same concepts are used with the adult. However, the child has a developing motor system and usually will show more progress than the young adult and adult. The infant under 1 year old will show the most progress.

Application of Basic Concepts

High Tone or Spasticity

The basis for treatment of the child with high muscle tone is the use of *movement to reduce tone.*[17] Initially, movement is passive to elongate the muscles in the trunk and extremities. This allows greater mobility, active movement, and decreased muscle tone. A ball or roll may be used. The child is picked up in the desired position and placed on the ball; he or she is not placed on the ball and then positioned. To position and pick up a child who is prone, the therapist places one arm under the child's thighs and one arm under the extended arms. This puts the child in an extended, elongated position. (It is easy to lose control of a wiggly child, nonetheless.) To reduce tone, the child is slowly rocked on the ball. The more proximally the child is held, the less trunk work he or she must do. As muscle tone is reduced, the child may be held further down on the legs.

If the child's trunk is asymmetrical or if the child pulls his or her arms down from the extended position, it may be necessary to further elongate the side. To passively move an arm, grasp it above the elbow and then move it. If the arm is grasped below the elbow, there is a tendency for the child to pull into flexion. (This should also be remembered when dressing and bathing a child.) With the arm on the shortened or tight side held over the head, the child may be rolled to that side to elongate the muscles. Gentle rocking may continue forwards, backwards, sideways, and diagonally. Care should be taken that the hip on the elongated side is in line with the body. If it is flexed, it will not allow full stretch. A flexed hip may be a compensation to avoid stretching and using that side. This type of elongation is especially beneficial for children with hemiplegic involvement. Additional elongation may be done by having the child prop up on an elbow when in a sidelying position. It is necessary to do all activities to both sides of the child's body. The child should be assisted to move in the appropriate sequential manner needed to assume elongation on the opposite side. This gives the child much-needed sensorimotor feedback. He or she should not be bodily lifted off a surface and placed into another position.

The child with high muscle tone needs *mobility with stability in larger ranges and movements.* This may be developed by using the basic concepts of weight shift and elongation. For example, a child is placed on the elbows when prone. He or she initially maintains the prone position with no weight shift. The child then either weight shifts to one elbow or is assisted to shift by movement of the therapy ball. The weight-bearing side is elongated, an early component of a balance response. The opposite and nonweight-bearing side becomes free to move in space. Depending on the placement of a toy or other stimulus, the child will reach out and develop larger ranges of movement. Mobility is increased through weight shift and elongation. Trunk mobility is increased through the prone-on-elbows position and later by the prone-on-extended-arms position. This will be discussed in more detail under gross motor development.

Verbal commands often make the child with high muscle tone tense. It is important to use other methods of communication such as touch, movement, and appropriate play to communicate.

Fluctuating Tone or Athetosis

The key to working with a child who has fluctuating tone or athetosis is to work on *steadying the tone and achieving midline orientation.* This may be done by giving the child firm, steady pressure through the joints with symmetical positioning. For example, a therapist may lay a child supine on a pillow so that the neck is slightly flexed, the shoulders are forward, and the arms are across the chest. The therapist sits in front of the child with his or her legs on either side of the child to help cradle the trunk and shoulders and to control movements. The child's hips and pelvis are positioned against the therapist's body. Steady, controlled pressure is given through the shoulders to steady muscle tone. The therapist grasps the child's pelvis and gives a downward stretch while flexing the child's trunk. This will elongate the child's neck and back and give him or her the feeling of steady, stable movement as the knees come into close reaching range of the already midline-oriented arms. The child with fluctuating muscle tone works well within small ranges and small movements. If midline control of head or arms is lost when attempting to touch knees, the therapist may use his or her feet or legs to bring the shoulders and arms symmetrically forward. This should also reorient the head. The therapist will usually be able to control arm use from the shoulders without actually moving the arms. The older child may not be interested in touching the knees and feet and will need an appropriate stimulus such as a toy or piece of food placed on the knees or feet. In the above activity, the therapist has given the child stability in conjunction with movement, increased trunk control, and practice of small movements within small ranges.

When a child is moved into more upright positions, more inner control is needed. From the curled-up position just described, the child is brought to a sitting position. The therapist lies back on an inclined plane and brings the child forward to sit with the child's legs either straddling the therapist's trunk, to put weight on his or her feet, or extending in a long sit. The therapist's legs are used as a back support. Side-to-side and forward-to-backward movements facilitate weight shift in the trunk. Another sequential movement from the curled-up position is to bring the child into a sitting position in front of the therapist. Weight shift may be done through the trunk and compression down from the shoulders to increase muscle stability. Midline orientation of the head and arms is necessary. The further down on the trunk, hips, or legs the child is held, the more trunk control he or she needs to use. If the child seems fearful and appears to be holding on tightly or fixing, it may be necessary to move up the trunk for support and to go back to some preparation activities such as elongation.

It is important to work on balance responses while the child is in an upright position (sitting, standing, or half-standing with the support of a piece of equipment). Balance responses develop through weight shift to a weight-bearing side that allows the other side and the trunk to be free to move and react.

The more stability the therapist gives the child with fluctuating muscle tone, the more the child uses and depends on it. The child should be given support only as needed. For this reason, the treatment must be active, with the therapist removing and replacing his or her hands often to encourage the child to develop inner control.

Oral commands work nicely with this child. The therapist states his or her intention before touching and moving the child. However, the child with fluctuating muscle tone is difficult to treat because he or she is always changing.

Low to Normal Muscle Tone or Ataxia

The ataxic child needs to have *movement with stability* (as opposed to the athetoid child who needs stability with movement). Because the ataxic individual wants to stay still, therapy involves increased trunk movement and assistance in developing righting and balance or equilibrium reactions. These are incorporated into small, slow movements. For example, the child can sit on a large ball without the feet touching the floor. At first, the therapist gives the child proximal hip support by either holding the child on either hip or holding him or her with one hand on the lower abdomen and one hand on the lower back. When the child is in this stable, supported position, the ball is moved in slow, small movements to encourage weight-shift reactions in the child's trunk. The child should feel comfortable and not have the need to stabilize abnormally by pulling into flexion or into any convenient surface. If this occurs, the treatment may be on too high a level, and it may be better to return to prone activities or to find a more

supported position. If the sitting position is tolerated and functional, the child can be held further down on the thighs. To help stabilize low to normal tone, the therapist gives compression down through the shoulders while controlling the legs with his or her elbows. This is done intermittently. The ataxic child uses the eyes to fix or stabilize by cuing in on a stable visual target.

During treatment, the child needs constantly changing intermittent support from the therapist: any consistent pressure or weight provides an opportunity for fixing. The child needs the opportunity to react to the movement that is imposed on him or her. For example, the moving surface of a roll or ball may be used. It is necessary to increase muscle tone but not to the point of making the child spastic. Careful monitoring of muscle tone can prevent this.

Low Muscle Tone or Floppy

The child with low muscle tone (the "floppy" child) needs *weight-bearing with movement* to stimulate tactile and proprioceptive input. Muscle tone must be increased. This is done through compression activities such as bouncing up and down and compressing the head into shoulders or the shoulders into trunk, arm into shoulder, and leg into hip. For example, the child can be placed over a roll, and passive compression can be applied to the joints. While the trunk is supported on the roll, the child is positioned to experience weight bearing on one arm. By assisting and maintaining the child's arm in alignment with the body, the trunk is moved over the arm to give joint compression and weight bearing with movement. This is done with each extremity, working from elbow and knee weight bearing to extended arm and leg weight bearing. Bouncing and compression can also be done while the child is sitting on the therapist's lap. When the child is sitting, the more the arms are used for support, the less the trunk is used. Positional stability of wide hip abduction and external rotation is often used to increase the base of support rather than active use of the trunk muscles. For this reason, it is important to keep the child's hips and legs in a more neutral and adducted position.

Specific Remediation Techniques

Preparation

The child needs to be prepared before treatment can be successful. Preparation refers to the steadying of muscle tone. Suggestions for reducing or increasing muscle tone in each diagnostic area were given under "Application of Basic Concepts." Preparation also includes elongation of muscles and full passive range of motion in a joint.

After the child has been prepared, the therapist uses

the normal developmental continuum as a basis for treatment planning. The type of preparation is specific to the abnormal muscle tone. It may be necessary to incorporate preparation activities into many parts of each treatment session, as the child may become tight and unstable and may need to have preparation activities repeated. The therapist's flexibility is essential to meet the specific needs of each child.

Gross Motor Movement

The treatment program follows the normal developmental sequence. Components of movement necessary for higher level functions are facilitated first.

One of the first gross motor tasks for the infant is lifting and turning the head. The same applies to the child with cerebral palsy. Normal positions must be studied and used. Because less gravitational pressure is exerted on an upright head, it is easier to raise the head from a vertical position. If a child is prone on a large ball, the ball may be rolled backwards to place the child upright. Pressure down through the shoulders and on the large proximal trunk muscles of the back will help to facilitate neck extension and to give a posterior weight shift. The heel of the therapist's hand is used for pressure or facilitation, as fingers could pinch the child's skin. If the child's elbows are adducted and behind the shoulders, trunk stabilizing of the proximal back muscles will be used to lift the head. This elongates the anterior trunk muscles and facilitates bringing the arms forward. If the child is placed on the ball with the elbows forward or under the shoulders, this mechanically elongates the trunk. This will help the child use neck extensors but may not facilitate stabilizing the scapula on the chest wall for later development of upper extremity dissociation and independent use. The therapist is cautioned that the unstabilized scapula may be torn from the chest wall if too much force is used to bring the elbows forward. This may hamper the development of fine motor skills.

While the child remains prone, the ball may be moved forward for more gravitational pressure and sideways or diagonally to bring in lateral head righting responses. If the child holds his or her head in an asymmetrical position, pressure over the pectoralis muscles in front of the shoulder will facilitate turning of the head toward the side facilitated. Pressure on either the flexor (front) and/or extensor (back) surface of the trunk will facilitate head and neck flexor or extensor movements. The therapist may need to maintain backward downward pressure on the child's shoulders and trunk to assist in holding up the head. Some children find that direct pressure on the shoulders is aversive. If this happens, the therapist may facilitate from the upper arm or the upper trunk. Gradually, shoulder pressure may be accepted.

As voluntary control begins to develop, facilitated or

stabilized control should be lessened. To voluntarily lift the head, the child needs a stable pelvis that is lower than the head. The therapist may need to place his or her hand on the child's buttocks to stabilize the pelvis. A toy, bright mobile, interesting book, or person may encourage visual attention and may interest the child in lifting the head. Midline placement of the head while the child is on the elbows will allow midline orientation for symmetrical bilateral upper extremity activities.

Head control may also be facilitated while the child is in a sitting position, because there is less gravitational pull. If the child has little or no neck control, the therapist needs to use his or her hands to support the head while also supporting the rest of the body. Firm cocontraction of the neck and trunk muscles and bouncing the child also builds up muscle tone. While fully supported and receiving intermittent facilitation, the child is moved forward, backward, and side to side to stimulate head and neck righting responses.

The therapist helps the child to lie prone on the elbows by facilitating the pectoralis muscles in front of the shoulder. His or her hands are placed under the child's chest, and pressure is applied in front of the shoulder. This also allows the therapist to shift the child's trunk to one side for weight shift. It is important to let the child experience the movement needed to achieve a position rather than to be placed in a static position. For this reason, the sequential transition from one activity to another is an integral part of treatment.

While the child is in a prone position and raised up on the elbows, the sideways movement of a ball facilitates lateral weight shift. The weight-bearing elbow is brought under the shoulder to provide increased proprioceptive and kinesthetic feedback. When the child is able to turn his or her head from side to side without looking to the weight-bearing or face side, an important milestone has been reached. Head movements are becoming dissociated from trunk movements. He or she is able to turn the head to either side while maintaining weight on one side. Side-to-side weight shift frees the nonweight-bearing side for other actions. The higher the child reaches, the greater the weight shift, weight bearing, and elongation on the opposite side. The child also experiences the upper-trunk rotation necessary for higher-level activities. Reaching higher helps the child push up on extended arms, which elongates the lower back and mobilizes the pelvis.

Developing an ability to shift weight from side to side when prone on the elbows helps the child to roll over. The child falls off balance and initiates a turn to the side by using the neck or shoulders. Pressure down through the shoulder and side facilitates a lateral righting response necessary for rolling. The child's legs must not be "frogged," or they will block the rolling pattern.

The child may be facilitated in moving from a prone position to a sitting position and back after having shown some early trunk rotation, such as reaching out in prone. Any piece of equipment may be used that will assist both therapist and child. With the child lying prone on the elbows, the therapist facilitates weight shifting by holding the child under the shoulder. The therapist facilitates a lateral righting response on the opposite side by pressing down through the side with his or her other hand. If the child has some hip stability, he or she is turned and brought into a sitting position with guidance only from the shoulder. The nonweight-bearing side leads. The child goes back into a prone position by reversing the process, in which case the weight-bearing side leads. A slow transition from one position to another facilitates the trunk muscles more; a fast movement uses momentum rather than muscle power.

The child may be brought to a sitting position from a sidelying position. The therapist places his or her right arm under the right shoulder and arm of the child and his or her left hand on the child's left hip. While leading with the hip or the nonweight-bearing side, the hip is rotated backwards, and the child is encouraged to push up on extended arms to rotate to a sitting position. Initial assistance at the weight-bearing shoulder may be necessary. This pattern of movement is easier when the child faces away from the therapist. The child is brought down to a sidelying position using the same basic pattern, except that the shoulders lead. When the child comes up to a sitting position, the hips or nonweight-bearing side lead. When going down to a sidelying or prone position, the shoulders or weight-bearing side leads. It is important to do the same activity on both sides of the body.

The child must use his or her muscles most in the transition stage from flexion to extension and from extension to flexion. He or she should be encouraged to "play" or move slowly within this transition to strengthen abdominal muscles, which are essential for a stable trunk. The oblique abdominal muscles need to be facilitated in order to develop both lower trunk rotation and stability. To facilitate the oblique abdominals, the therapist places the heel of his or her hand on the lower part of the abdomen just above the pubic bone. Pressure on the muscle and the pull of the therapist's hand guides the child in the desired direction. Depending on the child's diagnostic classification, the child is facilitated in using small or large movements.

When moving from the sitting position, placement of the child's arms and knee and the type of weight shift dictates whether he or she ends up side sitting, prone, or on hands and knees. Placement of toys can encourage rotation into a side sitting position. Facilitation of the oblique abdominals on the weight-bearing side increases trunk rotation. The more the abduction of the weight-bearing arm, the easier it is for the child to go into a sidelying and prone position. With the weight-bearing arm under the shoulder and the hip flexed, the child rotates to hands and knees by reaching out with the nonweight-bearing arm. The child may need elongation of the nonweight-bearing shoulder and side, and diagonal pressure on the abdominals of the weight-bearing side. When the child is on hands and knees, side-to-side weight shift of the upper or lower trunk brings the extremities into weight bearing in line with the body. The normal baby mobilizes the pelvis and increases balance by rocking on hands and knees. The child with cerebral palsy must do the same thing.

It is more important for the child to move in and out of the hands-and-knees and sitting positions than it is for him or her to move forward or to creep on hands and knees. The transition between these positions builds up the muscles needed to creep and to develop more upright skills. It also helps the child increase balance reactions. The transition phases may be facilitated on balls and bolsters that move with the child.

When the child moves from hands and knees to a half-kneel position, weight is shifted to one side. The opposite-side abdominals are facilitated to externally rotate and flex the nonweight-bearing leg. The weight-bearing leg is in line with the body. The child may stay on extended arms with weight on one knee and the opposite foot. Some children creep in this position. Side-to-side and forward-to-backward weight shift increases balance responses. Rotation of the nonweight-bearing side to further shift the weight over the weight-bearing knee will bring the child into a half-kneel position. Elongation of the nonweight-bearing side assists in standing up. Moving in and out of the different stages of movement builds and reinforces the components necessary for balance reactions to develop.

Fine Motor Movement

Fine motor movement (the basic hand skills of reaching, grasping, releasing, and fine prehension) is developed through weight bearing on the upper extremities. As this is incorporated into the treatment program, the child will show an increasing refinement of hand skills.

The basic concepts of establishing a treatment plan should be followed. The child needs full range of motion and elongation of the proximal areas before the distal areas can be free to function. The child may be placed over a bolster on his or her side with the arm over the bolster and the hip on the same side as extended as possible. Movement of the roll will give additional stretch to the side to decrease muscle tone and to increase range of motion. At the same time, the child may be encouraged to reach out to pop bubbles or bat a balloon for more extensor and rotational activities. He or she may play a game or read a book in front of the roll. When the therapist feels that the tone on the stretched side is reduced, the child may be rotated to sit while the elongated and extended side is maintained. The shoulder may then be given full range of motion, after which the child may go back into an upper extremity weight-bearing position. This may be done by having the child prop up on an extended arm in long or side sitting, push up on elbows or extended arms in a prone position, or side lie raised on an elbow or extended arm. Instead of coming to a sitting position after being stretched and elongated over the roll, the child may go into a prone position and onto the opposite side for elongation.

It is important that the scapula have full range of motion. The child's arm may be extended and externally rotated so that the palm is supinated or turned up while maintaining elbow extension; diagonal pressure is given from the shoulder to the opposite hip. This also elongates the tight and often ignored pectoralis muscles on the flexor side of the trunk. Individuals with hemiplegia respond well to facilitation of the scapula muscles.

Scapula stability may also be achieved through backward propping on the externally rotated arms. The child may pretend to sun bathe. Weight shift may be further achieved, when shoes are put on him or her.

If the therapist and child choose to stay in the sitting position, the child sits on the floor or on a movable object such as a bolster or smaller ball. To encourage bilateral shoulder movements, the child and therapist may place large necklaces and hats on each other. The child may reach to touch a light object such as a mobile or a bubble. The child may put his or her hands on the therapist's shoulders or head while being moved on the ball or bolster. These activities also reinforce trunk stability and balance.

While the child is prone and raised on the elbows, he or she receives the proprioceptive and kinesthetic feedback necessary to dissociate the elbow from the shoulder. Elbow movement is a necessary part of self-feeding and dressing.

As control develops in the shoulders, a change from internal to external rotation occurs. Corresponding to shoulder control, weight bearing on the heel of the hand progresses from the ulnar side to the radial, or thumb, side of the hand. Weight bearing facilitates an open hand. The weight-bearing side of the hand corresponds to the finer hand skills. Initially, there is an ulnar–palmar grasp: the fingers on the ulnar side of the hand flex to make contact with the palm. When the weight shifts to the radial side of the hand, a radial–palmar grasp develops: the fingers on the radial side flex to make contact with the palm of the hand. When the weight shifts to the thenar eminence, the thumb rotates into contact with the fingers in lateral prehension. As the thumb becomes more active, the finer prehensile skills of inferior and superior pinch develop.

A stable trunk, elongation and range of motion of the shoulders, and the facilitation of weight shift and weight bearing through the shoulders help the finer skills to develop. Following weight-bearing activities, the child may be given small objects to pick up and play with. These include raisins, Cheerios, and small, safe toys. A game may be made up using small wads of paper, cotton, or Styrofoam chips.

Handling

Good handling techniques are basic to a treatment program. A child who receives appropriate and consistent physical handling will more than likely do better than a child who receives poor, inconsistent handling and has a "good" treatment program. Good handling includes the way a child is picked up, carried, and positioned in sitting, prone, supine, and sidelying. Handling is an important part of the child's everyday world. When handling the child, it is important to inhibit primitive and abnormal patterns. For many children, a flexed position is the most functional.

To pick a child up from a supine position, the therapist should gather him or her into flexion. To do this, the lifter slides one arm under the child's shoulders and upper back, making sure that the neck is supported in flexion on the lifter's arm and the child's arms are forward. At the same time, the lifter slides the other arm under the child's knees and flexes both the hips and knees. In this gathered-up position, the child is lifted comfortably. It is important to keep the child's head and arms forward and the knees higher than the hips.

If the lifter needs to have a free arm, the initial lifting process is started. Then the child is shifted to the side of the lifter that controls the child's legs. The child faces forward and the upper trunk is controlled against the lifter's chest and arm. The child's legs may be held at one or both knees. This allows the lifter to use one arm to interact with the child. Older children and adults are lifted the same way, but two lifters may be needed.

If the child is carried facing out, it allows him or her to look at and interact with the world. To increase trunk rotation, one knee can be pulled up toward the opposite shoulder. If a child is prone, sidelying, or sitting, he or she is turned and lifted in the same gathered-up position.

When supine, the child with cerebral palsy usually needs a pillow under the head and shoulders to increase upper trunk flexion and to decrease muscle tone. Care is taken to ensure that the child brings the arms together at the midline. If he or she cannot do this voluntarily, small rolled-up towels are placed next to the trunk and under the shoulders. If the child has increased stiffness in the legs, a roll is placed under the buttocks to increase trunk flexion. The knees should be positioned higher than the hips. A "donut" may be used to provide the position: depending on the size of the infant or child, a towel or blanket may be rolled up lengthwise to form a long roll, which is shaped into a ring or donut to achieve the appropriate functional position.

Sidelying places the child in a position where primitive and abnormal patterns have the least effect. The head, hips, and knees are flexed. The arms are free to come together at the midline. The trunk is slightly flexed. If the top leg is flexed forward over the bottom leg, it is easier to maintain the position. A pillow may be placed at the back and/or under the upper trunk and head. A "side lier" is commercially available. It simulates a corner and provides both support and straps that help maintain the child's position.

Feeding (Oral–Motor)

Normal Reflexes

Normal oral–motor behavior begins prenatally at approximately 7½ weeks, menstrual age. (Menstrual age refers to age of the fetus as measured from the onset of the mother's last normal menstrual cycle.)[23] Tactile stimulation applied to the perioral area facilitates the first fetal oral reflex activity.[16]

Table 36-1 indicates fetal reflex activity of the face as a result of tactile stimulation applied to the area innervated by the trigeminal nerve, the fifth cranial nerve. During normal postnatal development, primitive oral reflexes can be observed in the newborn.

Rooting Reflex

This reflexive response persists from birth to 3 to 4 months of age and can be seen in sleeping infants up to 7 months of age.[12] The turning of the head in the direction of tactile stimulation that is applied in a light stroking manner at the corner of the infant's mouth is characteristic of this reaction. Touching the upper lip elicits lip and tongue elevation accompanied by mouth opening and head extension. The opposite reaction occurs when the lower lip is stimulated. The lip and tongue depress, the mouth opens, and the head flexes.[16] These reactions

Table 36-1. *Fetal Reflex Activity of the Face*

Response	Area Stimulated	Menstrual Age
Mouth opening	Lower lip	9½ weeks
Swallowing	Lips	10½ weeks
Momentary lip closure and, with repeated stimulation, swallowing	Lips (and/or tongue)	12½ weeks
Maintained lip closure	Lips	13 weeks
Protrusion of upper lip	Upper Lip	17 weeks
Protrusion of lower lip	Lower lip	20 weeks
Protrusion and pursing of both lips simultaneously	Lips	22 weeks
Audible sucking	Lips	29 weeks

Based on data from papers of Hooker, cited in Jacobs, MJ: Development of Normal Motor Behavior. Am J Phys Med 46:41–42, 1967

are thought to be associated with the infant's search for the nipple of the mother's breast.[10] The reflexive response may diminish immediately after feeding; therefore, it is observed best when elicited in a hungry infant.[10] In the newborn, most responses to direct tactile input take the form of avoidance or protective withdrawal reactions (*i.e.*, the infant moves as far away from the input as possible). The rooting response is one of the first reactions of the neonate that enables him or her to pursue tactile input, thus allowing the infant to make contact with the external environment.

Suck–Swallow Reflex

The normal duration of this primitive response is from the first or second day of life to 2 to 5 months of age.[19] Tactile stimulation applied to the infant's lips by the nipple of the mother's breast or bottle results in lip closure followed by a rhythmical movement of the tongue and jaw enabling the infant to obtain food. Usually, three repetitive sucks followed by swallowing make up the rhythmical pattern.[11] Sucking action is performed by the elevation and applied pressure of the anterior aspect of the tongue against the nipple. This movement elicits the release of the liquid. Transferring of the liquid to the back of the oral cavity and swallowing is the function of the posterior aspect of the tongue.[10] Nonnutritive sucking (sucking action in the absence of food) can also be observed in the neonate.

Protective Gag Reflex

This is an oral reflex normally present from birth that gradually becomes weaker when chewing occurs but does persist throughout life. Tactile input to the posterior aspect of tongue or soft palate will normally elicit a gag response. The gag response is thought to be hyperactive if it is facilitated in any other area of the oral cavity.[19]

Bite Reflex

This reaction can normally be seen from birth. It gradually diminishes around 5 to 6 months when rotary chewing develops. A rhythmic opening and closing of the mouth is elicited by direct application of a tactile input to gums, teeth, or tongue.[11] Normally, the infant is very sensitive to tactile stimulation in the oral area. From birth, the infant engages in hand-to-mouth activity.[9] By 6 months of age, the total patterns of either complete flexion or extension are modified by combined patterns of flexion and extension, enabling the infant to bring the feet to the mouth. Oral exploration of body parts is not only important for the development of body image but also helps to desensitize the low threshold to tactile input. Another important developmental milestone is the object-to-mouth exploration, particularly dominant in children 6 to 7 months of age.[14] This not only teaches the child about the external environment but also decreases oral sensitivity. When finger feeding begins and various consistencies of food are introduced, the infant will be able to accept food and spoons without facilitating the primitive oral reflexes, particularly gagging.[11]

Babkin Reflex

This reflex is a normal neonatal response characterized by the opening of the infant's mouth when pressure is applied to the palm of the hand.[16]

Mental Palmar Reflex

This normal reflexive response is characterized by observable movements of the infant's chin elicited by the light touching of the infant's palm.[10]

Normal and Abnormal Development

The feeding process includes all the components that are part of a normal feeding pattern, such as sucking, swallowing, biting, chewing, self-feeding, and accepting food texture and the many complicated and interrelated movements necessary to accomplish each one of these.

The individual with cerebral palsy may not be able to take food and liquids in the normal way or may not be able to feed himself or herself. He or she may have primitive and abnormal oral patterns resulting from high, low, or fluctuating muscle tone, causing a lack of balance between the extensor and flexor muscles. Such a balance is needed to produce normal stable head, shoulder, and trunk control, and it provides the basis for the development of the oral fine motor control necessary for eating. Many oral motor problems may be the result of or compensations for blocks in development causing abnormal oral characteristics.[1] Neck blocks may result in abnormal oral characteristics. There may be jaw thrust, in which there is a strong downward extension of the lower jaw. The jaw may appear to be stuck open, and the child may have difficulty closing his or her mouth.[18] Jaw thrust may occur during any phase of feeding.

The individual who maintains a neck block may exhibit lip and cheek retraction, in which there is a drawing back of the lips and cheeks so that they form a tight horizontal line over the mouth. This limits lip closure. The teeth usually show, and there is often a constant smile. The child may compensate by having a purse-string action of the lips and may try to counteract the basic tendency toward retraction by pursing or pulling the lips forward.[18]

Neck hyperextension and the pull of gravity may cause tongue retraction, in which there is a strong pulling back of the tongue into the pharyngeal space. The tip of the tongue is not even with the gums or in approximation with the lower lip as it should be. It is often pulled back toward the middle of the hard palate and may be in firm approximation with the hard or soft palate. This makes it difficult to place a nipple, cup, or spoon in the child's mouth or to initiate a swallowing response. The airway may also be obstructed by the tongue.

A tongue thrust may be a compensation for a neck block.[1] It may be defined as a forceful protrusion of the tongue from the mouth. It is frequently arrhythmic; its intermittent occurrence breaks a previously sustained rhythm.[18] The thrusting of the tongue may interfere with any phase of the feeding process. The individual may compensate for a neck block by having abnormally strong jaw closure. Such tight, involuntary closure of the jaw often makes opening the jaws difficult. This is related to excessive extensor tone throughout the body or to stimulation of a tonic bite reflex.[18]

A bite reflex is the rhythmic closing and opening of the jaws when the gums or teeth are stimulated. This may be in the form of an easy phasic bite with slight chewing motion during stimulation, or a strong tonic bite. In the tonic bite reflex, the jaw closes strongly and often does not open easily.

The cerebral palsied child may lack the ability to produce his or her own tactile stimulation. This may cause oral tactile hypersensitivity, which results in the child's resisting textured foods. It may also lead to a jaw thrust, tonic bite, lip and cheek retraction, lip purse, tongue thrust, and tongue retraction.

An individual with a neck block may further compensate by using strong shoulder elevation to help stabilize his or her head during oral activity. This may increase tightness throughout the chest, inhibiting breathing and feeding.

Shoulder blocks may result in other abnormal oral characteristics and compensations. Scapulohumeral tightness may cause the use of elevated, internally rotated shoulders to stabilize the head. Shoulder elevation increases neck hyperextension, which may cause the many problems associated with a neck block. Tightness in the upper chest limits both breathing and feeding. Scapular adduction does not allow the hands to come together at the midline, preventing the child from providing his or her own tactile oral desensitizing. Tension across the chest may limit breathing and feeding. Neck hyperextension may be increased, which may cause related oral problems.

The therapist may simulate each of the blocks and their oral consequences in order to experience personally a little of what the individual with cerebral palsy feels:

1. *Neck hyperextension.* Is it easy or hard to close the

mouth? If the jaw opens too wide, is a jaw thrust possible? Is there tightness across the mouth that could cause lip retraction and a purse-string compensation? What has happened to the tongue? Is it retracted? What if food is placed in the mouth? Does it cause a tongue thrust? Is there a tendency to use tongue retraction and elevation to the hard palate to keep food out of the air passage? Does an attempt to bite cause an abnormally strong response? Have the shoulders elevated to maintain stability?

2. *Neck asymmetry.* How does it feel to swallow? Try to close the mouth. Is there jaw deviation? Does the jaw want to snap shut, retract, or thrust?

3. *Scapulohumeral tightness.* With the shoulders elevated, how does it feel to swallow and breathe? Is there a tendency for the neck to hyperextend?

4. *Scapular adduction.* With the shoulders adducted and externally rotated, how does it feel to swallow and breathe? Is there a tendency for the neck to hyperextend?

The therapist may further experience oral motor problems by having someone else feed him or her while in these primitive abnormal positions.

Stability and Symmetry

Using a problem-solving model based on the abnormal oral characteristics as compensations for blocks in development, the components essential for a successful remediation program are *stability* and *symmetry.*

Stability may be both internal and external, as discussed under "Basic Components of Movement." Internal stability develops along a developmental continuum. An infant has a suckle pattern because of no jaw stability and a small oral cavity. A 2-year-old will bite on the rim of the cup because he or she does not have enough internal stability to hold the jaw steady as he or she drinks. A 3-year-old should have the internal jaw stability needed to hold the cup between the lips.

External stability is the additional control needed by, and/or given to, individuals who have not developed their own internal control. The child does this when biting on the cup rim. The therapist provides external stability until the child develops internal stability in oral as well as other motor skills.

Positioning

Two types of external stability will be discussed: *positioning* and *jaw control.* To position a child for feeding, stability and symmetry are essential. There are different ways to position a child. Common to all are the following components:

1. Head forward with the chin tucked or down
2. Head in the midline
3. Shoulders forward
4. Arms internally rotated
5. Hands in the lap
6. Trunk straight
7. Hips and knees flexed to at least 90°

The infant or baby may be cradled in the feeder's arms in the above position. This encourages eye contact and communication with the feeder. If the feeder needs both hands free to assist the baby, he or she may sit tailor or Indian fashion and cradle the baby in his or her lap. The baby's head is at the feeder's knee. The shoulders may be brought forward and internally rotated by the feeder's legs. The baby's hips may be flexed at a 90° angle in the center of the lap.

A young child may sit on the feeder's lap. One of the feeder's arms may be used to control the child's neck and upper trunk while feeding with the other arm.

The baby may be placed in an infant or car seat that has been adapted. A "Feeder Seat" by Tumbleforms may be used for a child who needs the support of a larger infant seat. This may be placed in a beanbag chair, regular chair, or against the wall. It may be reclined or positioned vertically, depending on the needs of the child. A beanbag chair may be arranged to position a child functionally. It may need to be overcorrected to allow for settling of the Styrofoam "beans." An inflatable infant bathtub called a "Tubby" may be used as a back support for the larger child in the beanbag chair. It centers the head and brings the arms forward. An adapted seating device such as a wheel chair or "care chair" may also be used for feeding. A high chair may be adapted to meet the above criteria.

The child may be placed supine on a firm inclined wedge placed on the feeder's lap and resting against a table edge. A very firm pillow may be used. The child faces the feeder. The hips and knees may be flexed and adducted with the feet resting on the feeder's abdomen, or else the hips may be abducted, with the legs straddling the feeder's hips. A child is never fed in a fully supine position.

Because mealtime is a time of direct communication, it is better to feed the child from the front. If this is not feasible, the therapist may feed the child from the side. The food should usually enter the child's mouth at the midline, although the side position may be necessary for certain types of jaw control. A child with excessive flexor tone may be fed in prone either on a wedge or bolster. He or she should be encouraged to lift his or her head to get the food. A severely involved child, who cannot be positioned in a seating device, may be fed in a sidelying position. A "Side Lier" by Tumbleforms may be used. The same basic criteria must be met.

It is often necessary to position the child functionally by adapting the child. To bring the head forward in a chin tuck in the midline, a rolled-up towel or small roll may be placed at the base of the skull. This must be high enough to elicit a chin tuck in which the neck is flexed. The chin must not jut forward, and the neck must not hyperextend over the top of the roll. A conveniently shaped stuffed animal such as a stuffed snake may be used. This acts as a neck roll but also may go behind the shoulders to bring them forward. The neck may be brought forward by appropriate placement of the head against the feeder's elbow or knee. A small wedge or molded head piece may be placed on a wheelchair or care chair. The occipital area of the skull should be avoided, as pressure on this area causes hyperextension of the neck.

To position the shoulders forward with the arms internally rotated and the trunk straight, a rolled-up towel may be placed on either side of the trunk and behind the shoulders. The thickness of the roll depends on the amount of internal rotation the child needs.

Before a child's hips and knees can be flexed to a 90° angle, the child must be positioned to sit on the buttocks or ischial tuberosities and not on the "tailbone" or sacrum. To do this, stand behind the child, grasp under the upper thigh, and roll the child's pelvis under and pull him or her back. A small roll may be placed under the knees to maintain the desired flexion.

The angle of feeding is important. The child should be as upright as possible but reclined enough to allow the child to keep the food in the mouth, chew it, and swallow it. Regardless of where the child is positioned, the angle should be no less than 45°. A more reclined position may cause aspiration.

The very hypotonic child who will not stay positioned long enough to eat may need some additional help. If the arms are elevated to the shoulder level, spinal extension will increase. This will help him or her stay in position and will also facilitate the entire feeding process by increasing general muscle tone. A towel or roll across the child's chest and under the arms will help to maintain the position. The child's arms may be placed over the edge of a high table. The feeder's arms may go across the chest to elevate the trunk. A child who seems to get "stuck" or who stops eating in the middle of a meal (and is not full) may be helped to resume the feeding process by elongating the trunk. He or she may be so tight that eating is no longer possible.

Jaw Control

When functional positioning does not provide enough stability, jaw control may be necessary. The child may not have enough internal stability to control the jaw because of high or low muscle tone and persistent primi-

tive, and abnormal, oral patterns. He or she may have jaw thrust, jaw retraction, jaw asymmetry, exaggerated opening or closing, poor lip closure, and/or tongue thrust.

There are two types of jaw control. One type uses two fingers and a front approach (Fig. 36-1). The distal phalanx of the feeder's thumb is placed in the center of the child's chin at the base of the chin. Inward and upward pressure is applied to control jaw opening and closing. The feeder's index finger is placed under the child's chin at the base of the tongue to control jaw movement. The feeder's wrist may be placed on the upper chest to facilitate upper trunk flexion and chin tuck.

The second type of jaw control uses three fingers and a side approach. The feeder stands to the side or behind the child (Fig. 36-2). The therapist's thumb is placed on the child's jaw line to control lateral jaw movements. The index finger is positioned on the child's chin. Inward and upward pressure is applied to control jaw and lip movements. The middle finger is placed under the chin to control jaw opening. This method allows more external control of chin tuck and neck elongation. The feeder's body against the child can be used for additional control.

Jaw control is not needed with every child. When it is used, the feeder must not get so caught up in controlling the jaw that he or she inadvertently puts a finger in the

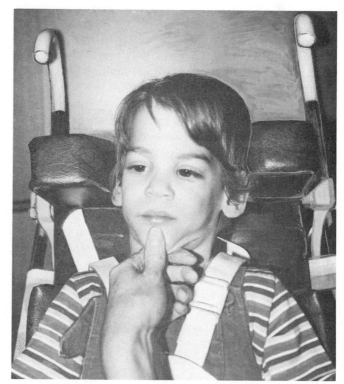

Figure 36-1. Jaw control: two fingers from the front.

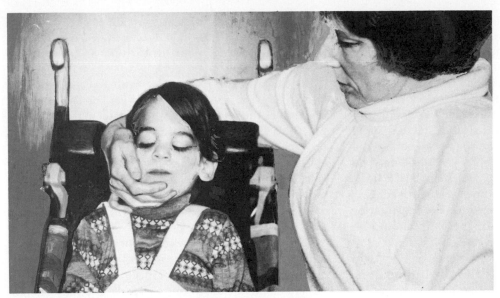

Figure 36-2. Jaw control: three fingers from the side.

child's eye or ear. The child should not be held so tightly that there is no independent jaw movement; he or she needs to move the jaw during the feeding process but at the same time to have enough stability to experience a more functional feeding pattern. This is especially important with infants who normally have an unstable jaw. The feeder should give the child only the amount of external stability necessary. Perhaps there is enough internal jaw control for the developmental level, and only lip control is needed. The program must be geared to the individual's needs.

Some children may be too sensitive in the oral area to accept jaw control. Compromise between the feeder and child may be necessary. In the meantime, an oral desensitizing program may be initiated. With the hypersensitive child, it may be possible to gradually "sneak in" and give light jaw control at an important feeding phase. Jaw control is increased as tolerance develops.

Treatment

When planning a feeding program, the therapist should be aware of the difference between a feeding management program and a therapeutic feeding program. A management program involves getting food into the child and includes optimum positioning. A therapeutic feeding program emphasizes righting and balance responses as the basis for feeding development; the child has a more active role. A treatment program seeks to increase oral–motor development, whereas a management program seeks to solve an immediate need. Both are important. The infant and young child may initially need both a management program and a therapeutic feeding program for development. The older child or adult may need a management program.

Using the developmental framework to analyze feeding activities is important. The size of the infant's oral area and the lack of stability greatly influence the ability to take foods. As the oral area grows, more tongue movement is possible. This necessitates more stability of the head, neck, and upper trunk for the finer oral skills of sucking, swallowing, biting, and chewing to develop. As textured foods are introduced, the child must use more refined feeding abilities.

To protect both the child and the feeder, disposable gloves should be used by the feeder.

Sucking

Sucking is the rhythmic method of drawing soft food or drink into the mouth with a negative pressure component. Tongue action is primarily up and down. Negative pressure builds up within the oral cavity because of firm approximation of the lips. This helps to pull soft food and liquid into the mouth.[18]

The early infantile method of sucking is called *suckling.* This involves a definite extension/retraction movement of the tongue. Liquid or soft food is obtained through a rhythmic licking action of the tongue combined with strong jaw opening and closing. There is frequently a rather loose approximation of the lips. The tongue does not protrude beyond the borders of the lips.[18] Tongue action in suckling should not be confused with the hard forceful protrusion of the tongue thrust.

An infant or child may have a weak or absent suck. It may be a medical necessity to tube-feed the infant to provide nourishment. A nasogastric (N/G) tube goes in one nostril and down to the stomach. The N/G tube may negate the child's gag response. This type of tube may be used for a temporary feeding problem.

Another type of feeding tube is the gastric (G) tube, which goes through the abdominal wall directly into the stomach. This requires a surgical procedure called a gastrostomy and is used with a child who has a long-standing feeding problem and who cannot take foods by mouth. A positive aspect of the G tube is that the child does not experience the negative oral input that he or she receives when an N/G tube is inserted or removed. An oral stimulation program may be used. The child is given some food by mouth, but the rest goes directly into the tube.

It is important for an individual to receive oral stimulation at the same time as he or she is tube-fed: the filling of the stomach should be associated with oral activity. If possible, he or she should be held while fed to communicate with the feeder. This early communication is essential for bonding with the feeder and for later communication skills.

The normal infant increases the suckle pattern by moving the tongue within the small oral cavity. The only way that the tongue can move is in an extension/retraction pattern as it rubs against the hard palate. Since all treatment is based on normal development, the therapist facilitates a suckle by rhythmically stroking the hard palate with his or her finger pad. It is important to find the individual's own rhythm for all phases of sucking. This includes sucking from the bottle, cup, and spoon. Rhythmic stroking of the spoon on the lower lip may increase the strength of the suck. The faster the food moves from the front of the mouth in a controlled pattern, the less likely the child is to choke. Slow transit time may cause choking.

A child with poor oral control may aspirate food into the lungs. This may cause aspiration pneumonia. A child who gurgles in his or her throat may aspirate. Using the chin-tuck head position should decrease this possibility. Feeding the child with the neck extended should be avoided, as this allows direct access from the oral cavity to the lungs. Giving oily liquids to children who may aspirate is not recommended. The body can absorb a water-based liquid, such as juices, more easily.

The infant or child with a poor suck needs many oral experiences. Because of blocks in development, the child may not have been able to put the hands in his or her mouth. The normal infant will first put the dorsum of his or her hand in the mouth. Later, he or she will turn the wrist to put a fist in the mouth. A child with a poor suck needs to experience the same sequence. This also helps to desensitize the mouth. The therapist may put his or her hand in the child's mouth. The child should be introduced to a pacifier and small, textured toys to chew and suck on. A weak suck may be facilitated by helping the child move his or her lips and cheeks in a rhythmic pattern. This may be done with toys as well as with a bottle.

When working with a bottle-fed infant with a weak suck, the therapist may want to experiment with different types of nipples. A "preemie" nipple with a cross-cut hole often works well. This is a soft rubber nipple used with premature infants. Some come with a small cross-cut hole, which may be enlarged with small scissors. (Small suture or nail scissors work well.) The "x" cut lets the child control the flow of liquid. As he or she sucks or bites on the nipple, the liquid flows into the mouth. When he or she releases the nipple, the liquid stops flowing. This allows time for the child to process what is in the mouth. It may be necessary to assist the infant with jaw control and/or cheek facilitation. A nipple with an enlarged hole is not good, as it will allow too much liquid to flow into the child's mouth. He or she may not be able to control and swallow the liquid and could aspirate some of it.

When high muscle tone is present, a child may have a hard, nonproductive suck. The child's position should be evaluated. The neck may be hyperextended. Repositioning the child in flexion will facilitate a functional suck. Jaw control may be needed to control ungraded jaw movements and to provide stability. The child may have a strong nonnutrient suck on a pacifier but may not be able to have a slower and deeper nutrient suck from a bottle or spoon. The two sucking patterns are different, and it is difficult for the child to generalize from one to the other. The child needs to build up confidence as he or she controls suck, swallow, and breathing in the nutrient suck.

Swallowing

Initially, swallowing is part of the suck–swallow or suckle–swallow pattern. The infant is dependent on the suckle or suck to trigger a swallow. He or she gradually dissociates swallowing and can swallow whenever food is in the mouth. This necessitates movements of the tongue, lips, and cheeks that help to form a bolus of food and to send it to the back of the mouth for the final swallow.[18]

A child may hold liquid or food in the mouth and may have a slow swallow. A quick, light touch between the child's upper lip and nose may facilitate a swallow. Some children will both suck and swallow slowly but automatically if they are given the time to do it. A feeder who is in too much of a hurry might not give this child enough time to organize the oral area to swallow. Gentle bouncing and rocking may provide vestibular stimulation, which might help the child to organize to swallow. There are times when a child may need the help of gravity to swallow. He or she may need to be in a semireclined position with the chin tucked. As the child gains control of swallowing, he or she may be brought into a more upright position. Children should not be fed in a fully supine position.

It is easier to form a bolus for swallowing if the food

is finely ground and a little dry. For this reason, textured foods should be used. Some children may scatter the food in their mouth and need liquids to either form a bolus of food or wash it down.

A child with low muscle tone may keep the mouth open. This makes swallowing difficult. This individual responds well to a therapeutic feeding program that builds up muscle tone. He or she needs oral play. Quick stretching of the lips and cheek may increase muscle tone. Jaw control during feeding, with emphasis on lip closure, is important. Light, quick tapping of the lips will facilitate lip closure. The therapist must be cognizant that some children have to breathe through their mouths and will need to keep them open.

A child with lip retraction may not be able to close his or her lips to suck or swallow. The upper lip may appear to be very thin. The teeth and upper gums may be visible. Stretching of the lip and cheek muscles may provide the range of motion needed for muscle activation. The therapist places the thumb and index finger of a supinated hand on the cheeks and gently pulls them forward so the child looks like a "chipmunk" with fat cheeks and full lips. The antiretraction position is maintained throughout the feeding session. If a strong suckle is present, the anti-retraction position needs modifying to prevent the cheeks from being bitten. An individual with lip retraction may also have a tonic bite reflex. The therapist needs to be cautious when placing a finger in the child's mouth. If the therapist is not quick enough and a child bites down on his or her finger, the child's jaws may be opened by flexing the child's head forward and opening the jaws with pressure on the outside, back part of the cheeks between the teeth.

Chewing and Biting

Chewing and biting are more voluntary aspects of feeding. Although they have their origins in early reflexive movement patterns that are triggered by stimulation of the gums and tooth receptors, they remain at a reflexive level for only a brief period. Munching is the earliest form of chewing and seems to evolve from a combination of the tongue pattern seen in a true suck and the jaw pattern seen in a phasic bite reflex. It involves a flattening and spreading of the tongue combined with an up-and-down movement of the jaw. The jaws make a definite biting or chewing rhythm. The tongue does not move in a lateral direction, which would be necessary to transfer food to the teeth for real chewing. Munching remains a part of the adult chewing pattern and is observed when food is not being transferred.[18] The untrained person may confuse a primitive phasic bite reflex with munching and chewing.

Chewing is the process of using the teeth and tongue to break up and pulverize pieces of food in preparation for swallowing. The chewing pattern progresses from the primitive phasic bite-and-release pattern, to a non-stereotyped vertical movement, and then to the diagonal rotary jaw movements that occur as food is transferred to the side or middle of the mouth by the tongue. These movements continue to be refined until they become smooth and well coordinated. They finally develop into the circular rotary jaw movements that occur as the child transfers food across the midline from one side of the mouth to another.[18] The development of gross motor extension and flexion, diagonal trunk patterns, and rotational trunk patterns needs to be well established before fine oral movements occur. Placement of food between the child's teeth facilitates chewing.

The phasic bite-and-release pattern is the first, primitive form of biting to occur. Next, the child learns to quiet the jaw and develops a holding posture. Later, the child will be able to bite soft food such as a soft cookie in a sustained, controlled manner. Still later, the child will be able to bite hard food such as a hard cookie in a sustained manner but with excessive overflow of movement to other body parts.[18] Finally, the child develops a sustained, controlled bite with the head in the midline and appropriate grading of jaw movements. Using food with different textures facilitates biting. The child progresses from a soft cookie to crisp food such as pretzels to hard cookies. Lunch meat, hot dogs, and other soft meats may be introduced.

Oral Sensitivity

Oral hypersensitivity negatively influences the feeding process. The child may not accept anything into the mouth or may refuse all lumps of food. There may be a history of not putting the hands or toys in the mouth. He or she may take objects to the lips without mouthing them. This child may have a very active gag reflex. The infant normally has a large gag-sensitive area. This may not yet have been integrated. The child may refuse to allow anyone to brush his or her teeth or wash his or her face. He or she may turn away when touched on the face. (There may be a difference between light and firm touch. Light touch is less acceptable than firm touch.) A dislike of being held and rocked may go with the syndrome.

The therapist should give the child firm tactile input to the trunk and then progress up to the arms and mouth. When this is tolerated, the child needs oral play around and inside the mouth similar to that discussed under "Sucking." The firm tactile input provided by swaddling and close-fitting knitted clothing may be helpful. After a bath, a brisk rubdown with a towel will provide input. The child needs to feel and experience many different textures and sensations on the body. The same progression of hands in his or her mouth working up to toys discussed under "Sucking" may be done. Flavors may be added to hands or toys.

Oral digital stimulation may be done after the child tolerates having his or her face touched. At first, the lips are touched and rubbed. Then he or she is touched and rubbed between the lips. When the child allows the therapist to put his or her finger in the child's mouth, the gums may be rubbed. One quarter of the mouth is done at a time. Starting at the back of the mouth, the finger makes small, firm circular movements. It is brought forward and out of the mouth at the midline. While maintaining external jaw and lip control, the therapist must wait for the child to swallow. Each quadrant is done in the same way. The inside of the gum ridge and cheeks may also be rubbed. The child should not be forced to accept the stimulation. If he or she resists, the child is saying that it is aversive. It is necessary to find compromise between the child's immediate needs and the therapeutic program.

Some children may be so sensitive to anything in their mouths that oral feeding is not practical for either the child or feeder. The child will need to be fed through a nonoral method such as a G tube. The occupational therapy program would emphasize oral desensitizing, oral play, and rhythm without the introduction of food. Later, taste and food would be introduced when the child is ready.

Gagging

A child who will not accept textured foods may gag and spit out the smallest lump. It is best to process table foods in a blender and gradually add thickening such as instant potato, baby cereal, or bran. Work up to fork-mashed foods. The child may find softer foods such as pasta more acceptable.

Some children may be hyporesponsive to oral stimulation. They may lack sensory awareness in the oral area. They need a sensory program similar to that needed by the hypersensitive child. The therapist should be aware that a child may have been so sensitive in the mouth that he or she needed to "shut down" his or her sensory system to survive. This defense mechanism may make him or her appear unresponsive.

Some children may gag and vomit frequently. Physical problems must first be ruled out. A common cause of vomiting is esophageal reflux. Here, the esophagus does not close off sufficiently to hold food in the stomach, and food or gastric juices flow back into the esophagus and may be vomited. Reflux is common in the infant who "spits" or vomits small amounts of food. Reflux can be surgically corrected. If the child might have this condition, he or she should be kept sitting for at least 3 minutes after feeding to allow gravity to help keep the food down. Alternatively, the child who vomits may be a "ruminator." Ruminators stimulate themselves by bringing up partially digested food that they may spit out or reswallow. A developmental psychologist is needed to help formulate a behavior-oriented program.

There are several ways to interrupt gagging. The child's head needs to be flexed forward. Rapid tapping under the chin at the base of the tongue and lips may reduce the muscle tone that has built up. The therapist must move quickly, cover the child's mouth, and move out of the "line of fire."

Drooling often occurs in individuals with cerebral palsy and may be mild to severe. Remediation is directly related to the development of upper trunk and head control. This is the foundation on which to build the sucking and swallowing components of oral movements. Lip and jaw closure are especially important. Drooling may also be a sensory problem, in which the child does not feel the need to swallow. Oral sensitizing may help the child become more aware of saliva in the mouth and be internally cued to swallow.

Food Intake

Until the child develops sufficient oral control, he or she should be fed. Self-feeding may cause associated abnormal reflexive movements in the oral area and in other areas of the body. Before one feeds a child, it is best to prepare the child as one does before a treatment session. It is hoped that this will help him or her to use innate abilities optimally. Symmetrical, stable, functional positioning is necessary.

A small, flat spoon is often easier for the child to accept. A small amount of food is placed on the end of the spoon. The spoon is presented to encourage chin tuck and midline orientation of the head. It should be placed about one-third of the way back on the tongue with slight downward pressure. Time should be allowed for the lips to close on the spoon and for the sucking process to begin. Jaw and lip control may be needed. Slight upward pressure on the skin of the chin will assist with lip closure on the spoon.

The child should use his or her lips to clean the spoon. The food should not be scraped on the upper teeth, as this may cause a tongue thrust and extension–retraction suckle pattern. To facilitate the use of both lips, the spoon may be withdrawn from the child's mouth using a slightly upward diagonal pattern. Sufficient time must be allowed for swallowing.

If chewing or increased lateral tongue movements are treatment goals, the food should be placed on the side of the child's tongue or between the teeth. Placement should facilitate the forming of a bolus for swallowing. The child with strong tongue thrust may benefit from placement of the food between the teeth or in the cheek pocket. Pressure on the lateral aspect of the tongue with the spoon as food is placed in the mouth may inhibit tongue thrust and protrusion and may facilitate tongue lateralization.

If more lip closure is needed, more food may be placed in the child's mouth. He or she may continue to chew with the mouth open but might close it to swallow so as to keep the food in the mouth. The therapist should look for pulling in of the corners of the mouth and cheeks and later for approximation of the lips at the midline.

Spoon-feeding may require compromises between the child and the feeder. A child with a tonic bite may need quick movement of the spoon in and out of the mouth to prevent a bite reflex. The child's teeth and gums should be avoided, as touching them could stimulate the reflex.

Most children are able to drink from a cup, even when they cannot drink from a bottle. It is essential that the child controls the amount of liquid that flows into the mouth. A cut-out cup works well. This is a soft plastic or paper cup that has been cut out on one side to accommodate the nose and to allow the feeder to closely monitor the child's drinking. Place the uncut edge of the cup on the child's lower lip and allow some liquid to flow to the lip. Wait for him or her to initiate a suck. Although he or she may be slow to start the process, the child may have the ability to do it. Liquids should not be poured into the child's mouth, as this makes it harder for the child to suck and swallow. If the child does not have the ability to initiate a suck, it may be necessary for the child to taste a small amount of liquid. Jaw and lip control may be necessary throughout the drinking sequence. It should be maintained until swallowing is completed. He or she may need to swallow several times for every mouthful. If the child swallows immediately, the feeder may leave the cup in place for several suck–swallow sequences before giving the child a short break to breathe. Symmetrical, stable, and functional positioning is necessary. The feeder must not let the child's head tip back, because this increases the possibility of aspiration. Downward pressure on the sternum or breastbone will help induce chin tuck.

If the feeding program is not working the way the therapist wishes, he or she should re-evaluate all areas of it. More preparation may be needed. The key areas of positioning should be reassessed. Is the child compensating with poor patterns? Are there too many distractions? Does he or she dislike the food?

The type of food used influences the feeding process. Thin liquids can be difficult to handle. Fruit nectars and juices thickened with fruit sauce might be easier to suck and swallow. Dehydrated baby foods, gelatin, and baby cereal may be used to thicken liquids.

Commerical baby foods are not recommended. It is cheaper and usually more appetizing to puree, grind,

mash, or chop table food. This also lets the child acquire the taste preferences of the rest of the family. Pureed foods tend to liquify in the mouth and to be drooled back. Finely ground foods are easier to process.

Milk may increase the thickness of mucus, so a non-dairy formula may be better for a baby who has difficulty handling secretions. Oily fluids such as beef and chicken broth may help to thin mucus, but they should be used with caution with children who may aspirate. As was previously mentioned, oily liquids are slower to be absorbed into the system if they get into a child's lungs.

Beef and pork may be difficult to chew. Softer meats, such as hot dogs, lunch meats, veal, lamb, and chicken, are easier. Chicken and turkey roll are especially good, as they are soft and easy to finger-feed. Cheese and boneless fish are usually even softer.

Foods combining several textures may be difficult for a child to process. These include soups with vegetables and noodles and vegetables with skins, such as corn, lima beans, and peas, which are soft inside but have a firm outer covering. Finger foods include the softer meats that have been cubed, rolled, or stripped. Vegetables, such as carrots, beets, potatoes, and green beans, may be cut and cooked in a shape that is easily finger-fed.

If the child is having difficulty forming a bolus to swallow, gummy, cakey foods should be kept to a minimum. Tepid foods are more readily accepted than hot or cold foods. This is especially true of the child with hypersensitivity in the oral area.

Self-Feeding

When the child has integrated primitive oral patterns and developed sufficient oral control, self-feeding may be initiated. A child may be motivated but may continue to have oral–motor problems. It may be necessary to make a compromise between the child's goal of self-feeding and the theapist's goal of developing better oral control. The therapist may therapeutically feed the child most of the meal and then allow him or her to self-feed one food such as dessert or a finger food.

Self-feeding may be started at snack time with the introduction of finger foods. The child must be in a symmetrical, stable, functional position at a table or in a high chair. The child's feet should also be supported. The same principles apply to self-feeding that apply to feeding in general.

A preparation period before feeding will increase the child's ability to eat. Self-feeding skills may develop parallel to fine motor skills. The foods offered should be appropriate for the child's type of grasp. If a child has a palmar grasp, rolled lunch meat or a slivered hot dog might be good. If he or she has a fine pincer grasp, raisins or Cheerios might be good. He or she may need to compensate and stabilize himself or herself by leaning on the elbows. A higher table can help stabilize the child's upper trunk.

Spoon-feeding will progress as with the normal child. A regular spoon should be tried first. If the child lacks the supination needed to place the spoon in the mouth, a spoon can be bent to accommodate his or her needs by twisting the bowl down. A few children may need a build-up spoon handle. The use of a swivel spoon, in which the bowl moves to remain level, is less common. A drawback of a swivel spoon is that it may continue to move as it nears the mouth, making it difficult for the child to place the spoon in the mouth. If the child cannot scoop with a spoon, stabbing the food with a fork may be more functional.

The therapist assists the child to fill and take the spoon to the mouth by holding the child's hand with his or her index finger in the palm and thumb on the back of the hand while maintaining the wrist in extension or in the functional position. The child's hand should not be covered by the therapist. "Backward chaining" is used (*i.e.*, when the child initiates putting the spoon into the mouth, the therapist releases the hand for the child to complete the task). When the bowl and spoon are presented to the child, the spoon is placed upright and perpendicular at the 12 o'clock position in front of the child. This allows the child a choice of which hand to use to grasp the spoon. It also exaggerates the scooping and filling process to establish the pattern.

The less special equipment used, the better. A lip on the child's plate may keep the food from slipping off. Scoop dishes that have a built-up side to assist with filling a utensil are available. They usually have a nonskid bottom that stabilizes them. A commercial product called "Dycem" is an excellent nonskid material to place under a plate. A flat, wet washcloth placed under a dish will provide some resistance to sliding. A small plastic cup without handles is the most functional for a child's use because it provides a larger surface to hold on to. Handled cups tend to reinforce scapular adduction and to increase muscle tone. Covered cups are often just a step up from a bottle. Straw-drinking seems to reinforce neck hypertension; as the liquid is sucked up a straw, the individual tends to go into hyperextension. Straw-drinking should be used with caution and carefully evaluated.

Dressing

The acquisition of dressing and undressing skills by the child with cerebral palsy should follow the same sequence as for the normal child (Table 36-2). However, whereas a normal child is most commonly dressed while supine, this position may make a cerebral palsied child more rigid and will unecessarily complicate the dressing process. Laying the small child across the therapist's

Table 36-2. *Acquisition of Dressing and Undressing Skills.*

Age	Skill
12 mo.	Cooperates with dressing; *i.e.*, extends arms to put in sleeve
18 mo.	Purposefully removes socks
2 yr.	Removes unlaced shoes
	Removes pants with assistance over hips
3 yr.	Removes clothes completely except for small buttons and back fastenings
	Unfastens medium-sized buttons
	Puts on underpants, socks, and shoes
4 yr.	Fastens large buttons
	Laces Shoes
5 yr.	Fastens medium-sized buttons
	Dresses self except for bows and small buttons
6 yr.	Ties bows

Adapted from Finnie N: *Handling the Young Cerebral Palsied Child at Home*, 2nd ed. New York, EP Dutton, 1975

knees or lap, prone with arms and legs extended, makes dressing much easier. The child's extremities can easily be manipulated into clothing, and the whole child is in a therapeutically functional position.

The best way of dressing a child is to sit the child between the therapist's legs with the child leaning forward at the hips, with legs abducted and knees flexed. This decreases extensor tone. One should describe and name each article of clothing as it is used and each part of the body as it is moved. At first, it may help to work in front of a mirror so that the child can see what is happening. When the child begins to assist the therapist, the mirror should be removed, as the reversed image may be confusing.

For the person dominated by flexor or extensor tone, the sidelying position seems to neutralize excess tone and facilitates dressing. When rolling an individual from side to side, the knees and hips should remain flexed to inhibit extensor tone. If the person must be supine, a hard pillow should be placed under the head and shoulders to break up the extensor tonus. Knees and hips should be flexed and abducted.

Whichever position is used for dressing the child, it should be symmetrical. Note the following suggestions:
1. Put the more affected limb in clothing first.
2. Straighten the arm before putting it in a sleeve.
3. Hold the arm at the elbow or above to move it. If resistance is felt, do not attempt to pull the arm through a sleeve by pulling on the hand. This causes the whole arm to flex and the shoulder to retract.

4. Before putting on shoes or socks, the leg should be flexed.

If the child wears braces, remove them by unfastening them at the most proximal point and work distally toward the feet. When putting braces on, be sure that the child's heel is placed firmly down into the shoe before lacing and securely tying the bow. Continue to work from distal to proximal. Two adult fingers should fit under each closure for a comfortable fit.

Some children can dress while sitting in a sturdy low chair. If the child does not have enough balance to lean forward when sitting, several alternatives may be used. The child may sit between the therapist's legs for support. A triangular chair may be used either on the floor (Fig. 36-3) or raised on a platform. A corner or wall may provide additional support (Fig. 36-4).

An older and more severely involved child may not be able to sit. If head control has been attained, he or she

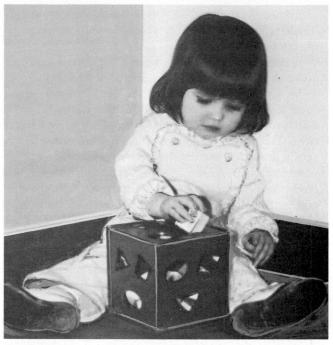

Figure 36-4. A corner may provide additional sitting support.

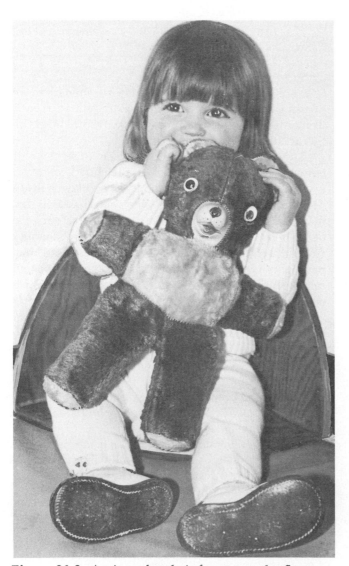

Figure 36-3. A triangular chair for use on the floor.

may be able to dress and undress from a side lying, prone, or supine position. A simple pants pusher or pants puller is often needed.

While sitting with hips and knees bent, the child may remove socks by pulling on the toe end or by sliding a thumb down the back of the leg and over the heel. The sock may also be rubbed off the toes either by using the other foot or against the floor. It is helpful to avoid stretch and elastic socks. Tube socks are easier to put on than those with a heel.

In order to put on socks, the child should have knees and hips bent. The sock is opened with two hands, and the child is encouraged to make a "big mouth with the opening" in order to put all toes in at one time. Some children will try to put the sock on the big toe first and will try to stretch it across to the little toe. This often leaves the little toes out of the sock or pops the sock off the foot. In this case, it helps to start with the little toe and stretch the sock over the big toe.

Removing underpants or trousers may be done while sitting or lying down. The child shifts his or her weight to push them over the hips and down the legs. To put underpants or trousers on, the child is flexed at the knees and hips. After the feet are in the correct holes, the child may stand up, kneel stand, or roll from side to side to pull them up.

Unlaced shoes may be kicked or rubbed off. Two colored laces may be used to encourage unlacing. When first putting shoes on the feet, the laces should be very loose. A flexed and abducted leg is necessary. A velcro closure simplifies this process. High-top shoes are easier to put on if loops are sewn on at the tops; these keep the back of the shoe from being crushed. Tying bows can be difficult to learn. When the child is ready for tying, the same words of instruction should be employed during each teaching session.

Many children seem to benefit from the backward-chaining method of instruction. The therapist ties the bow up to the last step and then asks the child to complete the process. As each step is mastered, the child continues working backwards until the entire process has been completed. It is important to follow the same process with each article of clothing.

Taking off pullover and front-opening shirts can be done in several ways. The usual way is to cross one's arms, grasp either side of the bottom, and pull the shirt up and over the head. One or both hands can be used to grasp the back of the collar and pull the shirt over the head. Children usually pull their nondominant arm out of the sleeve first. The dominant side sleeve is either shaken or pulled off by the other hand. Some children prefer to remove both arms from the sleeves, then pull the shirt off and over their heads. Another way to take off a shirt is to remove the nondominant arm from the sleeve and to pull the shirt over the head and off the opposite arm. Most methods can be used while lying supine or prone.

The process is reversed when a child puts a shirt on. The child's arms are put in first and then the shirt is pulled over the head, or vice versa. The more involved side goes in first, and the dominant arm in last. The "duck-the-head" method is helpful in putting on a front opening shirt or coat. The garment is positioned with the collar near the child, label side up. The arms are placed in the sleeves, and the whole shirt is tossed over the head.

Buttoning and unbuttoning should be learned on the child's own clothing or on a button vest (Fig. 36-5). Buttonboards are nonfunctional since they put the buttons in a position not related to the child's body.

Few clothing adaptations are necessary for individuals with cerebral palsy. Clothing should be loose fitting to facilitate putting on and removing. Velcro closures can be used if an individual's coordination is too poor

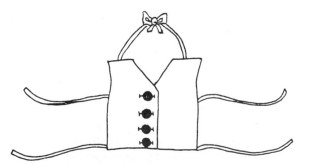

Figure 36-5. A button vest.

for handling buttons, zippers, or snaps. Sometimes, a buttonhook is helpful, and the addition of a large loop to a zipper may prove advantageous. Adolescents may need pants pushers or pullers. Trousers with elastic tops avoid waist-closure problems.

When older children are referred to occupational therapy for treatment, dressing is often something they need to learn. It often seems easier for a parent to dress a child than to take the time to teach the child how to do it. This may happen because parents have not been included in their children's treatment programs and do not know how to help. This exemplifies how essential it is for the occupational therapist to work with the parents.

Chair Adaptations

The basic principles of positioning and handling also apply to chair positioning. The child sits with the trunk straight, hips and knees flexed to beyond 90°, with the legs abducted. The ankles are at 90° and the feet are supported. The child's elbows rest comfortably on arm rests or lapboard. The occupational therapist needs to problem solve with the child and family to determine the most suitable seating device and if it is commercially available or needs to be custom made.

There are many seating devices available. A sturdy infant seat or car seat may be appropriate for a baby. A small child may use a regular stroller with or without adaptations. Specially designed inserts for strollers are available (Fig. 36-6). An older child or small adult may need a large stroller called a "Pogon buggy" with a specially designed insert. A care chair or travel chair may meet the needs of the child and the family. It has several positions that range from reclined to upright at table height. It folds to attach to a car seat and is used for safe transportation.

A wheelchair may be appropriate for some individuals. The same adaptations used in the stroller insert may provide proper fit in a wheelchair. Solid seat and back inserts keep the trunk straight and the shoulders forward. To increase trunk symmetry and midline orientation, long foam-padded wedges are added to the solid back. They are placed laterally and extend from under the arm to the waist or hip, fitting closely against the trunk.

The depth of the seat should come to an inch or two behind the child's knees to provide normal flexion. A pillow may be placed behind the child to push him or her forward to achieve this position. The seat upholstery may be removed and a specially made insert put in its place. This insert should be made to the child's dimensions and be of the proper depth to provide flexion for the knees. A firm wedge-shaped seat that is higher in the front than in the back may be used to increase hip flexion.

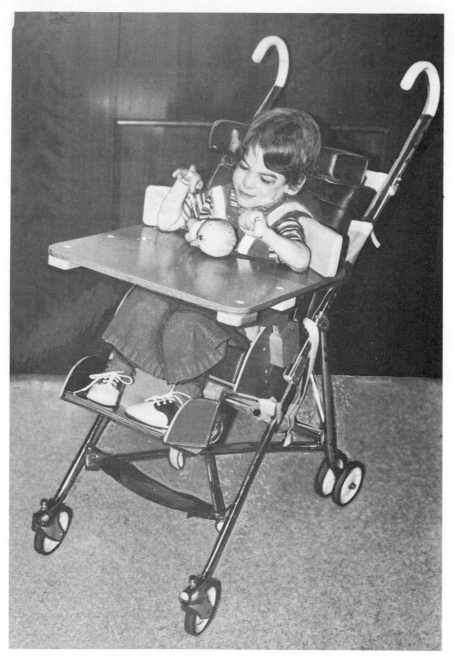

Figure 36-6. A stroller adapted with a specially designed insert.

To inhibit adduction of the legs, a molded seat insert may be made to fit the child. This insert places the pelvis in a neutral position, the hips in flexion, and the legs in abduction. It may have a built-in wedge shape. The back may incorporate lateral support wedges for the trunk. An individual with low muscle tone and excessive abduction may use a molded seat insert to provide more adduction of the hips and trunk control. A foot rest can be positioned so that the knees are slightly higher than the hips to decrease extensor tone. The entire sole of the foot should be supported to prevent extension (see Fig. 36-6).

A U-shaped head support is used for the child unable to hold his head up and in the midline. It is angled so that the center of the U is at the base of the skull. This elongates the neck extensor muscles. The side projections of the U are angled under the child's ears. This facilitates chin tuck as well as midline orientation.

A lapboard may be used to provide the individual with a stable surface on which to eat, play, and work (Fig. 36-7). It is positioned at elbow height for comfort and to assist external stability. For the baby and young child, a toy bar may be added. Objects may be hung directly in front of the child at a height which is easily accessible. The toys are always available to encourage reaching into space at the appropriate level for shoulder and back extension and eye–hand coordination. The

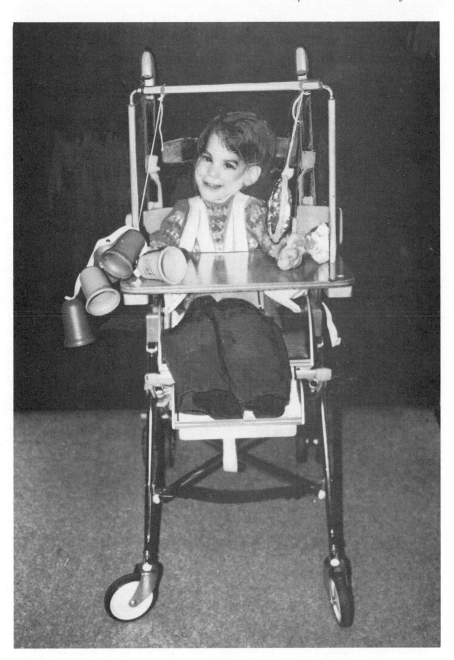

Figure 36-7. A lapboard and toy bar with suspended toys for ready access.

visually handicapped child will always have toys near him.

High chairs, commode or potty chairs, and other devices may be adapted using the same basic ideas.

A triangular chair provides good support for the individual with cerebral palsy. It rests on the floor, giving the child support while allowing him or her to experience the normal developmental activity of playing on the floor (see Fig. 36-3). The back of the chair comes to the child's shoulders to provide lateral and back support. The child's knees come to the edge of the seat to allow slight flexion while long sitting. The child is also able to circle sit in a triangular chair. Abductor wedges may be placed on the seat to inhibit adduction. A trian-

gular chair may also be raised on a platform and fitted with a small table. This gives back, side, and frontal support. The child's elbows rest comfortably on the table. One can sit in the chair to eat, play, or even complete schoolwork.

Communication

The basic human need to communicate one's joys, sorrows, needs, ideas, frustrations, anxieties, and sense of belonging may be thwarted in the cerebral palsied individual because he or she is unable to express himself or herself through the spoken word. The individual may be intelligent but too severely involved physically to talk or to control the head, trunk, and upper extremities. Oral control may be insufficient for speech. The occupational therapist, together with the speech therapist, can provide a means of nonverbal communication.

In the early stages of treating and handling the young infant, communication between mother and infant is stressed, just as it is with the normal child. Because of the added special needs of the infant with cerebral palsy, early communication skills are often overlooked. These skills usually begin with face-to-face contact between mother and infant. In order to gain and hold the infant's attention, good external control of the child's head and shoulders is necessary.

The occupational therapist should be sensitive to the subtle nonverbal messages that a child may give. Increased muscle tone may mean the child is upset, excited, or hurt; needs the bathroom; or wants attention. Darkness under the eyes may mean the child has a headache. Excessive drooling may mean the child is under emotional stress. Closing the eyes may mean the child is retreating from the environment.

For older children who still have not developed speech, alternate means of language expression are utilized. The simplest form of communication is indicating "yes" or "no" by moving a body part. This may be done by blinking the eyes, looking up, moving an arm or leg, or turning the head. Some intelligent children have learned to blink the Morse code in order to communicate.

The next level of communication for the nonverbal child may be the use of a language board or book. This may be a lapboard secured to a wheelchair or a book or card that is carried. A language board is covered with either Plexiglass or a clear plastic material to protect it from drooling and everyday wear. The child points to the board using fist, finger, elbow, eyes, paper straw, or headstick. A headstick may be fastened to a headband on the child's forehead.

Several types of boards are possible. A ring board has Plexiglass rings ⅝-inch to ½-inch thick. These are glued to the top of a Plexiglass board. Used to reduce involuntary movements, the rings can be large and spaced far apart or they can be small and spaced close together. The written insert is attached under the board. The writing shows through the rings. A ring board adapted for a headstick has smaller rings, about ¾-inch in diameter. These may be arranged like a typewriter keyboard or in a list form with phrases. The child points to the message with a headstick. Flat boards may list important words and phrases. The child points to the words or phrases in the appropriate column to convey the message.

A more sophisticated form of language board utilizes number and color coding of the words. Colors and numbers are spaced along the edges of the board. In the center, a color- and number-coded grid has many words

or phrases on it. The nonverbal child uses his or her eyes to point to an appropriate color first and then to a number. This locates a word on the grid to relay a message. Whole sentences, phrases, or individual words may be placed on the grid.

It is important that the material is positioned within the child's functional area of movement. Correct positioning maintains body symmetry and will not facilitate abnormal movement pattern.

The language board changes as the child's abilities develop. The first board may have objects on it, such as a toy toilet and small cup. The next board may have pictures on it. These may come from magazines or be familiar photographs or simple drawings. Pictures may depict needs such as the toilet, drink, food, bed, television, Mother, Father, places to go. As the child's reading skills develop, words replace pictures. Eventually, words may be arranged by parts of speech and increase in complexity. For some nonverbal individuals, an alphabet card and pointer may be sufficient to meet their communication needs. The letters may be arranged alphabetically or as on a typewriter keyboard.

Electronic aids are now available for the nonverbal individual. Three basic approaches with these aids are scanning, encoding, and direct selection. Scanning generally refers to the placing of appropriate phrases, letters, or symbols in a line or a grid configuration. The individual then controls a system that goes through each step until the desired message is completed. Encoding refers to a more complex system of controls in which a particular pattern of numbers or letters is used to relay a message. Usually, there is a series of activating switches. Direct selection refers to communication by direct input. An example would be a small calculator-type device that allows the individual to spell a word or message on the keyboard, which is then displayed on the device.

The rapid advances in the computer field have opened new ways of communication and learning for the cerebral palsied individual. Some devices actually talk for the person. Some allow him or her to draw electronically. Computers and electronic aids can be controlled using many different switches. A rocking lever may be activated by gross hand or arm movement or by a mouth- or headstick. A tongue switch may be activated by the tongue or lips. A pneumatic switch is activated by either blowing or sucking. A rocking level may be adapted to a chin switch. An arm slot control holds the arm on a desired switch without activating other ones. Some devices are activated by a beam of light.

Although electronic devices may help to meet many needs for the individual, the therapist is cautioned that they are not for everyone. The device and access switches must be specifically selected for the individual. An assistive devices center may facilitate the selection of an appropriate device.

References

1. Alexander R: Neurodevelopmental treatment: baby course. Unpublished class notes, 1980
2. Bayley N: Bayley Scales of Infant Development. New York, Psychological Corp, 1969
3. Berzins GF: Causes of cerebral palsy. Mimeographed handout, 1972
4. Bly L: Abnormal motor development: Blocks. Mimeographed, 1980
5. Bly L: Neurodevelopmental treatment: baby course. Unpublished class notes, 1980
6. Bly L: Normal motor development: The first twelve months. Mimeographed, 1980
7. Bobath K: The motor deficit in patients with cerebral palsy. Clin Dev Med No. 23, 1975
8. Bobath K, Bobath B: Cerebral palsy. In Pearson PH (ed): Physical Therapy Services in the Developmental Disabilities, pp 31, 33, 35, 36, 37. Springfield, Illinois, Charles C Thomas, 1972
9. Brazelton TB: Neonatal Behavior Assessment Scale. London, Spastics International Medical Publications, 1984
10. Colangelo C, Bergen A, Gottleib L: A Normal Baby: The Sensory–Motor Processes of the First Year, pp 5, 7. Valhalla, Blythedale Children's Hospital, 1976
11. Davis L: Pre-speech development. In Connor F, Williamson G, Siepp J (eds): A Program Guide for Infants and Toddlers with Neuromotor and Other Developmental Disabilities, pp 211–212. New York, Teachers' College Press, 1976
12. Fiorentino MR: Normal and Abnormal Development: The Influence of Primitive Reflexes on Motor Development, p 10. Springfield, Illinois, Charles C Thomas, 1972
13. Frankenburg WK, Dodds JB: Denver Developmental Screening Test, rev ed. Denver, La Doca Foundation, 1981
14. Gesell A, Halverson HM, Thompson H et al: The First Five Years of Life, p 23. New York, Harper & Row, 1940
15. Gordon N: Pediatric Neurology for the Clinician. Clin Develop Med No. 59/60, 1976
16. Jacobs MJ: Development of normal motor behavior. Am J Phys Med 46:41, 1967
17. Mohr J: Basic neurodevelopmental treatment course. Unpublished class notes, 1978
18. Morris SE: Pre-Speech Assessment Scale: A Rating Scale for the Measurement of Pre-Speech Behaviors from Birth Through Two years, revised ed. Milwaukee, Curative Rehabilitation Center, JA Preston, 1982
19. Mueller H: Facilitating feeding and pre-speech. In Pearson PH (ed): Physical Therapy Services in the Developmental Disabilities, p 287. Springfield, Illinois, Charles C Thomas, 1972
20. Nihira K, Foster R, Shellhaas M, Leland H: American Academy of Mental Deficiency Adaptive Behavior Scale, rev ed. Washington, DC, American Academy of Mental Deficiency, 1974
21. Rogers S, D'Eugenio D: Developmental Programming for Infants and Young Children: Assessment and Application. 2nd ed, vol 2, p 5. Ann Arbor, University of Michigan Press, 1981
22. Samilson RL (ed): Orthopaedic Aspects of Cerebral Palsy. Clin Dev Med No 52/53, 1975
23. Shepard T, Smith D: Prenatal life. In Smith D, Marshal R (eds): Introduction to Clinical Pediatrics. Philadelphia, WB Saunders, 1972

Bibliography

Apley J, Ounsted C (eds): One Child. London: Spastics International Medical Publications, 1982

Baird HW, Gordon EC: The Neurological Evaluation of Infants and Children. London, Spastics International Medical Publications, 1983

Bergen A: Selected Equipment for Pediatric Rehabilitation. Valhalla, Blythedale Children's Hospital, 1974

Bobath K: A Neurophysiologic Basis for the Treatment of Cerebral Palsy, 2nd ed. London: Spastics International Medical Publications, 1980

Braun M, Palmer M: Early Detection and Treatment of the Infant and Young Child with Neuromuscular Disorders. New York, Therapeutic Medica, 1983

Brazelton TB: Neonatal Behavioral Assessment Scale, 2nd ed. London, Spastics International Medical Publications, 1984

Carlsen PL: Comparison of two occupational therapy approaches for treating the young cerebral palsied child. Am J Occup Ther 29:267, 1975

Clark P, Allen A: Occupational Therapy for Children. St Louis, CV Mosby, 1985

Connor FP, Williamson GG, Siepp JM (eds): Program Guide for Infants and Toddlers with Neuromotor and Other Developmental Disabilities. New York, Teachers' College Press, 1978

Developmental disabilities: Current problems of early detection and management (clinical conference). Brain Dev 2:149, 1980

Drillien CM, Drummond M: Developmental Screening and the Child with Special Needs. London, Spastics International Medical Publications, 1984

Dubowitz L, Dubowitz V: The Neurological Assessment of the Preterm and Full-Term Newborn Infant. London, Spastics International Medical Publications, 1981

Dubowitz V: The Floppy Infant, 2nd ed. London, Spastics International Medical Publications, 1980

Erhardt R: Developmental Hand Dysfunction. Laurel, Maryland, Ramsco Publishing, 1982

Farber S: Neurorehabilitation: A Neurosensory Approach. Philadelphia, WB Saunders, 1982

Ferry PC, Banner W Jr, Wolf RA: Seizure Disorders in Children. Philadelphia, JB Lippincott, 1985

Fiorentino MR: Reflex Testing Methods for Evaluating C.N.S. Development. Springfield, Illinois, Charles C Thomas, 1979

Fiorentino MR: A Basis for Sensorimotor Development: Normal and Abnormal: The Influence of Primitive Postural Reflexes on the Development and Distribution of Tone. Springfield, Illinois, Charles C Thomas, 1981

Fulford FE, Brown JK: Position as a cause of deformity in children with cerebral palsy. Dev Med Child Neurol 18:305, 1976

King T: Plaster splinting as a means of reducing elbow flexor spasticity: A case study. Am J Occup Ther 36:671, 1982

Knobloch H: The Administration and Interpretation of the Revised Gesell and Amatruda Developmental and Neurologic Examination. Philadelphia, JB Lippincott, 1980

Knott GP: Attitudes and needs of parents of cerebral palsied children. Rehab Lit 40:190, 1979

Leiper CI, Miller A, Lang J, Herman R: Sensory feedback for head control in cerebral palsy. Physiotherapy, 61:512, 1981

Minde KK: Coping styles of 34 adolescents with cerebral palsy. Am J Psychiatr 135:1344, 1978

Morris SE: Pre-Speech Assessment Scale: A Rating Scale for the Measurement of Pre-Speech Behaviors from Birth Through Two Years, rev ed. Milwaukee, JA Preston, 1982

Morris SE: Program Guidelines for Children with Feeding Problems. Edison, New Jersey, Childcraft, 1977

Morris SE: The Normal Acquisition of Oral Feeding Skills: Implications for Assessment and Treatment, New York, Therapeutic Media, 1982

Scherzer A, Tscharnuter I: Early Diagnosis and Therapy in Cerebral Palsy: A Primer on Infant Developmental Problems. New York, Marcel Dekker, 1982

Slaton D (ed): Development of Movement in Infancy (Proceedings). Chapel Hill, University of North Carolina Division of Physical Therapy, 1981

Appreciation is extended to Joyce Perella, who contributed the section on oral reflexes.

CHAPTER 37

Occupational Therapy in the School System
Nancy Allen Kaufmann

The child's role as a student dominates a large percentage of time in the developmental years. The occupational therapist's task in this setting is to facilitate competencies that will help the child benefit from the total educational experience.

Private schools for the handicapped were the first educational programs to hire occupational therapists. By the early 1970s, therapists were being hired by public as well as private schools to evaluate and treat other children who previously had been excluded from public education; for example, the severely mentally retarded. By the 1980s, the behaviorally and emotionally disturbed were also included in some school therapists' caseloads, and more therapists worked with the moderately retarded or learning disabled and those with severe sensory impairments. By 1982, schools had become the second most common setting for employment of registered occupational therapists (OTR) and the third most common for certified occupational therapy assistants (COTA).[67]

A rapid expansion of occupational therapy services in schools was accompanied by a lack of uniformity of policy, problems of communication, and blurring of roles between educational, medical, and therapeutic personnel at state as well as local levels. In 1981, the American Occupational Therapy Association (AOTA)

conducted a comprehensive training program in every state to train occupational therapists to serve in educational settings.[24] In 1980, the Representative Assembly passed Standards of Practice for Occupational Therapy in Schools (see Appendix C), and, in 1981, prepared a position paper, The Role of Occupational Therapy as an Education-Related Service.[65] By the early 1980s, the World Federation of Occupational Therapists documented occupational therapists' growing involvement in educational settings abroad.[23]

By 1986, optional master's degree-level training for therapists interested in school employment became available because of the specialized skills and interdisciplinary practice required. The School System Task Force of the Council on Practice developed a document to help define the roles and responsibilities of the COTA in the public school setting and presented it for approval to the 1987 Representative Assembly.

To help with role delineation, attractive brochures were developed by the AOTA in the 1980s for therapists to distribute to parents and school personnel.[3,48] With the passage of federal legislation mandating appropriate personnel in every school district receiving federal funds, parent advocate groups became effective in creating occupational therapy positions in many states.

Legislation

In the early 1970s, there was a legislative trend at the state level initiating educational rights for the retarded and other handicapped persons. Section 504 of the Federal Rehabilitation Act of 1973 was intended to eliminate discrimination against handicapped citizens.

PL94-142

In 1975, the federal government responded further to state legislative changes, and President Gerald Ford signed into law the Education of the Handicapped Act, PL94-142. It required free and "appropriate" public education for all handicapped children including the learning disabled; speech, language, hearing, and vision impaired; or physically, mentally, or emotionally impaired. Education in its broadest sense was intended,[52] and many states implemented programs for children ages 3 to 21. The changes had a dramatic effect on occupational therapy that was specifically included as a "related service."

One emphasis of the law was the "mainstreaming" of as many handicapped children as possible into regular education classes, a concept commensurate with the normalization concept developed during the preceding decades. Normalization recommends conditions for the handicapped as close as feasible to the mainstream of society. The Cascade System (Fig. 37-1) is a theoretical prototype used in many states as a conceptual framework for providing educational services for the handicapped. Children are placed in "the least-restrictive alternative," or, in other words, the class that best fits their needs and is as close as possible to the everyday classroom. Also called the inverted pyramid, this system assumes the greatest number of handicapped children can be absorbed into mainstream education, thus allowing financial resources to be directed to the most handicapped. Ideally, support from counseling, educational, and therapeutic services is provided as needed to facilitate each transition, which is made as soon as educationally feasible.[49]

PL94-142 was amended in 1986 to include special education and related services to handicapped preschoolers, with emphasis on training family involvement in furthering the child's development (PL99-457). Grants were provided for programs for 3 to 5 year olds and helped establish new programs for disabled children from birth through age 2. Occupational therapy was identified as a primary early intervention service, independent of medical, health, and special education services.[42,51]

By the time 10-year anniversary celebrations of PL94-142 were held around the country during the 1985–1986 school year, 10.99% of the school population was receiving special education services. In keeping

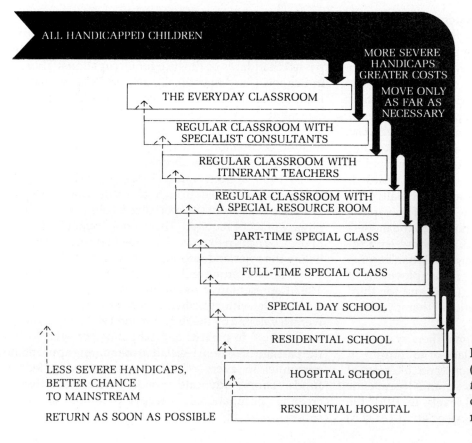

Figure 37-1. The Cascade System. (*One Out of Ten: School Planning for the Handicapped*, p 7, 1974. Courtesy of Educational Facilities Laboratories, New York.)

with the least-restrictive placement policy, 93% of these children were served in settings that included their non-handicapped peers.[50,63]

Due Process

Parents or guardians now have the legal right to examine all school records. They also participate with professionals in making educational placement decisions and in developing written diagnostic–prescriptive plans. These are called an Individualized Educational Program (IEP) for school-age children (must be revised annually) and an Individualized Family Service Plan (IFSP) for preschoolers (must be reviewed every 6 months). Parents may bring trained advocates to help them understand and protect the rights of their child at meetings of interdisciplinary teams that create these decisions and documents. They are entitled to due process of the law in safeguarding their child's rights. They may bring legal counsel and other professionals before an impartial Fair Hearing Officer of the state in order to question school decisions. Therapists must be prepared to present testimony at such a hearing and to be cross-examined by lawyers representing the parent and the school district (see box).

The law requires public participation in the development of educational policies, and occupational thera-

pists have presented testimony at state public hearings and federal House and Senate subcommittee hearings. They also participate in state task forces for determining the role of occupational therapists within school systems and in interagency coordinating councils of parents and providers of early intervention services for preschoolers.[54]

Additional Legislative and Judicial Changes

By 1981, many states had adopted statutes requiring an excess of the usual 180 school days if regression in skills following an extended vacation would be expected to be excessive, and recoupment or regaining of the lost abilities would be unduly slow, especially in self-care skills. Simultaneously, a movement was astir at the federal level to consider reducing the mandate for provision of related services to an optional status. Block grants were being considered, a policy in which large sums of federal money with few restrictions would be provided to state and/or more local educational administration. Since priorities would be established at state or local levels, some occupational therapists were apprehensive.

In June 1982, the Supreme Court ruled in one deaf student's case that local school districts were not obliged to provide all services that handicapped children need in order to reach their full academic potential. While they must provide free appropriate public education that "benefits" the handicapped child, no particular level of education was required.[26,53]

With assistance from the AOTA Government and Legal Affairs Division, the US Department of Education in 1985 initiated a 3-year survey to investigate the cost of providing special education and related services and to provide a basis for important policy decisions affecting occupational therapy and other related services.[45]

By the late 1980s, some states had developed new legislation in response to child sexual abuse cases involving a few adults working in day care centers and other programs for children. As a precautionary measure, these states required persons applying for positions in public and private schools to undergo criminal history checks.

Team Approach

Position of Occupational Therapy

It is important to understand the role of the occupational therapist within the particular local school system by first studying the state and local hierarchy of administration and service delivery. Does the therapist fit into the health chain of command or that of education? How

---

Tips to Help Reduce Anxiety in Preparing Testimony for a Due Process Hearing

Rely on the high standards of documentation you have maintained. They will help prove your testimony.

Organize your testimony carefully. Include treatment goals, objectives, and progress measured by pre- and post-testing.

Informally review your testimony with a co-professional who has testified or with a due process lawyer.

Read Bateman[9] or other introductory due process information.

Have in hand records that might help you document answers to questions posed during cross-examination.

Project confidence and self-assurance but not presumptuousness.

Use clear communication without therapy jargon. State observations and behaviors, not hypotheses (about causes of deficits).

Answer questions as asked by the lawyers. Do not say more than you are asked.

are therapy services provided locally and statewide? Are local parents strong advocates in favor of occupational therapy?

The occupational therapist functions often as a member of the local school system interdisciplinary committee, which makes decisions about placement of children in programs at various levels of the Cascade. These decisions are based on such things as developmental level, adaptive ability, academic performance, social maturity, and behavior, in addition to intelligence quotient (IQ). The primary cause of the child's learning problem determines placement; if a secondary problem, such as emotional overlay, has developed, appropriate education emphasizing treatment of the primary problem often eliminates it.

Gilfoyle emphasizes the importance of knowing how to participate effectively in the group decision-making process.[24] Communication skills should enhance understanding by other members of the team, and jargon specific to occupational therapy should be avoided so the team members receiving the information can process it.[24] Hypotheses regarding causes of deficits in observable behavior should be clearly stated as such.[14] It is important for therapists to become familiar with tests frequently used by each team member in order to better interpret results. A task analysis, after observing pertinent tests being administered, is one effective method.

The role of members who usually serve on the interdisciplinary committee within school systems will be described later. Others who may serve as committee members or who may provide consultation are medical, neurological, psychiatric, and optometric personnel. Important team members who do not serve on interdisciplinary committees are teachers of art, music, and physical education. These teachers may have been specially trained to work with handicapped children. The child, classroom aide, and volunteer also play important roles in the team effort of teaching the handicapped child.

The COTA carries out treatment programs under the supervision of the OTR. Although the school principal may be responsible for *administrative* supervision of the COTA (payroll, vacations, working hours), an OTR provides *professional* supervision (caseload determination, daily schedule, treatment activities).[66]

Interdisciplinary Team Members

Members of the interdisciplinary committee assist in formulating decisions on appropriate placement and educational programming for children:

School Principal or Program Director: These committee members interpret local administrative policies in special education.

Counselor: The counselor brings to the interdisciplinary committee awareness of both the child's family milieu and a variety of placement services within the community and the school system.

Parent: The parent, as the primary care-giver for the child, helps set goals commensurate with family expectations. Parents, with the help of their trained advocate or lawyer, may initiate suggestions regarding educational placement and programming or, through team meetings, may be better prepared to give informed consent. Under the 1986 amendment regarding preschool services (PL99-457), the family's strengths and needs are a major consideration in establishing intervention strategies, which may include parental training and counseling.[42]

Psychologist: The psychologist reports mental age or IQ scores, cognitive and adaptive functioning, and sometimes social and emotional information resulting from projective tests. Consideration of scores and quality of performance on tests and subtests given by the psychologist may give diagnostic information that can reduce the amount of time spent in evaluation by the therapist. Figure 37-2 and the accompanying box provide information to help with interpretation of subtest scores from two psychological tests. A breakdown of subtest scores may have to be specifically requested.

Educational Evaluator: This specially trained teacher reports results of standardized or criterion-referenced tests of academic, developmental, and readiness levels in number concepts as well as the sequence of listening, speaking, reading, and, finally, writing. The evaluator also makes observations about the child's learning style that may differ widely from the child's strengths and weaknesses in tactile, kinesthetic, visual, or auditory modalities. For example, the child may score low in tests of auditory processing but may learn to read better through listening than looking tasks.[46] The diagnostician may report on perceptual, language, and motor performance if they are not tested by other services.

Special Education Teacher: Next to the parent, the teacher probably has the most consistent contact with the handicapped child. This teacher makes recommendations about everyday social maturity and behavior as well as academic, perceptual, and language performance of children in the classroom. The resource room teacher sees mildly handicapped children for a portion of each day to work on specific deficit areas.

Physical Therapist: The physical therapist reports on quality of movement, reflex development, equilibrium reaction, gait, and gross motor development.

Speech and Language Clinician: This member of the interdisciplinary committee reports test results of the child's receptive language (comprehension or decoding of what is heard) and expressive language

THE TESTS	Spatial	Quantitative	Sequencing	Perceptual organization	Conceptualization and verbal comprehension	Ability to concentrate: Distractibility	Visual motor integration: Fine motor	Verbal expression
● VERBAL SCALE Information					✓			✓
Similarities					✓			✓
Arithmetic		✓			✓	✓		
Vocabulary					✓			✓
Comprehension					✓			✓
Digit Span		✓	✓			✓		
● PERFORMANCE SCALE Picture Completion	✓					✓		
Picture Arrangement			✓		✓			
Block Design	✓			✓				
Object Assembly	✓			✓			✓	
Coding	✓		✓				✓	
Mazes	✓						✓	

Figure 37-2. Content of test items of the Wechsler Intelligence Scale for Children (WISC-R). (Modified from Waugh KW, Bush WJ: *Diagnosing Learning Disorders.* Columbus, Charles Merrill, 1971.)

(encoding through the use of linguistic symbols). For both expressive and receptive language, consideration is given to the child's use of sounds (phonology), meaning (semantics or vocabulary and concepts), and grammar (syntax and morphology). Integration (inner associative language processing such as categorization and understanding of analogies) is also considered, as well as retention (memory) and such perceptual problems as auditory discrimination and speed of verbal response.

Occupational Therapist: The occupational therapist reports the quality and level of functioning of the child in the developmental areas evaluated. Consideration is also given to architectural planning, positioning for seatwork, assistive devices for eating and writing, and work-related programming (even from the earliest grade-school years). Service delivery may be provided through direct, hands-on intervention. However, an evaluation and treatment model that can be integrated right into the home and classroom environments (rather than the isolated once-a-week model in the artificial therapy environ-

ment) is recommended by Sternat and associates, particularly for the severely handicapped or preschool student.[62]

The therapist and teaching members of the team may provide itinerant services to numerous schools or, particularly in the case of preschoolers, to homes. There, occupational therapists either screen and treat children, or suggest to regular teachers academic intervention methods for mildly impaired children, or work with parents or special education teachers who carry out home or classroom programs.

Team members should make every effort to maintain close professional involvement with parents through telephone or personal contact, written test results or progress notes, and team meetings. Parents may appreciate guidance toward reading publications such as "The Exceptional Parent" magazine[56] and books written for parents, or joining such national organizations as the Association for Children with Learning Disabilities (ACLD), Association of Retarded Citizens (ARC), and Council of Exceptional Children (CEC) (see Glossary).

Subtests of the Kauffman Assessment Battery for Children (K-ABC)

Intellectual Functioning

Sequential Processing Scale

Hand movements .... Copying a movement series

Number recall .... Digit repetition

Work order .... Touching objects in sequence named

Simultaneous Processing Scale

Magic window .... Identifying picture moving behind screen

Face recognition .... Selecting from group photograph

Gestalt closure .... Naming partially completed inkblot drawing

Triangles .... Assembling to match pattern

Matrix analogies .... Completing visual analogies

Spatial memory .... Recalling picture placement

Photo series .... Sequencing photographs

Acquired Knowledge

Achievement Scale

Expressive vocabulary .... Naming object photograph

Faces & places .... Recognizing and naming pictures

Arithmetic .... School math abilities

Riddles .... Inferring concept when told its characteristics

Reading/decoding .... Recognizing letters and words

Reading/understanding .... Following commands

(Modified from American Guidance Service: *Important Advances in Individually Administered Measures of Intelligence, Achievement and Adaptive Behavior.* Circle Pines, MN, 1985.)

Assessment

Evaluation of handicapped school children provides the basis for planning treatment and, in some cases, identifies which children need special help. Children with severe handicaps tend to be placed in appropriate programs at an early age, but for others, the need for special education is not readily apparent.

The goal of screening is to identify children who need help without interfering in the lives of those who have only a mild and temporary developmental delay. Screening during the preschool years may allow early detection of children with attention-deficit disorder, mild mental retardation, or mild emotional disturbances. Early home programming, special class placement, or special help within the mainstream classroom helps prevent development of a secondary emotional overlay resulting from learning failure in later grades. It also provides intervention procedures at a critical time in the child's life when they will be most helpful. Preparing the child to succeed in a mainstream classroom at the earliest opportunity is currently considered most desirable.

In many school districts, preschool children are screened by age 3 based on referrals from parents, phy-

sicians, and community agencies. New school programs for even younger children are developing.

Thorough reviews of screening methods and tests for this age group are presented by Stangler and associates,[60] Lerner and coworkers,[38] and the Educational Staff of Chapel Hill.[21] The beginning therapist may wish to screen children with mild handicaps using the *Pre-School Screening System*[27] or the *Learning Accomplishment Profile.*[55]

Mildly impaired children having only subtle problems are difficult to identify before kindergarten. Occupational therapists, along with educators, language specialists, and medical personnel, may play a key role in district-wide and local school methods for finding such children and planning suitable programs for them. Several examples of group screening procedures will be discussed.

In one school district, teachers identified young children with suspected problems by color-coded name tags as occupational therapists led the whole class through informal screening tasks. The therapists observed especially carefully the children whose colored tag suggested the likelihood and severity of subtle problems in motor skills, perception, or sensory-based poor behavior. Classroom recommendations for training of problem children were made, and a small percentage of children was recommended for further standardized testing.

Another school district sent a team of medical and educational personnel to individually observe and screen a few problem children identified by each teacher. Recommendations were made to the teacher and parents for managing the specific educational and behavioral problems. Later, the team returned and used additional test measures for the one or two children who, in spite of several months of maturation and special teaching techniques, still had the greatest problems.

Volunteers were used in Fort Worth Public Schools to assist professionals in testing children using a locally developed screening instrument.[34]

The School District of Philadelphia developed a learning disabilities checklist to be marked by classroom teachers for each of their kindergarten or first-grade students.[64] It eliminated the need for screening by specialists. Although the attempt was made to write items observable during normal classroom activities, many teachers resisted the extra burden of evaluation. Such a checklist could be used for parent observation or for school use where teachers have been trained and motivated. The checklist, typical of many developed around the country, did serve one of its purposes: to familiarize teachers with behavioral and performance characteristics of young children with subtle learning problems. Easily understood phrases were checked as occurring frequently or seldom and cover these topics:

Behavior: Items in this section cover hyperactivity; distractibility and impulsiveness; overreaction to change, excitement or unexpected touch, sounds or smells; hypoactivity; focusing on irrelevant details; difficulty completing tasks; perseveration; inconsistent academic performance; and difficulty with peer relations.

Motor coordination: These items test for placing two feet per tread when climbing or descending stairs; clumsiness or awkwardness in moving or catching a ball; inability to hop three times or skip; difficulty copying pantomimed body positions especially when crossing the midline; difficulty touching the tip of the nose with the little finger with the eyes closed; inability or awkwardness in bead stringing, coloring, pasting, buttoning, cutting, or holding a pencil.

Orientation: Items tested are body image; drawing a person; underreaching or overreaching for objects or colliding with people or things; environmental disorientation; confusion of directional words such as up and before; inappropriate placement or size of drawings or writing on paper; and difficulty understanding schedules and elementary time concepts.

Visual motor integration: These include difficulty matching symbols or pictures and recognizing a figure when only fragments are presented; difficulty with puzzles or connecting dot patterns; switching of hand use while cutting, throwing, drawing, or eating; and inability to copy correctly a circle, cross, square, or X.

Language: These items test for poor auditory figure ground and discrimination; inability to categorize or classify objects ("mistakenly groups large with small, round with flat, toys with clothing, etc."); inability to reproduce simple sound rhythms; poor auditory sequencing of three spoken simple directions; inability to repeat the sequence of three words or numbers and to easily and rapidly recall words or names of familiar items (note: a combination of poor rote auditory memory plus difficulty with word calling in a child often means the child will need long-term special education services); avoidance of spoken language; inability to rhyme; difficulty communicating events sequentially or in complete sentences.

Using the Child Development Chart (Table 37-1), a therapist can quickly determine the normal age at which children acquire commonly tested abilities. The chart reads developmentally from the top to the bottom. It also reads across from left to right, as some developmental sequences on the right side of the chart may be interrupted because of deficits in developmental sequences on the left side. For example, equilibrium (in the fourth column) may not be developing properly because of poorly inhibited reflexes (first column). Body scheme and eye–hand coordination (columns three and seven) may be negatively affected by poor sensory development, which appears in an earlier column. Inadequate development of language (the last column) in some cases is a reflection of poorly integrated visual percepts or sensory information. The use of the chart is intended to promote continual awareness in the mind of the therapist of all the goals established for each child and their interrelationship. Also, the chart can be helpful in talking with parents, recommending developmental activities, or making general judgments about children's performance levels.

Following the use of such screening methods as those described above, or on the direct referral of educational or medical personnel, therapists will further evaluate children showing evidence of dysfunction. They may use informal functional assessments based largely on clinical impressions; or they may use standardized tests, which compare a child's performance with that of many other children. Standardized test administration methods must be followed exactly and may require special training, as for example the Sensory Integration and Praxis Tests.[6]

In addition to clinical impressions and standardized

(text continues on page 720)

Table 37-1. Child Development Chart

	General Reflex Development	Sensory Development	Body Scheme	Equilibrium
	Items closer to top of each column suggest remedial sequences for problems observed closer to bottom of column. Items in left hand columns suggest possible causes of problems in certain columns further to the right.			
0–3 mo.	• 0–2 mo. Phasic/movement spinal cord reflexes predominate. Limbs coordinated in total flexion or extension • 0–6 mo. Static, brain-stem-mediated reflexes are present. Stimulation of labyrinths or neck muscle feedback changes distribution of muscle tone throughout body	• 1–4 wk. Infant differentiates: tactile (touch, pressure) temp. (hot, cold) taste (sweet, sour, salty, bitter) vision (see vis. percept. column) • Infant also experiences vestibular input, internal chemical changes, audition	• 1 mo. Mass motor activity reaction to stimuli • 3 mo. Plays regarding hands	• 2 mo. Prone, head and chest up to 45° recurrently • Head bobs when sitting, back rounded
3 mo. to 1 yr.	• 4–15 mo. Midbrain-mediated reactions in all-fours position help child right self, turn over, assume crawl & sit positions. Maximum concerted effort 10–12 mo. • 6 mo. Equilibrium reactions under cortical control begin to gradually modify, inhibit, & dominate righting reactions if muscle tone is normal. Results in standing, walking, well-coordinated person	• 3 mo. Tickle reaction.	• 4–6 mo. Plays with hands and feet in supine. Hands come together in play • 5–6 mo. Pats mirror image • 7–8 mo. Plays peek-a-boo	• 3 mo. Prone, supports weight on forearms • 5 mo. Pull to sit. No head lag • 6–8 mo. Sit, head erect • 7–9 mo. 4-point kneel; rocks back and forth
1–2 yr.			• 12–18 mo. Points to 2 of own body parts	• 12–13 mo. Kneel/stands • 14 mo. Stands • 14–18 mo. Walks; feet wide apart, arms in primary blance role usually at or above shoulder height. • 17 mo. Stoops to pick up toy without losing balance

714

Age norms are approximate. Authors vary. Children vary. Development does not really occur in separate rows and columns. All parts of the nervous system influence each other.

Bilateral Integration	Visual Perception	Eye-Hand Coordination	Language
• 1–4 wk. Asymmetrical postures predominate • 2 mo. Supine, child can hold head in midline & extremities symmetrical • 2 mo. Eyes begin to follow past midline	• 3–4 wk. At 10" discriminates ⅛" stripes from plain surface • 1–2 mo. Discriminates stylized face from oval pattern. Also color • 2 mo. Visual size & near distance constancy developing. Unable to apply them simultaneously • 2 mo. Recognize visual cliff.	• 0–4 wk. Reflexive grasp. No eye–hand coordination. Touch tells when to grasp • 1–4½ mo. Fixates on light monocularly • 2 mo. Prone, head and chest up for forward vision • 3 mo. Eye follows across midline and past 90° • 3 mo. Plays regarding hands	• 1 mo. Responds to sound. Undifferentiated crying • 2 mo. Single vowel sounds, coos • 3 mo. Vocalizes pleasure in response to social stimuli. Vocal noises resemble speech • 2 mo. Discriminates intonations and 2 voices
• 4–6 mo. Hands together in play • 6 mo. Symmetrical arm use & postures predominate • 7 mo. Transfers toy 1 hand to the other. Hands cross midline • 7–8 mo. Creeps amphibian; tactile stim. to abdomen • 7–8 mo. Bunny hops • 7–9 mo. 4-point crawl; homolateral then heterolateral	• 6–7 mo. Discriminates + ○ □ △. 3-dimensional discrim. easier than 2-dimensional • 8–24 mo. Convergence to 2" from nose. Divergence to 20". Primitive depth perception • 9 mo. Recognizes danger of visual cliff	• 4 mo. Rotates head to inspect surroundings • 4–6 mo. Visually pursues lost toy • 6 mo. Eye–hand coord. begins • 6 mo. Palmar grasp • 10 mo. Crude release. Pokes finger in holes	• 3 mo. Chuckles • 4 mo. Turns to noise & voice • 6 mo. Distinguishes angry–friendly voices • 6 mo. Intonational jargon • 9 mo. Comprehends a few gestures, intonations, "no-no," "hot." Echolalia • 10 mo. Word-like syllables: ma-ma-ma, da-da-da. Comprehends & waves bye-bye
• 11–12 mo. Cruises sideways, holding furniture • Creeps up stairs • 15 mo. Creeps down stairs	• 15 mo. Looks selectively at pictures in book • 21 mo. Aligns 3 blocks for train • Object permanence	• Imitates scribble • 12 mo. Neat pincer grasp. Supinated grasp developing, wrist extended • 13 mo. Good release • Tower of 2 cubes • 15 mo. Places objects into & out of containers • Spontaneous scribble • 18 mo. Turns pages, 2 or 3 at a time • Uses spoon, cup well • 21 mo. Puts large pegs in pegboard	• 12 mo. First word, usually noun • Action response to commands • 1–5 word vocabulary • 1-word sentences • Can mentally perform behavior before physically performing • Produces all vowel sounds • 1½ yr. Extension of word meanings; overgeneralizations • 50-word vocabulary, mostly nouns

(continued)

715

Table 37-1. *Child Development Chart*   *(continued)*

	General Reflex Development	Sensory Development	Body Scheme	Equilibrium
2 yr.			• Identifies 2 body parts from picture • Touches tummy, cheek, arm, leg, mouth, hair	• Up & down stairs independently, 2 steps per tread holding on • 2½ yr. Jumps, 2-foot take off. Tiptoes briefly • Runs. Walks sideways & backwards • Kicks ball on request
3 yr.		• Vision occluded, matches grossly different textures, *e.g.,* sandpaper & satin	• Knows front, back, side of self. Also chin, neck, forearm	• Jumps from 12″ height, feet together or 1 foot lead • Upstairs 1 foot per tread, no support Down 2 steps per tread, no support • Hops 1 foot 2, 3 times • Climbs 3 rungs • Squats • 3½ yr. Tandem walks 10 ft
4 yr.		• Names heavier of 2 weights • Discriminates different scents • Compares different textures; *e.g,* soft, smooth	• Draws man with head and legs	• Stands on 1 foot 4 sec. Broad jumps . . . • standing—8–10″ • running—23–33″

Bilateral Integration	Visual Perception	Eye-Hand Coordination	Language
• Rhythmical bounce, sway, nod, swings arms	• Enjoys watching moving objects • Simultaneous visual size & distance constancy developing • 20/70 visual acuity • Points to pictures of familiar objects • 2½ yr. Adds chimney to 3-cube train ⌑ • Begins matching colors	• Hand preference beginning • Tower of 6–7 cubes • Strings large beads • Throws • Imitates / • 2½ yr. Imitates —, ○ • Copies / • Pours well, glass to glass	• 2-word sentences that are functionally complete • Imitates absent models; pretends; reconstructs memories • Knows "in" and "under" • Knows "I," "you," "me," "mine" • 2½ yr. Telegraphic speech • 3-word sentences
• Walks swinging arm with opposite leg, arms free of shoulder ht. balance position • Pedals tricycle • Weight shift in throwing. No step into	• Tends to react to entire stimulus rather than label separate parts, especially if unfamiliar • Picks longer line 3 of 3 times • Imitates cube bridge ⌒ • 3½ yr. Recognizes 2 colors named	• 10 pellets into bottle in 30 sec. • Tower of 9–10 cubes • Copies —, ○ • Simian pencil grasp (fist clenched) • Turns doorknob, forearm rotation • Unbuttons accessible buttons • May shift handedness • Catches large ball, arms extended • 3½ yr. Imitates X	• Has adult grammatical structure. Complete simple active sentences • Uses sentences to tell understandable stories • 3½ yr. Speech disfluency • "Why" questions • Names 1 color
• Runs with good arm–leg coordination • Up and down stairs 1 foot per tread • Gallops • 4½ yr. Skips, 1 foot only (lame duck skip)	• With increasing age child tends to differentiate stimuli in environment, esp. when specific language labels applied to them • Slow down of rapid visual acuity development since birth • Matches shapes (same color and size) • Can find simple familiar overlapping outline figures • Builds 6-block pyramid • 4½ yr. Copies gate ⌂	• Follows moving object smoothly with eyes ↔ ↕ ↘ ↗ ↺ • Copies + • Imitates □ • 10 pellets into bottle in 25 sec. • Bounces ball awkwardly • Tries to cut on straight line	• Transforms kernel sentences • 4-word sentences, some complex or compound • Intuitive thought begins, less concreteness • Little word analysis; deals with whole sentences • Counts 3 objects, though imperfectly • Uses slang • Understands syntax, grammatical contrasts beyond production ability • Repeats 3 digits • 4½ yr. Names primary colors • 4½ yr. Perceives differences in concrete events

(continued)

Table 37-1. *Child Development Chart* (continued)

	General Reflex Development	Sensory Development	Body Scheme	Equilibrium
5 yr.	• Primitive reflexes inhibited or dominated. In supine & all-fours child can turn head side-to-side, up, down without elbows, shoulders, or knees changing angle • Can flex in supine & extend in prone positions for 10 sec. • Sits and stands symmetrically from supine with only slight body rotation	Vision occluded . . . • discriminates ○□☆ blocks (stereognosis) • points to touched finger 1/2 times • points to within 3″ of stimulus spot on arm • points to hand &/or cheek touched singly or simultaneously	• Copies Simon Says postures • Draws 6-part unmistakable man with body • Points front, back, near, up, down, with eyes closed • Can clench and bare teeth • Aware of, but confuses left and right • In pictures identifies object that is beside, between, in middle, in front of	• Down stairs, alternating feet, no support • Stands 1 foot 6–8 sec. • Balances on tiptoe, 1/3 trials • Running broad jump 28–35″ • Jumps 10″ high hurdle • Begins balance beam backwards • Tries roller skates, jump rope, stilts
6 yr.				• Jumps over rope 20 cm. high • Standing broad jump 3 ft.
7 yr.	• Arises from supine to standing in 1–1.5 sec.	• Vision occluded, can reproduce - ✕ ○ drawn on back of hand 1/2 trials	• Good jumping jacks • Can knit eyebrows • 7½ yr. Stabilizes arms and trunk against much resistance • Knows left and right on self	• Stands on 1 foot, eyes closed, 3 seconds • Can hop and jump accurately into small squares • Walks 2″ wide balance beam
8 yr.			• Eyes closed, points right & left • Can wrinkle forehead	• Crouches on tiptoes without falling 1/3 trials
9 yr.			• 9½ yr. Discriminates left & right on facing person	• Runs 16–17 ft./sec. • Jumps over rope 15″ high 2/3 trials • Jump, clapping hands 3 times, 1/3 trials

Bilateral Integration	Visual Perception	Eye-Hand Coordination	Language
• Mimics pointing to ipsi- or contralateral ear or eye 2/3 trials • Can reproduce simple rhythmic clapping • Marches in time to music	• 20/30 visual acuity • Difficulty with orientation. Can detect ↕ reversals easier than ↔ reversals after instruction • Difficulty performing closure necessary to distinguish incomplete ○ □ ▭ • Simultaneous size constancy & form discrim. developing • Imitates 10-block pyramid • 5½ yr. Begins to mentally rotate simple shapes for solving puzzles	• Tripod pencil grip Begins flex IP joint • Copies / □ \ × • Imitates △ • Sequential finger opposition (1, 2, 3, 4) with visual regard and minor associative movements. Slow • Throws 16″ playground ball 10–11 feet. Catches bounced large playground ball	• Embeds phrases, clauses in sentences • Develops percepts of number, speed, time, space • Inner logic & imaginative thinking • Categorizes by likeness & difference • Marked increase in vocab. comprehension (not use) • Repeats 4 digits • 5½ yr. mean length of response = 4.9 words
• Skips alternately • Throws stepping with foot opposite throwing arm	• Begins to identify imbedded familiar outline figures • Recalls 3½ of the 9 Bender Gestalt figures • May still reverse some letters or numbers	• Copies △ ✳ • Ties shoelaces • 6½ yr. Hand dominance established	• Command every form of sentence structure • Mean sentence length rapidly increasing; now 6.5 words • Asks for and attempts to verbalize explanations, causal relationships
• Can tap floor alternately with feet	• 20/20 visual acuity • b-d, p-q confusions resolved • Builds 6-block pyramid from memory	• Grips pencil tightly, often close to tip. Pressure may be heavy • Good sequential finger opposition (1, 2, 3, 4) • Drops 20 coins, one at a time, into open box in 16 sec. • Accurately taps swinging suspended ball 2/5 tries • 7½ yr. Copies ◇ ◇	• Good speech melody & facial/hand gestures • Good inner language • True communication; shares ideas • Mean length of response = 7.2 words • Repeats 5 digits • 80% know comparative relationships (*e.g.*, bigger than)
• Good 2–2, 2–1, 1–2 hop • Can run into moving jump rope but cannot alter step	• Identifies heavily embedded familiar figures • Notices and labels component parts of stimulus more than does younger child • Capable of attending to both whole and part	• Laces 8 beads in 20 sec. • Places 10 pairs of matchsticks in box in 16 sec.	• Skilled use of grammatical rules • Acceptable articulation
	• Closure figure recognized and seen as incomplete • Notices wholes & parts simultaneously in figures composed of familiar objects		• 80% know passive relationships (*e.g.*, person was hit by) • 75% know familial relationships (*e.g.*, "your mother's father")

(continued)

Table 37-1. *Child Development Chart* (continued)

General Reflex Development	Sensory Development	Body Scheme	Equilibrium
10–12 yr.			• 10 yr. Hops 50 ft. on 1 foot in 5–6 sec. • 11 yr. Standing broad jump 4½–5 ft. • 12 yr. Standing high jump 3 ft.

Developed from Ayres, Banus, Beery, Berry, Bobath, Cattell, Colarusso & Hammill, Cratty, Dale, Denhoff, Erhardt, Fantz, Fiorentino, Frostig, Gardner, Gesell & Armatruda, Gilfoyle & Grady, Gibson, Hull & Hull, Kephart, Llorens, Miller, Moore, Norton, Oseretsky, Pearlson, Piaget, Wiig & Semel.

tests, the therapist may use criterion-referenced tests, some of which have instructional activities suggested to remediate each test item or section in which the child needs additional help. Criterion-referenced tests, now widely used to establish goals and objectives, evaluate performance on specifically described skills or knowledge without comparisons between individuals as in standardized testing. Skills are arranged in a sequence at the discretion of the test author, and an attempt is usually made to list skills in the order in which they are normally acquired. Specific skills on the test that have not yet been acquired are trained, and the criterion of the test is 100% mastery.[25] One example of a criterion-referenced test is the *Learning Accomplishment Profile.*[55]

Other chapters in this textbook suggest appropriate assessment tools for various types of handicaps found in the school-age population. They describe methods of testing range of motion, muscle strength, sensation, motor skills, sensory integration, cognition, developmental reflexes and reactions, eating, writing, activities of daily living, and prevocational and vocational skills. In addition, assessments are included for cerebral palsy (Chapter 36) and hand rehabilitation (Chapter 31). Lerner and associates[38] and Gilfoyle[24] give thorough annotated bibliographies of published screening and evaluation tools for children.

Lists of tests for screening and evaluating learning-impaired children are available from federally funded area learning resource centers and local centers, sometimes called Special Educational Instructional Materials Centers (SEIMC). These centers, in many locations around the country, also have samples and lists of educational curriculum materials. *The Mental Measurements Yearbook*, edited by the director of the Buros Institute of Mental Measurements,[43] and published every several years, is an important reference book that groups tests by topic and that includes several critiques of each one by authorities in the field.

When screening and testing children, constellations in the results of all testing must be considered rather than single low scores. Even normal children may fail in some aspect of motor, sensory, or psychosocial functioning. Plan goals and make recommendations that are relevant to the presenting educational problem,[14] because providing therapy to improve an irrelevant area in which the child happens to score low is not the goal. All the testing methods described are only as valuable as the program planning that results.

Program Planning and Documentation

Planning

After using assessment procedures such as those just described, the occupational therapist documents the test results in writing, including all the areas outlined in the AOTA "Uniform Occupational Therapy Evaluation Checklist" (see Appendix F). Information related to the client's personal data and history as well as the referral are included. The checklist also urges therapists to include skill/performance in independent living, sensorimotor areas, cognition, psychosocial areas, therapeutic adaptation, and prevention (see Uniform Occupational Therapy Evaluation Checklist[2] for details of subcategories). In addition to this initial evaluation report, the therapist keeps daily progress records of treatment programs and of recommendations made to teachers, administrators, parents, or volunteers. Once or twice a year, therapists send descriptive reports home and write formal progress notes that are added to the child's school records.

When planning a program, the occupational therapist considers all areas assessed that might be pertinent to quality of performance in the educational environ-

Bilateral Integration	Visual Perception	Eye-Hand Coordination	Language
	• 11 yr & above. Recalls 5½–6 of the 9 Bender Gestalt figures	• 10 yr. Draws 3-dimensional geometric figures:	
		• 10 yr. Judges & intercepts pathways of small balls thrown from a distance	
		• 12 yr. Linear perspective seen in drawings	
		• Anticipates locomotor & manual responses to rapidly moving objects; *e.g.*, where to catch ball whose complete trajectory is not observable	

ment. Specific documentation of planned treatment is now required by law, although school personnel are not held accountable for children's progress.

Often, the therapist is required to write a portion of the student's IEP (or IFSP for preschoolers). These include a statement of present educational levels, annual or semiannual long-term goals (a general statement of treatment intent), and short-term objectives. The latter are written in behaviorally observable (not theoretical) terms and include the conditions under which they will take place, terminal behavior, a measurable criterion level, and expected completion date[69] (see IEP, Fig. 37-3).

Figures 37-4 and 37-5, adapted from Llorens and Seig,[39] show a method of organizing treatment goals for whole classes or small groups of young children. Such an evaluation record provides a visual chart of assets and deficits. The therapist administers only those evaluation procedures most suitable to the age and capability of the child. Whereas one inadequate score within a particular heading is usually insignificant, clusters of low scores suggest treatment goals. Individual subtests cannot be considered separate entities, and caution should be used in determining the importance of any one subtest score, but listing them on such an evaluation record helps point out clusters of low scores.

Test results of 5½-year-old Richard, a student with attention-deficit disorder, are recorded in Figure 37-4 as an example of the use of this evaluation record. A diagnostic–prescriptive program for improving motor and perceptual functioning might be correlated as follows: through sensory-integrative techniques, the therapist or occupational therapy assistant would use vestibular and tactile stimulation and developmental activities to enhance motor planning, body scheme, reflex development, ocular control, and visual perception. Following three auditory sequential directions, using

the scooter board could frequently be included in the activities. The physical education teacher could emphasize prone extension and supine flexion along with games involving moving specific body parts. The classroom aide, volunteer, or resource room teacher could supervise Richard's copying of specifically selected inch cube and pegboard designs to help fine motor and prereading perceptual skills. Independent work could include worksheets or computer games emphasizing imbedded geometric shapes and alphabet letters for visual figure–ground discrimination. The parents could be providing daily tactile stimulation and discrimination at home. Such a complete program could be organized by the therapist or might be planned and agreed upon by all the professionals at a team meeting. The language therapist would be emphasizing Richard's associative language processing and the speed with which he makes oral responses. Awareness of the language problems helps all members of the team understand his learning style better.

The columns listed in Figure 37-4 are only examples of test results or developmental activities that could be listed. Other standardized or observational score items could be substituted; for example, pertinent subtests of the WISC-R or K-ABC psychological tests.

Figure 37-5 shows a similar group evaluation record designed for younger or more handicapped children. Rather than listing standardized tests, space is left under each heading for listing skills or clinical observations indicating strengths or deficits of each child. Red pencil hachures can be used to mark columns indicating current treatment objectives, as they do in Figure 37-4.

Interpreting Performance

Testing and treatment of the youngster in the special education setting may be complicated by undetected

(text continues on page 725)

Individualized Educational Program Plan (I.E.P.)
(abbreviated version)

Name___ Richard (R.)_____   Date of Birth_____
Address _____   Today's Date _____
School_____ Grade/Program_____   I.E.P. Review Date _____

	Date started	Frequency or % of time	Expected duration of services
Primary assignment Integration into regular education (opportunities for child to participate with mainstream children during school hours.) Related Services (e.g., transportation, O.T., P.T., speech, audiology, psychology, counseling, social work, etc.)		(e.g. 20% of each school day) (e.g. 30 minutes 2 times per week)	

Reason for assignment _____

Administrative person responsible for program _____

I.E.P. Planning Meeting Participants_____   _____

_____   _____

Present Educational Levels	Curricular Area	Assessment Procedure	Date	Program Planner
(Results of testing: clinical impressions, standardized tests, criterion referenced measures, etc.)		(tests used)		

Curricular Area (e.g. (1) gross motor)   Annual Goal (e.g. (1) improve motor planning)

(e.g. (2) fine motor)   (e.g. (2) improve eye–hand coordination)

Short Term Objectives	Criteria for Successful Performance
(e.g. (1) With eyes closed (R.) will correctly touch one body part to another on command . . . . (e.g. (2) With a ½-inch diameter pencil (R.) will maintain correct pencil grip while copying ○, □, & △	. . . . . 3 times in sequence on 3 successive days.) . . . . . with shapes clearly discernible.)

Figure 37-3. Individualized Educational Program Plan (IEP).

Head-ings	Column items		Test results			
	Classroom #					
	Age		5½			
	I.Q.		93 ok ok			
	Behavior		ok			
Reflex development	ATNR		ok			
	Prone Ext.	(Kep)	↓			
	Supine Flex.		↑↑			
	Cocontract'n		→			
	Postrot. Nystag.	(SIPT)	↑ ?			
	Sitt'g Blance		ok ok ok ok			
	Forw'd Bal. Beam	(Kep)				
	Sideway Bl. Bm.	(Kep)				
	Backw'd Bl. Bm.	(Kep)				
	Stand'g/Walk'g Bal.	(SIPT)	+!	‒?		
	Static Bal.	(Dev)	ok ok			
Bilateral integration	STNR creep	(Bndr)	→			
	Midline Xing	(SC)				
	Bilat. Mot. Cord.	(SIPT)				
	Dbl. Circles	(Kep)				
	Skip	(Kep)				
	2-2, 2-1 hop	(Kep)				
	Dominance Hand Eye Foot		R R R L			
Body scheme and tactile discrim.	Postural Prax.	(SIPT)	‒2d			
	Sequ. Prax.	(SIPT)				
	Perc. Mot.	(Dev)				
	Sequ. Mot.	(Dev)				
	Point Body Parts		↑			
	Angls in Snow	(Kep)				
	Kinesthesia	(SIPT)	‒1½			
	Man. Form.	(SIPT)				
	Fing. Identif.	(SIPT)	‒.9			
	Graphesthesia	(SIPT)				
	Locaiz'n Tac. Stim.	(SIPT)	‒1			
	Dbl. Tact. Stim.	(SC)	‒1½			
	Tactile Dfsirenes	(SC)	ok			

CLASS DAYS: _____

TIME: _____ TO _____

Richard

Figure 37-4. Evaluation Record for the Mildly Neurologically Impaired (*continues*).

Code for standardized tests indicated in parenthesis:

Kep — Kephart's Purdue Perceptual Motor Survey
SIPT — Sensory Integration and Praxis Tests
Dev — Devereux Test of Extremity Coordination
Beery — Beery–Buktenica Test of Visual Motor Integration
MVPT — Motor Free Test of Visual Perception
SC — Southern Calif. Sensory Integration Test
TVPS — Test of Visual–Perceptual Skills (Gardner)

Blank score indicates item not tested because (a) it was not age appropriate, or (b) new insight into deficit areas would not result.

Category	Test	Item	Richard			
Language	(SIPT)	Oral Praxis				
		Speed of Auditry Process'g	→			
		Sound-symbol assoc.				
		Word finding (naming)	→			
		Auditory Discrim.	ok			
		Integrative (Associative)				
		Expressive	ok ok			
		Receptive	ok ok			
Memory	Aud	Sequ. of 3 audit. directns	→ (hatched)			
		Repeat 3 wrds or #'s	→ (hatched)			
	Vis'l (TVPS)	Vis. Sequ. Mem.	73% 37%			
	(TVPS)	Vis. Memory				
		Sequ. of 3 vis. instrctns	ok ok			
		Sequence of 4 color beads				
Vis. discrim. whole/part	(TVPS)	Vis. Fig. Grnd.	→			
	(SIPT)	Fig. Grnd.	→			
	(TVPS)	Perceptual Quotnt	76% (hatched)			
	(MVPT)	Percept Quotnt	70% 84% (hatched)			
Spatial orientatn	(SC)	R-L Discrim.				
		Reading L. to R. direct.				
		Reversals: letter—word				
	(SIPT)	Space Visualiz.	-7 -7			
	(TVPS)	Vis.—Spat'l Relat.	-9 -7			
		Envirnmtl Disorientation	ok			
Fine motor	(Kep)	Ocular Converg.	→			
	(Kep)	Ocular Pursuit	→			
		Ocular Fixation	ok			
	(SIPT)	Constr. Praxis				
		Sequent. Fing. Tip Touch	→			
		Handwriting	→			
		Pencil Grip	→			
	(SIPT)	Design Copy				
	(Beery)	Vis. Mot. Integr.				
	(SIPT)	(non-domin.)				
	(SIPT)	Mot. Acc. (domin.)	-24			

After testing use soft pencil to fill in scores on pages 1 and 2 only for those items tested. Then with soft red pencil make hatch marks in boxes of pertinent low scores indicating current treatment objectives. Use the Evaluation Record to see goals common to the whole group, to zero in on particular children's deficits when part of the group is suddenly absent, and for ready reference when talking with parents and teachers. Erase and change scores often as children show progress.

Figure 37-4. (continued from preceding page)

Class	Gross motor and reflexes	PRNT	Equilibrium		Bilateral integration	Domin: Hand	Body scheme	Tactile and sensory	Self help	Social emotional
Names ↓		L	Dynamic	Static		Eye				
		R				Foot				

	Eye/hand coordination			Perception		Memory and speed of processing	Language	Cognitive adaptive	Age
	VMI	Dexterity	Ocular motility	Spatial orientation	Visual discrimination and figure ground				I.Q.

Figure 37-5. Evaluation Record for Young or Moderately to Severely Handicapped Children.

deficits in visual, auditory, or tactile acuity. On the other hand, a child may hear well and express himself well verbally but may have a severe impairment in auditory reception. In that case, automatic or learned reliance on visual cues may cause misinterpretation by the child unless gestural cues and body language accurately convey the therapist's intent. Instructions for tactile testing,

for example, may need to be demonstrated in order to be understood. In that case, the written report must reflect the deviation from standardized instructions and the possible educational significance of the language processing confusion.

In addition, "Do this, this, and this after you roll to the ladder," may be an impossible activity for the child who cannot remember the sequence of three visual stimuli or who does not understand the temporal concept "after." It is important to know a child's sensory, language processing, and cognitive deficits as well as to task analyze testing and treatment requirements in order to understand the full impact of a child's performance.

Implementing the Program

The value of occupational therapy treatment techniques in educational settings is a controversial issue among some educators and physicians, and strongly worded adverse opinions have appeared in print.[1,36,58] Therapists must be prepared to counter with research results and carefully compiled articles supporting the importance of sensory integration,[4,5,7,68] motor programs,[18] and other occupational therapy techniques.[32] Although special education classes and medication have consistently been shown to produce academic gains in learning-disabled children,[59] training visual perception[28] and motor performance have not. School therapists should be alert to relevant new scientific reporting in their own and other professional literature, and they should continually investigate and scientifically evaluate their own testing and treatment data.

The therapist is encouraged to update treatment skills often but to avoid applying one treatment method exclusively or following a bandwagon approach to solving children's problems. Drilling splinter skills should be avoided, and a broad developmental program should be emphasized.

OTRs and COTAs must be prepared to provide programs for a wide variety of handicapping conditions (see appropriate treatment sections of this textbook). The age of students served runs the gamut from infant stimulation and preschool programs through the grade-school years and on into secondary education programs and vocational high schools for special education students to age 21. For the mainstreamed population, the therapist must be able to suggest classroom or home activities to help the nonspecial education student who manifests mild motor or perceptual difficulties. Some therapists are employed by schools, whereas other school systems contract for occupational therapy services through private therapists, public health departments, or hospitals.

The occupational therapist's role may include: (1) direct treatment in one or several schools (including itinerant service in which therapy equipment may need to be transported in the therapist's car); (2) home treatment for preschoolers and their families; (3) treatment accompanied by personal or telephone monitoring and updating of recommendations suggested to parents, aides, or teachers (such as classroom, physical education, art, or vocational teachers); (4) supervising of COTAs, volunteers, or others who plan or carry out treatment; and (5) consultancy (Table 37-2).[37]

Occupational therapy treatment is intended to allow the child to be able to direct cognitive skills toward the academic task at hand rather than toward execution of balance, motor planning, fine manipulation, and so forth. Therapy prepares the preschool and school-age child to learn; however, it does not result in increased academic performance for school children unless accompanied by an appropriate academic program. The therapist should avoid removing a child from the classroom unless direct therapy is clearly warranted and ongoing assessment indicates progress is being made.

Direct Treatment

Improved quality of life is the goal in occupational therapy. Emotional and social factors as well as physical needs should be considered. Play, the primary occupation of the child, is an important consideration in program planning. Activities should be fun and should foster in the child a positive self-image. As one therapist put it, every pediatric occupational therapy treatment program should include Play, Pleasure, and Success. Clark and associates point out that play is intrinsically motivating, and self-direction by the child should play a major role in therapy, accompanied by artful vigilance by the observant therapist.[15] They point out that therapy is an art that is best carried out within a healthy helping relationship that values the child as an important contributor to the process. On the other hand, the child must not be permitted to misbehave, control, or misuse activities to the detriment of his or her own progress or that of classmates.

Hyperactivity often causes behavior management problems and inaccurate interpretation of performance capability, particularly for therapists and teachers working with several developmentally impaired children at once. Helping a child learn to manage his own behavior may be one goal of therapy. In addition, it is important for children to leave therapy quietly controlled and ready to resume desk work, preschool, or family activities without disruption.

The occupational therapist may employ such techniques as slow rocking, firm pressure on the skin, neutral warmth, or slow rotation for certain conditions associated with overactive behavior. Medications prescribed by the child's physicians may be helpful if the cause of the hyperactivity is organic, particularly in the presence of hyperactivity, poor impulse control, and short attention span. The central nervous system stimulant methylphenidate (Ritalin) is most often effective, while dextroamphetamine (Dexedrine) is a good second choice. It is thought that the stimulants may act on the reticular activating system, a part of the brainstem that receives and sorts out stimuli. In a few cases, the tran-

Table 37-2. *The Do's and Don't's of Consultancy.*

Do	Do Not
Keep record of consultancy contacts	
Recognize you hold an equal position with consultee socially, emotionally, administratively	Try to assume authority or take responsibility (that would be supervision, not consultation)
Evaluate needs	
Promote learning by consultee *and* yourself.	Act patronizing, benign, or aloof
Impart specialized knowledge; find solutions jointly	Make unilateral decisions
Suggest changes that are palatable and realistic	Expect consultee to modify behavior to please you
Enhance creative, self-directed implementing of your suggestions	Teach
Listen; expect 2-way communication	Ignore feedback
Be task oriented; delegate treatment	Be patient- or student-oriented or provide hands-on treatment
Recognize you are dealing with a whole social system	Be an *advisor* who does not become involved with the social system, but supervises, dictates authority
Be nonthreatening in your approach	Try to upstage the consultee or compete for attention from shared supervisors
Consider *who* asked you to consult, and *why*	Fail to try obtaining and maintaining sanction of people who opposed your appointment
Solve a problem or crisis. Recognize your involvement is likely to be temporary. Consultee may terminate your relationship at any time	Plan to stay in this position indefinitely
Recognize that a consultant's role may not establish deep personal relationships and provide deep personal gratification.	

Compiled from Leopold R: The techniques of consultation: Some thoughts for the occupational therapist. Presentation before Eastern Pennsylvania Occupational Therapy Association, Norristown, Pennsylvania, 1966.

quilizers chlorpromazine (Thorazine) and thioridazine (Mellaril) may help reduce anxiety.[30,35] The use of medication should be accompanied by special education, environmental control, and, sometimes, counseling.

Hyperactivity may also be psychogenic. It may be caused by emotional overlay secondary to a learning problem, or it may reflect an inconsistent child-rearing approach. In this case, the child is physically able to control his behavior but is preconditioned not to do so.[44]

Management of hyperactive behavior requires firmness, structure, and environmental controls. Reducing distractions, defining performance expectations clearly, and giving clear warnings of impending minor changes are helpful. Keeping an accurate daily record of the types and forerunners of inappropriate behavior in the classroom helps determine the cause of hyperactivity and the effectiveness of intervention procedures.[44]

Behavior modification, currently widely used in the field of education, is a particularly useful method of managing hyperactive behavior of psychogenic origin and of bringing about improvement in specific behaviors. Performance is assessed first, and terminal goals or "behavioral objectives," are established. Positive rewards or reinforcements that are important to the child are determined so that they may be given upon completion of each small step approaching the goal. Negative or incorrect behavior or performance are usually ignored and are not negatively reinforced by scolding or criticism. Primitive rewards are often edible. Interim rewards, such as paper tokens that can be traded in for treats or privileges, are more therapeutically desirable, and social rewards such as a handshake or a smile are the highest level. The frequency of rewarding is decreased as the child's performance improves.[47,61]

Mildly impaired school-age children, even the very hyperactive, learn to sit quietly on their special spots waiting for treatment to begin when they know the star they then receive can later be exchanged for free play time. They understand when newly performed activities are listed on an "I can do" sheet to take home. On individually written self-paced activity sheets, each step leading to correct skipping, for example, can be checked off as it is mastered.

Consistency of expectations and rewards is important, especially when working with a group. Motivating and allowing a child to make the decision to cooperate has more positive results than trying to force conforming behavior. Having a child help establish his own goals often fosters cooperative behavior.

In a difficult-to-control class, it may be necessary to

plan the same activities for the whole class. In that case, formal structure or calming activities, at least at the beginning and end of the session, may be necessary to establish control.

This finely delineated sequence of steps might be helpful when working with more than one or two students simultaneously:

1. Have equipment ready and highly motivating activities planned (some will have been selected by the students).
2. Position children with enough space between them to perform the task.
3. Gain the undivided attention of the group.
4. Introduce equipment and wait until reaction subsides.
5. Briefly and clearly explain the task using three or fewer sequential directions.
6. Demonstrate.
7. Gain undivided attention.
8. Have one or all children demonstrate verbally or physically that they understood directions.
9. Gain undivided attention.
10. Signal start of task.
11. Continually reward appropriate performance verbally or with a pat, handshake, star, privilege, or other reward.
12. Conclude task specifically by change in positioning of children or equipment or by some other specific means. Avoid the temptation of rushing into a new activity before the children have had time to "change gears."

The experienced therapist may wish to make efficient use of time with a well-controlled group of mildly impaired children by using "learning stations" or "circuit training." At several positions around the room, equipment or activities are placed for use by one or two children. It is important for each unsupervised activity to provide its own feedback so the child knows whether it was performed correctly. (Did the beanbags go in the can? Did you catch the ball?) Children change stations at their own volition, or as "the gong sounds," or as the therapist directs. With this method, all children are therapeutically engaged with activities or equipment that can be used by only one child at a time. The therapist stays with the station that is least safe or that needs to have feedback provided. Also, each child could be directed only to those particular stations within his or her treatment program. Classroom and physical education teachers are often experts in using this method and can be helpful models.

Expanding the Occupational Therapist's Role

In addition to seeking expertise in treating or consulting for various handicapping conditions, the therapist ex-plores novel roles when appropriate. One therapist in a private high school for the learning disabled and language impaired expanded her role as prevocational therapist to include curriculum development to promote work-related habits even in the early elementary school years, fund-raising for high school job-training equipment, grant writing, and public relations. She even wrote a textbook on work-related school programs.[8,31] Another therapist designed a school's aquatics program to include functional learning experiences as well as basic swim instruction and increased adult supervision by importing a group of occupational therapy students to work as aides.[40]

The well-prepared therapist keeps abreast of relevant publications and journals[13,33,57] and acquires information regarding the organizational and legal idiosyncrasies of educational systems (for example, through the training program "Occupational Therapy Educational Management in Schools" offered by AOTA).[24] Organizations such as ACLD, AAMD, ARC, and CEC (see Glossary) offer opportunities for sharing between educators, parents, and therapists. Increasing involvement and professional contributions by therapists in local chapters, national conventions, and journal or newsletter publications of these organizations help highlight the expanding role of the school therapist.

Collaboration with other disciplines and membership on school curriculum development committees are encouraged (for example, in curriculum design of a teaching unit prepared to accommodate severe physical impairments by use of a microcomputer headstick, key-guard, joystick, or specially programmed software). Therapists point out to others the unique contributions they are qualified to make within the total educational program while remaining open to opportunities for role release exchange with other educatioinal professionals. Role release for the therapist involves encouraging classroom faculty members to carry out therapeutic activities, sometimes in conjunction with achieving IEP objectives, and helps the therapy become an integral rather than a peripheral part of the learning process.[41]

Providing Developmental Program Planning Guidelines

The developmental sequences in the child development chart presented earlier provide a basis for creating non-academic school curriculum ideas to share with teachers, physical educators, parents, and aides. The program ideas on the next pages are based on that chart and are examples of developmental activities particularly suitable for the early elementary-school-age mildly impaired child. They are divided into four sections:

1. Body scheme (which includes sequenced items listed under Sensory Development on the Child Development Chart);

2. A combined section of reflex development and balance skills (the latter from the Equilibrium section);
3. Coordination of the two body sites (from the Bilateral Integration section of the chart);
4. Eye–hand coordination (which also includes some developmentally sequenced items under Visual Perception).

Behaviors in the left column of each of the four sections are arranged approximately developmentally, and some include approximate age norms. Therefore, they can be used by educational personnel for informal evaluation/data gathering to determine *general* areas that need remedial help, for developmental program planning, and for re-evaluation. This would not, of course, replace the standardized and developmental testing to be done by the therapist. Early "behaviors" are generally, though not absolutely, prerequisite to later behaviors, and they may have to be mastered before progress in later behaviors can be expected. Adjacent behaviors may be interchangeable.

The behaviors in the left column may also be stated in positive terms by therapists or educators for writing behavioral objectives as a part of diagnostic–prescriptive IEPs.

Body Scheme

Body scheme is the unconscious awareness of the physical and sensory components of one's self. It includes awareness of the physical structure, movement/functions, and positions of the body and its parts in relation to each other and to objects in the environment. As used here, it also includes the ability to recognize and interpret touch and pressure to the skin. Children with good body scheme accurately imitate new body postures or movements; have smoothly coordinated movements on the playground, particularly when trying new actions; adequately point to or name body parts (assuming that language comprehension and memory are adequate); usually draw human figures age appropriately; and interpret touch/pressure to the skin comfortably and accurately.

If these behaviors are observed	*Try these activities, strategies, or materials*
Cannot comfortably accept ordinary new or unexpected touch/pressure to skin. Has aversion to haircuts, new clothes, sand play, mudpies, love pat on shoulder, injections, bare feet in grass, wind through hair.	• Apply firm, well-modulated pressure in rapid rhythm. Teacher rubs back/arms during rest time.
	• "Time out" four times daily for child's *self*-rubbing of arms, tummy, legs, neck, and face. With rapid back-and-forth motions, use *child's* choice of soft or rough fabric, carpet piece, baby oil, hairbrush, or paint brush.
	• Present a variety of textures/sensations in calm, well-structured atmosphere: ice cubes, warm water, textured fingerpaints, sand play, rotary electric shoe polish brush, vibrator, tug-of-war on tummy in grass, electric hair dryer, inchworm race on back on grass or thick carpet.
	• Avoid unexpected touch by teacher/students. Encourage "thinking space" between children in line; position desk to avoid accidental touch; praise verbally rather than with love pats unless child sees the "pat" approaching.
	• Slowly encourage physical contact within child's toleration level—lapsitting, arm around shoulders, hand pat on hair.
Is unable to imitate simple body postures/movements accurately.	• Give visual, verbal, *and* tactile clues. Manually move child to appropriate position so movement/position can be felt and learned through experiencing it.
	• Encourage movement/contact of all body parts with different textures and surfaces: mat, shredded paper, blankets, floor, grass, brick wall, and smooth wall.
	• Mimetics, pantomime, obstacle courses, animal walks, Simon Says "do this," "See a Lassie."

If these behaviors are observed	*Try these activities, strategies, or materials*
	• Trampoline, cheerleader yells, signal flags, mat stunts.
	• Child wiggles through rungs of leaning, suspended, or sidelying ladder with predetermined movements or climbs in and out of holes cut into refrigerator shipping cartons.
	• Action songs: I'm a Little Teapot, Inky Dinky Spider, Two Little Ducks, Little Cottage in the Woods, My Hat It Has Three Corners.
	• Child performs familiar movements in slow motion: walking, especially against resistance, walking backwards, crawling, skipping.
	• Child reproduces silhouette of partner's body positions (use film projector light), then verifies by measuring/feeling silhouette against wall.
Inaccurately uses and points to own body parts as directed.	• Beginning with easiest to learn (facial features, arm, side, leg), teach body-part awareness, being alert to child whose problem is not poor body image but poor language comprehension or poor auditory–motor match (can understand words but can't carry out appropriate movement response without visual clue).
	• Then work on identification of more difficult body parts (wrist, knee, shoulder, elbow, ankle, neck, waist, etc.)

	• One sequence of teaching body parts (achieved over a long period of time) is to have child:
	    touch and move part while repeating the name of the part
	    touch and move part, eyes shut
	    touch part to object (from standing, sitting, lying down positions) while repeating the name of the part
	    touch part to object, eyes shut
	    touch part to part ("put your ankle on your knee")
	    touch part to part, eyes shut
	    name part independently
	    "place ankle higher than shoulder," or "back higher than head," or "ear lower than knee"

	• Refer to body image instructional sequences recommended in *Developmental Sequences of Perceptual Motor Tasks.*[17]

	• Child rapidly and firmly rubs body parts while naming:
	    "paint" with wet or dry brush
	    rub off "mud" or "ice cream" with hand-sized towel/carpet
	    wrap body part with yarn or bandage
	    at goal line, rub powder off "hurt" ankle or wrist held in air during lame puppy race.

	• Point out body parts and movements during doll play or on pop-singer posters.
	• Sing "Dem Bones," "Head and Shoulders—Knees and Toes," "Looby Loo," "Hokey Pokey."

If these behaviors are observed	*Try these activities, strategies, or materials*
	• Play Busy Bee (partners touch back-to-back, ankle-to-ankle, etc.) or Simon Says (naming one body part while teacher demonstrates the wrong one — for advanced players).
	• Be alert to the idea that pointing to or naming body parts is only one step in "knowing" body image.
With eyes closed, cannot point to location of one or two touches on body parts (approximately age 5).	• Emphasize identification of and tactile stimulation to body parts.
	• Emphasize activities suggested for imitation of simple body postures/movements.
Does not know meaning of in front, back, beside, in, up, above, out, by age 5. Has difficulty negotiating obstacles and judging distances, especially if blindfolded.	• Eyes closed, child points to objects in familiar room, then verifies by looking, approaching, and *touching* with specified body parts.
	• Place three to five 8-inch numbers around room. Eyes closed, children point to numerical answer to simple oral math problem, then verify.
	• Eyes closed, child touches one body part to another; touches body part to object in environment; goes through obstacle course; follows thick-rope path; touches environmental objects to front, side, top of body planes.
	• Child applies oral directional labels to gross body movements and fine manipulative placement of small objects.
	• Child uses beanbags or plastic or playground balls for target or goal throws or dodge ball. Increase spatial awareness through eye–body, eye–hand, and foot–eye coordination activities.
Is unable to draw six-part recognizable person with body (approximately age 5).	• Look for other indications of delayed eye–hand coordination.
	• Emphasize awareness of body parts and imitation of postures (above).
Cannot discriminate simple shapes traced on skin with eyes closed.	• Help child identify large simple shapes traced on back, hand, or tummy using "point to the answer" method instead of "draw the answer" (eye–hand coordination may be poor) or naming answer (language deficits may be present). Advance to more complex shapes and to naming shapes.
	• Set teams facing forward. Trace shape or letter on back of last child on each team. Each child traces on back of person in front. Child in front of each team traces that team's shape on chalkboard.
	• Identify hand-sized objects felt in bag but not seen.
	• Child identifies finger touched by partner when eyes closed or points to spot(s) touched by partner or by "it" in circle game.
Cannot name heavier of two weights (approximately age 4); with eyes closed cannot tell whether one finger has been moved to up or down position by partner/teacher by age 7½; cannot stabilize arms and trunk against much resistance.	• Children do tug-of-war while standing, sitting, and lying down.
	• Encourage pressure on joints through resistance: walrus, crab, seal walk, wheelbarrow race, crawling with partner facing child and pushing against shoulders, stretching inner tubes, partners trying to force wrists together or apart.

If these behaviors are observed	*Try these activities, strategies, or materials*
	• Compression of joints through jumping, leaping, trampoline, and bouncing board.
Has poorly developed sense of rhythm. Awkwardly performs rapid alternating motions using opposite muscle groups.	• Rhythm band, marching, dancing, musical activities, and Lummi sticks.
	• Provide definite, clear auditory rhythm signal (drum or triangle beat) with each separate motion response. This may need to be accompanied by touch-pressure clue. Example: angels-in-snow movements slowly to beat of metal triangle, with touch by teacher to appropriate limb for those children who need this extra clue.

	• Child performs rapid opposing motions on signal or to beat of music:
	    palms down, palms up
	    index finger touch tip of nose, tip of finger held at arm's length
	    tongue protrudes straight forward, retracts into mouth
	    protruding tongue touches one side of open mouth, then opposite side
	    child repeatedly says sound "puh, puh, puh" or "buh, buh, buh" or "tuh, tuh, tuh"
	    heel-toe, heel-toe tap while sitting, standing.

Does not know right/left on self with eyes closed (approximately age 8); right/left on facing person (approximately age 9½).	• Point out freckle or tiny scar on child's right or left hand to help in discrimination.
	• Child identifies randomly distributed right and left hand/foot cutouts.
	• Footsie game. Advance player on game board number of spaces written on correctly identified foot "playing card" drawn from pack.
	• Zip Zap. (Circle game. "Zip" means name right neighbor, "Zap" means name left neighbor. Encourage speed.)
	• Blindfold one child. Others give oral directions to lead child to target (*e.g.*, three steps to right, two steps backwards, two steps to left).
(If these advanced body scheme tasks are difficult for a child, return to "behaviors" and "activities" for younger children.)	• Use facing pairs of objects such as trucks, TV sets, chairs, to demonstrate and quiz diagonal aspect of right and left before applying labels to right or left of facing object. *Later,* teach right and left on facing person.

Reflex Development and Balance Skills

As early primitive postural reflexes decrease in importance, the normally developing child acquires more advanced balance skills, which allow automatic equilibrium responses. These responses first develop with the infant in a lying-down position, then in sitting and kneeling on hands and knees, and finally in standing and walking positions. Training for delayed balance skills should proceed in the same developmental sequence. Early "behaviors" are generally, though not absolutely, prerequisite to later behaviors and should be mastered first. Grade-school children with good balance skills have good head and trunk stability while sitting and/or standing. They can walk with feet close together and with hands swinging reciprocally at sides, and walk a balance beam, hop, jump, and leap comfortably.

If these behaviors are observed	*Try these activities, strategies, or materials*
Has very inadequate sitting balance and difficulty "leading with the head" when rolling.	• Log and egg rolls, somersaults on mats or down inclines. (Make more difficult up incline, against resistance, or holding beanbag between knees.) • Move head separate, from stable body in backlying position to look in various directions on cue, including looking at toes without lifting back.
Is unable to lie on abdomen on small pillow and hold head, shoulders, arms, knees and toes off floor for 10 seconds (by age 5½). Is unable to curl up in a ball while lying on back and hold head, arms, feet off floor for 10 seconds (by age 5½).	• Back raises with feet held; leg raises with trunk held. Kraus Weber position. Push ups. • Scooterboard activities on stomach. • With chin on chest and arms bent and folded, child kicks ball across floor with sole of foot, kicks balloon over short "net," rides bicycle motion with legs while hips off floor, blows tissue off chest. • Child rides gym scooter on back, with head and feet up, using hands to pull forward on suspended rope or ladder rungs. • On monkey bars and jungle gyms, child attains and then holds upside-down, curled-up position while looking forward.
Cannot stand from backlying position almost symmetrically by age 5½ or 6. Must turn nearly onto abdomen or hands–knees position before reaching standing.	• From backlying, child quickly jumps up and runs or moves to goal or target with minimal trunk rotation. • From standing position, child stoops, reaches for object across midline, picks it up from floor, and returns to standing position.
Squirms or readjusts posture often in sitting position. Has difficulty sitting on unsteady or tipsy equipment, especially if not holding on.	• Child seat-walks on buttocks—race or stunt. • Play musical chairs on tipsy seats, no hands. • Partners sit back to back, lock elbows, then try to stand. Partners face each other, hold hands, and touch soles of feet while rocking far forward and backward. • Child sits on and rides swing, seesaw, sliding board, barrel lying on its side, board with hubcap screwed under it so curve touches floor, scooterboard, one-rope swing.
Has difficulty balancing in hands-and-knees position on unsteady surface or in three-point position (one hand or foot raised), especially if head is turned toward one side.	• In hands-and-knees position, child rocks forward and backward, head facing forward. With forehead, child taps suspended ball so it hits target on wall or knocks over bowling pins on chair. • Vary head position during hands-and-knees balance activities so eyes look at targets forward and at either side. • In hands-and-knees position, child rocks side to side or uses one hand or knee to push ball or beanbag to goal. • Place color card (or vocabulary word, letter or number) under each hand and knee. Instruct child to "lift yellow (or #7) hand (knee) and hold for 5 seconds." Advance to lifting two limbs and later three.
Is unable to jump in place, climb stairs one foot per tread without holding on, squat, or briefly tiptoe (approximately age 4).	• Child jumps off short, then taller, objects, then jumps over flat, then taller, obstacles. • Child runs up incline and jumps off in various directions and postures. • All teachers and parents cooperate to remind child about one foot per stair tread.

If these behaviors are observed

Try these activities, strategies, or materials

Cannot heel-toe walk, broad jump, hop on one foot briefly, descend stairs one foot per tread without holding on (approximately age 5).

- Stunts or musical games encourage squatting (duck-like), walking on tiptoes (fairies and tall people), and jumping (over imaginary brooks, obstacles).
- Play potato-on-a-spoon race, dodgeball with plastic beach ball, hopscotch with two feet and later one foot, potato sack race, hopping tag, and trampoline.
- Child heel-toe walks on tape, fat rope, balance beam, and side of ladder.

Does not try roller skates, stilts, jump rope (approximately age 6). Cannot high jump 8 inches, broad jump 3 feet.

- Introduce skates, coffee-can stilts, wooden-pole stilts, jump rope (first teacher turns, later self-turning occurs).

Is unable to crouch on tiptoes (approximately age 8), jump clapping hands three times (approximately age 9), hop 50 feet in 5 seconds by age 12.
(If these advanced tasks are difficult for a child, return to "behaviors" and "activities" for younger children.)

- Advanced balance beam activities.
- Simple track and field events.

Coordination of the Two Body Sides

This skill indicates the body's motoric ability to function as a whole. Developing children first initiate purposeful movement with both arms/legs similarly and later reciprocally (*i.e.*, with one limb after another in steady rhythm). Children also first perform movements without crossing the body's midline (a theoretical plane or line drawn from the center of the forehead straight down to a point between the feet) and later with midline crossing. It is recommended that training of motorically delayed children proceed in the same sequence. Children having good coordination of the two body sides have adequately established hand dominance with adequate assist by the nondominant hand; spontaneous crossing of the midline when appropriate; and smooth, coordinated patterns of walking, running, and skipping (within age expectancy).

If these behaviors are observed

Try these activities, strategies, or materials

Is unable to creep, tummy off floor, with opposing hand and knee moving almost simultaneously before the age of 12 months.

- Bunny hopping with two knees moving ahead simultaneously is an immature pattern that should be discouraged in the school-age youngster.
- Child creeps facing target at eye level, hands and tops of feet flat on floor, and pointing straight (not away from or toward midline of body). See the *Bender–Purdue Reflex Test and Training Manual.*[10]
- As correct reciprocal pattern of arm/leg movement develops, add resistance to forward movement at the shoulders and ankles. Resist backward creeping at the buttocks.
- Introduce puppy, kitty, and wild animal walks and races and obstacle courses.

Walks and runs without opposing reciprocal arm and leg movements at age 4.

- If hands are held at shoulder level during walking/running, train balance skills.
- Invert tricycle. Child rotates wheel with reciprocal hand motion on pedals.
- Child pulls rope, hand-over-hand, to move gym scooter seat toward goal, to lift weighted pulley rope. "Pedal" gym scooter with hands moving reciprocally.
- Introduce tricycles, pedal cars, Big Wheels, Sit 'n' Spin, Irishmail cart.

If these behaviors are observed	*Try these activities, strategies, or materials*

Cannot gallop, sashay, slide-step well, or skip with one foot only (lame duck skip) (approximately age 5).

- Encourage reciprocal hand and foot rhythms: xylophone, bongo drums, Ali Babba and the Forty Thieves, wheelbarrow walk, step-together-step sideways to music.
- New skills may have to be taught and learned with two hands moving together first, later hands moving reciprocally.
- Teach component skill parts of gallop, sashay, slide-step, lame duck skip, and crab walk.

Inaccurately imitates pantomimed midline crossing postures (approximately age 5). Avoids spontaneous midline crossing.

- Play Simon Says with midline crossing, Lummi sticks, crepe paper humming, lasso motions, target throws across midline (also during scooter rides), partner hand-clap games (Peas porridge, Miss Mary Mack, Oh Little Playmate, Pretty Little Dutch Girl), folk dancing steps (heel-toe cross over; grapevine).
- Hurry-Hurry Relay (team game: pass each of many items, two hands together, sideways to team mates until all items reach winning bucket).
- Child taps suspended ball sideways with palms. Advance to backs of hands, then palms when arms crossed.
- Child creeps along rope or line with knees straddling, hands crossed to opposite side. If necessary, give touch clue to indicate next hand movement.

Cannot skip alternately and exhibits much difficulty learning to throw a ball with proper weight shift onto foot opposite the throwing arm (approximately age 6½).

- Skipping: teach slow step-hop pattern on each foot. Place straight rope between feet, or place one foot on board, one foot on floor. Thus child can see and feel difference between the two feet and can begin to predict the feel of the slow step-hop rhythm. (If the board on which one foot practices step-hop is unsteady and clatters on the floor with each step-hop, it gives an additional auditory clue.) Teach reciprocal arm rhythm simultaneous to step-hop by moving arms correctly for the child.
- Introduce component skills of throwing, pitching, and catching.

Has not established good hand dominance (approximately age 6½ or 7).

- Check for asymmetry of discrimination in identifying small objects by touch; in recognizing shapes drawn on hand; in recognizing which finger is touched. Train accordingly. (Hand that doesn't feel things adequately may "refuse" to accept dominant role.)
- Check again for midline crossing. If each hand works independently only on its own side of the body, neither accepts dominant role.

Cannot perform good jumping jacks or tap floor alternately with feet (approximately age 7). Cannot hop alternately 2 right – 2 left or 3 right – 1 left foot patterns (approximately age 8). Cannot throw small ball 40 to 60 feet (approximately age 9).

- Child performs angels in snow, jumping jacks, and commando crawl (tummy touching floor) with variety of specified arm/leg movements.
- Introduce advanced reciprocal hand/foot rhythms, slowly advancing up to need for balance while performing. Sample sequence:
  2 right, 2 left rhythm on xylophone
  2-2 stamp of feet while sitting
  2-2 stamp of feet while standing

If these behaviors are observed	*Try these activities, strategies, or materials*
(If these advanced tasks are difficult for a child, return to "behaviors" and "activities" for younger children.)	2-2 hop *once* while holding teacher's two hands 2-2 hop *once* without holding hands 2-2 hop several times, holding hands 2-2 hop several times, not holding hands • Child bounces ball in pattern or 2 right–2 left or 3 right–1 left.

Eye–Hand Coordination

Good eye–hand coordination is seen in the child who cuts, writes, works puzzles, manipulates small materials, and performs motor self-care activities age appropriately and with a good dominant/assistive hand use pattern. Behaviors are listed approximately by degree of difficulty (*i.e.*, in the sequence in which they are normally acquired). Success in more difficult classroom behaviors can be expected only if earlier levels have been mastered.

If these behaviors are observed	*Try these activities, strategies, or materials*
Is unable to focus on object with both eyes as it moves nearer to and farther from face (convergence).	• Teacher or other child slowly moves straw as child tries to put toothpick inside. • Child tries Forward Pass ball-on-rope toy by Developmental Learning Materials.[19]
Is unable to follow moving object (with eyes only, head not moving) thru 160° arc vertically, horizontally, diagonally, and in a circle. Eyes do not move smoothly and together. (Be sure visual acuity has been examined. Persistent or exceptional ocular problems should be referred to a vision specialist.)	• Child tries ball activities using first balloons, large plastic beach balls, whiffle balls and later large playground balls, then firmer balls, then smaller balls. • Coathanger bats for balloons can be made by stretching nylon stockings over hanger pulled to square shape.
Does not poke finger into small hole. Is clumsy in picking up small items between thumb and index finger.	• Child places small objects into and "fishes" them out of small necked container. This can be timed. • Child tears — tissue (easiest), paper, manila folder, rag (hardest) — while holding between thumb and index finger. • Pinch and squeeze seeds or small discs (toward target), clothespins, and metal clips.
Has difficulty using wrist in side-to-side movements and palms-up/palms-down rotation. Grasps without wrist slightly extended.	• Child rings handbells, turns doorknobs, and unlocks with keys. • Child unscrews nuts and bolts, bicycle spokes from their end-casings or lids from small photofilm can containers.
Balances poorly on floor and chair so hands and forearms are not free to develop manipulative skills.	• Train sitting balance.

Has difficulty rolling clay into snake shape, later ball shape. Is clumsy when pasting, gluing, using even large paint brush, throwing ball with voluntary release. Displays generally inadequate eye–hand coordination in spite of adequacy in previously mentioned eye–hand behaviors.	• Child practices spreading fingers apart and squeezing them together while they are *straight*.*
	  squeeze tiny sponges, eye droppers between fingers
	  squeeze cardboard between straight fingers or finger and thumb so it cannot easily be pulled away
	  spread rubberband wide with straight fingers
	  suddenly spread apart straight fingers without moving wrist, and knock beads or blocks off desk.

---

* Fine motor dexterity activities.

If these behaviors are observed   *Try these activities, strategies, or materials*

- Finger plays: Inky Dinky Spider; church and steeple.*
- Child walks balloon up and down wall with fingertips. Advance to small plastic ball, ping-pong, golf, and playground balls.*
- Look for body scheme difficulty and train accordingly.
- Introduce coloring accurately, dot-to-dot, tracing, mazes, lacing cards, pipe cleaners, beads, jacks, chalkboard road (trace on, wet fingers on, wet paintbrush on).†
- Child glues outline of letters, then sprinkles on glitter.†
- Squirts out lit candle with water pistol.†
- Pastes tiny things accurately (*e.g.,* holes punched) using toothpicks.†
- Try commercial games such as Perfection, Numbers Up, Drop in the Bucket, Pick Up Sticks, Operation, Etch a Sketch, Cross Fire.†
- Child traces on graph paper through empty squares as directed (right, left, up, down); guesses letter reproduced.† (Can be adapted to all later ages.)

Has not established use of one dominant hand at a time with other hand helping; for example, in stringing large beads, later small beads; folding paper with definite crease (although inaccurately).

Does not reach across midline of body spontaneously to pick up and put down objects.

Has difficulty making tower of 9- or 10-inch cubes or 3-cube bridge before age 4 or placing small pegs in pegboard holes.

Cannot copy |, –, or O holding crayon/pencil with appropriate grip and using good assistance of nondrawing hand before age 4.

- All of the above activities plus Origami paper folding.
- Look for and train problems in coordination of two body sides.
- Look for and train problems in coordination of two body sides.
- Child practices block building, pegboards, and copying simple models.
- Look for and train visual perception problems.
- Use plastic, three-sided pencil grippers for correct and comfortable pencil position (from Developmental Learning Materials).[19]
- Encourage correct grip in all pencil, crayon, and painting activities.
- Move arm, later hand, through correct motion on chalkboard, paper, and fingerpaint.

Cannot unbutton accessible buttons before age 4.

Does not use hands reciprocally.

- Emphasize self-help skills, breaking each into component parts.
- Look for and train coordination of two body sides difficulty.
- Child winds thread on spool evenly, sharpens pencil, uses manual egg beater.

Is unable to cut paper fringe before age 4. (All cutting activities are listed developmentally here. Actually, more advanced cutting skills develop in conjunction with more advanced eye–hand coordination skills.)

- Use four-holed scissors that can be held by both child and teacher.
- Introduce cutting tasks in sequence listed under Behaviors.
- Encourage:
    elbow near waist, not away from body
    wrist slightly extended, not slightly flexed

---

* Fine motor dexterity activities.

† Eye–hand coordination activities. (Can be adapted to all later age activities.)

If these behaviors are observed	*Try these activities, strategies, or materials*
	palm facing midline or face, not floor
	all fingers flexed while cutting, not extended and wide apart
	scissors held comfortably and consistently in thumb-finger position, preferably near knuckle of thumb but near middle of middle finger
	assisting hand adjusting paper position to scissors, not cutting hand adjusting position to paper.
Is unable to cut across paper, generally following straight, later curved, line.	• Prevent jagged edges by placing paper against center of X of scissors.
Is unable to cut out simple shapes having very wide outlines and no sharp angles.	• Child cuts *slowly*, down center of "road" (outline) while rotating paper *slowly* with nondominant hand. Success measured by half of "road" (outline) appearing on each side of cut.
Is unable to cut out small ○, △, ▭, □.	• Encourage accuracy.
Is unable to cut cloth.	• Grade up from thin to heavier cloth. Also try manila folder paper for heavy resistance.
Is unable to cut out complex pictures following outlines.	• Look for and train visual figure–ground problems.
Has great difficulty bouncing and catching large playground ball (approximately age 5); accurately tapping swinging suspended ball two out of five tries (approximately age 7).	• Teach handball skills in sequence of throw, catch, bounce and catch, toss and catch, and strike. • Teach foot–eye skills in sequence of kick nonmoving ball, kick moving ball, run and kick, and catch with feet.
Cannot put 10 pellets into bottle in 25 seconds before age 5; 20 coins into open box, one at a time, in 16 seconds (approximately age 7).	• Encourage speed of fine motor response.
Is unable to copy +, /, \, □, × (approximately age 7).	• Walk outlined shapes on floor. Then use templates of straight line plus simple geometric forms. Begin with chalkboard size; advance to desk size.
Cannot draw unmistakable six-part man including body (approximately age 5).	• Look for and train other indications of body image difficulties. • Encourage competency, later speed in this skill.
Cannot oppose thumb and each finger tip sequentially while looking at fingers, even slowly and with similar but incomplete movements of opposite hand (approximately age 5); is unable to do this competently—eyes open or closed with no overflow movements in the other hand (approximately age 7).	
With inch cubes, is unable to reproduce six-block pyramid and gate (approximately age 4½); copy △, ✳ (approximately age 6).	• Look for and train other indications of visual perception problems.
Hand dominance has not been established (approximately age 6½ or 7).	• Look for and train problems in coordination of two body sides.
Is unable to copy many letters and numbers (approximately age 6).	• Encourage correct position of pencil and child's body. Paper position may vary with child's hand preference but should be consistent. Elbow should be abducted from body sufficiently to allow slight wrist extension (not flexion) while writing. • For most learning-disabled children, cursive handwriting is easier to master than manuscript. • If child forms letters consistently better with eyes closed, allow child initially to learn feel of making each letter without the need for placing it on lines or

If these behaviors are observed	*Try these activities, strategies, or materials*
	tracing letter shapes. Later child can learn to visually direct hand.
	• Use salt tray, heavy crayon tracing, VAKT (Visual Auditory, Kinesthetic Tactile System developed by Fernald[22]).
	• Use Dubnoff School Programs 1, 2, and 3 by Teaching Resources Company.[20]
	• Read pages 107–122 in *Teaching Children with Learning and Behavior Problems.*[29]
Is unable to reproduce letters and numbers from memory.	• Encourage visual memory and imagery as well as adequate visual perception.
	• Read pages 191–247 in *Aids to Psycholinguistic Teaching.*[12]
	• Encourage right–left body part discrimination.
Has not resolved letter and number inversions (approximately age 6) or b–d, p–q reversals (approximately age 7). Tries to write or read in right to left direction.	• Mark frequently confused letters for easier discrimination; for example, put a "stinger" (b) on all b's to represent buzzing bee.
	• Use nondominant index finger to point out direction of pencil movement; for example, left index finger points toward round movement for right-hander's b (∩), 6 (⊂), 3 (∩).
(If these advanced tasks are difficult for a child, return to "behaviors" and "activities" for younger children.)	• Put arrow pointing to right in upper left-hand page corner indicating left–right progression.

References

1. Accardo PJ: A Neurodevelopmental Perspective on Specific Learning Disabilities. Baltimore, University Park Press, 1980
2. American Occupational Therapy Association: Uniform Occupational Therapy Evaluation Checklist. Rockville, MD, American Occupational Therapy Association, 1981
3. Answers to Questions About Occupational Therapy In the Public School System. Rockville, Maryland, American Occupational Therapy Association, 1982
4. Ayres AJ: A response to defensive medicine. Academic Ther 13:149, 1977
5. Ayres AJ: Improving academic scores through sensory integration. J Learn Disab 5:24, 1972
6. Ayres AJ: Sensory Integration and Praxis Tests. Los Angeles, Western Psychological Services (1984)
7. Ayres AJ: The Effect of Sensory Integrative Therapy on Learning Disabled Children. Pasadena, Center for the Study of Sensory Integrative Dysfunction, 1976
8. Balmuth D: A therapist with a working philosophy: Karen Jacobs. Occup Ther News 39(5):1, May 1985
9. Bateman B: So You're Going to a Hearing: Preparing for a Public Law 94-142 Due Process Hearing. Champaign, Illinois, Research Press, 1981
10. Bender M: The Bender–Purdue Reflex Test and Training Manual. San Rafael, California, Academic Therapy Publications (PO Box 899), 1975
11. Bruininks R: Bruininks–Oseretsky Test of Motor Proficiency. Circle Pines, MN, American Guidance Service, 1978
12. Bush WI, Giles M: Aids to Psycholinguistic Teaching. Columbus, Ohio, Charles E Merrill, 1969
13. Campbell SK (ed): Physical and Occupational Therapy in Pediatrics. New York, The Haworth Press (149 Fifth Ave, 10010)
14. Clark F: Advanced Interpretation Course: Moving Beyond Preliminaries. Pasadena, Center for the Study of Sensory Integrative Dysfunction, 1980
15. Clark F, Mailloux Z, Parham D: The Art of Therapy. Pasadena, The Center for the Study of Sensory Integrative Dysfunction, 1981
16. Colarusso R, Hammill D: Motor-Free Visual Perception Test. San Rafael, California, Academic Therapy, 1972
17. Cratty B: Developmental Sequences of Perceptual–Motor Tasks. Freeport, New York, Educational Activities, 1967
18. Cratty BJ: Motor development for special populations: Issues, problems, and operations. Focus Except Child 13:1, 1980
19. Developmental Learning Materials. 7440 Natchez Avenue, Niles, Illinois 60648
20. Dubnoff School Programs 1, 2, and 3. Boston, Teaching Resources Corporation (100 Boylston St), 1975
21. Educational Staff of Chapel Hill: Critical Review of Commonly Used Preschool Assessment Instruments: Resource Guide for Health Care Coordinators. Chapel Hill, NC, Resource Access Project, 1977
22. Fernald G: Remedial Techniques in Basic School Subjects. New York, McGraw-Hill, 1943
23. Flynn S: Pediatric care in occupational therapy in Ireland. In Davidson JE: Ways in which occupational therapy involves the community in treatment. World Fed Occup Ther Bull 5:9–13, 18–20, 1980

24. Gilfoyle EM: Training: Occupational Therapy Educational Management in Schools. OSERS Grant No. G007801499. Rockville, Maryland, American Occupational Therapy Association, 1980

25. Gillespie PH, Johnson L: Teaching Reading to the Mildly Retarded Child. Columbus, Charles Merrill, 1974

26. Greenhouse L: Schools backed on limiting aid to handicapped. New York Times, June 29, 1982, p 1

27. Hainsworth P, Hainsworth M: Pre-School Screening System. Pawtucket, Rhode Island, Pre-School Screening (Box 1635, 02862), 1974

28. Hammill DD: Thoughts to consider before beginning a visual perception program. In Hammill DD, Bartel NR: Teaching Children with Learning and Behavior Problems. Boston, Allyn and Bacon, 1975

29. Hammill DD, Bartel NR: Teaching Children with Learning and Behavior Problems. Boston, Allyn and Bacon, 1975

30. Haslam HA, Valletutti PJ (eds): Medical Problems in the Classroom, pp 294–297. Baltimore, University Park Press, 1975

31. Jacobs K: Occupational Therapy: Work-Related Programs and Assessments. Boston, Little, Brown, 1985

32. Kauffman NA, Kinnealey MS, Gressang JD: The Role of Occupational Therapy in the Education of the Learning Disabled Student. Philadelphia, Cornman Diagnostic Center, 1980 (out of print; available from the author of this chapter.)

33. Kratoville BL (ed): Academic Therapy. Novato, California, Academic Therapy Publications (20 Commercial Boulevard)

34. Kurko V, Crane LL, Willemin H: Preschool Screening Instrument. Fort Worth, Fort Worth Public Schools, 1973

35. Lecky P: Drug Management and Survival Techniques for Parents and Teachers. Presented at Programming for Learning Disabilities Conference, St Joseph's College, Philadelphia, 1974

36. Lehrer RJ: An open letter to an occupational therapist. J Learn Disab 14:3, 1981

37. Leopold RL: The techniques of consultation: Some thoughts for the occupational therapist. Presentation before Eastern Pennsylvania Occupational Therapy Association, Norristown, 1966

38. Lerner J, Mardel–Czudnowski, Goldenberg D: Special Education for the Early Childhood Years, pp 302–331. Englewood Cliffs, New Jersey, Prentice–Hall, 1981

39. Llorens LA, Seig KW: A profile for managing sensory integrative test data. Am J Occup Ther 29:205, 1975

40. Lottes L, LaVesser P: Occupational therapists design children's aquatics program. Occup Ther News 40(4):8, April 1986

41. Lyon S, Lyon G: Team functioning and staff development: A role release approach to providing integrated educational services for severely handicapped students. J Assoc Sev Handicap 5:250, 1980

42. Manes J: Education for handicapped children now includes preschoolers. The Mental Health Law Project's Update on Developments in Law and Policy of Concern to Mentally Disabled Children 5(4–5):1, 1985

43. Mitchell JV (ed): Mental Measurements Yearbook, 9th ed. Lincoln, University of Nebraska Press, 1985

44. Murray JM: Is there a role for the teacher in the use of medication for hyperkinetics. J Learn Disab 9:30, 1976

45. National study to examine cost of special education and related services. Occup Ther News 39(9):3, September 1985

46. Newcomer P, Hammill D: ITPA and academic achievement: A survey. The Reading Teacher, p 739, May 1975

47. O'Leary KD, O'Leary SG: Classroom Management: The Successful Use of Behavior Modification. Elmsford, NY, Pergamon Press, 1972

48. Occupational therapy makes learning possible. Rockville, Maryland, American Occupational Therapy Association, 1985

49. One Out of Ten: School Planning for the Handicapped. New York, Educational Facilities Laboratories (850 Third Avenue), 1974

50. PL 94-142 Tenth Anniversary Celebrated. Occup Ther News 39(12):6, December 1985

51. President Reagan signs P.L. 99-457, the Education for Handicapped Amendments of 1986. Government Legal Affairs Div Bull, Rockville, Maryland, American Occupational Therapy Association, 1986

52. Public Law 94-142: Education for All Handicapped Children Act. As reviewed in Legislative Alert. Rockville, Maryland, American Occupational Therapy Association, 1975

53. Rehnquist WH: Excerpts from justices' opinions in case of a deaf girl and school district. New York Times, June 29, 1982, p B4

54. Rourk JD: School Therapy Task Force recommends guidelines. Occup Ther News 39(11):5, November 1985

55. Sanford AR: Learning Accomplishment Profile and Manual. Winston–Salem, Kaplan School Supply Corp (600 Jonestown Road), 1974

56. Schleifer M (ed): The Exceptional Parent. 296 Boylston Street, Boston, Massachusetts

57. Senf GM (ed): Journal of Learning Disabilities. Chicago, Illinois, The Professional Press (101 East Ontario Street, 60611)

58. Sieben RL: Controversial medical treatments of learning disabilities. Academic Ther 13:133, 1977

59. Silver LB: Acceptable and controversial approaches to treating the child with learning disabilities. Pediatrics 55:406, 1975

60. Stangler SR, Huber CJ, Routh DK: Screening Growth and Development of Preschool Children: A Guide for Test Selection. New York, McGraw-Hill, 1980

61. Stephens TM: Directive Teaching of Children with Learning and Behavioral Handicaps. Columbus, Charles Merrill, 1970

62. Sternat J, Nietupski J, Lyon J, Messina R, Brown L: Occupational and Physical Therapy Services for Severely Handicapped Students: Integrated vs Isolated Therapy Models. Federal Contract No. CEC-0-74-7993. Madison, Wisconsin, Madison Public Schools, 1980

63. Tenth Anniversary of Handicapped Children Education Act Recognized. Occup Ther News 40(4):2, April 1986

64. The Cornman Diagnostic Center Learning Disabilities

Checklist for Kindergarten and 1st Grade, 2nd ed. Philadelphia, The School District of Philadelphia, 1975 (Out of print; available from the author of this chapter.)

65. The role of occupational therapy as an education-related service. Am J Occup Ther 35:811, 1981
66. Wendt W: I'm Glad You Asked. Occup Ther News 40(8):5, August 1984
67. Where occupational therapists are employed. Occup Ther News 38(10):9, October 1984

68. White M: A first-grade intervention program for children at risk for reading failure. J Learn Disab 12:321, 1979
69. Wilder JM, Wall C: Pennsylvania's Preschool Pilot Individualized Educational Program. Harrisburg, Pennsylvania, CONNECT Division of Special Education, 1976

Appreciation is extended to Richard, Philip, and Elizabeth.

CHAPTER 38

Gerontology* Linda J. Davis

America is aging. Life expectancy at birth has increased dramatically during the 20th century and continues to increase into the dawn of the 21st. Currently, about 80% of the population can expect to survive to the age of 75.[13] The explosion of medical technology and preventive health care has and is adding years to life. Moreover, the resulting reduction of related illness and degeneration promises an unprecedented number and percentage of older adults in the upper age categories. Whereas Americans of the past century who lived past 60 were a distinct and fortunate minority, Americans of the future will probably be planning for an expected life span of nine or more decades.

These changes in the population profile and individual expectancies for longer and healthier lives will profoundly influence many aspects of American life. Of particular concern is health care and the way the health care system will respond to promote and maintain a life of meaningful activity for those who are susceptible to the vicissitudes of aging.

In the US today, the chronic diseases and physical changes associated with age have replaced acute infectious disease as the major causes of death and disability.[16] Persons over the age of 65 comprise approximately 12% of the population yet account for a disproportionate 30% of health expenditures.[45] If the trend continues, at the turn of the 21st century, persons over age 65 will comprise 13% of the population, with the greatest growth in the older categories, and account for 50% of all health care expenses.[13] The costs are primarily related to acute care of the community elderly or to the institutional care of the 5% of the older population who reside in long-term care facilities. The vast majority of older adults are thus adapting idiosyncratically, and on a continuing basis, to the deleterious effects of chronic disorders and aging.[11]

Health care utilization statistics indicate that older people are receiving medical care primarily for acute exacerbations of chronic disease. Given the disabling nature of chronic disease, the great gap is in systematic services that support day-to-day self-management in health maintenance and independence in activities of daily living.[11] For many older people, this gap is partially filled by family members, friends, neighbors, privately paid community service providers, and partly reim-

---

*Some information in this chapter is modified from Davis LJ, Kirkland M: *Role of Occupational Therapy With the Elderly*. Rockville, MD, American Occupational Therapy Association, 1986.

bursed services such as homemakers or Meals-on-Wheels. Services are often fragmented and unstable, depending on the circumstances of the outside provider, creating even more hardship, as arrangements must be continuously altered.

The constellation of changing life expectancy; incomplete, costly health care; and unstable conditions for continuity of care foretell a pressing need for services that will maximize the independence of elderly individuals in their activities of choice and thus reduce inappropriate and unnecessary "doing for" and "doing to".[11] It is clear that most medical services for older adults are not focused on encouraging adaptation to challenges from the environment through therapeutic intervention for self-responsibility. Instead, the focus is on, and reimbursement incentive promotes, symptom-oriented treatment with an assumption that individuals and environments will interact and adapt through an unknown process of stress resolution.

In occupational therapy, health is defined as a status of "optimal functional capacity wherein the individual is able to perform effectively the roles and tasks that are expected."[20] Further, occupational therapy is based on a belief that involvement in a purposeful, self-directed "occupation" enhances functional capacity, adaptation, and performance in roles and tasks. As a profession, occupational therapy supports the concept that mastery of environment leads to feelings of usefulness and to resolution of developmental tasks throughout the life span. As professionals, occupational therapy personnel possess unique attitudes and skills for addressing dysfunction in daily living at the level of adaptation to environmental challenges in chosen activities. Rather than concentrating primarily on symptom-related deficit and treatment, occupational therapy strives to maximize self-responsibility through a focus on individual and environmental assets. Because of this holistic orientation, occupational therapy is in a significant position to contribute to the health care system in closing the gap between medical care and independent community living for both the disabled and the well elderly.

This chapter presents an overview of the domain of gerontic occupational therapy, the aging process, how gerontology can be applied to the occupational therapy process, and treatment approaches. The information is designed to introduce the reader to the scope of gerontology as it interacts with and is applied through occupational therapy practice. Gerontology, the study of aging, is an interdisciplinary area of great theoretical and practical breadth and depth. The growing body of knowledge in biological, psychological, and social aging processes is enormous, well beyond in-depth coverage in this chapter. Bibliographical resources are presented at the end of the chapter for those interested in pursuing particular facets of gerontology. The relationship of occupational therapy to the aging process is an exciting prospect for further study and application to practice.

As a final introductory note, it is important to clarify the terminology that will be used in regard to working with older adults. Several terms commonly used and often confused in the field of aging are: *geriatrics, gerontology, gerontological,* and *gerontic.* "Geron" is from the Greek, meaning old person. "Iatros," meaning healer or physician, combines as a suffix with "geron" to yield geriatrics. Geriatrics is defined herein as medical practice that deals with diseases associated with aging and old people. Gerontology is defined as the study of aging. Thus, the use of "geriatric" or "gerontological" with "occupational therapy" does not correctly describe this area of practice, which is neither primarily medical nor the study of aging.[11] For this reason, the term "gerontic," coined for nursing education by Gunter and Estes[18] and later discussed by Rogers[40] and Freeman[15] has been used to describe the practice of occupational therapy with older adults. Gerontic means "of or pertaining to old age."

The Domain of Gerontic Occupational Therapy

Gerontology and Occupational Therapy

Knowledge in occupational therapy and knowledge in gerontology interface for translation of theory into practice.[11] Multidisciplinary gerontological knowledge can be applied in planning gerontic occupational therapy programs and for utilization of special approaches and techniques in carrying out treatment. Gerontic occupational therapy thus interfaces with all disciplines encompassed in gerontology, such as medicine, sociology, psychology, and physiology. For example, occupational therapy is concerned with the family environment, with attitudes toward aging, and with the function of sensory organs in learning skills. Occupational therapists use theories from these disciplines in combination with occupational therapy models for practice, such as occupational behavior, cognitive disability, or the rehabilitation approach.

Figure 38-1 illustrates the domain of concern in gerontic occupational therapy. The interlocking circles represent occupational therapy, gerontology, and gerontic occupational therapy. Some competencies needed in gerontic practice are shared by all practitioners in gerontology, and some are shared with all practitioners in occupational therapy, and yet gerontic occupational therapy is a unique combination of both. Its domain, then, is *the scientific study of health–aging–illness interactions and their implications for occupational therapy practice.*

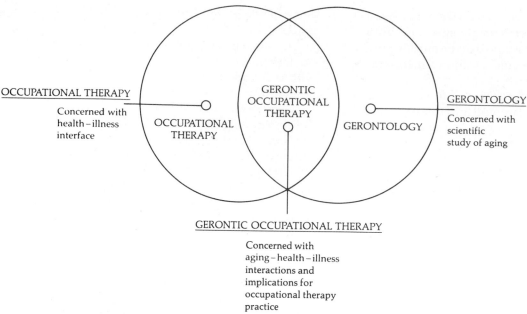

Figure 38-1. The domain of gerontic occupational therapy.

Objectives of Occupational Therapy in Gerontic Practice

Occupational therapy involves the use of goal-directed activity in the evaluation and treatment of persons whose independent functioning has been impaired by normal aging, illness, injury, or developmental disability. It also encompasses the use of preventive approaches, such as environmental modifications, to promote independence, maintenance of wellness, and minimization of disability.

Therapeutic activities are designed to assist individuals in adapting to their social and physical environment, given their functional capacity, through mastery of the tasks essential to their survival and lifestyle. This general objective does not differ from other areas of occupational therapy practice. However, there are services that are of particular importance in gerontic practice:

1. *Education and training in functional activities of daily living.* In addition to usual skills in personal care and household maintenance, special consideration is needed for self-management of nutrition and health regimens, mobility, leisure time, and stress.
2. *Therapeutic adaptations.* Assistive devices, adaptive equipment, and physical environment design need special consideration for their appropriateness for use with older adults.
3. *Compensation for sensory loss.* An area of extreme importance in all aspects of gerontic occupational therapy.

4. *Sensorimotor treatment.* This includes strengthening, endurance, range of motion, coordination, balance, and sensory stimulation.
5. *Cognitive treatment.* Of special importance are memory, orientation, and appropriateness of the level of activity for cognitive capacities.
6. *Prevention and health promotion.* Older adults are in particular need of attention to leisure interests, meaningful activity, self-management skills, socialization, the life review process, energy conservation, body mechanics, and joint protection.
7. *Care of the terminally ill.* Most patients encountered in hospice or other care programs for the terminally ill are in the older age categories. Maintenance of independent living skills, dignity, and comfort are important objectives.
8. *Preretirement education.* A new area of concern for middle-aged and late middle-aged persons, regardless of functional status. It involves preparation for leisure time, assumption of modified work roles, and a lifestyle of health promotion to reduce deleterious effects of aging.

Setting and Roles for Practice

In a recent federally funded project conducted by the American Occupational Therapy Association,* surveys were conducted to assess the extent to which the nearly 40,000 registered occupational therapy personnel work

*The Role of Occupational Therapy with the Elderly (ROTE) funded by the Department of Health and Human Services, Office of Human Development, Administration on Aging, Grant No. 90AT00B3, 1983–1986.

with older adults, the settings in which they work, and the roles and functions they carry out within those settings. Currently, approximately 50% of all occupational therapy personnel, including Registered Occupational Therapists (OTRs) and Certified Occupational Therapy Assistants (COTAs) work full- or part-time with older adults. They provide services in an ever-increasing variety of institutional and community-based settings for practice. These include acute-care hospitals, rehabilitation hospitals, long-term care facilities, outpatient facilities, day centers, home health agencies, senior centers, residential centers, hospices, private practice, health care corporations, and industrial settings.

The professional roles filled by occupational therapy personnel in gerontic practice are varied, overlapping, and often determined by the unique needs of the organization in which they serve. The following list describes each general role and examples of professional functions and positions within that role.

1. *Evaluator:* Screening, assessment, continued evaluation of individual patients. Examples: Clinical evaluator in a geriatric assessment unit; discharge planner in acute-care stroke unit.
2. *Implementer:* Designing and conducting the therapeutic treatment plan. Examples: Practitioners in home health; leader of an activity group in a long-term care facility.
3. *Planner:* Designing and developing new programs. Examples: Industrial preretirement program planner; senior center prevention and wellness program planner; program specialist with a government agency.
4. *Coordinator:* Identifying needs and brokering of services. Examples: Case manager; program coordinator in an adult day center.
5. *Administrator/manager:* Fiscal maintenance, staffing, supervision, quality review, documentation. Examples: Occupational therapy department head; occupational therapy program manager within a corporate health care organization.
6. *Educator:* Relating of professional knowledge and skills formally and informally. Examples: In-service trainer at a skilled nursing facility; patient and family education; university faculty member.
7. *Consultant:* Program-related problem solving. Examples: Consultant to a long-term care facility on activity programming; consultant to an area agency on aging for rehabilitation program planning.
8. *Researcher:* Basic and applied systematic investigation for theory building or validation of practice. Examples: Developer of assessment instruments; investigation in studies of efficacy of occupational therapy treatment.
9. *Advocate:* Promoting policy, legislative programs, and activities that enhance the goals of gerontic occupational therapy. Examples: Community networker; proponent of Medicare legislation that mandates reimbursement of occupational therapy services.

These roles are common to occupational therapy personnel in all areas of practice. It is their application and setting that differ in gerontic practice.

It should be noted at the conclusion of this section on the domain of gerontic occupational therapy that gerontic practice is not a clinical specialty. Rather, it is a generalist practice which manifests in a holistic approach to multifaceted age-related problems, with a special focus on expertise in applied gerontology. With that expertise, the professional practice of occupational therapy may in turn be applied to the older adult in the settings where services are most likely to be delivered.

The Aging Process
Gerontology, Aging, and Development

Philosophical and scientific interest in the unending cycle of birth, maturation, and death, and curiosity about aging processes dates back to ancient times.[42] The value of longevity and rejuvenation has been expressed throughout the ages in stories such as Ponce de Leon's legendary search for the Fountain of Youth and in modern-day promises of potions and mixtures to retard the inevitable aging process. However, prior to the 20th century, systematic study of aging was relatively unknown; rather, the meaning of aging was addressed in the philosophical reflections of poets, novelists, and other observers of life.

The first three decades of the 20th century marked the advent of modern gerontology with the works of Minto, *The Problems of Age, Growth and Death* (1908); Metchnikoff, *The Prolongation of Life* (1908); Hall, *Senescence: the Second Half of Life* (1922); and Cowdry, *Problems of Aging* (1939). E.V. Cowdry is recognized by some as the founding father of modern gerontology because of his book, his recognition of the interdisciplinary nature of gerontology, and his organizational skills in contributing to the establishment of the International Association of Gerontology in 1948.[42]

In the 1940s, scientific interest in aging gained momentum. The Gerontological Society of America, established in 1945, as well as other special-interest units in the public and private sectors, provided the forums in which the issues could be formulated and in which scientific inquiry could be nourished.

Today, gerontology, the scientific study of aging, is flourishing in a worldwide interdisciplinary context. Institutes and centers on aging abound in government, academic, and clinical settings. The ever-expanding literature provides a growing body of knowledge regarding every aspect of the aging process.

Among the questions addressed by gerontology is "What is aging?" Aging is a universal change process that occurs in all living organisms with the passage of time. In the purest sense, "normal" aging, or that which may be due to the passage of time alone, has not yet been distinguished from changes due to harmful life styles or diseases.[49] Evidence exists, however, for "normal" biological changes at the cellular level: in receptors to hormones, protein molecules, the structure of collagen, and nuclear chromosomes. These changes have implications for such outcomes as the different effects of drugs on older people and the stiffening of connective tissue. Nevertheless, much more knowledge of the facts of biological aging is needed before "normal aging" can be distinguished from preventable degeneration.

Senescence is the common term used to describe biological aging from maturation of the organ systems to death. During this period of adulthood, functional decline is observable in various organ systems, whether due to normal aging, disease processes, or the interaction of the two. The extent of functional decline differs dramatically among organ systems and, within a given system, differs equally dramatically among individuals.[26]

Aging as a process also involves widely diversified psychosocial and cognitive change among individuals. These are discussed in Chapter 4. Many view aging negatively as a time of progressive loss of physical and cognitive functioning, social role, meaningful relationships, and valued activities. It is true that profound life changes may occur with such late life events as retirement, geographic mobility of offspring, death of spouse and friends, and lessened ability to engage in certain physical or cognitive activities. However, profound life changes occur at all ages. When they occur at younger ages, they are often thought of as developmental tasks. Perhaps a more positive view of the "losses" commonly associated with old age is the perspective that they are events common in the final stages of a series of sequential developmental stages.

Scholars have only recently begun to focus on the patterns and processes of adult development. Early examples of this work include the "life stages" approach of Charlotte Buhler,[9] Erik Erikson,[14] and Robert Peck.[37] Working from the life stages approach, others, such as Gould,[17] Vaillant,[46] and Levenson[27] have described common developmental processes among specific study populations. What is known thus far is that the effects of late life events on the lifestyle of the individual are highly idiosyncratic and heavily influenced by variables such as attitudes, functional health, and socioeconomic status.

Concomitant with the negative view of aging are the myths and stereotypes that contribute to the pervasive gerontophobia that exists in American society today. Careful scientific study of aging, however, is currently revealing facts which may countermand many of these "common sense" observations. Gerontology may not yet have arrived at the point of clearly defining what aging is, but there is building evidence to refute common myths. For example, Williams[49] and the US Senate Special Committee on Aging report on *Aging America*[45] summarize several interesting points. First, among older persons up to age 80 who are free from identifiable diseases, various organ functions may remain similar to those of young adults, suggesting that preventable disease processes are the primary cause of functional loss. Second, careful longitudinal studies of intelligence demonstrate a consistent level of performance up to age 80, which is as far as research subjects have been followed thus far. Third, personality characteristics tend to remain stable over the years. Fourth, sexual functioning can and does continue in most older people, depending largely on social circumstances. Fifth, most older people stay in close contact with family members; about 80% see relatives at least once a week. Sixth, most older people continue to live in the community. Only 5% are living in a long-term care setting at any given time, and only 20% to 30% ever enter a nursing home. Finally, the majority of older people (65%) perceive themselves to be in excellent or good health compared with others of their own age.

These findings present a profile of promise for successful aging among most adults of today and future years. At the same time that myths are set aside, it should be noted that professionals working in the current health care system are more likely to be involved with the care of older adults who are the exception to these facts about aging. The special needs of the functionally disabled, socially isolated, or institutionalized members of this population are of paramount importance to the occupational therapist, as they are with those at high risk for dependence in any other age group.

Functional Disability and the Older Adult

Functional changes in organ systems, regardless of cause, lead to functional impairments in performance of the activities of daily living. It is not yet clear which changes and impairments of aging are preventable or modifiable by medical and rehabilitation intervention and which are not. Of importance to occupational therapy, however, is an awareness that four of five persons over the age of 65 have at least one chronic condition, with multiple conditions commonplace.[45] Chronic disabling conditions do increase with age, with arthritis, impaired hearing, atherosclerosis, hypertension, chronic heart conditions, and orthopedic impairments heading the list of causes of limitation in activities of daily living. The 1982 National Long-Term Care Survey[45] revealed that 19% of all noninstitutionalized persons over age 65 have some limitation. This percentage increases in a linear fashion with age. That is, among persons 65 to 74 years of age, 13% are limited. This percentage almost doubles to 25% of those between 75 and 84 and more than triples to 46% of those 85 years and older.

In addition to diagnosable chronic diseases, other degenerative conditions that commonly occur contribute to the functional limitations of the elderly. Knowledge of these common age-related changes are useful to occupational therapy personnel so their implications for practice can be taken into consideration. Of importance are changes in the efficiency of the cardiovascular, sensory, musculoskeletal, nervous, respiratory, skin and subcutaneous tissue, metabolic and endocrine, genitourinary, and gastrointestinal systems. Bibliographical resources are provided at the end of the chapter for those who wish to pursue these facts in depth. The general implications for practice include the following:[34]

1. There is a decrease in the speed of return to normal function following exertion.
2. The older body is less efficient in dealing with stress and so has to work harder and longer to adapt.
3. Endurance is diminished, so fatigue from overexertion may become a problem.
4. Exercise and activity of an appropriate intensity is beneficial.
5. Good nutrition is essential.
6. Safety in the environment warrants special attention, including mobility supports, nonslip flooring, and adequate lighting.
7. Compensation for sensory loss is essential, including lighting, glare reduction, contrast coloring, reduction of background noise, and sufficient tactile and olfactory stimulation to surpass the perception threshold.
8. Learning ability and response speed are related to sensory and neurological changes. Pacing, repetition, and multiple cues may be helpful.
9. Joint sensitivity, skeletal fragility, and postural changes should be taken into account when planning and positioning activities.
10. Sensitivity to temperature may cause older persons to become particularly uncomfortable or hypothermic in cool environments.

It is always important, when working with older adults, to remember that biological changes interact with and influence the psychological and social life of the individual. Enthusiasm and enjoyment of activity may be diminished because of pain and difficulty of performance.

Adaptation to biological change is basic in guiding older adults toward continued functional independence in all aspects of their life.

Although the majority of elderly are not disabled, as self-reported in national health surveys, degenerative aging, the high incidence of chronic disease, and the rapid expansion of the older population suggest that a large number of noninstitutionalized elderly are at risk of progressive loss of functional independence. Occupational therapy activities that focus on maintenance of independent living skills, environmental modification, and prevention of severe disability will become increasingly important as the health care system seeks to respond to the needs of this growing population.

Functional disability among older adults is not limited to degenerative and disease-related physical changes. The aging person is also exposed to developmental changes that involve social or cognitive loss during a period in life when support systems and coping mechanisms may be weakened or absent.[31] A variety of interactive physical and psychosocial events may thus seriously threaten the elderly person's emotional health. Further, it is often difficult to distinguish among physical, cognitive, and psychosocial factors in assessing dysfunction. For this reason, it is especially important to approach the older patient in a holistic fashion, attending to all aspects of adaptation to the environment for functional independence. As in physical change, it is also very difficult to distinguish between "normal" and pathological behaviors in the elderly.[19] To some, the term "pathological" or "abnormal" connotes deviance from the cultural norm; to others, it means maladaptive behavior that does not promote the well-being of the individual or the group in which he or she functions. In contrast to mental health, then, psychopathology is characterized by the inability to adapt successfully to life issues of change and concomitant dysfunction in maintenance of independent activity.[31]

Hayslip[19] has conceptualized mental health in the later years into ten factors:

1. Competence in adapting to environmental demands
2. Awareness of one's own changing needs
3. Utilization of opportunities for support
4. Desirability of control over one's environment
5. Willingness to change goals
6. Giving and receiving external rewards
7. Adjustment to the impact of external significant events
8. Willingness to acknowledge feelings about death and dying
9. Perceived family ties
10. Ability to make decisions that imply change

Mental health problems in older adults may be due to cognitive disorders, pre-existing conditions, inability to cope with multiple stresses accompanying the developmental stage, or any combination of these. Due to interactive effects of many factors, evaluation and accurate diagnosis is often difficult.[4,6]

Various estimates have been made regarding the prevalence of mental disorders among the elderly. Pfeiffer indicated that as many as 15% of the noninstitutionalized population suffer from actual psychopathology.[38] Statistics from the National Institutes of Mental Health (NIMH) suggest that older people have fewer mental impairments than other age groups.[45] That same survey found cognitive impairment in approximately 18% of the noninstitutionalized elderly. A similar survey of nursing home residents found that cognitive impairment is a principal cause of institutionalization: 20% of nursing home residents had a primary diagnosis of a mental disorder.

Kemp suggests that *disabled* older persons have a high prevalence of mental health problems that relate to their success in rehabilitation programs.[25] Those problems particularly relevant to occupational therapy include:

Affective disorders: Dysphoria, depression, mania, excessive worry, discouragement and passivity. Of these, depression is probably the most prevalent and damaging. Blazer estimates that 20% to 30% of the disabled elderly suffer from depression.[7] Among the general older population, the rate is estimated at 8% to 15%.[5]

Cognitive impairments: Acute and chronic organic brain syndrome, including drug reactions, Alzheimer's disease, arteriosclerotic dementia, and other degenerative diseases.

Motivational issues: Individual inability or passivity in knowing that what he or she wants and lack of expectation that it can be obtained. This often leads to a lack of adherence to suggested regimens.

Stress-related disorders: Excessive bodily concern, dependence, sick role behavior, and substance abuse.

Family problems: Lack of family support, health, or resources; negative attitudes; feelings of being overburdened; "old business," and open conflict or abuse may cause the older person to feel damaged, isolated, and alone. The family is so important in health care of the elderly that it should be considered the unit of treatment.

Social isolation: Little or no positive or meaningful interaction with friends, relatives, or visitors. This situation occurs in perhaps 15% to 20% of older persons who have a physical disability. Social isolation is strongly linked to functional deficit[8] and depression.[7]

Psychotic behavior: Schizophrenia, paranoia including delusional systems, hallucinations, disorientation, and memory loss are relatively rare but may accompany dementia. Schizophrenia is more often found in institutionalized elderly who were diagnosed earlier in life and have grown old in custodial care.

Special groups: Unique mental health problems may be found in several subgroups of the elderly population who have received little attention in gerontology research thus far. These include: (1) persons with early life disability or mental retardation who are now growing older and adapting to aging; (2) deinstitutionalized elderly who, after living for many years in custodial settings, are now adapting simultaneously to aging and to community life ("bag ladies" are included in this group); and (3) ethnic and racial minority aged who differ in their cultural adaptation to aging. Understanding of cultural variance is critical to appropriate mental health assessment, treatment, and support.

Occupational therapy personnel should be aware that physical, cognitive, and psychosocial dysfunction are closely related in the elderly. The inability to carry out expected roles and responsibilities may be both due to and result in mental health problems and dysfunction behavior. Occupational therapy can contribute in significant ways in the assessment and treatment of geriatric psychopathology. Drawing on knowledge of physical and psychosocial dysfunction, human development, and the use of activity, occupational therapy personnel offer unique and valuable therapeutic interventions that can significantly promote positive mental health and independent living.

Gerontology Applied to the Occupational Therapy Process

The occupational therapy process in gerontic practice includes assessment of the impact of disease, aging, and social change on the work, leisure, and self-maintenance activities of the elderly, and planning and implementation of interventions that maximize the older person's functional performance in basic daily living skills.[20,41] Terms synonymous with basic living skills are *activities of daily living* (ADL), *functional activities, functional capacity, routine tasks of daily living,* and *occupational performance.*[41] Occupational therapy personnel perform the basic roles of evaluator and implementer of therapeutic treatment, in the variety of settings described earlier, across the continuum of health care services. The increasing involvement of occupational therapy in these settings has resulted in additional diversified roles. In gerontic practice, these include but are not limited to interdisciplinary team member,[36] case manager,[43] consultant,[30] educator,[21] discharge planner, and program manager. Occupational therapy personnel often work closely with family and with members of other professional disciplines due to the complexity of ADL dysfunction in the elderly.[21,36]

In all settings, however, the overall goal of gerontic occupational therapy remains the same: facilitation of continued meaningful daily activity for promotion of well-being and "total optimal performance in life's tasks."[32] The basic occupational therapy process of assessment, treatment planning, treatment implementation, continuity of care, and documentation does not differ from that for other age groups. There are components of the process, however, that should be modified to take into consideration the special characteristics of older adults and application of gerontological knowledge in their care. These modifications are discussed in the following sections.

Assessment

Assessment of the health status of the elderly is conducted across all disciplines involved in geriatrics and gerontology. Kane and Kane, in a comprehensive analysis of important health indicators and instruments to measure them, state that: "Measures of functional status that examine ability to function independently despite disease, physical and mental disability are the most useful overall indicators to assist those who care for the elderly."[23] The occupational therapist's training and expertise in the assessment of independent living skills thus make a critical and unique contribution to a complex multidisciplinary process.[21]

Assessment in occupational therapy generally refers to the overall process of determining the need for treatment. Evaluation, a subcategory of assessment, refers to the gathering and interpretation of data necessary for treatment planning. In gerontic practice, assessment involves a description of the older adult's strengths and weaknesses in daily living skills. Rogers suggests that an occupational history obtained from the older adult, the caregiver, or both, provides necessary information on how the individual performs "routinely," satisfaction level with performance, and expectations for performance.[41] Information on the balance of leisure, work, and self-care; aging and disease processes that have led to current lifestyle; and environmental conditions that promote or hinder performance provide the therapist a general picture of the daily living situation.

In gerontic practice, it is important that data provided through such an assessment be supplemented by objective performance evaluations that test the individual's competence in biological and cognitive parameters and in daily living skills (see Kane and Kane for specific evaluation instruments.[23]) Discrepancies between what the person is doing, can do, wants to do, and has the potential to do then become the focal point of intervention.[41] In utilizing these evaluation instruments, it is important to obtain objective performance measures in the context of normal living situations, the physical and social environments in which daily living skills are routinely exercised. Also, in conducting evaluations of older adults, care should be taken to compensate for sensory loss, fatigue, and unfamiliar surroundings.

Hasselkus points out the challenge to occupational therapists in the struggle to identify and measure important components of functional activities of daily living.[21] With unique expertise in understanding objective versus subjective performance, and individualized versus standardized evaluation, the occupational therapist can contribute significantly to the development of sound, holistic approaches to measurement in this area of geriatric health care.

Treatment Planning

Treatment planning, based on assessment and evaluation, consists of two phases: problem identification and goal setting.[47]

As noted previously, sorting out the functional problems of the older adult is a complex challenge. Often, it is difficult to identify the specific problems at the individual and environmental levels that are most important to the individual and caregiver and are most amenable to intervention. Some problems are obvious, others subtle. Expectations for improvement differ among patient, caregiver, and care provider. Although all functional problems may be considered important by the therapist, those which create the most difficulty for patient and caregiver may be sorted out and addressed first. Remembering that gerontic occupational therapy personnel usually function with an interdisciplinary team, the therapist should consider whether the problem is within the domain of occupational therapy and, if so, how best to collaborate with patient, family, and other disciplines in goal setting and intervention.

Once shared problems are identified, occupational therapy goals are developed to give direction to expected short- and long-term efforts. In general, goal setting for the older adult should be appropriate to the condition but high. Wells points out that older adults may not be as fragile as they first appear and that with specific self-selected goals, they may accomplish more than believed possible.[47]

Treatment Implementation and Continuity of Care

Re-evaluation and follow-up activities are of particular importance in gerontic treatment implementation. Re-evaluation means continual analysis of the efficacy of treatment, a redefinition of problems, and resetting of more precise short- and long-term goals. Treatment progress may vary with the elderly for many reasons; perhaps the most important is the motivation of the patient to continue striving for functional goals in the face of fatigue, discouragement with slow progress, and the stress of adapting to multiple intrinsic changes and demands from the environment. Care should be taken to maintain goals at an achievable level, where the individual can perceive success and benefit from treatment and where the cost of the effort does not exceed and destroy the motivation toward functional independence.

Follow-up means continued contact with a patient outside the occupational therapy treatment setting to ensure continuity of therapeutic regimens and newly acquired adaptive skills.[47] Often, elderly patients "disappear" into institutional or community residential settings with little assurance of the linkages that will support gains made in the treatment setting. Follow-up is logistically difficult but strongly suggested in some form of continued contact for extending treatment into all aspects of the older patient's functional living environment.

Documentation

Fundamental principles of documentation, evaluation, and quality assurance do not vary according to the age of the client. Several issues important to gerontic occupational therapy should be considered, however, when planning documentation and patient care monitoring.[22] First, what are important monitors of care in gerontic occupational therapy? These include but are not limited to level of functional independence, degree of adherence to suggested regimens, understanding of condition, discharge destination, and most effective length of hospital stay or treatment period. Second, do standards for outcomes differ for the elderly compared with other age groups? An example of a likely difference is in adherence to therapeutic regimens: lower adherence might be expected due to negative side effects or cognitive problems. Third, under current funding mechanisms, what issues should receive priority for documentation and program evaluation? A demonstration of the efficacy of occupational therapy in cost containment, by preventing older adults from "excessive" acute hospitalization or by retaining full benefits of treatment through improved function in activities of daily living, would support continued funding for occupational therapy services.

As Joe points out, competition is keen among health care services for funding and reimbursement.[22] Perhaps this is especially true in the multidisciplinary climate of geriatric care. Having good evaluation systems in place will help to assure professional survival for gerontic practitioners.

Treatment Approaches

The chapter thus far has provided a broad description of gerontic practice, the roles and functions of practitioners, and the application of basic gerontology to the occupational therapy process. Because of the biopsychosocial origins of older adult dysfunction, gerontic occupational therapy requires a multifaceted approach using therapeutic procedures and techniques that are the intervention tools of the profession. As Rogers states, "gerontic practice integrates physical disabilities and psychosocial occupational therapy."[41]

Gerontic practice encompasses two general treatment approaches: *remedial* and *compensatory*.[41] Remedial treatment aims toward full restoration of function. When such outcomes cannot be expected, a compensatory approach is used to overcome the deficiency and dysfunction. Whether one approach or both are used, the success of treatment is measured by the effect on function rather than by the impact on dimensions of function. Often, treatment is a blend of remedial and compensatory techniques, with reciprocal influence of one on the other.

Several treatment approaches common to all occupational therapy practice are particularly appropriate in gerontic practice. These include activity programming, prevention, ADL, therapeutic adaptations (including compensation for sensory loss), cognitive treatment, psychosocial treatment, and care of the terminally ill. Sensorimotor treatment is also of importance, especially for techniques that address the dimensions of dysfunction, such as strength and range of motion. This area of practice, however, is in particular need of extensive review and definition of its optimal use in gerontic practice.

The following sections describe each treatment approach, its purpose, and the major considerations for gerontic practice. No attempt is made to relate specific techniques for implementation of each approach. References and bibliographical resources are provided for the reader who desires in-depth material or methods for practice.

Activity Programming

Activity programming is not a discrete treatment approach per se but is used across remedial and compensatory interventions. It is differentiated from "treatment" in that it is not focused on a treatment goal. Rather, it supports and supplements therapeutic objectives through reinforcement and enjoyment of skills.[10]

Activities are purposeful tasks that require skills and resources to meet intrapersonal and interpersonal needs through participation in the continuum of work and leisure.[24] Activity programming becomes necessary when daily living patterns of activity are no longer established by the individual. They enrich the environment and life of the older adult, not by providing passive "busy work," but by involving participants in every step of the process, from planning to implementation.

Activity programs are common in long-term care institutions, day programs, senior centers, and residential settings. They are often implemented by trained or untrained "activity directors." By virtue of their special expertise in the use of activity, occupational therapy personnel are important to these programs as consultants, planners, administrators, or direct service implementers.

Prevention

Prevention may be added to the two basic remedial and compensatory approaches. On the continuum of health care of the elderly, it may be used with both remedial and compensatory techniques in any setting for gerontic practice. Its *primary* aim, however, is reduction of the risk of disease or disability and prevention of dependence and institutionalization.[35] In practice, it includes interventions that focus on: (1) elimination of casual factors of dysfunction, such as architectural barriers, lack of transportation, and unusable consumer goods; (2) assisting the individual in avoiding dysfunction through behavioral changes, improved coping skills, and incorporation of external protective measures in ADL; and (3) preventing deterioration and dysfunction after the onset of disease among those who are particularly vulnerable to severe disability.

Interventions defined as prevention and health promotion are increasingly considered to be of paramount importance in the total rehabilitative care of the elderly.[1] Economic and demographic imperatives are bringing into sharp focus the need to support health care activities that allow older adults optimum achievement of age-specific developmental tasks with independence and competence. Occupational therapists, by virtue of their concern with daily living skills, are in perhaps the best professional position to assume leadership in preventing ADL dysfunction.

Activities of Daily Living and Therapeutic Adaptations

Interventions in ADL, including therapeutic adaptations as described previously throughout the chapter, are the heart of gerontic occupational therapy. ADLs with older adults must be considered, in a global sense, to include the whole spectrum of the individual's functional involvement with his or her environment.[48] Important basic activities, with the elderly as with all age groups, are *mobility* (including transportation and transfers), *eating, bathroom activities, dressing, communication, housekeeping, house repair, financial management,* and *obtaining goods and services.* Precautions and modifications are indicated to compensate for sensory loss, joint limitation, and cognitive changes such as confusion and memory loss. Several areas of ADL treatment warrant special attention in relation to the older adult:

posture, sleep and rest, proper nutrition, self-medication, and management of incontinence.[48]

Therapeutic adaptations in gerontic occupational therapy refers to the design or restructuring physical environmental supports to assist in self-care and work and leisure activities. Common interventions are orthotics, assistive/adaptive equipment, and environmental modification. Application is much the same as with other age groups. Special attention should be given to the effects of sensory loss, changes in integument with age, and the desirability to individual and family of suggested equipment or environmental changes.

In environmental modifications, changes are often disability specific but should always take into account sensory change deficits in mobility associated with the aging process. Lighting, contrasting colors and textures, visual cues, and arrangement of furniture and other possessions are important considerations.[28]

Cognitive Treatment

Cognitive treatment refers to the interventions addressing the dysfunction associated with senile dementia. Levy points out that in true irreversible dementia, nothing can be done to treat the disease itself. Instead, the treatment approach is "one of helping the afflicted individual maintain as much comfort and dignity as possible through the course of the disease."[29]

Helping each individual to optimize functional potential and supporting caregivers are both important. The most promising approach, however, involves modification of the environment to provide the "just right" stimulation to enable individual function at the best of capacity. This approach is effective in reducing confusion, agitation, and frustration and in enhancing individual satisfaction in functioning.[29] Sensory stimulation, activity stimulation, milieu approaches, group approaches, and behavioral approaches are all commonly used in the domain of gerontic occupational therapy. Reality orientation has been a favored approach since its inception in the 1950s. However, recent reports of its effectiveness, as reviewed by Levy.[29] suggest that it may not be as effective as originally believed and in fact may produce negative outcomes.

A frame of reference that has recently emerged in the occupational therapy literature, *cognitive disability,*[2] may prove extremely useful in providing guidelines for environmental modifications that are specific to cognitive deficit. Cognitive disability presents a much-needed theoretical basis of occupational therapists in planning the "just right" fit of individual and environment to help compensate for cognitive deficit and promote optimal function in daily living skills.

Psychosocial Treatment

An important factor in psychosocial treatment of the elderly is to remember that psychosocial components of well-being cannot be separated from successful independent functioning in ADL or from any other treatment approach. Gerontic occupational therapy settings that provide primarily psychosocial treatment are inpatient and outpatient psychogeriatric services, long-term care facilities, day treatment programs, home health programs, senior centers, and freestanding prevention programs.[33]

Two major occupational therapy goals that are effectively incorporated into psychosocial treatment are: (1) provision of a supportive environment for problem solving, self-expression, adaptation to functional living problems, learning new skills, and positive self-regard; and (2) emotional and social reintegration through individual activity. These goals are accomplished through treatment approaches similar to those listed for cognitive treatment.

It has been suggested in the literature on psychiatric care of the elderly that significant professional attitudinal barriers may exist regarding the worth of older people and older persons' ability to manage their own lives.[3] Therapists may underestimate the potential of older patients, may not understand the needs of the patient in the developmental context, may fail to comprehend the underlying reasons for dysfunctional behaviors, and may be negatively affected by the poor interpersonal behavior of some elderly people. To act as agents of change in reducing psychosocial dysfunction in elderly patients, occupational therapy personnel may have to challenge long-standing negative attitudes and myths. To succeed in confronting such attitudes, occupational therapy personnel must be willing to accept as biased the therapeutic pessimism that so often surrounds rehabilitation of the elderly. Commitment to treatment of the elderly depends on a belief that function and satisfaction can be maintained or improved throughout the life span.[33]

Sensorimotor Treatment

Sensorimotor treatment approaches include both neuromuscular treatment and sensory integration. In the neuromuscular component of treatment, which includes reflex integration, muscle testing, range of motion, and coordination and exercise tests, procedures used with all age groups can be adapted, taking into account the anatomical and physiological needs of the elderly. Several age- and disease-related problems are especially relevant to these adaptations:

1. Aeration: problems with shortness of breath, dizziness, dozing, and standing endurance may be related to poor posture and lack of oxygen.
2. Swallowing and coughing: head posture, tongue control, and reflexes may be impaired.
3. Positioning: exercise limitations, joint protection, and pain reduction are important in preventing

demineralization and joint deformity in osteoporosis and osteoarthritis.
4. Pain tolerance may be affected by edema, inflammation, and hypertonicity.
5. Balance: stable mobility may be affected by visual problems, antigravity muscle coordination, and vestibular function.
6. Trunk rotation: rigidity in turning and reaching and spasticity in the extremities are especially problematic in ADL.
7. Hand function: a multiplicity of factors may affect hand function, including tactile sensory loss, arthritis, intrinsic muscle coordination, flaccidity, spasticity, and lack of eye–hand coordination.

The influence of these and other age-related conditions on neuromuscular treatment are in need of definition and articulation in the gerontic occupational therapy literature.

The sensory integration component of sensorimotor treatment is frequently applied clinically but not well developed theoretically for application to the older adult. Sensory integration is often referred to as sensory stimulation in gerontic occupational therapy literature. It usually is comprised of therapeutic techniques that use sensory input to evoke a motor response, which, in turn, results in an adaptive functional performance. Most sensory stimulation programs thus described are concerned primarily with cognitive and psychosocial treatment of institutionalized older adults. Although these forms of sensory stimulation treatment are useful, applications of sensory integration should be carefully analyzed and synthesized for therapeutic use with the normal and pathological aspects of the aging nervous system. Only then can practitioners conceptualize appropriate, safe, and productive sensory integration treatment programs for older adults.

Care of the Terminally Ill

Terminally ill older people are assessed and treated by occupational therapy personnel in a variety of environments, including hospices, hospitals, the home, nursing homes, and day centers.[39] The important contribution of occupational therapy in this area is helping the individual to die with dignity by enhancing the control he or she wishes to exercise over what remains of life. The capacity to exercise control and the desirability of independence varies from one person to the next. Goals relevant to continued function in important living tasks should be articulated by the patient and should be short term in view of a limited time frame.[39] Occupational therapy has a role in supporting the family (which is regarded as the "unit" facing the terminal condition) by assisting them in reorganizing their own lives and in enhancing the care of the patient.

Hospice care is a setting for growing occupational therapy involvement. There are five basic tenets of hospice care: pain and symptom control; diagnostic honesty; quality of life; around-the-clock availability of staff with patients in home care; and 12-month bereavement follow-up.[44] In hospice care, occupational therapy personnel can make significant contributions in assessment and goal setting for patient and family, in facilitating ADL function, and in diagnostic honesty when temporarily improved physical function may blur the importance of realistic goal setting.

Hospice care is a difficult challenge that goes beyond working with any age group. As Tigges points out, it calls for working with people who know they are going to die and want professional help to support them in fulfilling their last desires.[44] Occupational therapy personnel can provide much to the terminally ill by helping them engage actively in what remains of their lives.

Conclusion

Gerontology and occupational therapy interface on all aspects of the developmental process and at all levels of practice. Much work remains, however, in precisely articulating those relationships and in validating gerontic occupational therapy practice. The focus of occupational therapy with older adults is daily living skills.[41] In order to function effectively, occupational therapy personnel need to acquire competencies in gerontological knowledge related to supporting living skills and its application to practice. These competencies include:

1. An understanding of aging as a normal development process
2. Knowledge of the basic biological and psychosocial aspects of the aging process
3. An awareness of the incidence, prevalence, and characteristics of diseases and psychosocial disorders associated with aging
4. An understanding of the roles and functions of occupational therapy personnel in a variety of gerontic practice settings
5. Application of principles of assessment, treatment planning, implementation, continuity, and evaluation to gerontic practice
6. An understanding of chronic illness and disability as an adaptive task for older adults
7. Development of effective gerontic occupational therapy programs in activity programming, prevention, activities of daily living, therapeutic adaptation, cognitive and psychosocial treatment, sensorimotor treatment, and care of the terminally ill
8. Ability to function on an interdisciplinary team in various capacities and models of service coordination
9. Patient and family education
10. Development of skills in consultancy and community networking.[12]

The magnitude and complexity of the subject matter that constitutes gerontic occupational therapy is a challenge worthy of continued study and careful consideration in program planning.

References

1. Abdellah FG: Public Health Aspects of Rehabilitation of the Aged, p 55. In Brody SJ, Ruff GE: Aging and Rehabilitation. New York, Springer, 1986
2. Allen C: Occupational Therapy for Psychiatric Diseases: Measurement and Management of Cognitive Disability. Boston, Little, Brown, 1985
3. Arie T: Prevention of mental disorders in old age. J Am Ger Soc 32:460, 1984
4. Birren JE, Renner VJ: Concepts and Issues in Mental Health and Aging. In Birren JE, Sloane RB (eds): Handbook of Mental Health and Aging. Englewood Cliffs, New Jersey, Prentice–Hall, 1980
5. Birren JE, Sloane RB: Handbook of Mental Health and Aging. Englewood Cliffs, New Jersey, Prentice–Hall, 1980
6. Blazer D: The Epidemiology of Mental Illness in Late Life. In Busse E, Blazer D (eds): Handbook of Geriatric Psychiatry. New York, Van Nostrand Reinhold, 1980
7. Blazer D: Depression in Late Life. St. Louis, CV Mosby, 1982
8. Brummel–Smith K: Training health professionals: A rehabilitation orientation could improve the gerontology field. Generations 8:47, 1984
9. Buhler C: The curve of life as studied in biographies. J Appl Psychol 19, 1935
10. Crepeau EL: Activity programming. In Davis LJ, Kirkland M (eds): Role of Occupational Therapy with the Elderly, p 199. Rockville, Maryland, American Occupational Therapy Association, 1986
11. Davis LJ: Introduction. In Davis LJ, Kirkland M (eds): Role of Occupational Therapy with the Elderly, pp 1,5. Rockville, Maryland, American Occupational Therapy Association, 1986
12. Davis LJ, Kirkland M (eds): Role of Occupational Therapy with the Elderly. Rockville, Maryland, American Occupational Therapy Association, 1986
13. Dychtwald K: Wellness and Health Promotion for the Elderly, p 2. Rockville, Maryland, Aspen, 1986
14. Erikson E: Childhood and Society, 2nd ed. New York, WW Norton, 1963
15. Freeman JT: Gerontism: A neologism. Exp Gerontol 20:71, 1985
16. Fries JF, Crapo LM: The elimination of premature disease. In Dychtwald K (ed): Wellness and Health Promotion for the Elderly, p 22. Rockville, Maryland, Aspen, 1986
17. Gould RC: The phases of adult life: A study in developmental psychology. Am J Psychiatr 129:521, 1972
18. Gunter L, Estes C: Education for Gerontic Nursing, p 31. New York, Springer, 1979
19. Hayslip B: Mental health and aging. In Ernst NS, Glazer–

Waldman JR (eds): The Aged Patient: A Sourcebook for the Allied Health Professional, pp 158–181. Chicago, Year Book Medical Publishers, 1983

20. Hasselkus BR: The occupational therapist. In Maguire GH (ed): Care of the Elderly: A Health Team Approach, pp 145–146. Boston, Little, Brown, 1986

21. Hasselkus BR: Patient education. In Davis LJ, Kirkland M (eds): Role of Occupational Therapy with the Elderly, pp 123, 126. Rockville, Maryland, American Occupational Therapy Association, 1986

22. Joe, BE: Quality assurance and accountability. In Davis LJ, Kirkland M (eds): Role of Occupationional Therapy with the Elderly, p 42. Rockville, Maryland, American Occupational Therapy Association, 1986

23. Kane RE, Kane RL: Assessing the Elderly: A Practical Guide to Measurement, p 1. Lexington, DC Heath, 1981

24. Kielhofner G, Burke JP: A model of human operation I: Structure and content. Am J Occup Ther 34:731, 1980

25. Kemp B: Psychosocial and mental health issues in rehabilitation of older persons. In Brody SJ, Ruff GE (eds): Aging and Rehabilitation, p 127. New York, Springer, 1986

26. Lakatta EG: Health, disease and cardiovascular aging. In Health in an Older Society, p 73. Institute of Medicine and National Research Council. Washington, DC, National Academy Press, 1985

27. Levenson DJ: The Seasons of a Man's Life. New York, Ballantine Books, 1978

28. Levy LL: Sensory change and compensation. In Davis LJ, Kirkland M (eds): Role of Occupational Therapy with the Elderly, pp 58–64. Rockville, Maryland, The American Occupational Therapy Association, 1986

29. Levy LL: Cognitive treatment. In Davis LJ, Kirkland M (eds): Role of Occupational Therapy with the Elderly, pp 193, 294, 303–305. Rockville, Maryland, American Occupational Therapy Association, 1986

30. Lewis SC: Consultation in gerontic occupational therapy. In Davis LJ, Kirkland M (eds): Role of Occupational Therapy with the Elderly, pp 385–392. Rockville, Maryland, American Occupational Therapy Association, 1986

31. Macdonald KC, Davis LJ: Psychopathology of aging. In Davis LJ, Kirkland M (eds): Role of Occupational Therapy with the Elderly, pp 103–104. Rockville, Maryland, American Occupational Therapy Association, 1986

32. Maguire GH: Occupational therapy: The role of education in occupational therapy for the aged. Gerontol Geriatr Educ 1:115, 1980

33. Mayer MA: Psychosocial treatment approaches. In Davis LJ, Kirkland M (eds): Role of Occupational Therapy with the Elderly, pp 329, 332. Rockville, Maryland, American Occupational Therapy Association, 1986

34. Menks F: Anatomical and physiological changes in late adulthood. In Davis LJ, Kirkland M (eds): Role of Occupational Therapy with the Elderly, p 46. Rockville, Maryland, The American Occupational Therapy Association, 1986

35. Miller PA: Preventive treatment approaches. In Davis LJ, Kirkland M (eds): Role of Occupational Therapy with the Elderly, p 227. Rockville, Maryland, American Occupational Therapy Association, 1986

36. Nystrom EP, Evans LS: The interdisciplinary treatment approach. In Davis LJ, Kirkland M (eds): Role of Occupa-

tional Therapy with the Elderly. Rockville, Maryland, American Occupational Therapy Association, 1986

37. Peck R: Psychological developments in the second half of life. In Neugarten BL (ed): Middle Age and Aging. Chicago, University of Chicago Press, 1968

38. Pfieffer E: Psychopathology and social pathology. In Birren JE, Schaie KW (eds): Handbook of the Psychology of Aging. New York, Van Nostrand Reinhold, 1977

39. Pizzi M: Care of the terminally ill, part I. In Davis LJ, Kirkland M (eds): Role of Occupational Therapy with the Elderly, pp 241, 243. Rockville, Maryland, American Occupational Therapy Association, 1986

40. Rogers JC: The issue—Gerontic occupational therapy. Am J Occup Ther 35:663, 1981

41. Rogers JC: Roles and functions of occupational therapy in gerontic practice. In Davis LJ, Kirkland M (eds): Role of Occupational Therapy with the Elderly, pp 118–119. Rockville, Maryland, American Occupational Therapy Association, 1986

42. Schwartz AN, Snyder CL, Peterson JA: Aging and Life: An Introduction to Gerontology, 2nd ed, p 10. New York, Holt, Rinehart and Winston, 1984

43. Snow TL: Case management. In Davis LJ, Kirkland M (eds): Role of Occupational Therapy with the Elderly, p 7. Rockville, Maryland, American Occupational Therapy Association, 1986

44. Tigges KN: Care of the terminally ill, part 2. In Davis LJ, Kirkland M (eds): Role of Occupational Therapy with the Elderly, pp 253, 260. Rockville, Maryland, American Occupational Therapy Association, 1986

45. US Senate Special Committee on Aging: Aging America: Trends and Projections, 1985–86 ed, pp 91, 103. Washington, DC, US Government Printing Office 498-116-814/42395, 1986

46. Vaillant GE: Adaptation to Life. Boston, Little, Brown, 1977

47. Wells MA: Treatment planning. In Davis LJ, Kirkland M (eds): Role of Occupational Therapy with the Elderly, pp 126, 133. Rockville, Maryland, American Occupational Therapy Association, 1986

48. Wells MA, Chew TA, Lang B, Campbell BA, Chenderlin JJ: Activities of daily living. In Davis LJ, Kirkland M (eds): Role of Occupational Therapy with the Elderly, pp 269, 279. Rockville, Maryland, American Occupational Therapy Association, 1986

49. Williams TF: The aging process: Biological and psychosocial considerations. In Brody SJ, Ruff GE (eds): Aging and Rehabilitation: Advances in the State of the Art, p 13. New York, Springer, 1986

Bibliography

Position Papers

Commission on Practice Hospice Task Force: Occupational therapy and hospice. Am J Occup Ther 40:839, 1986

Levy LL: Occupational therapy in adult day care. Am J Occup Ther 40:814, 1986

Macdonald KC, Epstein CF, Vastano S: Roles and functions of

occupational therapy in adult day care. Am J Occup Ther 40:817, 1986

Marshall E, Kerr J: The Role of the Occupational Therapist in Home Health Care. Rockville, MD, American Occupational Therapy Association, 1981

Rogers JC: Roles and Functions of Occupational Therapy in Long Term Care. *Ibid.*, 1983

Rogers JC: Occupational therapy services for Alzheimer's disease and related disorders. Am J Occup Ther 40:822, 1986

Standards of Practice

American Occupational Therapy Association: Standards of Practice for Occupational Therapy Services in a Home Health Program, 1978

Ellis NB: Sustaining the frail disabled elderly in the community: An innovative approach to in-home services. In Gerontological Social Work in Home Health Care. New York, Haworth Press, 1984

Ellis NB: Aging: Occupational therapy and the demographic imperative. Occup Ther News 39:4, 1985

Strasburg DM, Gingher MC: A review of entry-level education in gerontology. Am J Occup Ther 40:557, 1986

The Aging Process

Birren JE, Schaie KW (eds): Handbook of the Psychology of Aging. 2nd ed. New York, Van Nostrand Reinhold, 1985

Birren JE, Woodruff DS (eds): Aging: Scientific Perspectives and Social Issues. 2nd ed. Monterey, Brooks/Cole, 1983

Binstock RH, Shanas E (eds): Handbook of Aging and the Social Sciences. 2nd ed. New York, Van Nostrand Reinhold, 1985

Ebersole P, Hess P: Toward Health Aging: Human Needs and Nursing Response. St Louis, CV Mosby, 1981

Finch CE, Schneider EL (eds): Handbook of the Biology of Aging. 2nd ed. New York, Van Nostrand Reinhold, 1985

Kimmel DC: Adulthood and Aging. 2nd ed. New York, John Wiley & Sons, 1980

Lawton MP: Environment and Aging. Los Angeles, Brooks/Cole, 1980

Saxon SV, Etten MJ: Physical Changes and Aging: A Guide for the Helping Professions. New York, Teresias Press, 1978

Gerontic Treatment

Bachner SC: Retirement activity planning. In Davis LJ, Kirkland M (eds): Role of Occupational Therapy with the Elderly. Rockville, Maryland, American Occupational Therapy Association, 1986

Brever J: A Handbook of Assistive Devices for the Handicapped Elderly: New Help for Independent Living. New York, Haworth Press, 1982

Brody SJ, Ruff GE (eds): Aging and Rehabilitation: Advances in the State of the Art. New York, Springer, 1986

Butler RN: The life review: An interpretation of reminiscence in the aged. In Neugarten BL (ed): Middle Age and Aging. Chicago, University of Chicago Press, 1968

Butler RN, Lewis MI. Aging and Mental Health: Positive Psychosocial and Biomedical Approaches. 3rd ed. St Louis, CV Mosby, 1982

Crossman L, Kaljian D. The family: Cornerstone of care. Generations 8:44, 1984

Dychtwald K. Wellness and Health Promotion for the Elderly. Rockville, Maryland, Aspen, 1986

Ernst NS, Glazer–Waldman JR (eds): The Aged Patient: A Sourcebook for the Allied Health Professional. Chicago, Year Book Medical Publishers, 1983

Hartford ME: The use of group methods for work with the aged. In Birren JE, Sloane RB (eds): Handbook of Mental Health and Aging. Englewood Cliffs, New Jersey, Prentice–Hall, 1980

Hasselkus BR: Patient education and the elderly. Phys Occup Ther Geriatr 2:55, 1983

Kane RA, Kane RL: Assessing the Elderly. Lexington, Lexington Books, 1981

Kirchman M: The preventive role of activity: Myth or reality —A review of the literature. Phys Occup Ther Geriatr 2:39, 1983

Maguire GH (ed): Care of the Elderly: A Health Team Approach. Boston, Little, Brown, 1985

Oriol W: The Complex Cube of Long Term Care: The Case for Next Step Solutions—Now. Washington, DC, American Health Planning Association, 1985

Pizzi M: Hospice and the terminally ill geriatric patient. Phys Occup Ther Geriatr 3:45, 1983

Steinberg RM, Carter GW: Case Management and the Elderly: A Handbook for Planning and Administering Programs. Lexington, Lexington Books, 1982

Tickle LS, Yerxa EJ: Need satisfaction of older persons living in the community and in institutions 1: The environment. Am J Occup Ther 35:644, 1981

Tickle LS, Yerxa EJ: Need satisfaction of older persons living in the community and in institutions 2: Role of activity. Am J Occup Ther 35:650, 1981

Tigges K: Occupational therapy in hospice. In Corr CA, Corr DM (eds): Hospice Care: Principles and Practice. New York, Springer, 1983

CHAPTER 39

Community Home Health Care *Ruth Ellen Levine*

Today, many patients who were previously cared for as inpatients are now cared for at home. Examples include individuals who require intravenous solutions, chemotherapy, and respiratory treatment. In fact, home-care practitioners are frequently asked to treat patients in ways that require the use of complex equipment. This change occurred because of newly developed Medicare Diagnostic-Related Groups (DRGs), a system that uses statistical averages to determine the reimbursement for a hospital on the basis of a patient's diagnosis and age. Thus, many of the present population of homebound patients are more acutely ill and the family caregivers more anxious and taxed.

Home health services may be defined as an array of services provided to individuals and families in their places of residence or in ambulatory-care settings for purposes of preventing disease; promoting, maintaining, or restoring health; or minimizing the effects of disability.[1] Home care can be described as a holistic context for providing therapeutic services in the patient's home. A home-care agency offers skilled professional services, such as nursing; physical, occupational, and speech therapies; medical social service; laboratory testing; and other services such as light housekeeping, shopping, and personal care. Also available are counseling, specialized testing, and visits from other health specialists such as podiatrists, dentists, and respiratory therapists.

This chapter describes a growing area of occupational therapy practice—home care. In 1982, 4% of all American Occupational Therapy Association (AOTA) members worked in home care, in contrast to 1% in earlier years, and the numbers of home-care specialists continue to increase in this high-growth area of practice.[30] This chapter will explain why home-care practice is growing in popularity, offering an overview of home-care practice, defining frequently used terms and boundaries, presenting a theoretical overview, presenting a delivery process, and discussing current social issues that affect delivery.

Home-care delivery can take place in an urban, suburban, or rural setting. No matter where the service is delivered, the delivery principles and methods are the same. Also, 28% of one population of home-care therapists work in a combination of three geographic areas in a practice that includes urban, rural, and suburban patients; moreover, 21% work in both suburban and urban areas.[31] Thus, home-care therapists must learn to adjust to a variety of settings. Many therapists are entering home care as a full-fledged specialty area.

The average home-care therapist has worked for more than 12 years, 6 of them in home health. Just over half (53%) work part-time, and 24% have master's degrees. About half work for one agency, but many work for several. By working in home care, therapists find that they can augment a full-time position or devote full time to a practice. Fees range from $18 to $45 per visit.[31] A fictitious profile of a person who might enter home care is as follows:

Profile and Case Study

Stacy Reynolds, OTR, graduated from an entry-level program more than 10 years ago. She liked her job in a rehabilitation center but wanted to see patients in their own homes, since she felt that patients might be more motivated. Stacy also felt that home-care therapists have more control over scheduling and allocating treatment time. For these reasons, Stacy applied for a position with a private practice group where she would receive supervision, realizing she needed to learn more about delivery methods, documentation requirements, and patient and caregiver teaching. The private practice supervisor told Stacy that she would be an asset to the group since Stacy, like many home-care therapists, was an experienced OTR with knowledge of physical and psychosocial dysfunction. The supervisor explained that successful home-care therapists are organized, competent people who create their own schedules, complete their documentation accurately, adjust easily to a variety of social and environmental situations, work independently without direct supervision, and communicate ideas effectively. Because of diverse demands, Stacy would have to be flexible and adjust to a broad range of people, both professional and nonprofessional.

The interviewer asked Stacy about her stamina, since home care is demanding on three levels. First, the therapist must demonstrate the ability to transfer and to ambulate patients in less-than-ideal situations. At times, the therapist must teach reluctant family members and caregivers to execute difficult techniques. Second, therapists must be able to work and drive in extreme weather conditions, including rain, snow, ice, and hail. Patients may not live in conveniently located, temperature-controlled, accessible homes. Finally, home-care therapists must adjust to different social systems and cultural settings throughout the day as they move in and out of different homes. These shifts require the ability to interact with a variety of people successfully. Stacy asked the supervisor to describe a patient that a member of the group had treated recently.

> The supervisor described Mr. H, a 78-year-old black American who was discharged from a 27-day stay in a metropolitan hospital. Mr. H was admitted with a diagnosis of adenocarcinoma of the rectum, chronic obstructive pulmonary disease, a left temporal-lobe ce-

rebral vascular accident, glaucoma, anemia, and bladder outlet obstruction. The patient was also diabetic and almost blind. Mr. H underwent a resection with colostomy and was discharged to a home-care team consisting of a nurse, physical and occupational therapists, social worker, and home health aide. The occupational therapy orders were to instruct the patient in activities of daily living and to teach colostomy care.

> Mr. H lived with his wife, who was blind and hypertensive, in a modest two-story house in a densely populated area of the city. The therapist assessed the patient's environment and discovered a number of architectural barriers such as narrow hallways, steep stairs, a difficult-to-reach bathroom located on the second floor, and a difficult-to-reach kitchen. Mr. and Mrs. H had no relatives or friends well enough to help them. Mr. H had little endurance, was dependent in self-care, and demonstrated perceptual and sensory deficits. He also had little coordination and strength.

> The therapist assessed the patient and decided to make the next home visit with the nurse, since the patient had so many unmet medical and self-care needs. The nurse and therapist reviewed general colostomy care with the patient, and the nurse also evaluated the therapist's knowledge regarding the preparation and application of a colostomy bag. Occupational therapy treatment continued for 6 weeks consisting of upper-extremity resistive exercises and self-care activities such as shaving and dressing. Also reviewed were sensory and perceptual activities designed to maximize the patient's ability to identify objects in his paralyzed hand, since his vision was so limited.

> Mr. H attained independence in bathing, dressing, and light meal preparation; his incoordination precluded his success in colostomy care. The therapist tried to teach Mrs. H how to perform the colostomy care, and although she gained some proficiency on a model, she refused to attempt actual care on her husband because she feared that she might infect him. The therapist and nurse conferred with the family and decided to decrease other services so that visits for colostomy care could be continued.*

The supervisor explained that the case was illustrative because the patient and his wife had few resources, few family or interpersonal support systems, and multiple medical problems. The home-care team members had to communicate with each other and the family in order to make the difficult decision regarding Mr. H's continued care.

Stacy weighed the demands of the home-care delivery system with her desire to enter this growing area of practice. She decided to join the private practice group and to develop her expertise in home-care delivery. □

---

* The patient case study is a fictitious composite developed by Gregory Wilson, OTR/L, Community Occupational Therapy Consultants, Inc.

Overview of Home Care

Patients are referred to home care by their physicians. The referral may follow a hospitalization, a convalescence in a nursing home, or a stay in a rehabilitation center. In the majority of cases, a nurse visits the patient first and orders the other needed services. Where nursing services are not required, a physical therapist or speech pathologist may evaluate the patient and order other needed services. Recent changes in Medicare legislation will also permit occupational therapists to evaluate and treat patients as primary providers; however, other team members are still crucial to obtaining occupational therapy referrals.

The home health team works in conjunction with patients and their families to stabilize health needs and to increase functional abilities. Once a referral for occupational therapy is received, the therapist collaborates with the patient, family, and other team members to promote the patient's independence using functional exercises, sensory retraining, adaptive equipment, perceptual training, and energy conservation techniques. The therapist must consider the patient from a holistic perspective, because emotional, social, cultural, and environmental factors have as much influence on the outcome of care as do the medical prognosis and patient's present abilities.

Case Study

Mr. S, a 67-year-old former truck driver, suffered a cerebrovascular accident in March of 1986. He was rushed to the hospital, where his medical condition was stabilized by medication, rest, remedial diet, and bed exercises. After one week, he was transferred to a rehabilitation center. The staff there taught Mr. S to bathe from a basin while in bed, dress if supervised and assisted, eat using adapted equipment, transfer with supervision and assistance, and to perform selected joint range of motion exercises with his affected upper extremity. Mrs. S was involved in the rehabilitation program. Mr. S was fitted for a resting hand splint and arm sling. He was sent home with a tub transfer seat, wheelchair, walker, and raised toilet seat.

The rehabilitation center team thought that Mr. S could benefit from additional training; therefore, the physiatrist ordered a home program. Three days prior to discharge, a hospital social worker referred Mr. S to a home-care agency. The social worker described Mr. S's rehabilitation program and discussed his progress.

A home health agency nurse visited the day that Mr. S came home. Mr. S was lying in bed when she arrived. The nurse evaluated his condition, checked on the available medical equipment, and verified the need for other skilled services. She found that Mrs. S seemed anxious and threatened by her new responsibilities. The nursing supervisor referred the case to physical and occupational therapies. The patient's diagnosis, history, and address were given.

The occupational therapist visited the patient three days after he came home. The therapist found that Mr. S could eat cut-up food but was dependent on Mrs. S for all other aspects of his daily care. His impulsive behavior, short attention span, and left visual-field cut all limited his performance in daily self-care. The home visiting team continued services for the next 2 months.

The occupational therapist upgraded the therapeutic exercises initiated in the rehabilitation center. Mr. S could use his affected arm to stabilize objects. A complete review of dressing techniques was necessary because Mrs. S initially found it easier to dress her husband. The occupational therapist also taught Mr. S to compensate for his left field cut by using familiar cues from his environment.

After 2 months of training in occupational and physical therapy, Mr. S required minimal assistance to dress, eat, and do light housekeeping. He could ambulate to the front door and go down the front steps if assisted. □

In this case, the home-care team reinforced and completed the patient's rehabilitation program. Much therapy was initiated by the rehabilitation hospital staff; however, additional treatment was required to make the patient independent. The home visiting team could adjust Mr. S's program to the needs of his family by using the familiar setting of his home.

Home Health Team Defined

The *nurse* carries out skilled duties that include supervising medication, giving injections and nutritional advice, giving intravenous medication, caring for wounds and dressings, monitoring vital signs, and teaching and supervising the patient and caretakers regarding daily care. The nurse is usually the coordinator of the patient's care; he or she supervises other nursing personnel such as home health aides.

The *home health aide* carries out the nursing care plan. Duties include bathing, dressing, and feeding the patient; carrying out or reinforcing therapeutic activities and exercise regimes; maintaining the environment; assisting in the preparation of meals; and providing assistance with ambulation and self-administered medications. The home health aide also offers psychological support.

The *physical therapist* employs physical agents such as heat, light, water, electricity, massage, radiation, and exercise to restore patients to their maximum level of physical function.

The *speech therapist* uses knowledge about speech,

hearing, and language to plan and implement a realistic program to increase the patient's communication skills. The patient's emotions affect speech; thus, psychological aspects are an important consideration in speech therapy.

The *occupational therapist* uses specified therapeutic, self-care, homemaking, and creative activities to facilitate or maximize the patient's level of function. Both the phychosocial and the physical aspects of the patient's condition are assessed in terms of the total context for treatment.

The *social worker* uses a problem-solving approach to help patients help themselves. Options and resources are presented to the patient and caretakers in an attempt to maximize the patient's adjustment.

Not all of the possible home care professionals were presented in this section. Others may include a podiatrist, optometrist, dentist, homemaker, dietician, and home-visiting physician.

Home-bound patients cannot leave their homes without assistance. This is an important classification for third-party carriers (insurance coverage). *Ambulatory* patients may be asked to travel to outpatient therapy. Most carriers refuse to cover home services if patients can walk out of their house even if assistance is required. Some third-party carriers consider patients ineligible for homebound services if they can get to their front door. This means that therapists must consider this constraint when planning and documenting treatment progress, because patients can easily lose their classification as homebound. This issue will be addressed in the Documentation section of this chapter.

Resources are the patient's available human and physical assets. Assets can help to balance the debilitating effects of health problems. Resources can be categorized into human and material classes.

Human resources are caregivers — people who assist with the patient's daily care. Caregiver duties include such tasks as preparing meals; caring for the patient's wounds, and dressings; offering medication at the appropriate times; bathing the patient; cleaning the surrounding environment; and offering support, encouragement, and entertainment. At times, the caregiver assumes responsibility for the patient's financial obligations. The patient's skills determine the scope of the caregiver's responsibilities and the time required to complete the daily tasks. Human resources are so important that they frequently influence the overall course of the patient's progress.

There are three kinds of human resources. *Primary caregivers* assume full responsibility for all of the patient's needs. The amount of effort involved is determined by the extent of the patient's independence. If the patient is dependent in all aspects of self-care, primary care may be equivalent to a full-time job. In many cases, the burdens of patient care are added to the normal responsibilities of the caregiver, so that the caregiver has two jobs. The work load can become emotionally and physically draining. *Secondary caregivers* do not assume total responsibility for the patient's care. However, they frequently perform routine patient care tasks, thereby offering respite to the primary caretaker. *Tertiary caregivers* offer infrequent but welcome assistance. They visit the patient and provide emotional support and social contact. Also important is the periodic help given to the primary and secondary caregiver. Although tertiary caregivers are not available for daily rehabilitation training and personal care, they may perform duties such as shopping for food and medicine, transporting the patient to the doctor, and staying with the patient while the primary caregiver attends to other business.

Material resources consist of the patient's financial assets, including insurance coverage. Insurance coverage may consist of a private or governmental policy. Home care may be covered under Blue Cross, health maintenance organization (HMO), private carrier, or prospective payment organization (PPO). Furniture, equipment, supplies, clothing, medication, safety equipment, and aide services are other material assets which can be purchased if the patient has sufficient funds.

Boundaries of Home Care

There are four factors that make home-care delivery different from the care offered in an institution. These factors are the unique characteristics of the patient, home-care practitioners, the delivery system, and the importance of communication.

The Patient

The unique characteristics of the home-care patient are determined by factors such as the patient's medical condition, motivation, culture, emotions, resources, and environment.

Medical conditions

Individuals who are recovering from a variety of medical conditions can benefit from home-care services. The majority of patient are elderly adults who are recovering from fractures, heart or pulmonary diseases, cerebrovascular accidents, neurological disorders, decubitis ulcers, surgical wounds, burns, brain injury, spinal cord injuries, and arthritis.[31] Younger adults and children with similar medical conditions are also eligible for care.

Patients with acute medical problems should be medically stable before they are admitted to home-care services. Today, patients are discharged from hospitals earlier, and home-care team members are required to treat more acutely ill patients; however, these patients should not require acute care even though many home-care teams are now on call 7 days a week, 24 hours a day. If patients are medically unstable, the physician should be notified and the patient admitted to the hospital if necessary. Terminally ill patients may also be treated at home with the support of a hospice team.

Motivation, culture, and emotions

Patients can gain positive reinforcement from family and friends and from the objects in their own homes. Some patients find little comfort in the institutional environment, where their daily roles and habits are disrupted. Patients long for their own ways of life — their own home, bed, food, and pets. Also, the familiar habits that provide structure for daily life can soften the stressful results of illness. These factors will be considered in greater depth in the next section of this chapter.

Resources

Because the home-care patient requires supervision and direct care, available human and material resources become more important. Since patients are now being discharged earlier from acute-care settings, they require more attention when they arrive home. Family members and caregivers are frequently overwhelmed with the responsibilities of care, and home-care practitioners must be sensitive to stress caused by these added responsibilities. Therefore, from the start of care, relatives, friends, and neighbors should be encouraged to help with the patient's care. A secondary and tertiary support network can relieve the primary caregivers so they will be able to carry on better. Some tasks that secondary and tertiary caregivers can assume are providing a meal periodically, taking responsibility for the patient's care for a day, shopping for the primary caregiver, and taking the patient to the physician.

In a growing number of cases, the patient has no nearby relatives and no friends. Neighbors may not be close enough to offer emergency help. Isolation is especially problematic in rural towns and farms where children do not live near their parents and friends are inaccessible, deceased, or have moved away. To complicate matters further, there are few agencies or private groups that offer assistance. Private and religious groups sometimes are willing to deliver meals and encourage visits from volunteers who may provide assistance and transportation.

If support networks are lacking, home convalescence can be difficult and awkward. Unfortunately, there are fewer opportunities to substitute institutional care for informal support networks. This is especially true among Medicare and Medicaid patients, who are restricted by constraints on the duration of a patient's stay in an institution.

Therapists must also learn to work collaboratively with the hospital staff as patients who become ill repeatedly are admitted to the institution for a brief period of time, only to be discharged again because of regulations regarding the number of days that the hospital can be reimbursed for care. The patient is discharged and home-care treatment is resumed, but the disruption becomes another negative factor that must be considered in treatment planning.

Environment

The home-care therapist must be aware of the extensive influence of the environment on the patient's progress. Barris maintains that people reflect a combination of factors and circumstances as they explore and master their environment.[3] These ideas can be conceptualized as four concentric circles or layers. The core is comprised of objects and things from the nonhuman environment. The second layer comprises tasks that are carried out during self-care, work, or leisure activities. The third layer consists of social groups and organizations that influence an individual's roles, and the outermost layer is the culture, the pattern of beliefs and values that influence all of the other layers.[3]

The object layer consists of nonhuman *objects*, which includes everything in the home that is not human, such as plants, animals, and artifacts. Home-care therapists learn to observe and use objects as cues to understanding the patient's lifestyle; for example, furniture placement, the quality and quantity of ornaments, the availability of food, and the way that animals and plants are cared for. The significance of certain objects may also offer insight into family relationships, roles, and habits. The therapist observes, interprets the cues, and verifies ideas with the patient or caregivers, since interpretations are not always accurate.

The *task behavior* of the patient and caregivers includes task complexity, temporal boundaries, rules, level of playfulness, and social dimensions.[3] At first, task behavior is usually tentative and exploratory; then, after a period of practice, performance becomes routine. Habitual tasks do not require concentration. On the other hand, new tasks demand much more energy and attention.[3] A 45-year-old patient with a traumatic brain injury may find self-care activities taxing, because the memory loss complicates tasks that were once routine.

Social groups and organizations shape the patient's ability to interact with the environment. The size, function, permeability, and structural complexity of social groups and organizations all are relevant.[3] Many patients reside with relatives or friends, creating a family group that has certain interaction patterns, rules, norms, and rewards. Even patients who live alone interact with neighbors, tradepersons, and professionals. The size of the patient's support group can range from as few as two people to as many as fifty. If there is only one person caring for the patient, then the burden of care rests solely on that individual. On the other hand, a larger group can develop specialized roles so the primary caregiver is relieved of the responsibilities of daily care.

The purpose or function of the group may be the care of the patient. Usually, this new role is added to the group members' other daily responsibilities. Thus, some members may be more invested in the patient's progress than others. The therapist has to gauge the level of member commitment and direct program planning toward the capable and interested members. Sometimes, home-care teams can enlist the assistance of disinterested group members and involve them in the caregiver network.

Some families or caregivers are open and receptive to the home visiting team, whereas others remain cautious and guarded. An outsider, the therapist must determine the best ways to teach and offer suggestions. Some individuals need additional time to learn to trust the home-care therapist and to consider if they want help. Rural families may resist assistance from "strangers," and the therapist will have to learn to recognize these communication barriers and encourage the patient and caregiver to overcome their suspicions.[8] Changing a home into a convalescent center is not easy, and even the simple suggestions may be misunderstood by the patient or caregiver unless they trust the home-care therapist.

The last dimension of the environment is the patient's *culture.* Culture consists of the beliefs, perceptions, values, roles, customs, and way of life that are passed from one generation to the next through interrelationships.[13] Culture can be viewed as a multifaceted influence that is acquired by direct and indirect daily experiences based on what people do, say, make, and use.[35] Home-care therapists must realize that the patient's way of life cannot be changed easily by several months of teaching, even under ideal circumstances. Few home-care patients, individuals who have suffered functional losses, have the energy to make sudden major changes in their lifestyle, which now seems so fragile and precarious because of their illness. Therefore, it is important for therapists to introduce activities that emphasize the patient's functional abilities at the same time that dysfunction is reduced. The home-care therapist can never forget the extensive influence of the patient's culture during the delivery of care.

A typical but frustrating example of the effect of culture on planning may be a patient's refusal to accept labor-saving techniques. This rejection may be based more on the patient's need to resist further changes in the environment than on a negation of the therapist's ideas. The patient's illness has disrupted family roles and habits, and members may resist more change. Rather than push the family, the therapist should objectively select ideas that are both nonthreatening and helpful, such as the removal of throw rugs in hallways to prevent falls; the installation of a hospital bed, commode, and wheelchair in the dining room of a two-story house; or the placement of the patient in the family room during the day. If the caregivers continue to resist change, their wishes should be respected, and the therapist should not get involved in a competitive test of wills. One cannot expect to change complex patterns of living in a few months.

The Home-Care Practitioner

The unique characteristics of the home care practitioner are based on the ability to shift social roles, use available equipment creatively, combat professional isolation, balance teaching with direct care, organize and manage time, adjust to diverse cultural settings, develop a code of ethics, and set continuing education and professional goals.

Shift in Social Roles

The health care practitioner enters the social hierarchy of the patient's family and friends. The therapist is a guest in the patient's house, a visitor in his or her lifespace. The reverse is true with services offered in an institution: the patient enters the institution as a temporary member of the formal social hierarchy.

As a visitor in the patient's world, the practitioner must adjust to values, traditions, communication patterns, and environmental factors. The patient's lifestyle might be unfamiliar, but the practitioner must use verbal, nonverbal, and environmental cues to promote effective interaction. Successful home-care practitioners have the ability to interact in a variety of social systems. Communication skills must promote patient and caregiver cooperation.

Use available equipment creatively

Home-care practitioners cannot rely on the equipment and supplies that are commonplace in most institution-based clinics. Therapists carry a limited supply of evaluation tools and a few frequently used modalities in their car trunks. The selection of evaluation tools and modalities should be based on the patient's values, goals, interests, roles, habits, skills, and medical condition.

This does not mean that home-care therapists work without the benefit of any equipment. Instead, they adapt objects found in the patient's home. An old sock filled with a soup can and knotted at the top becomes a weight, a rolled washcloth or towel becomes a positioning tool, a chair becomes a bath seat. Home therapists monitor the patient's environment and select appropriate items to use in their treatment.

Combat professional isolation

Home-care practice can be a professionally isolating experience unless one deliberately seeks out other occupational therapists. Although there are opportunities to interact with other professionals, such as nurses and physical therapists, opportunities for interactions with other occupational therapists are limited. Therefore, although voluntary, membership in local, state, and national organizations becomes essential. These organizations have scheduled meetings, continuing education programs, occupational therapy newspapers for communicating ideas, as well as scholarly and practice-oriented journals. Meetings provide opportunities to discuss treatment ideas and to explore solutions to problems, newspaper articles offer new ideas and opportunities for professional growth, and journal articles validate practice through research.

Balance teaching with direct care

Since home-care practitioners commonly visit the patient only two or three times a week, with each visit averaging 35 to 45 minutes, effective teaching is especially important. Direct hands-on techniques are required for home-care practice. Of equal importance, however, is the therapist's ability to promote patient and family independence. Effective communication by home-care practitioners encourages carryover of skills taught during visits. Home-care practitioners realize that teaching skills either make or break the rehabilitation program. Thus, the practitioner must tailor each program to meet the unique needs of a particular family.

Therapists provide direct service and explain how and why a technique or activity is used. As soon as the patient and the caregiver become comfortable with it, the responsibility for the exercise or activity is turned over to the family. The patient can benefit from a daily treatment regime if the patient and caregivers are cooperative.

Home health aides may visit five times a week for a week or two until the family and caregiver network is fully developed. Therapists can train the aide to carry out routine tasks that will promote the patient's independence. Visits are decreased as the patient improves. If home health aide services are ordered, then these services must be supervised by the appropriate professional staff — the nurse, the physical therapist, and the occupational therapist must meet with the aide and the patient to evaluate the patient's progress and change the program if warranted.

Organize and manage time

Home-care therapists must be organizers and planners. Tasks must be prioritized and completed in an orderly fashion. Each therapist is responsible for the daily tasks of accepting new referrals, scheduling and making visits, documenting treatment progress, collaborating with other staff, and reporting any unusual situations or circumstances to the patient's nursing supervisor and physician.

Visits must be coordinated so patients are not seen by three people on one day and no one on another day. Therapists usually schedule visits in a selected area on certain days of the week. The selection is based on arrangements with other professional staff. The patient and caregivers may also have preferences for a certain time or day. These choices must also be considered by the home visiting team.

Home-care therapists are rigidly bound by regulations regarding the timeliness of calls to accept new referrals, the number of days that can lapse between referral and first visit, and the interval between a visit and when the agency receives the progress note. These rules will be discussed later in the chapter. Because therapists are commonly reimbursed by the visit, it is important to work efficiently so that time is devoted to patient care and not to peripheral concerns.

Adjust to diverse cultural settings

When working in an institution, the staff are part of the permanent social hierarchy, and the patients are visitors. The reverse is true in home care, where the therapist is a guest in the patient's home. Understanding the patient's view of reality is an important first step. This view is based on culture or way of life that is taught to individuals during childhood. Therapists must convey their understanding of the patient's values, goals, interests, and emotions gained from cues from the human and nonhuman environment. Home-care therapists learn to adapt their affect to the demands of different social situations. This requires the ability to analyze the meaning of different actions and words regardless of one's own culture.

Develop a Code of Ethics

Therapists who work without direct supervision need to develop a strong code of ethics. The AOTA has adopted an ethical code that has 13 principles related to the recipients of service, professional competence, records, reports, grades and recommendations, intraprofessional relationships, other personnel, employers and payers, education, evaluation and research, the profession, advertising, law and regulations, misconduct and bioethical issues, and problems of society. Therapists should read the *Principles of Occupational Therapy Ethics*, which are reprinted in Appendix B.

Home visiting professionals represent not only their own profession but in some instances all helping professionals. The unethical conduct of a therapist can create undue suffering for a number of patients and caregivers alike. Examples of such conduct are shortening treatment times even though the patient is capable of participating in longer treatments, evaluating patients and visiting them less frequently because the home is not conveniently situated or the neighborhood is unfamiliar, or offering substandard forms of treatment to minority patients or immigrants from different cultures. If any violation of standards is witnessed, the incident should be discussed with the supervisor or officer of the state association, because substandard treatment can only compromise the patient and the profession.

Set continuing educational and professional goals

The diverse pressures of home care need to be offset by a conscious decision to seek new ideas to improve one's clinical practice. Setting yearly goals for continuing education and professional growth and development ensures that one's knowledge and skills are current. Home care is a public arena for practice, and patients are becoming sophisticated and demanding consumers. Thus, therapists try to attend at least one continuing education program a year, and many are active in professional organizations.

Delivery System

The unique characteristics of the home-care delivery system are based on the setting. The home environment does not always afford optimal space, personnel, and equipment for rehabilitation. Use of complex tools, modalities, and techniques is limited by the home environment and the interest and motivation of the patient and caregivers. Even if the patient and caregiver want to participate in a home program, they may be overwhelmed by the burden of the patient's basic needs; this is work added to existing responsibilities.

Other factors that inhibit active participation in rehabilitation are the recent changes in Medicare legislation. DRGs were added to the Medicare laws to curb inflation in the health care industry. Reimbursement for hospital stays is now determined by statistical averages, and visit overruns become an additional expense for the institution. Prospective payment is becoming the norm for health care reimbursement, and patients are being discharged sooner. Thus, more cases are referred to home care.

At the same time, insurance carriers want to contain the cost of home care, so guidelines for covered services are becoming increasingly stringent. In fact, there seems to be a concerted effort to contain the growth of home care at the same time that patients are being discharged earlier from institutional care.[28,29] Although there are no recent major changes in Medicare home-care legislation or in the policies and procedures that govern practice, there is evidence that there is much more paperwork, that patients admitted to home care are much sicker, that more people who need help are not being treated, that payments for services are frequently denied, and that payments owed to agencies for services rendered are not paid promptly.[28]

Another problem is the interpretation of the patient's homebound status. Many home-care practitioners believe that fiscal intermediaries are adopting a restrictive interpretation of guidelines. For example, the term "homebound" is now being interpreted so that it means "bedridden." This interpretation reduces the number of patients eligible for rehabilitation care and the services that can be provided.[29] Even supportive insurance carriers or fiscal intermediaries will cover only 4 months of rehabilitation services or less unless extraordinary circumstances are cited and the company agrees that more services are warranted.

The administrators and staff of home health agencies are caught in a dilemma, because they feel that more services will help patients over a long period of time but the insurance carriers are focused on short-term costs. The insurance carriers are setting policies for patient care, because they can deny payments for services.[25] A representative from the National Association of Home Care testified before the Senate Finance Committee in 1985, emphasizing that when alternate forms of health care delivery are encouraged, the Health Care Financing Administration (HCFA) has curtailed "already limited Medicare home health benefits through a series of 'cost containment' measures which will result in more reliance on institutional care and defeat the purpose of the prospective payment system."[25]

Recently (October 1986), there have been several changes in the Medicare legislation. Occupational therapy will join nursing, physical therapy, and speech therapy as primary services. The rules and regulations that will govern these changes were not completed when this chapter was written. The changes will be operative July 1987. At present, the number of allowed visits, the medical diagnoses that make patients eligible for treatment by occupational therapy, and the duration of treatment varies by fiscal intermediary and geographic region, so it is best to check with a nursing supervisor who can offer current guidelines for care. These issues will be described in the section on documentation later in this chapter.

These problems in obtaining services are not unique to home-care practice, because the entire health care industry is in flux, as institutions discharge patients earlier and the responsibility for care shifts to the family. All health care practitioners are searching for ways to deliver services more efficiently and develop ways to curb rising costs.

Communication

Home-care therapists must be effective communicators, since they interact with many people. Formal and informal interactions using verbal, nonverbal, and written communication patterns are used. Practitioners must relate to family members, caregivers, other professionals, and nonprofessional staff. Thus, the ability to express knowledge in clear, concise language unencumbered by jargon is necessary.

Home-visiting occupational therapists must communicate with colleagues even though this is time consuming and requires planning. Telephone conferences and scheduled meetings are the only way that team members can share observations about the patient's progress. Calls can be exchanged at night or during weekends, when there is more time to express different ideas; meetings can be arranged when therapists and nurses are visiting patients in the same neighborhood. It is also essential for therapists to call other professionals before physicians' orders are renewed. The penalty for lack of communication may be an untimely termination of services, since the occupational therapist may have a different perspective on the patient's progress than other team members.[36]

Choosing a Theory Base

The need for a theory base in home care-practice cannot be overemphasized. A theory base consists of a conceptual model that organizes and guides the therapist to think about complex patient problems in a systematic fashion. This is important because services can become fragmented, and family members, caregivers, and professional colleagues can become confused. A clearly articulated theory or delivery model can explain occupational therapy services to professional and nonprofessional team members. Services that are clearly conceptualized and articulated are also easier to explain to managers and fiscal intermediaries.

A theory base consists of a philosophical base or belief system and a conceptual framework that is used to organize evaluation tools, goal selection, treatment modalities, and quality-assurance practices.

Philosophical base

A philosophical base consists of values that cannot be proved. Philosophy is defined as "a study of the processes governing thought and conduct; the general principles or essential elements that produce laws in a field of knowledge."[22] The philosophical base of a profession is based on fundamental ideas that govern practice, ideas that are beliefs or values about humankind, suffering, and life.[4] Members of a profession are united by their commitment to the ideas embodied in their philosophical base.

Because our profession developed as a reaction to the insensitive treatment of the chronically ill in the 1890s, therapists value the "essential humanity of a person in spite of severe and sometimes chronic disease."[37] Occupational therapists focus on the patient's pathology but also on the capacity of humans to adapt and adjust to internal and external demands.[20,33] Occupational therapists have long demonstrated their belief that individuals can "do for themselves and take responsibility for their own health."[37]

Occupational therapists focus on adaptation or what people *can do,* so this holistic approach requires an understanding of the individual's lifestyle, values, goals, interests, and culture. Yerxa maintains that this view of the patient contrasts with the segmented focus of other hospital-based professionals. At the core of our profession is the belief that an individual's active participation in a meaningful activity can promote health and well-being.[37] Reilly stated this succinctly when she maintained that humans, "through the use of their hands, as they are energized by mind and will, can influence the state of their own health."[27]

Philosophy encourages therapists to critically consider their own treatment, to compare values and beliefs about patient care, and to formulate questions regarding the patient's lifestyle. For example, how do we encourage individuals to overcome developmental, traumatic, socioeconomic, and pathological conditions? A technician can superficially select convenient exercises and crafts, but the therapist searches for activities that reflect the patient's values, goals, and interests. Thus, the philosophical base of occupational therapy practice includes the quest for meaningful existence.

Matching Philosophy and Values

The first step in establishing a theory-based practice is to explore one's own values. What are values? Rath developed criteria that qualify a belief or behavior as a value: the belief or behavior must be selected from alternatives, prized and cherished, chosen freely after a consideration of the consequences of holding the belief, publicly affirmed, and acted upon with some pattern of frequency.[26] Carl Rogers maintains that there are many definitions to describe values, but he finds the distinctions made by Morris[23] most useful. Morris identifies three types of values: operative, conceived, and objective. Operative values are preferences that lead to actions which may not involve any cognitive or conceptual thinking. Choices are made and carried out, one object is selected over another. For example, someone may decide to drive to the post office rather than walk. A preference created the tendency to act in one way instead of another. A conceived value requires consideration, since it is a preference for a symbolized object or action where the outcome of the choice is anticipated. For example, therapists frequently value independence in self-care, which is a conceived value. An objective value is not necessarily desirable, but it is an objective or ideal. Objective values are "preferable whether or not they are conceived of as desirable."[23] Objective values are not quite as important, since they require less commitment because they are convenient ideas.

Rogers explains the importance of operative and conceived values and scarcely discusses objective values, since they are not necessarily part of the individual's personal value system. Home-care therapists should identify their operative and conceived values concerning topics such as independence, work, family roles, religion, suffering, death, aging, illness, meaningful activity, and different cultural groups. In other words, a theory-based practice should be based on operative and conceived values rather than on objective values, which are abstract and removed from daily practice.

Engelhardt discussed conceived values when he urged occupational therapists to balance the technical aspects of occupational therapy with the belief that a patient is a person. The use of activities both as rituals designed to recapture pleasure and as significant experiences for individuals who are searching for a "sense of place, purpose and function" is an important part of the therapeutic process.[9] In home care, activities must be meaningful because daily care is delivered by the patient, caregivers, and family members as well as by the therapist. Therefore, activities must reflect patient and caregiver goals, be carried over with relative ease, and maximize the patient's functional abilities.

Therapists who understand their own values can identify disagreements and underlying reasons for the dissimilarities. They can redirect treatment toward the patient's goals, values, interests, and needs.

A commonplace example is a patient who does not want to learn how to dress. There are a number of reasons why this may occur, and the therapist must separate personal values from the needs of the patient. The following vignette is based on a potential values clash.

Case Study

Mrs. K, a 66-year-old obese woman, suffered from arthritis and a recent cerebrovascular accident, resulting in left-sided paralysis with little functional return in the upper extremity. The home-care therapist was referred to maximize the patient's functional status. During the evaluation, the therapist asked the patient about her performance in activities of daily living. The patient, a congenial person, jokingly stated that she alone had raised eight children and felt that some of the eight "could figure out how to take care of me." The therapist tried to convince Mrs. K that dressing would make her feel better. In fact, Mrs. K was enjoying her sick role, since she had never taken time to focus on herself.

At first, the therapist began to debate the importance of getting dressed with Mrs. K. The therapist identified her own objective values regarding the importance of being self-sufficient. She also realized her own conceived values regarding the importance of not depending on others for help. Mrs. K, on the other hand, valued interdependence and felt deserving of the attention and nurturing of her family. Mrs. K decided to concentrate on improving functional movement in her arm before learning how to dress independently. The therapist focused treatment on upper extremity retraining and noted that Mrs. K requested help with her bathing and dressing activities once her arm regained some movement. ☐

This vignette demonstrates that the patient directs the ultimate focus of care even when these goals are not shared by the therapist.

Importance of a conceptual model

Conceptual models, or frames of reference, are thought structures used to organize and guide clinical reasoning. Therapists should identify their own values concerning chronic illness, independence, pathology, and activities and then consider a theory or model that best reflects their beliefs. In home care, the conceptual model must be broad enough to encompass the patient's environment, culture, lifestyle, and functional needs. If the theory base is inclusive, the therapist can rely on the conceptual structure to organize treatment planning.

Model of Human Occupation

Keilhofner and Burke developed the model of human occupation based on the ideas of Mary Reilly.[19,20,33] Although there are a number of other useful theories that can be applied to home care, the model of human occupation offers a broad organizational framework so more specific treatment techniques and theories can be systematically applied to the patient's problems.

The model of human occupation is based on two major premises: individuals are open systems that both influence and are influenced by the environment, and the mind and body are interrelated.[18,19] The individual can be viewed as an interrelated three-tiered hierarchy consisting of the volitional, habituation, and performance subsystems.[20] The volitional subsystem consists of values, personal causation, goals, and interests; the habituation subsystem consists of roles and habits; and the performance subsystem consists of skills.[20] Home-care therapists direct attention to the patient's volitional (values, personal causation, goals and interests) and habituation (habits and roles) subsystems as well as the performance (skills) subsystem. Treatment should include more than deficits; therapists should also consider the functional aspects of the patient.[17]

Students interested in acquiring specific information on the application of the model of human occupation should consult the references cited. The text *A Model of Human Occupation: Theory and Application* is designed as an independent learning tool with a self-paced workbook.[16] Also useful is the case analysis format developed by Kaplan and Cubie, which is based on a systems perspective.[15] By posing a series of questions, therapists will be able to determine the patient's goals, values, interests, habits, and roles.

Therapists can use the model of human occupation in conjunction with other theories and treatment techniques. For example, a patient with hemiplegia can be treated using the model of human occupation, but specific techniques to treat the upper extremity must be drawn from other theorists.[21]

Delivery Process: A Model

There are several stages in the delivery of home services. After initial intervention, there is a period of gradual building, during which relationships and treatment regimes are established. After this period, a plateau frequently occurs, and fewer gains take place. During this time, learning and therapeutic patterns are reinforced. Finally, the patient and the caregiver return to their former lives, and the case is discharged.

The stages of this process are depicted in Figure 39-1. Each of the five divisions represents a phase in the treatment cycle. The umbrella of prevention arches over the entire model; this is a fundamental consideration throughout the delivery process. The five stages of this process are intervention, building a therapeutic relationship, carrying out the treatment program, discharge planning, and after-care. Each of the stages, as well as some of the issues that arise during the stage, will be discussed in detail later. In brief, characteristics of each stage include the following:

1. *Intervention.* This includes the referral, initial evaluation, and process of data collection.
2. *Building a therapeutic relationship.* In this period, the initial evaluation is completed. Long- and short-term goals are established, defining the focus of the occupational therapy care plan. The initial foundations for a trusting relationship are being built.
3. *Carrying out the treatment program.* This is a time to teach the patient and the caregivers how to maximize the patient's level of function. Meaningful, goal-directed activities are initiated, including therapeutic exercises, activities of daily living, crafts, and games. The goal is to integrate the patient's evolving skills into functional performance.
4. *Discharge planning.* During discharge planning, goals are reassessed and new resources are sought out. Preparation is made for the termination of direct services. The full responsibility for care shifts back to the patient and the caregivers.
5. *After-care.* There are few resources available to pay for follow-up. This is a time when therapists could offer sporadic help to reinforce the therapeutic program. It is also a time for therapists to evaluate the quality of their treatment.

How to Deliver Home-Care Services

The conceptual material presented earlier has been offered as a foundation for understanding the delivery of home-care services. At this point, we will consider some direct service issues. How does the occupational therapist obtain cases, and how is the occupational therapy program carried out?

This section can be compared to an orientation handbook. The information is useful as an introduction to home-care delivery. The material is divided into the five stages of the home care delivery model (Fig. 39-1), as follows:

Intervention—Referral, preparation, initial visit, evaluation

Building a therapeutic relationship—establishing rapport, reassessing goals, and initiating programs

Treatment program—activity choices, teaching and learning, coordination, architectural barriers, body mechanics, transfer techniques, and home modalities

Discharge planning—reinforcing program

After-care and program evaluation—voluntary patient contact and program evaluation.

Intervention

Intervention includes the therapist's preparation for and entry into a new case. The agency personnel intervene and offer direct patient services. The process begins with a telephoned referral to the home health agency. Patients must be under the care of a physician, who may refer the case to the agency. Social workers, nurse coordinators, rehabilitation teams, family members, and friends may also make a home-care referral.

The first agency contact is usually made by a nurse. If there is no need for skilled nursing services, a physical therapist or a speech pathologist may open the case.

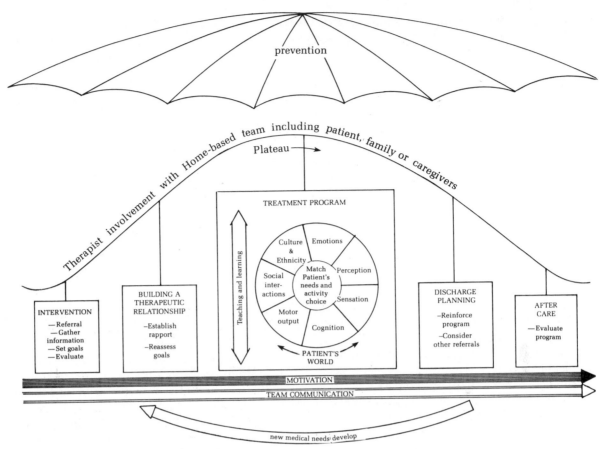

Figure 39-1. A home care schematic.

(Occupational therapists could not open cases until recently; when the Medicare law was changed. Previously, occupational therapists were not classifed as primary providers.) Referrals to occupational therapy may be included in the physician's original orders. If not, and the patient could benefit from occupational therapy, the coordinating nurse will contact the patient's physician, verify the request, and obtain written occupational therapy orders.

Information commonly given in the referral includes the patient's: (1) location—name, address, telephone number, and zip code, (2) date of birth, (3) primary and secondary diagnoses and treatment precautions, (4) recent hospitalization dates, if applicable, (5) physician's name, address, and telephone number, and (6) name, address, and telephone number of the primary caregiver. Also listed are the date the agency started care, the name of the person who opened the case, the other services the physician ordered, the frequency of visits if specified, and physician's orders.

If the patient was treated in a hospital or rehabilitation facility, the former therapist may be contacted to ensure continuity of the occupational therapy program. The referral must be answered within 72 hours of receipt.

Preparation

Preparation for the intitial visit involves three steps: locating the patient's house, scheduling the visit, and selecting appropriate modalities for the evaluation. Planning maximizes the time spent with the patient, as one minimizes the time wasted on nonproductive concerns. It is best to make the shortest trips between patient houses. Using a detailed map will make routing easier.

The new patient must next be contacted by telephone. Offer an introduction and ask for permission to visit. Emphasize the time and day of the visit, verify the address, and discuss directions to the house that will help in avoiding traffic obstacles.

Most therapists carry a bag with evaluation tools and common modalities. The bag may contain a stereognosis testing kit (box of familiar objects), perceptual test materials (may be formal or informal tests), goniometer, watch with a second hand (pulse rate measurement), safety pin (test for neurological deficits), a blindfold (testing for proprioception), and household items (paper towels, soap, crayons, scissors, pens, pencils, and masking tape). Some therapists also carry exercise putty, rubber bands, Theraplast, stacking cones, foam rubber, surgical tubing, and equipment catalogs. Splinting materials, crafts, weights, pulleys, and other equipment may be required later.

Initial Visit

The initial visit is crucial to the treatment process. The therapist evaluates the patient's abilities, establishes a baseline for measuring treatment progress, and determines the goals of the program. Also important is the assessment of the entire environment, including the caregiver and resources. Finally, the therapist must determine how to interact effectively within the patient's social system. The therapist takes in as much information as possible.

There are six tasks that must be completed during the initial session:
1. Evaluation of the patient's motor, sensory, perceptual, and cognitive abilities
2. Exploration of the patient's present ability to perform life tasks
3. Assessment of human and nonhuman resources
4. Establishment of long- and short-term goals for the occupational therapy program
5. Projection of the time it will take to achieve the goals
6. Consideration of the lifestyle of the patient and caregivers: their values, goals and interests, roles and habits.

Other objectives of the initial visit are to verify information about the patient's medical history, diagnoses, and treatment precautions, and to meet the caregivers.

The therapist must determine the treatment goals and the duration of services during the initial visit. Goals must include independence in self-care and upper extremity retraining. Most funding sources require evidence of *measurable, practical* progress in a reasonable period of time.

Long-term goals establish the desired outcome of the therapy regime. The success of the patient's progress will be measured in terms of the expected therapy outcome. *Short-term goals* are the graded steps to attainment of long-term goals. Short-term goals are part of the mastery process.

Evaluation

The evaluation form must be completed. A case study and blank evaluation form and care plan are included here and on the following pages. Read the case study below and develop your own treatment plan.

Case Study

Mrs. U, an 81-year-old woman with a right above-elbow (AE) amputation, right cerebral vascular

accident with residual left hemiparesis, and rheumatoid arthritis, lives with her son, daughter-in-law, and granddaughter in a walk-up apartment above a neighborhood tavern. Her son owns the tavern, and the daughter-in-law helps him with cooking and serving and assumes responsibility for Mrs. U's care. The granddaughter is mentally retarded and requires supervision and care. Mrs. U has been set up in a rented hospital bed in the living room of the apartment; a commode and wheelchair are also available. The daughter-in-law suffers from cardiac problems and is always guilt-ridden, harried, and stressed. The case was referred to occupational therapy because the patient wanted to learn how to eat independently. Her AE amputation occured in 1946. She had no prosthesis but had been totally independent until recently, when she suffered a cerebrovascular accident that abolished isolated movement in her left arm. Tone in the extremity was increased, and sensation was impaired. Mrs. U has good cognitive skills.

Initially, the OTR found Mrs. U totally dependent in all aspects of self-care with the exception of transfers, where she requires moderate assistance. The left upper extremity is spastic, and the elbow is usually held flexed. The therapist and patient agreed that Mrs. U will increase her independence in self-care; this is the long-term goal. The short-term goal is to teach the use of a universal cuff and improve ability to transfer during self-care activities and to eat independently if set up.* □

What would you do if you were the therapist? Use the evaluation form that is included here and establish goals and a treatment plan.

Mrs. U's occupational therapy treatment program was as follows. The therapist taught the patient how to use a universal cuff and sandwich holder and how to exercise her left upper extremity. The therapist worked with the patient to create a work area that was built-up, and Mrs. U was able to turn pages of book placed on a slant board using a mouth page turner. The therapist made 16 visits, and the patient achieved the long- and short-term goals.

Consider the complexity of Mrs. U's home situation. What factors would you consider as most significant? Note how the environment and available human and nonhuman resources influence treatment planning and outcome. Do you agree with the therapist's choice of activities?

---

* This case study is a fictitious composite of several patients that was developed by Renee Baumblatt-Magida, OTR/L, Community Occupational Therapy Consultants, Inc., Philadelphia.

OCCUPATIONAL THERAPY EVALUATION AND CARE PLAN

Name _____ H.I.C. No. _____

Date of Evaluation _____ Age _____ Medical Record No. _____

_____ Date of Onset _____

Diagnosis _____

_____

_____

Communication Ability _____

_____

HOME SITUATION

Architectural
Consideration _____

_____

Family Members _____

Daily Routine _____

PHYSICAL CAPACITY

	Right	Left	COMMENTS
RANGE OF MOTION/UE			
Active	___	___	
Passive	___	___	
MUSCLE TONE	___	___	
STRENGTH	___	___	
HAND CAPACITY			
Appearance	___	___	
Hook Grasp	___	___	
Lateral Pinch	___	___	
Palmar Grasp	___	___	
3-Jaw Pinch	___	___	
Opposition	___	___	
COORDINATION			
Gross	___	___	
Fine	___	___	
Bilateral	___	___	
PRONATION/SUPINATION	___	___	
SENSORY			
Sharp/Dull	___	___	
Stereognosis	___	___	
Proprioception	___	___	

Physical Endurance _____

Visual Deficits/Aids _____

_____

Hearing Deficits/Aids _____

Visual Motor Perception _____

Hand Dominance _____ Change Required? _____

Comments from Perceptual Evaluation: _____

OCCUPATIONAL THERAPY EVALUATION AND CARE PLAN (Continued)

Name _____ Medical Record No. _____

ACTIVITIES OF DAILY LIVING

I—Independent   M—Maximum Assistance
A—Minimal Assistance   D—Dependent

Feeding: Dressing:
  Eat with Fork _____   UE Dressing _____
  Cut Meat _____   UE Undressing _____
  Butter Bread _____   LE Dressing _____
  Drink from Glass _____   LE Undressing _____
Hygiene: Buttons _____
  Comb Hair _____   Fasteners _____
  Brush Teeth _____   Shoes/Braces _____
  Cosmetics/shave _____   Ties/Laces _____
  Wash Upper Body _____   Sling _____
  Wash Lower Body _____   General Abilities:
  Shower/Tub _____   Phone _____
  Nails _____   Turn Pages of Book _____
  Urinal/Toilet _____   Wristwatch _____
Transfers: Doorknob/Key _____
  Chair _____   Writing _____
  Bed _____   Open/Close Drawers _____
  Toilet _____   Operate TV _____
  Tub/Shower _____   Lights _____
  Car _____   Faucets _____
                                              Flush Toilet _____
Ambulation   Pick Up Articles
Ability _____   From Floor _____

Patient's Homemaker Skills (Meals prepared by) _____
_____

Medical Equipment Available _____
Additional Equipment Needed _____
Comments _____
_____
_____
_____

Short Term Goals _____
_____
Long Term Plans _____
Treatment Frequency
and Duration _____

_____
OCCUPATIONAL THERAPIST

(Developed by Ruth Levine, Lynn Marcus, Jane Roda, and Carmella Strano, Community Occupational Therapy Consultants, Inc.)

Building a Therapeutic Relationship

In the second stage of home-care delivery, the therapist must establish a good rapport, refine treatment planning, and initiate the treatment program. Communication must be effective. The human and nonhuman environment provide information. The case study offered here demonstrates the importance of using cues from the environment to enhance communication.

Case Study

The occupational therapist walked up a flight of freshly scrubbed marble steps and rang the doorbell of a twin house. Peering through the double glass doors of the glass-enclosed porch, he noted an orderly, modestly furnished porch and living room. Starched, white, ruffled curtains stood out from the window sills. Crocheted doilies adorned the dated, overstuffed sofa and arm chairs. Tiny, delicate china *objets d'art* were displayed on the sofa endtables. The focal point of the living room was a religious statue on an altar. The front windowsill was lined with large potted plants. The potting soil in several pots was decorated with china figurines and large satin bows.

A neatly attired elderly woman hobbled to the door; she seemed hesitant and fearful. The therapist displayed his arm patch and loudly mentioned his name and their earlier telephone call. The woman could see the agency insignia on the therapist's car door. She smiled and opened the door.

The therapist analyzed his observations. Signs indicated that the family might have little contact with young men. If he made enthusiastic gestures, for example, they might be unfamiliar and arouse suspicion. The orderly rooms implied a formal, respectful demeanor, a boisterous person might not be well received in this home. One might also speculate that changes should be introduced gradually; abrupt decisions should be avoided. The therapist used these cues from the nonhuman environment to enhance the effect of his communication. □

A home-care therapist needs to develop the ability to establish a rapport with people in various social systems. Developing this kind of skill depends on making good observations and evaluating what is observed. The therapist must also be aware of his or her own value systems and how they affect the perception of others.

Once communication patterns are established, the therapist may discover information that will affect the outcome of therapy. The therapist addresses the altered goals and changes the treatment plan accordingly.

The treatment regime can now be given full attention. The program is introduced to the patient and the caregiver. Once the treatment program is underway, the program moves to the third stage in home-care delivery.

Carrying Out the Treatment Program

Most patient learning takes place during the third stage of the delivery process. There are seven concerns that one must address during this stage: the activity choice, the teaching and learning process, coordination among team members, communication, architectural barriers, body mechanics and transfer techniques, and home modalities. Each topic will be discussed.

Activity Choice

Curiosity about the activity base of occupational therapy has increased. The home setting offers an excellent example of the positive effects that can be derived from goal-directed activities. Few individuals will work at a task that they neither understand nor find pleasurable, whereas a match between patient needs and an activity can stimulate and motivate the patient.

An easy way to begin the search for a relevant activity is to ask patients about the former life. What tasks did they perform in their house? How did they manage daily life? Were they interested in any particular activities? A formal activity history might help to organize your thoughts. Another strategy is to ask the patient to describe a typical day.

The occupational therapist tries to find an activity that will motivate the patient. Motivation is self-directed behavior that an individual pursues for internal or external reinforcement.[10] The individual moves toward a goal. Occupational therapy relies on both extrinsic and intrinsic motivation.

Goal-directed behavior stimulated by rewards outside of an organism can be called extrinsic motivation. Intrinsic motivation, on the other hand, is dependent on an internal reward system. The individual will pursue an idea or task to fulfill an inner need. This need is not based on the satisfaction of basic drives, such as hunger, thirst, or libido. "Intrinsic motivation builds toward self-reward in independent action that underlies competent behavior."[10] Crucial factors in the environment determine the extent to which an individual is motivated by intrinsic rewards.

Successful home-care programs are carried over when the occupational therapist is not present. The choice of activity promotes the patient's goals, ideally generating some intrinsic rewards.

Teaching and Learning

If you are a student, you are engaged in teaching and learning. Although the complexity of teaching and learning is seldom acknowledged, every person has unique learning needs. Thus, there are no definitive rules that can be used as a guide to success. Nevertheless, there are some basic tenets that might serve the home-care practitioner. First, center the learning on the patient's goals and expectations. Second, modalities should promote goal attainment. Third, activities must have a moderate degree of difficulty, but the choice should not foster anxiety. Fourth, the occupational therapist slowly increases the patient's level of participation. Fifth, the responsibility for a daily program will ultimately rest with the patient and the caregivers. Finally, feedback is offered to help the patient learn how to self-monitor.[24]

Programs should be written out so that other caregivers and team members can follow the instructions. Teaching aides—pictures, samples, demonstrations, and cues—help facilitate teaching and learning.

Coordination

Coordination determines the degree to which the home-care team is able to work together. The home-care team has two parts: the patient and caregivers, and the professional staff. This diverse group is most effective when it functions as a unit. Although the patient is the focal point of the delivery process, each individual views the patient's condition from a different perspective, and all views must be respected. Diverse *opinions* must be organized into a unified effort (Fig. 39-2).

It is difficult to create a home-care team. However, if several professionals assume the responsibility for coordination, the communication channels can begin to open. The patient, who is the focus, should be informed of and included in all communication. No decision can be made without his or her participation. If the patient is unable to take part in decision making, a family member or caregiver should be included in the discussions. In keeping with this spirit of family participation, conferences can be held in the patient's house.

A healthy team may have conflicts and problems. Issues should be identified and aired. Skilled group members are able to separate subjective issues from objective goals. This is why the home-care practitioner needs to understand group dynamics. Such knowledge can be gleaned from a balance of practical experience and a theoretical base.

The patient and the caregiver, who are together for most of the day, form the hub of the wheel of effort. The wheel cannot roll forward unless all of the team members that operate around it move in the same direction (Fig. 39-2). The team must work toward similar goals.

It will be remembered that primary, secondary, and tertiary caregivers constitute the caregiver network. The caregiver network, or the hub of the wheel of effort, is the bedrock of effective home care. Cooperative participants reduce the stress of caring for the ill family member. On the other hand, the stress of illness taxes the family's resources. If some of the family members are uncooperative, the wheel of team effort cannot move forward.

Patient care requires time and effort. Eventually, stress may tax communication among the closest family

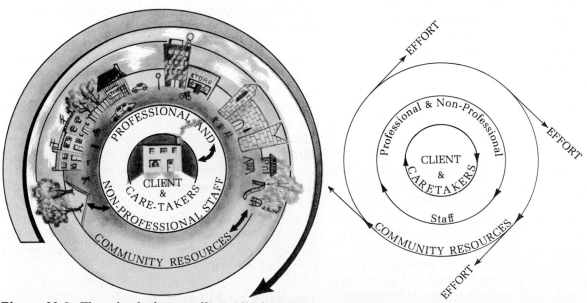

Figure 39-2. The wheel of team effort. All of the unique goals and skills of all the team members must be organized into a unified effort. All members must move in one direction so that the treatment can move forward.

members and friends. Specialists should assist the family and help members with any interaction problems. This assistance should be offered before the situation deteriorates and family members have no energy left to invest in cooperation.

It is helpful to discuss the patient's assets and strengths as well as liabilities and weaknesses. The patient's premorbid lifestyle should be explored in an effort to understand the present situation. New information may alter the thrust of care and reorder treatment priorities. Professionals may also encourage increased use of secondary and tertiary caregivers. No caregiver should feel overburdened. Family members may be reluctant to admit that they need help. The next case study is an example of a functional caregiver network.

Case Study

The S. family has a network of caregivers. Mr. S. suffered a fracture of his right humerus and hip one month ago. He was treated in the hospital and discharged to his own home. Mrs. S. is the primary caregiver. She oversees the exercise regime, dressing, and bathing activities. All this is done at the same time that she continues her normal household and shopping chores.

Mr. S.'s brother Stephen and his wife Maria are the secondary caregivers. They live five miles from the patient. They visit Mr. S. almost every night on their way home from work. They assist with shopping, heavy cleaning, and occasionally with the exercise programs.

The patient's daughter, Lydia H., lives 30 miles away. She is a working mother with house, work, and family responsibilities. Lydia stops to see her parents every other week. Her mother asks her to complete selected errands—shopping for special equipment, drycleaning, and staying with her father when her mother goes out to Bingo once a month. ☐

Communication

In the home setting, there are three basic forms of communication—face-to-face, telephone, and written.

Face-to-face communication takes place in the patient's home or in the agency. This type of interaction may be difficult to arrange for a team because each member has a different schedule and visits the patient at a different time. Team goals and roles must be clarified early in the treatment process, because confusion could block communication and progress.

Written communication may be used in lieu of a face-to-face interaction. On an informal level, notes may be left in the patient's house for other team members. Telephone discussions may be a more effec-

tive method of exploring issues and potential areas of confusion.

Another form of written communication takes place after each patient visit—the progress note. The importance of documentation cannot be overemphasized in the home situation. Many fiscal intermediaries have stringent requirements for documentation that must be followed to qualify for reimbursement.

Communication creates a sense of teamwork that is satisfying to all members. The following quotation underscores the effort that one must invest to develop a team:

> It is naive to bring together a highly diverse group of people and expect that, by calling them a team, they will in fact behave as a team. It is ironic indeed to realize that a football team spends 40 hours per week practicing teamwork for those two hours on Sunday afternoon when their teamwork really counts. Teams in organizations seldom spend two hours per year practicing when their ability to function as a team counts 40 hours per week.[12]

Architectural Barriers

Physical factors affect the outcome of home-care programs. For example, architectural barriers can impede patient progress. However, economic factors limit large-scare changes in many homes, yet few people have access to the resources needed to renovate basic structures such as the bathroom and kitchen fixtures. Therefore, the therapist must assess the type of changes that would be helpful and possible; little is gained from exploring changes that can never come about.

Another less-obvious factor is cultural. Although some people enjoy change that will facilitate their daily performance, others regard adjustment with new discomfort. The total expenditure of energy needed for change is not considered possible; the daily, smaller energy expenditure attached to the current inconvenience seems more acceptable. Sometimes, the only stable part of the patient's world is the unchanging nonhuman environment. The illness may have upset and altered everything else, including roles and relationships. To such people, investment in the secure and unchanging environment may be more reasonable.

The therapist who blindly suggests extensive change in this type of situation may encounter a brittle and resistant audience. It seems logical to suggest minor changes, such as moving a bookcase 1 foot to the left to free a passage for wheelchair accessibility. However, the patient may not wish to crowd the picture that hangs next to the bookcase. The nonhuman world may be the last place that remains unscathed by illness.[34]

The best approach for the therapist to use cannot be precisely outlined. Patients must be assessed in the context of their nonhuman environment and social interaction patterns. There is no need for the therapist to invest energy in attempting to foster change when the patient or caregiver do not think that any benefit can be gained from the alterations. Some ideas may be accepted at a later date.

Change was precluded in the next example because of cultural and economic factors. This family was limited in income and provincial in outlook. They could not value the suggestions of an "outsider." The therapist could raise questions but could never expect to see immediate results. The therapist's role regarding changes to the environment was, at best, that of a catalyst. The only change that was considered was the addition of a snack table to the right side of the refrigerator. Any others would have been too costly. The family seemed to accept the idea, but the item was never purchased. Possibly after the patient was discharged, the family was able to develop its own solution to the problem.

Case Study

The H. family has resided in their small row house for 30 years. The brick house is more than 150 years old; it is situated in a blue-collar residential district in a large metropolitan area.

Mrs. H. is 54 years old. She has a residual left hemiparesis. Her recovery is complete except for a decrease in shoulder function. A Winter–Haven perceptual test revealed a possible deficit in visual memory and spatial relations. She can dress independently, although her performance is slow. The occupational therapist has been active with Mrs. H.'s training for 1 month. The long-term goal is to "maximize independent functioning." The short-term goal is to "help Mrs. H. be independent in the kitchen and increase left upper extremity function."

The therapist found that Mrs. H. used her disabil-

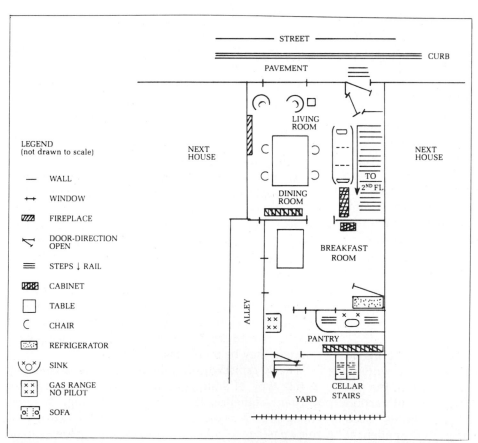

Figure 39-3. Floor plan of the first floor of the H. family's house. The floor plan depicted here is common in a blue-collar neighborhood near the industrial center of a large city. The houses are more than 150 years old. Streets are narrow and barren. Small yards extend for 15 to 20 feet from the back doors. The average income is $25,000 a year for a family of four. This particular neighborhood is close-knit and insular. Relatives live "two doors" away or "around the corner."

ity. She could now garner the sympathy and support of her two teenaged children. She agreed to try to work in the kitchen only because her children could not cook very well. The biggest problem that hindered progress was the layout of the kitchen and the breakfast room (see floor plan in Fig. 39-3). Whenever Mrs. H. wishes to take things out of the refrigerator, she has to walk back several feet to place the objects on the table. The food then must be transferred into the pantry. Mrs. H. refused to consider carry-all baskets; she felt that they "looked funny." The therapist suggested that a snack table be placed next to the refrigerator. The patient agreed but never was able to procure the item. The stove is also a problem; it does not have an automatic pilot light. After a few unsuccessful attempts at cooking, Mrs. H. was willing to turn this responsibility over to her oldest daughter. "I guess that she is old enough after all," she said.

The H. family could not afford any extensive changes. Their culture did not support do-it-yourself innovations. The nonhuman environment was one of the only stable things in their lives. There was little energy left to invest in change.   □

Body Mechanics and Transfer Techniques

All home-care personnel must be skilled in transferring patients under less-than-ideal circumstances. Caregivers are unfamiliar with the process; they may fear that they will injure the patient or themselves. Also, the occupational therapist must frequently position the patient for activities. This is commonly done without assistance, and principles of good body mechanics must be used. Since caregivers and neighbors frequently observe therapy, good technique and an air of competence are essential.

Home Modalities

Modalities and tools must be suited to the home environment. One patient may welcome special equipment and tools, while another may refuse to learn new methods to cope with the disability. The lack of material resources may be inconvenient, but this lack should not alter the progress of a rehabilitation program. If equipment is not available, therapists learn to improvise. Commonplace objects can be substituted for "special" equipment. Examples of such improvisions follow:
1. *Weight*—place canned goods in a zippered pocketbook or knotted sock
2. *Stablizer*—put a damp cloth under the plate or tray
3. *Elastic shoe laces*—use 1/8-inch elastic cut to shoe lace size
4. *Skateboard*—place a towel under the affected arm; use on a smooth table top

5. *Bathtub transfer seat*—two chairs, one placed inside and one placed outside of the tub.

Discharge Planning

There are two types of discharge, planned and unplanned. Planned discharges take place after 2 to 4 months of treatment. Once the patient's performance in activities of daily living and upper extremity retraining reaches a plateau for two or three visits, the occupational therapist must prepare the patient for discharge. This decision should be discussed with the patient and caregivers and the other home-care team members. If circumstances warrant additional visits, the therapist should contact the case coordinator and discuss the reasons why visits should continue. Occupational therapists can visit a patient even if all other services are discontinued. In cases where the other team members feel that the patient still has unmet needs, the team can act as the patient's advocate by working with the case coordinator, who can contact the fiscal intermediary and discuss the interpretation of the guidelines. On the other hand, it is well to remember that fiscal intermediaries will not reimburse agencies for maintenance-level treatment.

If discharge is appropriate, at least two visits should include information on a home program that the patient and caregivers can pursue. The information should be stated in clear, jargon-free language that caregivers can use with ease. When appropriate, diagrams are useful to clarify a point.

Unplanned discharges occur more frequently now than in the past, since patients may be sicker when they are discharged from hospitals. Their medical conditions are more acute, which means that their medical conditions change and may necessitate inpatient services. This means that communication among the patient, family, and caregivers, as well as with the home health agency and hospital staff, becomes even more important.

After-Care and Evaluation

At present, there are no resources channeled into after-care. Ideally, each patient would be followed using telephone and brief visits designed to reinforce the rehabilitation program and to offer updated information. Insurance carriers do not recognize the value of after-care, since they are devoting their limited resources to acute patient needs.

Some therapists feel, however, that select cases require after-care. Using their own time and resources, they telephone the patient, family, and caregivers to see how well they are managing. At times, a strategically planned visit may boost morale and encourage the patient to continue working toward his or her goals. Although this type of follow-up is rare, therapists find that they can help the occasional family to cope with emerging needs. This type of maintenance service should be provided as a form of preventative care.

Another aspect of after-care is a critical evaluation of the occupational therapy services the patient received. A questionnaire covering the quality of occupational therapy services is directed to the patient, family, and caregiver. Outcome studies where the final outcome of the patient's care is weighed against the initial goals are also important. It is essential that occupational therapists compare the patient's progress with the cost of care. Where resources used wisely? Quality assurance has long been a concern of members of the AOTA, and they have developed information on how to design studies to determine the benefit of occupational therapy services. (See the Quality Assurance chapter in this text.) Home-care patients frequently develop a need for service at a later date. Hospitalizations, relapses, and changes in residences may necessitate additional treatment. If so, the patient is referred to a home health agency again, and the delivery cycle is initiated again.

The mechanical aspects of home-care delivery were presented in this section. Unfortunately, the fun, excitement, and fascination of home visiting is not easily conveyed in a written narrative. During a home visit, the therapist enters the patient's sanctum—his or her home. The therapist becomes privy to confidential information, environmental cues, and emotional displays that are frequently hidden from the professional person's view. This information shapes the quality of care that is offered to the patient and the family.

Outside Issues Affecting Home-Care Delivery

There are four factors that directly affect the type of service given in the home: reimbursement, documentation, continuing education, and present practice.

Reimbursement

Home health agencies are funded by both public and private sources, including insurance companies, health care corporations, religious groups, charities, endowments, hospitals, and fees collected from patients. In the US, most home-care programs receive some of their funds from Medicare reimbursement. Since this program is national, guidelines for other reimbursement may be based on this legislation. It is important for practitioners to have a broad-based knowledge of reimbursement principles.

Medicare

Title XVIII of the Social Security Act provides legislation for Medicare funding. Medicare provides medical benefits primarily for older Americans, but persons who have been disabled for more than 24 months can also qualify for benefits. Specific requirements are established for all of the services that Medicare will fund. Not only do these guidelines influence current practice, but they will also affect the future. The importance of Medicare extends beyond funding; it sets national standards for practice. In short, Medicare establishes national priorities regarding the services that will be covered, the quality and nature of those services, and the degree to which the practitioner and the agency will be held accountable for the care they give.

The responsibility for administering the Medicare program was given to the Secretary of Health and Human Services and, within this authority, the Health Care Financing Administration (HCFA). To accomplish this huge task, the US is divided into HCFA regions, and each regional staff develops agreements with public or private organizations to serve as payment "intermediaries." These companies or intermediaries use HCFA guidelines to establish the "services covered, amounts payable, and payments to be paid to beneficiaries and providers such as home health agencies and hospitals."[7] The intermediary becomes HCFA's representative in the region by supervising and overseeing the disbursement of benefits. In effect, this means that there are differences in the interpretation of the guidelines and regulations among the intermediaries.[7] To qualify for home-care services, patients must be homebound, which means they must be unable to walk and get out of their homes. Patients must also require skilled levels of care, since maintaining function is not covered under the law. Skilled services are nursing and physical and speech therapies. As of October 1986, occupational therapy also is recognized as a skilled service. The new occupational therapy extension of services went into effect in July 1987. HCFA staff must develop regulations and intermediary instructions. Thus, at this time, the exact meaning of the legislation is still unclear.[5]

Medicare requirements for occupational therapy are centered on the expectation that the patient will benefit from the services and make significant practical improvement in functional abilities in a reasonable period of time.[11] If the patient does not make progress, services must be curtailed, because the fiscal intermediary may refuse to pay for the service. This action is usually taken retroactively, so therapists must learn to monitor their own cases to prevent costly denials.

Medicaid

Medicaid, or Medical Assistance, Title XIX of the Social Security Act, is a program for people who have no other means to pay for medical care. The program is based on a formula for matching federal and state dollars. For example, the state must contribute a percentage of its per capita income. The ratios for the contributions are set by law. Some states do not contribute large sums of money to this program. Their reimbursement rates for home care may not cover even half of the actual cost of the services. If services are rendered, the agency must deal with the resulting deficit. If no alternative income is generated, the agency assets will be eaten away. Usually, monies from other sources are used to reduce the loss. However, this solution creates a complex and, at times, precarious funding situation. This is one of the reasons for establishment of rigid eligibility criteria. States may also develop their own criteria for eligibility.

Most states are required to provide home health services to Medicaid beneficiaries who are also eligible for skilled nursing care. Occupational therapy coverage varies, since it is an optional service.

There are strict limitations on the resources available to Medicaid patients. Thus, the nursing supervisor usually works out a rigid schedule of visits so the ceiling is not exceeded.[36] Agencies try to cope with this situation by providing fewer services over a shorter period of time. In rare cases, agencies use private donations to subsidize patients whose benefits have expired. As resources for the poor are stretched further and further, there are fewer sources to tap for providing services for people who have dire needs.

Other Sources

Other sources of revenue include third-party carriers such as private insurance companies. For example, most of Blue Cross policies cover home-care benefits.[36] Third-party carriers are slowly recognizing the benefits of using home care instead of in-hospital services; however, coverage still differs even among policies offered by the same carrier. Many prepayment plans — HMOs and PPOs — also cover home-care services. These programs are new, and the guidelines and standards for coverage are not always clear.

Many hospitals are developing their own home-care organizations, and the number of privately owned home health agencies has grown drastically in the past few years.

There are a number of private agencies that try to augment home health services. Funded by private donations and combinations of federal and state funds, some of these agencies offer creative solutions for patient problems. Specific services such as the loan of hospital equipment may be available. Religious groups may also offer patient visiting services or meal delivery to the chronically disabled.

Another emerging source of referrals and financial support for home care is the federally approved HMO. All federally approved HMOs must offer home-care services. The HMO is a prepaid group practice. Each subscriber pays a fee which entitles him or her to receive a wide range of health services. Some services that are covered are routine checkups, eye examinations, and prenatal care. All are oriented toward the maintenance of health. If a member becomes ill, the HMO provides complete medical care. Therefore, it behooves the HMO to utilize preventative rather than remediation services. If not, all of the practice finances will be absorbed by medical costs.

Documentation

Health care providers sometimes forget that documentation is a form of communication. Home-care delivery is not easy to observe because of the number of patients' residences that are visited. Documentation therefore becomes an important tool to measure the quality of patient care. There is an adage that is frequently repeated by nursing supervisors — "if it isn't written, it hasn't been done." This statement reflects the stringent demands of the majority of fiscal intermediaries. Most fiscal intermediaries demand adherence to their guidelines; if not satisfied, a carrier will refuse to reimburse the agency for the visits. Organized, goal-oriented, concise notes that clearly convey the patient's status to the reviewer are essential. Most fiscal intermediaries demand measurable progress in a reasonable period of time.[6] There are few funding sources for extended maintenance-level care.

Most fiscal intermediaries rely on Medicare standards for their reimbursement guidelines. These guidelines determine the thrust of covered services and the diagnoses and care that will be covered. These guidelines establish the narrowest definition for occupational therapy services. Therefore, it seems reasonable to outline this base, although it is hoped that therapists will be able to deliver broader services. In general, Medicare coverage dictates that the patient must be able to improve significantly in a *reasonable* and generally predictable period of time. Claims for reimbursement for custodial care or maintenance are not accepted by Medicare.

On the first visit, the patient must be evaluated, treatment goals must be established, the total number of treatment visits required to attain the goals must be projected, and the patient must be given treatment. An evaluation form was presented earlier. The therapist must inform the supervisor about the treatment frequency and plans. The therapist must also fill out a certification form. Every evaluation, certification form, or progress note must demonstrate to a person who is not an occupational therapist how the patient will progress and complete the established goals. Some agencies require a treatment plan for every scheduled visit. If plans change, the therapist must explain why.

The patient's progress is reviewed every 60 days, when a certification and plan of treatment form must be completed. This is the same form that was completed after the evaluation. This justification has three parts: a certification component, a medical and patient information update, and an addendum for additional information. Information commonly given in the recertification includes the patient's: (1) name and address; (2) health insurance number; (3) medical record number; (4) start of care (SOC) date; (5) how long treatment can continue; (6) name of home health agency; (7) principal diagnosis using code numbers; (8) surgical procedure code if relevant; (9) other pertinent diagnoses; (10) functional limitations (*e.g.*, contracture, endurance, mental, vision, speech) and activities permitted (*e.g.*, bedrest, transfer to bed/chair, partial weight bearing, cane, or no restrictions); (11) safety measures; (12) orders for services and treatments, which must specify modality, amount, and frequency; (13) medications, including doses, frequency, and route; (14) mental status; (15) nutritional requirements; (16) medical supplies; (17) allergies; (18) goals for rehabilitation and patient's potential and, if pertinent, discharge plans; (19) significant clinical findings with a summary from each discipline; (20) prognosis; (21) attending physician's name and address; (22) physician certification regarding need for treatment; and (23) physician's signature and date signed.[11]

At present, Medicare defines occupational therapy as a "medically prescribed treatment concerned with improving, or restoring functions which have been impaired by illness or injury or, where function has been permanently lost or reduced by illness or injury, to improve the individual's ability to perform those tasks required for independent functioning."[6] Services may include:

1. The evaluation and re-evaluation as required of a patient's level of function by administering diagnostic and prognostic tests
2. The selection and teaching of task-oriented therapeutic activities designed to restore physical function
3. The planning, implementing, and supervising of individualized therapeutic activity programs as part of an overall active treatment program for a patient with a diagnosed psychiatric illness
4. The planning and implementing of therapeutic tasks and activities to restore sensory–integrative function
5. The teaching of compensatory techniques to improve the level of independence in the activities of daily living
6. The designing, fabricating, and fitting of orthotic and self-help devices
7. Vocational and prevocational assessment and training.[6]

There are other restrictions: services must be prescribed by a physician and performed by a qualified occupational therapist or certified occupational therapy assistant who works under the therapist's supervision. The most important clause in the criteria for coverage is that services are considered "reasonable and necessary" only where the patient's condition indicates that there will be a significant practical improvement in the level of function in a "reasonable" period of time.[6] Occupational therapy must be goal-directed, purposeful activity that can maximize the patient's level of function in a predetermined period of time.

Not all programs are governed by Medicare, but the number of older Americans increases daily, and this will in itself expand Medicare services. Recent changes in the legislation offer three opportunities for occupational therapists to increase their practice. The legislation was part of budget-deficit reduction legislation (HR 5300) that was signed by President Reagan on October 22, 1986, after a number of years of intense educational efforts directed by the members of AOTA under the leadership of the Government and Legal Affairs Division of the Association. The new amendment will impact on three areas. First, occupational therapy services will be covered under Part B, outpatient programming and private practice. Part A covers inpatient, skilled nursing facility, and home health care for 100 days, and occupational therapy services were covered except when the patient had exhausted his or her coverage. Occupational therapy services then had to be terminated even if they were needed. Now, occupational therapy would be covered under the Part B coverage, since this part includes outpatient services and home health care as well as physician's office visits and some durable medical equipment.

The second part of the new law deals with outpatient programming for occupational therapy services. Such services will be covered in rehabilitation agencies, including satellite centers, in skilled nursing facilities, or in the patient's home. Occupational therapy can enter a case without the necessity of another skilled service.

Finally, private practice in occupational therapy will be improved by the last change in the law. Effective July 1, 1987, occupational therapy will join physical therapy as the only nonphysician providers. This means that therapists will be assigned a provider number and can bill Medicare directly for services rendered to beneficiaries in the office, skilled nursing facility, home, or any other appropriate setting. There is a $500 limit per beneficiary under this provision.[2]

In some settings, the value of custodial and maintenance services are recognized, and undiagnosed mental illness may also be treated.

The boundaries of Medicare coverage are presented here to establish a base for home-care practice. Services should not be narrowed further. The home-care therapist should define the role of occupational therapy so that the maximum number of patients can be reached. However, if the role were too broadly defined, other services could be duplicated, and the unique focus of occupational therapy could be lost. A balanced, well-defined role should be developed and should function within the boundaries of the home-care agency's financial resources.

Continuing Education

Home-care practitioners function independently. Although they work on patient-care teams, they rarely work with other occupational therapists. The practitioner's knowledge and skills can become dated by this isolation, as there are few opportunities for discussion regarding new treatment ideas and modalities in the daily home care routine. For this reason, home-care practitioners must create their own educational opportunities. One way to expand learning is to take advantage of continuing education programs. Advertisements appear in occupational therapy journals and newspapers. Participation in occupational therapy organizations also promotes the sharing of ideas. One should never feel that one works alone, separated from new ideas. Some agencies require that the occupational therapist attend one professional program a year. The future of any specialty practice rests on the continued excellence of the practitioners.

Present Practice

The recent changes in the Medicare law, the increased numbers of experienced therapists who want to own their own practice, and the numbers of patients who need care make private practice a fast-paced area for personal growth. Students who are interested in a private practice are advised to work for a year or two in a facility which offers a broad range of learning opportunities under the supervision of an experienced practitioner before entering home care. The more knowledgeable and skilled the practitioner, the more advanced the level of care offered to patients. The home setting is not an arena to develop basic knowledge and skills, because care is isolated from other occupational therapy practitioners.

Private Practice

Some therapists are engaged in private practice. They divide their time among several agencies or settings. These practitioners may also receive private referrals. Payment may be a combination of part-time salary and fees-for-service. A fee-for-service is a lump sum of money paid to the therapist for each visit. The therapist is not a bona fide member of the agency; no benefits are paid. Note-writing and travel time is included in the fee.

At times, the agency will pay for attendance at staff meetings and conferences.

One advantage of private practice is the freedom that it affords the therapist. Treatment times and hours and patient load and demands can be varied. Practice can be carried out in several specialty areas; programs that could not afford occupational therapy can begin to offer the service. This modest beginning does not put the service in a make-it-or-break-it position. Some therapists are combining part-time institutional work with private practice.

Group Practice

Another convenient way to develop part-time occupational therapy is in a group practice with one therapist acting as coordinator. A registry of local therapists who wish to pursue part-time work is compiled. Once the names are organized, the process is not complex. State laws must be researched for local requirements. This is usually a simple matter for a lawyer to handle. When the group is organized, referrals can be received. Contracts can be signed with several agencies, or single referrals can be accepted. Individual therapists are assigned to a location near their home or work. Referrals are assigned by location. At least one member must be available during the day for phone calls, referrals, and attendance at meetings.

The benefits of a group practice are numerous. The agency can deal with one coordinator instead of several part-time workers. A broad geographical area can be serviced without wasting time in travel. The group seeks its own members and is better able to evaluate member skills. Service to patients is not interrupted by vacations, illness, and other obligations—the group and not just one person is responsible for the referrals.

The group members benefit because the work is part time. More therapists can participate in home-care delivery. Agencies with small case loads can still provide occupational therapy services. Therapists can join or leave the group without any major disruption of service. The group name becomes familiar to agencies and community centers even if individual therapists have to drop out of the group.

References

1. Administrator's Handbook of Community Health and Home Care Services, p 95. New York, National League of Nursing Publication No. 21-1943, 1984
2. American Occupational Therapy Association: Occupational Therapy Medicare Amendment fact sheet. Rockville, Maryland, The American Occupational Therapy Association, undated
3. Barris R, Kielhofner G, Levine R, et al: Occupational as interaction with the environment. In Kielhofner G (ed): A Model of Human Occupation: Theory and Application, pp 42, 49–55. Baltimore, Williams & Wilkins, 1985

4. Brameld T: Philosophies of Education in a Cultural Perspective. New York, Dryden Press, 1955 (quoted in Yerxa EJ: The philosophical base of occupational therapy. In Occupational Therapy: 2001 A.D., p 26. Rockville, Maryland, American Occupational Therapy Association, 1979

5. Congress approves the occupational therapy Medicare amendments. Occup Ther News 40:1, 1986

6. Coverage of services: Occupational therapy. In Medicare Home Health Agency Manual, Section 205.2, p 15.1 US Dept. of Health and Human Services, HCFA Publication No. 11. Washington, DC, 1982

7. DePaoli TL, Zenk–Jones P: Medicare reimbursement in home care. Am J Occup Ther 38:739, 1984

8. Devereaux EB: Community home health care—In the rural setting. In Smith H, Hopkins H (eds): Willard and Spackman's Occupational Therapy, 6th ed, pp 779–795. Philadelphia, JB Lippincott, 1982

9. Engelhardt TH Jr: Occupational therapists as technologists and custodians of meaning. In Kielhofner G (ed): Health Through Occupation: Theory and Practice in Occupational Therapy, pp 139–145. Philadelphia, FA Davis, 1983

10. Florey LL: Intrinsic motivation: The dynamics of occupational therapy theory. Am J Occup Ther 23:319, 1969

11. Form HCFA-485(C4)(4-85). Washington, DC, US Dept. of Health and Human Services Health Care Financing Administration, approved 1985

12. Fry RE, Lech BA, Rubin I: Working with the primary care team: the first intervention. In Wise H, Beckhard R, Rubin I, et al: (eds): Making Health Teams Work, p 56. Cambridge, Massachusetts, Ballinger Publishing, 1974

13. Hall ET: The Hidden Dimension. Garden City, New York, Anchor Books, 1969

14. Health Insurance System, p 12–2. Washington, DC, US Dept. of Health and Human Services Health Care Financing Administration, Publication No. 10013-81, 1981

15. Kaplan K, Cubie SH: A case analysis method for the model of human occupation. Am J Occup Ther 36:645, 1982

16. Keilhofner G (ed): A Model of Human Occupation: Theory and Application. Baltimore, Williams & Wilkins, 1985

17. Kielhofner G: Occupational function and dysfunction. In Kielhofner G (ed): A Model of Human Occupation: Theory and Application, pp 63–75. Baltimore, Williams & Wilkins, 1985

18. Kielhofner G: General systems theory: Implications for theory and action in occupational therapy. Am J Occup Ther 32:637, 1978

19. Keilhofner G, Burke JP: A model of human occupation 1: Conceptual framework and content. Am J Occup Ther 34:572, 1980

20. Kielhofner G, Burke JP: Components and determinants of human occupation. In Kielhofner G (ed): A Model of Human Occupation: Theory and Application, pp 12–36. Baltimore, Williams & Wilkins, 1985

21. Kielhofner G, Shepherd J, Stabenow CA, et al: Physical disabilities In Kielhofner G (ed): A Model of Human Occupation: Theory and Application, pp 170–247. Baltimore, Williams & Wilkins, 1985

22. McKechnie JL: Webster's New Twentieth Century Dictionary of the English Language, p 1347. Williams Collins, 1980

23. Morris CW: Varieties of Human Value. Chicago, University of Chicago Press, 1956 (quoted in Rogers CR: Freedom to Learn, pp 241–242. Columbus, Charles E Merrill, 1969)

24. Mosey AC: Activities Therapy. New York, Raven Press, 1973

25. National Association for Home Care: Testimony to US Senate Finance Committee on cost limits. The Association Report No. 140, p 3, September 17, 1985

26. Rath L (cited in Kirschenbaum H: Beyond values clarification. In Simon SB, Kirschenbaum H (eds): Readings in Values Clarification, p 93. Minneapolis, Winston Press, 1973)

27. Reilly M: Occupational therapy can be one of the great ideas of 20th century medicine. Am J Occup Ther 16:1, 1962

28. Report No. 166: NAHC survey of all HHA's in Rhode Island confirms drastic administration cutbacks in Medicare Home Health Benefit, p 10. Washington, DC, National Association for Home Care, June 6, 1986

29. Report No. 149: Special report, p 3. Washington, DC, National Association for Home Care, January 17, 1986

30. Research Information Division: Dataline. Occup Ther News 39:7, October 1985

31. Research Information Division: Dataline. Occup Ther News 40:8, September 1986

32. Rogers J: Order and disorder in medicine and occupational therapy. Am J Occup Ther 36:29, 1982

33. Rogers JC: The study of human occupation. In Kielhofner G (ed): Health Through Occupation: Theory and Practice in Occupational Therapy, pp 93–124. Philadelphia, FA Davis, 1983

34. Searles HF: The Nonhuman Environment. New York, International Universities Press, 1960

35. Spradley JP, McDurdy DW (eds): Conformity and Conflict, p 2. Boston, Little, Brown, 1980

36. Trossman PB: Administrative and professional issues for the occupational therapist in home health care. Am J Occup Ther 38:726, 1984

37. Yerxa EJ: Audacious values: The energy source for occupational therapy practice. In Kielhofner G (ed): Health Through Occupation: Theory and Practice in Occupational Therapy, pp 151–152. Philadelphia, FA Davis, 1983

Appreciation is extended to the following individuals who offered feedback on current home-care practice: Claire Lozowicki, President, Community Occupational Therapy Consultants, Inc. and members of the group; Gregory Wilson, Marlene Basiago, and Reneé Baumblatt–Magida who provided case studies and a critical analysis of current practice; and Terri Healey, Director of Home Care, Thomas Jefferson University, who offered an administrator's perspective on current administrative issues.

APPENDICES

Occupational Therapy Definition for Purposes of Licensure*

Occupational therapy is the use of purposeful activity with individuals who are limited by physical injury or illness, psychosocial dysfunction, developmental or learning disabilities, poverty and cultural differences or aging process in order to maximize independence, prevent disability and maintain health. The practice encompasses evaluation, treatment and consultation. Specific occupational therapy services include: teaching daily living skills; developing perceptual-motor skills and sensory integrative functioning; developing play skills and prevocational and leisure capacities; designing, fabricating, or applying selected orthotic and prosthetic devices or selective adaptive equipment; using specifically designed crafts and exercises to enhance functional performance; administering and interpreting tests such as manual muscle and range of motion; and adapting environments for the handicapped. These services are provided individually, in groups, or through social systems.

Principles of Occupational Therapy Ethics†

Preamble

The American Occupational Therapy Association (AOTA) and its component members are committed to furthering man's ability to function fully within his total environment. To this end the occupational therapist renders service to clients in all stages of health and illness, to institutions, other professionals, colleagues, students and to the general public.

In furthering this commitment the American Occupational Therapy Association has established the Principles of Occupational Therapy Ethics. The Principles are intended for use by all occupational therapy personnel, including practitioners in all settings, administrators, educators, and students. Licensure laws and regulations should reflect and support these Principles which are intended to be action oriented, guiding and preventive rather than negative or merely disciplinary. The Principles, likewise, should influence the consulting, planning, and teaching of occupational therapists.

It should be noted that these Principles are intended only for internal use by the American Occupational Therapy Association as a guide to appropriate conduct of its members. The Principles are not intended to define a standard of care for patients or clients of a particular community.

Professional maturity will be demonstrated in applying these basic Principles while exercising the large measure of freedom which they provide and which is essential to responsible and creative occupational therapy service.

For the purpose of continuity the following definitions will support information in this document: Occupational therapist includes registered occupational therapists, certified occupational therapy assistants, occupational therapy students; Clients include patients, students, and those to whom occupational therapy services are delivered.

I. Related to the Recipient of Service

The occupational therapist demonstrates a beneficent concern for the recipient of services and maintains a goal-directed relationship with the recipient which furthers the objectives for which it is established. Services are evaluated against objectives and accountability is maintained therefore. Respect shall be shown for the recipients' rights and the occupational therapist will preserve the confidence of the client relationship.

---

* Adopted by the Representative Assembly, American Occupational Therapy Association, March 7, 1981. Published in 1981 Representative Assembly Minutes. Am J Occup Ther 35:798, 1981. Reprinted with permission of the American Occupational Therapy Association.

† Adopted by the Representative Assembly, American Occupational Association, April 1, 1977; revised April, 1980. Am J Occup Ther 34:896–899, 1980.

Guidelines: Recipients of occupational therapy services refer to clients, patients, students and the employers of occupational therapists; *i.e.* agencies, facilities, institutions, etc.

It is the professional responsibility of occupational therapists to provide services for clients without regard to race, creed, national origin, sex, handicap or religious affiliation. Occupational therapists recognize each client's individuality and worth as a unique person.

Services provided should be planned in concert with clients' involvement in goal-directed activities, in accordance with the overall habilitation or rehabilitation plan. Treatment objectives and the therapeutic process must be measurable to insure professional accountability.

Clients' and students' rights are to be protected as stipulated in the Federal Privacy Act of 1974, in addition to any specified rules, regulations or procedures as may be required by the employer.

The financial gain of occupational therapists should never be paramount to the delivery of services. Those occupational therapists who are compensated by virtue of being a direct service provider or vendor have the right to assess reasonable fees for profit.

Occupational therapists are obligated to provide the highest quality of service to the recipient. If further services would be beneficial to the client, the referring practitioner should be informed. It is also incumbent upon occupational therapists to recommend termination of services when established goals have been met, or when further services would not produce improved recipient performance.

Occupational therapy educators are obligated to provide the highest quality educational services supporting the AOTA "Essentials" and the current theory that supports service delivery.

II. Related to Competence

The occupational therapist shall actively maintain and improve one's professional competence, represent it accurately, and function within its parameters.

Guidelines: Occupational therapists recognize the need for continuing education and where relevant, they obtain training, experience, self-study or counsel to assure competent occupational therapy services.

Occupational therapists accurately represent their competence, education, training, and experience. Occupational therapists must accurately represent their skills and should not provide services or instructions, either for pay or in a voluntary capacity, that are not within their demonstrated competencies.

Occupational therapists must recognize the skills necessary to manage a client or a position. If client needs exist that the therapist cannot effectively manage, the

therapist should seek consultation or refer the client to an occupational therapist or another professional who can provide the required service.

III. Related to Records, Reports, Grades and Recommendations

The occupational therapist shall conform to local, state and federal laws and regulations and regulations applicable to records and reports. The occupational therapist abides by the employing institution's rules. Objective data shall govern subjective data in evaluations, grades, recommendations, records and reports.

Guidelines: Occupational therapists realize that reports are a required function of any position. Occupational therapists accurately record information and report information as required by AOTA standards, facility standards and state and national laws.

Occupational therapists fulfilling a teaching role utilize objective data in determining student grades.

All data recorded in permanent files or records should be supported by the occupational therapist's observations or by objective measures of data collection.

Students' records can only be divulged as authorized by law or the students' consent for release of information.

IV. Related to Intra-Professional Colleagues

The occupational therapist shall function with discretion and integrity in relations with other members of the profession and shall be concerned with the quality of their services. Upon becoming aware of objective evidence of a breach of ethics or substandard service, the occupational therapist shall take action according to established procedure.

Guidelines: Information gained or data gathered on a client shall only be divulged as expedient to other professional colleagues, students, referring practitioner, and employer. This includes data used in the course of in-service programs, professional meetings, prepared papers for presentation or publication, and educational materials. Undue invasion of privacy should be of utmost concern. Any reference to quality or service rendered by, or the integrity of a professional colleague will be expressed with due care to protect the reputation of that person.

It is the obligation of occupational therapists with first-hand knowledge of a breach of the ethical principles of this Association, by a colleague or student, to attempt to rectify the situation. If informal attempts fail, such activities or incidents against the ethical principles of this Association should immediately be brought to the attention of the appropriate local, regional or national Association committee/commission on ethical standards. Designated procedures should be followed and at all times the confidentiality of the information must be respected to protect the alleged party.

Practices by an employer that are in conflict with the ethical principles of this Association should also be brought to the immediate attention of the appropriate body(ies).

Information gained in peer review procedures should be held within the realm of confidentiality and be dealt with according to established procedures.

Publication credit for material developed by colleagues must be given. Also, credit for materials used in the classroom, manuals, in-service training, and oral or written reports, for example, should acknowledge the name of the individual or group who developed the material.

V. Related to Other Personnel

The occupational therapist shall function with discretion and integrity in relations with personnel and cooperate with them as may be appropriate. Similarly, the occupational therapist expects others to demonstrate a high level of competence. Upon becoming aware of objective evidence of a breach of ethics or substandard service, the occupational therapist shall take action according to established procedure.

Guidelines: Occupational therapists understand the scope of education and practice of related professions, and make full use of all the professional, technical and administrative resources that best serve the interests of consumers.

Occupational therapists do not delegate to other personnel those client-related services where the clinical skills and expertise of an occupational therpist is required. Other personnel or student may support treatment or educational goals, but must have demonstrated competency in each aspect of service to the occupational therapist before the responsibility can be delegated.

Occupational therapists who employ or supervise other professionals or technicians, or professionals or technicians in training, accept the obligation to facilitate their further development be providing suitable working conditions, consultation and experience opportunities.

Occupational therapists protect the privacy of all persons with whom professional collaboration occurs. If, however, an occupational therapist has first-hand knowledge of a colleague's performance which is in conflict with ethical standards, the therapist shall attempt to rectify the situation. Failing an informal solution, the occupational therapist shall utilize procedures established within the facility or agency, or to call the behavior to the attention of management, or utilize pro-

cedures established by the profession to handle such situations. Under no circumstances should the occupational therapist remain silent when a client, student or facility's status is in jeopardy.

VI. Related to Employers and Payers

The occupational therapist shall render service with discretion and integrity and shall protect the property and property rights of the employers and payers.

Guidelines: Occupational therapists function within the parameter of the job description or the goals established mutually between the employer or agency, and the occupational therapist. Occupational therapists use the utmost integrity in all dealings with the facility, university/college or contracting agency. Established procedures are followed regarding purchasing and bids.

Occupational therapists recommend appropriate fees for services and gain necessary acceptance for fees from the facility, agency and payers. Fees must be based upon cost analysis or a factor that can be justified upon request.

Occupational therapists shall not use the property, such as supplies and equipment, of the employer for their own personal use and aggrandizement.

VII. Related to Education

The occupational therapist implements a commitment to the education of society and the consumer of health services as well as to the education of health personnel on matters of health which are within the purview of occupational therapy.

Guidelines: Occupational therapists do not only provide direct service to alleviate specific problems with clients, programs or a community, but in addition, include education of all phases of services which can be provided to the public. This should include education of situations and conditions for which the competency of occupational therapists is recognized to assist in alleviating barriers limiting a persons' ability to function socially, emotionally, cognitively, or physically.

The public includes not only individuals concerned with the well-being of a member of their family, but also federal, state and local governmental agencies, educational systems and social agencies dealing with the health and well-being of the public.

VIII. Related to Evaluation and Research

Occupational therapists shall accept responsibility for evaluating, developing and refining service and the body of knowledge and skills which underlie the education and practice of occupational therapy and at all times protects the rights of subjects, clients, institutions and collaborators. The work of others shall be acknowledged.

Guidelines: Clients' families have the right to have, and occupational therapists have the responsibility to provide explanations of the nature, the purposes, and results of the occupational therapy services unless, as in some employment or treatment settings, there is an explicit exception to this right agreed upon in advance.

In reporting test results, occupational therapists indicate any reservations regarding validity or reliability resulting from testing circumstances or inappropriateness of the test norms for the person tested.

In performing research and reporting research results, occupational therapists must use accepted scientific methodology.

IX. Related to the Profession

The occupational therapist shall be responsible for gaining information and understanding of the principles, policies and standards of the profession. The occupational therapist functions as a representative of the profession.

Guidelines: Occupational therapists should provide accurate information to the public about the profession and the services that can be provided. Occupational therapists should remain informed about changes in the profession and represent the profession accurately to the consumer.

Occupational therapists may provide information to the public about available services through procedures established by the employing facility or contracting agency. When an occupational therapist provides an independent service, it is appropriate to advertise those services in accordance with AOTA established policy.

Occupational therapists should conduct themselves in a manner befitting professionals. The profession is judged in part by the conduct of its members as they carry out their functions.

Occupational therapists should show support and loyalty to the Association by cooperating with the Representatives in collecting information regarding proposed Association policy, replying to official requests for information and supporting the policies of the Association. It is the member's duty if he disagrees with an Association policy to work through existing channels to effect change.

Occupational therapists who engage in work or volunteer activities in addition to professional occupational therapy responsibilities, shall not violate the ethical principles of the Association in such activities.

X. Related to Advertising

Advertising by therapists under their professional title shall be in accordance with propriety and precedent in health professions.

Guidelines: Occupational therapists may provide information to the public about available services through procedures established by the employing facility or contracting agency. If an occupational therapist provides an independent service, it is appropriate to advertise those services.

The occupational therapist shall not use, or participate in the use of, any form of communication containing a false, fraudulent, misleading, deceptive, self-laudatory or unfair statement or claim. Testimonials or statements which promise a favorable result shall be avoided.

XI. Related to Law and Regulations

The occupational therapist shall seek to acquire information about applicable local, state, federal and institutional rules and shall function accordingly thereto.

Guidelines: Occupational therapists are obligated to function professionally as a practitioner within the limits of all laws related to the delivery of health services, and applicable to the practice of occupational therapy. Occupational therapists will not engage in any cruel, inhumane or degrading practices in the treatment of clients or in the education of students, or in supervision of others or in peer relationships.

It is the responsibility of occupational therapists to make known to their employers, employees and colleagues, those laws applicable to the practice of occupational therapy and education of occupational therapists.

XII. Related to Misconduct

The occupational therapist shall not appear to act with impropriety nor engage in illegal conduct involving moral turpitude and will not circumvent the principles of occupational therapy ethics through actions of others.

Guidelines: As employees, occupational therapists refuse to participate in practices inconsistent with legal, moral and ethical standards regarding the treatment of employees or the public. For example, occupational therapists will not condone practices that are inhumane, or that result in illegal or otherwise unjustifiable discrimination on the basis of race, age, sex, religion, handicap or national origin in hiring, promotion or training.

In providing occupational therapy services, occupational therapists avoid any action that will violate or diminish the legal and civil rights of clients or of others who may be affected.

As practitioners and educators, occupational therapists keep abreast of relevant federal, state, local and agency regulations and American Occupational Therapy Association Standards of Practice and education essentials concerning the conduct of their practice. They are concerned with developing such legal and quasi-legal regulations that support the interests of the public, students and the profession.

XIII. Related to Bioethical Issues and Problems of Society

The occupational therapist seeks information about the major health problems and issues to learn their implications for occupational therapy and for one's own services.

Guidelines: The principle is a philosophical statement that encourages occupational therapists to be global in their views of health in relationship to society.

APPENDIX

Standards of Practice for Occupational Therapy*

Preface

These standards will assist AOTA members in the management of occupational therapy services and will serve as a minimum standard for occupational therapy practice that is applicable to all client populations and the programs in which clients are served.

These standards are for qualified occupational therapists (OTRs) that are currently certified or licensed where required by the state.

Standard I: Screening

1. Occupational therapists have the responsibility to identify clients who may present problems in occupational performance (work, self-care, and play/leisure) that would require an evaluation.
2. Occupational therapists screen independently or as members of a team.
3. Screening methods shall be appropriate to the client's age, education, cultural background, medical status, and functional ability.
4. Screening methods may include interview, observation, testing and record review.
5. Occupational therapists shall communicate the screening results and recommendations to all appropriate individuals.

---

* Compiled by: Doris J. Shriver, OTR, Mary Foto, OTR, and members of the AOTA Commission on Practice for the AOTA Commission on Practice, John Farace, OTR, Chair.

Standard II: Referral

1. A client is appropriately referred to occupational therapy for remediation, maintenance, or prevention when the client has, or appears to have, a dysfunction or potential for dysfunction in occupational performance (work, self-care, play/leisure) or the performance components (sensorimotor, cognitive, psychosocial).
2. Clients shall be referred to occupational therapy for evaluation, design, contruction of, or training in therapeutic adaptations that include, but are not limited to, the physical environment, orthotics, prosthetics, and assistive and adaptive equipment.
3. Occupational therapists respond to a request for service and enter a case at their own professional discretion and on their own cognizance, and then assume full responsibility for the determination of the appropriate type, nature, and mode of service.
4. When physician referral is necessary to meet regulations (facility, state, federal, Joint Commission for Accreditation of Hospitals, licensure) or is required for third-party payment, the registered occupational therapist enters a case at the request of a physician; assumes full responsibility for the occupational therapy assessment; and, in consultation with the physician, establishes the appropriate type, nature, and mode of service.
5. Registered occupational therapists shall refer clients to other appropriate resources when, in the judgment of the occupational therapist, the knowledge and expertise of another professional is required.
6. Occupational therapists have the responsibility to

teach appropriate persons how to make occupational therapy referrals.

Standard III: Evaluation

1. Occupational therapists shall evaluate the client's performance according to the *Uniform Occupational Therapy Checklist* (AOTA-adopted, 1981).
2. Initial occupational therapy evaluations shall consider the client's medical, vocational, educational, activity, social history, and personal/family goals.
3. The occupational therapy evaluation shall include assessment of the functional abilities and deficits as related to the client's needs in the following areas:
   a. Occupational Performance: work, self-care, and play/leisure.
   b. Performance Components: sensorimotor, cognitive, psychosocial.
   c. Therapeutic adaptations and prevention.
4. Initial occupational therapy evaluations shall be completed and results documented within the time frames established by facilities, government agencies, and accreditation programs.
5. All evaluation methods shall be appropriate to the client's age, education, cultural and ethnic background, medical status, and functional ability.
6. The evaluation methods may include observation, interview, record review, and the use of evaluation techniques or tools.
7. When standardized evaluation tools are used, the tests should have normative data for the client characteristics. If normative data are not available, the results should be expressed in a descriptive report.
8. Collected evaluation data shall be analyzed and summarized to indicate the client's current status.
9. Occupational therapists shall document evaluation results in the client's record and indicate the specific evaluation tools and methods used.
10. Occupational therapists shall communciate evaluation results to the appropriate persons in the facility and community.
11. If the results of the evaluation indicate areas that require intervention by other professionals, the occupational therapist should refer the client to the appropriate service or request consultation.

Standard IV: Individual Program Planning

1. Occupational therapists shall use the results of the evaluation to develop an individual occupational therapy program that is:
   a. Stated in measurable and reasonable terms appropriate to the client's needs and goals and expected prognosis.
   b. Consistent with current principles and concepts of occupational therapy theory and practice.
2. The planning process shall include:
   a. Identifying short- and long-term goals.
   b. Collaborating with client, family, other professionals, and community resources.
   c. Selecting the media, methods, environment, and personnel needed to accomplish goals.
   d. Determining the frequency and duration of occupational therapy services.
3. The initial program plan shall be prepared and documented within the time frames established by facilities, government agencies, and accreditation programs.

Standard V: Individual Program Implementation

1. Occupational therapists shall implement the program according to the program plan.
2. Occupational therapists shall formulate and implement program modifications consistent with changes in the client's occupational performance and performance components.
3. Occupational therapists shall periodically re-evaluate and document the client's occupational performance and performance components.
4. Occupational therapists shall document the occupational therapy services provided and the frequency of the services within time frames established by facilities, government agencies, and accreditation programs.

Standard VI: Discontinuation of Services

1. Occupational therapists shall discontinue services when the client has achieved the goals or has achieved maximum benefit from occupational therapy.
2. Occupational therapists shall document the comparison of the initial and current state of functional abilities and deficits in occupational performance and performance components.
3. Occupational therapists shall prepare a discharge plan that is consistent with the occupational therapy, client interdisciplinary team, family and goals, and the expected prognosis. Consideration should be given to appropriate community resources for referral and environmental factors or barriers that may need modification.
4. Occupational therapists shall allow sufficient time for the coordination of and the effective implementation of the discharge plan.
5. Occupational therapists shall document recommendations for follow-up or re-evaluation.

Standard VII: Quality Assurance

1. The occupational therapist shall periodically and systematically review all aspects of individual occupational therapy programs for effectiveness and efficiency.
2. Occupational therapists shall periodically and systematically review the quality and appropriateness of total services delivered, using predetermined criteria that reflect professional consensus and recent developments in research and theory.

Standard VIII: Indirect Services

1. Occupational therapists shall provide supervision of other personnel as assigned in accordance with the AOTA *Guide for Supervision* (AOTA-Adopted, 1981).
2. Occupational therapists shall maintain records to meet facility, government agency, and accreditation program requirements.
3. Occupational therapists shall maintain a level of professional knowledge and skills to assure continued competency.
4. Occupational therapists shall facilitate research as it applies to the active practice of occupational therapy.
5. Occupational therapists shall provide administration and management services that ensure the use of AOTA standards.
6. Occupational therapists shall provide consultation services in order to develop or coordinate occupational therapy services, provide in-service education, adapt environments, and promote preventive health care in the home, client care facility, or community.

Standard IX: Legal/Ethical Components

1. Occupational therapists shall maintain current AOTA certification or licensure where required by the state.
2. Occupational therapists shall practice and manage occupational therapy programs as defined by federal and state laws and regulations.
3. Occupational therapists shall be familiar with and abide by the ethical practices of the specific facility or system in which the service is provided.
4. Occupational therapists shall observe the ethical practices as defined by the American Occupational Therapy Association, Inc., *Principles of Ethics* (AOTA, Revised 1980).
5. Occupational therapists shall provide all aspects of direct and indirect services according to Standards

and Policies of The American Occupational Therapy Association, Inc.

Glossary*

Occupational therapy assessment. The process of determining the need for, nature of, and estimated time of treatment, determining the needed coordination with other persons involved; and documenting these activities.

Evaluation. The process of obtaining and interpreting data necessary for treatment. This includes planning for and documenting the evaluation process and results. These data may be gathered through record review, specific observation, interview, and the administration of data collection procedures. Such procedures include, but are not limited to, the use of standardized tests, performance checklists, and activities and tasks designed to evaluate specific performance abilities.

Maintenance of function. The process of preserving and supporting an individual's current abilities to engage in interpersonal relationships and to manipulate the nonhuman environment.

Occupational performance. Life tasks (self-care, work play/leisure) that are all those activities that individuals must perform to meet their own needs and to be contributing members of the community.

Performance components. The skill areas (sensorimotor, cognitive, psychosocial) a person develops to facilitate carrying out self-care, work, and play/leisure.

Program planning. The development of an individual client's treatment plan.

Screening. The review of the potential client's case to determine the need for evaluation and treatment.

Therapeutic adaptations. The design and restructuring of the physical environment to assist self-care, work, and play/leisure performance. This includes selecting, obtaining, fitting, and fabricating equipment, and instructing the client, family, and staff in proper use and care of equipment. It also includes minor repair and modification for correct fit, position, or use. Categories of therapeutic adaptations consist of: orthotics, prosthetics, and assistive and adaptive equipment.

---

* Uniform Terminology for Reporting Occupational Therapy Services, adopted March 1979 by The Representative Assembly, AOTA

Adopted April 1983 by the Representative Assembly, The American Occupational Therapy Association, Inc.

Standards of Practice for Occupational Therapy Services for Clients with Physical Disabilities*

Preface

These standards are intended for internal use by the AOTA as guidelines to assist members in the practice of their profession. These standards by themselves cannot be interpreted to constitute a standard of care in any particular locality.

Standard I: A Referral for Occupational Therapy Services Must Be Based Upon the Provisions as Outlined in the Statement on Occupational Therapy Referral.

1. When a referral is received, the therapist shall document:
   a. The date of receipt and referral source
   b. The services requested
   c. The above (a & b) within one working day of receipt of the referral.

Standard II: The Occupational Therapist Shall Evaluate the Client's Performance.

1. The therapist shall orient the client, family, and/or significant others to the purposes and procedures of the occupational therapy evaluation.
2. An initial evaluation shall be completed at least 5 working days after acknowledgment of referral receipt.
3. The initial evaluation shall include an initial assessment of the client's goals, and functional abilities and deficits in:
   a. Occupational performance (ADL)
      1) Self-care skills
      2) Home–work–school skills
      3) Play/leisure skills
   b. Motor skills
   c. Sensory integration.
4. If the results of the above evaluation indicate possible deficits in psychological/social and/or cognitive skills, the therapist should evaluate these areas and document any functional deficits; or should refer the client to the appropriate service.
5. If any of the above evaluation results indicate the client's need for referral to community services or

programs, the therapist should determine the availability of such community resources; or should refer the evaluation to the appropriate service.
6. The therapist should obtain information about the client's medical history, education, work history, avocational interest, family, and cultural background. This information may be obtained through client interview, record review, and/or discussion with informed sources.

Standard III: The Therapist Shall Prepare and Document a Program Plan Based Upon an Analysis of the Occupational Therapy Evaluation Data and the Client's Expected Prognosis.

1. The therapist shall document the program plan within six working days after the acknowledgment of the referral receipt.
2. The documented program plan should consist of a statement of:
   a. achievable program goals
   b. methods to achieve the goals
3. The program plan goals and methods should be consistent with:
   a. the evaluative results and expected prognosis
   b. the goals of the client and/or family
   c. the program plans of other health care practitioners
4. The program plan methods may include, but need not be limited to, the use of:
   a. adaptive equipment and techniques
   b. passive, assistive, active and/or resistive activities and exercises
   c. counseling techniques
   d. facilitation/inhibition techniques
   e. joint protection techniques
   f. orthotic and/or prosthetic devices
   g. work simplification techniques

Standard IV: The Therapist Shall Implement the Occupational Therapy Program According to the Program Plan.

1. The therapist shall routinely document the occupational therapy services provided, the frequency of the services, and the client's progress toward goals. The timing of documentation shall be based upon frequency of contact with the patient/client and the significance of change in the client's condition.
2. The therapist shall periodically re-evaluate and

---

* Adopted May 1978 by the Representative Assembly, AOTA.

document the changes in the client's occupational performance and/or performance component skills.

   a. if the client's program exceeds a three-month period, the client should be re-evaluated at least every two months.

   b. if the client's program is less than three months, the client should be re-evaluated at least once per month

3. The therapist shall formulate, document and implement program changes consistent with changes in the client's occupational performance and performance-component-skills.

Standard V: The Therapist Shall Prepare and Document the Occupational Therapy Discharge Plan.

1. The discharge plan shall be consistent with the client's goals, functional abilities and deficits, community resources, and expected prognosis.
2. The discharge plan shall be consistent with the discharge plans of the other health care practitioners.
3. In preparation of the discharge plan, the therapist should allow enough time for coordination, acceptance, and effective implementation of the discharge plan.
4. The therapist shall document within two days following discharge, the client's functional abilities and deficits in occupational performance and performance component skills at time of discharge.
5. The therapist shall recommend discontinuation of occupational therapy services when the client has achieved the program goals and/or has achieved maximum benefit from the services.

Standard VI: The Therapist Should Re-evaluate the Client with Chronic Conditions at an Appropriate Time Interval Following Discharge.

1. The re-evaluation results shall be documented.
2. If the client needs further service, the therapist shall refer the client to the services needed.

Standard VII: The Occupational Therapist Shall Systematically Review the Quality, Including Outcomes, of their Services, Using Predetermined Criteria Reflecting Professional Consensus and Recent Developments in Research and Theory.

1. If actual care does not meet the criteria, it may be justified by peer review.

2. If justification by peer review fails, a program to improve care shall be planned and implemented.
3. Patient care review will be repeated to assess the success of the corrective action.

Standards of Practice for Occupational Therapy Services in a Mental Health Program*

Preface

These standards are intended for internal use by the AOTA as guidelines to assist members in the practice of their profession. These standards by themselves cannot be interpreted to constitute a standard of care in any particular locality.

Standard I: A Referral for Occupational Therapy Services Must be Based Upon the Provisions as Outlined in the Statement on Occupational Therapy Referral.

1. When a referral is received, the therapist shall:
   a. document the date of receipt and referral source
   b. document the occupational therapy services requested in the referral

Standard II: The Occupational Therapist Shall Evaluate the Client's Performance.

1. The therapist shall evaluate and document the client's goals, functional abilities and deficits in occupational performance (activities of daily living):
   a. self-care skills
   b. work skills
   c. play/leisure skills
2. The therapist shall evaluate and document the client's goals, functional abilities and deficits in the following performance component areas:
   a. psychological/intrapersonal skills
   b. social/interpersonal skills
   c. cognitive skills
3. If the results of the occupational performance evaluation indicate possible deficits in the client's motor and/or sensory–integrative skills, the therapist should evaluate these areas and document any functional deficits; or should refer the client to another practitioner for evaluation.
4. If any of the above evaluation results indicate the client's need for referral to community services or programs, the therapist should determine the

---

* Adopted May 1978 by the Representative Assembly, AOTA.

availability of such community resources; or should refer the evaluation to another.

Standard III: The Therapist Shall Prepare and Document a Program Plan Based Upon an Analysis of the Occupational Therapy Evaluation Data and the Client's Expected Prognosis.

1. The documented program plan shall consist of a statement of achievable program goals and the methods to achieve the goals.
2. The program plan goals and methods shall be consistent with the evaluation data on the client's goals, functional abilities and deficits, community resources, and expected prognosis.
3. The program plan goals and methods shall be compatible with the program plans of the other health care practitioners.

Standard IV: The Therapist Shall Implement the Occupational Therapy Program According to the Program Plan.

1. The therapist shall periodically document the occupational therapy services provided and the frequency of the services.
2. The therapist shall periodically re-evaluate and document the changes in the client's occupational performance and performance component skills.
3. The therapist shall formulate, document and implement program changes consistent with changes in the client's occupation, performance and performance component skills.

Standard V: The Therapist Shall Prepare and Document the Occupational Therapy Discharge Plan.

1. The discharge plan shall be consistent with the client's goals, functional abilities and deficits, community resources, and expected prognosis.
2. The discharge plan shall be consistent with the discharge plans of the other health care practitioners.
3. Sufficient time should be allowed for coordination, acceptance and effective implementation of the discharge plan.
4. The therapist shall document the client's functional abilities and deficits in occupational performance and performance component skills at time of discharge.
5. The therapist shall terminate occupational therapy services when the client has achieved the goals, or

when the client has achieved maximum benefit from occupational therapy.

Standard VI: The Therapist Should Re-evaluate the Client with Chronic Conditions at an Appropriate Time Interval Following Discharge.

1. The re-evaluation results shall be documented.
2. If the client needs further service, the therapist shall refer the client to the services needed.

Standard VII: The Occupational Therapist Shall Systematically Review the Quality, Including Outcomes, of their Services, Using Predetermined Criteria Reflecting Professional Consensus and Recent Developments in Research and Theory.

1. If actual care does not meet the criteria, it may be justified by peer review.
2. If justification by peer review fails, a program to improve care shall be planned and implemented.
3. Patient care review will be repeated to assess the success of the corrective action.

Standards of Practice for Occupational Therapy Services for the Developmentally Disabled Client*

Preface

These standards are intended for internal use by the AOTA as guidelines to assist members in the practice of their profession. These standards by themselves cannot be interpreted to constitute a standard of care in any particular locality.

Standard I: A Referral for Occupational Therapy Services Must be Based Upon the Provisions as Outlined in the Statement on Occupational Therapy Referral.

1. A client should be referred to the occupational therapist for evaluation when the client has or appears to have a dysfunction, or has a predisposition towards dysfunction in any of the following areas:

---

* Adopted May 1978 by the Representative Assembly, AOTA.

a. occupational performance (activities of daily living):
  1. self-care activities
  2. home–school–work activities
  3. play/leisure activities
  b. performance components:
  1. neuromuscular development
  2. sensory–integrative development
  3. psychological development
  4. social development
  5. cognitive development
2. When a referral is received, the therapist shall document:
  a. the date of receipt and referral source
  b. services requested in the referral.

Standard II: The Occupational Therapist Shall Evaluate the Client's Performance.

1. The occupational therapy evaluation shall include an assessment of the developmental levels, as well as the functional abilities and deficits in the following areas:
  a. Occupational performance (activities of daily living):
  1. self-care skills
  2. home–work–school skills
  3. play/leisure skills
  b. motor skills
  c. sensory integration
2. If the results of the above evaluation indicate possible deficits in psychological/social and/or cognitive skills, the therapist should evaluate these areas and document any functional deficits; or should refer the client to the appropriate service.
3. If any of the above evaluation results indicate the client's need for referral to community services or programs, the therapist should determine the availability of such community resources; or should refer the evaluation to the appropriate service.
4. All evaluation methods shall be appropriate to the chronological age and functional level of the client. The methods may include, but need not be limited to, observation of activity performance, interview, record review and testing.
5. If standardized evaluative tests are used, the tests should have normative data for the age of the client. If normative data are not available for the age range of the client, the standardized test results should be expressed in relation to the normative data that are available.
6. The therapist shall document the evaluation results in the client's record. Indicating evaluation tools.

Standard III: The Therapist Shall Prepare and Document a Program Plan Based Upon an Analysis of the Occupational Therapy Evaluation Data and the Client's Expected Prognosis.

1. The documented program plan shall consist of a statement of achievable program goals and the methods to achieve the goals.
2. The program plan goals and methods shall be consistent with:
  a. established principles of normal growth and development
  b. the evaluative results and expected prognosis
  c. the goals of the client, the client's family and significant others
  d. the program plans of the other health care practitioners
3. When the occupational therapy program goal is to prevent or diminish dysfunction in occupational performance (activities of daily living) or to enhance occupational performance, the program plan shall include the use of one or more of the following types of activities:
  a. self-care activities; may also include instruction in the use of adapted methods and/or equipment
  b. home–work–school activities; may also include instruction in the use of adapted methods and/or equipment
  c. play/leisure activities; may also include instruction of family in play activities appropriate for child's developmental level: instruction in the use of adapted methods and/or equipment
4. When the goal is to prevent or diminish neuromuscular dysfunction or enhance neuromuscular development, the program plan shall include (but not be limited to) the use of one or more of the following types of activities:
  a. activities which maintain or increase range of motion and/or muscle strength
  b. activities which facilitate integration of developmentally appropriate reflex behavior
  c. activities which provide appropriate sensory stimulation
  d. activities which promote the development of normal movement patterns and motor control
  e. activities which maintain or increase coordination
  f. instruction in use of proper positioning techniques
  g. provision of and instruction in the use of adaptive equipment and/or orthotic devices
5. When the goal is to prevent or diminish sensory–integrative dysfunction or to enhance sensory–integrative development, the program plan shall

include (but need not be limited to) the appropriate use of:
a. sensory input techniques for visual, auditory, gustatory, olfactory, tactile, proprioceptive/kinesthetic, and vestibular stimulation
b. facilitation techniques
c. inhibition techniques
d. activity to promote adaptive motor response
6. When the goal is to prevent or diminish psychological dysfunction or to enhance psychological development, the program plan shall include (but need not be limited to) the use of activities which assist the client in learning to:
a. experience and cope with competition, frustration, success, failure
b. identify and respond appropriately to feelings
c. develop or refine self-esteem; self-identity
7. When the goal is to prevent or diminish social dysfunction or to enhance social development, the program plan shall include (but need not be limited to) the use of activities which assist the client in learning to:
a. initiate and develop appropriate social behavior
b. listen and communicate
c. develop sensitivity to other person's feelings and behavior
8. When the goal is to prevent or diminish cognitive dysfunction or to enhance cognitive development, the program plan shall include (need not be limited to) the use of the following activities which assist the client in developing:
a. concentration/attention span
b. memory/recall
c. decision making and problem-solving skills

Standard IV: The Therapist Shall Implement the Program According to the Program Plan.

1. The therapist shall periodically document the occupational therapy services provided and the frequency of the services.
2. The therapist shall periodically re-evaluate and document the changes in the client's occupational performance and performance components.
3. The therapist shall formulate, document and implement program changes consistent with changes in the client's occupational performance and performance components.

Standard V: The Therapist Shall Prepare and Document the Occupational Therapy Discharge Plan.

1. The discharge plan shall be consistent with the client's goals, functional abilities and deficits,

expected prognosis, and the goals of the client's family. Consideration should be given to community resources and other environmental factors.
2. The discharge plan shall be consistent with the discharge plans of the other health care practitioners.
3. Sufficient time should be allowed for coordination, acceptance and effective implementation of the discharge plan.
4. The therapist shall document the client's functional abilities and deficits in occupational performance and performance components at time of discharge.
5. The therapist shall terminate occupational therapy services when the client has achieved the goals; or when the client has achieved maximum benefit from occupational therapy.

Standard VI: The Therapist Should Re-evaluate the Client with Chronic Conditions at an Appropriate Time Interval Following Discharge.

1. The re-evaluation results shall be documented.
2. If the client needs further service, the therapist shall refer the client to the services needed.

Standard VII: The Occupational Therapist Shall Systematically Review the Quality, Including Outcomes, of Their Services, Using Predetermined Criteria Reflecting Professional Consensus and Recent Developments in Research and Theory.

1. If actual care does not meet the criteria it may be justified by peer review.
2. If justification by peer review fails, a program to improve care shall be planned and implemented.
3. Patient care review will be repeated to assess the success of the corrective action.

Standards of Practice for Occupational Therapy Services in a Home Health Program*

Preface

These standards are intended for internal use by the AOTA as guidelines to assist members in the practice of their profession. These standards themselves cannot be interpreted to constitute a standard of care in any particular locality.

---

* Adopted May 1978 by the Representative Assembly, AOTA.

Standard I: A Referral for Occupational Therapy Services Must Be Based Upon the Provisions as Outlined in the Statement on Occupational Therapy Referral.

1. Within one working day of receipt of a referral, the therapist shall document:
   a. the date of receipt and referral source
   b. the services requested
2. Within seven working days of receipt of referral, the therapist shall:
   a. review client's records
   b. discuss case with other home health team members
   c. document the acceptance/rejection of referral or the referral of client to other resources

Standard II: The Occupational Therapist Shall Evaluate the Client's Performance.

1. The therapist shall orient the client, family and/or significant others to the purpose and procedures of the occupational therapy evaluation.
2. An initial evaluation shall be completed and the results documented within five working days after acceptance of referral.
3. The initial evaluation shall include an initial assessment of the client's goals, functional abilities and deficits in:
   a. occupational performance (activities of daily living):
      1) self-care skills
      2) work skills
      3) play/leisure skills
   b. motor skills
4. The initial evaluation should include an initial assessment of the client's goals, functional abilities, and deficits in the following performance component skills, if the evaluation of occupational performance (ADL) skills and/or motor skills, or referral indicates possible deficits in these areas.
   a. sensory–integrative skills
   b. psychological/intrapersonal skills
   c. social/interpersonal skills
   d. cognitive skills
5. The therapist should evaluate these areas and document any functional deficits; or should refer the client to the appropriate service/individual for evaluation if the evaluation is beyond the therapist's expertise.
6. If any of the above evaluation results indicate the client's need for referral to community services or programs, the therapist should determine the availability of such community resources and/or

should refer the evaluation to the appropriate service.

7. If the evaluation results indicate deficits in occupational performance skills, motor skills, sensory–integration, and/or cognitive skills, the therapist should evaluate the client's environment in relation to architectural barriers and safety factors. The evaluation results should be documented.
8. The therapist should obtain information about the client's medical history, education, work history, avocational interests, family, and cultural background. This information may be obtained through client interview, record review and/or discussion with informed sources.
9. The therapist should evaluate the ability of the client, family, and/or significant others to implement the home health program.

Standard III: The Therapist Shall Prepare and Document the Program Plan.

1. Seven working days after the acceptance of the referral.
2. The documented program plan should consist of a statement of:
   a. client's projected goals
   b. achievable occupational therapy program goals
   c. methods to achieve the goals
   d. frequency of visits
   e. projected length of occupational therapy program
   f. expected need for equipment
3. The program plan goals and methods should be consistent with:
   a. the evaluative results and expected prognosis
   b. the goals of the client and/or family
   c. the program plans of other home health team members
   d. client's economic resources and available home health resources
4. The program plan methods may include, but need not be limited to, the use of:
   a. activities of daily living
   b. assistive, active and or resistive activities and exercises
   c. adaptive equipment and environmental modifications
   d. facilitation/inhibition techniques
   e. joint protection techniques
   f. orthotic and/or prosthetic devices
   g. work simplification techniques
   h. sensory–integration techniques
   i. cognitive skill development techniques
   j. counseling techniques

Standard IV: The Therapist Shall Implement the Therapy Program According to the Program Plan.

1. The program should begin within five working days after the documentation of the program plan.
2. The therapist shall document for each home visit: the occupational therapy services provided, the length of the service and other pertinent information as required by the home health agency.
3. The therapist shall communicate problems or program changes to the physician, client, family and other home health team members.
4. The therapist shall document pertinent information obtained through sources other than home visits; e.g., telephone calls.
5. The therapist shall re-evaluate and document the changes in the client's occupational performance and performance component skills:
   a. if the client's program exceeds a three-month period, the client should be re-evaluated at least every two months.
   b. if the client's program is less than three months, the client should be re-evaluated at least once per month
6. The therapist shall formulate, document and implement program changes consistent with changes in the client's occupational performance/component-skills.
7. When dealing with the medical problem, the therapist shall work in collaboration with the physician managing the case.

Standard V: The Therapist Shall Prepare and Document the Occupational Therapy Discharge Plan.

1. The discharge plan shall be consistent with the client's goals, functional abilities and deficits, community resources, and expected prognosis.
2. The discharge plan should be consistent with the discharge plans of the other home health team members.
3. In preparation of the discharge plan, the therapist should allow enough time for coordination, acceptance, and effective implementation of the discharge plan.
4. The therapist shall document within two days following discharge, the client's functional abilities and deficits in occupational performance and performance component skills at the time of discharge, reason for discharge, number and length of treatment.
5. The therapist shall recommend discontinuation of

occupational therapy services when the client has achieved the program goals and/or has achieved maximum benefit from the services.

Standard VI: The Therapist Should Re-evaluate the Client With Chronic Conditions at an Appropriate Time Interval Following Discharge.

1. The re-evaluation results shall be documented.
2. If the client needs further service, the therapist shall refer the client to the services needed.

Standard VII: The Occupational Therapist Shall Systematically Review the Quality, Including Outcomes, of Their Services, Using Predetermined Criteria Reflecting Professional Consensus and Recent Developments in Research and Theory.

1. If actual care does not meet the criteria, it may be justified by peer review.
2. If justification by peer review fails, a program to improve care shall be planned and implemented.
3. Patient care review will be repeated to assess the success of the corrective action.

Standards of Practice for Occupational Therapy in Schools*

These guidelines are to assist AOTA members and school administrators in the management of occupational therapy in the school systems. These standards by themselves cannot be interpreted to constitute a standard of care in any particular locality.

The occupational therapist shall manage the therapy program in accordance with all available Standards of Practice, as defined by the American Occupational Therapy Association, Inc.

The purpose of the Occupational Therapy program in the school system is to enable the student to gain optimum benefit from the educational program.

Direct Services

Direct services include screening, referral systems, evaluations, program planning, program implementation, re-evaluation and termination of services.

* Adopted April 1980 by the Representative Assembly, AOTA

Standard I: Screening
The occupational therapist should be involved in the screening process

1. The screening process should allow the therapist to identify those students who need further educational and/or related service evaluation.
2. All screening methods shall be appropriate to the chronological, educational and/or functional level of the student, and shall not be racially or culturally discriminatory.
3. The occupational therapist should refer the results and recommendations to the appropriate school educational planning committee.

Standard II: Referral
A referral for occupational therapy must comply with the AOTA statement on referral.

1. A student should be referred to the occupational therapist for evaluation when the student has or appears to have a dysfunction in any of the following areas:
   a. occupational performance (activities of daily living); self-care activities; home–school–work activities; play/leisure activities; and/or prevocational/vocational activities/skills.
   b. performance components: neuromuscular development; sensory–integrative development; psychological development; social development; and/or cognitive development.
2. A referral may originate through the individual education plan or educational planning committee (including teachers, other student services staff, parents, physicians, etc.).
3. When a referral is received, the therapist shall document:
   a. the date of receipt and referral source; and
   b. services requested in the referral.
4. If in the therapist's judgment there is the need for medical management of the student, the therapist shall immediately apprise the student's parent/guardian or appropriate person and recommend physician involvement, or the therapist shall, after parental/guardian written permission or release has been obtained, contact the physician.

Standard III: Evaluation
The occupational therapist shall evaluate the student's performance.

1. The initial occupational therapy evaluation shall be completed and results documented according to the time frames established by federal and/or state rules and regulations.
2. The occupational therapy evaluation shall include

assessment of the developmental leval as well as the functional abilities/capacities and deficits/limitations as related to the student's educational level and needs in the following areas:
   a. occupational performance: self-care activities; home–school–work activities; pre-vocational/vocational activities/skills; and/or play/leisure activities.
   b. performance components: neuromuscular development; sensory–integrative development; psychological development; social development and/or cognitive development.
3. If the results of the above evaluation indicate possible deficits in psychological/social, cognitive, physical/medical, speech/language areas, the therapist should refer the student to the appropriate service and/or request consultation if necessary.
4. All evaluation methods shall be appropriate to the chronological age and/or functional level of the student and identify baseline behaviors. The methods may include, but need not be limited to, observation of activity performance, interview, record review, testing and individual/group screening.
5. If standardized evaluative measurements are used, the tests should have normative data for the age range of the student. If normative data are not available for the age range of the student, the results should be expressed in a descriptive report and standardized scales not used.
6. Tests and other evaluation material used in placing handicapped students will be prepared and administered in such a way as not to be racially or culturally discriminatory, and they will be presented in the child's native tongue.
7. As part of the evaluation process, the therapist may make clinical judgments based on observations and recorded progress during intervention programs.
8. The therapist shall document evaluation results in the student's record, indicating evaluation instruments and procedures and also communicate these findings via written reports, oral conferences, and staffings to the appropriate persons and/or community resources.

Standard IV: Program Planning and/or Individual Education Plan
The therapist shall prepare and document a program plan based upon an analysis of the data from the occupational therapy and other education planner's evaluation results.

1. The initial program plan shall be prepared and documented according the the time frames estab-

lished by federal and/or state rules and regulations.

2. The therapist shall utilize the results of the evaluation process to prepare an occupational therapy program that is:
   a. stated in practical outcomes applicable to the student's needs and educational goals,
   b. consistent with principles and concepts of growth and development; and
   c. consistent with expected behavior/progress for the student's defined educational/health problems and needs.

3. The planning process shall include:
   a. identifying short term and long term (annual) goals;
   b. collaborating with child/family/staff to establish appropriate goals to enhance education;
   c. participation in staffings to coordinate the occupational therapy program with the other programs within the educational setting;
   d. documenting of practical outcomes to be achieved;
   e. selecting the media, methods, environment and personnel to accomplish goals; and
   f. monitoring and modifying the program to meet the established goals.

4. The documented educational program plan shall consist of a statement of when these services will be provided and how long they will last.

5. When the occupational therapy program goal is to prevent or diminish dysfunction in occupational performance and learning or to enhance occupational performance, the program plan shall include the use of one or more of the following types of activities:
   a. self-care activities; may also include instruction in the use of adapted methods and/or equipment, energy conservation, joint protection techniques.
   b. home–work–school activities; may also include instruction in the use of adapted methods and/or equipment.
   c. prevocational/vocational activities/skills may also include improvement of standing or sitting tolerance, general endurance, or awareness and utilization of community resources; and
   d. developmental play/leisure activities; may also include instruction of family in activities appropriate for student's developmental level; instruction in the use of adapted methods and/or equipment.

6. When the goal is to prevent or diminish neuro-muscular dysfunction or enhance neuromuscular development and learning, the program plan shall include, but need not be limited to, the use of one or more of the following types of activities:
   a. activities which maintain or increase range of motion and/or muscle strength;
   b. activities which facilitate integration of developmentally appropriate reflex/reaction behavior;
   c. activities which provide appropriate sensory stimulation;
   d. activities which promote the development of normal postural tone, movement patterns and motor control;
   e. instruction in the use of proper positioning and handling techniques;
   f. provision of and instruction in the use of adaptive equipment; and/or
   g. fabrication/recommendation of splints or orthotic devices/equipment.

7. When the goal is to prevent or diminish sensory–integrative dysfunction or to enhance sensory integrative development, the program plan shall include, but need not be limited to, the appropriate use of:
   a. sensory facilitation and/or inhibition techniques for vestibular, tactile, proprioceptive/kinesthetic, visual, auditory, gustatory and olfactory stimulation; and/or
   b. activities to promote adaptive sensorimotor response.

8. When the interdisciplinary educational evaluation results indicate goals to prevent or diminish psychological or social dysfunction, or enhance psychological or social development, the occupational therapy program shall include, but need not be limited to, the appropriate use of activities which assist the student in learning to:
   a. experience and cope with competition, frustration, success and failure;
   b. identify and respond appropriately to feelings;
   c. develop or refine self-esteem or self-identity;
   d. imitate and develop appropriate social behaviors;
   e. listen and communicate; and
   f. develop sensitivity to other persons' feelings and behaviors (interpersonal relationships).

9. When the interdisciplinary education team evaluation results indicate goals to prevent or diminish cognitive dysfunction or to enhance development in the cognitive areas, the occupational therapy program shall include, but need not be limited to, the appropriate use of activities which assist the student in developing:
   a. concentration/attention span;
   b. memory/recall;
   c. decision making and/or problem solving.

The purposes of the occupational therapy program in the above stated areas, (#8 and #9), are not intended to replace academic or other programming. The purposes are to assist the child to receive maximum benefit from educational programming.

Standard V: Program Implementation
The therapist shall implement the program according to the program plan.

1. The therapist shall periodically and on an ongoing basis document the occupational therapy services provided (including techniques utilized and the results) and the frequency of the services.
2. The therapist shall periodically re-evaluate and document the changes in the student's occupational performance and performance components.
3. The therapist shall formulate, document and implement program changes consistent with changes in the student's occupational performance and performance components.

Standard VI: Re-Evaluation
The therapist shall re-evaluate the student receiving occupational therapy on a yearly basis.

1. The re-evaluation results shall be documented.
2. If the client needs further service, the therapist shall make appropriate recommendations.
3. A re-evaluation does not necessarily constitute a referral for services.

Standard VII: Termination of Services
The therapist shall prepare and document the occupational therapy discharge plan.

1. The discharge plan shall be consistent with the student's goals, functional abilities and deficits, expected prognosis and the goals of the educational planners. Consideration should be given to appropriate community resources for referral and environmental factors/barriers that may need modification.
2. The discharge plan shall be consistent with the discharge plans of the other educational planners and appropriately documented through the individual educational planning process.
3. The therapist shall document the comparison of the initial state of functional abilities and deficits in occupational performance and performance components and the current state of these abilities and deficits at the time of discharge.
4. The therapist shall terminate occupational therapy services when the student has achieved the goals,

or has achieved maximum benefits from occupational therapy.
5. Recommendations for follow-up or re-evaluation, if appropriate, shall be documented.

Indirect Services

With the provision of indirect services, the occupational therapist in a school-based program performs supervision, consultation and administration/management roles.

Standard VIII: Administration/ Management
The occupational therapist shall provide appropriate management and administrative services.

The management and administrative functions for the school-based therapist shall include:
1. Supervision of other personnel as assigned.
   a. informal and formal training of personnel and volunteers assigned to occupational therapy.
   b. reviewing performances (self and others) and providing evaluations.
2. Design of the occupational therapy program with periodic reviews of all aspects of the total occupational therapy program to determine its effectiveness and efficiency.
3. Occupational therapists shall systematically review the quality, including outcomes, of services delivered, using predetermined criteria reflecting professional consensus and recent developments in research and theory:
   a. To determine if actual service may be justified by peer review.
   b. If justification by peer review fails, a program to improve services shall be planned and implemented.
   c. Review will be repeated to assess the success of the corrective action.
4. Maintaining current certification as required by state regulations and AOTA.
5. Maintaining current records and files to meet school requirements and professional standards.
6. Participating in budget planning and is responsible for budget implementation.
7. Responsibility for knowledge, including use of, and utilizing community resources.
8. The therapist shall maintain and update professional knowledge and skills and seek consultation/supervision from others when necessary to assure continued competency.

Standard IX: Consultation
The therapist shall provide consultation services when appropriate.

In the consultation role, the therapist is one member of an interdisciplinary educational team collaborating with a variety of professional personnel to assist students with special needs. The practice of consultation shall include when appropriate:

1. Developing and coordinating occupational therapy programs with the total educational curriculum.
2. Provide consultation for classroom environmental adaptation to enhance the learning potential of students.
3. Provide consultation to teachers and staff regarding the identified special needs of students.
4. Collaborate with the educational team regarding the student's program including the IEP (Individualized Education Program).
5. Provide in-service education.
6. Provide consultation for appropriate programs outside the school program.
7. Provide consultation and education to parents to help them understand the special needs of their child.
8. Provide consultation for home environmental adaptation to enhance independent functioning.
9. Provide consultation to school administrators and staff regarding preventive health education and activities to enhance the educational environment and learning potential of students.

Standard X: Legal/Ethical Components
The occupational therapist shall provide all aspects of direct and indirect services according to legal regulations and ethical standards.

1. The occupational therapist shall practice and manage occupaptional therapy programs as defined by federal and state laws or legal principles as they apply to issues or situations when relevant to students or themselves in school systems.
2. The therapist shall observe the ethical practices as defined by the American Occupational Therapy Association Standards and Ethics Commission.
3. The therapist should be familiar with and abide by the ethical practices of the specific school district or system in which the therapist serves.

APPENDIX

Uniform Terminology for Reporting Occupational Therapy Services*

Occupational Therapy Function

Occupational Therapy is the application of purposeful, goal-oriented activity in the evaluation, problem identification, and/or treatment of persons whose function is impaired by physical illness or injury, emotional disorder, congenital or developmental disability, or the aging process, in order to achieve optimum funcitoning, to prevent disability, and to maintain health. Specific occupational therapy services include, but are not limited to the following:

> education and training and evaluation of performance capacity in activities of daily living (ADL); the design, fabrication, and application of orthoses (splints); sensorimotor activities; guidance in selection and use of adaptive equipment; therapeutic use of activities and the *activity process* to develop/restore function performance; prevocational evaluation and training; consultation concerning the ad-

aptation of physical environments for the handicapped; involvement in discharge planning and community reentry; time/space/role management; and opportunity for self-expression and communication. These services are provided to individuals, groups, and to the community.

Description of Occupational Therapy Services

In selecting items and defining terms, the following criteria were taken into consideration:

1. Emphasis on description of treatment outcomes rather than treatment procedures.
2. Reflection of Medicare and Medicaid guidelines in terminology and category selection and definition.
3. Comprehensive description of occupational therapy services/product.
4. Reflection of the uniqueness of occupational therapy services/product in comparison with the services of other professions.

---

* Adopted April 1979 by the Representative Assembly, AOTA.

5. Coverage of recognized occupational therapy role in medical practice rather than all possible occupational therapy roles.

I. Occupational Therapy Assessment

Occupational therapy assessment refers to the process of determining the need for, nature of, and estimated time of treatment, determining the needed coordination with other persons involved; and documenting these activities.

A. *Screening*

Screening refers to the review of potential patient's client's case to determine the need for evaluation and treatment. It includes discussion with other professionals and/or patient advocate, and patient/client interview or administration of screening tool.

B. *Patient-Related Consultation*

Patient-related consultation refers to the sharing of relevant information with other professionals of patients/clients who are not currently referred to occupational therapy. This may include but is not limited to discussion, chart review, treatment recommendation, and documentation.

C. *Evaluation*

Evaluation refers to the process of obtaining and interpreting data necessary for treatment. This includes planning for an documenting the evaluation process and results. This data may be gathered through record review, specific observation, interview, and the administration of data collection procedures. Such procedures include but are not limited to the use of standardized tests, performance checklists, and activities and tasks designed to evaluate specific performance abilities. Categories of occupational therapy evaluation include independent living/daily living skills and performance and their components:

1. Independent Living/Daily Living Skills and Performance (see II A).
2. Sensorimotor Skill and Performance Components (see II B).
3. Cognitive Skill and Performance Components (see II C).
4. Psychosocial Skill and Performance Components (see II D).
5. Therapeutic Adaptations (see II E).
6. Specialized Evaluations. Specialized evaluations refer to evaluations or tests requiring specialized training and/or advanced education to administer and interpret. Examples of specialized evaluations are employment preparation, evaluation (prevocational testing), sensory–integration evaluation, prosthetic evaluation, driver's training evaluation.

D. *Reassessment*

Reassessment refers to the process of obtaining and interpreting data necessary for updating treatment plans and goals. This frequently involves administering only portions of the initial evaluation, documenting results, and/or revising treatment.

II. Occupational Therapy Treatment

Occupational therapy treatment refers to the use of specific activities or methods to develop, improve, and/or restore the performance of necessary functions; compensate for dysfunction; and/or minimize debilitation; and the planning for an documenting of treatment performance. The necessary functions treated in occupational therapy are the following.

A. *Independent Living/Daily Living Skills*

Independent living/daily living skills (including self-care) refer to the skill and performance of physical and psychological/emotional self-care, work, and play/leisure activities to a level of independence appropriate to age, life-space, and disability. Life-space refers to an individual's cultural background, value orientation, and physical and social environment.

1. *Physical Daily Living Skills*

Physical daily living skills refer to the skill and performance of daily personal care, with or without adaptive equipment. It includes but is not limited to:

a. *Grooming and Hygiene*

Grooming and hygiene refer to the skill and performance of personal health needs, such as bathing, toileting, hair care, shaving, applying make-up.

b. *Feeding/Eating*

Feeding/eating refers to the skill and performance of sequentially feeding oneself, including sucking, chewing, swallowing, and using appropriate utensils.

c. *Dressing*

Dressing refers to the skill and performance of choosing appropriate clothing, dressing oneself in a sequential fashion, including fastening and adjusting clothing.

d. *Functional Mobility*

Functional mobility refers to the skill and performance in moving oneself from one position or place to another. It includes skills necessary for activities such as bed mobility, wheelchair mobility, transfers (bed, car, tub, toilet, chair), and functional ambulation, with or without adaptive aids. It also includes use of public and private travel systems, such as driving own automobile and using public transportation.

e. *Functional Communication*
Functional communication refers to the skill and performance in using equipment or systems to enhance or provide communciation, such as writing equipment, typewriters, letterboards, telephone, braille writers, artificial vocalization systems, and computers.

f. *Object Manipulation*
Object manipulation refers to the skill and performance in handling large and small common objects, such as calculators, keys, money, light switches, doorknobs, and packages.

2. *Psychological/Emotional Daily Living Skills*
Psychological/emotional daily living skills refer to the skill and performance in developing one's self-concept/self-identity, coping with life situations, and participating in one's organizational and community environment. It includes but is not limited to:

a. *Self-concept/Self-identity*
Self-concept/self-identity refers to the cognitive image of one's functional self. This includes but is not limited to:
(1) clearly perceiving one's needs, feelings, conflicts, values, beliefs, expectations, sexuality, and power.
(2) realistically perceiving others' needs, feelings, conflicts, values, beliefs, expectations, sexuality, and power.
(3) knowing own's performance strengths and limitations.
(4) sensing one's competence, achievement, self-esteem, and self-respect.
(5) integrating new experiences with established self-concept/self-identity.
(6) having a sense of psychological safety and security.
(7) perceiving one's goals and directions.

b. *Situational Coping*
Situational coping refers to skill and performance in handling stress and dealing with problems and changes in a manner that is functional for self and others. This includes but is not limited to:
(1) setting goals, selecting, harmonizing, and managing activities of daily living to promote optimal performance.
(2) testing goals and perceptions against reality.
(3) perceiving changes and need for changes in self and environment.

(4) directing and redirecting energy to overcome problems.
(5) initiating, implementing, and following through on decisions.
(6) assuming responsibility for self and consequences of actions.
(7) interacting with others, dyadic and group.

c. *Community Involvement*
Community involvement refers to skill and performance in interacting within one's social system. This includes but is not limited to:
(1) understanding social norms and their impact on society.
(2) planning, organizing, and executing daily life activities in relationship to society, including such activities as budgeting, time management, social role management, arranging for housing, nutritional planning, assessing and using community resources.
(3) recognizing and responding to needs of families, groups, and complex social units.
(4) understanding and responding to organizational/community role expectations as both recipient and contributor.

3. *Work*
Work refers to skill and performance in participating in socially purposeful and productive activities. These activities may take place in the home, employment setting, school, or community. They include but are not limited to:

a. *Homemaking*
Homemaking refers to skill and performance in homemaking and home management tasks, such as meal planning, meal preparation and clean-up, laundry, cleaning, minor household repairs, shopping, and use of household safety principles.

b. *Child Care/Parenting*
Child care/parenting refers to skill and performance in child care activities and management. This includes but is not limited to physical care of children, and use of age-appropriate activities, communication, and behavior to facilitate child development.

c. *Employment Preparation*
Employment preparation refers to skill and performance in precursory job activities (including prevocational activities). This includes but is not limited to:
(1) job acquisition skills and performance.
(2) organizational and team participatory skills and performance.

(3) work process skills and performance.

(4) work product quality.

4. *Play/Leisure*

Play/leisure refers to skill and performance in choosing, performing, and engaging in activities for amusement, relaxation, spontaneous enjoyment, and/or self-expression. This includes but is not limited to:

a. Recognizing one's specific needs, interests, and adaptations necessary for performance.

b. Identifying characteristics of activities and social situations that make them play for the individual.

c. Identifying activities that contain those characteristics.

d. Choosing play activities for participation, such as sports, games, hobbies, music, drama, and other activities.

e. Testing out and adapting activities to enable participation.

f. Identifying and using community resources.

B. *Sensorimotor Components*

Sensorimotor components refer to the skill and performance of patterns of sensory and motor behavior that are prerequisites to self-care, work, and play/leisure performance. The components in this section include neuromuscular and sensory–integrative skills, including perceptual motor skills.

1. *Neuromuscular*

Neuromuscular refers to the skill and performance of motor aspects of behavior. This includes but is not limited to:

a. *Reflex Integration*

Reflex integration refers to skill and performance in enhancing and supporting functional neuromuscular development through eliciting and/or inhibiting stereotyped, patterned, and/or involutary responses coordinated at subcortical and cortical levels.

b. *Range of Motion*

Range of motion refers to skill and performance in using maximum span of joint movement in activities with and without assistance to enhance functional performance. The standard levels of performance include:

(1) active range of motion: movement by patient, unassisted through a complete range of motion.

(2) passive range of motion: movement performed by someone other than patient or by a mechanical device, requiring no muscle contraction on the part of the patient.

(3) active-assistive range of motion: move-ment performed by the patient to the limit of his/her ability, and then completed with assistance.

c. *Gross and Fine Coordination*

Gross and fine coordination refers to skill and performance in muscle control, coordination, and dexterity while participating in activities.

(1) *muscle control*

Muscle control refers to skill and performance in directing muscle movement.

(2) *coordination*

Coordination refers to skill and performance in gross motor activities using several muscle groups.

(3) *dexterity*

Dexterity refers to skill and performance in tasks using small muscle groups.

d. *Strength and Endurance*

Strength and endurance refers to skill and performance in using muscular force within time periods necessary for purposeful task performance. This involves but is not limited to progressively building strength and cardiac and pulmonary reserve, increasing the length of work periods, and decreasing fatigue and strain.

2. *Sensory Integration*

Sensory integration refers to skill and performance in development and coordination of sensory input, motor output, and sensory feedback. This includes but is not limited to:

a. *Sensory Awareness*

Sensory awareness refers to skill and performance in perceiving and differentiating external and internal stimuli, such as:

(1) tactile awareness: the perception and interpretation of stimuli through skin contact.

(2) stereognosis: the identification of forms and nature of objects through the sense of touch.

(3) kinesthesia: the conscious perception of muscular motion, weight, and position.

(4) proprioceptive awareness: the identification of the positions of body parts in space.

(5) occular control: the localization and visual tracking of stimuli.

(6) vestibular awareness: the detection of motion and gravitational pull as related to one's performance in functional activities, ambulation, and balance.

(7) auditory awareness: the differentiation and identification of sounds.

(8) gustatory awareness: the differentiation and identification of tastes.

(9) olfactory awareness: the differentiation and identification of smells.

b. *Visual-Spatial Awareness*

Visual-spatial awareness refers to skill and performance in perceiving distances between and relationships among objects, including self. This includes but is not limited to:

(1) figure–ground: recognition of forms and objects when presented in a configuration with competing stimuli.

(2) form constancy: recognition of forms and objects as the same when presented in different contexts.

(3) position in space: knowledge of one's position in space relative to other objects.

c. *Body Integration*

Body integration refers to skill and performance in perceiving and regulating the position of various muscles and body parts in relationship to each other during static and movement states. This includes but is not limited to:

(1) *body schema*

Body schema refers to the perception of one's physical self through proprioceptive and interoceptive sensations.

(2) *postural balance*

Postural balance refers to skill and performance in developing and maintaining body posture while sitting, standing, or engaging in activity.

(3) *bilateral motor coordination*

Bilateral motor coordination refers to skill and performance in purposeful movement that requires interaction between both sides of the body in a smooth, refined manner.

(4) *right–left discrimination*

Right-left discrimination refers to skill and performance in differentiating right from left and vice versa.

(5) *visual–motor integration*

Visual-motor integration refers to skill and performance in combining visual input with purposeful voluntary movement of the hand and other body parts involved in an activity. Visual–motor integration includes eye–hand coordination.

(6) *crossing the midline*

Crossing the midline refers to skill and performance in crossing the vertical midline of the body.

(7) *praxis*

Praxis refers to skill and performance of purposeful movement that involves motor planning.

C. *Cognitive Components*

Cognitive components refer to skill and performance of the mental processes necessary to know or apprehend by understanding. This includes but is not limited to:

1. *Orientation*

Orientation refers to skill and performance in comprehending, defining, and adjusting oneself in an environment with regard to time, place, and person.

2. *Conceptualization/Comprehension*

Conceptualization/comprehension refers to skill and performance in conceiving and understanding concepts or tasks such as color identification, word recognition, sign concepts, sequencing, matching, association, classification, and abstracting. This includes but is not limited to:

a. *Concentration*

Concentration refers to skill and performance in focusing on a designated task or concept.

b. *Attention span*

Attention span refers to skill and performance in focusing on a task or concept for a particular length of time.

c. *Memory*

Memory refers to skill and performance in retaining and recalling tasks or concepts from the past.

3. *Cognitive Integration*

Cognitive integration refers to skill and performance in applying diverse knowledge to environmental situations. This involves but is not limited to:

a. *Generalization*

Generalization refers to skill and performance in applying specific concepts to a variety of related situations.

b. *Problem Solving*

Problem solving refers to skill and performance in identifying and organizing solutions to difficulties. It includes but is not limited to:

(1) defining or evaluating the problem.

(2) organizing a plan.

(3) making decisions/judgments.

(4) implementing plan, including following through in logical sequence.

(5) evaluating decision/judgment and plan.

D. *Psychosocial Components*

Psychosocial components refer to skill and performance in self-management, dyadic and group interaction.

1. *Self-management*
   Self-management refers to skill and performance in expressing and controlling oneself in functional and creative activities.
   a. *Self-expression*
      Self-expression refers to skill and performance in perceiving one's feelings and interpreting and using a variety of communication signs and symbols. This includes but is not limited to:
      (1) experiencing and recognizing a range of emotions.
      (2) having an adequate vocabulary.
      (3) having writing and speaking skills.
      (4) interpreting and using correctly an adequate range of nonverbal signs and symbols.
   b. *Self-control*
      Self-control refers to skill and performance in modulating and modifying present behaviors and in initiating new behaviors in accordance with situational demands. It includes but is not limited to:
      (1) observing own and others' behavior.
      (2) conceptualizing problems in terms of needed behavioral changes or action.
      (3) imitating new behaviors.
      (4) directing and redirecting energies into stress-reducing activities and behaviors.

2. *Dyadic Interaction*
   Dyadic interaction refers to skill and performance in relating to another person. This includes but is not limited to:
   a. Understanding social/cultural norms of communication and interaction in various activity and social situations.
   b. Setting limits on self and others.
   c. Compromising and negotiating.
   d. Handling competition, frustration, anxiety, success, and failure.
   e. Cooperating and competing with others.
   f. Responsibly relying on self and others.

3. *Group Interaction*
   Group interaction refers to skill and performance in relating to groups of three to six persons or larger. This includes but is not limited to:
   a. knowing and performing a variety of task and social/emotional role behaviors.
   b. understanding common stages of group process.
   c. participating in a group in a manner that is mutually beneficial to self and others.

E. *Therapeutic Adaptations*
   Therapeutic adaptations refer to the design and/or restructuring of the physical environment to assist self-care, work, and play/leisure performance. This includes selecting, obtaining, fitting, and fabricating equipment, and instructing the client, family, and/or staff in proper use and care of equipment. It also includes minor repair and modification for correct fit, position, or use. Categories of therapeutic adaptations consist of:
   1. *Orthotics*
      Orthotics refer to the provision of dynamic and static splints, braces, and slings for the purpose of relieving pain, maintaining joint alignment, protecting joint integrity, improving function, and/or decreasing deformity.
   2. *Prosthetics*
      Prosthetics refer to the training in use of artificial substitutes of missing body parts, which augment performance of function.
   3. *Assistive/Adaptive Equipment*
      Assistive/adaptive equipment refers to the provision of special devices that assist in performance and/or structural or positional changes such as the installation of ramps, bars, changes in furniture heights, adjustments of traffic patterns, and modifications of wheelchairs.

F. *Prevention*
   Prevention refers to skill and performance in minimizing debilitation. It may include programs for persons where predisposition to disability exists, as well as for those who have already incurred a disability. This includes but is not limited to:
   1. *Energy Conservation*
      Energy conservation refers to skill and performance in applying energy-saving procedures, activity restriction, work simplification, time management, and/or organization of the environment to minimize energy output.
   2. *Joint Protection/Body Mechanics*
      Joint protection/body mechanics refers to skill and performance in applying principles or procedures to minimize stress on joints. Procedures may include the use of proper body mechanics, avoidance of static or deforming postures, and/or avoidance of excessive weight bearing.
   3. *Positioning*
      Positioning refers to skill and performance in the placement of a body part in alignment to promote optimal functioning.
   4. *Coordination of Daily Living Activities*
      Coordination of daily living activities refers to skill and performance in selecting and coordinating activities of self-care, work, play/leisure, and rest to promote optimal performance of daily life tasks.

III. Patient/Client-Related Conferences

Patient/client-related conferences include participating in meetings to discuss and identify needs, treatment program, and future plans of referred client, and documenting such particpation. Patient/client may or may not be present. Categories of conferences include:

A. *Professional Conferences*

Professional conferences refer to participating in meetings with a group or individual professionals to discuss patient's/client's status, and to advise/consult regarding treatment needs. Synonymous terms for professional conferences include initial conference, interim review, discharge planning, case conference, and others.

B. *Agency Conferences*

Agency conferences refer to participating in meetings with vocational, social, religious, recreational, health, educational, and other community representatives to assess, implement, or coordinate the use of services.

C. *Client-Advocate Conferences*

Client-advocate conferences refer to participating in meetings with client advocate (*e.g.*, family, guardian, or others responsible for patient/client) to assess patient's/client's situation, set goals, plan treatment and/or discharge; and to instruct client advocate to support or carry out treatment program.

IV. Travel: Patient-Treatment Related

Travel: Patient-treatment related refers to travel by therapists, with or without patient; that is, related to direct patient treatment.

The Following Items Do Not Involve Direct Patient Care

V. Service Management

Service management refers to planning, leading, organizing, and controlling the occupational therapy facility and service.

A. *Quality Review/Maintenance of Quality*

Quality review/maintenance of quality refers to those phases of departmental management that serve to assure and document normative standards to occupational therapy service.

1. *Development of Standards of Quality Treatment/ Services*

Development of standards of quality treatment/services refers to the development, implementation, evaluation, and documentation of departmental policy and procedures for the purpose of assuring standardized and quality treatment. This policy includes but is not limited to those procedures governing standards of occupational therapy practice, health and safety, infection control, and ethical behavior.

2. *Chart Audit*

Chart audit refers to the evaluation of documentation based on criteria developed within the facility, the profession, Health Systems Agency (Health Planning Act) and/or Professional Standards Review Organizations for a specified geographical area.

3. *Accrediting Reviews*

Accrediting reviews refer to those activities that are necessary to routinely document the meeting of the standards of a recognized accrediting body such as State Department of Health, Joint Committee on the Accreditation of Hospitals, Commission on Accreditation of Rehabilitation Facilities; or other accreditation procedures, voluntary or mandated by state or local law, and/or by the administration of a particular institution.

4. *Occupational Therapy Care Review*

Occupational therapy care review refers to the ongoing evaluation and documentation of the quality of care given. Three review programs may be included in the care review process: pre-admission screening, concurrent review, and retrospective studies.

5. *Inservice Education*

Inservice education refers to the participation of regularly employed occupational therapy personnel (*e.g.*, OTR, COTA, OT Aide, or OT orderly) in regularly scheduled classes, in-house seminars, and special training sessions, either in or outside the facility.

B. *Departmental Maintenance*

Departmental maintenance refers to activities to maintain the physical environment of the occupational therapy department so as to assure the health and safety of patients and staff. Some of these activities are mandated by accrediting agencies, state or local law, or administration of the facility, whereas others may be developed by the occupational therapy service.

C. *Employee Meetings*

Employee meetings refer to meetings of occupational therapy departmental staff for the purpose of disseminating and receiving information, conveying information concerning the administrative policies of the institution and/or conditions of employment, and discussing issues relevant to the management of the program, the development of the department and/or institution, and its relationship to total health care.

D. *Program-Related Conferences*

Program-related conferences refer to interdepartmental meetings for the purpose of disseminating and receiving information and discussing issues relevant to program planning, development, and management.

E. *Supervision*

Supervision refers to activities to enhance the performance of departmental employees through appraisal of their effectiveness, evaluation of their conformance to departmental standards, and/or evaluation of their adherence to specific institutional policies.

VI. Education

Education refers to the dissemination and collection of knowledge pertaining to occupational therapy and health care by means of lecture, demonstration, observation, or direct participation.

A. *Occupational Therapy Clinical Education: Occupational Therapy Students*

Occupational therapy clinical education: occupational therapy students refer to the orientation, instruction, supervision of student involvement in the occupational therapy program. This may include preclinical, fieldwork professional, and/or technical level occupational therapy students.

B. *Occupational Therapy Clinical Education: Others*

Occupational therapy clinical education: others refers to the orientation of nonoccupational therapists to occupational therapy treatment principles and theories and to interprofessional working relationships by occupational therapy departmental staff.

C. *Occupational Therapy Clinical Education: Continuing Education*

Occupational therapy clinical education: continuing education refers to ongoing educational experiences beyond basic education. The purpose of continuing education is to enrich or improve the occupational therapist's knowledge, skills, and attitudes in his/her work performance. Continuing education is designed for therapists interested in maintaining and updating themselves in the field of occupational therapy and in its related aspects such as research, consultation, education, administration, and supervision.

VII. Research

Research refers to formalized investigative activities for the purpose of improving the quality of occupational therapy patient care by means of recognized scientific methodologies and procedures.

APPENDIX

Occupational Therapy Product Output Reporting System*

Determination of Relative Value Units

To determine the relative value units which should be assigned to each category of service, five factors which affect cost and productivity levels of occupational therapy services were identified: expertise, equipment and supplies, patient–therapist interaction, facility, and interpretation and analysis. In turn, the four levels were identified for each factor.

A. Factor 1: Expertise

Level 1: omitted
Level 2: performed by an occupational therapist (OTR

and COTA) who meets the basic entry levels for the profession of occupational therapy.
Level 3: performed by an Occupational Therapist, Registered, who is experienced in the specific area of occupational therapy practice
Level 4: performed by an Occupational Therapist, Registered, who has specialized training and/or advanced education in the specific area of occupational therapy practice.

B. Factor 2: Equipment and Supplies

Level 1: requires no specific equipment and/or less than $5.00 worth of supplies
Level 2: requires equipment valued at $1.00 to $100.00 and/or supplies worh $5.01 to $10.00
Level 3: requires equipment valued at $101.00 to

---

* Adopted April 1979 by the Representative Assembly, AOTA.

$1,000.00 and/or supplies worth $10.01 to $50.00

Level 4: requires equipment valued in excess of $1,000.00 and/or supplies in excess of $50.01

C. Factor 3: Patient–Therapist Interaction

Level 1: requires preparation, planning, and minimal supervision of a patient, or group supervision of six or more patients

Level 2: requires preparation, planning, and intermittent supervision of a patient or group supervision of three to five patients

Level 3: requires preparation, planning, and constant supervision of one to two patients

Level 4: requires one-to-one interaction between patient and therapist with preparation, planning, and continuous attention and/or supervision.

D. Factor 4: Facilities

Level 1: performed in facilities which are not designated specifically to the occupational therapy department (*e.g.*, patient care unit, hospital day room)

Level 2: performed in designated occupational therapy facilities in which concurrent treatments may take place (*e.g.*, general clinic)

Level 3: performed in a designated occupational therapy facility in which concurrent treatments do not take place (*e.g.*, occupational therapy evaluation room)

Level 4: performed in specifically designed or specialized facility necessary for carrying out specific occupational therapy evaluation and/or treatment (*e.g.*, wheelchair accessible kitchen)

E. Factor 5: Interpretation and Analysis

Level 1: recording patient performance by daily attendance, census, and/or check-sheet

Level 2: reporting patient performance in the form of daily or weekly progress notation

Level 3: integrating and summarizing evaluation and treatment results in the form of a summary and/or consultation report

Level 4: interpreting test results, analyzing patient performance, and writing a formalized report specifying treatment goals and objectives and results

Each service category was assigned a level on each factor. This was done by consensual agreement of the opinions of the professional experts on the Task Force. An example is shown in the chart on this page.

The numerical values (levels) of the assignments on each factor were summed to give a total score for each category of service. Values across all categories of services were found to range from 8 through 18. These numbers were then multiplied by 10/8 to convert the scale to whole numbers beginning with 10—a scale which was considered to be easier to work with but which preserved the original relative weights between categories. This scale then became the relative value unit assignments for the service categories for individual evaluation and treatment. Readjustment factors were superimposed to bring group evaluation and treatment into a productivity measure realistically proportional to individual evaluation and treatment. Four categories of patient–therapist ratios were designated: (1) one patient per therapist; (2) two to four patients per therapist; (3) five to eight patients per therapist; and (4) nine or more patients per therapist. The readjustment factors were 50% of the individual RVU scale for the two to four patient category, 30% of the individual RVU scale for the five to eight patient category, and 10% of the RVU scale for the nine or more patients category. All RVUs

Category: Treatment, Independent Living, Work, Homemaking

Levels	Expertise	Equipment & Supplies	Patient-Therapist Interaction	Facility	Interpretation & Analysis
1					
2	X				X
3		X	X		
4				X	

Total Score $= 2 + 3 + 3 + 4 + 2 = 14$

Relative Value Units $= (14)(10/8) = 14$ RVUs for first patient category are based on a 15-minute interval of time, or multiples thereof.

provided to individuals or groups, and to both inpatients and outpatients.

Description of Accounts — Occupational Therapy

Function

Occupational Therapy is the application of purposeful, goal-oriented activity in the evaluation, diagnosis, and/or treatment of persons whose function is impaired by physical illness or injury, emotional disorder, congenital or developmental disability, or the aging process, in order to achieve optimum functioning, to prevent disability, and to maintain health. Specific occupational therapy services include, but are not limited to, education and training in activities of daily living (ADL); the design, fabrication, and application of orthoses (splints); guidance in the selection and use of adaptive equipment; therapeutic activities to enhance functional performance; prevocational evaluation and training; and consultation concerning the adaptation of physical environments for the handicapped. These services are

Description

This cost center contains the direct expenses incurred in maintaining an occupational and patient–therapist ratio categories. Each RVU is measured in 15-minute intervals, or multiples thereof.

Occupational Therapy Relative Values as developed by the American Occupational Therapy Association shall be used to determine the units related to product output of the Occupational Therapy Service Center. Relative Value Units for unlisted procedures or services are reasonably estimated on the basis of other comparable procedures or services.

Count units for all procedures or services rendered.

Data Source

The number of Relative Value Units shall be obtained from an actual count maintained by the Occupational Therapy Service Center.

Occupational Therapy Relative Values

| Code Number* | Occupational Therapy Service Category | | RVUs per 15 minute time interval Patient–Therapist Ratio Categories | | | |
			1 pt.	2–4 pts.	5–8 pts.	9 or more pts.
	I. Occupational Therapy Assessment					
98001-03	A. Screening		11	5.5	3.3	—
98004	B. Patient Related Consultation		14	—	—	—
	C. Evaluation					
98005-06		1. Independent Living/Daily Living Skills & Performance	18	9.0	—	—
98010-11		2. Sensorimotor Skill & Performance Components	21	10.5	—	—
98015-16		3. Cognitive Skill & Performance Components	20	10.0	—	—
98020-21		4. Psychosocial Skill & Performance Components	18	9.0	—	—
98025-26		5. Therapeutic Adaptations	19	—	—	—
98030-32		6. Specialized Evaluation	23	11.5	6.9	—
98035-36	D. Reassessment		18	9.0	—	—

* Only one code number may be used for a given category. Thus, where a series of code numbers are listed, each code number in the series is to be used for a different patient-therapist ratio category. For example, code numbers 98001 through 98003 are given for Screening. 98001 would be used for screening one to two patients, 98002 for screening a group of three to five patients, and 98003 for screening a group of six to eight patients.

(Continued)

Code Number*	Occupational Therapy Service Category	RVUs per 15 minute time interval Patient – Therapist Ratio Categories			
		1 pt.	2–4 pts.	5–8 pts.	9 or more pts.
	II. Occupational Therapy Treatment				
	A. Independent Living/Daily Living Skills & Performance				
98040-42	1. Physical Daily Living Skills	13	6.5	3.9	—
98045-47	2. Psychosocial/Emotional Daily Living Skills	13	6.5	3.9	—
	3. Work				
98050-52	a. Homemaking	15	7.5	4.5	—
98055-57	b. Child Care/Parenting	18	9.0	5.4	—
98060-62	c. Employment Preparation	19	9.5	5.7	—
98065-67	4. Play/Leisure	14	7.0	4.2	—
	B. Sensorimotor Components				
	1. Neuromuscular				
98070	a. Reflex Integration	18	—	—	—
98075-78	b. Range of Motion	13	6.5	3.9	1.3
98080-83	c. Gross and Fine Coordination	13	6.5	3.9	1.3
98085-88	d. Strength and Endurance	13	6.5	3.9	1.3
98090-92	2. Sensory Integration	16	8.0	4.8	—
	C. Cognitive Components				
98095-98	1. Orientation	10	5.0	3.0	1.0
98100-01	2. Conceptualization/Comprehension	14	7.0	—	—
98105-06	3. Cognitive Integration	14	7.0	—	—
	D. Psychosocial Components				
98110-13	1. Self-Management	14	7.0	4.2	1.4
98115-16	2. Dyadic Interaction	14	7.0	—	—
98120-23	3. Group Interaction	10	5.0	3.0	1.0
	E. Therapeutic Adaptation				
98125	1. Orthotics	20	—	—	—
98130-31	2. Prosthetics	16	8.0	—	—
98135-36	3. Assistive/Adaptive Equipment	16	8.0	—	—
98140-43	F. Prevention	13	6.5	3.9	1.3
98145	III. Patient/Client Related Conferences	14	—	—	—
98150-53	IV. Travel: Patient Treatment Related	12	6.0	3.6	1.2

Uniform Occupational Therapy Evaluation Checklist*

Application

The following Uniform Occupational Therapy Evaluation Checklist is designed as a generic occupational therapy guide for baseline data gathering. In order to use this checklist, each therapist will need to select the specific method of evaluation to be utilized. Data may be gathered through such means as suggested in the *Uniform Terminology System for Reporting Occupational Therapy Services;* for example, record, review, specific observation, interview, and the administration of data-collecting procedures. Such data collecting procedures include, but are not limited to, use of standardized tests, performance checklists, and activities designed to evaluate specific performance abilities. The occupational therapist should use evaluation procedures that reflect the philosophical base of occupational therapy.

Occupational therapists need to thoroughly understand how to use the Uniform Occupational Therapy Evaluation Checklist. The therapist should:
1. compare/overview the client in all areas,
2. determine areas that require specific tests,
3. select specific tests (for example, client may not need Activities of Daily Living, but only tests for sensory–integration function; this must be stated in the report),
4. report on all major categories (I A,B,C — II A,B,C,D,E,F) even though all subcategories may not apply,
5. document the type of evaluation used (*i.e.*, record review, standard tests, etc.).

Procedure

I. Demographic Information

A. Personal Information
   1. Name
   2. Address
   3. Telephone
   4. Date of Birth
   5. Age
   6. Sex
B. Referral Related Information
   1. Date of Referral
   2. Reason for Referral
   3. Referral Source

4. Date client first seen by OT
5. Diagnosis
6. Presenting problems/symptoms
7. Date of onset
8. Medications
9. Precautions/complications
10. Date of evaluation
11. Evaluator
C. Personal History
   1. Developmental History
   2. Educational History
   3. Vocational History
   4. Socio-economic History
   5. Medical History

II. Skills and Performance Areas†

(See the AOTA *Uniform Terminology System for Reporting Occupational Therapy Services,* January 1979, for definition of categories.)
A. Independent Living/Daily Living Skills and Performance
   1. Physical Daily Living Skills
      a. Grooming and Hygiene
      b. Feeding/Eating
      c. Dressing
      d. Functional Mobility
      e. Functional Communication
      f. Object Manipulation
   2. Psychological/Emotional Daily Living Skills
      a. Self-concept/self-identity
      b. Situational Coping
      c. Community Involvement
   3. Work
      a. Homemaking
      b. Child Care/Parenting
      c. Employment Preparation
   4. Play/Leisure
B. Sensorimotor Skills and Performance Components
   1. Neuromuscular
      a. Reflex Integration
      b. Range of Motion
      c. Gross and Fine Coordination
      d. Strength and Endurance

---

* Adopted March 1981 by the Representative Assembly, AOTA.

† This outline was taken and adapted from the AOTA Uniform Terminology System for Reporting Occupational Therapy Services, prepared by AOTA Commission on Uniform Reporting System Task Force, Rockville, AOTA, January 7, 1979.

2. Sensory Integration
   a. Sensory Awareness
   b. Visual-Spatial Awareness
   c. Body Integration
C. Cognitive Skill and Performance Components
   1. Orientation
   2. Conceptualization/Comprehension
      a. Concentration
      b. Attention Span
      c. Memory
   3. Cognitive Integration
      a. Generalization
      b. Problem Solving
D. Psychosocial Skills and Performance Components

1. Self-Management
   a. Self-Expression
   b. Self-Control
2. Dyadic Interaction
3. Group Interaction
E. Therapeutic Adaptation
   1. Orthotics
   2. Prosthetics
   3. Assistive/adaptive Equipment
F. Prevention
   1. Energy Conservation
   2. Joint Protection/Body Mechanics
   3. Positioning
   4. Coordination of Daily Living Skills

APPENDIX

Guidelines for Occupational Therapy Documentation

These guidelines are provided to assist members of the American Occupational Therapy Association (AOTA) in documenting occupational therapy services. Occupational therapy personnel shall document the type and frequency of services provided within the time frames established by facilities, government agencies, and accreditation organizations.

The purpose of documentation is to do the following:
1. Provide a serial and legal record of the patient's condition and the course of therapeutic intervention from admission to discharge.
2. Serve as an information source for patient care.
3. Facilitate communication among health care professionals who contribute to the patient's care.
4. Furnish data for use in treatment, education, research, and reimbursement.

Types of Documentation

The various types of documentation are
1. initial note
2. assessment notes and reports
3. treatment plans and goals

4. progress notes
5. treatment records
6. discharge summaries
7. consultation reports
8. special reports (*e.g.*, referrals to other programs and agencies, summary reports for legal reasons, home programs, and correspondence)
9. critical incidents reports or notes

Protocol for Documentation

Each patient referred to occupational therapy must have a case record maintained as a permanent file. The record should be:
1. organized
2. legible
3. concise
4. clear
5. accurate
6. complete
7. current
8. objective (clear distinction made between facts and opinions)
9. correct in grammar and spelling

Fundamental Elements of Documentation

The following ten elements should be present:
1. patient's full name and case number on each page of documentation;

Prepared by the Documentation Task Force (Linda Kohlman McGourty, MOT, OTR, chair; Mary Foto, OTR: Susan Kronsnoble, OTR; Carole Lossing, OTR; Sharon Rask, OTR; and Christine de Renne Stephan, OTR) for the Commission on Practice (Esther Bell, MA, OTR, FAOTA, chair).

Approved by the Representative Assembly, April 1986.

(list continues on page 813)

Table 1.   *Components of Total Occupational Therapy or Facility Record for Each Patient*

Content	*Clarifications*
A. Identification and Background Information	
1. Name, age, sex, date of admission, treatment diagnosis, and date of onset of current diagnosis.	Name may be omitted depending on the facility and department policies and procedures
2. Referral source, services requested, and date of referral to occupational therapy.	Include who requested occupational therapy services, what specific services were requested, and the date.
3. Pertinent history that indicates prior levels of function and support systems	Include applicable developmental, educational, vocational, socioeconomic, and medical history (may be brief).
4. Secondary problems or preexisting conditions	Include any additional problems or conditions that may affect patient function or treatment outcomes.
5. Precautions and contraindications.	May be identified by referral source or occupational therapy staff.
B. Assessment and Reassessment	
Refer to the Uniform Occupational Therapy Checklist (AOTA, 1979) for specific skills and performance.	Independent living/daily living skills and performance components Sensorimotor skills and performance components Cognitive skills and performance components Psychosocial skills and performance components Therapeutic adaptations and prevention
1. Tests and evaluations administered and the results.	State name and type of evaluation, date administered, and results and whether assessment or reassessment.
2. Summary and analysis of assessment findings.	State facts in an objective manner. Analysis of objective findings should include measurable data to define the patient's assets and deficits.
3. References to other pertinent reports and information.	Include any additional sources of data or evaluation results that help formulate the total assessment of the patient.
4. Occupational therapy problem list.	This list should be compatible with a master problem list developed by the health care team or other health care professionals (when available).
5. Recommendations for occupational therapy services.	State whether occupational therapy services are recommended or not.
C. Treatment Planning	
1. Short- and long-term goals.	Define clearly the goals established by the patient, family, and therapist. These goals should be measurable and related to the occupational therapy problem list.
2. Activities and/or treatment procedures.	State clearly the specific methods to be used in the intervention and relate the methods to the problems identified on the occupational therapy problem list.
3. Type, amount, and frequency of treatment.	State skill and performance areas to be addressed and estimate the number, duration, and frequency of treatment sessions to accomplish goals.
4. Anticipated time to achieve goals.	State the anticipated number of therapy sessions or days of therapy to reach the desired outcome. This information may be an overall statement not necessarily written for each goal.
5. Statement of potential functional outcome.	State the anticipated outcome and clearly relate it to the long-term goals.
D. Treatment Implementation	
1. Activities, procedures, and modalities used.	State the specific media and methods used.
2. Patient's response to treatment and the progress toward goal attainment as related to problem list.	State the patient's physical and behavioral response to therapy and whether the goals are being achieved.
3. Goal modification when indicated by the response to treatment.	If the goals have been modified in the treatment process, state the new goals and rationale for changes.
4. Change in anticipated time to achieve goals.	If for any reason the treatment time frame is altered, include the reason for the change and the new anticipated time frame.

(continues)

Table 1. *Components of Total Occupational Therapy or Facility Record for Each Patient (continued)*

Content	*Clarifications*
D. Treatment Implementation	
5. Attendance and participation with treatment plan (attendance could be a check format).	State if the patient is following through with treatment plan.
6. Statement of reason for patient missing treatment.	Write the reasons for treatment not occurring as scheduled.
7. Assistive/adaptive equipment, orthotics, and prosthetics if issued or fabricated, and specific instructions for the application and/or use of the item.	State the device, note whether it was fabricated, sold, rented, or loaned, and state the effectiveness of the device.
8. Patient-related conferences and communication.	If occupational therapy personnel participated in a conference of made a pertinent contact with a family member, agency, or health care professional, state this information with a brief summary of the conference or communication.
9. Home programs.	Include a copy of the home program as established with the patient in the patient record.
E. Discontinuation of Services	
1. Summary of assessment and treatment implementation.	State clearly and concisely a summary of the total occupational therapy intervention process, the number of sessions, the goals achieved, and the functional outcome. Compare the initial and discharge status.
2. Home programs.	Include the actual written home program that is to be followed after discharge.
3. Follow-up plans.	State the schedule and specific plans.
4. Recommendations.	State any recommendations pertaining to the patient's future needs.
5. Referral(s) to other health care providers and community agencies.	Make referral(s) or recommendations for referral(s) when additional or new services are needed.

2. date stated as month, day, and year for each entry;
3. identification of type of documentation and department name;
4. signature with a minimum of first name, last name, and professional designation;
5. signature of the recorder directly at the end of the note without space left between the body of the note and the signature;
6. countersignature by a registered occupational therapist (OTR) on documentation written by students and certified occupational therapy assistants (COTA) if required by law or the facility;
7. compliance with confidentiality standards;
8. acceptable terminology as defined by the facility;
9. facility approved abbreviations;
10. errors corrected by drawing a single line through an error, and the correction initialed (liquid correction fluid and erasures are not acceptable), or facility requirements followed.

Content of Documentation

The following components should be included in the total occupational therapy or facility record for each patient (see Table 1). Each occupational therapy department must determine the type and frequency of documentation and must abide by the written policies and procedures of the individual facility.

Reference

American Occupational Therapy Association. (1979). Uniform Terminology for Reporting Occupational Services. Rockville, MD, AOTA

Entry-Level Role Delineation
for OTRs and COTAs*

Introduction

This role delineation is intended for internal use by the American Occupational Therapy Association, Inc. as a guide to assist members in the practice of their profession. The role delineation may be used to assist in the development of entry-level educational Essentials and certification criteria, but may not be used (except with the written permission of the AOTA) to draft legal documents of any kind such as licensure bills or private contracts.

The contents of this document are not to be construed as entirely original, but represent a compilation of resource materials and professional judgment. Resource documents used were:

1. AOTA Entry Level Functions of the Registered Occupational Therapist, Certified Occupational Therapy Assistant and Occupational Therapy Aide: AOTA; 1972.

2. Task Inventory for Entry Level Occupational Therapy Personnel in Direct Service Roles: NIH Contract No. 72-4172; AOTA; June 1973.

3. Phase 1—Delineation of the Role of Entry Level Occupational Therapy Personnel: Contract #231-76-0052; AOTA; July 1, 1976–February 1, 1978.

4. AOTA Standards of Practice for Occupational Therapy Services for the Developmentally Disabled Client; Clients with Physical Disabilities; in a Mental Health Program; and in a Home Health Program; AOTA; January 1979.

5. Essentials of an Accredited Educational Program for the Occupational Therapist; June 1972; and Essentials of an Approved Educational Program for the Occupational Therapy Assistant; April 1975.

6. AOTA Resolutions #533-79 (Funding for 518-77), #535-79 (Role Delineation Concept and Use), #552-79 (Strategy to Educate Independent Health Professionals), #551-79 (Position on Proficiency Testing for Individuals Outside the Field of Occupational Therapy), and proposed Resolution "J"-1980 (Strategy for Determining the Place of the COTA in the Profession of Occupational Therapy).

7. Entry Level Study Committee Memo; AOTA; April 7, 1980.

8. Essentials Review Committee Report; Recommendation #1; AOTA; 1980.

9. Components and Interrelationships of a Competency Assurance System. Chart #1 and Management of the AOTA Competency Assurance System. Chart #2; AOTA; 1979.

10. *AOTA Uniform Terminology for Reporting Occupational Therapy Services*; AOTA; 1979.

The following principles/concepts were used in the development of the role delineation document:

1. OTRs must be able to call COTA roles and functions.

2. The role delineation reflects present and future practice of occupational therapy.

3. The role delineation reflects entry-level practice only and may be used only for that level when used to develop educational Essentials or certification requirements.

4. Entry-level is defined as the first year of practice.

5. Entry-level COTAs must receive direct supervision by an OTR during the first year of occupational therapy practice. COTAs are encouraged to participate in continuing education programs provided by agencies and professional associations and to pursue other continuing education opportunities.

6. Entry-level OTRs are certified for general practice and are able to independently provide services. Entry-level OTRs are encouraged to pursue continuing education, consultation and other collaborative activities in their professional role.

7. Employers should provide appropriate personnel for the supervision of new graduates.

8. The role delineation addresses tasks and not "professional" behaviors that reflect ethical or value judgments.

Refer to the Role Delineation Glossary and *AOTA Uniform Terminology System for Reporting Occupational Therapy Services* for definitions of terms used in this document.

---

* Approved by the Representative Assembly AOTA, March 1981.

Entry Level Role Delineation Committee:

Jay Bullock, OTR	Gladys Masagatani, OTR	Nancy Prendergast, OTR
Sr. Miriam Joseph Cummings, OTR	Linda McGourty, OTR	Sally Ryan, COTA
Jeanne Madigan, OTR	Nancy Moulin, OTR	Javan Walker, Jr., OTR

AOTA Staff

Madelaine Gray, OTR
Carole Hays, OTR
Stephanie Presseller, OTR

The Entry-Level OTR	**The Entry-Level COTA**

I. **Referral:** the initiation or acknowledgment of a referral may be before initial screening or after. A referral for occupational therapy service must be based upon the provisions as outlined in the AOTA Statement of Referral.

A. Responds to request for service, whatsoever its source

A. Responds to a request for service by relaying information or formal referral to supervising OTR

B. Initiates referrals when appropriate

B. Initiates referrals for independent living/daily living skills intervention

C. Supervises documentation and filing of referrals according to department standards

C. Enters case as appropriate to standards of department and profession when authorized by supervising OTR

D. Delegates case to COTA, as appropriate, according to standards of department and profession

II. **Occupational Therapy Assessment:** Occupational therapy refers to the process of determining the need for, nature of, and estimated time of treatment, determining the needed coordination with other persons involved, and documenting these activities.

A. *Screening*: determine client's need for occupational therapy services; may occur before or after referral

A. *Screening*: determine client's need for occupational therapy services in collaboration with OTR; may occur before or after referral

1. Collect data:
   a. identify type and sources of information that are needed

   b. obtain and review information and identify pertinent details about client; or plan and supervise data collection
   c. explain overall occupational therapy services to client, family, and significant others

   d. observe and interview client, family, and significant others to obtain general history and information
2. Analyze data:
   a. organize data
   b. summarize data
   c. interpret data

1. Collect data:
   a. obtain and review information as determined by OTR and identify pertinent details about client
   b. explain overall occupational therapy services to client, family and significant others

   c. observe and interview client, family, and significant others *using a structured guide* to obtain general history and information

2. Organize data:
   a. summarize *own* data
   b. record and report *own* data to OTR

The Entry-Level OTR	The Entry-Level COTA

3. Formulate recommendations
4. Document and report occupational therapy screening data, interpretation, and recommendations

B. *Evaluation*: obtain and interpret data necessary for treatment. This includes planning for and documenting the evaluation process and results. The OTR is responsible for the evaluation process.

B. *Evaluation*: The COTA contributes to the evaluation process under the supervision of the OTR.

1. Select appropriate area(s) to evaluate
  a. independent living/daily living skills
    (1) Physical Daily Living Skills
      (a) Grooming and Hygiene
      (b) Feeding/Eating
      (c) Dressing
      (d) Functional Mobility
      (e) Functional Communication
      (f) Object Manipulation
    (2) Psychological/Emotional Daily Living Skills
      (a) Self-concept/Self-identity
      (b) Situation Coping
      (c) Community Involvement
    (3) Work
      (a) Homemaking
      (b) Child Care/Parenting
      (c) Employment Preparation
    (4) Play/Leisure
  b. sensorimotor components
    (1) Neuromuscular
      (a) Reflex Integration
      (b) Range of Motion
      (c) Gross and Fine Coordination
      (d) Strength and Endurance
    (2) Sensory Integration
      (a) Sensory Awareness
      (b) Visual-Spatial Awareness
      (c) Body Integration
  c. cognitive components
    (1) Orientation
    (2) Conceptualization/Comprehension
      (a) Concentration
      (b) Attention Span
      (c) Memory
    (3) Cognitive Integration
      (a) Generalization
      (b) Problem Solving
  d. psychosocial components
    (1) Self-management
      (a) Self-expression
      (b) Self-control
    (2) Dyadic Interaction
    (3) Group Interaction

The Entry-Level OTR	The Entry-Level COTA

2. Plan evaluation methodology

3. Explain evaluation plan to client, family, significant others, and other health professionals

4. Interview client, family, and significant others for information about:
   a. medical history and current health status
   b. developmental milestones
   c. social and family history
   d. self-care abilities
   e. academic history
   f. vocational history
   g. play history
   h. leisure interests and experiences
   i. future plans and goals
   j. accessibility of home environment
   k. accessibility of work or school system
   l. accessibility of community support system

       1. Assist OTR by interviewing client, family, and significant others *using a structured format* as determined by OTR for information about:
       a. family history
       b. self-care abilities
       c. academic history
       d. vocational history
       e. play history
       f. leisure interests and experiences

5. Observe client while engaged in individual and/or group activity to collect data and report on: (refer to areas in Section II.B.1 for specifics in each area)
   a. independent living/daily living skills
   b. sensorimotor skills

   c. cognitive skills
   d. psychosocial skills

       2. Assist OTR by observing client while engaged in individual and/or group activity to collect general data and report on: (refer to areas in Section II.B.1 for specifics in each area)
       a. independent living/daily living skills
       b. selected sensorimotor skills:
         (1) Gross and fine coordination
         (2) Strength and endurance
         (3) Tactile awareness
       c. cognitive skills
       d. psychosocial skills

6. Administer standardized and non-standardized assessments in the following areas: (refer to areas in Section II.B.1 for specifics in each area)
   a. independent living/daily skills and performance
   b. sensorimotor skills and performance

   c. cognitive skills and performance

   d. psychosocial skills and performance
   e. therapeutic adaptations
      (1) Orthotics
      (2) Prosthetics
      (3) Assistive/Adaptive Equipment

       3. Administer *structured* tests as directed by the OTR to collect data on:

       a. independent living/daily living skills and performance
       b. sensorimotor skills and performance in the following areas of:
         (1) Gross and Fine Coordination
         (2) Tactile Awareness
       c. cognitive skill and performance in the area of orientation

7. Analyze and synthesize evaluation data:
   a. state evaluation findings
   b. analyze, interpret, and synthesize scores or results of tests and assessments
   c. state client's assets and deficits

The Entry-Level OTR	The Entry-Level COTA
8. Document evaluation data and interpretation	4. Summarize, record and report *own* evaluation data to OTR supervisor
9. Report evaluation data	5. Report evaluation data as detemined by OTR
10. Develop recommendations as to the continuation or discontinuation of occupational therapy services and/or referral to other type of service	6. Make recommendations to the OTR supervisor as to the continuation or discontinuation of occupational therapy services and/or referral to other type of service

III. Program Planning: Planning refers to the identification of achievable program goals and the methods to those goals.

A. Develop long- and short-term goals (in collaboration with client, family, and significant others) to develop, improve, and/or restore the performance of necessary functions; compensate for dysfunction; and/or minimize debilitation, in the areas of: (refer to areas in Section II.B.1 for specifics in each area)
  1. Independent living/daily living skills and performance
  2. Sensorimotor skills and performance
  3. Cognitive skills and performance
  4. Psychosocial skills and performance
	A. Assist OTR with the development of long- and short-term goals (in collaboration with client, family, and significant others) to develop, improve, and/or restore the performance of necessary functions; compensate for dysfunction; and/or minimize debilitation, in the areas of:
	  1. Independent living/daily living skills and performance
	  2. Sensorimotor skills and performance in the following areas:
	    a. gross and fine coordination
	    b. strength and endurance
	    c. range of motion
	    d. tactile awareness
	  3. Cognitive skills and performance
	  4. Psychosocial skills and performance

B. Refer client to experienced OTR for specialized evaluation and services Examples of specialized evaluations are employment preparation, evaluation (prevocational testing), sensory integration evaluation, prosthetic evaluation, driver's training evaluation	
C. Select occupational therapy techniques, media, and determine sequence of activities to attain goals in all areas	B. Assist OTR in selecting occupational therapy techniques, media, and in determining sequence of activities to attain goals in areas designated above

D. Analyze components which make up tasks and activities	C. Analyze activities in the following areas:
	  1. Relevance to client's interests and abilities
	  2. Major motor processes
	  3. Complexity
	  4. Steps involved
	  5. Extent to which it can be modified or adapted

E. Adapt techniques/media to meet needs, capacities and roles of the client	D. Adapt techniques/media, under the supervision of the OTR, to meet client needs

The Entry-Level OTR	The Entry-Level COTA
F. Discuss occupational therapy goals and methods with client, family, significant others and other staff	E. Discuss occupational therapy program goals and methods with client, family, significant others, and staff
G. Document and report program plan	F. Document and report program plan as directed by the OTR
H. Coordinate the program with staff and other services	
I. Determine point of termination	

IV. **Occupational Therapy Treatment:** Occupational therapy treatment refers to the use of specific activities or methods to develop, improve, and/or restore the performance of necessary functions; compensate for dysfunction; and/or minimize debilitation.

The Entry-Level OTR	The Entry-Level COTA
	• In situations where patient conditions or treatment settings are complex (involving multiple systems) and where conditions change rapidly, requiring frequent or ongoing reassessment and modification of treatment plan, the COTA is required to have close supervision by the OTR.
	• In situations where patient conditions or treatment settings are more singular or stable so that decisions regarding program revision are required less frequently, the COTA may function independently as directed by the OTR.
A. Engage client in purposeful activity, in conjunction with therapeutic methods, to achieve goals identified in the following areas:	A. Under the direction of the OTR, engage client in purposeful activity, in conjunction with therapeutic methods, to achieve goals identified in the program plan in the following areas:
I. Independent living/daily living skills a. physical daily living skills (1) Grooming and Hygiene (2) Feeding/Eating (3) Dressing (4) Functional Mobility	1. Independent living/daily living skills a. physical daily living skills (1) Grooming and Hygiene (2) Feeding/Eating (3) Dressing (4) Functional Mobility: (a) Bed Mobility (b) Wheelchair Mobility (c) Transfers (d) Functional Ambulation (e) Public Transportation
(5) Functional Communication (6) Object Manipulation b. psychological/emotional daily living skills (1) Self-Concept/Self-Identity (2) Situational Coping (3) Community Involvement	(5) Functional Communication (6) Object Manipulation b. psychological/emotional daily living skills (1) Self-Concept/Self-Identity (2) Situational Coping (3) Community Involvement

The Entry-Level OTR	The Entry-Level COTA

c. work
  (1) Homemaking
  (2) Child Care/Parenting
  (3) Employment Preparation
    (a) Work Process Skills and Peformance
    (b) Work Product Quality
d. play/leisure
	c. work
	  (1) Homemaking
	  (2) Child Care/Parenting
	  (3) Work Process Skills and Performance
	
	d. play/leisure

2. Sensorimotor components
  a. neuromuscular
    (1) Reflex Integration
    (2) Range of Motion
    (3) Gross and Fine Coordination
    (4) Strength and Endurance
  b. Sensory integration
    (1) Sensory Awareness
    (2) Visual-Spatial Awareness
    (3) Body Integration
	2. Sensorimotor components
	  a. neuromuscular
	
	    (1) Range of Motion
	    (2) Gross and Fine Coordination
	    (3) Strength and Endurance
	  b. Tactile Awareness
	  c. Postural Balance

3. Cognitive components
  a. orientation
  b. conceptualization/comprehension
    (1) Concentration
    (2) Attention Span
    (3) Memory
  c. cognitive integration
    (1) Generalization
    (2) Problem Solving
	3. Cognitive components
	  a. orientation
	  b. conceptualization/comprehension
	    (1) Concentration
	    (2) Attention Span
	    (3) Memory

4. Psychosocial components
  a. self-management
    (1) Self-Expression
    (2) Self-Control
  b. dyadic interaction
  c. group interaction	

5. Therapeutic adaptation
  a. orthotics
    (1) Static Splints
    (2) Slings
  b. assistive/adaptive equipment
	4. Therapeutic adaptation
	  a. orthotics
	    (1) Static Splints
	    (2) Slings
	  b. assistive/adaptive equipment

6. Prevention
  a. energy conservation
  b. joint protection/body mechanics
  c. positioning
  d. coordination of daily living activities
	5. Prevention
	  a. energy conservation
	  b. joint protection/body mechanics
	  c. positioning
	  d. coordination of daily living skills

B. Orient and instruct family, significant others and non-OT staff in activities which support the therapeutic program	B. Orient and instruct family and significant others in activities which support the therapeutic program
C. Observe medical and safety precautions	C. Observe medical and safety precautions

The Entry-Level OTR	The Entry-Level COTA

D. Prepare and instruct a program with client, family and significant others to implement at home

D. Assist in instruction of client, family and significant others in implementation of home program developed by OTR

E. Monitor client's program
1. Observe client's response to program
2. Summarize and analyze client performance
3. Document response to program
4. Discuss client performance with client, family, significant others and staff
5. Reassess client's performance
6. Modify goals
7. Modify program
8. Coordinate program modifications with other services

E. Monitor client's program
1. Observe client's performance as directed by OTR
2. Summarize client's performance as directed by OTR
3. Document client's performance as directed by OTR
4. Discuss client performance with client, family, significant others, and staff as directed by OTR
5. Discuss need for reassessment with OTR
6. Assist OTR in identifying program changes
7. Coordinate program modifications with other services.

V. **Program Discontinuation:** Program discontinuation refers to the termination of occupational therapy services when the client has achieved the program goals and/ or has achieved maximum benefit from the services.

A. Formulate, in collaboration with client, family, significant others and staff, discharge and follow-up plan

A. Discuss need for program discontinuation with OTR

B. Recommend termination of occupational therapy services

B. Assist OTR in preparing program for implementation at home

C. Prepare program for implementation at home

C. Assist OTR in recommending adaptations in client's everyday environment

D. Recommend adaptations in client's everyday environment

D. Assist OTR in identifying community resources

E. Refer client and/or family to another occupational therapist or other service provider

E. Assist in summarizing and documenting outcome of the OT program

F. Recommend community resources

G. Summarize and document outcome of the OT program

H. Terminate program

VI. **Service Management:** Service management refers to planning, leading, organizing and controlling the occupational therapy facility and service.

A. Maintain service
1. Plan daily schedule according to assigned workload
2. Prepare and maintain work setting, equipment, and supplies

A. Maintain service
1. Plan daily schedule according to assigned workload
2. Prepare and maintain work setting, equipment, and supplies

The Entry-Level OTR	The Entry-Level COTA
3. Order supplies and equipment according to established procedures	3. Order supplies and equipment according to established procedures
4. Determine space, equipment and supply needs	4. Maintain records according to department procedure
5. Prepare and maintain records and budget	5. Ensure safety and maintenance of program areas and equipment
6. Ensure safety and maintenance of program areas and equipment	6. Assist with compiling and analyzing data of total OT service
7. Compile and analyze data of OT service	7. Follow reimbursement procedures
8. Follow reimbursement procedures	8. Participate in employee meetings
9. Conduct and participate in employee meetings	9. Participate in program-related conferences
10. Participate in program-related conferences	10. Receive supervision from immediate supervisor in order to enhance self-performance
11. Receive supervision from immediate supervisor in order to enhance self-performance	11. Comply with departmental standards and/or evaluate adherence to institutional policies
12. Comply with established standards and/or evaluate adherence to institutional policies	
13. Seek and use consultation	
B. Recruit, select, orient, train, supervise, and evaluate:	B. Assist with other personnel:
1. COTAs	1. Orient, supervise aides and assist in their training
2. Support staff such as secretary, aide, transport personnel	2. Recruit, select, orient, train, supervise and evaluate volunteers under direction of OTR
3. Volunteers	
C. Plan, direct, coordinate and evaluate service programs	C. Assist OTR with evaluation of service program
D. Determine service and personnel needs	
E. Assure collaboration, coordination, and communication	
F. Develop and implement quality review program including:	D. Participate in quality review program
1. Standards of quality treatment/services	
2. Chart audit program	
3. Occupational therapy care review	
4. Inservice education program	
G. Participate in accrediting reviews	E. Participate in accrediting reviews
H. Supervise Level I fieldwork students, and non-OT students	F. Supervise Level I OTA fieldwork students as assigned by OTR
I. Develop, through the use of statistics, the justification for having or increasing OT services	

The Entry-Level OTR	The Entry-Level COTA

VII. **Continued Education:** Continued education refers to ongoing educational experiences beyond basic education.

The Entry-Level OTR	The Entry-Level COTA
A. Participate in continuing education programs	A. Participate in continuing education programs
B. Participate in inservice programs	B. Participate in inservice programs
C. Plan and provide inservice education	C. Assist OTR in planning and providing inservice education

VIII. **Public Relations:** Public relations refers to promoting awareness and understanding of the profession of occupational therapy.

The Entry-Level OTR	The Entry-Level COTA
A. Identify the need for and explain occupational therapy services and profession to public and professional groups	A. Explain occupational therapy services and profession to public groups
B. Serve as a representative of the profession and the association	B. Serve as a representative of the profession and the association

Definitions

Independent living/daily living skills refer to the skill and performance of physical and psychological/emotional self-care, work, and play/leisure activities to a level of independence appropriate to age, life-space, and disability. Life-space refers to an individual's cultural background, value orientation, and physical and social environment.

Physical daily living skills refer to the skill and performance of daily personal care, with or without adaptive equipment. It includes but is not limited to:

Grooming and hygiene refer to the skill and performance of personal health needs, such as bathing, toileting, hair care, shaving, applying make-up.

Feeding/eating refers to the skill and performance of sequentially feeding oneself, including sucking, chewing, swallowing, and using appropriate utensils.

Dressing refers to the skill and performance of choosing appropriate clothing, dressing oneself in a sequential fashion, including fastening and adjusting clothing.

Functional mobility refers to the skill and performance in moving oneself from one position or place to another. It includes skills necessary for activities such as bed mobility, wheelchair mobility, transfers (bed, car, tub, toilet, chair), and functional ambulation, with or without adaptive aids. It also includes use of public and private travel systems, such as driving own automobile and using public transportation.

Functional communication refers to the skill and performance in using equipment or systems to enhance or provide communication, such as writing equipment, typewriters, letterboards, telephone, braille writers, artificial vocalization systems and computers.

Object manipulation refers to the skill and performance in handling large and small common objects, such as calculators, keys, money, light switches, doorknobs, and packages.

Psychological/emotional daily living skills refer to the skill and performance in developing one's self-concept/self-identity, coping with life situations, and participating in one's organizational and community environment. It includes but is not limited to:

Self-concept/self-identity refers to the cognitive image of one's functional self. This includes but is not limited to:

- clearly perceiving others' needs, feelings, conflicts, values, beliefs, expectations, sexuality, and power
- realistically perceiving others' needs, feelings, conflicts, values, beliefs, expectations, sexuality, and power
- knowing one's performance strengths and limitations
- sensing one's competence, achievement, self-esteem, and self-respect
- integrating new experiences with established self-concept/ self-identity
- having a sense of psychological safety and security
- perceiving one's goals and directions.

Situational coping refers to skill and performance in handling stress and dealing with problems and changes in a manner that is functional for self and others. This includes but is not limited to:

- setting goals, selecting, harmonizing, and managing activities of daily living to promote optimal performance
- testing goals and perceptions against reality
- perceiving changes and need for changes in self and environment
- directing and redirecting energy to overcome problems
- initiating, implementing, and following through on decisions
- assuming responsibility for self and consequences of actions
- interacting with others, dyadic and group.

Community involvement refers to skill and performance in interacting within one's social system. This includes but is not limited to:

- understanding social norms and their impact on society
- planning, organizing, and executing daily life activities in relationship to society, including such activities as budgeting, time management, social role management and using community resources
- recognizing and responding to needs of families and groups
- understanding and responding to organizational/community role expectations as both recipient and contributor.

Work refers to skill and performance in participating in socially purposeful and productive activities. These activities may take place in the home, employment setting, school, or community. They include but are not limited to:

Homemaking refers to skill and performance in homemaking and home management tasks, such as meal planning, meal preparation and clean-up, laundry, cleaning, minor household repairs, shopping, and use of household safety principles.

Child care/parenting refers to skill and performance in child care activities and management. This includes but is not limited to physical care of children, and use of age-appropriate activities, communication, and behavior to facilitate child development.

Employment preparation refers to skill and performance in precursory job activities including prevocational activities. This includes but is not limited to:

- job acquisition skills and performance
- organizational and team participatory skills and performance
- work process skills and performance
- work product quality.

Play/leisure refers to skill and performance in choosing, performing, and engaging in activities for amusement, relaxation, spontaneous enjoyment, and/or self-expression. This includes but is not limited to:

- Recognizing one's specific needs, interests, and adaptations necessary for performance
- Identifying characteristics of activities and social situations that make them play for the individual
- Identifying activities that contain those characteristics
- Choosing play activities for participation, such as sports, games, hobbies, music, drama, and other activities
- Testing out and adapting activities to enable participation
- Identifying and using community resources.

Sensorimotor components refer to the skill and performance of patterns of sensory and motor behavior that are prerequisites to self-care, work, and play/leisure performance. The components in this section include neuromuscular and sensory integrative skills, including perceptual motor skills.

Neuromuscular refers to the skill and performance of motor aspects of behavior. This includes but is not limited to:

Reflex integration refers to skill and performance in enhancing and supporting functional neuromuscular development through eliciting and/or inhibiting stereotyped, patterned, and/or involuntary responses coordinated at subcortical and cortical levels.

Range of motion refers to skill and performance in using maximum span of joint movement in activities with and without assistance to enhance functional performance. The standard levels of performance include:

- active range of motion: movement by patient, unassisted through a complete range of motion
- passive range of motion: movement performed by someone other than patient or by a mechanical device, requiring no muscle contraction on the part of the patient
- active-assistive range of motion: movement performed by the patient to the limit of his/her ability, and then completed with assistance.

Gross and fine coordination refers to skill and performance in muscle control, coordination, and dexterity while participating in activities

- muscle control: skill and performance in directing muscle movement
- coordination: skill and performance in gross motor activities using several muscle groups
- dexterity: skill and performance in tasks using small muscle groups.

Strength and endurance refers to skill and performance in using muscular force within time periods necessary for purposeful task performance. This involves but is not limited to progressively building strength and cardiac and pulmonary reserve, increasing the length of work periods, and decreasing fatigue and strain.

Sensory integration refers to skill and performance in development and coordination of sensory input, motor output, and sensory feedback. This includes but is not limited to:

Sensory awareness refers to skill and performance in perceiving and differentiating external and internal stimuli, such as:

- tactile awareness: the perception and interpretation of stimuli through skin contact
- stereognosis: the identification of forms and nature of objects through the sense of touch
- kinesthesia: the conscious perception of muscular motion, weight, and position
- proprioceptive awareness: the identification of the positions of body parts in space
- ocular control: the localization and visual tracking of stimuli
- vestibular awareness: the detection of motion and gravitational pull as related to one's performance in functional activities, ambulation, and balance
- auditory awareness: the differentiation and identification of sounds
- gustatory awareness: the differentiation and identification of tastes
- olfactory awareness: the differentiation and identification of smells

Visual-spatial awareness refers to skill and performance in perceiving distances between and relationships among objects, including self. This includes but is not limited to:

- figure-ground: recognition of forms and objects when presented in a configuration with competing stimuli
- form constancy: recognition of forms and objects as the same when presented in different contexts
- position in space: knowledge of one's position in space relative to other objects

Body integration refers to skill and performance in perceiving and regulating the position of various muscles and body parts in relationship to each other during static and movement states. This includes but is not limited to:

- body schema: the perception of one's physical self through proprioceptive and interoceptive sensations
- postural balance: skill and performance in developing and maintaining body posture while sitting, standing, or engaging in activity
- bilateral motor coordination: skill and performance in purposeful movement that requires interaction between both sides of the body in a smooth, refined manner
- right-left discrimination: skill and performance in differentiating right from left and vice versa
- visual-motor integration: skill and performance in combining visual input with purposeful voluntary movement of the hand and other body parts involved in an activity. Visual-motor integration includes eye-hand coordination
- crossing the midline: refers to skill and performance in crossing the vertical midline of the body
- praxis: refers to skill and performance of purposeful movement that involves motor planning.

Cognitive components refer to skill and performance of the mental processes necessary to know or apprehend by understanding. This includes but is not limited to:

Orientation refers to skill and performance in comprehending, defining, and adjusting oneself in an environment with regard to time, place, and person.

Conceptualization/comprehension refers to skill and performance in conceiving and understanding concepts or tasks such as color identification, word recognition, sign concepts, sequencing, matching, association, classification, and abstracting. This includes but is not limited to:

Concentration refers to skill and performance in focusing on a designated task or concept.

Attention span refers to skill and performance in focusing on a task or concept for a particular length of time.

Memory refers to skill and performance in retaining and recalling tasks or concepts from the past.

Cognitive integration refers to skill and performance in applying diverse knowledge to environmental situations. This involves but is not limited to:

Generalization refers to skill and performance in applying specific concepts to a variety of related situations.

Problem solving refers to skill and performance in identifying and organizing solutions to difficulties. In includes but is not limited to:

- defining or evaluating the problem
- organizing a plan
- making decisions/judgments
- implementing plan, including following through in logical sequence
- evaluating decision/judgment and plan.

Psychosocial components refer to skill and performances in self-management, dyadic and group interaction.

Self-management refers to skill and performance in expressing and controlling oneself in functional and creative activities.

Self-expression refers to skill and performance in perceiving one's feelings and interpreting and using a variety of communication signs and symbols. This includes but is not limited to:

- experiencing and recognizing a range of emotions
- having an adequate vocabulary
- having writing and speaking skills
- interpreting and using correctly an adequate range of nonverbal signs and symbols.

Self-control refers to skill and performance in modulating and modifying present behaviors, and in initiating new behaviors in accordance with situational demands. It includes but is not limited to:

- observing own and others' behavior
- conceptualizing problems in terms of needed behavioral changes or action
- imitating new behaviors
- directing and redirecting energies into stress-reducing activities and behaviors

Dyadic interaction refers to skill and performance in relating to another person. This includes but is not limited to:

- Understanding social/culture norms of communication and interaction in various activity and social situations
- Setting limits on self and others
- Compromising and negotiating
- Handling competition, frustration, anxiety, success, and failure
- Cooperating and competing with others
- Responsibly relying on self and others.

Group interaction refers to skill and performance in relating to groups of three to six persons, or larger. This includes but is not limited to:

- Knowing and performing a variety of task and social/emotional role behaviors
- Understanding common stages of group process
- Participating in a group in a manner that is mutually beneficial to self and others.

Therapeutic adaptations refer to the design and/or restructuring of the physical environment to assist self-care, work, and play/leisure performance. This includes selecting, obtaining, fitting, and fabricating equipment, and instructing the client, family, and/or staff in proper use and care of equipment. It also includes minor repair and modification for correct fit, position or use. Categories of therapeutic adaptations consist of:

Orthotics refer to the provision of dynamic and static splints, braces, and slings, for the purpose of relieving pain, maintaining joint alignment, protecting joint integrity, improving function, and/or decreasing deformity.

Prosthetics refer to the training in use of artificial substitutes of missing body parts, which augment performance of function.

Assistive/adaptive equipment refers to the provision of special devices that assist in performance, and/or structural or positional changes such as the installation of ramps, bars, changes in furniture heights, adjustments of traffic patterns, and modifications of wheelchairs.

Prevention refers to skill and performance in minimizing debilitation. It may include programs for persons where predisposition to disability exists, as well as for those who have already incurred a disability. This includes but is not limited to:

Energy conservation refers to skill and performance in applying energy-saving procedures, activity restriction, work simplification, time management, and/or organization of the environment to minimize energy output.

Joint protection/body mechanics refers to skill and performance in applying principles or procedures to minimize stress on joints. Procedures may include the use of proper body mechanics, avoidance of static or deforming postures, and/or avoidance of excessive weight bearing.

Positioning refers to skill and performance in the placement of a body part in alignment to promote optimal functioning.

Coordination of daily living activities refers to skill and performance in selecting and coordinating activities of self-care, work, play/leisure, and rest to promote optimal performance of daily life tasks.

Reassessment refers to the process of obtaining and interpreting data necessary for updating treatment plans and goals. This frequently involves administering only portions of the initial evaluation, documenting results, and/or revising treatment.

Development of standards of quality treatment service refers to the development, implementation, evaluation, and documentation of departmental policy and procedures for the purpose of assuring standardized and quality treatment. This policy includes but is not limited to those procedures governing standards of occupational therapy practice, health, and safety, infection control, and ethical behavior.

Chart audit refers to the evaluation of documentation based on criteria developed within the facility, the profession, Health Systems Agency (Health Planning Act), and/or Professional Standards Review Organizations for a specified geographical area.

Occupational therapy care review refers to the ongoing evaluation and documentation of the quality of care given. Three review programs may be included in the care review process: preadmission screening, concurrent review, and retrospective studies.

Inservice education refers to the participation of regularly employed occupational therapy personnel (e.g., OTR, COTA, OT Aide, or OT orderly) in regularly scheduled classes, in-house seminars, and special training sessions, either in or outside the facility.

Accrediting reviews refer to those activities that are necessary to routinely document the meeting of the standards of a recognized accrediting body such as State Department of Health, Joint Commission on the Accreditation of Hospitals, Commission on Accreditation of Rehabilitation Facilities; or other accreditation procedures, voluntary or mandated by state or local law, and/or by the administration of a particular institution.

ROLE DELINEATION GLOSSARY

1. *structured assessment*: an assessment instrument or form that is constructed and organized to provide guidelines for the content and process of the assessment: e.g., Interest Inventory.

2. *standardized assessment*: an assessment that provides for measurement against a criterion or norm. The assessment must be done according to the testing protocol; e.g., ROM assessment; Southern California Sensory Integration Tests.

3. *non-standardized assessment:* an assessment that provides information but with no precise comparison to a norm; e.g., Social History.

4. *therapeutic activities in occupational therapy:* self-care, work, home management, child care, educational, play/leisure, and cultural activities that have been selected and adapted to meet specific occupational therapy goals.

5. *significant others:* refers to persons, excluding the indi-

vidual's family and health professionals, who have an important relationship to the individual.

6. *OT Program:* refers to the delivery of occupational therapy services to a client.

7. *OT service:* refers to the organizational structure and

system within which occupational therapy programs are provided.

8. *Level I Fieldwork:* is that which occurs as an integral part of didactic course work.

Approved by Representative Assembly March 1981

Hierarchy of Competencies Relating to the Use of Standardized Instruments and Evaluation Techniques by Occupational Therapists

Approved by the Representative Assembly, May 1984 Developed by Patti Maurer, PhD, OTR; Roann Barris, EdD, OTR; Betty Bonder, PhD, OTR; and Nedra Gillette, MEd, OTR.

This hierarchy of competencies has been developed by the AOTA/AOTF Committee on Standardized Assessments/Evaluations in an effort to establish the range of knowledge and skills required of occupational therapists. The hierarchy is intended to provide guidance for educators in the preparation of scholarly practitioners at several levels of practice.

Responding to a charge from the Representative Assembly to design a plan for the development of standardized evaluations for use by occupational therapists, the committee recognized as a first step the need for some agreement across the profession as to the scope and nature of the competencies required in assessment and evaluation. This proposed hierarchy represents the committee's efforts to obtain agreement regarding this aspect of practice.

By definition, items at the beginning (or lower level) of a hierarchy are implied as necessary for later (or higher) level functions. Thus, all members of a profession must demonstrate each Basic Competency, in each aspect of practice.

Entry-level competencies of the COTA may be presumed as competencies of the entry-level OTR, and so forth. Higher-level competencies are built on and incorporate the lower-level competencies which precede them. Higher-level competencies may be acquired through practice and experience, or through advanced education. Some competencies at Level IV, and all at Level V, would require advanced education.

Terminology for Assessment Competencies

Assessment: refers to the process of determining the need for, nature of, and estimated time of treatment, as well as determining the needed coordination with other persons involved[1].

Clinical Reasoning: the process of systematic decision-making based on an identifiable professional frame of reference and utilizing both subjective and objective data accrued through appropriate assessment/evaluation processes.

Entry-level competencies: minimal competence acceptable upon completion of technical or professional education program.

Evaluation: refers to the process of obtaining and interpreting data necessary for treatment. This includes planning for and documenting the evaluation process and results. These data may be gathered through record review, observations, questioning, and testing. Such procedures include but are not limited to the use of standardized tests, performance checklists, interviews, and activities, and tasks designed to evaluate specific performance abilities. Categories of occupational therapy evaluation include independent daily living skills and performance, and their components[1].

Hierarchy: the basic hierarchical scheme used in this document is the level of professional competence required by the COTA and the OTR.

Instrument: a device for recording or measuring; especially such a device functioning as a control system.

Norms: a standard, a model, or pattern for a specific

group; an expected type of performance or behavior for a particular reference group of persons.

Objective: facts or findings which are clearly observable to and verifiable by others, as reflecting reality.

Reliable: the degree to which a test's results may be expected to be consistent.

Standardized: made standard or uniform; to be used without variation; suggests an invariable way in which a test is to be used, as well as denoting the extent to which the results of the test may be considered to be both valid and reliable.

Subjective: an observation not rigidly reflecting measurable reality; may imply observer bias; may not be verifiable by others in the same situation.

Valid: the degree to which a test's results are actually measures of the characteristics it claims to measure.

I. Basic Competencies in Assessment

A. recognizes the importance of using standardized, reliable, and valid instruments whenever such are appropriate.

B. distinguishes between subjective and objective data, and uses each accordingly.

C. distinguishes the critical differences between standardized and nonstandardized instruments.

D. recognizes the need to use standardized instruments according to the instructions given in the test administration manual.

E. recognizes that using standardized instruments in an unstandardized (or adapted) manner may result in an invalid assessment.

F. recognizes that specialized training may be necessary to administer certain instruments correctly and to interpret the data appropriately.

G. uses assessment data to document work with client so as to provide a logical, continuous record of performance, therapeutic goals and media, and outcomes.

H. follows ethical practices in the use of assessments: recognition of copyright, protection of the security of tests, protection of the confidentiality of test results, use of assessments for which one's education and experience is sufficient.

II. Entry-Level Competencies, Technical Education

A. uses a structured interview format as directed by the OTR to elicit background information on family history, self-care function, and leisure interests and experiences.

B. administers other structured instruments as supervised by the OTR.

C. combines information collected through assessment procedures with standards of customary practice and collaborates with the OTR to develop a treatment plan for the client.

D. informs OTR supervisor when client performance seems to indicate need for reassessment or evaluation.

III. Entry-Level Competencies, Professional Education

A. identifies available instruments in one's area of practice.

B. identifies behavioral dimension measured by specific instruments.

C. interprets information on reliability, validity, and norms of instruments used.

D. selects instruments based on a clinical/theoretical rationale for their use.

E. identifies areas of practice where instrument development is needed.

F. administers and interprets standardized and other instruments which assess the client's occupational performance and performance components with relation to the given environment.

G. identifies need for further specific assessment of function.

H. integrates data from assessments to formulate a treatment plan using principles derived from theory to show coherence between findings and treatment goals and media.

I. recognizes the need for reassessment or evaluation of client performance.

J. supervises assessments and evaluations done by a COTA in conformance with state and federal laws and regulations.

IV. Advanced-Level Competencies

A. critiques existing instruments on the basis of reliability, validity, norms, and relationship to theory in occupational therapy.

B. contributes to the development, field testing, and dissemination of instruments clearly linked to theory in occupational therapy.

C. obtains specialized training to use instruments critical to one's area of practice.

V. Scholarly Research Competencies

A. designs new instruments in accordance with principles of instrument development, and plans research to field tests and standardize the instrument.

B. obtains funding for the development of a new instrument.

C. articulates the need for such an instrument and the rationale for its design so as to increase proper use of it within the profession.

D. designs research linking assessments/evaluations to theory development in occupational therapy.

References

1. Uniform Terminology for Reporting Occupational Therapy Services. Rockville, MD, The American Occupational Therapy Association, Inc, Approved by the AOTA Representative Assembly, March 1979
2. The American Heritage Dictionary of the English Language, New College Edition. Boston, Houghton Mifflin, 1976

APPENDIX **J**

Directory of Resources

The following are addresses that professionals and families can use to obtain information and support. This list provides major sources of information; there are other national organizations not listed that provide services. In addition to these addresses, information and support can be obtained locally through community-supported United Way organizations, local federal agencies, hospitals and health-related agencies, religious centers, and other community groups.

Miscellaneous Resources

American Academy of Physical Medicine and Rehabilitation
30 N Michigan Ave, Suite 922
Chicago, IL 60602

American Association for World Health
2121 Virginia Ave NW
Washington, DC 20037

American Congress of Rehabilitation Medicine
30 N Michigan Ave
Chicago, IL 60602

American National Standards Institute
1430 Broadway
New York, NY 10018

American Occupational Therapy Association, Inc.
1383 Piccard Drive
Rockville, MD 20850

American Physical Therapy Association
111 N Fairfax St
Alexandria, VA 22314

Centers for Disease Control
Atlanta, GA 30333

Goodwill Industries of America, Inc.
9200 Wisconsin Ave
Bethesda, MD 20814

National Foundation — March of Dimes
Box 2000
White Plains, NY 10602

National Institutes of Health
Bethesda, MD 20014

National Rehabilitation Association
633 S Washington St
Alexandria, VA 22314

National Rehabilitation Information Center
4407 Eighth St NE
Washington, DC 20017

Rehabilitation International
22 East 21st St
New York, NY 10010

Roosevelt Warm Springs Foundation
530 S Omni International
Atlanta, GA 30303

World Health Organization
Geneva 27, Switzerland

Aging

American Association of Retired Persons
1909 K St NW
Washington, DC 20049

American Society on Aging
833 Market St, Suite 516
San Francisco, CA 94103

Gerontological Society of America
1411 K St NW, Suite 300
Washington, DC 20005

National Association of Area Agencies on Aging (AAA)
600 Maryland Ave SW, Suite 208
Washington, DC 20024

National Association of State Units on Aging
600 Maryland Ave SW, Suite 208
Washington, DC 20024

National Council on the Aging, Inc
600 Maryland Ave SW, West Wing 100
Washington, DC 20024

US Administration on Aging
330 Independence Ave SW
Washington, DC 20201

Burns

American Burn Association
Good Samaritan Medical Center
1130 East McDowell Road, Suite B-2
Phoenix, AZ 85006

Jobst Institute
653 Miami Street
Toledo, Ohio 43694
(visual aids and educational material)

Phoenix Society, Inc
11 Rust Hill Road
Levittown, PA 19056

Chronic Health Problems

American Brittle Bone Society
1415 E Marlton Pike
Cherry Hill, NJ 08077
(osteogenesis imperfecta)

American Cancer Society
777 Third Ave
New York, NY 10020

American Diabetes Association
600 Fifth Ave
New York, NY 10020

American Heart Association
7320 Greenville Ave
Dallas, TX 75231

American Hospital Association
840 North Lake Shore Drive
Chicago, IL 60611

American Lung Association
1740 Broadway
New York, NY 10019

American Parkinson Disease Association
116 John Street
New York, NY 10038

Arthritis Foundation
1314 Spring Street NW
Atlanta, GA 30309

Arthritis Information Clearinghouse
PO Box 34227
Bethesda, MD 20034

Asthma and Allergy Foundation of America
19 W 44th St
New York, NY 10036

Epilepsy Foundation of America
4351 Garden City Dr
Landover, MD 20785

Guillain–Barré Syndrome Support Group
PO Box 262
Wynnewood, PA 19096

Leukemia Society of America, Inc
800 Second Ave
New York, NY 10017

Muscular Dystrophy Association of America, Inc
810 Seventh Ave
New York, NY 10019

Myasthenia Gravis Foundation, Inc.
15 East 26th St, Suite 1603
New York, NY 10010

National ALS Foundation
185 Madison Avenue
New York, NY 10016

National American Diabetes Association
600 Fifth Ave
New York, NY 10020

National Association for Sickle Cell Disease, Inc
945 S Western Ave, Suite 206
Los Angeles, CA 90006

National Cystic Fibrosis Research Foundation
3379 Peachtree Rd NE
Atlanta, GA 30326

National Diabetes Information Clearinghouse
NIMANCD–DEMD
Westwood Bldg, Rm 603
Bethesda, MD 20205

National Epilepsy League
6 N Michigan Ave
Chicago, IL 60602

National Kidney Foundation
2 Park Ave
New York, NY 10016

National Multiple Sclerosis Society
205 East 42nd St
New York, NY 10017

National Parkinson Foundation, Inc
1501 NW Ninth Ave
Miami, FL 33136

United Cerebral Palsy Association
66 E 34th St
New York, NY 10016

Learning Disabilities

Association for Children with Learning Disabilities
4156 Library Rd
Pittsburgh, PA 15234

Directory of College Programs for Learning Disabled Students
Loyola Academy
Wilmette, IL 60091

National Aid to Retarded Citizens
2709 East St
Arlington, TX 76011

National Association for Retarded Citizens
2709 Avenue E East
Arlington, TX 76011

National Society for Autistic Children
169 Tampa Ave
Albany, NY 12208

Parents of Down Syndrome Children
11507 Yates St
Silver Spring, MD 20902

Scholastic Aptitude Test (SAT)
Services for Handicapped Students
Institutional Services
Box 592
Princeton, NJ 08541

Mental Health

National Center on the Rights of the Mentally Impaired
1600 20th St NW
Washington, DC 20009

Neurologic Impairment

Architectural and Transportation Barriers Compliance Board
330 C Street SW
Washington, DC 20201

Association for Persons with Severe Handicaps
7010 Roosevelt Way NE
Seattle, WA 98115

Clearinghouse on the Handicapped
Office of Special Education and Rehabilitative Services
US Department of Education
Room 3106 Switzer Building
Washington, DC 20202

Coordinating Council for Handicapped Children
407 S Dearborn
Chicago, IL 60605

Disability Rights Center, Inc
1346 Connecticut Avenue NW, Suite 1124
Washington, DC 20036

International Center for the Disabled
340 E 24th St
New York, NY 10010

National Center for Law and the Handicapped
University of Notre Dame
PO Box 477
South Bend, IN 46656

National Head Injury Foundation
18A Vernon St
Framingham, MA 01701

National Information Center for the Handicapped
Box 1492
Washington, DC 20013

National Paraplegia Foundation
333 N Michigan Ave
Chicago, IL 60601

National Spinal Cord Injury Foundation
149 California St
Newton, MA 02158

Office for Handicapped Individuals
330 Independence Ave SW
Washington, DC 20201

Paralyzed Veterans of America
801 18th St NW
Washington, DC 20006

President's Committee on Employment of the Handicapped
Washington, DC 20210

Pediatrics

Association for the Care of Children in Hospitals
3615 Wisconsin Ave
Washington, DC 20016
(202) 244-1801

Department of Health and Human Services
National Center of Child Abuse and Neglect
US Children's Bureau
Office of Child Development
PO Box 1182
Washington, DC 20013

National Center for Child Advocacy
PO Box 1182
Washington, DC 20013

National Center for the Prevention and Treatment of Child Abuse and Neglect
Department of Pediatrics
University of Colorado Medical Center
1205 Oneida St
Denver, CO 80220
(National Child Protection Newsletter)

National Committee for Prevention of Child Abuse
Suite 510
111 East Wacker Dr
Chicago, IL 60601

Prosthetics

American Orthotic and Prosthetic Association
717 Pendelton St
Alexandria, VA 22314

Child Amputee Prosthetic Project (CAPP prosthesis and components)
University of California at Los Angeles
Los Angeles, CA

Fidelity VA-NU Myoelectric Hand System and Cosmetic Components
Fidelity Electronics, Ltd
5245 West Diversey Ave
Chicago, IL 60639

Hosmer Dorrance Corporation (conventional, modular, and external power components)
PO Box 37
561 Division St
Campbell, CA 95008

Motion Control (Utah Artificial Arm; myoelectric elbow)
1005 South 300 West
Salt Lake City, UT 84101

National Amputation Foundation, Inc
12-45 150th St
Whitestone, NY 11357

Northwestern University Medical School Prosthetic–Orthotic Center
345 East Superior St
Chicago, IL 60611

Otto Bock Orthopedic Industry, Inc (conventional, myoelectric, and endoskeletal components)
4130 Highway 55
Minneapolis, MN 55422

Pope Brace (Accru-Hook system)
197 South West Ave
Kankakee, IL 60901

Prosthetics and Orthotics
New York University Post-Graduate Medical School
317 E 34th St
New York, NY 10016

Prosthetic Research Laboratory at Northwestern University Medical School
Michigan Department of Public Health
Area Child Amputee Center
Grand Rapids, MI

Realistic Cosmetic Prosthetics
Emerald Road
PO Box 368
Greenwood, SC 29646

Therapeutic Recreation Systems (prehensile hook terminal device)
1280 28th St, Suite 4
Boulder, CO 80303

United States Manufacturing Co (Pope Brace Orthotics and Fracture Products)
180 N San Gabriel Blvd
PO Box 5030
Pasadena, CA 91107

Variety Village Electro Limb Production Centre (myoelectric and cosmetic components)
3701 Danforth Ave
Scarborough (Toronto) Ontario
Canada M1N 2G2

Recreation

National Amputee Golf Association
5711 Yearling Ct
Bonita, CA 92002

National Center for Therapeutic Riding
9244 E Mansfield Ave
Denver, CO 80237

National Easter Seal Society
2023 West Ogden Ave
Chicago, IL 60612

National Handicapped Sports and Recreation Association
PO Box 33141 Farragut Station
Washington, DC 20033

National Recreation and Park Association
3101 Dart Center Dr
Alexandria, VA 22302

Sensory Impairment

American Deafness and Rehabilitation Association
814 Thayer Ave
Silver Spring, MD 20910

American Foundation for the Blind
15 W 16th St
New York, NY 10011

American Printing House for the Blind
1839 Frankfort Ave
Louisville, KY 40206

American Speech and Hearing Association
10801 Rockville Pike
Rockville, MD 20852

Association for Education of Visually Handicapped
919 Walnut St
Philadelphia, PA 19107

Association for the Visually Handicapped
1839 Frankfort Ave
Louisville, KY 40206

Centers & Services for Deaf – Blind Children, Bureau of Education for Handicapped
US Office of Education
400 Maryland Ave SW
Donohoe Bldg, Rm 3155
Washington, DC 20202

Helen Keller National Center for Deaf – Blind Youths & Adults
111 Middle Neck Rd
Sands Point, NY 11050

International Association of Parents of the Deaf
814 Thayer Ave
Silver Spring, MD 20910

John Tracy Clinic
806 W Adams Blvd
Los Angeles, CA 90007
(Has correspondence courses for families of deaf and deaf – blind infants and children.)

National Association of the Deaf
814 Thayer Ave
Silver Spring, MD 20910

National Association for Hearing and Speech Action
814 Thayer Ave
Silver Spring, MD 20910

National Association for Visually Handicapped
305 E 24th Street
New York, NY 10010

National Library Service for the Blind and Physically Handicapped
Library of Congress
1291 Taylor Street NW
Washington, DC 20542

National Society for Prevention of Blindness, Inc
79 Madison Ave
New York, NY 10016

Optacon (electronic reading device for the blind)
Telesensory Systems Inc
Palo Alto, CA 94302

The University of Wisconsin–Stout
Menomonie, WI 54751

The National Center for Research in Vocational Education The Ohio State University
1960 Kenny Rd
Columbus, OH 43210–1090

Vocational Education

Materials Development Center
Stout Vocational Rehabilitation Institute, School of Education and Human Services

Glossary

AAMD. American Association on Mental Deficiency

Accommodation. The response or the motor process of adjusting the body to react to incoming stimulation

Achievement motivation. The will to perform or to achieve, using some standard.

Low-achievement motivation: minimal will to try

High-achievement motivation: high level of performance

ACLD. Association of Children with Learning Disabilities; a nonprofit organization whose purpose is to advance the education and general welfare of children with normal or potentially normal intelligence who have learning disabilities of a perceptual, conceptual, or coordinative nature.

Acquisitional. Referring to behaviors, attitudes, and ideas that have been learned through experience

Acting out. Action rather than verbal response to unconscious drives or impulses; brings temporary relief of tension situation; may be a substitute for the impulse that originally gave rise to the action

Active listening. In conversation or interview, attending carefully to what is said by the other—awareness of both verbal and nonverbal communication

Acuity. Sharpness of perceptual ability; how well or clearly one can see or hear or use other senses

Adaptation. Any change in structure, form, or habits of an organism to suit a new environment. In reflex action, decline in the frequency of impulses when the sensory nerve is stimulated repeatedly. In psychiatry, those changes experienced by an individual that lead to adjustment

Adaptive behavior. Manner with which the individual deals with the cultural, social, physical, and mental demands of the environment.

Adaptive skills. Learned patterns of behavior that enable the individual to fulfull his/her own needs and the needs of others

Addiction. Habit of drug or alcohol use, in which the individual has symptoms of distress when deprived of the drug and the irresistible impulse to take the drug

Adolescence. Stage of life between onset of puberty and psychological and biological maturity

Adulthood. Stage of life that begins when the individual attains biological and psychological maturity and ends with the gradual onset of old age

AE. Above elbow

Affect. Emotional feeling or tone (inner feelings) and external manifestation (mood)

Affiliations. A relationship(s) that helps one to see through the eyes of another and to confirm or reject our own experiences in a warm and accepting way

Aggression. Forceful goal-directed behavior

Agitation. Motor restlessness with anxiety

Agnosia. Loss of comprehension of auditory, visual, or other sensations although the sensory sphere is intact; inability to recognize an object

Agonist. The muscle directly engaged in contraction, as distinguished from muscles that have to relax at the same time

AJOT. *American Journal of Occupational Therapy*

AK. Above knee

Akinesia. Absence or diminution of voluntary motion

Alienation. Feelings of detachment from self, others, or society in general; avoidance of emotional experiences

Alimentation. Giving nourishment

Alloplastic. Changing or moving things other than self; the external environment

Amaurosis. Partial or total blindness from any cause

Amblyopia. Lazy eye; dimness of vision, especially that not caused by refractive errors or organic disease of the eye; may be congenital or acquired

Amnesia, anterograde. Loss of memory of events after an injury

Amnesia, retrograde. Loss of memory of events immediately preceding injury

Amniocentesis. Removal of fluid containing fetal cells from the amniotic sac for chemical and chromosomal analysis to detect certain fetal abnormalities

Amphetamine. A central nervous system stimulant drug

Amputation. Cutting off a limb or part of a limb, the breast, or other projecting part

Amyotrophic lateral sclerosis (ALS). A degenerative disease of the pyramidal tracts and lower motor neurons characterized by motor weakness and a spastic condition of the limbs associated with muscular atrophy, fibrillary twitching, and final involvement of nuclei in the medulla

Anal phase. Second stage of psychosexual development (ages 1–3); interests, activities, and pleasure centered in anal zone (Freud)

Anastomosis. A natural communication, direct or indirect, between two blood vessels or other tubular structures; an operative union of two hollow or tubular structures, as divided ends of intestine or blood vessels

Anergia. Lack of energy, passivity

Aneurysm. Circumscribed dilation of an artery or a blood-containing tumor connecting directly with the lumen of an artery

Animism. Belief that inanimate objects are alive

Ankylosis. Natural fixation of a joint; abnormal immobilization of a joint caused by destruction of articular cartilage, enabling bony surfaces to fuse

Anoxia. Oxygen deficiency

ANSI. American National Standards Institute

Antagonist. Certain muscles opposing or resisting the action of others

Antecedent. That which goes before; preceding circumstance, event, or condition

Anxiety. Unpleasurable affect, with physiological and psychological changes; feelings of impending danger, powerlessness, tension, and readiness for expected danger in absence of objective danger or threat

Apgar test. Objective test of newborn's health

Aphasia. Impairment or loss of ability to receive or to express verbal symbols or ideas; speech and hearing mechanism may be intact

Apnea. Cessation of breathing, usually temporary

Appendicular. Relating to the limbs, as opposed to axial (trunk and head)

Apraxia. Inability to perform purposeful voluntary movements, the nature and mechanism of which are understood in the absence of motor or sensory impairment

ARC. Association of Retarded Citizens; a parent-founded nonprofit association that promotes the general welfare of retarded citizens by encouraging research, advising parents, developing better understanding of retardation by the public, distributing information, and raising funds

Arteriosclerosis. "Hardening of the arteries"

Arthrodesis. Fusion of a joint by removing the articular surfaces and securing bony union; operative ankylosis; surgical fixation of a joint

Arthroplasty. Surgical formation of a joint

Artificialism. Belief that an action was a result of an outside agent

Art therapy. Treatment technique using spontaneous creative work of patients to explore, analyze, express underlying emotional problems

Assimilation. Sensory process of "taking in" or receiving information that is external to or within the self system

Association. The organized process of relating the sensory information with the motor act or relating present and past experiences with each other

Astereognosis. Loss of the power of judging the form of an object by touch

Asymmetrical. Denoting a lack of symmetry between two or more parts

Ataxia. Incoordination of voluntary muscle movements, particularly those used in reaching and walking

Atresia. Congenital absence or pathological closure of a normal opening, passage, or cavity

Atrophic, atrophy. Pertaining to a wasting of tissues, organs, or the entire body

Audiometrist. One who evaluates a person's hearing

qualitatively and quantitatively by use of an audiometer

Audit. An official examination and verification of accounts and records

Autition. Acoustic ability; hearing

Autogenic. Autogenetic; self-producing

Autocosmic play. Play centered on infant's body

Autonomic nervous system (ANS). Part of nervous system functioning outside of consciousness — directs, for example, breathing, heart rate, and digestion

Autonomy. Quality of being self-governing and self-determining (striving toward independence)

Autoplastic. Changing or moving one's self

Aversive. Causing strong feelings of repugnance, distaste, dislike, or displeasure

Axial. Relating to or situated in the central part of the body, in the head or trunk, as distinguished from the extremities

Axon. Essential conduction portion of a nerve fiber continuous with the cytoplasm of a nerve cell

Barbiturate. Highly addictive CNS depressant (ex. phenobarbital, thiopental)

Basal ganglia. Basal nuclei of the endbrain (telencephalon)

BE. Below elbow

Biofeedback. Technique in which patient is made aware of unconscious or involuntary physiological processes and learns to control them

BK. Below knee

Body image. Conscious or unconscious image of one's body (including function); sum of all feelings concerning the body

Body language. System by which a person expresses feelings and thoughts through posture, gesture, or movement

Body scheme. Perception of one's physical self through proprioceptive and interoceptive sensations.

Bolus. Round mass; *e.g.,* of masticated food that is ready to be swallowed

Boutonnière deformity. PIP flexion with DIP hyperextension

Breech delivery. Presentation of the buttocks instead of the head in childbirth

Bruxism. Grinding of the teeth, especially during sleep

Carpal tunnel syndrome. Compression of the median nerve in the carpal tunnel at the wrist causing thenar atrophy and paralysis as well as trophic changes of the finger tips and sensory disturbances of the first three fingers

Catabolic phase; catabolism. Breaking down by the body of complex chemical compounds into simpler ones, often accompanied by the liberation of energy

Cataracts. Partial or complete opacity of the crystalline lens of the eye or its capsule

Catchment area. Defined geographical area representing a specified number of people to be served by a mental health center

Catharsis. Release of ideas, thoughts, repressed materials from the unconscious, with emotional responses and release of tension (psychoanalytical term)

Causalgia. Neuralgia distinguished by a burning pain along certain nerves

CEC. Council of Exceptional Children; an associated organization of the National Education Association for the advancement of education of exceptional children and youth, both gifted and handicapped

Centering. Ability to focus on only one aspect of situation

Cerebellum. Posterior brain mass; it consists of two lateral hemispheres united by a narrow middle portion

Cerebral contusion. Bruising of brain causing diffuse disturbance with edema and hemorrhage and destruction of brain tissue

Cervical. Pertaining to the neck and its eight vertebrae

Cesarean section. Removal of the fetus by means of an incision into the uterus, usually by way of the abdominal wall

Chaining. In behavior therapy, the process by which behavioral patterns are learned by reinforcements given for behaviors that are associated or related to an established behavior

Childhood. Stage of life lasting from the end of infancy until the onset of puberty

Chorea movements. Irregular and uncontrollable movements of muscles of the limbs and face

Chromosomes. Bodies in the cell nucleus that carry the genes

Circolectric bed. Circular frame containing a bed on which a patient can lie and be passively positioned from supine to prone on a 180° axis by an electric mechanism. The patient can be tilted at any angle on the axis.

CMHC. Community mental health center

CNS. Central nervous system

Cocontraction. Simultaneous contraction of the agonist and antagonist muscles to provide stability

Cognition. Conscious process of awareness and knowledge of objects through perception, memory, and reasoning; mental process of knowing and understanding; an ego function — thinking, judgment

Cognitive development. Development of a logical method of looking at the world; knowing and understanding

COJ. Classification of jobs according to worker trait factors

Collagen. Protein of the white fibers of connective tissue, cartilage, and bone

Combinational analysis. Systematically isolating all

the individual variables of a situation plus all possible combinations of these variables

Compensation. Process in which a tendency for change in a given direction is counteracted by another change so that the original change is not evident; an unconscious mechanism by which an individual tries to make up for fancied or real deficiencies

Competence. Quality of adequacy or possession of required skill, knowledge, or capacity

Conceptual. Formation or construct of ideas and thoughts

Conceptual model. Organization of theoretical constructs or of knowledge upon which a frame of reference for action can be based

Concrete operations. Third stage in Piagetian theory during which the 7- to 11-year-old begins to think logically although thinking is still limited to what is seen

Conditioning. Procedure used to alter behavior. *classical:* through pairing of stimuli to evoke response. *operant:* through presentation of reinforcements

Confidentiality. Medical ethics; keeping secret information that a patient has divulged

Conflict. Clash of opposing emotional forces

Conjugate deviation. Forced and persistent turning of the eyes and head toward one side; observed with some lesions of the cerebrum

Conscious (noun). That part of the mind that is experienced in awareness (psychoanalytical)

Consensual validation. Comparison of thoughts, feelings, and perceptions with others — results in effective reality testing (Harry Stack Sullivan term)

Conservation. Cognitive ability described by Piaget as occurring with concrete operations; the time when a child begins to understand physical properties of matter equivalence

Constancy. Property of remaining the same, as in perceptual constancy, in which things are perceived as unchanged in form even if position or distance may change

Contract. Explicit agreement to a well-defined course of action, as in therapy or in supervision

Contracture. Permanent muscular contraction resulting from tonic spasm or loss of muscular equilibrium, the antagonists being paralyzed

Contralateral. Originating in or affecting the opposite side of the body

Coordination. Harmonious working together of several muscles or muscle groups in the execution of complicated movements; the working together of different systems of the body in a given process, as in the coordination between the system of glands and involuntary muscles in digestion

Cortex. Layer of gray matter that invests the surface of the cerebral hemispheres and the cerebellum

Countertransference. Conscious or unconscious responses of therapist to the patient determined by therapist's need; transferred feelings, not necessarily relevant to the real situation (psychoanalytical)

Creativity. Quality of being productive and imaginative

Crisis intervention. Brief therapeutic encounter in time, with limited structure, aimed at amelioration of symptoms

Criterion reference test. Oral performance on specifically described skills or knowledge without comparisons between individuals

Crossed diagonal. Highly integrated pattern with flexion of the upper extremities and extension of the lower extremities on the face side with extension of the upper limbs with flexion of the lower limbs on the opposite side (reciprocal)

Crystallized intelligence. Cognitive skills such as verbal comprehension and word relationships

Cutaneous. Relating to the skin

CVA. Cerebrovascular accident; a lesion in the brain resulting in paralysis of contralateral side of the body

Cyanosis. Dark bluish or purplish discoloration of the skin and mucous membrane resulting from deficient oxygenation of the blood

Cytomegalic inclusion disease. Infection caused by cytomegalovirus; may be transmitted transplacentally to the fetus from a mother, producing a latent infection

Dance therapy. Technique of using movement and nonverbal communication to aid in rehabilitation; may be group or individual

Debride. To remove foreign or devitalized tissue surgically

DB-decibel. Tenth of a bel; a unit frequently used to measure the intensity of sound

Decerebrate rigidity. Forceful extension of all joints of the lower extremities and extension and internal rotation of the upper extremities; caused by brainstem contusion

Decubitus ulcer. Defect of the surface of an organ or tissue caused by prolonged pressure (also known as a bedsore or a pressure sore)

Deductive reasoning. Reasoning or thought by hypothesis and adult logic

Defense mechanism. Unconscious intrapsychic process (ego defenses) to relieve anxiety and conflict from unconscious drives that are not acceptable; includes conversion, denial, displacement, dissociation, idealization, identification, incorporation, intellectualization, introjection, projection, rationalization, reaction formation, regression, repression, sublimation, substitution, symbolization, transference, and undoing

Deformity. Congenital or acquired unnatural distortion or malformation of a part of the body

Degenerative disease. Progressive deterioration of tissue, particularly in diseases of the central nervous system

Degenerative joint disease. Degenerative, noninflammatory, localized form of arthritis that causes breakdown of cartilage and results in limitation of motion and formation of body outgrowths at the joints affected; osteoarthritis

Dementia. Irreversible organic brain pathology characterized by a slowly progressive loss of mental capacity including memory, orientation, and ability to do serial tasks. Diagnosis can be made properly only after other causes are ruled out by adequate history, examination, and laboratory analyses

Denial. Unconscious defense mechanism in which an aspect of external reality is blocked from awareness

Dependency. The state of needing someone or something for support

Depersonalization. Sense of unreality about self, others, and environment

Deprivation. Negative reinforcement used to weaken or eliminate an undesired action

Desensitization. Reciprocal inhibition (Wolpe); conditioning a person to associate comfortable, supportive surroundings with anxiety-producing stimuli so gradually reducing the adverse effects.

Development. Changes in the structure, thought, or behavior of a person as a function of both biological and environmental influences (which may be quantitative or qualitative)

Developmental disability. Result of any condition, trauma, deprivation, or disease that interrupts or delays the sequence and rate of normal growth, development, and maturation

Developmental sequence. Established progression pattern of growth and development

Differentiation. Process of discriminating those essential elements of a specific behavior that are pertinent to a given situation from those that are not and thereby modifying or altering the behavior in some manner

DIP joint. Distal interphalangeal joint

Diplegia. Paralysis of similar parts on both sides of the body

Diplopia. Perception of two images of a single object (double or binocular vision)

Disability rating. Classification of loss of function

Disequilibrium. Lack or destruction of equilibrium

Disintegration. Psychic disorganization

Dislocation. Displacement of a bone from its normal position in the joint

Disorientation. Inability to judge time, space, and personal relationships

Displacement. Unconscious defense mechanism in which the feeling-laden part of an unacceptable idea or object is transferred to an acceptable one

Dissociation. Unconscious defense mechanism in which an idea is separated from its accompanying feeling tone

DOT. Dictionary of Occupational Titles

Dramatic play. Symbolic play used to display creative ability and physical prowess. It combines reality with magic to fulfill wishes and needs

DRGs. Diagnosis-related groups

DSM. Diagnostic and Statistical Manual of Mental Disorders of the American Psychiatric Association

Dyadic. One-to-one relationship, as between two people

Dynamic splint. Splint that allows for or provides motion. Motion is provided by transfer of motion from other body parts or by use of outside forces such as springs, rubber bands, carbon dioxide, or electricity

Dysarthria. Motor speech deficit

Dysfunction. Inability to perform and interact effectively with the environment; impairment of normal function of a body part or organ

Dyskinesia. Impairment of voluntary movement

Dyspnea. Shortness of breath

Dyspraxia. Difficulty in performing purposeful voluntary movements, the nature and mechanism of which are understood in the absence of motor or sensory impairment.

Echolalia. Involuntary repetition of words; may be accompanied by twitching of muscles

Eclectic. Choosing from various sources; not following any single system or frame of reference; selecting and using elements of several systems

Edema. Condition in which the body tissues contain an excessive amount of tissue fluid; it may be local or general

Efferent. Conducting (fluid or a nerve impulse) outward or centrifugally

Ego. One of three components of psychic structure (with id and superego); mediates between instinctual drives and external reality demands (Freud)

Egocentric. Preoccupied with one's own needs; self-centered; lacking interest in others

Ego functions. Ego's management of defense mechanisms to meet person's needs—defense mechanisms mediating between id, superego, and reality; reality testing

Ego strength. Effectiveness of ego functions. Strong ego can mediate between id, superego, and reality with enough flexibility to retain energy for creativity and other needs

Embolus. Clot brought from a larger vessel to a smaller one causing obstruction

Empirical. Founded on practical experience but not proved scientifically; based on observable fact or objective experience

Encephalitis. Inflammation of the brain

Encopresis. Incontinence of feces

Encounter group. Form of sensitivity training, experiencing individual relationships within a group; focuses on present (J. L. Moreno)

Endocept. Intrapsychic primitive organization of perceptions, memory traces, and images; preverbal; cannot be shared; experienced vaguely (Arieti)

Engrams. Mnemic hypothesis — the theory that stimuli or irritants leave definite traces on neurons

ENT. Ears, nose, and throat

Enuresis. Bedwetting

Environment. Composite of all external forces and influences affecting the development and maintenance of an individual

Epicritic function. Denoting a set or system of sensory nerve fibers supplying the skin and oral mucosa enabling one to appreciate the finer degrees of the sensation of touch, pain, and temperature and to localize same; distinguished from protopathic

Epithelium. Tissue composed to contiguous cells with a minimum of intercellular substance

Equilibration. Process of finding a balance between accommodation and assimilation

Equilibrium. State of balance or equality between opposing forces; bodily stability or balance

Equilibrium reactions. Bodily reactions to retain state of balance in relation to gravity

Erythema. Redness of the skin occurring in patches of variable size and shape

Erythemia. Condition characterized by an increased number of red blood cells; polycythemia

Eschar. Thick coagulated crust or slough that develops following a thermal burn or cauterization of the skin

Escharatomy. Incision in a burn eschar to lessen constriction of a distal part

Etiology. Study of causes of a disease

Euphoria. Sense of well-being; the absence of pain or stress that might be exaggerated

Exacerbation. Aggravation of symptoms of a disease

Excitatory. Stimulating; increasing the rapidity of the physical or mental processes

Existential psychotherapy. Treatment that emphasizes here-and-now — confrontation and feeling experiences; based on philosophy that one has responsibility for one's own existence

Exocepts. Intrapsychic images of actions, movement; kinesthetic–proprioceptive images (Arieti)

Expressive aphasia. Impairment of the ability to use speech and to write communicatively

External powered flexor-hinge splint. Use of an outside source to provide power for prehension

Exteroceptive. Outside the organism; *e.g.,* sense organ of the skin located on the surface of the body

Extrapyramidal. Central nervous system control of involuntary motor behavior

Extrinsic motivation. Will to act based on external standards or incentives

Extrinsic muscles. Muscles whose origin lies outside the part moved

Facilitator. Person who helps make a process easier, assists progress toward a goal

Family of origin. Family into which one is born

Family therapy. Treatment of family in conflict; focus is on interactions among all members, not on pathology of one

Fasciotomy. Incision through a fascia; used in the treatment of certain vascular disorders when marked swelling is anticipated that could compromise blood flow.

Fatigability. Susceptibility to fatigue

Fear. Unpleasurable feeling with psychological and physical changes in response to realistic threat or danger

Febrile. Pertaining to or characterized by fever

Feedback. Response to behavior

Festination gait. Small-stepped shuffling gait seen in Parkinson's disease; involuntary increase in momentum to compensate for displaced sense of center of gravity

Fetus. Unborn child from eighth week of gestation to birth

Fibrillation. Small local involuntary contraction of muscle fibers

Fibroblasts. Cells that synthesize mucopolysaccharides and collagen fibers necessary for the development of new connective tissue

Fibrotic. Pertaining to or characterized by formation of fibrous tissue, usually as a reparative or reactive process

Field dependent. Highly motivated to conform to standards or pressures that are external

Flaccid. Relaxed; flabby; having defective or absent muscular tone

Flexor hinge. Splint or operation used to provide grasp function of the hand through stabilization of the interphalangeal joints of the first two fingers in slight flexion, the thumb in opposition, and providing movement at the metacarpophalangeal joint to effect prehension

Fluid intelligence. Cognitive capabilities such as associative memory, inductive reasoning, and figural relationship

Forearm orthosis. Ballbearing feeder

Formal operations. Fourth and final stage of Piagetian theory beginning at 12 to 15 years and characterized by logical thinking and a grasp of abstract concepts

Formative evaluation. Along the way

Frame of reference. Belief system based on conceptual models; in therapy, organized basis of theory, delineation of function and dysfunction, evaluation and treatment approaches, postulates regarding change

Froment's sign. Flexion of the distal phalanx of the

thumb when a sheet of paper is held between the thumb and index finger in unlar nerve palsy

Functional treatment. Relates to a specific function that has been lost and is being relearned or to a function that is being learned for the first time

Gastroschisis. Congenital defect in the abdominal wall, usually with protrusion of the viscera

Gavage feeding. Feeding by a stomach tube

Gender identity (core). Identification of oneself as male or female

Gender identity. Convictions one has about one's gender and its associated role

Gender orientation. Stable, subjective sense of comfort and liking for one's sex and for those functions that are "sex specific"

Gender preference. Gender role an individual finds most desirable, regardless of compatibility with his/her own core gender identity

Gender role. Clusters of behaviors or characteristics that are associated with one gender more frequently than the other; a set of cultural prescriptions and prohibitions

Gene. Unit of the chromosome that transmits a hereditary characteristic

Generativity. Concern with the establishment and guidance of future generations

Genital phase. Final stage of psychosexual development, during puberty; pleasure centered on genital to genital contact (Freud)

Geriatrics. Physiology and pathology of old age

Gerontology. Study of later maturity and old age in its biological, psychological, and sociological aspects

Geropsychiatry. Branch of psychiatry dealing with problems of the aged

Gestalt. Organized field that has unique properties that cannot be devised merely from the sum of its various component parts; the whole or total quality of the image

Gestalt therapy. Psychotherapeutic technique focusing on treatment of person as a whole; focuses on here-and-now experience. Use of role playing to promote individual or group growth (Frederick S. Perls)

Gestation. Period of fetal development from conception to birth

Glaucoma. Disease of the eye marked by heightened intraocular tension; may lead to blindness

Gliosis. Proliferation of neurological tissue in the central nervous system

Grand mal. Complete epileptic seizure

Graphesthesia. Recognition of the form of a number or letter drawn on the skin

Gray matter. Substantia grisea; the ganglionic or cellular portion of the brain and spinal cord

Growth. Biological/structural changes of the body; increase in size, function, or complexity up to some optimal point

GTO. Golgi tendon organ

Guillain–Barré syndrome. Spreading paralysis, sometimes reversible, with involvement of nerves, nerve roots, cord, brain, and meninges, separately or in combination

Gustatory. Pertaining to the sense of taste

Habilitate. To educate or train (the mentally or physically handicapped, the disadvantaged) to function better in society

Habituation. Ability to become used to certain stimuli and no longer respond to them

Hallucination. False sensory perception without concrete external stimulus; may be visual, auditory, olfactory, gustatory, or tactile

Haptic. Pertaining to touch; tactile

Hematoma. Accumulation of blood within a tissue

Hemianopsia. Blindness in one half of the visual field; may be bilateral or unilateral; also called hemiopia, hemianopia

Hemiparesis. Muscular weakness of one side of the body

Hemiplegia. Paralysis of one side of the body

Hemorrhage. Bleeding; escape of blood from the vessels

Heuristic. Quality that encourages further discovery or investigation

Histologic. Dealing with the science of the structure of cells, tissues, and organs in relation to their function; microscopic anatomy

HMO. Health maintenance organization

Homeostasis. Maintenance of steady states in the organism by coordinated physiologic processes

Homolateral. Ipsilateral pattern, with the head, thorax, and pelvis turned toward the flexing upper and lower extremities with extension of the contralateral extremities (camel walk)

Hyaline membrane disease. Airlessness of the lungs, seen especially in premature neonates with respiratory distress; pulmonary collapse

Hydrocephalus. Condition marked by excessive accumulation of fluid dilating the cerebral ventricles, thinning the brain, and causing a separation of cranial bones

Hydroureter nephrosis. Distention of the ureter and renal pelvis with urine because of blockage from any cause

Hyperactivity. Excessive or increased activity

Hyperalimentation (HA). Overfeeding, superalimentation, forcing of food upon a patient in excess of the demands of the appetite or of the nutritional needs of a person in health. Also, intravenous administration of nutrients

Hyperesthesia. Increased sensitivity to touch

Hyperplasia. Rapid growth; abnormal increase of cells without formation of a tumor but with increase in size of an organ or part

Hypertension. Tension or tonus above normal; a condition in which patient has a higher blood pressure than normal for his or her age

Hyperthermia. Abnormally high fever; also hyperexia

Hypertonicity. Hypertonia; an increased effective osmotic pressure of body fluids

Hypertrophic scarring. Enlargement of the scar; excessive growth of the scar

Hypertrophy. Enlargement or growth of an organ or other part of the body; the growth is independent of natural growth and is caused by unnatural increase in the size of cells

Hypoesthesia. Dulled sensitivity to touch

Hypotension. Decrease of systolic and diastolic blood pressure below normal; deficiency in tonus or tension

Id. One of three components of psychic structure (with ego and superego); unconscious, unorganized, the seat of basic instinctual drives and energy (Freud)

Idealization. Unconscious or conscious defense mechanism; person overestimates an attribute or aspect of another person

Ideational apraxia. Inability to correlate purpose and accomplishment of tasks

Identification. Unconscious defense mechanism in which a person patterns himself/herself after another (distinguished from imitation, which is a conscious process)

Identity. Sense of self

Ideomotor apraxia. Inability to imitate gestures or perform purposeful activities on command while retaining ability to perform automatic routine activities

Imitation. Conscious patterning of oneself after another

Impotence. Inability to perform sexual intercourse; may be erective (inability to achieve erection); ejaculatory (inability to expel seminal fluid); or orgastic (inability to attain full orgasm)

Imprinting. Process by which animals develop a social attachment for a particular object

Incontinence. Inability to retain urine or feces through the loss of sphincter control

Inductive reasoning. Ability to use concrete events, objects, perceptions, or representations to solve a problem

Indwelling catheter. Catheter left in place; *e.g.*, in the bladder

Infancy. Stage in the life cycle lasting from birth until approximately 18 to 24 months

Inhibitory. Restraining; tending to inhibit

Integration. (1) Organization and incorporation into the personality and functioning of the individual of data and experience gained. (2) Reflex inhibition or excitation by higher centers or increasingly complex networks that modify a reflex in such a way that the response is not noticeable; a reflex may work in concert with others to produce movement; primitive reflexes can reappear as a result of brain damage or under stress

Integrative. Helping toward wholeness, organization of thoughts, feelings, and actions

Intelligence quotient. Number assigned to express intellectual capacity, obtained by multiplying mental age by 100 and dividing by chronological age

Intension tremor. Tremor precipitated or increased by attempt to perform a voluntary coordinated movement

Interoceptive. Within viscera; inside the organism

Interpersonal thought. Orientation toward the possible and hypothetical; the ability to explore all possibilities by subjecting the problems to combinational analysis

Interstitial. Situated between important parts; occupying the interspaces or interstices of a part

Intimacy. Ability to make and abide by commitment to affiliations and partnerships

Intrinsic marriage. Marriage based solely on the relationship between two people

Intrinsic motivation. Will to act based on personal internal standards, incentives, desires, and needs

Intrinsic muscles. Muscles of the extremities whose origin and insertion are both in the same part of the limb (*e.g.*, hand)

Intuitive thought. Part of the preoperational period (approximately 5 to 7 years of age) when a child is able to separate mental from physical reality and to understand multiple points of view

Invariant clauses. Segments of thought processes that are unaffected by mathematical or logical operations

Ipsilateral. On the same side; denoting especially paralytic or other symptoms occurring on the same side as the brain lesion causing them

Ischemia. Local anemia or diminution in the blood supply resulting from obstruction of inflow of arterial blood or to vasoconstriction

Isolation. Sense of separateness and self-absorption

Jacksonian. Spasmodic contractions in certain groups of muscles or paroxysmal paresthesias in certain skin areas as a result of local disease of the cortex

Jargon. Unintelligible speech

Jaundice. Condition marked by yellow skin and eye whites, caused by changes in the liver cells or obstruction which causes the bile pigment, bilirubin, to be diffused into the blood

Job satisfaction. Sense of well-being about one's work resulting from a feeling of commitment based on one's personal and interpersonal goals

Job tryout. Placement of client on actual job in industry

Kinesthesia. Conscious perception of movement, weight, resistance, and position of a body part; also kinesthesis

Kirshner wire. Apparatus for internal fixation of a long bone fracture

Kyphosis. Convex backward curvature of the spine; humpback

Lability. State of being unstable, changeable, or having lack of emotional control

Laminectomy. Surgical removal of the lamina or posterior arch of the vertebrae

Latency. State of inactivity, where potential is hidden or dormant

Latency phase. Stage of psychosexual development (age 5 to puberty) with apparent cessation of sexual preoccupation (Freud)

LE. Lower extremity

Learning. Relatively permanent change in behavior or in the capacity for behavior resulting from experience or practice

Lesion. Structural or functional alteration of a part caused by injury or disease

Libido. Basic psychological energy inherent in every person; the energy supplies the sexual drive whose goal is to obtain pleasure (Freud)

Life satisfaction. Subjective sense of well-being

Locus of control. Source or origin of direction of events (Rotter). *External locus of control:* control of life events from outside oneself. *Internal locus of control:* control of life events by one's own thoughts, abilities, and actions

Lordosis. Hollow back; anteroposterior curvature of the spine

Lower motor neuron lesion (LMN). Lesion occurring in the anterior horn cells, nerve roots, or the peripheral nerve system resulting in flaccid paralysis

Ludic. Playful; expressing frivolity, excitement, joy, and celebration

Lumbar. Pertaining to the lower back and its five vertebrae

Macrosphere stage. In play, stage when a child begins to share with others on a broader scale

Malignancy. Condition of being resistant to treatment; severe; and frequently fatal. Also, ability to metastasize (said of tumor)

Mastery. Command or grasp of a subject

Maturation. Emergence of an organism's genetic potential; includes a series of preprogrammed changes that comprise changes in the organism's structure for form as well as in its complexity, integration, organization, and function

MBD. Minimal brain dysfunction; diagnostic and descriptive category of neurodevelopmental lags

Menopause. Cessation of menses

Microsphere stage. In play, stage when a child masters and manipulates the world on a small scale

Microthorax. Abnormally small chest

Micturition. Urination

Milieu. Surroundings; social and physical environment

Milieu therapy. Treatment using manipulation of the socioenvironmental setting to benefit the patient

Modeling. Setting an example for imitation

Monoplegia. Paralysis of one limb

Morality. Sense of what is right and wrong

Morality of reciprocity. Parallels the advanced level of abstract thought; the sense of morality enables one to develop a new conscientious, internally sensitive changing of rules (primarily internally monitored value responses)

Morphology. Structure and form of an organism, excluding its functions

MP joint. Metacarpophalangeal joint

Multi-infarct dementia. Deterioration of personality and intellect as a result of a series of small strokes; it results in a stepwise deterioration in intellectual function (not uniformly progressive) with some intellectual functions relatively intact early in its course (patchy deterioration)

Multiple sclerosis (disseminated) (MS). Patches of demyelination in the white matter of the nervous system, sometimes in the gray matter; progressive disease of the nervous system

Muscular dystrophy (MD). Progressive, hereditary disorder marked by atrophy and stiffness of the muscles and observed when voluntary action is first attempted

Music therapy. Use of music as treatment modality

Myasthenia gravis. Disease characterized by an abnormal exhaustibility of the voluntary muscles manifest in a rapid diminution of contractility, both when the muscle is activated by the will and when stimulated by electric current

Myelination. Myelinization; the process of supplying or accumulating myelin during the development or repair of nerves

Myelin sheath. Sheath formation of myelin substance that covers axons and nerve fibers

Myelomeningocele (MM). Spina bifida with protrusion of both the cord and its membranes

Myoneural junction. Point at which a motor nerve joins with the muscle it innervates

Myopia. Defect in vision so that objects can be seen distinctly only when very close to the eyes

NARC. National Association for Retarded Citizens

NASA. National Aeronautics and Space Administration

Necrotic eschar. Dead scar tissue

Neonate. Newly born individual, especially an infant during his/her first month of life

Neoplasm. New formation of tissue abnormally, as a tumor or growth

Nephrostomy. Establishment of an opening between the pelvis of the kidney and the external surface of the body

Neuritis. Inflammation of a nerve or nerves, usually associated with degenerative processes

Neurodevelopmental treatment approach. Movement as primary modality of treatment (Bobaths)

Neuromuscular spindle. Muscle proprioceptor

Neuron. Unit of the nervous system consisting of the nerve cell body and its various processes, the dendrites, axon, and ending

Neurophysiological treatment approach. Activation, facilitation, and inhibition of voluntary and involuntary muscle action through the reflex arc (Rood)

Neurotendinous organ. Proprioceptive sensory nerve ending in which branching nerve fibers are spread over a bundle of encapsulated fibers near their attachment to muscle; Golgi's organ

NIMH. National Institute of Mental Health

NMS. Coordinated actions of the nervous, muscular, and skeletal systems

Nociceptive response. Response to stimuli that could cause harm, injury, or pain

Normal development. Determined by wide range of data collected for a particular population within a given time and culture, referring to a specific area or segment of development

Normalization. Part of the rehabilitation process emphasizing the patient's ability to grow, adapt, and change as he/she moves toward healthfulness, self-directed behavior, and independence of function

Nuclear family. Natural parents and children

Nystagmus. Involuntary rapid movement of the eyeball; may be congenital or acquired

Object permanence. Assumption that objects continue to exist when they are out of sight, touch, or some other perceptual contact

Object relations. Emotional attachment for another person or object (that which is other than self)

Occiput. Occipital area of the skull; the back of the head

Occlusion. Act of closing or the state of being closed

Occupational behavior. Organization and action based on skills, knowledge, and attitudes to make functioning possible in life roles (Reilly)

Occupational performance skills. Skills required for successful performance of the roles that are assumed by individuals in their lives. Most human roles fall into the categories of play, self-care, and work

Oedipal conflict. Conflict that appears during the phallic stage. It consists of sexual attraction to the parent of the opposite sex and hostility toward the parent of the same sex (Freud)

Olfaction. Sense of smell; the act of smelling

Ontogeny, ontogenetic. Relating to the biological development of the individual (distinguished from phylogeny)

Operant conditioning. Procedure through which subject is conditioned by use of reinforcement techniques to learn a desired behavior (B. F. Skinner)

Opisthotonic. Relating to a tetanic spasm in which the spine and the extremities are bent with convexity forward, the body resting on the head and heels

Optometrist. One who measures the degree of visual powers; a refractionist

Oral phase. Earliest stage of psychosexual development (to 18 months); oral zone is pleasure center (Freud)

Orthotics. Science that deals with the making and fitting of orthopedic appliances

Osteoarthritis. Degenerative, noninflammatory, localized form of arthritis that causes breakdown of cartilage and results in limitation of motion and formation of bony outgrowths at the joints affected

Osteosclerosis. Osteopetrosis; a rare developmental error of unknown cause but of familial tendency characterized by excessive radiographic density of most or all of the bones

Otologist. One versed in the science of the ear, its anatomy, functions, and diseases

Otosclerosis. Characterized by chronic progressive deafness, especially for low tones

Paleo-. Prefix meaning older; *e.g.*, paleocortex, the older portion of the cerebral cortex

Paralinguistics. Communication through intonation, gestures, and other nonverbal aspects of speech

Paralysis. Loss or impairment of motor and/or sensory function of a part caused by injury to nerves or neurons

Paranoid. Psychiatric syndrome characterized by delusions

Paraparesis. Partial paralysis or weakness in lower extremities

Paraplegia. Paralysis of muscles in lower extremities

PARC. Pennsylvania Association for Retarded Citizens

Parkinson's disease. (Synonymous with parkinsonism, Parkinson's syndrome). Neurological symptom complex characterized by four major symptoms: rigidity, tremor, akinesia, and loss of spontaneous and automatic movement

Peer. Another person of one's own age or status

Perception. Mental process by which intellectual, sensory, and emotional data are organized meaningfully; the process of conscious recognition and interpretation of sensory stimuli

Peripatologist. One who teaches a blind person to travel

Peripheral. Located or pertaining to an outer portion of the body away from the center, such as the extremities

Petit mal. Brief lapse in consciousness

Phallic phase. Third state of psychosexual development (ages 2 to 6); interest, curiosity, and pleasure centered on penis or clitoris. The oedipal conflict is present during this phase (Freud)

Phasic reflexes. Observable movements in response to a touch, pressure, or movement of the body or to sight or sound received

Phenomenology. Study of consciously reported experiences

Phenylketonuria (PKU). Genetic disorder of metabolism leading to presence of phenylketone in the urine

Phonology. Science of vocal sounds

Phylogeny, phylogenetic. Evolutionary development of any plant or animal species; ancestral history of the individual; distinguished from ontogeny, the development of the individual

Physical impairment. Weakening, damage, or deterioration; *e.g.,* as a result of injury or disease

PIP joint. Proximal interphalangeal joint

Plateau. Period or state of relative stability following or preceding fluctuating change

Play. Activity voluntarily engaged in for pleasure

Pleasure principle. Notion that a person tries to gain pleasure and avoid pain (psychoanalytical)

PNS. Peripheral nervous system

Poliomyelitis. Common virus disease of man that may involve the central nervous system and result in a nonparalytic or paralytic form, the latter being the classical form of acute anterior poliomyelitis

Polyneuritis. Simultaneous inflammation of many nerves, usually in a symmetrical pattern

POMR. Problem-oriented medical record

Postulate. Theoretical proposition assumed without proof

Postural adaptation. Righting; midline; stability; equilibrium

Pragmatic. Practical; concerned with actual practice

Praxis. Performance of a purposeful movement or group of movements; ability to motor plan

Preconceptual. First part of the preoperational period lasting from age 2 to 4 in which there is new use of symbols and symbolic play

Prefrontal lobotomy. Neurosurgical procedure in which one or more nerve tracts in the prefrontal area of the brain are severed (also called leukotomy)

Prehominids. Ancestors of the human species from which humans evolved

Presbyopia. Inability of the eye to focus sharply on nearby objects, resulting from hardening of the crystalline lens with advancing age

Prevocational evaluation. Evaluation of activities of daily living (ADL), educational abilities, and physical capabilities and deficits as required for participation in vocational activity

Primary circular reaction. Action on the part of the infant that fortuitously leads to an event that has value and is centered about his or her body. The infant learns to repeat the behavior in order to reinstate the event. The culmination of the process is an organized scheme.

Primary degenerative dementia. Also called senile dementia, Alzheimer type (SDAT); characterized by the same brain pathology as Alzheimer's presenile dementia (senile plaques, neurofibrillary tangles, granulovascular degeneration); meets the DSM III criteria for dementia but has an insidious onset and uniformly progressive deteriorating course; other causes have been eliminated by history, examination, and laboratory investigation

Prism glasses. For use by the patient lying supine to prevent eye strain by enabling the patient to see ahead by looking up to the ceiling

PRN. Abbreviation of Latin *pro re nata;* according to needs; sometimes used in prescriptions or written orders

Prodromal. Early or premonitory symptoms of disease

Prognosis. Predicted course of an illness over a given period of time

Projection. Unconscious defense mechanism in which person attributes ideas and feelings to another; the ideas, feelings, and impulses that are his/her own but that are unacceptable to him/her

Projective techniques. Loosely structured procedures in which the patient reveals feelings, personality, and unconscious material

Prophylactic. Preventing disease; an agent (*e.g.,* vaccine) that acts as a preventive against a disease

Proprioception. Appreciation of position, balance, and changes in equilibrium of a body part during movement as a result of stimulus within body tissue such as muscles, tendons, and joints

Protopathic function. Denoting a set or system of peripheral sensory nerve fibers furnishing a low order of sensibility, enabling one to appreciate pain and temperature but not to a very delicate extent and definitely not localized; distinguished from epicritic

Pseudobulbar paralysis. Paralysis resembling bulbar paralysis but caused by lesion of cortical centers

Pseudohypertrophy. Increase in size of an organ without increased size of one or more of its components

Pseudostupidity. Interpretation of a situation at a more complex level than is warranted

PSNS. Parasympathetic nervous system; the craniosacral division of the autonomic nervous system

PSRO. Professional Standards Review Organization

Psychomotor. Combination of physical and emotional activity

Psychopharmacology. Study of drugs and their effects on psychological and behavioral processes

Psychotherapy. Treatment of mental disorder in which trained person interacts with patient on the basis of a therapeutic contract; treatment is based on communication

Ptosis. Drooping of the upper eyelid; abnormal prolapse or falling down of an organ or part

Puberty. Period of life when an individual's sexual organs become functional and secondary sex characteristics appear

Pubescence. Period of about 2 years prior to puberty; it is a period of physiological change that triggers the emergence of primary and secondary sexual characteristics

Pulmonary stenosis. Narrowing of the opening into the pulmonary artery from the right ventricle

Purposeful activity. Treatment directed to a response that enhances neural integration.

Quadriparesis. Partial paralysis or weakness in all four extremities

Quadriplegia. Paralysis of muscles in all four extremities

Qualitative changes. Subjective elements; no scale to measure

Quantitative change. Measurable and thus easily understood

Rapport. Conscious, harmonious accord or relationship between people

RAS. Reticular activating system

Rationalization. Unconscious defense mechanism; person uses a feasible, acceptable reason to explain irrational behavior, motives, or feelings

Reactions. Complex and inconstant responses developing from integration of simultaneous sensory stimulation such as tactile, vestibular, visual, and auditory

Reality testing. Fundamental ego function; objective evaluation of world outside self; testing of real world — human, nonhuman, concrete, ideational

Reality therapy. Treatment method in which milieu and therapeutic relationships are based on real and present situations and cause and effect relationships (Glasser)

Recapitulation of ontogenesis. Repetition of passage through stages of human development

Receptive aphasia. Impairment in interpretation of the meaning of spoken and written words

Reciprocal innervation. Contraction in a muscle accompanied by a loss of tone or by relaxation in the antagonistic muscle

Re-enactment. Acting out of a past experience as if it were happening in the present — person can feel, perceive, and act as he/she did the first time

Reflex. Fetal or neonatal responses that are simple and predictable resulting from tactile and vestibular stimulation

Reflex action. Immediate unconscious, involuntary response of a limb or organ to stimulation of the sensory branch of a reflex arc

Reflex arc. Pathway from the receptor in the skin to the effector organ through which an impulse travels

Reflexes. Automatic response of an organism to a specific event in the environment

Regression. Unconscious defense mechanism; person returns to earlier patterns of adaptation

Rehabilitation. Restoration to a disabled individual of maximum independence commensurate with his limitations by developing his residual capacities

Reinforcement. In behavior therapy, strengthening a response by using a stimulus immediately after the response (may be positive or negative)

Reliability. Degree to which a test produces the same results on repeated administrations

Remission. Abatement or lessening of symptoms of a disease

Repression. Unconscious defense mechanism; removal from consciousness, usually of ideas, impulses, and feelings that are not acceptable (Freud)

Respiratory distress syndrome (RDS). Condition (usually present at birth) of unknown cause formerly known as hyaline membrane disease; clinical signs include delayed onset of breathing

Reticular formation. Fine network formed by cells or by certain structures within cells or of connective tissue fibers between cells

Retinitis pigmentosa. Slowly progressing connective tissue and pigment cell proliferation of the entire retina with wasting of its nerve elements

Retrolental fibroplasia. Blinding disease of the eye affecting premature infants

Reversible dementia. Symptomatic dementia, prompt treatment of which will reverse or alleviate it; untreated, it becomes a true dementia

Reward. Positive reinforcement used to strengthen a desired action

Rh factor. A human blood antigen; its presence or absence is referred to as Rh positive and Rh negative

Rheumatoid arthritis. Chronic progressive inflammatory systemic disease that causes pain, swelling, limitation, and deformity in the joints with accompanying involvement of tendons and sheaths, nerves, and muscles

Righting reactions. Reflexes that through various receptors in the labyrinth, eyes, muscles, or skin tend to bring an organism's body into its normal position in space and which resist any force acting to put it into a false position; *e.g.,* on its back

Rigidity. Inflexible and tonic contraction of muscles giving consistent resistance to passive movement through total range of movement

Role diffusion. Identity confusion; discontinuity in both experience and in how others perceive oneself

Rorschach test. Projective test in which subject reveals attitudes and emotions through response to inkblot pictures

Rote. Habit performance, without meaning; in a mechanical way

Rubella. German measles; an acute, contagious eruptive disease capable of causing serious birth defects in child infected prenatally; also called epidemic roseola, French measles

Rural. Counties with populations up to 10,000 (additional population begins to be semirural) accompanied by geographic isolation; cultural and economic isolation are likely as well

SAR—sexual attitude reassessment. Workshop designed to desensitize and resensitize participants to their sexuality and the sexuality of others, particularly the disabled

Schedule of reinforcement. Pattern set up for presentation of reinforcers in behavior therapy

Schemata. Piagetian term that refers to the structure or framework into which one's experiences are integrated

Schwann cell. One of the cells of the neurolemma; a cell that enfolds myelinated and unmyelinated nerve fibers

Sclerosis. Hardening of a part with growth of fibrous tissue resulting from atrophy or degeneration of nerve elements

Scoliosis. Lateral curvature of the spine

Scotoma. Abnormal blind spots

Sealing over. Covering up unconscious material

Sebaceous glands. Composed of fat, keratohyalin, granules, keratin, and cellular debris

Secondary circular reaction. Actions involving events or objects in the external environment; the ability to develop schemes that reproduce interesting events that were initially discovered by chance in the external environment

Secular trend. Recent generations tend to be more intelligent, taller, and stronger than previous generations; a generational shift

Sedative. Drug that produces calming, relaxing effect; CNS depressant

SEIMC. Special education instructional materials centers

Selective inattention. Blocking out stimuli that generate anxiety; failing to notice, see, or hear things that the individual may not wish to deal with

Semidomesticated. Refers to the situation of wild animals who have an adequate food supply provided artificially and who are relatively free from predators but who roam a relatively unrestricted territory

Senility. Gradual loss of physical and/or mental function and well-being of an aged person resulting in withdrawal, apathy, personal neglect, blunting of memory and cognitive abilities, weakness, poor appetite, and sleep disorders

Sensibility. Ability to perceive, appreciate, and transmit nerve impulses

Sensorimotor stage. First stage of Piaget's cognitive theory in which the child from birth to 2 years of age seeks to integrate perceptions and bodily motions

Seriation. Arranging or organizing in orderly series

Sex typing. Process of acquiring the behavior and attitudes regarded by the culture as masculine or feminine

Sexuality. Integration of physical, emotional, intellectual, and social aspects of an individual's personality that expresses maleness or femaleness

Shaping. In behavior therapy, system of establishing desired behavior patterns through reinforcement given for each successive approximation—moving closer to goal

Shearing. Distortion of a body to two oppositely directed parallel forces

Shock treatment. Psychiatric treatment through use of chemicals or electric current (insulin–ECT or EST)

Significant other(s). Human(s) or animal(s) of particular importance to the well-being of another

Situational or simulated job tryout. Placement of client in actual work situation in a sheltered workshop or other such institution

SMS. Sensory–motor–sensory; sensory feedback integration with the initial sensory input and motor accommodation

SNS. Sympathetic nervous system

SOAP. Subjective, objective, assessment, plan; used in problem-oriented medical record

Social bond. Underlying quality of attachment between two persons

Social interaction. Active affectionate reciprocal relationship between two persons

Social-technical evolution. Term referring to changes in human evolution that are not biological in nature. This includes the technology, culture, and social relations that have come about as a function of evolution

Sociodramatic play. Voluntary social play with at least one other child wherein a child imitates the actions and speech of others

Somatosensory. Concerning sensation of the body, as distinguished from the viscera or mind

Spasm. Sudden involuntary contraction of muscle or group of muscles

Spastic. Characterized by spasms and resulting in hypertonia and awkward movements from stiff muscles

Spasticity. State of hypertonicity, involuntary resistance of weak muscle caused by passive range of motion followed by sudden relaxation of muscle, associated with exaggeration of reflexes and loss of voluntary muscle control; increased muscle tone

Spatial relations. Relationship of the skeletal parts of the body to each other and to objects in the environment

Spatiotemporal adaptation. Continuous, ongoing state or act of adjusting those bodily processes required to function within a given space at a given time

Standardized. Having established and tested norms

Static splint. Splint with no moving parts; maintains a joint in desired position

Stereognosis. Perception and identification of the form and nature of an object through the sense of touch

Stereoscopic. Vision in which things have the appearance of solidity and relief as seen in three dimensions

Strabismus. Deviation of the eye that the individual cannot overcome

Stress. Physical, emotional, or intellectual strain or tension disturbing normal equilibrium

Stroke. Sudden and severe seizure or fit of disease; a popular term for cerebral vascular accident (CVA)

Stryker frame. Bed-turning frame that enables a patient to be rotated from front to back but does not allow tilting

Sublimation. Unconscious defense mechanism; replacement of unacceptable wishes, drives, feelings, or goals with those that are acceptable

Subluxation. Incomplete or partial dislocation of a joint

Superego. One of three components of psychic structure (with id and ego); (Freud) incorporates standards, moral attitudes, and conscience

Support system. People, agencies, or institutions that serve to help sustain a person in stress or problems

Supportive. Reinforcing the patient's defenses and reassuring him/her (as opposed to probing into conflicts)

Supportive treatment. Relates to the psychological and emotional needs and problems

Supression. Conscious act of controlling unacceptable impulses, feelings, or behavior (different from repression, which is unconscious)

Suprapubic catheter. Catheter positioned above the pubic arch

Surrogate mother. Someone or something that takes the place of a mother in an organism's life

Symbol. Something used for or representing an object, idea, image, or feeling

Symbolization. Unconscious defense mechanism; idea or object comes to stand for another, based on similarity or association

Synapse. Point at which an impulse passes from one neuron to another

Synergies. Combined or correlated actions of different organs of the body, as of muscles working together

Synoptic. Affording or taking a general view of the whole or of the principal parts of a subject

Synovectomy. Surgical excision of the synovial membrane

Synovial membrane. Connective tissue that lines a synovial joint

Synthesize. To form by combining parts into a single whole

Tactile. Pertaining to touch

Tactile defensiveness. Quality of being unable to tolerate touch; resistive and uncomfortable at certain kinds of touch (believed to be a form of sensory integrative dysfunction)

Tactile localization. Ability to determine the location of a cutaneous stimulus

Task-oriented group. Group whose focus is on reaching a goal, finding a solution to a problem, or making a product

Tay–Sachs disease. Amaurosis; a familial disease occurring almost exclusively in Jewish children characterized by flaccid muscles, convulsions, decerebrate rigidity, and blindness

TD. Terminal device in upper extremity prosthetics

Tenodesis splint. Functional handsplint that operates on the tenodesis principle of wrist extension and finger flexion

Term infant. Infant born after gestation of 38–42 weeks

Tertiary circular reaction. Interest in novelty and curiosity about an object; the child no longer relies on previous schemes.

Thematic apperception test. Projective psychological test; subject looks at series of ambiguous pictures and interprets what he/she sees; interpretation will be based on subject's own feelings and attitudes

Theory. Set of logically interrelated statements used to explain observed events; a proposed explanation whose status is still conjectural, in contrast to well-established propositions that are regarded as reporting matters of fact

Therapeutic recreation. Utilization of recreational experiences for the prevention and/or amelioration of handicapping conditions

Thoracic. Pertaining to the chest and ribs and the 12 chest vertebrae

Thrombus. Collection of blood or a clot causing vascular obstruction

TIA. Transient ischemic attack

TLC. Tender loving care

Toxoplasmosis. Disease caused by infection with the protozoan, *Toxoplasma gondii*; in the congenital form it, causes destructive lesions of the central nervous system, jaundice, and anemia

Tracheostomy. Surgical formation of an opening into the trachea and suturing of the edges to the skin in the neck for an airway or passage of a tube

Tranquilizer. Psychotropic drug inducing calming, soothing effect without clouding consciousness—major tranquilizers, antipsychotic drugs; minor tranqulizers, anti-anxiety drugs

Transaction. Interaction between two or more people

Transactional analysis. System centering on study of interactions between people in treatment—four parts: (1) structural analysis of intrapsychic processes; (2) determination of dominant ego state (parent, child, adult); (3) game analysis; and (4) script analysis (finding causes of problems); used in both group and individual psychotherapy (Eric Berne)

Transductive reasoning. Preoperational child's tendency to use associative reasoning rather than inductive or deductive thought (Piaget)

Transference. Projection of feelings, thoughts, or

wishes on to another who has come to represent someone from the past; inappropriate applied in present context; used in therapeutic process (psychoanalytical)

Trapeze bar. Triangular bar attached to a traction frame on the bed so that the patient lying in bed can reach the bar to assist in rolling over, coming to a sitting position, or transferring from the bed to a chair

Trauma. Injury as a result of physical or emotional means or insult

Tremor. Alternate contraction and relaxation of opposing groups of muscles resulting in involuntary rhythmic and oscillating movements such as quivering or trembling

Trophic changes. Changes in function concerned with nourishment of tissues caused by vascular, neurological, nutritional, or endocrine problems or inactivity (disuse)

Trouble team. Team composed of two or three people specially trained in crisis intervention and face-to-face counseling skills; usually sent out to meet with the caller when the situation (runaways, attempted suicides, etc.) seems to require more intervention that can be accomplished on the phone

UE. Upper extremity

Unconditional positive regard. Quality of accepting another person and communicating that acceptance regardless of what that person says or does (Rogers)

Unconscious. Part of the mind in which psychic material—primitive drives, repressed desires, and memories—is not directly accessible to awareness (psychoanalytical)

Underactive. Lacking or slow in taking the initiative to act

Underreactive. Responding minimally or slowly to stimuli

Upper motor neuron lesion (UMN). Lesion occurring in corticospinal or pyramidal tract located in brain or spinal cord resulting in paralysis, increased muscle tone, and pathological reflexes

Utilitarian marriage. Marriage not necessarily based on the couple's relationship; purpose of the marriage varies (*i.e.*, from pure physical relationship to raising family)

Validity. Statistical term; the degree to which a given measure indicates quality or attribute it attempts to measure

Values. Ideals, feelings, and beliefs that are acted upon

Vascular. Containing blood vessels

Ventricular septal defect. Flaw or defect in wall between ventricles of the heart

Viscera. Organs of the digestive, respiratory, urogenital, and endocrine systems as well as the spleen, heart, and great vessels

Visual accommodation. Ability to focus on an object at varying distances

Vocalization. Utterance of sounds

Vocational evaluation. Assessment of all factors (medical, psychological, educational, social, environmental, cultural, and vocational) that affect successful employment

Volition. Will or purpose

WHO. World Health Organization

WISC. The Wechsler Intelligence Scale for Children; well-known American IQ test that includes both verbal and performance (nonverbal) subtests.

Work evaluation. Evaluation of vocational strengths and weaknesses through utilization of work (real or simulated)

Work hardening. Therapeutic technique that moves the worker from a submaximal level of performance to a level adequate for entry or reentry into the work force.

Work sample evaluation. Sample of actual job tasks or a mock-up of actual tasks to determine client's job skills and abilities

Wrist driven flexor hinge splint. Use of wrist entension to provide prehension

Index

Page numbers followed by "t" denote tables;
page numbers in italics denote figures.